MOSBY'S

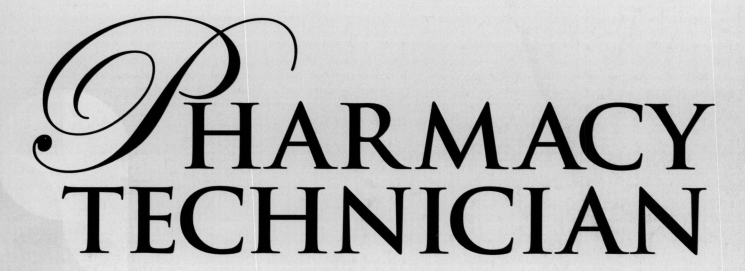

PHARMACY TECHNICIAN

Principles and Practice

FOURTH EDITION

MOSBY'S PHARMACY TECHNICIAN

Principles and Practice

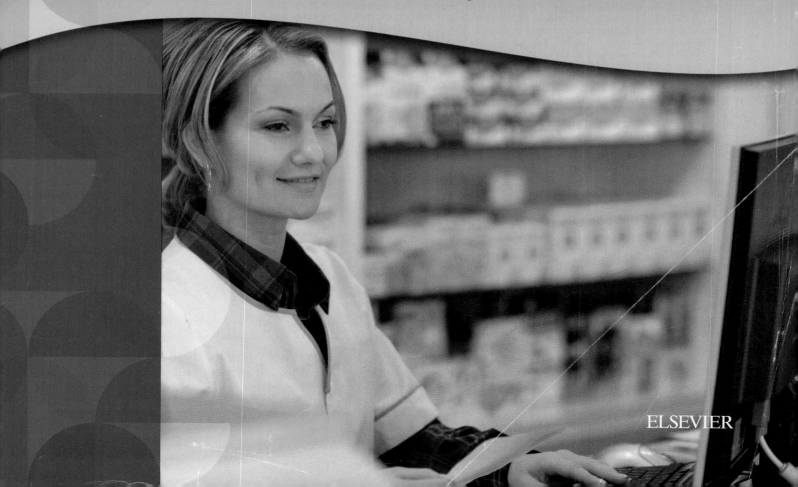

ELSEVIER

ELSEVIER

3251 Riverport Lane
St. Louis, Missouri 63043

MOSBY'S PHARMACY TECHNICIAN: PRINCIPLES AND PRACTICE, FOURTH EDITION

ISBN: 978-1-4557-5178-5

Notice

Knowledge and best practice in this field are constantly changing. As new research and experience broaden our understanding, changes in research methods, professional practices, or medical treatment may become necessary.

Practitioners and researchers must always rely on their own experience and knowledge in evaluating and using any information, methods, compounds, or experiments described herein. In using such information or methods, they should be mindful of their own safety and the safety of others, including parties for whom they have a professional responsibility.

With respect to any drug or pharmaceutical products identified, readers are advised to check the most current information provided (i) on procedures featured or (ii) by the manufacturer of each product to be administered, to verify the recommended dose or formula, the method and duration of administration, and contraindications. It is the responsibility of practitioners, relying on their own experience and knowledge of their patients, to make diagnoses, to determine dosages and the best treatment for each individual patient, and to take all appropriate safety precautions.

To the fullest extent of the law, neither the Publisher nor the authors, contributors, or editors assume any liability for any injury and/or damage to persons or property as a matter of product liability, negligence or otherwise, or from any use or operation of any methods, products, instructions, or ideas contained in the material herein.

Previous editions copyrighted 2012, 2007, 2004

International Standard Book Number: 978-1-4557-5178-5

Executive Content Strategist: Jennifer Janson
Content Development Manager: Luke Held
Senior Content Development Specialist: Jennifer Bertucci
Publishing Services Manager: Julie Eddy
Senior Project Manager: Rich Barber
Designer: Julia Dummitt

Printed in Canada

Last digit is the print number: 9   8   7   6   5   4   3   2   1

Working together to grow libraries in developing countries

www.elsevier.com • www.bookaid.org

Authors

Joshua J. Neumiller, PharmD, CDE, FASCP
Assistant Professor
College of Pharmacy, Department of
    Pharmacotherapy
Washington State University
Pullman, Washington

Bobbi Steelman, CPhT
Pharmacy Technician Program Leader
Daymar College–Bowling Green
Bowling Green, Kentucky

Karen Davis, AAHCA, CPhT
Accreditation Alliance Consulting Services
Pharmacy Tech Program Instructor
Society for the Education of Pharmacy Technicians
    (SEPhT)
Consultant for Pocket Nurse and Custom
    Solutions
Former Corporate Dean for Pharmacy and Surgical
    Tech (ECA) Virginia Colleges
Lyons, Georgia

Elaine Beale, RPh
Pharmacy Technician Program Director/Instructor
Paul D. Camp Community College
Division of Workforce Development
Franklin, Virginia

James J. Mizner, Jr., MBA, BS, RPh
Principal Owner
Panacea Solutions Consulting
Reston, Virginia

Julie Beccarelli, CPhT
Gatekeeper (Pharmacy Technician)
Pipeline Rx
Chicago, Illinois

Technical Reviewer

Anthony Guerra, PharmD, RPh
Chair, Pharmacy Technician Program
Des Moines Area Community College
Ankeny, Iowa

You are about to embark on an exciting journey into one of today's fastest-growing fields in health care. Whether you end up working in a hospital pharmacy, community pharmacy, mail-order pharmacy, Internet pharmacy, or another location, the knowledge you will gain from this textbook and its supplements will prepare you well for your new career. The contributors and publisher have made every effort to equip you with all the background knowledge and tools you need to succeed on the job. *Mosby's Pharmacy Technician: Principles and Practice* was designed as a fundamental yet comprehensive resource that represents the very latest information available for preparing pharmacy technician students for today's challenging job environment.

Who Will Benefit from This Book?

Pharmacy technicians are increasingly called upon to perform duties traditionally fulfilled by pharmacists. This development has occurred because federal regulations now require pharmacists to spend more time with patients providing patient education. As the number of pharmacy technicians in the United States and Canada continues to grow, the need to outline a scope of practice for the pharmacy technician profession has become more urgent. *Mosby's Pharmacy Technician: Principles and Practice* provides students with solid coverage of the information they need to be successful, while also giving the instructor the tools required to present the information effectively and easily.

Why Is This Book Important to the Profession?

This textbook maps directly to the Pharmacy Technician Certification Examination (PTCE) and to the American Society of Health-System Pharmacists (ASHP) Curriculum. The Pharmacy Technician Certification Board (PTCB) set forth its blueprint for the PTCE, and the blueprint was implemented in exams administered to candidates who applied for certification on or after November 1, 2013. The blueprint divides the information into nine Knowledge Domains and Areas: Pharmacy for Technicians, Pharmacy Law

and Regulations, Sterile and Non–Sterile Compounding, Medication Safety, Pharmacy Quality Assurance, Medication Order Entry and Fill Process, Pharmacy Inventory Management, Pharmacy Billing and Reimbursement, and Pharmacy Information System Usage and Application. ASHP's current Model Curriculum, finalized and approved in April 2013, provides details on how to meet the goals defined in the *ASHP Accreditation Standard for Pharmacy Technician Education and Training Programs*. It includes objectives and instructional objectives for each of the goals, in addition to examples of learning activities for each portion of the program, including the didactic, simulated (lab) and experiential program components. In total, the ASHP Model Curriculum has 45 goals, each with its own objectives. The goals are categorized into sections: Personal/Interpersonal Knowledge and Skills; Foundational Professional Knowledge and Skills; Processing and Handling of Medications and Medication Orders; Sterile and Non–Sterile Compounding; Procurement, Billing, Reimbursement, and Inventory Management; Patient and Medication Safety; Technology and Informatics; Regulatory Issues; and Quality Assurance. The criteria defined in the PTCB Blueprint (the foundation of the PTCE) and the ASHP Model Curriculum are designed to help pharmacy technicians work more effectively with pharmacists, provide greater patient care and services, and create a minimum standard of knowledge across all 50 states in the United States and the provinces throughout Canada, to help employers determine a knowledge base for employment.

Organization

For this edition, *Mosby's Pharmacy Technician: Principles and Practice*, has been completely reworked to relate to the PTCB Blueprint (the foundation of the PTCE) and ASHP Model Curriculum. This textbook remains a reliable and understandable resource, written specifically for the pharmacy technician student and for technicians already on the job, including those preparing for the certification examinations. In this fourth edition, the chapters and content have been reorganized, extensively revised to include the most up-to-date information and presented in a way that leads the student to a better understanding of pharmacological information. The writing style, content, and organization guide today's pharmacy technician student to a better understanding of anatomy and physiology, diseases, and, most important, the drugs and agents used to treat those diseases. The textbook is divided into two sections, **Pharmacy Practice** and **Pharmacology and Medications,** and also includes three appendices and a glossary.

Section One, Pharmacy Practice, provides an in-depth overview of pharmacy practice as it relates to pharmacy technicians. Highlights of Section One include the history of medicine and pharmacy; law and ethics (and regulatory agencies); competencies, associations, and settings for pharmacy technicians; communication; dosage forms (and routes of administration); conversions and calculations; drug information references; community pharmacy practice (including prescription interpretation); institutional pharmacy practice (including long-term care and medication order interpretation); additional pharmacy practice settings (including managed care, mail-order pharmacy, and pharmaceutical industry); bulk repackaging and non–sterile compounding; aseptic technique and sterile compounding; pharmacy stock and billing; and medication safety and error prevention. This section gives the pharmacy technician student a full, comprehensive look at the vast world of pharmacy practice today.

Section Two, Pharmacology and Medications, provides an overview of each body system and the medications used to treat common conditions that afflict these systems. Highlights of Section Two include therapeutic agents for all the body systems (i.e., nervous; endocrine; musculoskeletal; cardiovascular; respiratory; gastrointestinal; renal; reproductive; immune; eyes, ears, nose, and throat; dermatological; and hematological), in addition to over-the-counter (OTC) medications. It also covers the emerging world of complementary and alternative medicine (CAM). Unique to this section are detailed discussions of anatomy and physiology and photographs of a number of drugs used to treat various conditions of each body system.

Three appendices are included in this edition. Appendix A, Review for the Pharmacy Technician Certification Board (PTCB) Examination, presents 90 review questions that are directly indicative of the type of questions on actual PTCB examinations. This review is designed to help students assess their knowledge and readiness to sit for the examination. Appendix B, Top 200 Prescription Drugs, lists the 200 most commonly prescribed legend drugs, their classifications, and the indications for their use. Appendix C, Top 30 Herbal Remedies, lists some of the more popular herbal remedies and their commonly reported uses. The Glossary contains all key terms and definitions listed in the textbook.

Distinctive Features of This Edition

Learning Objectives

The organizational format of this textbook facilitates the learning process by providing students and educators with detailed learning objectives that address the cognitive knowledge required to master each chapter's content. These learning objectives are listed at the beginning of each chapter, giving both students and instructors definitive evaluation tools to use as each chapter's content is covered.

Key Terms

Key terms are identified and defined at the beginning of each chapter, providing students with a valuable terminology overview for the chapter. These key terms are included in the Glossary at the back of the book and are provided in flashcard form on the Evolve site to allow students to test their knowledge of the chapter's terms and definitions.

Scenario

In Section One (Pharmacy Practice), pharmacy technician scenarios are provided at the beginning of each chapter, and scenario check-ups appear throughout the chapter. These scenarios provide practical applications for pharmacy technician students and allow them to "connect" with their future beyond the classroom. The scenarios in the chapters often involve authentic pharmacy technicians sharing their fears, likes, hopes, and aspirations, providing a "real-world" feel to the book and inspiration for the student.

Tech Notes

Helpful pharmacy technician notes are interspersed throughout the chapters, providing interesting historical facts, drug cautions, hints, and safety information. These notes enhance students' acquisition of the practical information they will need to know in a pharmacy setting.

Tech Alerts

Tech alert boxes highlight important information the pharmacy technician needs to remember when in the pharmacy. In many instances, the Tech Alert functions as a medication safety reminder or presents proper drug names.

Technician Profile

In Section One (Pharmacy Practice), technician profiles are shared to help pharmacy technician students "connect" with their future beyond the classroom. These profiles provide insight into life after graduation and often show students the different types of jobs and responsibilities they may take on once they enter the real-life profession of pharmacy technician.

Mini Drug Monographs

Drug monographs with pill photographs are provided in Section Two (Pharmacology and Medications), where each body system is discussed. In addition to a photograph of the drug, these monographs include the drug class, generic and trade names, indication, route of administration, common adult dosage, mechanism of action, side effects, and any required auxiliary labels. The monographs provide students with quick, easy-to-understand information about specific drugs.

Do You Remember These Key Points?

These chapter summaries are placed at the end of every chapter to recap the highlights and most important topics covered in the chapter. These brief summaries of each chapter's key points can serve as a study tool, reminding students of the subject areas they may need to review before taking an examination on the chapter's content.

Review Questions

Multiple-choice review questions are included at the end of every chapter (and also, in interactive form, on the Evolve site). This section provides students with a unique review tool as they prepare both for classroom examinations and for certification examinations, once they're ready to begin their professional lives as pharmacy technicians. Just as the key points serve as a study tool and chapter summary, these review questions give students a chance to quiz themselves on the chapter content, assess their knowledge of important chapter topics, and evaluate which topics need follow-up review.

Technician's Corner

The Technician's Corner, which appears at the end of every chapter, provides critical thinking questions to help students prepare for on-the-job experiences.

New Chapters in This Edition

Chapter on the Technician's Role in Customer/Patient Communication

Chapter 4, Communication and Role of the Technician with the Customer/Patient, gives pharmacy technician students invaluable information about communication (verbal, nonverbal, and written), the communication cycle, telephone and cell phone etiquette, communicating with the health care team, communicating with special populations, and ways to optimize their communication methods. This chapter is essential for students to learn about professionalism and how to communicate with a variety of people, skills that are crucial to their success on the job.

Chapters on Community Pharmacy Practice, Institutional Pharmacy Practice, and Additional Pharmacy Practice Settings

Chapters 8, 9, and 10 give students a focused approach to the various types of pharmacy practice settings available to them after they graduate from a pharmacy technician program and pass their certification examination. Chapter 8, Community Pharmacy Practice, includes prescription interpretation and discusses the many types of community pharmacies: independent, franchise, and chain pharmacies. Chapter 9, Institutional Pharmacy Practice, includes medication order interpretation and the ins and outs of working in the challenging area of institutional (hospital) pharmacy practice. Chapter 10, Additional Pharmacy Practice Settings, covers long-term care, home infusion, managed care, mail-order pharmacy, and the pharmaceutical industry. It is important that students learn about all of these types of pharmacy practices, and the in-depth coverage in these chapters gives students a comprehensive view of all sides of each practice setting.

Chapter on Therapeutic Agents for the Hematological System

Chapter 26, Therapeutic Agents for the Hematological System, presents detailed coverage of the anatomy and physiology of the hematological system, including the major components of blood, conditions affecting the hematological system, and the drugs most commonly used to treat the conditions described. As with the other chapters the completely revised Section Two, Chapter 26 includes drug monographs for many medications.

Ancillaries for this Edition

Considering the broad range of students, instructors, programs, and institutions for which this textbook was designed, an extensive package of supplements has been designed to complement this fourth edition of *Mosby's Pharmacy Technician: Principles and Practice*. Each of these comprehensive supplements has been thoughtfully developed with the shared goals of students and instructors in mind; that is, to produce students who are well equipped for a career in pharmacy and well prepared to earn their certification. All of these supplements and their inventive features (with the exception of the Workbook/Lab Manual) can be found on the Evolve site (http://evolve.elsevier.com/Mosby/pharmtech). They include the following materials.

For the Instructor

TEACH Instructor Resource

TEACH for *Mosby's Pharmacy Technician* is designed to help the pharmacy technician instructor prepare for class by reducing preparation time, providing new and innovative ideas to promote student learning, and helping to make full use of the rich array of resources available. This completely revised manual includes:

- Detailed Lesson Plans that map to the chapter objectives (as well as the PTCE [Pharmacy Technician Certification Examination] and ASHP Model Curriculum)
- PowerPoint presentations
- Answer Keys for the Chapter Review Questions, as well as Workbook/Lab Manual exercises

Additional Instructor Ancillaries

- Correlation Grids
  - ASHP Curriculum
  - Pharmacy Technician Certification Examination (PTCE)
- Image Collection
- ExamView Test Bank
- Interactive Skill Check-off Sheets

For the Student

Ancillaries Available on the Evolve Site

- Interactive flashcards with each chapter's key terms and definitions
- Interactive Chapter Review Questions
- Mosby's Essential Drugs for Pharmacy Technicians
- Appendices from the textbook

Student Workbook/Lab Manual

The student workbook/lab manual has been completely revised to correspond to the vast amount of changes made in the textbook. This resource is a unique blend of a traditional workbook combined with lab exercises that enhance the student's ability to perform in class. This valuable product includes:

- Exercises to reinforce key concepts taught in this textbook
- Skill Check-off Sheets to correspond to textbook procedures
- Opportunities for students to reflect critically on topics as they develop critical thinking and decision-marking skills
- Complete lab activities that will relate to practice

Contents

SECTION TWO
Pharmacology and Medications

SECTION 1
Pharmacy Practice

SECTION OUTLINE

History of Medicine and Pharmacy

Bobbi Steelman

OBJECTIVES

Upon completing this chapter, you should be able to do the following:

1. Discuss ancient beliefs of illness and medicine from 440 BC through AD 1600.
2. List common ancient treatments that prevailed in Western civilization.
3. Describe nineteenth-century medicine and identify influences that major wars had on medicine.
4. Describe the wide use of opium and the problems surrounding opium use.
5. Differentiate between opiates and opioids.
6. Describe how the first pharmacies began in the United States.
7. Identify the role that early pharmacists played in society.
8. Describe the first technicians in pharmacy.
9. List major ways pharmacy has changed over the past 100 years.
10. List important current trends in pharmacy in relation to pharmacy technicians.

IMPORTANT PEOPLE

Aristotle	Greek scientist, philosopher
Asclepius	Greek god of healing and medicine
Bacon, Roger	English scientist responsible for scientific methods
Crick, Francis	Co-discoverer of the molecular structure of DNA, the double helix
Domagk, Gerhard	Developed sulfonamides and synthetic antibiotics
Fleming, Alexander	Discovered penicillin, the first antibiotic
Galen, Claudius	Greek physician
Hippocrates	Greek physician and philosopher, considered to be the father of medicine
Mendel, Gregor	Scientist and monk, known as the father of genetics
Nightingale, Florence	Nurse who was responsible for improving the unsanitary conditions at a British base hospital during the Crimean War, reducing the death count
Paracelsus	Swiss physician, philosopher, and scientist
Pasteur, Louis	French scientist, discovered several vaccines and invented pasteurization
Watson, James	Co-discoverer of the molecular structure of DNA, the double helix

TERMS AND DEFINITIONS

Apothecary Latin term for pharmacist; also, a place where drugs are sold

Bloodletting The practice of draining blood; believed to release illness

Caduceus Often confused as the symbol of the medical field; it is a staff with two entwined snakes and two wings at the top

Dogma A principle or set of principles laid down by an authority as incontrovertibly true

Herbals A substance made from or using herbs

Hippocratic Oath An oath taken by physicians concerning the ethics and practice of medicine

Inpatient pharmacy A pharmacy in a hospital or institutional setting

Laudanum A mixture of opium and alcohol used to treat dozens of illnesses through the 1800s

Leeches A type of segmented worm with suckers that attaches to the skin of a host and engorges itself on the host's blood

Maggots Fly larvae that feed on dead tissue; used in medicine to clean wounds not responding to routine antibiotics

Medicine The science and art dealing with the maintenance of health and the prevention, alleviation, or cure of disease

Opioid Any agent that binds to opioid receptors

Opium An analgesic that is made from the poppy plant

Pharmacist Person who dispenses drugs and counsels patients on medication use and any interactions it may have with food or other drugs

Pharmacy A place where drugs are sold

Pharmacy clerk Person who assists the pharmacist at the front counter of the pharmacy; the person who accepts payment for medications

Pharmacy technician Person who assists a pharmacist by filling prescriptions and performing other nondiscretionary tasks

Pharmacy Technician Certification Board (PTCB) Issues a national exam for pharmacy technicians

Shaman A person who holds a high place of honor in a tribe as a healer and spiritual mediator

Staff of Asclepius The symbol of the medical profession; it is a wingless staff with one snake wrapped around it

Trephining A practice of making an opening in the head to allow disease to leave the body

History of Medicine

Scenario:

Kelly is a new pharmacy technician student at a local career college. She begins her course of study by learning about the history of pharmacy. Why is this an important part of Kelly's education?

Ancient Beliefs and Treatments

Medicine has been practiced for thousands of years. Archaeological discoveries have unearthed civilizations that have documented the use of minerals, animals, and plant parts to heal the sick. Certain remedies, such as **herbals**, have been used consistently throughout history. For example, herbs have been used for centuries for minor ailments such as intestinal problems, arthritis, and gout.

Many ancient treatments for illness were based on the dreams or visions of the believers. A **dogma**, such as gods being able to both cause and cure illnesses, is based on a set of principles (e.g., religious or ideological doctrines) proposed by authoritarians. These principles are based on writings from respected spiritual authorities rather than scientific evidence. One belief about healing the sick was that severe illness was caused by evil spirits. To rid a person of an evil spirit, a cut was made into the skull to give the spirit a portal through which to leave. This type of treatment was called **trephining** and often was performed by a tribal **shaman** (a spiritual person in a tribe who cares for the spiritual, medicinal, and physical health of the tribe). Tribal shamans were believed to have the gift of being able to communicate with spirits. Other shamans believed that they were connected with a special spirit who helped them render the evil spirits harmless through the use of prayer, herbs, or potions. Shamans were prevalent throughout societies in ancient times. Some still exist in various societies throughout the world. In North America, various Eskimo and Native American tribes held shamans in high esteem. However, many of the popular beliefs of the past have mostly disappeared.

The Medical Staff

The **staff of Asclepius** is the formal symbol of medicine and is associated with **Asclepius**, the Greek god associated with healing. The staff of Asclepius is a wingless walking stick with a single serpent wrapped around it. Because snakes shed their skin, the snake was believed to signify renewal of youth. The **caduceus** is often mistakenly used as a symbol of medicine. The caduceus is the staff of Hermes, a Greek god; the staff represented magic and had two serpents wrapped around it, usually with two wings at the top (Figure 1-1). For example, in 1902 the U.S. Army erroneously adopted the caduceus as an emblem of the Medical Corps, leading to its mistaken use as a symbol of medicine. Although many organizations still use the caduceus to represent medicine, the true staff of Asclepius has been adopted as a symbol by authoritative health organizations, such as the World Health Organization and the American Medical Association.

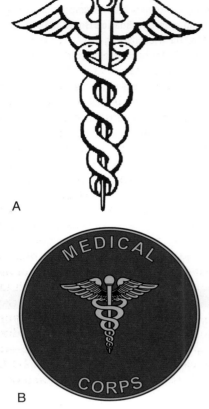

FIGURE 1-1 **A,** Caduceus. **B,** Army Medical Corp emblem.

The Evolution of Medicine

The early path of medicine was not a smooth road. Throughout the ages, many plagues killed thousands of people. The existence of microbes, unseen by the eye, was not known to be responsible for many of the diseases that caused death and despair. Despite advances made through early history, most remedies for physical ailments tended to be extreme. Other ancient remedies have been used for hundreds of years. Prevalent thoughts included the belief that sickness was an entity within the body that needed a means to leave the body. Another widely held belief was that spirits were responsible for illness. In many cultures, the most common form of treatment, prayer, has remained as the only way to cure illness.

Hippocrates (460-357 BC), born on the small island of Cos near Greece, was a third-generation physician. He taught at a school of medicine on Cos, which was one of the first medical schools established. He believed in the prevailing concept of that era: life consisted of a balance of four elements that were linked to qualities of good health. These four qualities were wet, dry, hot, and cold. In addition, he believed that illness resulted from an imbalance of the four humors of the body system: blood, phlegm,

yellow bile, and black bile. These four humors were linked to the four basic elements: blood is air, phlegm is water, yellow bile is fire, and black bile is earth. Methods used to treat imbalance of the humors included bloodletting and natural laxatives.

Hippocrates was responsible for many advances in the world of medicine. Some of his observations included the effects of food, climate, and other influences on illness. He was one of the first physicians to record his patients' medical illnesses. This new way of viewing the causes of illnesses eventually led to the belief that sickness originated from something other than the supernatural. Hippocrates believed that the spirit of the patient should be as important as the condition being treated, and he promoted kindness to the sick. He also believed in letting nature do the healing and promoted resting and eating light foods. He taught that doctors needed to rebalance the four humors. Most of his teachings have been documented in a collection of books called the *Corpus Hippocraticum.* Although many of the writings are now believed to be from different authors, they still reflect the teachings of Hippocrates.

Today's medical schools still use the **Hippocratic Oath** as part of their graduation ceremony. Box 1-1 presents the revised version of the Hippocratic Oath used today. The Hippocratic Oath outlines the physician's responsibility to the patient. Hippocrates practiced what he preached with respect to exercise, rest, diet, and overall moderation in lifestyle. Various records have documented his death as occurring in 377 BC, whereas others record his death has having occurred in 357 BC. Because of the advances he promoted in the world of medicine, it is not surprising that Hippocrates is known as the father of medicine. Before the existence of Hippocrates and other innovative scientists, people believed that they were at the mercy of the gods or supernatural forces.

 Tech Note!

The origin of the term "black humor" stems from the belief that too much of the black bile humor resulted in a person showing signs of melancholy.

Later in history, the Greek philosopher and scientist **Aristotle** (384-322 BC) was responsible for many advances in the areas of biology and medicine. His main area of interest was biology and the study and classification of various organisms. He classified human beings as animals. Because the Grecian belief system in those times did not allow dissection of the dead, he described much of human anatomy from observations he made from dissections of other

BOX 1-1

The Hippocratic Oath*

I swear to fulfill, to the best of my ability and judgment, this covenant:

I will respect the hard-won scientific gains of those physicians in whose steps I walk, and gladly share such knowledge as is mine with those who are to follow.

I will apply, for the benefit of the sick, all measures [that] are required, avoiding those twin traps of overtreatment and therapeutic nihilism.

I will remember that there is art to medicine as well as science, and that warmth, sympathy, and understanding may outweigh the surgeon's knife or the chemist's drug.

I will not be ashamed to say I know not, nor will I fail to call in my colleagues when the skills of another are needed for a patient's recovery.

I will respect the privacy of my patients, for their problems are not disclosed to me that the world may know. Most especially must I tread with care in matters of life and death. If it is given me to save a life, all thanks. But it may also be within my power to take a life; this awesome responsibility must be faced with great humbleness and awareness of my own frailty. Above all, I must not play at God.

I will remember that I do not treat a fever, chart a cancerous growth, but a sick human being, whose illness may affect the person's family and economic stability. My responsibility includes these related problems, if I am to care adequately for the sick.

I will prevent disease whenever I can, for prevention is preferable to cure.

I will remember that I remain a member of society, with special obligations to all my fellow human beings, those sound of mind and body as well as the infirm.

If I do not violate this oath, may I enjoy life and art, respected while I live and remembered with affection thereafter. May I always act so as to preserve the finest traditions of my calling and may I long experience the joy of healing those who seek my help.

*Written in 1964 by Louis Lasagna, Academic Dean of the School of Medicine at Tufts University, and used in many medical schools today.
http://ethics.ucsd.edu/journal/2006/readings/Hippocratic_Oath_Modern_Version.pdf

animals. This included in-depth descriptions of the brain, heart, lungs, and blood vessels.

Claudius Galen (129-210) began to study medicine at the age of 16. He attended medical schools in Greece and the famous Alexandria School of Medicine in Egypt. He later resided in Rome and was the personal physician of the Roman imperial family. Although he was born nearly 600 years after Hippocrates, he followed many of the same beliefs, such as eating a balanced diet, exercising, and practicing good hygiene. He contributed greatly to the study of medicine, writing more than 100 books on topics such as physiology, anatomy, pathology, diagnosis, and pharmacology. Many of his books were used in medical schools for 1,500 years. He proved that blood flowed through arteries rather than air.

Philosopher and alchemist **Roger Bacon** (1214-1294) further refined and explained the importance of experimental methods, which focused on observation, hypothesis, experimentation, and verification. During Bacon's time most explanations were based on tradition, not fact. He preferred to rely on mathematics and measurement to prove his theories. He is considered an important contributor to what is now known as the scientific method.

Paracelsus (1493-1541), a Swiss physician and alchemist, believed that it was important to treat illness with one medication at a time. At the end of the Middle Ages, it was a common practice to give multiple remedies or large quantities of agents that had not been tested previously. Through experimentation and documentation of the effectiveness and dosage of each individual agent, Paracelsus was able to produce many medications. He introduced one of the most popular tonics of that time—laudanum, which was used to deaden pain. Table 1-1 lists major figures and their influences throughout medical history.

Ancient Herbal Remedies

Over the millennia, some prevalent treatments consisted of multiple mixtures of plants, roots, and other concoctions. Digestion of the type of plant that resembled the organ affected by disease also was believed to cure illnesses. For example, those with liver problems ingested a plant called liverwort (named because the leaves were shaped like a liver). Other popular treatments included using garlic for inflammation of the bronchial tubes, wine and pepper for various stomach ailments, onions for worms, and tiger fat for joint pain. It was difficult to detect which, if any, of the ingredients administered actually worked because many concoctions contained a multitude of ingredients. As strange as many of these archaic remedies seem, there were many people who were "cured" because of their strong belief in the treatment given or their belief in the person treating them.

Throughout history, popular religious beliefs revolved around the idea that evil spirits were the cause of illness in a person who had sinned. This belief may have persisted partly because no one had the slightest idea about germs or genetics. Many times, through trial and error (error sometimes causing death), certain treatments were found to be fairly effective.

Anytime new theories are proposed, they can be met with some skepticism and disbelief. Eventually,

TABLE 1-1

Advances in Medicine

Name	Year	Medical Advance
William Harvey	1628	Writes first book on blood circulation through the heart
James Lind	1747	Discovers that citrus fruits prevent scurvy
Rene Laennec	1816	Invents stethoscope
James Blundell	1818	Performs first blood transfusion
Crawford W. Long	1842	Uses ether as a general anesthetic
Joseph Lister	1867	Publishes *Antiseptic Principle of the Practice of Surgery*
Louis Pasteur	1870s	Establishes germ theory of disease
Wilhelm Roentgen	1895	Discovers x-rays
Ronald Ross	1897	Demonstrates that malaria is transmitted by mosquitoes
Felix Hoffman	1899	Develops aspirin
Karl Landsteiner	1901	First describes ABO, B, AB, and O blood groups
Sir Frederick Gowland Hopkins	1906	Suggests existence of vitamins and concludes they are essential to health
Dr. Paul Dudley White	1913	One of the first cardiologists; pioneers use of electrocardiograph
Edward Mellanby	1921	Discovers that lack of vitamin D causes rickets
	1922	First uses insulin to treat diabetes
Sir Alexander Fleming	1928	Discovers penicillin*
Gerhard Domagk	1932	Discovers sulfonamides
Dr. John H. Gibbon, Jr.	1935	Successfully uses heart-lung machine (on cat) to continue circulating blood while patient was in surgery
Selman A. Waksman	1943	Discovers streptomycin
Paul Zoll	1952	Develops first cardiac pacemaker
James Watson, Francis Crick	1953	Describe double-helical structure of DNA
Dr. Joseph E. Murray	1954	Performs first kidney transplant
Dr. Luc Montagnier, Dr. Anthony Galo	1983	Discover the human immunodeficiency virus (HIV), the virus that causes acquired immunodeficiency syndrome (AIDS)
James Thomson	2007	Scientists discover how to use human skin cells to create embryonic stem cells; study was performed in laboratory at University of Wisconsin
Laurent Lantieri	2008	Performed the first full face transplant
Deborah Persaud	2013	First baby cured of HIV in the United States
Researchers at Massachusetts General Hospital in Boston	2013	Produced first kidney grown in vitro in the United States

*Although discovered in 1928, it was not isolated and used as an antibiotic until 1938.

Scenario CHECK UP 1-1

Kelly is assigned to create a poster board showing the advances of medicine throughout ancient history. What should she focus on when creating her poster? What important pieces of information from ancient history relate to today's pharmacy practice that Kelly could show on her poster?

medicine and science discovered methods to answer this need for corroboration, leading to modern approaches and effective treatments for disease. A new hypothesis should be treated as a possible answer that has not been disproved. As new sciences emerge and new methods are devised to test hypotheses, the results can lead to medical advances. This was especially evident throughout the golden age of microbiology.

Eighteenth- and Nineteenth-Century Medicine

From the time of Galen, it was widely believed that the four humors could be rebalanced through the use of cathartics to clean out the bowels; diuretics to lessen the imbalance of body fluids; emetics to empty the stomach; and bloodletting to lessen body fluids, heart rate, and temperature. Physicians brought this theory to America, where such techniques were widely used, especially **bloodletting**.

Bloodletting had its origins in Egypt more than 3,000 years ago and later spread into all areas of Europe through the Middle Ages. Just as trephination of the skull was believed to release evil spirits, bloodletting was thought to be an effective way of lessening excess body fluids that were believed to cause illness. Artifacts such as sharp bones, sharks' teeth, thorns, and sharpened sticks were believed to be the earliest instruments used in bloodletting. During the nineteenth century some even used bloodletting as preventive medicine to ensure good health. A well-known victim of bloodletting in America during the eighteenth century was George Washington, who suffered from an infection and died of complications from bloodletting. At that time, it was wrongly believed that the body contained 12 quarts of blood; however, it contains only 6 quarts, and President Washington was bled of 4 quarts over a 24-hour period.

One bloodletting treatment involved using **leeches**. These blood-sucking worms were gathered, stored, and used to remove blood from patients. The leech has the ability to latch onto the skin with sharp, teethlike appendages and engorge itself to nearly twice its size on a person's blood. Leeches also emit a natural anticoagulant, hirudin, that allows the blood to flow freely. Leeches were used in specific places, such as the vagina to treat menorrhea. Once the leeches were finished eating, they would normally detach themselves; if not, they were encouraged to detach with the use of salt. Bleeding would continue until it was necessary to manually stop the flow of blood with bandages.

Another form of bloodletting, venesection (phlebotomy, or drawing blood) was widely used in the 1700s and 1800s for those who did not want leeches applied. The physician would heat the air inside a small cup and place it on the skin, which would draw up the skin tissue, along with its blood flow (called "wet cupping"). At this point, a lancet would be used to cut into the skin, the cup would be removed, and 1 to 4 ounces of blood would be collected. Many patients succumbed to this procedure until the early 1900s, when this type of treatment was declared quackery.

Fortunately, medicine did advance through the nineteenth century in many ways. Medical schools arose throughout Europe, specifically in France and Germany. Many of the doctors trained in these schools came to America and brought with them this European influence in medicine. Medicinal recipes were written in Latin until the 1900s. Box 1-2 presents an example of a commonly compounded prescription. Because Latin was used in medicine and **apothecary** products, this order could be interpreted by most practitioners. Although there have been many changes in the accepted abbreviations

BOX 1-2

Example of a Prescription Compound from the 1900s

Infusion of Dandelion, &c.	Interpretation of Order
Infusi Taraxaci, f℥iv	4 fluid ounces of infusion of dandelion
Extracti Taraxaci, f℥ij.	2 fluid drachms of extract of dandelion
Sodæ Carbonatis, ℨβ.	½ drachm of sodium carbonate
Potasse Tartratis, ℨiij.	3 drachms of potassium tartrate
Tincturæ Rhei, f℥iij.	3 fluid drachms of tincture of rhubarb
Hyoscyami, gtt. xx.	20 drops [19] of henbane tincture

Signa.—One third part to be taken three times a day. In dropsical and visceral affections.

and weights in medicine, the fluid ounce can still be seen on pharmacy bottles. Several important medical advances that have changed medical treatments and lengthened the human life span are listed in Table 1-1.

Throughout the nineteenth century, the church became active in scientific research as well. A monk named **Gregor Mendel** experimented on plants and noticed the changes from generation to generation with respect to color, size, and appearance. He used pea plants to determine how traits were transferred from one to another and in doing so determined the basics of genetics. In 1822, he determined how stronger plants could be propagated through heredity. It was not until the 1900s, however, that other scientists were able to continue his work and enlighten the scientific world with the theory of genetics. As a result of his work, Mendel became known as the father of genetics.

Florence Nightingale was born in Florence, Italy, in 1820 and is best known as a nurse who spent her career caring for the wounded. She believed in cleanliness and its benefits to the medical field. She started a hospital and founded a school for nurses. Her writings sparked worldwide health care reform.

North American Medicine

In early North America, as new immigrants brought their families from Europe and other parts of the world, disease followed. At that time, doctors were responsible not only for diagnosing conditions, but also for preparing the necessary remedies to cure patients. Disease was widespread in the colonies, and many people did not survive the voyage across the sea from Europe, succumbing to diseases such as scurvy and severe intestinal infection. Patients were at a disadvantage throughout the colonies because there were few doctors and even fewer hospitals. The first pharmacists, known as druggists at the time, were doctors until pharmacy became a specialty. The term "druggist" was widely used from the 1700s until the mid-1800s to describe the practitioners of pharmacy, eventually leading to the title *pharmacist*.

Remedies used in early American history included cinchona bark (quinine) for the treatment of malaria. More unconventional and dangerous treatments also were used; for example, mercury was used to treat syphilis. Many people died of mercury poisoning because of its toxicity. Many people also died of typhoid fever, malaria, diphtheria, and dysentery. The need for doctors and treatments increased dramatically. The average life expectancy was approximately 40 years, and many families lost several children to childhood diseases, such as smallpox, for which no vaccines were available. Most treatments were concoctions handed down through family tradition. If a person were to use a doctor, he or she most likely would be treated at home or in the doctor's office, with treatments ranging from minor procedures to surgery. Box 1-3 presents some typical remedies used in the 1800s in the United States.

Tech Note!

Vaccines did not develop until 1796, with the first immunization against smallpox in England. Smallpox vaccination was stopped in 1971 because the disease had been eradicated worldwide. Polio is another serious illness that has been eradicated in developed countries through the use of an effective vaccination strategy. However, childhood immunization remains important to prevent the spread of wild-type polio infection worldwide. Countries such as Nigeria, India, Pakistan, and Afghanistan have been experiencing a resurgence of polio, which makes all countries that no longer immunize for this disease vulnerable to infection.

Opium and Alcohol. One of the most popular tonics made for medicinal use in early America contained opium and alcohol. Its effectiveness was surpassed only by its addictiveness. This tonic was given as a sedative and to dull the sensation of pain. Paracelsus (as mentioned earlier in this chapter) introduced the opium-alcohol mixture called **laudanum** in the sixteenth century, and laudanum was used as a medicinal remedy. Laudanum was used widely throughout Europe in the Victorian era. During the Civil War, laudanum not only was used to treat painful wounds from the battlefield (Box 1-4), it also found its way into households throughout the United States for

BOX 1-3

Typical Remedies during the 1800s in America

To stop earaches	Blow tobacco smoke into the ear.
To treat a cold	Combine a mixture of sugar, mineral oil, sulfur, ginger, lemon, and whisky in 8 oz. of water; drink this and go to bed.
For baldness	Rub the head with an onion in the morning and at night before bed until the skin becomes red, and then rub it with honey.
For worms	Take a tablespoon of molasses and mix it with tin rust and ingest.
For stomach aches	Mix strychnine and other alkaline additives into an oral solution.
For cough and cold	Mix terpin of hydrate with codeine or heroin into an oral solution.
For eye infections	Add mercury to other ingredients such as eye drops.

BOX 1-4

The Civil War

From 1861 through 1865 the Civil War claimed more lives than any other war in American history. More than 1 million soldiers died on the battlefield. Soldiers who did not die of their wounds succumbed to tuberculosis, typhoid fever, dysentery, and a host of other diseases, including measles, mumps, and chickenpox. Diseases spread rapidly as a result of the overcrowded and close quarters of men who had never been exposed to these diseases. Field hospitals were unsanitary and overcrowded. Many men died of infections caused by amputations and gunshot wounds. Medication was not available most of the time, and anesthesia was limited to chloroform, from which many men died as a result of an overdose of the drug. Those who were hurt on the battlefield received care from undertrained medical staff with less than adequate equipment in nonsterile conditions. Most of the doctors (in the states) had minimal training; usually they completed an apprenticeship in lieu of formal training.

less severe problems. Laudanum was used mostly by white middle- to upper-class women for a host of problems, including nervousness, diabetes, diarrhea, gastric problems, menstrual pain, and even morning sickness. Laudanum was also used to calm screaming babies. Individuals became addicted at an alarming rate. Many mortalities and miscarriages were attributed to this agent. Even though it was

BOX 1-5

Laudanum Recipe from 1669

16 ounces of sherry wine
2 ounces of opium
1 ounce of saffron
1 ounce powder of cinnamon
1 ounce powder of cloves

well-known by the eighteenth century that opium and alcohol were addictive, alternative remedies were hard to find. Box 1-5 presents an example of a laudanum recipe from 1669 that was used as a remedy for dysentery. Another alcohol-based liquid was absinthe. The herb *Artemisia absinthium* was mixed with alcohol and other additives. Absinthe was served with water and sugar and was purported to rid a person of tapeworms, among other ailments.

 Tech Note!

Alcohol use has been dated back to 3500 BC in Egypt. Opium has long been a part of human history; opium plants have been found as part of Neolithic burial sites. Cultivated opium made its appearance in Egypt about 1300 BC; from Egypt, opium was traded to Greece and eventually other parts of Europe.

Origin of Opium (Opiates). **Opium** has a long history in the medicinal relief of pain and in recreational use. Opium is a byproduct of the plant *Papaver somniferum,* commonly known as the opium poppy. The sap is taken from the head of the poppy. The raw opium then is precipitated from the sap. The result of this process is a potent drug that causes an analgesic effect. Although "opiate" was a term used for a drug derived from opium, the more common term is **opioid**, which refers to both synthetic and semisynthetic medications. Opiates and opioids react on the same opioid receptor sites, which are located in the central nervous system and gastrointestinal tract (see Chapter 15). The effects associated with the opioid receptors include analgesia, respiratory depression, pupil constriction, reduced gastrointestinal motility, euphoria, dysphoria, sedation, and physical dependence. Opioids and opiates have many of the same side effects, including nausea and vomiting. When used properly, the opioid drugs are effective and help many patients who otherwise would suffer extreme pain. Not until 1909, under the Opium Exclusion Act, did the prohibition of opium importation (except for medicinal purposes) begin in the United States (see Chapter 2).

Twentieth-Century Medicine

In the 1900s many new medicines were discovered; some of the earlier, groundbreaking discoveries were for medicines that were useful in treating infections. The Scottish physician and bacteriologist **Alexander Fleming** accidentally contaminated a plate of bacteria with mold while working in his laboratory in 1928; the mold inhibited the growth of the bacteria, and he named the mold "penicillin." Many years of failed and successful experimentation by many scientists followed before penicillin was recognized as a useful medicine. It was not until after 1938 that penicillin would undergo mass production and be used worldwide as a helpful antibiotic. Penicillin was the first antibiotic discovered and is still in use today. The first synthetic drug, a sulfonamide, was discovered by **Gerhard Domagk** in 1938 and was derived from a chemical dye found to inhibit bacterial growth. This sulfonamide was used extensively during World War II to treat infections that were a result of battle wounds. Today, sulfonamides are primarily used to treat urinary tract infections. Many antibiotics were discovered in the years after penicillin and sulfa.

Also in the twentieth century, a very important discovery was made by **James Watson** and **Francis Crick**. In April, 1953, they published a scientific paper presenting the structure of the DNA helix, the molecule that carries genetic information from one generation to another. They ultimately received the Nobel Prize in Physiology or Medicine, along with Maurice Wilkins, for their important contributions to science.

Advances in Drug Therapy and Vaccinations

Many of the most famous chemists, biologists, and doctors who contributed to science were from European countries, such as Germany, England, France, and Poland. **Louis Pasteur** (France), who is best known for the pasteurization process, also was responsible for discovering vaccines, such as the anthrax vaccine. Table 1-2 provides a list of pathogens and diseases that were discovered, along with the vaccines administered to prevent these diseases.

Are Old Remedies Making a Comeback?

Many archaic treatments fell out of favor during the middle to late nineteenth century, yet certain ones prevail. For instance, patients are bled daily in all types of medical settings. For example, if a physician orders a blood test to be done on a patient, up to 30 mL of blood will be taken from the patient's vein.

TABLE 1-2

Examples of Important Vaccine Advances in Medicine*

Scientist	Year of Discovery	Organism/Disease Identified	Vaccine
Edward Jenner (England)	1796 (acknowledged in 1800)	Smallpox	Smallpox vaccine
Robert Koch (Germany)	1876	Anthrax, tuberculosis	BioThrax[†] vaccine[‡]
Louis Pasteur (France)	1877-1887	*Staphylococcus, Streptococcus, Pneumococcus*	Rabies, chickenpox, cholera, anthrax vaccines
Emil von Behring (Germany)	1890	Discovers antitoxins	Tetanus/diphtheria/typhoid fever vaccine (DPT)
	1896	Typhoid fever	
	1926	Whooping cough	Pertussis vaccine
	1945	Influenza	Various vaccines used currently: Fluarix, Fluvirin, Fluzone, FluLaval intranasal, FluMist
Jonas Salk (U.S.)	1955	Polio	First polio vaccine
Albert Sabin (U.S.)	1962	Polio[§]	First oral polio vaccine
	1964	Measles	Vaccine combo (measles, mumps, rubella [MMR])
	1967	Mumps	Vaccine combo (MMR)
	1970	Rubella	Vaccine combo (MMR)
	1974	Chickenpox[¶]	Varicella (Varivax) vaccine
	1977	Pneumonia	Pneumovax vaccine
	1978	Meningitis	Menactra, Menomune vaccines
	1981	Hepatitis B	HepB (Engerix-B, Recombivax HB)
	1992	Hepatitis A	HepA (Havrix, Vaqta) HepA/HepB combo (Twinrix)
	1998	Lyme disease	Vaccine removed from U.S. market in 2002 because of low demand
	2003	Influenza	FluMist (first nasal vaccine for influenza approved in the United States)
	2006	Human papillomavirus	HPV (Gardasil)
	2006	Varicella-zoster virus (shingles)	Zostavax vaccine
	2009	Swine flu	H1N1 vaccine
	2010-2011	Influenza	H3N2 vaccine
	2010	*Streptococcus pneumoniae*	Prevnar 13 vaccine
	2013	Enterovirus 71	Hand-foot-mouth disease vaccine

*For more information on vaccines, refer to Chapter 23.
[†]For military use only.
[‡]Not used in the United States.
[§]Oral polio vaccine is no longer used for routine vaccination in United States because the disease has been eradicated in that country.
[¶]Given to individuals born after 1956.

This, of course, is used to diagnose an illness rather than as a curative measure, yet these techniques originated in the distant past, and today no one would question such a technique. The disorder hemochromatosis is a hereditary condition in which the body absorbs too much iron, which is stored in organs and can cause serious damage. The current treatment for this disorder is to remove blood (phlebotomy) on a regular basis.

The U.S. Food and Drug Administration (FDA) approved the use of both leeches and maggots in the medical setting in 1976. This may seem strange and not much of an advance in medicine. The origins of this type of treatment stem from research in the repair of tissue that has been severely damaged, such as that found in patients who have undergone reconstructive surgery or skin grafts or who have infections. However, surgical reattachment of veins can cause coagulation before blood flow is reestablished to the affected part, killing the affected tissues. Leeches are used to siphon excess blood from the area and prevent coagulation from taking place too soon. They are applied one at a time over 20 minutes for up to 2 days as necessary. Leeches are cared for and stored in the refrigerator in the pharmacy. They may not be the first choice of a physician, but they have been used successfully in many cases as a means of avoiding amputation.

Because dead skin is the main dietary intake of **maggots**, they can be used to remove dead skin. Antibiotics are normally used as the first course of treatment; however, when they are ineffective, physicians have used maggots to do the manual work of restoring the wound to a recoverable stage. Maggots not only eat the dead tissue, they also have the ability to kill the bacteria that are the cause of the infection. Treatments involving both leeches and maggots are very inexpensive compared with other treatments.

Other remedies are being studied, such as the honey produced by some bees (manuka honey). The medicinal attributes of this type of honey include the ability to heal wounds. Manuka honey keeps the wound moist, is bacteria free, and has a high sugar content, along with minerals, vitamins, and amino acids that are thought to promote healing. In 2007 the FDA and Health Canada approved its use for wounds and burns. In 2010, it was approved to treat leg ulcers and diabetic foot ulcers. In 2012, the FDA approved manuka honey wound dressings to treat over-the-counter abrasions, lacerations, and minor cuts. As medicine advances, it is wise not to forget the past because many historical treatments and remedies may be the answer for future cures. Pharmacy plays a part in both the historical and future advances in medicine and treatments because the roots of medicinal knowledge run deep.

History of Pharmacy

Early Pharmacists

The expanding population and the subsequent increasing need for trained medical personnel influenced the need for specialists such as veterinarians, eye doctors, and **pharmacists**. In addition, the shipping of medicines to America from England was becoming difficult as the colonies separated from England. After the Civil War, apothecaries (pharmacies) began to emerge in towns across America. Manufacturing plants were built, and people were trained to prepare medications accurately. As the physician's role changed from distributing drugs to diagnosing disease and performing surgery, the role of the pharmacist emerged. The first pharmacy school opened in

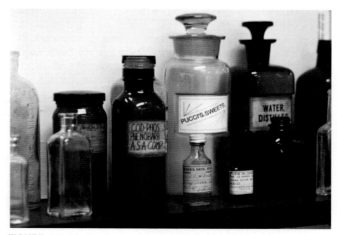

FIGURE 1-2 Medications were compounded by hand using a variety of compounds.

1821 at the College of Pharmacy and Sciences in Philadelphia. The school is now called the University of the Sciences in Philadelphia. Through the 1800s, pharmacists compounded nearly every drug ordered by physicians. Various sizes of ornate apothecary jars were used to store herbs and ingredients (Figure 1-2). The instructions for preparing remedies were contained in medical recipe books. Ingredients such as chalk for heartburn; rose petals for headaches; and oils, herbs, and spices filled containers in the apothecary. Although many of the ingredients in early compounded remedies are no longer used, several are still in use today, such as aspirin, digoxin, and others.

Another type of interesting container associated with the pharmacy was the show globe. Show globes have been the beacons for pharmacies dating back as far as the early 1600s. It is believed that they were placed in the apothecary stores of the town to let visitors know the status of the health of the town. Red meant there was illness or that the town was in quarantine because of disease, whereas green meant the town was healthy and thus it was safe to come into the town. It is also said that signs were posted on the doors of the contagious individuals, rather than relying only on the globes. Decorative globes (Figure 1-3) showed patrons the pharmacist's competencies in chemical mixtures. More ornate globes were layered in various colors, resulting in a striped appearance. This was done by using various liquids of differing densities, causing a layered effect. These types of jars are now displayed in many pharmacies, along with other artifacts from the past.

Early Pharmacy in America

The first **pharmacy** managed by a registered pharmacist opened in New Orleans in 1823. Starting in the mid-1800s and early 1900s, the soda fountain

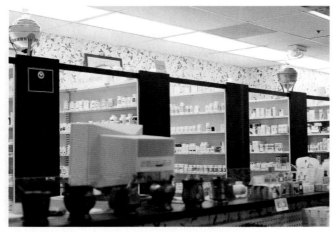

FIGURE 1-3 Large show globes (seen on top of shelf). An assortment of different mortars and pestles (seen on countertop).

BOX 1-6
Famous Pharmacists

Charles Alderton: Invented Dr Pepper
Caleb Bradham: Invented Pepsi-Cola
Susan Hayhurst: First woman to graduate from the Philadelphia School of Pharmacy
Charles Elmer Hires: Invented Hires Root Beer
John Pemberton: Invented Coca-Cola
William Proctor, Jr.: Father of American Pharmacy; founded American Pharmaceutical Association in 1852
Ella Phillips Stewart: One of the first African American female pharmacists in the United States
James Vernor: Invented Vernors Ginger Ale
Harvey A.K. Whitney: Founder and first president of the American Society of Hospital Pharmacists in 1942

became an extension of the town drugstore. The first soda fountain pharmacy began in the mid-1800s and gained popularity in the early 1900s. Prohibition in 1919 also helped with the proliferation of soda fountains. With the invention by a pharmacist, Jacob Baur (1921), of a soda fountain that dispensed carbon dioxide, soda fountain units could easily prepare all types of carbonated drinks.

Pharmacists would make and market their own recipes to be used for various treatments. It was common to find drugs mixed with flavorings, along with effervescent soda water, to treat ailments or provide a boost of energy. Both caffeine and cocaine were also often used in sodas. Some of the many conditions mineral water was supposed to cure were obesity, upset stomach, depression, and nervous disorders. Pharmacists sold phosphate sodas and ice cream favorites, worked the lunch counter, and filled the prescriptions for the day. The first 7-Up drink was made with lithium and was sold from soda fountains for conditions such as gout, uremia, and rheumatism. In 1886, Coca-Cola was invented by John Pemberton, a pharmacist in Georgia. The soft drink was marketed as a tonic and contained extracts of cocaine and caffeine until 1905, when cocaine was removed from the recipe because of changing public opinion regarding its use. It was not until later, after the Harrison Narcotic Drug Act of 1914 (see Chapter 2), that pharmacists were prohibited from making cocaine-containing preparations and began to sell plain soda drinks.

Box 1-6 presents a list of pharmacists/inventors. By the late 1800s, the soda shop/pharmacy was so popular that people came to drink the sweet concoctions whether they were ailing or not. This type of pharmacy setting undoubtedly added to the image of the friendly neighborhood pharmacist as a person who could be trusted. The stereotypic local neighborhood pharmacist who wore a white jacket, packaged medications, and sometimes worked the soda machine has all but disappeared, except in a few shops where a person may still purchase an old-fashioned malt or shake while waiting for a prescription to be filled.

Early Pharmacy Technicians

The first **pharmacy technicians** were those enlisted in the military because of the high demand for medications to treat injuries and illness. These individuals were trained on the job not only to fill prescriptions, but also to perform many of the functions of a pharmacist. To this day, military technicians have a broader scope of training than civilian technicians. Technicians also were employed by pharmacists who owned drugstores. Family members helped behind the counters, filled stock, and waited on customers. These early **pharmacy clerks** then moved on to become what we now call pharmacy technicians.

An urgent need for standardized training arose in the 1960s as pharmacist organizations, such as the American Society of Health-System Pharmacists (ASHP), the Michigan Pharmacists Association (MPA), and the American Pharmacists Association (APhA), realized that technicians would be able to better serve the patient with additional training. Technicians play such an important role in the health care of patients, it is important that they understand all aspects of their required tasks in the pharmacy. At the first conference on pharmacy technicians held by the ASHP in 1988, although many of the topics involved pharmacy technician training, other important aspects of the pharmacy setting, such as the lack of technician involvement in the workplace, were also discussed. In 1995 the **Pharmacy**

Technician Certification Board (PTCB) was formed, which was responsible for creating a national examination for technicians (see Chapter 3).

Although the transition from clerk to technician is fairly recent in history, forecasts indicate that the pharmacy technician will play a critical role in the future pharmacy setting. New job positions are constantly being created for technicians who have the necessary skills and knowledge to fill them. Clinical technicians now assist the pharmacist with a variety of tasks, such as anticoagulation monitoring. They may also manage the automation and pharmacy coordination systems in certain pharmacies. Table 1-3 presents an outline of the important chronological events that have transformed the position of pharmacy technician into its current role.

As of December 31, 2013, the PTCB had certified more than 525,365 technicians nationwide. This demonstrates the seriousness of this profession and the need for standardized competencies in the workplace. Up until the PTCB exam was established, most technicians had a high school diploma, although it was not mandatory; also, background checks were not done in every state. After the PTCB was established, not only were educational standards instituted, but also salaries were increased for many certified technicians. Attitudes have changed over time as well. Technicians once were viewed as incompetent in many areas of pharmacy but nonetheless a threat to replace pharmacists with cheap labor. Views now have changed because even with the increase in technicians in the workplace, pharmacists still are in high demand. Technicians are now a part of the health care team, and most pharmacists are confident they can delegate tasks to technicians knowing that the job will be done correctly. It is no coincidence that as higher standards and educational requirements have been set for the pharmacy technician, the pharmacists' trust in technicians has increased.

Changing Pharmacy Requirements

Times have changed and so have the requirements of today's pharmacist. For licensure, most states now require new pharmacists to obtain a doctor of pharmacy degree (PharmD). College students can start a 4-year pharmacy program after successfully completing 2 to 4 years of undergraduate coursework and earning a passing score on the Pharmacy College Admissions Test (PCAT). Coursework usually includes biology, chemistry, anatomy, and physics. Additionally, PharmD students must complete rotations in a variety of clinical and pharmaceutical settings.

Pharmacists who received a Bachelor of Science in pharmacy before this change have been allowed to

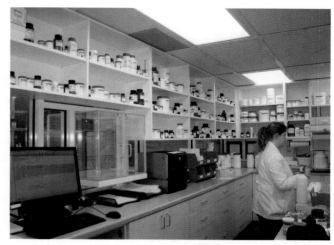

FIGURE 1-4 Pharmacy technician working in the pharmacy.

work in pharmacy without obtaining a Doctor of Pharmacy degree. Pharmacist licensure also requires examination through the National Association of Boards of Pharmacy (NABP), in addition to examination according to the state's pharmacy laws; candidates for licensure must demonstrate competency by passing these examinations. Today's pharmacist also needs in-depth and broad communication skills to communicate effectively with doctors and with customers.

Today's typical pharmacy technician is required to do an array of tasks, all of which require competencies in many areas. Therefore, in some states, technicians are required to complete additional education as well as on-the-job training. Currently, there are no nationally standardized requirements for pharmacy technicians. Technicians help the pharmacist by preparing prescriptions and compounding (Figure 1-4). In a hospital setting, also known as an **inpatient pharmacy**, tasks include supplying floor stock to the hospital floors, preparing parenteral medications, transcribing physicians' orders, and filling patients' medication cassettes. Other, specialized technicians may be responsible for ordering all drugs and supplies. In all pharmacy settings, technicians require strong communication skills (see Chapter 4).

Pharmacists can obtain specialty certifications and may participate in providing specialty services. In some cases, participation may be governed by state law, professional licensing boards, and certifying bodies. For example, some pharmacists participate in anticoagulation or pharmacokinetics services, in which they interpret patients' laboratory results to determine the drug concentration and its relation to the therapeutic response of the patient. These pharmacists then are allowed to write the necessary change in medication strength based on the laboratory results. Other specialty duties include, but are

TABLE 1-3

Advances in the Field of Pharmacy Technology

Date	Description of Change in Pharmacy
1940s	The origins of a training program for technicians are established in the military (U.S. Army).
1968	National support and development of a curriculum in junior colleges and other institutions are initiated by the Bureau of Health Manpower (U.S. Department of Health).
1969	The American Society of Health-System Pharmacists (ASHP) begins to establish national guidelines for pharmacy technicians to improve standards.
1973	The National Association of Chain Drug Stores (NACDS) begins support of technicians and on-the-job training programs.
1975	The ASHP creates a set of guidelines for the hospital pharmacy technician.
1977	The ASHP creates competencies for technicians in organized health care settings and qualifications for entry-level technicians in hospitals.
1979	The Massachusetts College of Pharmacy starts a pharmacy technician training program.
1979	The American Association of Pharmacy Technicians (AAPT) is formed.
1981	The Michigan Pharmacists Association (MPA) starts the first examination program for certifying pharmacy technicians. The ASHP creates a bulletin for technical assistance on training guidelines for pharmacy technician training programs.
1982	The ASHP creates accreditation standards for training programs.
1987	The Illinois Council of Hospital Pharmacists (ICHP) begins an examination program to certify technicians.
1988	The ASHP Research and Education Foundation holds a conference on the use of technicians in pharmacy. The conference addresses on-the-job training, quality care, voluntary certification of technicians, and the roles and responsibilities of a pharmacy technician in the hospital setting.
1991	The Pharmacy Technician Education Council (PTEC) is formed.
1994	A project called The Scope of Pharmacy Practice Project is completed. The project addresses task analysis of pharmacy technicians.
1995	The Pharmacy Technician Certification Board (PTCB) is created by the ASHP, American Pharmacists Association (APhA), ICHP, and MPA.
1996	The ASHP and APhA publish the first *White Paper on Pharmacy Technicians*. It addresses the need for national standards in training pharmacy technicians.
1997	The ASHP, APhA, American Association of Colleges of Pharmacy (AACP), AAPT, and PTEC collaborate on a model curriculum for training courses for pharmacy technicians.
1999	The National Pharmacy Technician Association (NPTA) is founded in Houston, Texas.
2000	The PTCB updates the task analysis of pharmacy technicians.
2001	The second edition of the *Model Curriculum for Pharmacy Technician Training* is published.
2002	The second *White Paper on Pharmacy Technicians: Needed Changes Can No Longer Wait* is published
2004	Major online search engines select PharmacyChecker.com to verify the validity of online pharmacies.
2008	Congress passes the Ryan Haight Online Consumer Protection Act banning online pharmacies from selling controlled substances based on online patient consultations.
2009	The Task Force on Pharmacy Technician Education and Training Programs meets in Rosemont, Illinois. It was established by the National Association of Boards of Pharmacy (NABP) to review the existing state requirements for technician education and training and to recommend national standards.
2010	At its 106th Annual Meeting in Anaheim, California, the NABP passes resolution No. 106-7-10, resolving to continue to encourage states to adopt uniform standards for pharmacy technician education and training programs.
2010	Google removes PharmacyChecker.com as a certifying authority for online pharmacies. Currently, online pharmacies can be verified by Verified Internet Pharmacy Practice Sites (VIPPS).
2011	The CPE Monitor is launched as a collaborative effort by the NABP and the Accreditation Council for Pharmacy Education (ACPE).
2011	The PTCB launches the CREST Initiative by hosting a summit focused on the areas of consumer awareness, resources, education, state policy, and testing as they relate to pharmacy technicians.
2013	The PTCB announces certification program changes.

not limited to, oncology, pediatrics, geriatrics, and compounding services. New specialty certifications and opportunities for technicians also are available. The National Pharmacy Technician Association (NPTA) offers specialized training in sterile products and extemporaneous compounding. Many hospitals allow technicians to prepare chemotherapy drugs and offer advanced positions as anticoagulant technicians (see Chapter 10 for more information on the advanced practice setting for pharmacy technicians).

Trust in Pharmacists and Technicians

Over the decades the pharmacist has become known as a person who can be trusted to provide truthful information, someone in whom a person can be comfortable confiding. Although some traditions continue, times have changed concerning the role of the pharmacist. The most prevalent change can be seen in the inpatient setting of the hospital. As the competency of a pharmacist has become more "clinical," pharmacists are becoming more involved, alongside physicians, in the appropriate prescribing of medications and their dosages. These clinical pharmacists are found in the community pharmacy and in hospital settings.

Another important change in pharmacy concerns the laws governing patient consultation. The Omnibus Budget Reconciliation Act of 1990 (OBRA '90; see Chapter 2) addressed several issues concerning patient education and monitoring of medications. Although initially consultation was required to be offered only to Medicaid patients, most states have developed statutes that require pharmacists to provide written and/or oral consultation to all patients who are prescribed new or changed medications. Consultation is meant to inform and educate the patient about the medication he or she is taking. Because of these changes in the way pharmacies function, virtually every pharmacy employs pharmacy technicians. Thousands of technicians help lighten the load of filling prescriptions and performing other nondiscretionary tasks. Therefore, it is important for the patient to be able to trust a technician to provide the best care by filling the correct medication and referring the patient to the pharmacist for appropriate counseling. Most pharmacists agree that it is important for pharmacy technicians to maintain a standard of knowledge about pharmacy practice. Thus far, national certification is one of the best markers for ensuring a minimum level of competency in pharmacy.

Pharmacists have earned the trust of their patients over many decades, and it will take time for technicians to earn the same trust. This requires a true commitment to the profession of pharmacy on the part of the pharmacy technician. Through education, training, and good communication skills, technicians can gain the trust of the patients whom they serve.

> **❯ TECHNICIAN PROFILE**
>
> As a pharmacy technician for 3 years at a community hospital, Julia has learned how to build trust with her colleagues in and out of the pharmacy. She is required to fill orders in a fast-paced but exciting environment. She works alongside a pharmacist, Dr. Ellen, to whom Julia has proven that she can do her job competently. Dr. Ellen hired Julia after she finished her pharmacy technician training at a local college and received her national certification. Julia has gained Dr. Ellen's trust and the trust of the nurses and physicians who rely on her to fill the medication orders in the busy hospital setting. She is careful, efficient, and friendly and thoroughly enjoys her career.

Technicians of the Twenty-First Century and Beyond

In the new millennium, with the roles of pharmacists and technicians becoming more clearly defined, new concerns arise. We must be aware that just as the advances of medicine through the ages met with much resistance, so has the profession of pharmacy. Changes in the roles of pharmacists, technicians, and even clerks have met their share of obstacles, mostly from within the medical community. Some physicians are not eager to have pharmacists writing orders, even if the medications are simple. Likewise, technicians have been perceived as posing a threat to pharmacy. Some pharmacists believe that technicians may take jobs away from pharmacists or may increase the pharmacist's liability if someone who is not properly trained makes a mistake. Therefore, there is disparity across the United States regarding the duties of a pharmacy technician. In some states, pharmacies limit technicians' duties to a clerical level. In other states, technicians are required to be certified as pharmacy technicians before they are employed. All technicians must be aware of the laws in their state. (To find out more about the laws in your state pertaining to pharmacy technicians, visit the website *www.nabp.net*.) Each year more pharmacies are requiring a certain level of education from their technicians. This in turn allows expansion of job duties and possibly higher pay for the technicians.

Technicians' duties continue to expand and change. In some pharmacies, technicians regularly enter new prescription orders into the computer. This task previously was done exclusively by a pharmacist. The pharmacist is moving into a more highly clinical role, not only counseling patients, but also working with the medical staff. To a degree, the technician now does what the traditional pharmacist did: a health professional who transcribed orders, pulled medications, and filled prescriptions. Some colleges are offering specialized training programs for pharmacy technicians. Education in understanding trade and generic drug names and instruction in billing procedures are some of the courses provided specifically for future pharmacy technicians.

Scenario CHECK UP 1-2

As Kelly reads this chapter, she wonders what her role will be like in the pharmacy as a pharmacy technician. What would you tell her? How would you tell her about the role of the pharmacy technician and how it has evolved over time? What would you tell her about how to maintain a professional image?

 DO YOU REMEMBER THESE KEY POINTS?

- Terms and definitions used in this chapter
- Common ancient beliefs, including the dogmas of those eras
- Common treatments used for conditions in earlier times
- Early American medical practices and challenges during the Civil War
- The use of opium in the nineteenth century

- Advances in medicine over the centuries
- Major figures who influenced the changes in the dogmas of medicine
- The use of leeches and maggots throughout history
- The beginnings of the roles of pharmacists and pharmacy technicians
- How the roles have changed for pharmacists and pharmacy technicians

Scenario FOLLOW UP

Kelly has learned that the history of medicine and pharmacy has provided a strong foundation for the career field she is pursing. There have been clear medical advances throughout history that have had an important impact on the pharmacy profession of today. Kelly will be better prepared to enter the workplace as a result of her knowledge of the evolution of the pharmacy technician's duties and responsibilities.

REVIEW QUESTIONS

Multiple Choice Questions

1. During the Civil War, many soldiers died as a result of:
   A. Unsanitary conditions
   B. Postsurgical infections
   C. Gunshot wounds
   D. All of the above
2. Which of the following choices best describes sources of materials for remedies in ancient times?
   A. Chemicals, minerals, vitamins
   B. Minerals, animals, prayer
   C. Minerals, animals, plants
   D. Plants, seeds, minerals
3. Which of the following statements is *not* true?
   A. Sulfonamides are synthetic antibiotics.
   B. Sulfonamides are used for urinary tract infections.
   C. Gerhard Domagk discovered sulfonamide.
   D. Sulfonamide was one of many new antibiotic classes discovered in the 1800s.

4. Taking new prescriptions over the phone and entering them into the computer are tasks a _____ can do.
   A. Pharmacist
   B. Pharmacy technician
   C. Pharmacy clerk
   D. All of the above
5. The PTCB was founded by the following entities:
   A. ASHP, MPA, CPhA, PTEC
   B. MPA, ICHP, APhA, ASHP
   C. NAPB, ASHP, MPA, ICHP
   D. APhA, ASHP, NABP, PTEC
6. Opium and alcohol were once used to:
   A. Desensitize a person to pain
   B. Help ease depression
   C. Treat anxiety
   D. All of the above

7. The word *apothecary* means:
   A. Pharmacist
   B. Store
   C. Drug
   D. Both A and B
8. The first pharmacy technicians were:
   A. Family members
   B. Clerks
   C. Military technicians
   D. All of the above

9. Pharmacy technicians perform the following functions *except:*
   A. Filling prescriptions
   B. Compounding medications
   C. Counseling patients
   D. Ordering medications
10. The PTCB is an organization that:
    A. Regulates all pharmacy technicians
    B. Gives a national exam for pharmacy technicians
    C. Was founded by several pharmacist associations
    D. Both B and C

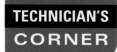

TECHNICIAN'S CORNER

Discuss why pharmacists consistently rank among the most trusted professionals. Research the 2013 annual poll conducted by Gallup to find out what percentage of respondents rated pharmacists "Very High" on honesty and ethical standards. Do technicians benefit from these statistics?

Bibliography

Anderson MJ, Stephenson KF: *Scientists of the ancient world*, Springfield, NJ, 1999, Enslow.

Ballington DA: *Pharmacy practice for technicians*, ed 3, St Paul, Minn, 2006, EMC/Paradigm.

Moulton C, editor: *Ancient Greece and Rome*, vol 3, New York, 1998, Simon & Schuster.

Narcto D: *The complete history of ancient Greece*, San Diego, 2001, Greenhaven.

Suplee C: *Milestones of science*, Washington, DC, 2000, National Geographic.

Websites Referenced

Asclepius: Encyclopedia Mythica. 2009. Encyclopedia Mythica Online. 23 Aug. 2009 (Referenced July 28, 2013.) www.pantheon.org/articles/a/asclepius.html

Asclepius: Mythology, Cult, the Staff of Asclepius and the Hippocratic Oath. (Referenced July 28, 2013) www-structmed.cimr.cam.ac.uk/Asclepius.html

Centers for Disease Control and Prevention: List of Vaccines used in United States. Last reviewed August 18, 2011. (Referenced July 28, 2013.) www.cdc.gov/vaccines/vpd-vac/vaccines-list.htm

Ella Phillips Stewart. (Referenced July 29, 2013.)

Florence Nightingale. (Referenced July 29, 2013.) www.biography.com/people/florence-nightingale-9423539

Gardasil Vaccination. (Referenced July 28, 2013.) www.fda.gov/BiologicsBloodVaccines/Vaccines/ApprovedProducts/UCM094042

Hemochromatosis: Mayo Clinic staff. 9/12/08 Mayo Foundation for Medical Education and Research. (Referenced July 17, 2013.) www.mayoclinic.com/health/hemochromatosis/DS00455/

http://en.wikipedia.org/wiki/Timeline_of_medicine_and_medical_technology. (Referenced July 29, 2013.)

http://explorepahistory.com/displayimage.php?imgId=1-2-189F

http://ptcb.org/about-ptcb/news-room/news-landing/2013/02/27/ptcb-announces-certification-program-changes#.UeVBkI1QGjk

Melancholy and black humor: Mirrors of Melancholy: Models, History and Reception (Referenced July 28, 2013.) http://web.uvic.ca/~histmed/mirrors.pdf

Prevnar vaccine. (Referenced July 17, 2013.) www.fda.gov/BiologicsBloodVaccines/Vaccines/ApprovedProducts/ucm201667.htm

PTCB. (Referenced July 29, 2013.) PTCB Announces Certification Program Changes by PTCB Staff. Feb. 27, 2013.

PTCB website: Active PTCB CPhTs and State Regulations as of June 30, 2011. (Referenced July 28, 2013.) www.ptcb.org

Sultz S: Epidemics in Colonial Philadelphia from 1699-1799 and the Risk of Dying. Archiving Early America. (Referenced July 28, 2013.) www.earlyamerica.com/review/2007_winter_spring/epidemics.html

Susan Hayhurst. (Referenced July 29, 2013.)

The Discovery of the Molecular Structure of DNA: The Double Helix. (Referenced July 29, 2013.) www.nobleprize.org/educational/medicine/dna_double_helix/readmore.html

The National Alliance of Advocates for Buprenorphine Treatment: Opiates/Opioids. 5/10/2008. (Referenced July 17, 2013.) www.naabt.org/education/opiates_opioids.cfm

The Top 100 Heroes of Western Culture. (Referenced July 29, 2013.) www.westerncultureglobal.org/roger-bacon.html

University of Wisconsin-Madison: "Scientists Guide Human Skin Cells to Embryonic State." ScienceDaily 21 November 2007. (Referenced July 17, 2013.) www.sciencedaily.com/releases/2007/11/071120092709.htm

Vivian J, Fink J: OBRA90 at Sweet Sixteen: A Retrospective Review, *US Pharm* 2008: 33(3):59-65. 3/20/08. (Referenced July 17, 2013.) www.uspharmacist.com/content/t/pain_management, miscellaneous/c/10126/

www.bbc.co.uk/news/health-22689593 Hand, foot and mouth disease: First vaccine, by James Gallagher, BBC News, 28 May 2013. (Referenced July 17, 2013.)

www.bgsu.edu/colleges/library/cac/ms/page44338.html; http://voices.yahoo.com/ella-phillips-stewart-pharmacist-business-woman-civil-11031410.html

www.cdc.gov/mmwr/preview/mmwrhtml/mm5518a4.htm; Vaccine Preventable Deaths and the Global Immunization Vision and Strategy, 2006-2015, *Weekly* 55(18):511-515, 2006. (Referenced July 17, 2013.)

Zostavax vaccine. (Referenced July 28, 2013.) www.fda.gov/NewsEvents/Newsroom/PressAnnouncements/2011/ucm248390.htm

2

Pharmacy Law, Ethics, and Regulatory Agencies

Bobbi Steelman

OBJECTIVES

Upon completing this chapter, you should be able to do the following:

1. List the history of federal drug laws in chronological order.
2. Describe the implications of the Health Insurance Portability and Accountability Act (HIPAA).
3. Explain how the Patient Protection and Affordable Care Act (ACA) and the Drug Quality and Security Act (DQSA) have changed health care.
4. Define the functions of the Food and Drug Administration (FDA) and Drug Enforcement Administration (DEA).
5. Describe the process for reporting any problems with a drug or any adverse reactions to the FDA.
6. Explain the three classes of drug recalls defined by the FDA.
7. Describe the proper handling of controlled substances.
8. Explain the necessary forms and regulations used for controlled substances.
9. List the basic information contained in a drug monograph.
10. Explain the purpose of boxed warnings and MedGuides.
11. List and explain the five pregnancy categories established by the FDA.
12. List who can prescribe medications and medical devices.
13. Describe prescription orders and prescription labels.
14. Perform the function of verifying a DEA number.
15. Explain the purpose of risk management programs for prescription drugs.
16. Explain the verification process for Internet pharmacies.
17. Explain the Occupational Safety and Health Administration (OSHA) guidelines as they pertain to pharmacy.
18. Explain the purpose of the Joint Commission.
19. Explain why pharmacy technicians must be knowledgeable about the law when performing nondiscretionary duties.
20. Discuss the differences between morals and ethics.

TERMS AND DEFINITIONS

Act A statutory plan passed by Congress or any legislature that is a "bill" until it is enacted and becomes law

Adulteration The mishandling of medication that can lead to contamination or impurity, falsification of contents, or loss of drug quality or potency. Adulteration may cause injury or illness to the consumer

Amendment A change in the original act or law

Barbiturate A drug derived from barbituric acid; a barbiturate acts as a central nervous system depressant. Barbiturates are often used in the treatment of seizures and as sedative and hypnotic agents

Board of pharmacy (BOP) State board that regulates the practice of pharmacy within the state

Boxed warning Drug warning that is placed in the prescribing information or package insert of the product and indicates a significant risk of potentially dangerous side effects. It is the strongest warning the FDA can give. It is common in the pharmacy profession to call these warnings "Black Box Warnings" because of their appearance in a drug label; the warning is often enclosed in a black outlined box to draw attention to the content

Controlled substance Any drug or other substance that is scheduled I through V and regulated by the Drug Enforcement Administration

Drug diversion The intentional misuse of a drug intended for medical purposes; the Drug Enforcement Administration usually defines diversion as the recreational use of a prescription or scheduled drug. Diversion can also refer to the channeling of the prescription drug supply away from legal distribution and to the illegal street market

Drug Enforcement Administration (DEA) Federal agency within the U.S. Department of Justice that enforces U.S. laws and regulations related to controlled substances

Drug utilization evaluation (DUE) A process that ensures that prescribed drugs are used appropriately. The main desired outcome of any DUE program is an increase in medication-related efficacy and safety

Ethics The values and morals used within a profession

Food and Drug Administration (FDA) The agency within the U.S. Department of Health and Human Services that is responsible for assuring the safety, efficacy, and security of human and veterinary drugs, biological products, medical devices, the national food supply, cosmetics, and radioactive products

Health Insurance Portability and Accountability Act of 1996 (HIPAA) Federal act that protects patients' rights, establishes national standards for electronic health care communication, and ensures the security and privacy of health data

Legend drug Drug that requires a prescription for dispensing; these drugs carry the federal legend: "Federal law prohibits the dispensing of this medication without a prescription"

Medicaid Federal- and state-operated insurance program that covers health care costs and prescription drugs for low-income children, adults, and elderly and those with disabilities

Medicare Federal- and state-managed insurance program that covers health care costs and prescription drugs for individuals older than 65, persons younger than 65 with long-term disabilities, and individuals with end-stage renal disease

Misbranding Labeling of a product that is false or misleading; label information must include directions for use; safe and/or unsafe dosages; manufacturer, packer, or distributor; quantity; and weight

Monograph Comprehensive information on a medication's actions within that class of drugs. Also lists generic and trade names, ingredients, dosages, side effects, adverse effects, how the patient should take the medication, and foods or other drugs (e.g., over-the-counter [OTC] medications, herbals) to avoid while taking the medication

Morals Standards concerning or relating to what is right or wrong in human behavior

Narcotic A nonspecific term used to describe a drug (such as opium) that in moderate doses dulls the senses, relieves pain, and induces profound sleep but in excessive doses causes stupor, coma, or convulsions, and may lead to addiction. From the standpoint of U.S. law, opium, opiates (derivatives of opium), and opioids, in addition to cocaine and coca leaves, are "narcotics"

National Drug Code (NDC) A 10-digit number that indicates specifics of a prescription drug or an insulin product. The NDC specifies the drug manufacturer, the drug product (drug strength, dosage form, and formulation), and the package size

Negligence A legal concept that describes an action taken without the forethought that should have been taken by a reasonable person of similar competency

Occupational Safety and Health Administration (OSHA) U.S. government–managed agency that oversees safety in the workplace; created Safety Data Sheet (SDS) requirements

Omnibus Budget Reconciliation Act of 1990 (OBRA '90) Congressional act that changed reimbursement limits and mandated drug utilization evaluation, pharmacy patient consultation, and educational outreach programs

Over-the-counter (OTC) Describes medication that can be purchased without a prescription; nonlegend medications

Physicians' Desk Reference (PDR) One of the many reference books on medications; it compiles and publishes select manufacturer-provided package inserts and prescribing information useful for health professionals

Pregnancy Category A system used by the FDA to describe five levels of assessment of fetal effects caused by a drug; a required section of current prescription drug labeling. First introduced in 1979, the system is being reevaluated for usefulness and inclusion in the prescription label

Protected health information (PHI) A term used to describe a patient's personal health data. Under HIPAA, this information is protected from being shared or distributed without permission

Safety Data Sheet (SDS) (formerly known as MSDS sheets) A document providing chemical product information. An SDS includes the product name, composition (chemicals in the product), hazards, toxicology, and other information about the proper steps to take with spills, accidental exposure, handling, and storage of the product. Filing of an SDS in the pharmacy or workplace is usually a requirement for meeting Occupational Safety and Health Administration (OSHA) standards

The Joint Commission (TJC) An independent, nonprofit organization that accredits hospitals and other health care organizations in the United States. Accreditation is required to be eligible for Medicare and Medicaid payments

Tort An act that causes harm or injury to a person intentionally or because of negligence

United States Pharmacopeia (USP) An independent, nonprofit organization that establishes documentation on product quality standards, drug quality and information, and health care information on medications, over-the-counter products, dietary supplements, and food ingredients to ensure that they have the appropriate purity, quality, and strength

United States Pharmacopeia–National Formulary (USP-NF) A publication of the USP that contains standards for medications, dosage forms, drug substances, excipients, medical devices, and dietary supplements

Introduction

Scenario:

Laura is a new technician at a local chain pharmacy. She graduated from an accredited technician training program in which she learned about her roles and responsibilities as a pharmacy professional. As she begins her career, she thinks about her legal liabilities. Does she need malpractice insurance in case she makes a medication error? What if she unknowingly violates a HIPAA regulation?

The practice of pharmacy is governed by a series of laws, regulations, and rules enforced by federal, state, and local governments. The practice of pharmacy is also subject to policies and procedures established by institutions and/or pharmacy management at each pharmacy site. The number of rules and regulations is staggering, and most of us cannot easily decipher the legal tangle of words; however, we are required to follow these rules and regulations. This chapter presents the most basic laws and regulations that pertain to pharmacy, pharmacists, and especially the technician. A good understanding of these laws is necessary to pass the Pharmacy Technician Certification Board examination; more important, it is necessary to know your responsibilities when working in pharmacy. An overview of the history of the **Food and Drug Administration (FDA)** is given, and its present-day functions are described. The laws are listed in chronological order, along with a short description of how and why each was enacted. Common record-keeping practices are covered. The legal liabilities of pharmacists and technicians are explained. Morals and ethics are discussed at the end of this section because they play a vital role in the decisions technicians make in pharmacy practice.

FDA History

The FDA was established in 1862, along with the U.S. Department of Agriculture. The FDA is the oldest consumer protection agency in the U.S. federal government. The FDA's Division of Chemistry consists of a staff from several disciplines, including chemists, physicians, veterinarians, pharmacists, microbiologists, and lawyers. Until 1901 the Division of Chemistry evaluated applications for new drugs for use in humans or animals, food and color additives, medical devices, and infant formulas. The chief chemist in the Division of Chemistry at that time, Harvey Wiley, changed the direction of the division, establishing scientific authority by researching the effects of chemical preservatives used in the production of foods and drugs, exposing potential hazards in products, focusing on consumer safety, and eventually paving the way for government regulation. Inspectors in the department visited thousands of food and other manufacturing facilities each year. In 1901 the Division of Chemistry was renamed the Bureau of Chemistry. Wiley's efforts led to the first passage of major legislation, the **Pure Food and Drug Act of 1906**. The new agency was to make many more changes in its authority and scope as it grew. In 1927 the agency's name was changed to the Food, Drug, and Insecticide Administration, and in 1930 the name was shortened to the Food and Drug Administration (FDA). The FDA remained under the authority of the U.S. Department of Agriculture until 1940, when the agency became part of the Federal Security Agency. As the FDA continued to regulate new applications for drugs, devices, and other products, the agency was transferred to the Department of Health, Education, and Welfare (HEW) in 1953 and eventually was placed under the authority of the U.S. Public Health Service within HEW in 1968. In 1980 the FDA was moved from HEW to the newly created U.S. Department of Health and Human Services.

Early Activity of the FDA

Since the FDA's founding, the agency has investigated the **adulteration** and **misbranding** of agricultural goods used for food and drugs. Hundreds of bills were introduced in Congress to establish standards to protect the health of consumers, yet the FDA's ability to regulate and enforce these standards remained limited, leaving the primary control of domestically produced food and drugs to the individual states. The laws varied widely from state to state. Meanwhile, horrible incidents continued to occur, such as the deaths of 13 children and nine babies in 1902 after they were injected with a tainted batch of tetanus diphtheria antitoxins. In June, 1906, President Theodore Roosevelt signed the Pure Food and Drug Act of 1906, also known as the Wiley Act. This important act gave the government the power to administer and prohibit the interstate transport of unlawful food and drugs. Drugs had to meet the standards of strength, quality, and purity established by the **United States Pharmacopeia (USP)** and the **National Formulary (NF)** guidelines; any variations from the guidelines had to be plainly listed on the product label. The label could not mislead the consumer, and all ingredients had to be listed on the label. The law also prohibited the addition of any ingredients to a food that would substitute for the food, conceal damage, pose a health hazard, or constitute a filthy or decomposed substance.

Wiley's authority was challenged and undercut many times by the Supreme Court as attempts were made to form standards affecting food and drug manufacturers. The FDA suffered a severe setback in 1912 when the Supreme Court determined that the law enforcing the regulation of drugs did not apply to false therapeutic claims. The controversy lay in the attempt to prove that the drug companies "intended" to defraud the consumer. This Supreme Court ruling undermined the Wiley Act, and many manufacturers won court cases, allowing their products to be sold to consumers. In 1912 Wiley resigned from the FDA, and at this point the bureau focused more closely on drug regulation because this was a great concern.

With a new presidential administration taking over in 1933 under Franklin D. Roosevelt, the FDA was able to change its authority to include both quality and identity standards for food and drugs, prohibition of false therapeutic claims for drugs, and coverage of cosmetics and medical devices. The FDA had the right to inspect factories and control the advertising of products. The FDA countered advertisements of drug claims by exposing the horrible but true results of certain drugs. For example, an eyelash dye that blinded some women as a result of dangerous additives had been widely advertised to consumers. A medication tonic made with radium as an additive was found to cause a slow and painful death for the user. All products were protected under the previous laws. For the next 5 years, a bill that would replace the 1906 revised law was stalled in Congress. It took tremendous effort to pass new standards enforceable by the FDA. In 1937 a Tennessee drug company advertised a new sulfanilamide elixir specifically intended for children. The toxic solvent was untested (per then current laws), and more than 100 people died, mostly children. It was later determined that the solvent was similar to antifreeze, which is fatal to humans and animals. Unfortunately, this type of deadly scenario was repeated several times before the necessary changes in the laws of that time were made. As a result of public pressure, Congress finally passed the 1938 Federal Food, Drug, and Cosmetic Act. The act required manufacturers to prove to the FDA that a drug was safe for use before marketing it, and the manufacturers had to provide directions on the drug's label for its safe use. The act also mandated standards for foods, set tolerances for certain poisonous substances, and authorized factory inspections. The FDA was given authority to enforce the standards. Just a few months after passage of the act, the FDA determined that sulfa and other drugs required a prescription from physicians before they could be purchased. Clarification of what constituted a prescription drug versus an over-the-counter drug was established in 1951 with the enactment of the Durham-Humphrey Amendment. Other laws passed in the 1950s banned carcinogenic additives to foods.

Another potential tragedy was averted in the United States in the 1960s when the drug thalidomide, a sedative used in Europe, was found to cause severe birth defects, including grossly deformed limbs, when administered during pregnancy. The drug was never approved for use in the United States. The Kefauver-Harris Drug Amendments of 1962 were revolutionary in their scope for ensuring the safety and effectiveness of medications in the U.S. market. Another growing concern was the use and abuse of amphetamines, **barbiturates**, and other potentially addictive agents. The FDA was given more control over these agents with the enactment of the Drug Abuse Control Amendments of 1965. This control was eventually delegated to the Drug Enforcement Administration (DEA) in 1968. In 1973 some of the responsibilities of the FDA were given to the Consumer Product Safety Commission. These included oversight of hazardous toys, flammable fabrics, and potential poisons in consumer products. Other provisions in the 1960s allowed for greater FDA oversight to ensure the safety and effectiveness of veterinary drugs and additives to animal feed.

Before 1938 the Post Office Department and Federal Trade Commission were in charge of ensuring the safety of cosmetics and medical devices; after 1938 regulating cosmetics and medical devices became the responsibility of the FDA. The advertising of various quack products was widespread throughout the country; claims such as increasing the life span, curing conditions, and protecting one's health were unfounded in many cases. However, in 1976 another disaster occurred when an intrauterine device, which claimed to prevent pregnancy, caused serious injury to thousands of women. Only then did the **1976 Medical Device Amendments** allow the FDA to regulate and approve these types of devices and to recall ineffective or dangerous devices.

With continued consumer and political pressure, the FDA has influenced new laws, such as the **Orphan Drug Act**, which was passed in 1983 and targeted all rare diseases. The Orphan Drug Act influenced expanded research and availability of new treatments for acquired immunodeficiency syndrome (AIDS), cancer, and genetic diseases. (An overview of several acts and **amendments** is presented in the following section, Description of Laws.) In recent years the FDA has continued its mission to ensure public safety, including the oversight of dietary supplements that present safety problems, make false or misleading claims, or are otherwise adulterated or misbranded.

Description of Laws

What is an **act**? An act is a statutory plan passed by Congress or any legislature that is called a "bill" until it is enacted, at which point it becomes a law. An amendment is a change in the original act or law. The following examples are brief because the various acts and amendments encompass broader descriptions. Further reading is suggested to gain a deeper insight into the laws that pertain to pharmacy and patients' rights. Box 2-1 presents a list of well-known federal laws, in chronological order, that are discussed in this chapter.

BOX 2-1

Well-Known Federal Food and Drug Laws

1906	Pure Food and Drug Act
1912	International Opium Convention
1914	Harrison Narcotics Act
1938	Federal Food, Drug, and Cosmetic Act
1951	Durham-Humphrey Amendment
1962	Kefauver-Harris Amendments (thalidomide disaster)
1970	Comprehensive Drug Abuse Prevention and Control Act
1970	Poison Prevention Packaging Act
1972	Drug Listing Act
1983	Orphan Drug Act
1987	Prescription Drug Marketing Act
1990	Anabolic Steroids Control Act
1990	Omnibus Budget Reconciliation Act of 1990 (OBRA '90)
1994	Dietary Supplement Health and Education Act (DSHEA)
1996	Health Insurance Portability and Accountability Act of 1996 (HIPAA)
2000	Drug Addiction Treatment Act (DATA 2000)
2003	Medicare Modernization Act (MMA)
2005	Combat Methamphetamine Epidemic Act (CMEA)
2006	Dietary Supplement and Nonprescription Drug Consumer Protection Act
2010	The Patient Protection and Affordable Care Act (ACA)
2013	The Drug Quality and Security Act (DQSA)

1906 Pure Food and Drug Act

The 1906 Pure Food and Drugs Act was one of the first laws enacted to stop the sale of inaccurately labeled drugs. All manufacturers were required to have truthful information on the label before selling their drugs. Although this act was well intentioned, there were many drugs that still made their way onto the market because of continued false claims regarding their effectiveness. Additional changes were made to this act that ultimately required manufacturers to prove the effectiveness of the drugs through methods such as scientific studies.

1914 Harrison Narcotics Act

By 1912 international meetings were being held to curb the increase in trafficking of highly addictive substances. The International Opium Convention of 1912 was one of these meetings. Limitations on opium transport and recreational use were attempted. The Harrison Narcotics Act of 1914 was enacted in the United States in parallel with international treaties to curb recreational use of opium. Individuals could no longer purchase opium without a prescription, and

it became harder to obtain opium for nonmedical purposes. The Harrison Narcotics Act required practitioner registration, documentation regarding prescriptions and dispensing, and implementation of restrictions regarding the importation, sale, and distribution of opium, coca leaves, and any derivative products.

1938 Federal Food, Drug, and Cosmetic Act

The 1938 Federal Food, Drug, and Cosmetic Act was enacted because the earlier Pure Food and Drug Act of 1906 was not worded strictly enough and did not include cosmetics. Two important concepts introduced in this new act were adulteration and misbranding. For example, false or exaggerated claims commonly were placed on new drug labels and often misled the consumer. This was considered misbranding. All addictive substances were required to be labeled "Warning: May be habit forming." This act also provided the legal status for the FDA. Adulteration deals with the preparation and/or storage of a medication. Mishandling of the food or drug may cause injury or even death to a consumer. This act described the exact labeling for products and defined misbranding and adulteration as illegal. The new law also required drug companies to include package inserts and directions to the consumer regarding safe use (see Food and Drug Administration/Drug Enforcement Administration, later in the chapter).

1951 Durham-Humphrey Amendment

The 1951 Durham-Humphrey Amendment added more instructions for drug companies and required the labeling "Caution: Federal law prohibits dispensing without a prescription." Under this amendment, certain drugs require a physician's order and supervision. This amendment also made the initial distinction between **legend drugs** (by prescription only) and **over-the-counter (OTC)** medications that do not require a physician's order (also known as *nonprescription drugs*).

1962 Kefauver-Harris Amendments

The Kefauver-Harris Amendments enacted in 1962 were groundbreaking in their attempts to ensure the safety and effectiveness of all new drugs on the U.S. market. The amendments gave the FDA specific authority to approve a manufacturer's marketing application before a drug could be made available for commercial use. Firms now had to prove safety and provide substantial evidence of effectiveness for the drug's intended use. The required evidence had to consist of adequate and well-controlled studies. The amendments helped establish rules of clinical drug investigation and required the informed consent of study subjects. The amendments also required that drug-related adverse events be reported to the FDA. The regulation of prescription drug advertising was transferred from the Federal Trade Commission to the FDA, and the burden was put on the drug manufacturing companies to ensure quality as "good manufacturing practice" (GMP) standards were established. One example of the effectiveness of the FDA is illustrated by its role in preventing the sale of thalidomide in the United States. In Europe, people were taking this new medication to help them sleep. In the early 1960s, European women who had taken thalidomide while pregnant gave birth to children with severe defects, including the absence of limbs. The FDA postponed approving thalidomide until just before the birth defects across Europe were reported. Very few cases were reported in America; those reported were due to women obtaining thalidomide from outside the United States. Consumers became aware that drug companies were not doing enough to test the drugs they were marketing. More laws ensued after the thalidomide tragedy to better safeguard the public; this also greatly increased the time and money spent on testing a drug for safety and effectiveness.

1970 Comprehensive Drug Abuse Prevention and Control Act (also known as the Controlled Substance Act)

The **Drug Enforcement Administration (DEA)** was formed to enforce the laws concerning controlled substances and their distribution. A stair-step schedule of controlled substances was introduced, based on the drug's intended medical use, the propensity of a drug to be abused, and safety and dependency concerns. The five-level stair-step schedule of controlled substances requires stricter rules for low numbered classifications and less strict rules for higher numbered categories. Schedule I is the most restrictive and is defined as drugs with no medically accepted use in the United States. The prescription of a schedule V drug is less restricted and requires less documentation than that for a schedule II drug.

1970 Poison Prevention Packaging Act (PPPA)

The Poison Prevention Packaging Act of 1970 required manufacturers and pharmacies to place all medications in containers with childproof caps or packaging. This includes both over-the-counter and legend drugs. The standard specifies that medication should not be able to be opened by at least 80% of children under the age of 5 and that at least 90% of

adults should be able to open the medication within 5 minutes. Exceptions to this act include physician requests for non-childproof caps for their patients, certain legend medications, hospitalized patients, or a specific request by the patient.

Before the implementation of this act, there were hundreds of unintentional deaths of children under the age of 5 years as a result of ingestion of either drugs or household chemicals. The first attempt to prevent these tragedies was the Hazardous Substances Labeling Act of 1960. Pharmacist Homer George of Mississippi was the driving force behind the first National Poison Prevention Week (occurring yearly in March). Individual states followed by implementing poison control centers. It was not until 1970 that the PPPA was enacted; it is now under the authority of the Consumer Product Safety Commission (CPSC). It was estimated that more than 1.4 million childhood deaths have been prevented annually because of childproof caps (for more information, see the CPSC website at *www.cpsc.gov/cpscpub/pubs/384.pdf*). Box 2-2 presents PPPA guidelines for exempt drugs.

1972 Drug Listing Act: National Drug Code (NDC)

In 1972 the Drug Listing Act (**National Drug Code [NDC]**) was implemented under the authority of the FDA. Every drug has a unique 10-digit number divided into three segments. The numbers identify the labeler, product, and trade package size (Figure 2-1). The first set of numbers (labeler code) is assigned by the FDA. The second set (product code) identifies the specifics of the product. The third set of numbers (package code) identifies the specifics of the package size and types. Both product and package codes are set by the drug company. The example in Box 2-3 presents a specific overview of each part of the code.

1983 Orphan Drug Act (ODA)

The 1983 Orphan Drug Act encouraged drug companies to develop drugs for rare diseases by providing research assistance, grants, and cost incentives to manufacturers. Before this act, companies had no incentive to develop medications and spend millions of dollars and many years of trials to treat a disease that affected a small portion of the population. Therefore, several regulatory restrictions were waived for diseases that affected fewer than 200,000 people in the United States. The act also covered diseases that affected more than 200,000 people if it could be proved that the cost of developing and testing a drug could not be recovered by the eventual sales. In addition, the act encouraged manufacturers to develop drugs for rare diseases by providing marketing

BOX 2-2

Poison Prevention Packaging Act Guidelines (Exempt Drugs)*

All medications must be dispensed with a childproof cap, with the exception of the following:

Anhydrous cholestyramine powder

Betamethasone tablets, 12.6 mg or less contained in dispenser packages

Colestipol, no more than 5 g

Conjugated estrogens containing no more than 32 mg

Contraceptives in daily dispensing sets

Erythromycin ethylsuccinate tablet packages not containing more than 16 g

Hormone replacement therapy products that contain one or more progestin or estrogen substances

Mebendazole containing no more than 600 mg in dispenser packages

Medroxyprogesterone tablets

Methylprednisolone tablets containing no more than 84 mg

Norethindrone mnemonic (memory-aid) packages containing no more than 50 mg

No more than 8 g of erythromycin granules in suspension

Pancrelipase powder, capsule or tablet forms

Prednisone package containing no more than 105 mg

Sacrosidase preparations in glycerin and water

Sodium fluoride containing no more than 264 mg per package

Sublingual forms of isosorbide dinitrate 10 mg or less

Sublingual forms of nitroglycerin

or

All medications dispensed in a hospital or nursing home do not require childproof packaging

or

Customer requests medication not be dispensed with childproof cap; may be a "blanket" request for all prescription medications

or

Physician requests medication not be dispensed with a childproof cap; may be a "blanket" request for all prescription medications

---

U.S. Consumer Product Safety Commission, Washington, D.C.; Poison Prevention Packaging: A Guide for Healthcare Professionals (revised 2005) http://www.cpsc.gov/PageFiles/114277/384.pdf (Referenced July 17, 2013.)

*The National Capital Poison Control Center can be contacted at 1-800-222-1222 or at the website www.poison.org

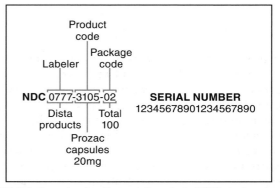

FIGURE 2-1 Example of a National Drug Code (NDC), broken down by section.

BOX 2-3

NDC Number Specifics

NDC 50580-449-05

50580: First five positions indicate the **labeler code**; this identifies any firm that manufactures or distributes (under its own name) the drug (includes **repackers** or **relabelers**).

449: Second set of numbers indicates the **product code**; this identifies a specific strength, dosage form, and formulation for a particular drug. Examples include active ingredients and size, shape, color, or imprinted code on drug, in addition to any other distinguishing markings on the drug.

05: Third set of numbers indicates the **package code** and identifies package types and sizes. For example, drug is in a bottle, vial, or box; drug's quantity or amount, such as in milliliters, ounces, or pints for liquids.

If the NDC number contains **two asterisks** at the end, this identifies the product as a bulk, raw, nonformulated controlled substance.

Although the NDC directory is limited to both prescription and insulin drugs, certain products may not be listed. Reasons include the following:

- The product is not a prescription drug or insulin.
- The manufacturer has notified the FDA that the drug is no longer being produced.
- The manufacturer has not complied with all requirements; the drug is not included until all information has been provided to the FDA.

---

exclusivity for orphan drugs for a period of 7 years after FDA approval.

1987 Prescription Drug Marketing Act (PDMA)

The 1987 Prescription Drug Marketing Act (PDMA) addressed issues related to the distribution and wholesale pedigree of human prescription drugs. The intent of the act was to solidify the legal supply channel of prescription drugs from manufacturers to authorized distributors and wholesalers. The act helps to prevent counterfeit drugs and ingredients in the supply chain and to limit diversion of pharmaceutical samples and prescription drugs.

1990 Omnibus Budget Reconciliation Act (OBRA '90)

The origins of the **Omnibus Budget Reconciliation Act** date to 1987, when Congress addressed the problems regarding health care quality for the elderly. With increasing numbers of elderly entering nursing homes, great concern arose over the substandard care being provided, the high nursing personnel-to-patient ratios, and the unhealthy conditions present. OBRA '87 set requirements for facilities participating in Medicare and Medicaid programs and addressed enforcement mechanisms. A minimum standard of care was required, and a change began to take place, transitioning nursing homes from uncomfortable institutions to comfortable, homelike environments providing higher quality care. However, the provisions of OBRA '87 did not address individual privacy rights. The **Omnibus Budget Reconciliation Act of 1990 (OBRA '90)** affected the responsibilities of practicing pharmacists and health care personnel in general. The act outlines specifics for pharmacies to participate in the Medicaid Drug Rebate Program. Medicaid is a state- and federally managed program that provides medical coverage for low-income individuals. OBRA '90 has profoundly affected pharmacy responsibilities. This act states that a pharmacist must offer to counsel (at the time of purchase) all Medicaid patients who receive new prescriptions. OBRA '90 also requires **drug utilization evaluation (DUE)**. The intent of DUE under OBRA '90 is to ensure that all medications being prescribed to patients would be reviewed for appropriateness. Three important provisions of OBRA '90 include:

1. Evaluation of drug therapy: This must be completed before a prescription is filled (prospectively). Pharmacists must review drugs for appropriateness, possible drug interactions, contraindications, and correctness of drug dosage and duration of therapy to ensure the patient's safety.
2. Review of drug therapy: This is a long-term review of provision 1 through the use of software programs and includes educational interventions intended to ensure the quality of prescribing by physicians.
3. DUE board review: The board reviews, evaluates, and develops strategies to improve patient care and reduce costs for those covered by the Medicaid program.

In addition, the DUE must include systems such as computer programs that alert the pharmacist to possible drug interactions, precautions, and other pertinent information that the patient should know. Pharmacies must document and maintain records to track consultations and outcomes. Although OBRA '90 is specific to **Medicaid** coverage, pharmacies usually now counsel all patients on medications that have been prescribed. If these provisions are not met, the pharmacy cannot receive federal reimbursement for medication and may face civil liability proceedings. The board of pharmacy in each state oversees OBRA '90 compliance. It can also impose fines on both pharmacies and pharmacists for noncompliance, although a patient may refuse counseling.

1996 Health Insurance Portability and Accountability Act (HIPAA)

The Health Insurance Portability and Accountability Act of 1996 (HIPAA) established the principle of **protected health information (PHI)**. HIPAA's privacy rules are meant to protect certain health information. Standards of PHI address the use and disclosure of an individual's health information. Entities that are covered by PHI are obligated to comply with all requirements in the rules of HIPAA, which became effective in 2003. A HIPAA-covered entity is a health care provider, a health plan, or a health care clearinghouse. This includes entities that process nonstandard health information they receive from another entity into a standard format (e.g., standard electronic format or data content, or vice versa).

All covered physicians were required to update their HIPAA policies and procedures and otherwise implement the changes required by these regulations no later than the September 23, 2013, compliance date. These new rules meant physicians needed to update their Business Associate Agreements (BAAs) and their Notices of Privacy Practices (NPPs). The rules also required them to understand the importance of encryption of electronic protected health information.

Scenario CHECK UP 2-1

Laura continues to work at the local chain pharmacy. She is able to put into practice the skills she learned in school. One day she finds herself filling a prescription for her daughter's fiancé. She recognizes the drug as a maintenance medication for individuals infected with the human immunodeficiency virus (HIV). Should she share this information with her daughter? Why or why not? Is this a legal or an ethical dilemma?

Patient Confidentiality

Confidentiality is another aspect of ethical work. The definition of confidentiality is to keep privileged information about a customer from being disclosed without his or her consent. This includes information that may cause the patient embarrassment or harm.

Under federal law, patients have the right to privacy concerning their medications, treatment, or any aspect of their health care. These laws affect all areas of medicine, including pharmacy, concerning issues of obtaining, transferring, and accessing patient information. Changes have been made throughout all medical facilities and medical information centers that limit access to patient information in charts and computer databases. A patient's approval is required for the release of any information about the patient to any third party, including insurance companies, physicians, and pharmacies. Because pharmacy technicians and other health care professionals have access to information about a patient's condition, medications, and other personal information, they are responsible for keeping the patient's information confidential.

What Information Is Protected?

The HIPAA Privacy Rule protects all *"individually identifiable health information"* held or transmitted by a covered entity or its business associate, in any form or media, whether electronic, paper, or oral.

What Does This Mean for the Pharmacy?

Patient information must be communicated on a need-to-know basis, with the provision that the entity is covered under the HIPAA health information rules and regulations. This means that the physician can call and request information about his or her patient. The patient's health insurance company can request information on the participant. The pharmacist can share information with the patient about his or her own coverage or medications.

How Is Information Protected on the Computer?

Several safeguards help protect electronically transmitted patient information. The sender of electronic PHI is required to use encryption to convert the information into a nonreadable format. Decryption is the reverse process. The encryption technology must be approved by the National Institute of Standards and Technologies to ensure its effectiveness in protecting patients' rights.

What Are the Rights of the Patient?

Under HIPAA, patients have the following rights:

- The right to ask to see and obtain a copy of their health records.
- The right to have corrections added to their health information.
- The right to receive a notice that tells them how their health information may be used and shared.

- The right to decide whether they want to give their permission before their health information can be used or shared for certain purposes, such as for marketing.
- The right to obtain a report on when and why their health information was shared for certain purposes.
- If patients believe that their rights are being denied or their health information is not being protected, they can:
  - File a complaint with their provider or health insurer
  - File a complaint with the U.S. government
  - Either authorize or not authorize any sharing of their personal or medical information
  - Change or rescind this permission any time they desire

The HIPAA Privacy Rule specifically permits certain persons identified by the patient, such as a spouse, family members, or friends, to receive information that is directly relevant to the patient's care or the patient's payment for health care. If the patient is present or is otherwise available before the disclosure and has the capacity to make health care decisions, the covered entity may discuss this information with the family and these other individuals if the patient agrees or, when given the opportunity, does not object.

For example, when a person comes to a pharmacy and requests to pick up a prescription on behalf of an individual he or she identifies by name, a pharmacist, based on professional judgment and experience with common practice, may allow the person to do so.

Examples of What the Technician Cannot Do

As a pharmacy technician, you may not do the following:

- Offer any personal or medical information pertaining to the patient to any entity not covered under HIPAA rules and regulations
- Share any information with any family member or friend, co-worker, manager, or any entity not covered under the HIPAA rules and regulations

Box 2-4 presents additional examples.

Examples of What Is Not Covered under HIPAA Patients' Rights

If you work as a pharmacy technician for a health plan or covered health care provider:

- The Privacy Rule does not apply to your employment records.
- The rule does protect your medical or health plan records if you are a patient of the provider or a member of the health plan.

BOX 2-4

Examples of Breaching Confidentiality

Explain why the following examples are in violation of HIPAA regulations.

Example 1: Ms. K has cancer. Two pharmacy technicians discuss her condition and the medications she is taking. A co-worker of Ms. K overhears this information and tells her employer.

Example 2: A computer screen is left on that shows a patient's health information and can be seen by other patients.

Example 3: A regular customer of the pharmacy asks the technician for another patient's phone number; the customer knows that patient.

Example 4: A technician looks up personal patient information because the technician is curious about the patient.

Example 5: A technician gives drug information over the phone to a family member of the patient.

Public Health Activities

Covered entities may disclose protected health information to the following:

1. Public health authorities authorized by law to collect or receive such information for preventing or controlling disease, injury, or disability and to public health or other government authorities authorized to receive reports of child abuse and neglect
2. Entities subject to FDA regulation regarding FDA-regulated products or activities for purposes such as adverse event reporting, tracking of products, product recalls, and post-marketing surveillance
3. Individuals who may have contracted or been exposed to a communicable disease when notification is authorized by law
4. Employers, regarding employees, for information concerning a work-related illness or injury or workplace-related medical surveillance to comply with the Occupational Safety and Health Administration (OHSA) or similar state law

Law Enforcement Purposes

Covered entities may disclose protected health information to law enforcement officials for law enforcement purposes under the following six circumstances, and subject to specified conditions:

1. As required by law, such as court orders
2. To identify or locate a suspect, fugitive, material witness, or missing person

3. In response to a law enforcement official's request for information about a victim or suspected victim of a crime
4. To alert law enforcement of a person's death, if the covered entity suspects that criminal activity caused the death
5. When a covered entity believes that protected health information is evidence of a crime that occurred on its premises
6. By a covered health care provider in a medical emergency not occurring on its premises, when necessary to inform law enforcement about the nature of a crime, the location of the crime or crime victims, and the perpetrator of the crime

Examples

1. Can I have a friend pick up my medications and medical supplies for me?
   - Yes; under HIPAA, pharmacists are allowed to give prescription medications and supplies to a family member, friend, or any person you send to pick up the medications or supplies.
2. If my daughter calls the pharmacy to ask about whether my medications are ready, can they tell her?
   - Yes; but no other information can be given out.
3. If I cannot speak the language and a stranger offers to interpret the exchange between myself and the pharmacist, is this okay?
   - Yes; as long as you do not object.
4. Is a pharmacist permitted to have the customer acknowledge receipt of the notice by signing or initialing the log book when picking up prescriptions?
   - Yes; provided the individual is clearly informed on the log book of what he or she is acknowledging and the acknowledgment is not also used as a waiver or permission for something else that also appears on the log book (such as a waiver to consult with the pharmacist). The HIPAA Privacy Rule provides covered health care providers with discretion to design an acknowledgment process that works best for their businesses (see the website *www.hhs.gov/ocr/privacy/psa/understanding/index.html*).

2000 Drug Addiction Treatment Act (DATA 2000)

The Drug Addiction Treatment Act of 2000 permits physicians to prescribe controlled substances (preapproved by the DEA) in schedules C-III, C-IV, or C-V to individuals suffering from opioid addiction for the purpose of maintenance or detoxification treatments. This act is different from the regulations that oversee methadone maintenance treatments for opioid addiction. Certain controlled substances have been found to effectively attenuate the craving for opioids and also prevent withdrawal symptoms.

Patients must be in a treatment program that provides additional support services. Physicians must complete a training course and must be registered with and certified by the DEA to prescribe these agents. If the physician is in private practice, he or she may treat only up to 30 patients at one time. After 1 year the physician may apply to treat up to 100 patients.

2003 Medicare Modernization Act (MMA)

Medicare is a government-managed insurance program that provides assistance to people older than age 65. In addition, those who are younger than age 65 with disabilities and individuals with end-stage renal failure are covered under this program. Medicare has a long history, starting in 1965. In 2003 a major change took place for millions of Americans with the passage of the Medicare Modernization Act. This revision provided a drug discount card to beneficiaries with low incomes who require pharmacy company assistance for obtaining medications. The new program is administered under the Medicare Advantage program, which began in 2006. This allows Medicare participants to offset high drug costs, which should also reduce preventable hospitalizations resulting from lack of medication treatment.

Scenario CHECK UP 2-2

Laura is assigned to cover the register in addition to performing her regular prescription-filling duties at a local chain pharmacy. It is a particularly busy day, and two technicians have called in sick during her shift. A customer comes to the register and asks to purchase two boxes of Sudafed. Laura has the person sign the log book but does not ask for identification. What are the possible negative implications for Laura in this transaction? What are the laws regarding the purchase of pseudoephedrine in your state?

2005 Combat Methamphetamine Epidemic Act

Until 2004 the drug pseudoephedrine (PSE) was sold OTC as a decongestant and was not limited in quantity for purchase by the consumer. Several different manufacturers produce this drug, and it was stocked outside the pharmacy on the shelves of every store that carried cold remedies. The OTC status of pseudoephedrine was changed when the U.S. government became aware of its diversion and use as an ingredient in the preparation of methamphetamine (Figure 2-2).

BOX 2-5
Combat Methamphetamine Epidemic Act 2005

Pseudoephedrine storage: Behind the counter or locked in a cabinet.

The maximum amount sold may not exceed 3.6 g in a calendar day or 9 g per 30 days retail, and 7.5 g per 30 days via mail order.

Purchaser's identification must be provided.

Documentation may be done electronically or via log book. If a log book is used, it must be a bound book.

Records of all information must be kept for at least 2 years.

Documentation required:
    Drug name
    Drug strength
    Drug amount
    Date/time of sale
    Customer's name
    Customer's address
    Customer's signature

In 2005 Congress passed the Combat Methamphetamine Epidemic Act (CMEA) in response to this problem. The bill addressed all areas of the manufacturing, law enforcement regulations, and sale of this drug. Although pseudoephedrine is still labeled as a "non–controlled substance," the manufacture, distribution, and sale of this drug must follow several strict guidelines. According to these guidelines, only a licensed pharmacist or technician may dispense, sell, or distribute this drug (Box 2-5). According to the Government Accountability Office (GAO) 2013 report, approximately 19 states have implemented electronic reporting to track PSE sales. Seventeen of the 19 use the tracking system called the National Precursor Log Exchange (NPLEx). Two states, Oregon and Mississippi, along with 63 Missouri counties and cities now require a prescription for PSE products. Many states, such as Alabama, Arizona, Georgia, Illinois, Kentucky, Tennessee, Washington, and Wyoming, restrict sales of pseudoephedrine products to pharmacies and require customers to show a photograph ID and sign a log book during purchase. States such as California, Maryland, Maine, and New Mexico have enacted degrees of controlled access to OTC pseudoephedrine products.

According to the GAO report, electronic tracking systems have helped enforce sales limits but have not reduced "meth lab" incidents. Statistics show that the meth lab count nationwide dropped to a low of 6,951 in 2007. Unfortunately, this number has been on the rise since. In 2010, there were 15,314 reported meth labs, more than double the number in

U.S. Department of Justice
Drug Enforcement Administration
Office of Diversion Control

Problem

Pseudoephedrine and ephedrine, both List 1 chemicals, are highly coveted by drug traffickers who use them to manufacture methamphetamine, a Schedule II controlled substance, for the illicit market. The diversion of over-the-counter, pseudoephedrine-containing products is one of the major contributing factors to the methamphetamine problem in the United States. Inappropriate retail level purchases by individuals attempting to procure pseudoephedrine for the illicit manufacture of methamphetamine have been documented as a source of much of the pseudoephedrine found in clandestine methamphetamine laboratories. These purchases, which are accomplished by methods such as "*smurfing*" and *shelf sweeping*, violate Federal law and may expose the seller to criminal and civil penalties.

Common Pseudoephedrine Products

Common cold products including, but not limited to Sudafed®, Tylenol®Cold, Advil®Cold, Drixoral®, Benadryl® Allergy & Cold Tablets, Robitussin®Cold Sinus & Congestion, as well as many generic brands.

Retail Thresholds

The Methamphetamine Anti-Proliferation Act (MAPA) limits the thresholds of pseudoephedrine drug products to 9-gram single transactions with the package size not to exceed 3 grams.

Nine (9) Gram Single Transactions--Three (3) Grams per Package

- 120 mg pseudoephedrine HCl = 92 tablets
- 120 mg pseudoephedrine HCl = 31 tablets
- 60 mg pseudoephedrine HCl = 184 tablets
- 60 mg pseudoephedrine HCl = 62 tablets
- 30 mg pseudoephedrine HCl = 367 tablets
- 30 mg pseudoephedrine HCl = 123 tablets

Common Methods of Diversion

- *Smurfing* involves the retail purchase of sub-threshold amounts by organized groups of individuals that either send in multiple purchasers into the same location or visit a large number of different locations.
- *Shelf sweeping* occurs when individuals or groups remove all the shelf stock and exit the store, similar to a "smash and grab" shoplifting technique.
- *Shoplifting* occurs when individuals remove stock from the shelves and exit the store without paying.

All of the above methods can be prevented by limiting access to products or by utilizing mirrors or other surveillance equipment such as cameras.

Suspicious Purchase Items

Camping fuel, lithium batteries, large quantities of matches, iodine, coffee filters, rock salt, battery acid, swimming pool acid (when purchased in unusual quantities or under unusual circumstances).

Theft or Loss of List I Chemicals

The DEA reminds List I chemical handlers of the regulatory requirement: "A regulated chemical handler must immediately report thefts or losses to the nearest DEA office and should notify state/local law enforcement and regulatory agencies. A written report must be submitted to the DEA within 15 days of discovery of the theft or loss." (CFR 21 §1310.05)

Improper Sales

"Any person who possesses or distributes a listed chemical knowing or having reasonable cause to believe that the listed chemical will be used to manufacture a controlled substance, except as authorized by this title, shall be fined in accordance with Title 18, or imprisoned not more than 20 years, or both." (Title 21 U.S.C. 841 (c)(2))

FIGURE 2-2 DEA poster on the misuse of pseudoephedrine. (Courtesy Drug Enforcement Administration, Washington, DC.)

2007. Interestingly, the number of meth lab incidents in Oregon and Mississippi declined after the implementation of the prescription-only approach; Mississippi declared a 66% decline from 2010 to 2011.

Table 2-1 presents an overview of other pharmacy-related acts.

2010 Patient Protection and Affordable Care Act (ACA)

In March, 2010, President Obama signed into law the Patient Protection and Affordable Care Act. This comprehensive health care reform makes preventive care more accessible and affordable for many Americans. The ACA has a number of provisions that will be phased in over a period of years, beginning in 2010 and continuing through 2020. The law requires insurance companies to cover all applicants with new minimum standards, including individuals with pre-existing conditions. Many components of the ACA involve pharmacy professionals, such as:

- Electronic health record (EHR) incentives and e-prescribing
- Medication therapy management (MTM)

- Accountable care organizations (ACOs)
- The Independence at Home Demonstration Project

Pharmacy technicians need to be knowledgeable about the ACA and the changes dealing with medication management and Medicare Part D. Well-informed technicians build credibility for the profession and for themselves as an important part of the pharmacy team.

More information on the ACA can be obtain at the website *www.hhs.gov/opa/affordable-care-act/index.html*.

2013 Drug Quality and Security Act (DQSA)

In November, 2013, President Obama signed into law a bill that gives the Food and Drug Administration greater oversight of bulk pharmaceutical compounding and enhances the agency's ability to track drugs through the distribution process. This legislation was prompted by the deadly fungal meningitis outbreak in the fall of 2012 that resulted from unsanitary conditions at a compounding facility in

TABLE 2-1

Additional Pharmacy-Related Laws

Date	Act	Abbreviation	Description
1967	Fair Packaging and Labeling Act	FPLA	Label must show net contents; name and place of business of manufacturer, packer, or distributor; and net quantity of contents in terms of weight, measure, or numeric count. Measurement must be in metric and U.S. units.
1972	Drug Listing Act	DLA	Provides the FDA with an accurate list of all drugs manufactured, prepared, propagated, compounded, or processed by a drug establishment regulated under the FDA. This act amends the Federal Food, Drug, and Cosmetic Act and prevents unfair or deceptive packaging and labeling.
1990	Anabolic Steroids Control Act	ASCA	Because of anabolic steroid misuse by athletes, this act helps enforce regulations on abuse.
1990	The Humanitarian Device Exemption—Safe Medical Devices Act	SMDA	This act encourages discovery and use of devices intended to benefit patients in treatment and diagnosis of diseases or conditions that affect fewer than 4,000 individuals in the United States.
1990	Nutrition Labeling and Education Act	NLEA	This act covers food items and their labeling; vitamins, minerals, or other nutrients are on the label and in some cases are highlighted.
1994	Dietary Supplement Health and Education Act	DSHEA	This act better defines the term *dietary supplements* to include herbs such as ginseng, garlic, fish oil, psyllium, enzymes, glandulars, and mixtures of these. Consumers must be informed of health-related benefits. Manufacturers of these supplements are held to the same regulations. Labels cannot mislead consumers. Labels must include nutritional values.
1997	Food and Drug Administration Modernization Act	FDAMA	New drugs are being reviewed and released into the public faster. Millions of persons have a wider and more timely access to information on new medications.
2010	Combat Methamphetamine Enhancement Act of 2010	CMEA	This act amended the Controlled Substance Act to increase the compliance of retailers and distributors of pseudoephedrine products. All persons engaged in the sale of pseudoephedrine must self-certify that they have trained personnel to comply with the Combat Methamphetamine Act. Also, distributors can sell only to retailers who are registered with the DEA.

Massachusetts. The DQSA comprises two separate acts: the Compounding Quality Act and the Drug Supply Chain Security Act.

The Compounding Quality Act creates a new class of compounding manufacturers that voluntarily register with the FDA as an "outsourcing facility." These manufacturers will be regulated similar to traditional pharmaceutical manufacturers and will be able to sell to hospitals in bulk.

The Drug Supply Chain Security Act addresses concerns relating to counterfeit, falsified, and substandard prescription medication. This act requires the FDA to create and implement a national tracking system to be used by manufacturers. Bar coding technology will be used to introduce pharmaceutical products into the supply chain. This new track-and-trace pedigree system for drugs will be phased in over 10 years.

In 2012, counterfeit vials of Avastin, a cancer medication, were found in the United States. They were introduced from Britain and traced back to a Turkish wholesaler. The vials had no active ingredient.

Food and Drug Administration/Drug Enforcement Administration

Two government agencies that are important in the practice of pharmacy are the FDA and the DEA. The FDA now is an agency of the U.S. Department of

Health and Human Services (see the discussion of the history of the FDA presented earlier in this chapter). The main function of the FDA is to enforce the guidelines for manufacturers to ensure the safety and effectiveness of medications. The Federal Food, Drug, and Cosmetic Act established standards that prohibit misbranding, adulteration, and misleading labeling of any products before they are provided to consumers. Any food, drug, or product that contains any avoidable, added, poisonous, or harmful substance is unsafe and is considered adulterated. To prevent misbranding, manufacturers must meet the following packaging standards under the Federal Food, Drug, and Cosmetic Act:

1. Mandatory drug labeling (see Drug Monographs, later in the chapter)
2. Standards of identity
3. Imitation foods
4. Nutritional information for special dietary foods
5. Manufacturers may not advertise false or misleading statements about their product

Examples of misleading information on product labeling include:

1. Incorrect, inadequate, or incomplete identification
2. Unsubstantiated claims of therapeutic value
3. Inaccuracies concerning condition, state, treatment size, shape, or style
4. Substitution of parts or material
5. Ambiguity, half-truths, and trade puffery
6. Failure to reveal material facts, consequences that may result from use, or existence of difference of opinion

The other enforcement department is the DEA. This agency was created later under the Department of Justice. The function of the DEA is to prevent illegal distribution and misuse of controlled substances. The DEA also issues licenses to practitioners, pharmacies, and manufacturers of controlled substances. The DEA's primary role is to enforce the nation's federal drug laws.

FDA Reporting Process and Adverse Reactions

The FDA has a toll-free number (1-800-FDA-1088) for reporting any defect found in OTC medications or any drug problem noted by a person. A technician or pharmacist also may use this number to report any problems with a drug, whether it is OTC or legend (prescription). A product that looks different from its normal package should be reported. Adverse reactions also should be reported to the FDA's MedWatch program. Any medication reaction that may cause disability, hospitalization, or death should be reported, along with any less-disabling type of reaction, such as fainting, or other types of reactions

that may not have been listed in the drug monograph. MedWatch is the program under the FDA that allows consumers and health care professionals to report discrepancies or adverse reactions to medications. The MedWatch form for such reports can be found in many drug reference publications and drug compendia databases or online at the website *www.fda.gov/medwatch/how.htm*. The patient and reporting person's identities are kept confidential (Figure 2-3).

 Tech Note!

Follow MedWatch on Twitter to keep up with the latest drug safety information and adverse event reporting! US FDA MedWatch @FDAMedWatch or the website *https://twitter.com/FDAMedWatch.*

Recalled Drugs

The FDA does not typically order recalls but instead may request (in writing) a recall by the manufacturer. Only if the manufacturer refuses and there is clear evidence of a risk to human health may the FDA enforce such a request. The manufacturer can voluntarily recall items that have been found to be defective or somehow tainted. This is done by several means, such as television news or newspapers, and recall notifications can be downloaded from the FDA website. In addition, the manufacturer must notify by e-mail, phone, or fax all entities that may have dispensed the product and must include instructions on how to handle each type of recall (Box 2-6). Once the product has been recalled, it is destroyed, and an investigation is conducted to determine why the product was defective.

All stock must be pulled from the shelves according to the guidelines of the manufacturer. The manufacturer supplies a return form with instructions for reimbursement. The three classes of recalls are as follows:

- Class 1: The highest level of recall; it deals with products that could cause serious harm or prove fatal. This includes life-saving drugs. This level also includes foods that contain toxins or labels that do not list ingredients that may cause allergies.
- Class 2: The next level, which deals with products found to cause a temporary health problem or to pose a slight threat of serious harm. This level includes drugs that are dispensed at less than the strength labeled on the container; it does not include drugs used in life-threatening events.
- Class 3: The lowest level, which is used for products that may have a minor defect or other condition that would not harm the patient but

DEPARTMENT OF HEALTH AND HUMAN SERVICES
Food and Drug Administration

Form Approved: OMB No. 0910-0291
Expiration Date: 6/30/2015
*(See PRA Statement on preceding
general information page)*

MEDWATCH Consumer Voluntary Reporting
(FORM FDA 3500B)

Section A – About the Problem

What kind of problem was it? *(Check all that apply)*

☐ Were hurt or had a bad side effect *(including new or worsening symptoms)*

☐ Used a product incorrectly which could have or led to a problem

☐ Noticed a problem with the quality of the product

☐ Had problems after switching from one product maker to another maker

Did any of the following happen? *(Check all that apply)*

☐ Hospitalization – admitted or stayed longer

☐ Required help to prevent permanent harm *(for medical devices only)*

☐ Disability or health problem

☐ Birth defect

☐ Life-threatening

☐ Death *(Include date)*: _____

☐ Other serious/important medical incident *(Please describe below)*

_____

_____

_____

Date the problem occurred *(mm/dd/yyyy)*

Tell us what happened and how it happened. *(Include as many details as possible)*

_____

_____

_____ | Continue Page |

List any relevant tests or laboratory data if you know them. *(Include dates)*

_____

_____

_____ | Continue Page |

For a problem with a product, including

- prescription or over-the-counter medicine
- biologics, such as human cells and tissues used for transplantation (for example, tendons, ligaments, and bone) and gene therapies
- nutrition products, such as vitamins and minerals, herbal remedies, infant formulas, and medical foods
- cosmetics or make-up products
- foods (including beverages and ingredients added to foods)

⇨ **Go to Section B**

For a problem with a medical device, including

- any health-related test, tool, or piece of equipment
- health-related kits, such as glucose monitoring kits or blood pressure cuffs
- implants, such as breast implants, pacemakers, or catheters
- other consumer health products, such as contact lenses, hearing aids, and breast pumps

⇨ **Go to Section C
(Skip Section B)**

For more information, visit *http://www.fda.gov/MedWatch*

Submission of a report does not constitute an admission that medical personnel or the product caused or contributed to the event.

FORM FDA 3500B (4/13)   **MedWatch** Consumer Voluntary Reporting   Page 1 of 3

EF

FIGURE 2-3 FDA MedWatch form. (Courtesy Drug Enforcement Administration, Washington, DC.)

Section B – About the Products

Name of the product as it appears on the box, bottle, or package *(Include as many names as you see)*

Name of the company that makes the product

Expiration date *(mm/dd/yyyy)*	Lot number	NDC number

Strength *(for example, 250 mg per 500 mL or 1 g)*	Quantity *(for example, 2 pills, 2 puffs, or 1 teaspoon, etc.)*	Frequency *(for example, twice daily or at bedtime)*	How was it taken or used *(for example, by mouth, by injection, or on the skin)?*

Date the person first started taking or using the product *(mm/dd/yyyy)*: _____

Date the person stopped taking or using the product *(mm/dd/yyyy)*: _____

Why was the person using the product *(such as, what condition was it supposed to treat?)*

_____

_____

_____

Did the problem stop after the person reduced the dose or stopped taking or using the product? ☐ Yes ☐ No

Did the problem return if the person started taking or using the product again?

☐ Yes ☐ No ☐ Didn't restart

Do you still have the product in case we need to evaluate it? *(Do not send the product to FDA. We will contact you directly if we need it.)*

☐ Yes ☐ No

⇨ **Go to Section D (Skip Section C)**

Section C – About the Medical Device

Name of medical device

Name of the company that makes the medical device

Other identifying information *(The model, catalog, lot, serial, or UDI number, and the expiration date, if you can locate them)*

_____

_____

_____

Was someone operating the medical device when the problem occurred?

☐ Yes

☐ No

If yes, who was using it?

☐ The person who had the problem

☐ A health professional *(such as a doctor, nurse, or aide)*

☐ Someone else *(Please explain who)*

_____

For implanted medical devices ONLY *(such as pacemakers, breast implants, etc.)*

Date the implant was put in *(mm/dd/yyyy)*	Date the implant was taken out *(If relevant) (mm/dd/yyyy)*

⇨ **Go to Section D**

For more information, visit *http://www.fda.gov/MedWatch*

Submission of a report does not constitute an admission that medical personnel or the product caused or contributed to the event.

FORM FDA 3500B (4/13)   **MedWatch** Consumer Voluntary Reporting   Page 2 of 3

FIGURE 2-3, cont'd

Continued

Section D – About the Person Who Had the Problem

Person's Initials	Sex	Age *(at time the problem occurred)* or Birth Date	Weight *(Specify lbs or kg)*	Race
	☐ Female ☐ Male			

List known medical conditions *(such as diabetes, high blood pressure, cancer, heart disease, or others)*

_____

_____

Please list all allergies *(such as to drugs, foods, pollen, or others).*

List any other important information about the person *(such as smoking, pregnancy, alcohol use, etc.)*

List all current prescription medications and medical devices being used.

_____

_____ | Continue Page |

List all over-the-counter medications and any vitamins, minerals, supplements, and herbal remedies being used. | Continue Page |

⇨ **Go to Section E**

Section E – About the Person Filling Out This Form

We will contact you only if we need additional information. Your name will not be given out to the public.

Last name	First name
Number/Street	City and State/Province
Country	ZIP or Postal code
Telephone number	Email address	Today's date *(mm/dd/yyyy)*

Did you report this problem to the company that makes the product (the manufacturer)? ☐ Yes ☐ No	May we give your name and contact information to the company that makes the product (manufacturer) to help them evaluate the product? ☐ Yes ☐ No

Send This Report by Mail or Fax

Keep the product in case the FDA wants to contact you for more information. Please do not send products to the FDA. Mail or fax the form to:

Mail: MedWatch Food and Drug Administration 5600 Fishers Lane Rockville, MD 20857	**Fax:** 1-800-332-0178 (toll-free)

Thank you for helping us protect the public health.

For more information, visit *http://www.fda.gov/MedWatch* | Submission of a report does not constitute an admission that medical personnel or the product caused or contributed to the event.

FORM FDA 3500B (4/13)   **MedWatch** Consumer Voluntary Reporting   Page 3 of 3

FIGURE 2-3, cont'd

BOX 2-6
Sample Recall Notification

The FDA posts press releases and other notices of recalls and market withdrawals by the firms involved as a service to consumers, the media, and other interested parties. The FDA does not endorse either the product or the company.

Recall—Firm Press Release
Baxter Initiates Nationwide Voluntary Recall of One Lot of Nitroglycerin in 5% Dextrose Injection
Contact
Consumer:
1-888-229-0001

Media:
Deborah Spak, John O'Malley
224-555-5353
media@baxter.com

FOR IMMEDIATE RELEASE—November 27, 2013—
Baxter International Inc. announced today it has initiated a voluntary recall of one lot of Nitroglycerin in 5% Dextrose Injection due to particulate matter found in one vial. If infused, particulate matter could lead to potential venous and/or arterial thromboembolism (blockage of blood vessels). Other adverse events associated with injection of particulate matter include inflammation due to foreign material, particularly in the lungs, and local irritation of blood vessels.

There have been no reported adverse events associated with this issue to date. The financial impact of this recall is not material to Baxter.

Nitroglycerin in 5% Dextrose Injection (Intravenous) is indicated for treatment of peri-operative hypertension (treatment of high blood pressure before, during and after surgery); for control of congestive heart failure in the setting of acute myocardial infarction (during a new onset heart attack, a weakness of the heart muscle may cause fluid to build up in the lungs and other body tissues); for treatment of angina pectoris (chest pain) in patients who have not responded to sublingual nitroglycerin and β-blockers (beta blocker drugs); and for induction of intraoperative hypotension (low blood pressure during surgery).

Baxter's Nitroglycerin in 5% Dextrose Injection is packaged in 250-mL glass containers, with 12 glass containers per carton. The affected product code is 1A0694, and the affected lot number is G105197. Product affected by this recall was distributed to healthcare centers and distributors in Colombia, Saudi Arabia, and the United States.

Baxter is notifying customers, who are being directed not to use product from the recalled lot. Customers should locate and remove all affected product from their facility. The affected lot was distributed to customers between January 17, 2013, and October 10, 2013. Unaffected lot numbers can continue to be used according to the instructions for use. Affected product should be returned to Baxter for credit by contacting Baxter Healthcare Center for Service at 1-888-229-0001 between the hours of 7:00 a.m. and 6:00 p.m., Central Time. Unaffected lots of product are available for replacement.

Adverse reactions or quality problems experienced with the use of this product may be reported to the FDA's MedWatch Adverse Event Reporting program either online, by regular mail or by fax.
- Online: www.fda.gov/medwatch/report.htm
- Regular Mail: Use postage-paid, preaddressed Form FDA 3500 available at: www.fda.gov/MedWatch/getforms.htm. Mail to address on the preaddressed form.
- Fax: 1-800-FDA-0178

This recall is being conducted with the knowledge of the U.S. Food and Drug Administration.

U.S. Food and Drug Administration, Safety Alerts; Baxter initiates nationwide voluntary recall of one lot of nitroglycerin in 5% dextrose injection. http://www.fda.gov/Safety/Recalls/ucm376942.htm (Referenced July 17, 2013.)

that prevents the drugs from being resold. This level includes a drug container defect (e.g., a faulty cap), a product with a strange color or taste, or the lack of English labeling on retail food items.

Controlled Substances

Controlled substances, such as barbiturates, opioids, benzodiazepines, and central nervous system stimulants, are substances that are addictive and have the potential to be abused. Opioids, such as codeine and morphine, are substances created from opium and are addictive. When consumed over time, a person can build up a tolerance to their effects and require increased doses. Each type of controlled substance is assigned a rating that depends on its addictive and abuse potential. Figure 2-4 presents an example of a labeled **narcotic**.

Ratings of Scheduled (Controlled) Substances

The letter C (meaning controlled substance) is used in addition to Roman numerals to indicate the addictiveness and abuse potential of controlled substances. In 1970 Congress established five levels of control based on the potential for abuse. The strongest level in terms of abuse potential are C-I drugs. These drugs have been determined to have a high potential for abuse and to have no acceptable medical purpose; they also are deemed unsafe for use under medical

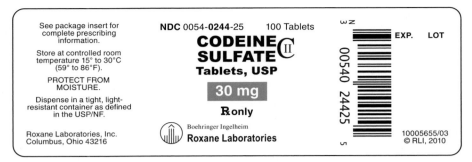

FIGURE 2-4 Codeine label showing C-II imprint.

supervision. This category includes such drugs as D-lysergic acid diethylamide (LSD) and heroin. Pharmacies do not stock drugs in the C-I class because they do not have any medicinal use in the United States. Therefore, physicians cannot prescribe C-I drugs for their patients. All medicinal controlled substances are placed in the following four categories: C-II, C-III, C-IV, and C-V. Table 2-2 shows the schedule, types of medications, and abuse potential for each level of controlled substances.

Individual states establish rules concerning controlled substances, such as storage and record keeping. Schedule C-V medications (referred to as *exempt controlled substances*) may be kept OTC in some states because of their low potential for abuse. However, even for exempt controlled substances, specific rules govern the quantity kept on hand and the records that must be retained by the pharmacy when these substances are purchased by consumers. Many states require C-II drugs to be kept (before filling) in locked storage areas because of their high potential for abuse.

The U.S. Attorney General has the authority to decide under which schedule a drug should be placed. The decision is made after careful consideration of the scientific findings and recommendations from various authorities on the dependency potential for each agent. Some drugs may be labeled under two different schedules because the dose may alter the dependency of the drug. Sometimes controlled substances can be reevaluated. For example, dronabinol (Marinol) previously was classified as a C-II drug but now is a C-III drug. In contrast, certain narcotics are used primarily for procedures in hospitals; for example, topical cocaine is used locally to stop bleeding and provide anesthesia before suturing.

Tamper-Proof Prescriptions

Many states have changed to a new type of prescription for controlled substances. These new prescriptions have up to eight different tamper-proof security marks on them. These features were designed to protect a prescriber's intended order from forgery and fraud. Several features eliminate the usefulness of photocopying the prescription order. The prescription forms can be ordered with any or all of the features. The DEA must approve the printer company that prints the new prescriptions, but no specific format has been established because each state may adopt its own features, colors, or size (check with your individual state board of pharmacy for more information). The individual features of these tamper-proof forms are listed in Box 2-7, and Figure 2-5 shows a sample prescription form.

Registration Requirements for Maintaining Narcotics

The DEA uses three main registration forms in the regulation of controlled substances. Only Form 224 is needed by the pharmacy to dispense controlled substances. The following is a list of form numbers issued by the DEA, along with additional requirements:

- To manufacture or distribute controlled substances: Form 225.
- To manage a controlled substances treatment program or compound controlled substances: Form 363.
- To dispense controlled substances: Form 224 (must be renewed every 3 years using Form 224a).
- To order or transfer schedule II substances: Form 222. This must be done by the receiving registrant to the registrant transferring the drugs. A final count of the drugs must be completed on the day of transfer. No copy needs to be sent to the DEA, but a copy should be kept on file for 2 years for DEA inspection.
- Authorization to destroy damaged, outdated, or unwanted controlled substances: Form 41. Retail pharmacies can request this form from the DEA only once a year. (Hospitals may

TABLE 2-2

Typical Controlled Substances

| Drug Level | Type of Medication | | Potential for Abuse |
	Generic Name	Trade Name	
C-I		LSD Cocaine (crack or street) Mescaline Heroin	Drugs that have no accepted medical use in the United States and have very high abuse potential
C-II	Meperidine Oxycodone/APAP Oxycodone/ASA Hydromorphone Methylphenidate Fentanyl Codeine Morphine Amphetamines Methadone Opium Hydrocodone/APAP Hydrocodone/ibuprofen	Demerol Percocet Percodan Dilaudid Ritalin Duragesic Vicodin Vicoprofen	High potential for abuse; used for medicinal purposes; abuse may lead to severe psychological or physical dependence
C-III	Acetaminophen/codeine #2, #3, #4	Tylenol/codeine	Potential for abuse under this schedule is less than that of controlled substances under C-II; abuse may lead to moderate or low physical dependence or high psychological dependence; most schedule III drugs are combination narcotics
C-IV	Diazepam Lorazepam Pentazocine Chlordiazepoxide Flurazepam Phenobarbital	Valium Ativan Talwin Librium Dalmane	Potential for abuse is low compared with C-III drugs; abuse may lead to limited physical or psychological dependence
C-V	Diphenoxylate/atropine Guaifenesin/codeine Promethazine/codeine	Lomotil Robitussin AC Phenergan/codeine	Low potential for abuse compared with C-IV drugs; abuse may lead to limited physical or psychological dependence

APAP, Acetyl-*p*-aminophenol (acetaminophen); *ASA*, acetylsalicylic acid (aspirin).

BOX 2-7

Tamper-Proof Features

- Tamper-resistant background ink shows attempts to alter script by patient.
- Thermochromatic ink box shows "SECURE" when rubbed or heated.
- Each prescription sheet has an individual numeric identifier so that lost or stolen prescription pads can be invalidated.
- Each sheet is sequentially numbered for internal and state-mandated record keeping.
- Security feature warning bands are on the front of each script to detail security features.
- Penetrating magnetic ink is used to print the prescriber's information on the script, preventing chemical "lifting" of information during forgery.
- Secure prescriptions have "coin reactive" ink; message appears when the back of the pad is rubbed with a coin.

- Photocopied features:
  - Hidden security "VOID" appears when photocopied on most high-end photocopiers.
  - Reverse printed RX (lighter colored) notations in upper corners of pad drop out when photocopied to appear white.
  - All secure prescriptions have a high-security watermark on reverse side that cannot be copied and can be seen only when held to a light source at an angle.
  - MicroPrint security borders are present, which are tiny printings of a security message along the edges of a pad that combine to form a solid line when digitally scanned or copied.

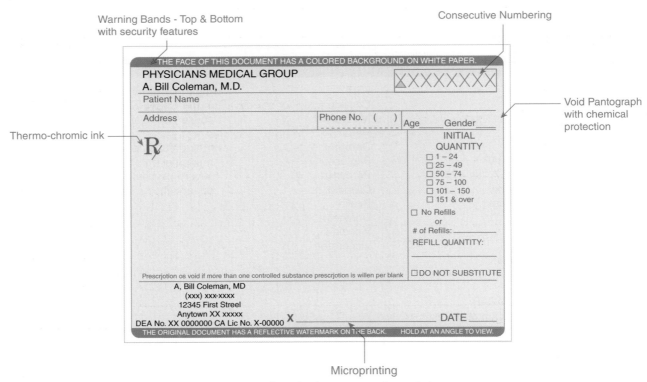

Warning Bands - Top & Bottom
with security features

Consecutive Numbering

Thermo-chromic ink

Void Pantograph
with chemical
protection

Microprinting

FIGURE 2-5 Example of a tamper-proof prescription.

request a "blanket destruction" permission form, which allows them to destroy a controlled substance multiple times throughout the year.) For retail pharmacies, a letter must be sent to the DEA for approval, along with the completed Form 41, at least 2 weeks before destruction. The request letter must contain the names of at least two people who will witness the destruction and the proposed date and method of destruction. The disposal of the scheduled drug or drugs must be witnessed by a licensed physician, pharmacist, registered nurse (RN), or law enforcement officer. Signed copies of Form 41 must then be forwarded to the DEA.

- Retail pharmacies that want to engage in wholesale distribution of bulk quantities of drugs containing pseudoephedrine, phenylpropanolamine, or ephedrine must register with the DEA: Form 510.
- For loss or theft of a controlled substance: Form 106. Required information includes the name and address of the pharmacy, DEA registration number, date of loss or theft, police department notified, type of loss or theft, drug name, and symbols or cost codes used by the pharmacy in marking containers (if applicable).

Refilling Controlled Substances

The DEA guidelines for C-II substances allow physicians to write up to three separate prescriptions at one time for multiple drugs, to be filled sequentially over 90 days. The date of each subsequent prescription must be written on the order, and the prescription cannot be filled before that date. Each state's **board of pharmacy (BOP)** may implement additional guidelines that control the amount of controlled substances that can be refilled.

Most states limit refills of schedule C-III through C-V drugs to a maximum of five times or within 6 months from the original order, whichever comes first. In addition, the amount ordered on the refills may not exceed the original order. The length of time for keeping records may also vary by state, but a record must be kept of controlled substance refills showing the pharmacist's initials and the date the refill was dispensed. (A list showing each state's BOP can be found at the website *www.nabp.net*.)

Ordering Controlled Substances

A pharmacy has two ways to obtain *schedule II* controlled substances from a distributor: electronic or paper filing of DEA Form 222. Form 222 (Figure 2-6) *must be signed* by the pharmacist who signed Form 224 or a person who has been *legally assigned* power of attorney by that pharmacist. This triplicate form must be completed only with a pen, a typewriter, or an indelible pencil. The top copy, or Copy 1, and the middle (DEA) copy, or Copy 2, with the carbon paper, are sent to the supplier or manufacturer by the pharmacy *receiving/ordering* the drugs.

Sample DEA Form 222

See Reverse of PURCHASER'S Copy for Instructions	No order form may be issued for Schedule I and II substance unless completed application form has been received (21 CRF 1305.04)	OMB APPROVAL NO. 1117-0010

TO: STREET ADDRESS

CITY AND STATE	DATE	TO BE FILLED IN BY SUPPLIER
		SUPPLIER DEA REGISTRATION NO.

	TO BE FILLED IN BY PURCHASER					
	No. of Packages	Size of Package	Name of Item	National Drug Code	Packaging Shipped	Date Shipped
1						
2						
3						
4						
5						
6						
7						
8						
9						
10						

◄ LAST LINE COMPLETED   *(MUST BE 10 OR LESS)* | SIGNATURE OF PURCHASER OR ATTORNEY OR AGENT

Date Issued	DEA Registration No.	Name and Address of Registrant
Schedules		
Registered as a	No. of this Order Form	

DEA Form 222 (Oct. 1992)   US OFFICIAL ORDER FORMS - SCHEDULES I & II
DRUG ENFORCEMENT ADMINISTRATION
SUPPLIER'S Copy 1

FIGURE 2-6 Drug Enforcement Administration Form 222. (Courtesy Drug Enforcement Administration, Washington, DC.)

The pharmacy retains the bottom copy (Copy 3). When the medication is shipped to the pharmacy, the middle (DEA) copy is forwarded to the DEA to prove that the medication has been properly received. When the pharmacy receives the controlled substances, the pharmacist compares the pharmacy's copy of Form 222 with the invoice and signs and dates both. The invoice and the form are stapled together and retained for 2 years. If any error is made, the form becomes invalid but must be retained for reference; therefore, the pharmacy cannot erase mistakes or throw away the form. When returning any C-II drugs, the pharmacy must have the manufacturer or wholesaler fill out the same form (Form 222) to request the controlled substance; the pharmacy then is the provider who retains the top copy and sends the middle copy to the DEA. Other controlled substances (C-III, C-IV, and C-V) are ordered on normal invoice forms, but invoices must be filed and retained for possible DEA or state board of pharmacy inspection. These should be kept separate from other nonscheduled drugs for easy retrieval. Once the scheduled drugs have been received, the invoice forms for schedules III through V must be kept for no less than 2 years.

 Tech Note!

Under the authority of the Controlled Substances Act of 1970, the Controlled Substances Ordering Systems (CSOS) now allows electronic filing of DEA Form 222. This allows more stock to be ordered than is possible using the paper form. A smaller amount of controlled stock usually must be kept in the pharmacy because ordering is quicker and stock can be ordered more often.

Record Keeping

A pharmacy has three methods of filing controlled substances and legend drugs (Table 2-3). Although federal law allows any one of these three methods to be used, a state's board of pharmacy may require a specific method. Each time a controlled substance is issued to a patient or nursing station, it must be logged out of the pharmacy stock (Figure 2-7) as required under state law. Levels are first counted; the amount of each drug must be correct. Then the technician or pharmacist subtracts the amount taken. The remaining stock is double-checked for accuracy. This same standard holds for returning items or adding new stock to the inventory.

TABLE 2-3

Three Methods of Filing Controlled Substances and Legend Drugs

System	Drawer I	Drawer II	Drawer III
1	C-II separate	C-III, C-IV, C-V	All other prescriptions
2	C-II separate	C-III, C-IV, C-V,* and all legend drugs	
3	C-II, C-III, C-IV, C-V†		All other prescriptions

*If any C-III, C-IV, or C-V controlled drugs are kept with non–controlled drugs (system 2) or mixed with C-II drugs (system 3), they must be stamped with a red C for easy identification. All records must be kept on site for no less than 2 years. Many states, however, have requirements for keeping records longer; remember that the strictest law is the one that must be followed. When taking inventory, the technician must have exact counts of C-II substances at all times. The final count can be inventoried only by a *licensed pharmacist*.
†Technicians should consult the regulations of the individual state.

Oxycodone/APAP 5/325mg Tablets

Date	Prescription/Invoice#	Quantity	Patient/Supplier	Balance	Initials	Current Inventory Count	Discrepancy
4/8/xx	Rx#12345	25	10	15	JJ	15	0
4/9/xx	Invoice# 9876	100	Glaxo	115	KB	115	0

A

Date	Patient	Dispensed	Oral — Codeine 30mg	Diazepam 5mg	Hydrocodone/ APAP 5/325mg	Lorazepam 5mg	Oxazepam 15mg	Oxycodone ER 10mg	Inj — Meperidine 25mg/mL	Meperidine 75mg/mL	Diazepam 5mg/mL	Hydromorphone 5mg/5mL	Morphine 1mg/mL	Morphine 10mg/mL	SIGNATURE
Previous Days Count			20	15	35	2	12	9	21	25	5	19	4	16	
9/21/xx	Jane Smith	10mg Meperidine							20						Paul James RN
9/21/xx	Add to stock-	John Whey CPhT		25		27	24				25		29		Sean Ray RN

B

FIGURE 2-7 A, Pharmacy log sheet. **B,** Nursing floor log sheet.

Narcotic Inventory

Narcotics are at high risk for **drug diversion** and must be inventoried differently from normal nonscheduled drugs. The pharmacy maintains a perpetual inventory of these medications. This means that once the inventory is started, it does not end; instead, it continues until the drug is no longer stocked. The basic principle is to identify an initial count of all controlled substances and to monitor the count as drugs are dispensed by subtracting the amount taken out of stock; this also involves adding to the count all drugs received by the pharmacy and placed into stock. This can be done either in pen in a ledger or through the use of software. The type of ledger or software used differs between community and institutional pharmacies, although basic information is required. Although the technician may be responsible for keeping track of all transactions, a pharmacist must validate all counts. In addition, overall periodic counts are done weekly or monthly by pharmacists. The DEA requires an inventory to be taken every 2 years; the DEA does not require a copy of the inventory taken. Any discrepancies that are identified must be investigated and explained.

Reverse Distributor

The term *reverse distributor* indicates all controlled substances that are unwanted, unusable, or outdated that are returned to the distributor. These must be dealt with in accordance with DEA regulations. All transactions must be under the control of a person authorized by the DEA to handle controlled substances; this process is meant to deter the loss or misuse of drugs, also known as *drug diversion*. If a controlled substance becomes outdated or damaged, the pharmacy must return the substance to the manufacturer or return the substance to a company that collects controlled substances and then either returns them to the manufacturer or arranges for their disposal. These authorized companies may call themselves reverse distributors or returns processors. If a nurse or pharmacy personnel uses a partial dose of a controlled substance, two parties are required to witness and sign off on the destruction or waste of the drug. All liquid and solid medications must have proper documentation, which is kept for 2 years. To destroy medication, DEA Form 41 must be filed. This is determined by an agent of the DEA, who instructs the applicant how to proceed. The completed form must include the following:

- Date
- Name of substance
- Dosage form
- Number of units
- Reason for destruction
- Manner of destruction
- Applicant's signature

Records must be kept on all drugs destroyed as determined by state law.

 Tech Note!

Because opioids in general are widely used to treat patients for pain, technicians, pharmacists, and nurses come in contact with these drugs daily. This has led to many cases of addiction in health care workers. All narcotics such as opioids and other controlled medications must be accounted for and must not be left out in the open, where they could be misused. All controlled substances must be signed into and out of stock in pen to create a permanent record.

Filling, Refilling, and Transferring Prescriptions for Controlled Drugs

Original Filling of C-II through C-V Drugs

Schedule II through V drug prescriptions can be accepted by the pharmacy in written, oral, or fax form according to certain DEA provisions and/or circumstances. A schedule C-II order may be called or

faxed ahead of time, but the original prescription, signed by the prescriber, must be presented before it is actually dispensed. Although the following regulations are outlined according to the DEA, each state normally has additional restrictions that must be followed. For information on your specific state's guidelines, visit your state's board of pharmacy website, which can be found at the National Association of Boards of Pharmacy website (*www.nabp.net*).

Emergency Filling of C-II Drugs

An oral order in place of a written prescription is permitted only in emergency situations. The guidelines are as follows:

1. The physician determines that the patient needs the C-II drug and considers it to be an emergency, with no alternative treatment possible.
2. The physician cannot give a written prescription to the pharmacist. This may be because the physician is away from the office.
3. The pharmacist must obtain all information from the physician, including the drug name, strength, dosage form, and route of administration. The physician's name, address, phone number, and DEA number are required. All information must be recorded in written form.
4. The amount of the drug can be only enough to sustain the patient through the emergency period. The pharmacist should indicate on the prescription that it is being filled because of an emergency.
5. The pharmacist must make every effort to verify the physician's authority unless he or she knows the physician personally.
6. The prescriber has 7 days to produce the written and signed prescription to the pharmacist. Each state may impose shorter time limits. In addition, the prescription must have written on its face "Authorization for Emergency Dispensing." If this is not done, the pharmacist must notify

the DEA. The written prescription must be attached to the oral record of the prescription.

7. There is no time limit when a C-II drug must be filled after being signed by the prescriber; however, the pharmacist must determine whether the patient still needs the medication (e.g., a drug filled several weeks after the order was written).
8. No limits are placed on the quantity of C-II drugs.
9. There may be additional provisions established by state BOP regulations.

Schedule C-III, C-IV, and C-V drugs may be reduced to written form if called into the pharmacy. All required prescription information must be obtained by the pharmacist, including the prescriber's DEA number.

Refilling of C-II through C-V Drugs

For refilling prescriptions according to DEA regulations, controlled substances are placed into three categories: C-II; C-III and C-IV; C-V.

1. Schedule C-II drugs may not be refilled.
2. Schedule C-III and C-IV drugs may be refilled only up to five times or within 6 months after the date the prescription was written, whichever occurs first. Patients are allowed to request refills by e-mail or by phone.
3. Schedule C-V drugs can be refilled as often as prescribed on the prescription.

When C-III, C-IV, and C-V drugs are refilled, the following required information must be provided on the back of the prescription: pharmacist's initials, refill date, and the amount of drug that is refilled. In addition, a pharmacy may use a data-processing system to store and retrieve C-III, C-IV, and C-V prescription refill information. To meet DEA regulations, the following criteria must be met:

1. Pharmacies must use one of two methods: manual or computerized log for refills.
2. A daily hard copy is printed, and pharmacists verify all refills they have authorized.
3. A log book is kept in which all controlled refills are verified by the pharmacist.
4. A computer system is used to print a refill-by-refill audit for any specific strength, dosage, or form, retrievable by either generic or trade name.
5. In case the computer system is not functioning, the pharmacy must have an alternative procedure for authorizing documentation. These data are entered into the computer system as soon as possible.

Partial Filling of C-II through C-V Drugs

Schedule III, IV, and V drugs may be partially filled if the pharmacist does not have enough in stock. The pharmacist must note on the prescription the amount filled, and the remaining amount must be dispensed within 6 months.

Schedule II drugs may be partially filled if the pharmacist does not have the full quantity in stock. The pharmacist must note on the prescription the amount filled, and the remaining amount may be dispensed within 72 hours of the first fill. If the amount cannot be filled within 72 hours, the pharmacist must notify the prescribing physician because no further quantity may be supplied after this time.

Transferring Controlled Drug Prescriptions (C-II through C-V Drugs)

Schedule III, IV, and V prescriptions may be transferred to another pharmacy one time only. The receiving pharmacy must have all of the information required on an original prescription, including the prescriber's DEA number, and the information must be transcribed into written form. Schedule II prescriptions are not transferrable because they can be filled only once.

Dispensing Without a Prescription

Schedule V drugs that are sold over the counter in some states are required to be dispensed by the pharmacist. The pharmacist must determine whether the medication is necessary and must follow these guidelines:

1. The purchaser must be at least 18 years of age.
2. The purchaser must show identification, including proof of age.
3. No more than 240 mL or 48 solid doses of opium can be sold.
4. No more than 120 mL or 24 solid doses of any other controlled substance can be sold.
5. No more than a 48-hour supply may be sold without a prescription to any one purchaser.
6. A schedule V log book is kept with the purchaser's name and address, name and quantity of medication sold, date dispensed, and pharmacist's initials.
7. The log book must be kept for 2 years.
8. If there are no federal or state laws that require a prescription to dispense schedule V drugs, then dispensing without a prescription is permitted.

Lending or Transferring C-II through C-V Drugs to Another Pharmacy

A pharmacy may lend scheduled drugs to another pharmacy as long as the following guidelines are met:

1. The pharmacy to be lent the medication is registered with the DEA to dispense controlled substances.

2. The lending pharmacy must record that it lent the medication, and the receiving pharmacy must record that it obtained the medication.

3. If a schedule II drug is lent, it must be documented on a DEA Form 222 by the pharmacy lending the C-II drug. The form must indicate the name, dosage form, and quantity of the drug, and the name, address, and DEA registration number of the pharmacy receiving the drug.

4. No more than 5% of the total number of dosage units of controlled substances can be dispensed by a pharmacy within a calendar year unless the pharmacy is registered as a distributor.

Mailing Controlled Substances (C-II through C-V Drugs)

A pharmacy is allowed to mail any controlled substance as long as it is mailed in a container that is not marked with the contents' information. The inner container must be labeled to indicate the name and address of the dispensing pharmacy.

Drug Monographs

Under the FDA labeling regulations, the following information must be available in **monographs**, also known as package inserts or official prescribing information, because of the lack of space on most drug containers. Physicians often refer to this information as published in the ***Physicians' Desk Reference*** **(PDR)**. It also is available from free online resources, such as the National Library of Medicine's DailyMed website (*http://dailymed.nlm.nih.gov/dailymed/about.cfm*), which provides files from the FDA database. The information in the package labeling is also found in the monographs published in many print and online nationally recognized drug compendia. All official label information is required to give the date of the most recent revision. As new information emerges or is reported, new monographs is written or revised. Therefore, it is important to have an updated copy of the required information in the pharmacy's referencing materials. If an updated copy is not available, the package insert from the medication container can be consulted for the most recent information. The following is the type of information contained in a package insert.

- FDA monograph information
- FDA prescription drug labeling, containing a summary of the essential scientific information for the safe and effective use of the drug; it should meet the following specific requirements:
  - Be informative and accurate
  - Use language that is not promotional in tone, false, or misleading

- Not make claims or suggested uses for drugs when there is insufficient evidence of safety and unsubstantiated evidence of effectiveness
- Contain information based whenever possible on data derived from human experience
- The information on prescription drug labeling is also referred to as:
  - Prescribing information
  - Package insert
  - Professional labeling

The Highlights section of the official prescribing information is approximately one-half page in length and provides a quick reference summary of the most important information about the prescription drug. The drug manufacturer is required to include a list of all changes made within the past year to ensure that the most updated information is available for the prescriber. The Highlights of the label cover the following topics and are cross-referenced to the corresponding full prescribing information section for additional details:

- Boxed Warning
- Major Recent Changes
- Indications and Usage
- Dosage and Administration
- Dosage Forms and Strengths
- Contraindications
- Warnings and Precautions
- Adverse Reactions
- Drug Interactions
- Use in Specific Populations
- Patient Counseling Information Statement

Full prescribing information now includes the following:

- Table of contents section (recent change). This easy-to-use reference helps practitioners quickly locate specific information rather than having to scan the whole document.
- Generic and trade names and date of initial U.S. approval.
- Boxed warning section: each drug may or may not have one.
- The use of bullets is limited to 20 lines for ease of reading.
- Complete prescribing information can be accessed using a cross-referencing number or the hyperlink given (see Boxed Warning, later in the chapter).

1. Indications and Usage

The following information may be found in this section:

- The conditions the drug is approved to treat, listed in bulleted form for ease of reading
- Pharmacological class of the drug (to remind the prescriber of the drug's mechanism of action)

- All limitations, such as patients who should not use the drug

2. Dosage and Administration

This section includes the recommended dosage regimen, dosage range, the manner in which the medication should be administered, and pharmacological information.

3. Dosage Forms and Strengths

This section lists all the dosage forms and their strengths. Product identification information, such as color and scoring, is also listed in the "How Supplied" section.

4. Contraindications

This bulleted section lists clear situations in which the drug should absolutely not be used. It describes specific conditions in which the risk of taking the medication clearly outweighs any possible therapeutic benefit, in addition to known hazards of the drug. The order in which contraindications are listed is based on the likelihood of occurrence and the size of the population studied.

5. Warnings and Precautions

This section is an abbreviated summary of the most clinically adverse reactions and also actions to take when such reactions occur. Additionally, information is given on the monitoring parameters of these side effects.

6. Adverse Reactions

This section lists the most commonly occurring adverse reactions and the incidence of these effects. Separate listings are required for adverse reactions reported from clinical trials or from post-marketing experience. Additional details are given on the nature, severity, and frequency of adverse reactions and the relationship to dose and demographics. This section also provides advice on how to report adverse reactions to manufacturers via telephone or electronically (or both) by using MedWatch to record reactions.

7. Drug Interactions

Both food and drug interactions are listed, as are instructions on how to prevent or lessen the interaction. Also included in this section are conditions in which the drug interaction necessitates a dosage adjustment (also found under Clinical Pharmacology).

8. Use in Specific Populations

This section is a bulleted summary of the use of the medication in various patient populations, including the following: pregnant patients (see Pregnancy Categories, later in the chapter), patients in labor and delivery units, pediatric patients, geriatric patients, patients with renal impairment, and patients with hepatic impairment. Also included are cross-references to sections that can be reviewed to determine necessary prescribing adjustments.

9. Drug Abuse and Dependence

If patients have shown any tendency to become addicted to the medication or if the medication has been found to be abused by patients, the information is listed in this section.

10. Overdosage

Information on toxicity and the use of antidotes is provided in this section.

11. Description

This section lists specifics about chemical agents and ingredients, such as the drug's chemical formula.

12. Clinical Pharmacology

This section describes how other drugs can interact with the medication, and alerts the prescriber to adverse reactions. Also included is a Microbiology data subsection for the drug, if applicable. Drug interaction data also may be found in section 7 (Drug Interactions).

13. Nonclinical Toxicology

This section contains information on studies conducted during the development of the drug, including in vitro studies (i.e., performed in test tubes), drug formulation, and in vivo efficacy studies (e.g., performed in live animals).

14. Clinical Studies

This section summarizes the most important studies that establish the effectiveness and safety of the drug in humans. Not all studies are included.

15. References

A list of reference materials that may be accessed for further information specific to the drug is presented in this section.

16. How Supplied/Storage and Handling

Information about how the medication is supplied often is given in chart format because it lists the varying strengths, amount of drug per container, and dosage form, and whether the medication has any special requirements, such as protection from light or storage in a refrigerator.

17. Patient Counseling Information

This section contains suggested pertinent information about the drug that professionals should convey to their patients. The FDA-approved patient labeling is written for a lay audience. Even drugs given in the hospital by a health care professional may have patient counseling information.

Hyperlinks can be used to access specific information. The FDA requires structured product labeling in a standardized electronic file format and the use of embedded computer tags to help health professionals improve patient care.

The FDA and the National Library of Medicine created the DailyMed labeling resource; it can easily be downloaded and is available to professionals and patients electronically free of charge (see *http:// dailymed.nlm.nih.gov*). Figure 2-8 shows a sample of important information found in a drug monograph.

Boxed Warning

A **boxed warning** is encased in a bold border in the manufacturer's insert; health care professionals often refer to the boxed warning as a Black Box Warning, even though this is not the official labeling term for the warning. This type of warning is required on medications and other products that carry a high risk potential for the consumer. The label indicates the proper use of a drug to avoid or decrease the possibility of serious or even life-threatening side effects. Warnings can be very specific or may include an entire class of drugs, such as antidepressants. Antidepressants have been found to cause an increase in suicidal behavior in adolescents, especially those with prior psychiatric disorders. Box 2-8, Part A, presents an example of a boxed warning; Part B presents a sample list of agents with boxed warnings.

MedGuides

MedGuides are paper handouts that are available with many prescription medicines. Many medications with boxed warnings also come with Med-Guides. The guides address issues specific to particular drugs and drug classes, and they contain

---

BOX 2-8
Boxed Warnings

(A) Special Warnings and Information
Explanation of the types of serious side effects that may occur
Monitoring recommendations, such as blood tests and pregnancy tests before and while using the medication; signs and symptoms that may occur during treatment
Indication of other medications that cannot be taken at the same time
Instructions to the prescriber regarding information that must be given to the patient before dosing
The steps to be taken if an adverse reaction may have occurred (MedWatch: 1-800-FDA-1088)

(B) Example of Drugs Requiring Boxed Warning
Amitriptyline
Antidepressants
Bupropion
Clozapine
Estrogens
Fenoprofen
Fluoroquinolones
Nonsteroidal antiinflammatory drugs (NSAIDs)
Pioglitazone, rosiglitazone
Stavudine
Tamoxifen
Zidovudine

FDA-approved information that can help patients avoid serious adverse events. A MedGuide is distributed by the pharmacy with each prescription and each prescription refill because the information for the patient may change frequently.

The FDA requires that MedGuides be issued with certain prescribed drugs and biological products when the agency has determined the following:
- Certain information is necessary to prevent serious adverse effects.
- The patient should be informed about a known serious side effect of a product.
- Patient adherence to directions for the use of a product is essential to the product's effectiveness.

Pregnancy Categories

A pregnant woman's fetus is susceptible to the effects of drugs taken by the mother. The drug may be transmitted to the fetus during its developmental stages, causing birth defects. The FDA established five **pregnancy categories** that indicate the potential of a drug to cause fetal defects; the categories are based on the ratio of risks to benefits (Box 2-9).

HIGHLIGHTS OF PRESCRIBING INFORMATION

These highlights do not include all the information needed to use Imdicon safely and effectively. See full prescribing information for Imdicon.

IMDICON

® (cholinasol) CAPSULES

Initial U.S. Approval: 2000

WARNING: LIFE-THREATENING HEMATOLOGICAL ADVERSE REACTIONS

See full prescribing information for complete boxed warning.

Monitor for hematological adverse reactions every 2 weeks for first 3 months of treatment (5.2). Discontinue Imdicon immediately if any of the following occur:

- Neutropenia/agranulocytosis (5.1)
- Thrombotic thrombocytopenic purpura (5.1)
- Aplastic anemia (5.1)

─────────────────RECENT MAJOR CHANGES─────────────────

Indications and Usage, Coronary Stenting (1.2) 2/200X

Dosage and Administration, Coronary Stenting (2.2) 2/200X

─────────────────INDICATIONS AND USAGE─────────────────

Imdicon is an adenosine diphosphate (ADP) antagonist platelet aggregation inhibitor indicated for:

- Reducing the risk of thrombotic stroke in patients who have experienced stroke precursors or who have had a completed thrombotic stroke (1.1)
- Reducing the incidence of subacute coronary stent thrombosis, when used with aspirin (1.2)
  Important limitations:
- For stroke, Imdicon should be reserved for patients who are intolerant of or allergic to aspirin or who have failed aspirin therapy (1.1)

─────────────────DOSAGE AND ADMINISTRATION─────────────────

- Stroke: 50 mg once daily with food. (2.1)
- Coronary Stenting: 50 mg once daily with food, with antiplatelet doses of aspirin, for up to 30 days following stent implantation (2.2)

Discontinue in renally impaired patients if hemorrhagic or hematopoietic problems are encountered (2.3, 8.6, 12.3)

─────────────────DOSAGE FORMS AND STRENGTHS─────────────────

Capsules: 50 mg (3)

─────────────────CONTRAINDICATIONS─────────────────

- Hematopoietic disorders or a history of TTP or aplastic anemia (4)
- Hemostatic disorder or active bleeding (4)
- Severe hepatic impairment (4, 8.7)

─────────────────WARNINGS AND PRECAUTIONS─────────────────

- Neutropenia (2.4% incidence; may occur suddenly; typically resolves within 1-2 weeks of discontinuation), thrombotic thrombocytopenic purpura (TTP), aplastic anemia, agranulocytosis, pancytopenia, leukemia, and thrombocytopenia can occur (5.1)
- Monitor for hematological adverse reactions every 2 weeks through the third month of treatment (5.2)

─────────────────ADVERSE REACTIONS─────────────────

Most common adverse reactions (incidence 2%) are diarrhea, nausea, dyspepsia, rash, gastrointestinal pain, neutropenia, and purpura (6.1).

To report SUSPECTED ADVERSE REACTIONS, contact (manufacturer) at (phone # and Web address) or FDA at 1-800-FDA-1088 or ***www.fda.gov/medwatch***.

─────────────────DRUG INTERACTIONS─────────────────

- Anticoagulants: Discontinue prior to switching to Imdicon (5.3, 7.1)
- Phenytoin: Elevated phenytoin levels have been reported. Monitor levels. (7.2)

─────────────────USE IN SPECIFIC POPULATIONS─────────────────

- Hepatic impairment: Dose may need adjustment. Contraindicated in severe hepatic disease (4, 8.7, 12.3)
- Renal impairment: Dose may need adjustment (2.3, 8.6, 12.3)

See 17 for PATIENT COUNSELING INFORMATION and FDA-approved patient labeling

Revised: 5/200X

FIGURE 2-8 Highlights of a drug monograph.

FULL PRESCRIBING INFORMATION: CONTENTS*
WARNING—LIFE-THREATENING HEMATOLOGICAL ADVERSE REACTIONS
1 INDICATIONS AND USAGE
   1.1   Thrombotic Stroke
   1.2   Coronary Stenting
2 DOSAGE AND ADMINISTRATION
   2.1   Thrombotic Stroke
   2.2   Coronary Stenting
   2.3   Renally Impaired Patients
3 DOSAGE FORMS AND STRENGTHS
4 CONTRAINDICATIONS
5 WARNINGS AND PRECAUTIONS
   5.1   Hematological Adverse Reactions
   5.2   Monitoring for Hematological Adverse Reactions
   5.3   Anticoagulant Drugs
   5.4   Bleeding Precautions
   5.5   Monitoring: Liver Function Tests
6 ADVERSE REACTIONS
   6.1   Clinical Studies Experience
   6.2   Postmarketing Experience
7 DRUG INTERACTIONS
   7.1   Anticoagulant Drugs
   7.2   Phenytoin
   7.3   Antipyrine and Other Drugs Metabolized Hepatically
   7.4   Aspirin and Other Non-Steroidal Anti-Inflammatory Drugs
   7.5   Cimetidine
   7.6   Theophylline
   7.7   Propranolol
   7.8   Antacids
   7.9   Digoxin
   7.10 Phenobarbital
   7.11 Other Concomitant Drug Therapy
   7.12 Food Interaction
8 USE IN SPECIFIC POPULATIONS
   8.1   Pregnancy
   8.3   Nursing Mothers
   8.4   Pediatric Use
   8.5   Geriatric Use
   8.6   Renal Impairment
   8.7   Hepatic Impairment
10 OVERDOSAGE
11 DESCRIPTION
12 CLINICAL PHARMACOLOGY
   12.1 Mechanism of Action
   12.2 Pharmacodynamics
   12.3 Pharmacokinetics
13 NONCLINICAL TOXICOLOGY
   13.1 Carcinogenesis, Mutagenesis, Impairment of Fertility
14 CLINICAL STUDIES
   14.1 Thrombotic Stroke
   14.2 Coronary Stenting
16 HOW SUPPLIED/STORAGE AND HANDLING
17 PATIENT COUNSELING INFORMATION
   17.1 Importance of Monitoring
   17.2 Bleeding
   17.3 Hematological Adverse Reactions
   17.4 FDA-Approved Patient Labeling

*Sections or subsections omitted from the full prescribing information are not listed.
http://www.fda.gov/ohrms/dockets/ac/06/briefing/2006-4210b_13_01_physician%20labeling%20rule.pdf

FIGURE 2-8, cont'd

BOX 2-9
Pregnancy Categories

Category A
Adequate and well-controlled studies have failed to demonstrate a risk to the fetus in the first trimester of pregnancy (and there is no evidence of risk in later trimesters).

Category B
Animal reproduction studies have failed to demonstrate a risk to the fetus, and there are no adequate and well-controlled studies in pregnant women.

Category C
Animal reproduction studies have shown an adverse effect on the fetus, and there are no adequate and well-controlled studies in humans, but potential benefits may warrant use of the drug in pregnant women despite potential risks.

Category D
There is positive evidence of human fetal risk based on adverse reaction data from investigational or marketing experience or studies in humans, but potential benefits may warrant use of the drug in pregnant women despite potential risks.

Category X
Studies in animals or humans have demonstrated fetal abnormalities, and/or there is positive evidence of human fetal risk based on adverse reaction data from investigational or marketing experience, and the risks involved in use of the drug in pregnant women clearly outweigh potential benefits.

BOX 2-10
Prescribing Authority

Except for the following footnoted prescribers, each state has its own regulations regarding prescriber authorization, in addition to specific exceptions, requirements, and limitations for prescribing medications.
Advanced practice registered nurse (RN)
Certified RN anesthetist
Chiropractors*
Clinical RN specialist
Dentist[†]
Doctor of homeopathy
Doctor of osteopathy
Doctor of podiatry[†]
Doctor of veterinary medicine (DVM)[†]
Emergency medical technician–paramedic
Licensed certified social worker (LCSW)
Medical physicians[‡]
Midwife, nurse-midwife
Neuropathic MD
Nurse practitioner
OB/Gyn RN
Optometrist
Pediatric RN practitioners
Pharmacists (have prescriptive authority agreements in certain states)
Physician assistants
Psychiatric RN practitioners
Psychologists

*Have no prescribing authority in any state.
[†]Has independent prescribing authority limited to their specific course of practice in every state.
[‡]Has unlimited, independent prescribing authority in every state.
For a list of specifics, refer to the National Board of Pharmacy website at *www.nabp.net*.

These categories are set for each drug based on extensive clinical trials by the manufacturer. Both the prescriber and the pharmacist must counsel the patient to make sure the patient understands the risks involved before taking the agent.

Prescription Regulation

Who Can Prescribe?

The FDA and DEA have no authority in determining prescribers. Physicians and other medical prescribers are licensed by their individual state boards. The scope of practice is determined by the person's degree. For example, a podiatrist, a physician who treats conditions of the feet, can prescribe medications and devices that are used in treating foot conditions; a podiatrist would not and should not prescribe heart medication. The same is true for dentists, veterinarians, and optometrists because each is an expert in their specialty and not in others. Prescribers can vary from state to state (Box 2-10); therefore, the specific laws governing them are not covered. However, more states allow professionals such as nurse practitioners and physician assistants to prescribe a limited number of medications and/or devices. These practitioners are regulated at the state level; some are required to be supervised by a physician, who assumes responsibility for their prescribing methods and scope of knowledge. In 12 states nurse practitioners are allowed to prescribe medications independently (including controlled substances). Each state also regulates whether it will accept out-of-state prescriptions written by practitioners who are not licensed in the state. Individuals who can prescribe controlled drugs must be registered as a midlevel practitioner with DEA Form 224. In some states, pharmacists are granted prescribing privileges under a collaborative drug therapy management agreement. This agreement is between a physician and a pharmacist and entails allowing the pharmacist to initiate, modify, and continue medication regimens; order laboratory tests; and perform patient assessments under a defined protocol. Montana, New Mexico, and North Carolina give pharmacists extended authority. Five other states (California, Massachusetts, Minnesota, North Dakota, and Washington) allow pharmacists to obtain a DEA number.

Who Can Receive a Prescription?

Clearly, a pharmacy technician takes in prescriptions, enters them, and fills them; the pharmacist is responsible for interpreting and reviewing the prescription before dispensing the medication. Most states prohibit pharmacy technicians from taking phone orders for **legend drugs**. All states require a pharmacist to authorize a phoned-in prescription for a controlled substance per DEA regulations. Often prescriptions are called in, faxed, or transmitted by computer from the physician's office by the physician or nurse. A pharmacist must translate any verbal orders into written form. Also, if a patient wants a prescription transferred to another pharmacy, this transaction must be done between licensed pharmacists or pharmacy interns under the supervision of a pharmacist. A pharmacy intern also can receive prescriptions by phone.

 Tech Note!

In the state of Tennessee, additional functions of a certified pharmacy technician include receiving new or transferred oral medical and prescription orders. However, this is uncommon at this time, and most states do not allow technicians to take verbal orders.

Prescription Labels and Prescription Orders

The information on a prescription label is different from that required on a prescription order, although both must have patient and medication information (Figure 2-9). The components of a prescription order and a prescription label are as follows.
- Prescriber's prescription order
  1. Name of prescriber
  2. Address and phone number of prescriber

Dr. Tracy Crum
DEA#AC1243170
LIC#44550

11287 E Villanova Drive
Aurora, CO 30358
Phone: 303-555-1212

Date: *12/12/XX*

Patient's name: Billie Jones   Age: *83 yrs*
Address: 125 Grand Canyon Drive, Tucson, Arizona 85707

Rx:

K-Dur 20 mEq tab
1 daily   #90

Substitution permitted Y N
Refills 1 2 3 4 5 6 7 8 9   Signature____Tracy L Crum, MD

A

Thomas Pharmacy
519 Barney Lane
Clarksville, TN 03542
Phone: 931-555-1122

Patient: Christopher Gilbert
RX # G03011984

Dosage: Clonazepam 1mg tablets   Quantity #30

Take 1 tablet by mouth at bedtime

Refills 0
Filled: 12/12/XX   Expiration date: 09/25/XX
Dr. Ronald Belham

B

FIGURE 2-9   A, Sample of the information required on a physician's prescription order. **B,** Sample of the information on a medication label.

BOX 2-11

Drugs Requiring Additional Information

- Estrogens
- Injectable contraceptives
- Oral contraceptives
- Fertility drugs
- Retinoids

3. License number of prescriber (DEA number if applicable)
4. Date prescription was written
5. Prescriber's signature
- Prescription label
  1. Name of pharmacy
  2. Address and phone number of pharmacy
  3. Name of prescriber
  4. Date prescription was filled
  5. Prescription number
  6. Any cautions described or provided on auxiliary labels

Special Labeling

Certain drugs require that additional, manufacturer-provided information be given to a patient because of the possibility of adverse effects from the medication; interactions between food, drugs, and/or supplements; and teratogenicity (genetic harm) to an unborn fetus. These instructions are known as *patient package inserts* and are distributed by the prescriber or the pharmacy dispensing the medication or device (Box 2-11).

Records and Labeling Requirements

Hospitals and community pharmacies differ in the length of time patient records must be kept. Record keeping is regulated by state law. Both hospitals and community pharmacies are required to keep complete and accurate records of patients. For the purpose of simplicity, Table 2-4 lists community patient information separately from institutional requirements.

Repackaging

Unit dose medication that is prepared in the pharmacy requires the following record-keeping rules. Technicians traditionally prepare most of the unit dose medications in a pharmacy setting; the pharmacist verifies the preparations (except in states that allow tech-check-tech). Any medication taken from bulk packages and placed in blister packs or unit-dosing devices (e.g., oral syringes) must have the following information on each individual label:

1. Drug name (trade/generic)
2. Strength
3. Dosage form
4. Manufacturer
5. Lot number
6. Expiration date

All information must be logged into a binder or a system in which such information can be retrieved easily. More information on repackaging is presented in Chapter 11.

Drug Enforcement Administration Verification

All prescribers must be registered with the DEA to write prescriptions for controlled substances. When approved, the prescribers are given a nine-character identification code. This code is different for each prescriber. There is a method of verifying DEA numbers. The first two characters are composed of letters. The first letter is an A, B, F, M, or X, followed by the first letter of the prescriber's last name. Prescribers who are qualified to order medications to treat opioid addiction are assigned an X. The letter M is assigned to midlevel practitioners (MLPs) such as nurse practitioners. For example, for Dr. D. Wong, MD, the DEA number could begin with AW or BW. The next seven digits are composed of numbers that form an equation. Procedure 2-1 presents the steps for verifying a DEA number.

 Tech Alert!

Hospital physicians are assigned an internal code number that is attached to their DEA registration number. This information must be kept by the institution for verification purposes (e.g., AB1234567-045).

Non–Child-Resistant Caps

Most medications are required to be packaged in containers that are exceptionally difficult for children to open. Hence, childproof caps were created. Unfortunately, the caps also can be difficult for some adults to open. Therefore, some exceptions to this regulation were made because of patients' need to access their medications easily (Table 2-5). In addition to these exceptions, medications can be packaged in non–child-resistant containers if certain requirements have been met. Either the prescriber, such as a physician, orders the medication to be filled without a childproof cap or the patient requests that the medication be filled without a childproof cap. Usually this information is entered into the patient's medical record for future reference. Some

TABLE 2-4

Required Prescription Information*

Type of Facility	Patient's Full Name	Prescriber's Name	Name and Strength of Drug	Date of Issue	Prescription Number	Expiration Date	Lot and Control Number of Drug	Manufacturer	Name of Drug Dispensed
Hospital	X	X	X	X	—†	X	—†	—†	X
Community	X	X	X	X	X	X	X	X	X
Home health	X	X	X	X	X	X	X	X	X

*Each medication sent to the floor has the manufacturer's name, the lot number, and the expiration date on each unit dose of medication. Hospital patients are not given prescription numbers; instead, orders are listed in the computer under a patient's medical record number, and a hard copy, often called the *medication administration record* (MAR), of all medications is made daily for the patient's chart.
†This information is not transcribed into the patient's electronic medical record.

▶ TECHNICIAN PROFILE

Avery is a lead controlled substance pharmacy technician at a Veterans' Health Administration hospital. He has worked in the pharmacy for 5 years. Controlled substance distribution is a highly visible and sensitive area for the facility. Avery's position requires an individual who is willing to accept increased responsibility and at the same time pay close attention to details. Most of Avery's duties are performed in the pharmacy vault, setting up controlled substances for dispensing, making appropriate record entries, and reviewing controlled substance administration records. Avery is expected to maintain a high degree of accurate productivity and performance while being extremely sensitive to his contribution to total patient care. He checks in shipments of drugs and supplies, verifies the accuracy of those shipments, and assures the proper storage of all items. All of Avery's activities are supervised by the Pharmacy Operations Manager and the controlled substance pharmacist on duty. Because of his increased responsibilities and the serious nature of his position, Avery is classified as a level 3 technician, which has a higher pay scale. He finds his job very challenging and rewarding.

TABLE 2-5

Prescription Drugs That Can Be Packaged in Non–Child-Resistant Bottles

Drug	Dosage Form
Betamethasone	Tablet
Cholestyramine	Powder
Colestipol	Powder
Erythromycin (EES)	Tablet, granules
Isosorbide dinitrate (less than 10 mg)	Sublingual, chewable tablets
Mebendazole	Tablet
Methylprednisolone	Tablet
Nitroglycerin*	Sublingual
Prednisone	Tablet
Sodium fluoride	Package

*Nitroglycerin is the only medication that does not have a dosage limit for filling the prescription without a childproof cap.

pharmacies may require the patient to sign a release form that is kept in the patient record.

Special Prescribing Programs

Programs for Opioid Maintenance

Methadone Maintenance Treatment (MMT)

Methadone is a schedule II controlled substance and is used to treat individuals addicted to opiates. Patients are to receive specialized treatment while taking this medication. No more than 1 day's supply may be filled by a pharmacy, and the medication must be taken in a physician's office or drug treatment center. Other brand names for methadone include Dolophine and Methadose. Although metha-done is more commonly used to treat opioid addiction, it can also be prescribed by physicians (with appropriate DEA registration) as an analgesic to treat chronic pain and to alleviate pain in cancer patients.

Suboxone and Subutex

Suboxone and Subutex, which are sublingual tablets, are schedule III controlled substances that require special consent forms to be completed by the patient. Although most treatments are supervised either in a physician's office or in a clinical setting, a pharmacy may receive orders for small amounts to be delivered to a physician's office or to be picked up by a family member of the patient. Under federal law, prescribers must meet certain criteria. When the prescriber has met all conditions, the DEA issues him or her a special number with an X, identifying the individual as a qualified prescriber.

PROCEDURE 2-1

Verification Process for Prescriber's DEA Number

GOAL: To be able to determine whether a DEA number on a prescription is valid or a forgery.

EQUIPMENT AND SUPPLIES

- Paper, pencil, and a calculator may be used.

Example

Dr. Tom Johnston writes an order for Tylenol #3. The physician's DEA number is AJ1234892.

PROCEDURAL STEPS

1. Verify that the first letter of the DEA number is A, B, F, or M (for nurse practitioners).

PURPOSE: To confirm that the doctor or nurse practitioner has the authority to prescribe controlled substances.

2. Determine whether the second letter is the first letter of the prescriber's last name (in this case, J for Johnston).

PURPOSE: To make certain that the letters match to prevent possible forgeries.

3. Use the formula: First, add the first, third, and fifth numbers in the DEA set (1 + 3 + 8 = 12).

PURPOSE: To make certain the DEA number is valid.

4. Continue the formula: Second, add the second, fourth, and sixth numbers and then multiply by 2 (2 + 4 + 9 = 15; 15 × 2 = 30).

PURPOSE: To verify that the DEA number is authentic.

5. Complete the formula: Finally, add the two sums together (12 + 30 = 42).

PURPOSE: To complete the process and determine whether the DEA number is valid or a forgery.

6. Compare the results. If the last digit from your total (i.e., 2), matches the last number in the DEA set, the number is valid. In this case, all steps match; therefore, the number is valid. If any of the key elements do not match, alert your pharmacist; the DEA number is invalid.

PURPOSE: To continually be on the lookout for forged prescriptions and to use your skill in determining whether DEA numbers are valid or invalid.

Risk Management Programs for Prescription Drugs

The Food and Drug Administration Amendments Act of 2007 gave the FDA the authority to require a Risk Evaluation and Mitigation Strategy (REMS) from manufacturers to ensure that the benefits of a drug or biological product outweigh its risks. Certain drugs are placed in a restricted status for use.

iPledge Program under the FDA

The FDA regulates isotretinoin (Accutane, Amnesteem, Claravis, Sotret) under a special program called iPledge because of the severe adverse effects of the drug. It causes birth defects; therefore, it is important that female users understand that they must take precautions to avoid becoming pregnant. In addition, possible side effects of suicidal thoughts and signs of depression are now associated with this drug. This agent requires a boxed warning. iPledge is a computer-based risk management program designed to increase awareness of the dangers of isotretinoin in an effort to eliminate fetal exposure to the drug. There are restricted distribution guidelines that must be followed before a patient can receive a prescription for isotretinoin.

Restricted drugs have different levels of restrictions based on REMS. Previously, the restriction for dispensing rosiglitazone-containing drugs consisted only of ensuring that the patient received a copy of the medication guide. The new restrictions require health care providers and patients to enroll in a special program for those prescribing and those receiving rosiglitazone-containing medicines.

Additional information about REMS and restricted drugs can be found on the FDA website at *www.fda.gov*.

 Tech Alert!

The special programs listed previously are not all inclusive. These are examples of the most common programs found in either the hospital or retail setting.

Pharmacy Sites

Brick and Mortar and Mail-Order Pharmacies

The term *brick and mortar* refers to a building, such as a retail pharmacy. A common practice is to mail medications through the post office or other authorized mailing system. This option has become even more accessible to patients because of the introduction of online pharmacies and mail-order pharmacies. Rules govern the way in which drugs are mailed. Prescription drugs can be mailed only by DEA-registered entities.

Online Pharmacies (E-Pharmacies)

In the 1990s e-pharmacies began to appear on the Internet, which led to the opportunity for drugs to be ordered illegally. In addition, consumers could be defrauded because some e-pharmacies charged credit cards but did not mail the drugs ordered. The National Association of Boards of Pharmacies (NABP) began to accredit sites in 1999 to allow consumers to distinguish between legal and illegal sites. The label Verified Internet Pharmacy Practice Sites (VIPPS) indicates to the public that the website from which they are ordering drugs is both legitimate and licensed (more information is available at the website *www.awarerx.org/*). When linking to a pharmacy Internet site, the customer should click on the label for authentication. At this time VIPPS is a voluntary accreditation. Although verification is done by the NABP, the organization does not regulate the sites; instead, the websites are regulated by the state in which the pharmacy is physically located, along with federal guidelines. E-pharmacies have the same regulations as retail and mail-order pharmacies with regard to dispensing to out-of-state pharmacy locations, and they are also required to adhere to HIPAA regulations.

There are many advantages to ordering medications via the Web, including ease of ordering, lower prices, and easy accessibility to online information, which lessens wait time when trying to ask a pharmacist for information. However, identifying illegal pharmacies is a constant struggle for both state and federal agencies. If a suspicious e-pharmacy is found, it should be reported to the NABP. If the wrong medication or label is dispensed, this should be reported to the state's board of pharmacy.

Signs that a pharmacy site probably is illegal include the following:

- Dispensing medications without having the customer mail in the prescription
- Faxing a prescription that cannot be confirmed as a valid prescription
- Dispensing medications upon completion of a questionnaire
- Not having a preexisting examination or patient-prescriber relationship
- Inability to contact a pharmacist at the website for consultation

Occupational Safety and Health Administration

The purpose of the **Occupational Safety and Health Administration (OSHA)** is to make the workplace safe for employees. Box 2-12 presents an outline of common safety and health topics. A safe workplace involves having safe equipment and materials, being able to safely perform tasks, and ensuring that the policies and procedures of a company (including pharmacies) are safe. OSHA requires

---

BOX 2-12

Common Safety and Health Topics

- Hazard communication standards
- Hazardous drugs during preparation
- Hazardous drugs during storage
- Hazardous drugs during administration
- Hazardous drugs during care giving
- Handling practices
- Disposal of hazardous drugs
- Latex allergy
- Ergonomics
- Workplace violence

Safety Data Sheet (SDS) information on all potentially dangerous chemicals used in the workplace.

Safety Data Sheets (SDS)

Almost all chemicals can be dangerous if ingested or spilled. In all workplaces, including pharmacies, all chemicals must have an SDS on file in an SDS binder, or the SDS must be available electronically through a database. The binders are normally bright yellow and black. The information on these sheets includes the storage requirements, handling procedures, and actions to take if the chemical is either spilled or sprayed into the eyes or comes in contact with the skin. It is important to know where the binder or database is kept and to ensure that every chemical has a sheet on file. For example, phenol is a very dangerous antiseptic agent often used in nerve blocks; it is stored in many institutional pharmacies. If it is spilled, it is important not to breathe in the fumes but to contain the spill as quickly as possible and call the appropriate department for cleanup. Normally, environmental services in a hospital will respond and handle the cleanup. It is extremely easy to get SDS information to protect the employees who will handle the agent. The phone number is always given by the manufacturer, who is required by law to distribute the information to the requesting party within 24 hours. Usually the manufacturer faxes the SDS directly to the business (more information can be obtained on OSHA's website at *www.osha.gov*). The SDS information not only is important, but also is required by law.

The Joint Commission

In 1951 several medical associations created the Joint Commission on Accreditation of Healthcare Organizations (JCAHO) as an independent, nonprofit organization that voluntarily accredited hospitals. In 1959 Canada withdrew from JCAHO to form its own accrediting organization. It was not until 1964 that JCAHO began to charge for its surveys. The following year, hospitals were required to be accredited to participate in the Medicare and Medicaid programs. Over the following years, JCAHO expanded its range of compliances over hospitals and institutions. In 2007 JCAHO changed its branding to The Joint Commission (TJC). The Joint Commission meets three times annually and has 32 voting board members, consisting of physicians, administrators, nurses, employers, a labor representative, health plan leaders, quality experts, ethicists, educators, and a consumer advocate. The TJC accredits more than 20,000 health care organizations and programs throughout the United States, including 9,500 hospitals and home care facilities. Organizations must be surveyed at least every 3 years. Once accredited, the organization may display the TJC seal of approval. Ratings of all institutions can be found on the TJC website at *www.jointcommission.org*. The benefits of accreditation and certification include the following:

- It provides the community with confidence in the quality and safety of care, treatment, and other institutional services
- It identifies and addresses risk management and reduction
- It provides professional advice and staff education to improve services
- It is recognized by many health care insurers and other third parties (Medicare and Medicaid)
- It meets regulatory requirements in specific states

The Joint Commission surveys all aspects of hospital services, including pharmacy services. Areas of concern in the pharmacy include how look-alike, sound-alike drugs are identified, communication, allergy notification, conflicting prescriptions, verbal orders, and other areas that may create an avenue for errors. All employees should be knowledgeable about the pharmacy's policies and procedures so that they can answer any questions asked by representatives of the TJC. If a technician is asked a question to which he or she does not know the answer, the technician should give an honest answer and should not try to make one up. The TJC representatives may collect pharmacy data to monitor the pharmacy's performance, identify adverse drug reactions, and determine how the pharmacy identifies and has attempted to improve problems in these areas. In 2004 the TJC created the "Do Not Use" list of abbreviations as a requirement. However, this requirement has met with resistance because surveys reveal that as of 2006, 22% of accredited organizations were still noncompliant with this standard. In 2010, the "Do Not Use" list was integrated into the National Patient Safety Goal as a part of the Information Management standards.

Legal Standards
State Laws

Each state has its own set of laws that pharmacists, interns, pharmacy technicians, and clerks must follow when working in the pharmacy. You must know the regulations of your state. All pharmacy personnel should become familiar with the laws by obtaining the regulations booklet from their state board of pharmacy. You will notice that many states have laws that differ from federal law. Remember that the strictest law is the one you follow. Therefore, if the FDA states that you must keep records for no less than 2 years but your state regulations require 7 years for inpatient records, you would follow the strictest regulation, in this case your state regulation. To learn more about your specific state regulations and laws, go to your state's board of pharmacy website, which can be found at *www.napb.net*.

Liabilities

You also should be aware of federal and state liability laws pertaining to pharmacy technicians. A patient can make various charges against a pharmacy technician if the pharmacy technician caused damage because of **negligence** or intentional action in the workplace. A **tort** is defined as an act causing injury to a person intentionally or because of negligence. The word *negligence* may describe an action taken without the forethought that should have been applied by a reasonable person of similar competency; a mistake was made. For an intentional mistake, the penalty can range from criminal charges to the awarding of damages, which usually means that money is paid to the person or persons who were wrongly affected. A negligent mistake can affect a person's ability to continue to work as a technician and also may result in punitive damages (i.e., monetary payment).

Mistakes occur for many reasons. Some happen because of an excessive workload or possibly staffing shortages, which can lead to a mishap and could be classified as a negligent tort. Criminal behavior, such as false insurance claims or diverting drugs, could be called an intentional tort and could result in imprisonment. One of the questions you should ask your employer is whether you are covered under the company's legal department. If a lawsuit were to be filed with you as the plaintiff, do you know who would represent you? Many companies have lawyers who represent the company, although you should not assume that they would represent you. If you are not covered by your employer, you may want to purchase malpractice insurance. Most technicians do not have such insurance; it is a personal preference. At the very least, be aware of what your rights and responsibilities are, including legal considerations, before entering a workplace. Depending on the state in which the technician works, laws vary as they pertain to the liability of the technician. Therefore, you must check your state laws as they pertain to you. If you are involved in or witness any incidents in the workplace, you should follow these guidelines:

1. Review your state's regulations.
2. Understand your employer's rules and practices.
3. Define your scope of employment.

 Tech Alert!

More states are enacting laws to make technicians accountable for their actions in the pharmacy. Previously, pharmacists had to take responsibility for any mistakes, even if the mistake was made by the technician. This is no longer true. A technician can lose his or her license, certification, and job and may have to pay court fees; in addition, he or she may face jail time if a criminal act was involved. Examples of such cases are listed in pharmacy journals and on the FDA website.

If an "event" occurs in the pharmacy, you should be prepared in the following ways:

1. Know the name of your attorney.
2. Always be careful of what you say and to whom you say it if you are ever questioned by state or federal investigators pertaining to an incident.
3. Write down in-depth notes on the facts of the event (as soon as possible) and keep them for reference.

Both federal and state laws change frequently; it is your responsibility to keep up with the current regulations. Pharmacy departments keep close track of these changes and notify employees of changes, but you are the one who carries out these laws on a daily basis. Be sure to learn the specifics of a new rule or regulation and obtain clarification if necessary because not understanding a new rule or regulation and not seeking further guidance are unacceptable excuses. Because pharmacy technicians can be held accountable for their actions, this is a fundamental competency of all pharmacy technicians. In addition, the Pharmacy Technician Certification Board (PTCB) requires at least one continuing education (CE) unit in current law to be taken for recertification within a 2-year period.

Ethics and Morals in the Workplace

Ethics are the values and morals that are used within a profession. **Morals** are a person's beliefs

concerning what is right or wrong in human behavior. Work ethics are a set of standards that should be followed by anyone working in a field. Work ethics are often outlined in the pharmacy protocol. One important factor that the pharmacy technician must remember is that he or she has a clear responsibility to the patient on many levels. Patients are consumers, and as consumers they have the right to receive goods that have been handled properly and are in good condition. They also trust the pharmacy personnel with their personal information, expecting that their information will be treated as confidential. Many times in a pharmacy, or any work setting, employees express their opinions concerning various medical procedures such as abortion, surgery, or a type of treatment. These are controversial topics, and the opinions that each person has are a part of personal morals or beliefs. Although each person has his or her own set of morals, many morals tend to coincide with the beliefs of others (e.g., stealing is wrong).

In the workplace, however, technicians, pharmacists, and other health care workers are faced with patients who might have different morals. In these situations, ethics include the professional behavior of a technician regardless of a patient's morals. Ethics tend to overlap many morals and need to be separated in the workplace and in the public domain. When you assume the responsibility of serving the public in a setting such as the pharmacy, you accept work ethics that guide your behavior. For instance, in a hospital, there may be a need for medication that is used for the termination of pregnancy, emergency contraception, or other controversial treatments. The responsibility of the pharmacy staff is to provide services for all patients. If providing the service conflicts with your morals or your beliefs prohibit you from participating in servicing patients, you must communicate this to your supervisor.

For many decisions, just keeping small matters in perspective can help you make the right choice. Keeping patients' information confidential and working within the pharmacy's rules and guidelines, including policies and procedures, ensure that patients receive the best service possible. The technician should always remember that pharmacists,

BOX 2-13

Pharmacy Technicians' Code of Ethics

Preamble

Pharmacy technicians are health care professionals who assist pharmacists in providing the best possible care for patients. The principles of this code, which apply to pharmacy technicians working in any and all settings, are based on the application and support of the moral obligations that guide the pharmacy profession in relationships with patients, health care professionals, and society.

Principles

- A pharmacy technician's first consideration is to ensure the health and safety of the patient, and to use knowledge and skills to the best of his/her ability in serving patients.
- A pharmacy technician supports and promotes honesty and integrity in the profession, which includes a duty to observe the law, maintain the highest moral and ethical conduct at all times, and uphold the ethical principles of the profession.
- A pharmacy technician assists and supports the pharmacist in the safe, efficacious, and cost-effective distribution of health services and health care resources.

- A pharmacy technician respects and values the abilities of pharmacists, colleagues, and other health care professionals.
- A pharmacy technician maintains competency in his/her practice and continually enhances his/her professional knowledge and expertise.
- A pharmacy technician respects and supports the patient's individuality, dignity, and confidentiality.
- A pharmacy technician respects the confidentiality of a patient's records and discloses pertinent information only with proper authorization.
- A pharmacy technician never assists in dispensing, promoting, or distribution of medication or medical devices that are not of good quality or do not meet the standards required by law.
- A pharmacy technician does not engage in any activity that will discredit the profession, and will expose, without fear or favor, illegal or unethical conduct in the profession.
- A pharmacy technician associates with and engages in the support of organizations that promote the profession of pharmacy through the utilization and enhancement of pharmacy technicians.

The Institute for the Certification of Pharmacy Technicians (2007); Code of Ethics for Pharmacy Technicians—adapted from the American Association of Pharmacy Technicians Code of Ethics, published. *Am J Health-Syst Pharm* 60:37-51, 2003. www.nationaltechexam.org/pdf/code-of-ethics.pdf. (Referenced July 17, 2013.)

technicians, and clerks are present to serve patients and customers in a professional manner at all times, as outlined in the pharmacy technician's code of ethics (Box 2-13).

Professional Ethics

Professional ethics are systematic rules or principles governing right conduct. Each practitioner has the duty to adhere to the standards of ethical practice and conduct set by the profession. Pharmacy technicians have a responsibility to make informed decisions based on their specialized training. Professional codes of conduct must be followed. Respect is a key component of professional behavior in the pharmacy. Technicians should always display a sincere respect for the pharmacist, the patient, and their health care colleagues. Being honest, trustworthy, and an all-around team player demonstrates professional ethics.

DO YOU REMEMBER THESE KEY POINTS?

- Terms and definitions covered in this chapter
- Major federal laws affecting pharmacists and pharmacy
- The differences between the functions of the DEA and FDA
- The process for reporting any problems with a drug or any adverse reactions to the FDA
- The three classes of drug recalls defined by the FDA
- The proper handling of controlled substances, including the necessary forms and regulations
- The basic information contained in a drug monograph

- The purpose of boxed warnings and MedGuides
- The five pregnancy categories established by the FDA
- Who can prescribe medications and medical devices
- How to decipher a DEA number
- Risk management programs and their purpose
- Regulation and authentication of Internet pharmacies
- OSHA guidelines as they pertain to pharmacy
- The purpose of the Joint Commission
- The legal limitations of pharmacy technicians
- The difference between morals and ethics

Scenario FOLLOW UP

As Laura continues in her retail pharmacy career, she has learned that it is imperative to keep abreast of the state and federal laws and regulations affecting her position. She understands that she can be held accountable for HIPAA violations and any medication errors in which she may be involved. Laura uses her continuing education courses to stay up-to-date on changes in the pharmacy profession. She also regularly checks websites maintained by the FDA, the DEA, and her state BOP for changes or legislation related to pharmacy law.

REVIEW QUESTIONS

Multiple Choice Questions

1. The amendment that required the labeling "Caution: Federal law prohibits dispensing without a prescription" was the:
   A. Durham-Humphrey Amendment
   B. Kefauver-Harris Amendments
   C. OBRA '90
   D. None of the above
2. What is the purpose of the Orphan Drug Act?
   A. It enacts stricter rules concerning sales and distribution of controlled substances.
   B. It allows drug companies to bypass lengthy testing to treat persons who have a rare disease.
   C. It stops the use of drug testing in animals.
   D. It ensures the safety and effectiveness of manufacturing practices.
3. The law that requires pharmacists to counsel patients on new medications is:
   A. OBRA '90
   B. Comprehensive Drug Abuse Prevention and Control Act
   C. Prescription Drug Marketing Act
   D. Durham-Humphrey Amendment
4. The primary purpose of the FDA is to:
   A. Make arrests
   B. Ensure that safety and effectiveness standards for medications are met by manufacturers
   C. Prevent the distribution and illegal use of controlled substances
   D. Make sure all laws pertaining to physicians and pharmacists are followed
5. A pharmacy that will be dispensing controlled drugs must have which one of the following forms on file with the DEA?
   A. Form 222
   B. Form 224
   C. Form 363
   D. Form 225

6. The five categories of controlled substances are rated on the basis of:
   A. Cost
   B. Strength
   C. Conditions that they treat
   D. Potential for abuse
7. Which of the following health care providers is *not* one of the standard practitioners that all states accept?
   A. Doctor of podiatry
   B. Dentists
   C. Chiropractors
   D. Veterinarians
8. Safety data sheets (SDS) contain information on:
   A. Storage of a chemical
   B. Actions to take in case of a spill
   C. The combustion and stability of a chemical
   D. All of the above
9. Which classification of drug recall could cause a temporary health problem or a slight threat of serious harm?
   A. Class I
   B. Class II
   C. Class III
   D. Class IV
10. What is the maximum legal amount of pseudoephedrine that can be purchased per day?
    A. 7.5 g
    B. 3.6 g
    C. 9 g
    D. 62 tablets

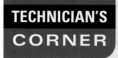

Dr. Beth Golden writes an order for the following prescription:
DEA#AG1958366
Disp: hydrocodone/acetaminophen tablets #50
Sig: Take 1 tablet q8h prn severe pain
0 refills
Determine whether this DEA number is correct and explain each step of the checking process.

Bibliography

Andrews S: The Affordable Care Act, *Todays Technician* 13:17, 2012.

Ballington DA: *Pharmacy practice for technicians*, ed 2, St Paul, Minn, 2002, EMC/Paradigm.

Gray Morris D: *Calculate with confidence*, ed 6, St Louis, 2013, Elsevier.

National Association of Boards of Pharmacy: *Survey of pharmacy law*, Mount Prospect, Ill, 2005, The Association.

Nielsen JR, James JD: *Handbook of federal drug law*, ed 2, Philadelphia, 1992, Williams & Wilkins.

Potter PA, Perry AG: *Fundamentals of nursing*, ed 8, St Louis, 2013, Elsevier.

Shargel L, Mutnick A, Souney P et al: *Comprehensive pharmacy review*, ed 8, Baltimore, 2012, Lippincott Williams & Wilkins.

Websites Referenced

American Family Physician: April 1, 2005. Methadone use. (Referenced June 10, 2013.) www.aafp.org/afp/20050401/1353.html

democrats.energycommerce.house.gov/index.php?q=bill/hr-2923-the-combat-methamphetamine-enhancement-act-of-2010

Encyclopedia of Surgery: Barbiturates. (Referenced July 28, 2013.) www.surgeryencyclopedia.com/A-Ce/Barbiturates.html

FDA website: National Drug Code Directory. (Referenced August 12, 2013.) www.fda.gov/Drugs/InformationOnDrugs/ucm142438.htm

FDA website: New Requirements for Prescribing Information. (Referenced August 12, 2013.) www.fda.gov/Drugs/GuidanceComplianceRegulatoryInformation/LawsActsandRules/

FDA website: Recall Firm Press Release. (Referenced August 12, 2013.) www.fda.gov/Safety/Recalls/ucm179943.htm

Gieringer D: The Safety and Efficacy of New Drug Approval. (Referenced August 9, 2013.) www.cato.org/pubs/journal/cj5n1/cj5n1-10.pdf

Life Science Services: Outsourcing-Pharm.com. Pseudoephedrine drugs still OTC. (Referenced August 9, 2013.) www.outsourcing-pharma.com/Contract-Manufacturing/Pseudoephedrine-drugs-still-OTC

OTC-Meds.com. Home: Controlled Substances Act: Federal Regulation of Pseudoephedrine. (Referenced August 12, 2013.) www.otcmeds.com/Controlled_Substances_Act::Federal_regulation_of_pseudoephedrine/encyclopedia.htm

Perrone M: New restrictions on hydrocodone to take effect, USA Today, August 2014. Retrieved from http://www.usatoday.com (Accessed October 28, 2014.)

Safety Emporium: Sample SDS for Benzoic Acid. (Referenced August 9, 2013.) www.ilpi.com/msds/benzoic.html

Schedules of controlled substances: Rescheduling of hydrocodone combination products from Schedule III to Schedule II (2014, August 22). 79 Federal Register. No. 163, 49661. (to be codified at 21 CFR Part 1308). Retrieved from: https://www.federalregister.gov/articles/2014/08/22/2014-19922/schedules-of-controlled-substances-rescheduling-of-hydrocodone-combination-products-from-schedule, Accessed October 28, 2014.

The FDA law blog; GAO report assesses state approaches to control pseudoephedrine, by Larry K. Houck—February 26, 2013. (Referenced July 1, 2013.) www.fdalawblog.net/fda_law_blog_hyman_phelps/2013/02/gao-report-assesses-state-approaches-to-control-pseudoephedrine.html

USP information: (Referenced July 10, 2013.) www.usp.org/aboutUSP/

USP_NF website: (Referenced June 10, 2013.) www.usp.org/USPNF/whocancerpain.wisc.edu/?q=node/180   (Referenced August 12, 2013.)

WHO Pain & Palliative Care Communications Program: Expanding nurses' role in pain management: International news on nurse prescribing. (Referenced August 12, 2013.)

www.fda.gov/downloads/BiologicsBloodVaccines/Vaccines/ApprovedProducts/ucm294307.pdf (Referenced February 7, 2014.)

www.fda.gov/Safety/Recalls/ucm376942.htm

www.hhs.gov/opa/affordable-care-act/index.html   (Referenced August 12, 2013.)

www.jointcommission.org/facts_about_the_official/   (Referenced August 12, 2013.)

www.medscape.com/viewarticle/754690 (Referenced August 12, 2013.)

www.nejm.org/doi/full/10.1056/NEJMp1314691   (Referenced January 1, 2014.)

Competencies, Associations, and Settings for Technicians

Bobbi Steelman

OBJECTIVES

Upon completing this chapter, you should be able to do the following:

1. Describe the competencies needed for technicians to be successful in various pharmacy settings.
2. Explain the term *nondiscretionary duties.*
3. Describe different nondiscretionary duties in inpatient, outpatient, and closed door pharmacy settings.
4. Discuss the American Society of Health-System Pharmacists (ASHP) Model Curriculum and how it relates to pharmacy technician training programs and certification.
5. State the differences between certification, licensure, and registration.
6. Explain the benefits of obtaining technician certification.
7. Explain the process by which a person can become a nationally certified pharmacy technician.
8. Describe the various national certification examinations and their requirements.
9. List ways in which the Pharmacy Technician Certification Board (PTCB) national exam differs from the National Healthcareer Association (NHA) national exam.
10. Describe the requirements technicians must meet to maintain their national certification.
11. Explore the various websites that can be used to obtain continuing education credits.
12. List advanced positions and specialty certifications available for technicians in the health care field.
13. List the various professional associations pharmacy technicians can join.
14. Explain the importance of professionalism in the workplace.
15. Explain the importance of networking as it relates to the job search.

TERMS AND DEFINITIONS

Accreditation Council for Pharmacy Education (ACPE) National agency for the accreditation of professional degree programs in pharmacy and providers of continuing pharmacy education

American Association of Pharmacy Technicians (AAPT) First pharmacy technician association; founded in 1979

American Pharmacists Association (APhA) Oldest pharmacy association; founded in 1852

American Society of Health-System Pharmacists (ASHP) Pharmacy association founded in 1942

American Society of Health-System Pharmacists (ASHP) Model Curriculum for Pharmacy Technician Education and Training A program that provides details on how to meet the ASHP goals for pharmacy technician training curricula

Board of pharmacy (BOP) A state-managed agency that licenses pharmacists and may either register or license pharmacy technicians to work in pharmacy

Certified pharmacy technician A technician who has passed the national certification examination; the technician can use the abbreviation CPhT after his or her name

Closed door pharmacy A pharmacy in which medications are called in from institutions, such as long-term care facilities, and are then delivered; closed door pharmacies are not open to the public

Communication The ability to express oneself in such a way that one is readily and clearly understood

Community pharmacy Also known as an *outpatient* or a *retail pharmacy;* these pharmacies serve patients in their communities;

consumers can walk in and purchase a prescription or over-the-counter (OTC) drug

Competency The capability or proficiency to perform a function

Confidentiality The practice of keeping privileged customer information from being disclosed without the customer's consent

Continuing education (CE) Education beyond the basic technical education, usually required for license or certification renewal

Hyperalimentation Parenteral (intravenous) nutrition for patients who are unable to eat solids or liquids; also known as total parenteral nutrition (TPN)

Inpatient pharmacy A pharmacy in a hospital or institutional setting

Licensed pharmacy technician A pharmacy technician who is licensed by the state board; licensing ensures that an individual has at least the minimum level of competency required by the profession, unlike a registered pharmacy technician

National Association of Boards of Pharmacy (NABP) National organization for members of state boards of pharmacy

National Healthcareer Association (NHA) Certification organization for a variety of health care careers, including the Institute for the Certification of Pharmacy Technicians (ICPT)

National Pharmacy Technician Association (NPTA) Pharmacy association primarily for technicians; founded in 1999

Nondiscretionary duties Tasks that do not require professional judgment such as repackaging medications, managing inventory, filling automated dispensing machines, and billing

Outpatient pharmacies Pharmacies that serve patients in community or ambulatory settings

Parenteral medications A term most commonly used to describe medications administered by injection, such as intravenously, intramuscularly, or subcutaneously

Pharmacy Technician Certification Board (PTCB) National board for the certification of pharmacy technicians

Professionalism Conforming to the right principles of conduct (work ethics) as accepted by others in the profession

Registered pharmacy technician A pharmacy technician who is registered through the state board of pharmacy; the registration process helps maintain a list of those working in pharmacies and may require a background check through the legal system; the registration process does not guarantee the level of the registrant's knowledge or skills

Total parenteral nutrition (TPN) Large-volume intravenous nutrition administered through the central vein (subclavian vein), which allows for a higher concentration of solutions

Introduction

Scenario:

Olivia is a newly hired technician at an independently owned pharmacy. She is required to register with the state board of pharmacy, but certification is not mandated. She is a graduate of a technical career college and remembers her instructor discussing the benefits of association membership. What are Olivia's membership options and how can she find more information on this subject?

Technician qualifications and job descriptions vary from state to state. Currently, there are no mandatory national standards or requirements pertaining to technician duties or training needed. Therefore, each state board of pharmacy determines the standards required and how they are to be met by technicians.

Due to the rapidly changing health care system, the job descriptions and educational requirements of pharmacy technicians are quickly changing. Among the changes are increased responsibilities, the need for higher education, more legal responsibility, and certification mandates. This trend can be seen across the United States. Many boards of pharmacy now require completion of a program accredited by the American Society of Health-System Pharmacists (ASHP) for a person to become a registered technician. Currently, several states require Pharmacy Technician Certification Board (PTCB) or National Healthcareer Association (NHA) certification and

have accepted it as their measure of the knowledge base of pharmacy technicians. Positive aspects of these changes include a wider range of jobs available, bonuses, salary increases, and better benefits for technicians.

This chapter begins with an overview of the history of pharmacy technicians' duties and then explores important attributes for a successful career in pharmacy. Necessary job qualifications, expectations, and trends in pharmacy are explored, along with the importance of national pharmacy organizations and the benefits of pharmacy technician certification. This chapter also provides information about the preparation necessary to conduct a successful job search and explores the exciting advanced roles now available to the pharmacy technician. This information can help the student technician determine the best career path to follow, understand the various positions available, and attain the ultimate goals and benefits of this profession.

Historical Data

Historically, technicians have answered to a variety of titles. These include pharmacy clerk, pharmacist assistant, or pharmacy aide. Technicians have held a variety of positions. Some of the job responsibilities have been billing, ordering, stocking medications, typing, answering the phone, greeting customers, troubleshooting, cashiering, and running errands. Technicians have been a part of the pharmacy field since the beginning of pharmacy (see Chapter 1). However, more recently, pharmacy managers and their respective state boards of pharmacy have been attempting to classify and clearly define the role of the pharmacy technician as the needs of pharmacy change.

Technicians' duties focus on tasks that do not require professional judgment, but rather concentrate on their technical skills and training. Pharmacists' duties have moved from filling prescriptions and compounding simple agents to counseling patients and interacting with other medical professionals, such as physicians and nurses. This change can especially be seen in the hospital setting, where pharmacists are responsible for managing dosing of medications and participating on committees. The change in responsibility has been addressed many times over the course of pharmacy technician history by the **American Society of Health-System Pharmacists (ASHP)**, the **American Pharmacists Association (APhA)**, and other pharmacy associations. The need for skilled personnel has never been greater.

One significant contribution to the improvement of the pharmacy technician profession was the development of the *white paper*. In 2002 the *American Journal of Health-System Pharmacists* addressed many of the challenges pharmacy faces by publishing the *White Paper on Pharmacy Technicians 2002: Needed Changes Can No Longer Wait*. A white paper argues a specific position or solution to a problem. The paper explores the diversity of pharmacy technicians' qualifications, knowledge, and responsibilities (Box 3-1). The white paper was endorsed by a panel of pharmacy organizations and comprehensively discussed issues pertinent to the promotion and growth of a competent pharmacy technician workforce.

In 2009 the Task Force on Pharmacy Technician Education and Training Programs met in Rosemont, Illinois. It was established by the National Association of Boards of Pharmacy (NABP) and was charged with the following mission:

1. Review the existing state requirements for technician education and training requirements for national technician training program accrediting organizations, such as the ASHP

BOX 3-1

White Paper on Pharmacy Technicians 2002

1. *Education and training:* Encompasses the history of training techniques and programs. Explores the need for adjusting the length of the training program based on the functions of the technician. Course curriculum adjustments and adequacy are discussed.
2. *Accreditation of training programs and institutions:* Describes the types of training programs and the need for institutional accreditation. Explains why it is important to oversee these programs because there are no nationally recognized ones.
3. *Certification:* Covers the history and growth of the national certification process; describes the importance of certification, both for the establishment of minimum levels of competency and for the recognition of pharmacy technicians as paraprofessionals.

http://www.ashp.org/DocLibrary/BestPractices/HREndWPTechs.aspx

---

and the Accreditation Council for Pharmacy Education (ACPE) Core Competencies
2. Recommend national standards for technician education and training programs and encourage boards of pharmacy to recognize them

The NABP executive committee accepted the following recommendations from the task force:

- NABP should encourage boards of pharmacy to require as an element of pharmacy technician certification completion of an education and training program that meets minimum standardized guidelines.
- NABP should encourage boards of pharmacy to require as an element of pharmacy technician certification completion of an accredited education and training program by 2015.
- NABP should assist in developing a national accreditation system for pharmacy technician education and training programs that is based within the profession of pharmacy and utilizes a single accrediting agency by 2015.
- NABP should encourage ACPE and ASHP to work collaboratively to develop an accreditation system for pharmacy technician education and training programs that reflects all pharmacy practice settings and, if feasible, to consolidate the activities into one accrediting body, preferably ACPE.
- NABP should encourage PTCB to change the process by which it determines who is qualified to sit for its examination to include completion of an accredited pharmacy technician education

and training program and high school diploma or GED verification.

- NABP should encourage PTCB to provide NABP with information on its certified pharmacy technicians so that NABP may enhance the pharmacy technician data contained in the NABP clearinghouse to provide the information necessary for the state boards of pharmacy to protect the public health.
- NABP should encourage ASHP to revise its current accreditation standards for pharmacy technician education and training programs to require accredited providers to inform potential program applicants of applicable state requirements for registration or licensure.

In 2010, at its 106th Annual Meeting in Anaheim, California, the NABP passed resolution No. 106-7-10, resolving to continue to encourage states to adopt uniform standards for pharmacy technician education and training programs.

In 2011, the PTCB launched the CREST Initiative by hosting a summit focused on the areas of consumer awareness, resources, education, state policy, and testing as they relate to pharmacy technicians. Summit participants made recommendations during the meeting pertaining to additional requirements for a candidate to sit for the Pharmacy Technician Certification Exam (PTCE). The following changes were made:

- By 2014, PTCB should require a minimum period of practical experience to be eligible for the PTCE.
- By 2015, mandatory criminal background checks should be required for all PTCE candidates.
- By 2020, all PTCE candidates should be required to complete a training program accredited by the ASHP.

Additional recommendations were made related to requirements for recertification. By 2015, it is recommended that PTCB change the current requirements for Certified Pharmacy Technician (CPhT) recertification to:

- Accept only pharmacy technician–targeted and/or ACPE "T" and/or "P/T" designated continuing pharmacy education (CPE) credits for a total of 20 hours every 2 years.
- Require at least 15 of the 20 hours of CPE to be provided through the state boards of pharmacy, NABP, employer-accredited programs, or programs accredited by ACPE. The allowable continuing education (CE) hours from college courses will be reduced from 15 to 10 by 2016, and allowable in-service hours will be phased out by 2018.
- Five hours of practical/employer-based CPE may be allowed as part of the 20-hour CPE requirement every 2 years.

- Maintain the requirement that one of the 20 required CPE credits be in pharmacy law.
- Require one of the 20 required CPE credits to be in medication/patient safety (effective in 2014).

In March, 2012, the CREST Initiative steering committee, composed of 10 leaders in pharmacy, developed and launched a profession-wide survey on these recommendations. The survey was completed by more than 17,000 pharmacy technicians and pharmacists nationwide. Results from the survey will provide the PTCB Board of Governors and Certification Council with important input from the profession on advancing the work of pharmacy technicians and the future of the PTCB certification program.

In February, 2013, the PTCB announced that these changes will be phased in over the next 7 years. The board of governors conducted a 90-day open online comment period to allow members of the pharmacy community to share their best practices for implementing the new requirements. The PTCB began releasing the policies and procedures on the implementation of these decisions in late 2013. More information on this topic can be found at the PTCB's website at *www.ptcb.org*.

The Pharmacy Technician Career

Pharmacy technician is one of the hottest careers for individuals interested in working in the health care industry. Pharmacies all over the country need technicians. According to Yahoo Education, pharmacy technician was one of the top five growing health care careers in the United States in 2013. More than 93,000 new technicians are expected to obtain jobs between 2008 and 2018.

Competencies

Competency can be defined as the capability or proficiency to perform a function. The practice of pharmacy includes a wide variety of settings. Technicians must have many different technical skills to function in each area. Box 3-2 lists chapters that cover common responsibilities and competencies. These competencies outline the roles and responsibilities that pharmacy technicians perform, which include specific job-related knowledge and skills needed to ensure patient safety.

State and National Boards of Pharmacy

Each state in the United States has its own **board of pharmacy (BOP)**, which is overseen by the **National Association of Boards of Pharmacy**

BOX 3-2

Chapter References Citing Common Responsibilities and Competencies of a Pharmacy Technician

Pharmacy Law, Ethics, and Regulatory Agencies	Chapter 2
Dosage Forms and Routes of Administration	Chapter 5
Conversions and Calculations	Chapter 6
Drug Information References	Chapter 7
Community Pharmacy Practice	Chapter 8
Institutional Pharmacy Practice	Chapter 9
Bulk Repackaging and Non-Sterile Compounding	Chapter 11
Aseptic Technique and Sterile Compounding	Chapter 12
Pharmacy Stock and Billing	Chapter 13
Medication Safety and Error Prevention	Chapter 14

BOX 3-3

Examples of Federal Laws Governing Pharmacy

Prescription Records

A record of all prescriptions dispensed should be maintained for 2 years after the last refill.

All systems used for maintaining records of any prescriptions must include the following:

- Prescription number
- Date of issuance
- Patient's identification (name, address)
- Name, strength, dosage form of medication
- Quantity dispensed
- Practitioner's identification (DEA registration, if applicable)
- Pharmacist's identification

Patient Consultation (OBRA '90)

Pharmacists must screen the entire drug profile of all Medicaid recipients before their prescriptions are filled. Each patient must be given counseling on the medication that has been prescribed, including topics such as how to take the drug, storage of the drug, and side effects of the medication. Most states have passed regulations that require counseling of all patients according to the same processes, although the requirements for the provision of written and/or oral consultation may be different among the states.

For more information on pharmacy law, refer to Chapter 2.

(NABP) (*www.nabp.net*). Each state's BOP serves many functions, including registering technicians and licensing pharmacists. The board also provides consumers with a way to file a complaint or report any problems or illegal actions they have experienced in a pharmacy. BOPs also review and update current rules and regulations pertaining to pharmacy practice. When new standards are implemented, BOP inspectors may visit any pharmacy to determine its compliance with these new standards. If the pharmacy is found to be in noncompliance, the BOP has the authority not only to impose fines but also to close the pharmacy until compliance is attained. If a pharmacy technician is found guilty of a violation of pharmacy law, the BOP can revoke his or her registration or license, depending on the state regulations.

The NABP and state BOPs are currently studying the expanded use of technicians in the pharmacy field. For example, technicians in California who have achieved a specific level of competency are granted the additional job duty of monitoring other pharmacy technicians. In Tennessee, technicians can take physicians' verbal orders over the phone. More states are requiring technicians to be registered, certified, and/or licensed. This examination of the current uses of technicians no doubt will reveal the skill level necessary for various types of pharmacy tasks, and ultimately changes will be made by each state board of pharmacy. Boards of pharmacy also may change technician-to-pharmacist ratios in pharmacy settings. A knowledge of pharmacy law (Box 3-3) is essential before a person can work in a pharmacy environment. Federal laws govern all 50 states. In addition, each state's BOP has specific laws, regulations, and guidelines that pertain to pharmacy practice in that state (Box 3-4). When state laws differ from federal laws, the strictest law should be enforced. (For more information on the legal requirements of pharmacy technicians, see Chapter 2.)

Scenario CHECK UP 3-1

Olivia is enjoying in her new position at the family-owned pharmacy. She is counting pills, reconstituting medications, and checking out customers at the register. She is allowed to answer the phone and take refill orders. Olivia has been on the job for approximately 3 months. She wonders why she has not been allowed to input prescriptions on the computer yet. Her typing speed is 28 words per minute. Why do you think the pharmacist has not put her on the computer yet? What steps can she take to gain this additional responsibility?

Nondiscretionary Duties

Technicians perform many **nondiscretionary** duties in the pharmacy setting. These are tasks that do not require professional judgment. Examples include repackaging medications, managing inventory, filling automated dispensing machines, and billing. All of

BOX 3-4

Pharmacy Technician State Requirements

Alabama—Must currently work in a pharmacy and be registered with the state board.

Alaska—Must be employed as a pharmacy technician in a training capacity under the guidance of a licensed pharmacist and registered with the state board.

Arizona—Pharmacy Technician Certification Board (PTCB) certification required.

Arkansas—Must currently work in a pharmacy, pass the test provided by the state through your employer, and obtain certification from the PTCB.

California—Several choices are available; you can do any of the following:
- Earn an associate's degree in pharmacy technology
- Finish a course that provides a minimum of 240 training hours or complete the American Society of Health-System Pharmacists (ASHP) training course
- Graduate from a pharmacy school accredited by the ASHP
- Complete training through the U.S. armed services
- Become PTCB certified

Colorado—No current regulations for pharmacy technicians. Those with certifications and additional education will have preference at the entry level.

Connecticut—Must be trained by a pharmacy manager, and the training must be documented. You must then apply for state certification. You can also obtain PTCB certification or another certification approved by Connecticut's Department of Certification of Pharmacy.

Delaware—No current regulations for pharmacy technicians.

Florida—Must complete a board-approved training program.

Georgia—Must register with the state board of pharmacy.

Hawaii—No current regulations for pharmacy technicians.

Idaho—Must have National Healthcareer Association (NHA) and/or PTCB certification.

Illinois—Must complete an on-the-job training program and obtain PTCB certification, or you can finish a pharmacy technician training program.

Indiana—Must complete a board-approved training program or obtain the PTCB certification.

Iowa—Must register with the state board of pharmacy and obtain either NHA or PTCB certification within a year.

Kansas—Must be currently employed as a technician and pass a test provided by the state through your employer.

Kentucky—Must be currently employed as a technician and must register with the state board of pharmacy. Hospital technicians are required to be certified by the NHA or PTCB.

Louisiana—Must have a job in a pharmacy; you must then apply for the Pharmacy Technician Candidate certificate from the state board. After obtaining that certificate, you must complete a state-approved training program within a year and a half. You must acquire 600 hours of practical experience, 200 of which must be through a training program. Finally, you must pass a board-approved certification exam.

Maine—Must have on-the-job training and register with the state board.

Maryland—Must obtain PTCB certification, or you can complete a board-approved training program involving at least 160 hours of work experience and that is no longer than 6 months' duration.

Massachusetts—Must complete an ASHP-accredited program, a program offered by the U.S. armed services, or one that has been approved by the state board. If you have 500 hours of work experience documented by your employer, you may take a state-approved exam or the PTCB.

Michigan—No current regulations for pharmacy technicians.

Minnesota—Must be currently employed as a technician and must register with the state board of pharmacy.

Mississippi—Must apply for certification with the state board and then take either the NHA or PTCB exam.

Missouri—Must get a job in a pharmacy and then register with the state board.

Montana—Must register with the state board and obtain NHA or PTCB certification within a year and a half of employment.

Nebraska—Must register with the state board.

Nevada—Must complete an ASHP-accredited training program or obtain 1,500 hours of experience and training that is documented by your employer. You can also complete a training program offered by the U.S. armed services. None of these options is required if you already have PTCB certification from another state; you can also transfer your registration from another state.

New Hampshire—Must get a job in a pharmacy, complete on-the-job training, and register with the state board before 30 days of employment have lapsed.

New Jersey—Must register with the state board.

New Mexico—Must register with the state board as non-certified, complete documented on-the-job training with a pharmacist, apply for certification, and obtain NHA or PTCB certification.

New York—No current regulations for pharmacy technicians.

North Carolina—Three options are available. (1) You may obtain on-the-job training, which must be completed within the first 6 months of being employed, and register with the state board; (2) you

BOX 3-4

Pharmacy Technician State Requirements—cont'd

may complete a training program for pharmacy technicians offered by a community college; or (3) you can get your PTCB certification and register with the state board of pharmacy.

North Dakota—Must complete a program accredited by the ASHP or complete your training on the job under the supervision of a licensed pharmacist.

Ohio—Must register with the state board and obtain NHA or PTCB certification within the first 210 days of employment at a pharmacy. Alternatively, you can obtain on-the-job training and then pass a test given by the employer.

Oklahoma—Must obtain a job in a pharmacy and complete on-the-job training provided by the pharmacist in charge or a staff pharmacist.

Oregon—Must obtain a job in a pharmacy and register with the state board. You must pass a national certification exam before a year has passed from the time of registration. You can also obtain NHA or PTCB certification and then do on-the-job training, which is documented by the pharmacist doing the training.

Pennsylvania—No current regulations for pharmacy technicians.

Rhode Island—Must complete a training program accredited by the AHSP. You can also finish a training program offered by the U.S. armed services. Finally, you can complete a program offered at a community college or earn NHA or PTCB certification.

South Carolina—Must register with the state board.

South Dakota—Must obtain a job in a pharmacy and then register with the state board, or you can participate in a training program and then register with the state board just before starting on-site work.

Tennessee—Must obtain a job in a pharmacy and then register with the state board.

Texas—Must register as a technician still in training. Then you must obtain PTCB certification and complete on-the-job training.

Utah—Must earn NHA or PTCB certification and complete a board-approved training program involving 180 hours of practical experience.

Vermont—Must register with the state board.

Virginia—Must complete a board-approved training program and sit for the state exam to obtain registration, or you may earn PTCB certification and register with the state board of pharmacy.

Washington—Must pass a national certification exam and then complete a board-approved program for training.

West Virginia—Must complete on-the-job training and pass a state test. You can also earn PTCB certification and complete 20 hours of on-the-job training.

Wisconsin—No current regulations for pharmacy technicians.

Wyoming—Must earn PTCB certification.

Washington, D.C.—No current regulations for pharmacy technicians.

---

these tasks are clearly defined and should be easy to follow. This does not mean that anyone can do the job, however, because prior knowledge of pharmacy terms, drugs, and procedures is required. As job classifications in pharmacy expand, so will the level of pharmacological knowledge required for pharmacy technicians. Historically, the pharmacist was responsible for the final approval of any task completed in a pharmacy setting, although this is also changing. Some states now permit "tech-check-tech" approval procedures; this allows a certified technician, rather than a pharmacist, to check another technician's order-filling accuracy. Nondiscretionary duties prohibit technicians from interpreting scientific studies, counseling patients about medications, and conferring with other medical personnel about proper treatments.

Basic Nondiscretionary Skills

Typing

The number of prescriptions processed per day in a pharmacy directly relates to the speed and accuracy of the typist. This makes a fast and accurate pharmacy technician, with a good working knowledge of medications, a great asset.

Computers

Pharmacies use computers for many jobs, including dispensing medications and maintaining inventory. Dispensing systems accurately count and dispense medications, which reduces the rate of errors. Although these systems increase accurate dosing, human error still occurs. A knowledge of dispensing machines and computer programs, such as Microsoft Word and Excel, is essential to creating various reports, ordering, filling prescriptions, and maintaining inventory. Nothing replaces the knowledge of a skilled pharmacy technician to reduce error rates.

Reports and Documentation

Many pharmacies expect technicians to prepare various reports. A knowledge of computers and programs such as Microsoft Word and Excel can make a technician a valuable asset to the pharmacy. Because all pharmacies have integrated computers into their ordering, filling, and documentation procedures, technicians must be computer savvy.

Ordering Supplies

The task of ordering stock is the responsibility of a specific person in the pharmacy, although everyone should know how to order stock when necessary. Ordering stock, returning expired or damaged stock, and handling recalled items are duties in which pharmacy technicians should be competent. This skill is normally taught on the job because each pharmacy has its own way of handling stock inventory. An important aspect of an inventory technician is the storage requirements of the medications that arrive in pharmacy. For more information on this topic, refer to Chapter 13.

Tech Note!

Technology is constantly changing! A technician must continually update and improve his or her computer skills to remain a valuable pharmacy team member.

Inpatient Setting Requirements

Inpatient pharmacy usually refers to pharmacies located in hospitals or institutions in which patients stay overnight or longer, depending on the procedures they require. Most departments in a hospital have medications and supplies that are specific to their department. These are supplied by the inpatient pharmacy. Therefore, inpatient pharmacies traditionally have a wider range of stock than outpatient pharmacies so that they can provide all the supplies required by each department. For example, the labor and delivery unit stocks a large amount of the drug oxytocin (which induces labor), whereas the intensive care unit and coronary care unit require a wide variety of cardiac medications in their stock areas. The cancer units may stock large amounts of morphine and other analgesics, and the pediatrics department stocks many drugs in liquid form for children. Stocking all of these areas is just one of the responsibilities of an inpatient pharmacy technician.

Other important tasks include preparing intravenous (IV) medications and **hyperalimentation** products (i.e., total parenteral nutrition) and performing non–sterile compounding of ointments and creams. The pharmacy loads patient medication drawers and/or automated dispensing systems that allow nurses to access medications. Various individuals in the health care institution are responsible for proper documentation of controlled substances and floor stock disposition; however, the inpatient pharmacy oversees the process. (For more information on

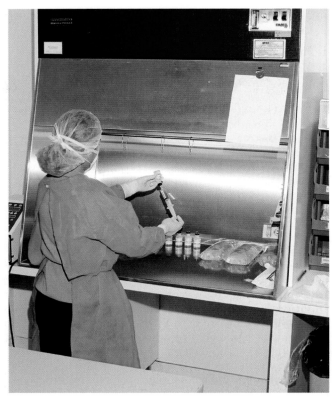
FIGURE 3-1 Room for preparing intravenous solutions for inpatients.

hospital job descriptions and competency requirements, see Chapter 9.)

In addition to knowing the various drugs, strengths, and dosage forms, the technician must be able to immediately and appropriately react when emergency (stat) orders are received by the pharmacy. The dynamics of an inpatient pharmacy can fluctuate minute to minute, depending on the flow of patients into and out of the hospital. "Stat" doses are to be delivered within 15 minutes or less to the area requesting them, such as the emergency department, operating room, intensive care unit, or cardiac care unit. This duty often includes preparing IV solutions (Figure 3-1).

Tech Note!

The bottom line when working in any area of pharmacy is this—always make sure the pharmacist has checked all drugs and/or devices before they leave the pharmacy. If this step is taken, the technician is working within his or her scope of practice, and fewer mistakes will occur.

Another aspect of the inpatient pharmacy is the preparation of unit dose medications (see Chapter 11), which are widely used in many hospital settings. Medications need to be repackaged because either (1) the drug companies do not have the medication available in unit dose or (2) the hospital has chosen to prepare its own unit dose medication for cost-saving reasons.

The following are common duties, roles, and responsibilities of technicians working in a hospital, nursing home, or other inpatient facility. Most inpatient pharmacy technicians who are interested in the following areas in pharmacy receive additional on-the-job training to prepare them for these additional tasks.

- *Inventory technician:* Orders all stock, handles billing, talks to drug representatives, and may be responsible for ordering lowest cost items.
- *Robot filler:* Many pharmacies are installing robots to fill patient medication drawers each day. Technicians must be trained to load these million-dollar mechanical robots and to keep them running smoothly.
- *IV technician:* Interprets orders and prepares all **parenteral medications**, in both large and small volumes, including controlled substance drips, **total parenteral nutrition (TPN)** products, insulin drips, and any other special-order intravenous or intramuscular drugs.
- *Chemotherapy technician:* Receives orders and prepares all chemotherapeutic agents and their adjunct medications, such as antiemetics.
- *Anticoagulant technician:* Assists the anticoagulant pharmacist in contacting patients when patient follow-up is necessary or the patient's anticoagulation medication (e.g., warfarin) or dosage needs to be changed.
- *Technician verifiers:* As a part of the tech-check-tech program, this specially trained technician checks the work of other technicians, including filling patient cassettes (plastic containers) and preparing floor stock. He or she performs the final verification of medication orders and identifies orders on a routine basis that need the pharmacist's intervention to improve the administrative experience.
- *Clinical technician:* Assists the clinical pharmacist with tracking patients' medications. The clinical technician may compile important data (e.g., patient demographics, medication records, laboratory results) that the pharmacist needs to monitor and evaluate patient outcomes or the appropriateness of drug therapies or to monitor formulary compliance.
- *Pharmacy informatics analyst:* This specially trained technician works with the clinical applications specialists to maintain pharmacy software and computers, coordinate hardware and software updates, and work with the pharmacy informatics team (see the sample job description in the box).
- *Supervisory technician:* Schedules other technicians and may even hire prospective technicians by reviewing their skills and backgrounds.

Community (Outpatient) Setting Requirements

Working in an **outpatient pharmacy** is one of the most difficult tasks in pharmacy because of the close interaction with patients. This job tests the **communication** skills and stress levels of the technicians who work with the public. The job has a high volume of interaction on the telephone; these technicians register refill prescriptions and answer questions pertaining to various types of insurance coverage. Computer skills are often necessary to find specific patient information and to assist the customer over the phone or in person. Many neighborhood pharmacies fill a high volume of prescriptions daily (Figure 3-2). It is not uncommon for a midsize pharmacy to fill 300 or more prescriptions a day, answer phone calls, and address patients' problems. In addition to filling prescriptions, the outpatient technician must be able to order stock in a timely manner. Smaller community pharmacies may keep minimal stock because of limited space and the limited variety of drugs prescribed by physicians in the area. The billing of various insurance companies is another skill the outpatient technician must master. This includes understanding the various rules, regulations, and special codes that may accompany each type of prescription claim.

The following list includes descriptions of the jobs performed by outpatient pharmacy technicians, in addition to descriptions of some of the new positions being filled by technicians in community pharmacies. Larger drug companies that are community based also have recognized the positive aspects of hiring technicians to fill certain positions.

- *Insurance billing technician:* This person must know the guidelines of Medicare, Blue Cross, Medicaid, and other insurance companies (see sample job description in the following box).
- *Retail technician:* This person must have excellent communication skills, phone skills, and prescription-filling abilities.

Sample Job Description

Pharmacy Informatics Analyst—Pharmacy Technician
If you are a Pharmacy Informatics Analyst with 3+ years of experience, please read on!
What you need for this position:

- Pharmacy Technician licensed in the State of South Carolina
- Experience with Cerner Software!!!
- At least 3 years of experience in EMR pharmacy and clinical computer applications. This will include: upgrades and implementations of new systems and providing staff education.
- Microsoft Office and Project Management software experience
- Knowledge of clinical pharmacy workflow and how computer applications would assist the pharmacy in these workflows.

What you'll be doing:

- Supports implementation, integration, and maintenance of technology to optimize medication use process.
- Organizes and completes the validation of changes to the pharmacy modules, including testing, coordinating training, functional support, auditing and documentation.
- Identifies computer applications and needs of the pharmacy and clinical departments.
- Assures that the objectives and goals of the clinicians are communicated and supported by the system as well as process improvements that are implemented.
- Communicates and coordinates with other I.S. clinical systems, applications analysts, and customers about changes and issues impacting pharmacy systems.
- Documents general functional requirements and detailed technical specifications for pharmacy applications as well as test scripts.
- Interacts with customers through various phases of implementation and maintenance.
- Monitors industry trends and technology advancements as they apply to the pharmacy and medication processes.
- Coordinates problem resolution with support services and vendors.
- Works closely with financial areas for modifying and updating charges.
- Assists in investigating and responding to billing and charge audits.
- Produces reports as requested.
- Maintains **confidentiality** of records.

What's in it for you:

- Competitive salary with a comprehensive benefits package
- Solid PTO package, including personal time, sick time, and vacation time
- Offers extended illness bank, education and training, tuition reimbursement
- Great work environment!

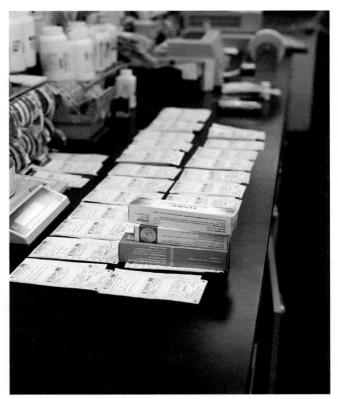

FIGURE 3-2 Outpatient filling station.

 Tech Note!

Did you know that technicians can work in the oncology field? Oncology pharmacy technicians assist pharmacists in caring for patients with various types of cancer. Typical duties include preparing chemotherapy IV admixtures, maintaining safety data sheet (SDS) information, calculating correct dosage volumes, and making sure that all guidelines for the handling of hazardous materials are followed. Oncology technicians work closely with patients and the pharmacist to provide optimal care. Job requirements include a high school diploma with a minimum of 2 years' experience in a pharmacy and also IV skills. IV certification is preferred, along with PTCB or NHA certification. In addition, many facilities have specific levels for technicians' responsibilities. The lowest level is tech I, followed by tech II, and then tech III. Each level requires a minimum amount of time spent working in the previous level. This type of structure allows for career advancement and salary increases based on responsibilities. In the community pharmacy, the structure of responsibilities is quite different.

- *Inventory/stock technician:* This person must know contacts for fast service, be able to obtain products and drugs as soon as possible, and perform proper billing functions for the pharmacy, including processing returns, recalled drugs, and controlled substances.

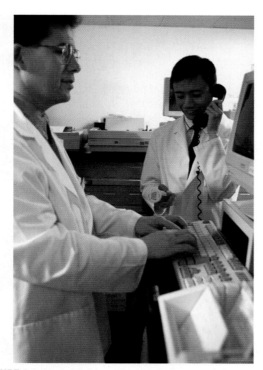

FIGURE 3-3 Home health and long-term pharmacy industry setting.

- *Technician recruiter:* Some outpatient pharmacies and/or temporary agencies employ these technicians to recruit other technicians into their company.
- *Technician trainer:* Various outpatient pharmacies employ technicians to train newly hired technicians on computer programs and to master other necessary skills relevant to their specific pharmacy.
- *Technician manager:* Many retail pharmacies promote technicians to managerial positions. Their job is to supervise the pharmacy technician staff. The technician manager is responsible for interviewing possible new employees, developing and maintaining work schedules, making sure registrations and certifications are current, and working with the pharmacists to continually train and update the skills of the pharmacy technician employees.

Closed Door Pharmacy Requirements

A **closed door pharmacy** is exactly what its name implies. These pharmacies are not open to the public, and they are normally based away from institutional sites (Figure 3-3). Depending on the types of service the closed door pharmacy provides, couriers deliver the medications to home health clients, inpatient hospital pharmacies, specialty clinics, and assisted living or long-term care facilities. The job descriptions of home health pharmacy technicians

Sample Job Description

Third Party Billing Rejection Specialist—Pharmacy Technician
Company: Brown County Nursing Home
Facility: Long-term health care pharmacy
Schedule: Full-time
Shift: Days/evenings
Job Details:
- State and national certified and licensed pharmacy technician
- Pharmacy technician
- Third-party billing rejection specialist to join our team.
- This is a full-time position. Hours and days of the position vary, and qualified candidates should be able to work day or evening shifts. Some weekends may be required.

Qualified Candidates Will Have:
- Strong knowledge of third-party plans and insurance processors.
- Previous technician experience (2+ years) working with prior authorizations, overrides, and rejection experience with various insurances.
- Knowledge of billing procedures for Medicaid, private insurance, and Medicare Part D plans.
- Current state Pharmacy Technician licensure—REQUIRED.
- Prior lead or supervisory experience.
- Excellent customer service skills and phone etiquette.

Other qualifications we look for in candidates include, but are not limited to:
- Excellent verbal and written communication skills
- Ability to work in a fast-paced environment
- Strong organizational skills
- Detail oriented and good problem-solving skills
- Computer knowledge—experience with Microsoft programs

Pharmacy offers competitive compensation, benefit packages, and outstanding growth opportunities.

incorporate some of the duties of both inpatient and outpatient pharmacy technicians. The technicians usually are processing prescription medications for patients weekly or monthly, which is similar to an outpatient setting. However, there are no patients, physicians, nurses, or other health care providers in the facility. Closed door pharmacies are different in that the oral prescriptions usually are packaged differently. Flat cardboard blister packs are prepared by technicians for use by nurses, who administer the drugs in the assisted living, long-term care, and home health settings (see Chapter 11).

Other technician responsibilities include preparing parenteral medications. Usually a few days to a 1-month supply is filled each time instead of only a

---

Sample Job Description

Pharmacy Technician (Closed Door Facility)
Job Snapshot

Employee Type:	Full time
Location:	Main facility
Job Type:	Pharmaceutical, Science, Health Care
Experience:	1 to 2 years
Date Posted:	1/22/2015

Certified Pharmacy Technician
Job Description
We have an opening for a certified pharmacy technician within a closed door pharmacy. As a member of our team, you'll enjoy a customized approach to your career needs as well as comprehensive benefits! Join our dynamic team, apply today!

Certified Pharmacy Technician (Closed Door Facility)
Job Responsibilities
As a certified pharmacy technician, you will be responsible for maintaining productivity and quality standards as well as legal and company compliance as you enter in new prescriptions and assist in the preparation of prescriptions. Your responsibilities will include:
- Item entry
- Establishing or maintaining patient profiles, including lists of medications taken by individual patients
- Answering telephones, responding to questions or requests
- Assisting customers by answering simple questions, locating items, or referring them to the pharmacist for medication information

Job Requirements
- 1 to 2 years of recent pharmacy experience
- Must have PTCB certification
- Must have excellent data entry skills
- Ability to successfully complete background check and drug screen
- Pay: depending on experience
- Schedule: to be determined

Benefits
- Health insurance with prescription coverage
- Vision/dental
- 401(k) and deferred compensation programs
- Cafeteria plans
- Free CE
- Low-cost group health benefits for part-time associates

24-hour dose of medication. A licensed pharmacist checks all medications filled for a home care patient before they are delivered. Home health nurses may receive supplies from the pharmacy clinic, or the patient's family may pick up or have the supplies delivered. Examples of patients who may receive care at home include kidney dialysis patients undergoing peritoneal dialysis and hospice patients. Nuclear pharmacies are considered closed door pharmacies and offer a unique work environment for pharmacy technicians. A Nuclear Pharmacy Technician (NPT) is a highly specialized type of pharmacy technician who has specialized training and education in a clinical setting for nuclear pharmacy. An NPT works under the direct supervision of a licensed nuclear pharmacist.

Mail-Order Pharmacy and E-Pharmacy

Mail-order and e-pharmacies are growing as the "baby boomers" reach maturity. The need to fill prescriptions expeditiously has increased as more medications have become available to treat commonly acquired illnesses specific to older persons. Large distribution centers process new prescriptions and refills. Technicians are also used in these settings.

This is a relatively new area of pharmacy that is growing steadily. This growth is occurring partially because many aging Americans are living longer and are taking multiple medications that can be costly. By using mail order, they often can receive drugs at a lower cost.

In 2004, due to Congress' concern about counterfeit drugs, the major online search engines selected PharmacyChecker.com to verify the validity of online pharmacies. In 2005 an investigation by the U.S. Food and Drug Administration (FDA) revealed that many drugs promoted online as "Canadian" were counterfeit and actually originated from other countries. In 2008, Congress passed the Ryan Haight Online Consumer Protection Act banning online pharmacies from selling controlled substances based on online patient consultations. In 2009 a report from LegitScrip found that 80% to 90% of search engine–sponsored advertisements of online drug pharmacies (verified by PharmacyChecker.com) violated federal and state laws. In 2010 Google removed PharmacyChecker.com as a certifying authority for online pharmacies. Currently, online pharmacies can be verified by Verified Internet Pharmacy Practice Sites (VIPPS).

Scenario CHECK UP 3-3

Olivia's pharmacist, Karen, invites her to attend the local pharmacy association meeting as a guest. This group meets once a month, and its membership consist of pharmacists and certified pharmacy technicians. Olivia is so impressed, she joins the group that very night. She enjoys participating in various continuing education sessions and networking with other professionals. What do you see as the benefits Olivia might gain from her association with this group?

Training Programs for the Pharmacy Technician Student

Since 1982, when pharmacy technician accreditation programs were first established, the ASHP has been the leader in providing course curriculum and standards and offering students the best foundation for becoming technicians. Before the formation of technician schools, the ASHP's training guidelines and standards were used in hospitals for training pharmacy interns. ASHP accreditation is a voluntary process at this time. Program accreditation is given to colleges and technical schools that apply and meet the requirements set by the ASHP. An outline of topics for the **ASHP Model Curriculum for Pharmacy Technician Education and Training** is provided in Box 3-5. The ASHP designed this model to aid programs that are just starting up, in addition to current programs that are reviewing their curriculum. The ASHP used the PTCB's scope of practice analysis data to determine the required outcomes for the programs. The ASHP's new standard has six components:

- Administration
- Program faculty
- Education and training
- Students
- Evaluation and assessment
- Graduation and certificate

According to this standard, a program must require a minimum of 600 hours: 160 hours of didactic training; 80 hours of simulation (laboratory) training; 160 hours of experiential training in at least two different practice sites, one of which must be a dispensing pharmacy; and 200 hours spent at the program's discretion.

The PTCB's CREST Initiative in 2011 proposed new pharmacy technician roles and responsibilities. These new roles included medication safety positions, tech-check-tech, providing operational support for clinics, participating in medication reconciliation, and maintaining and optimizing technology. To help prepare technicians for these expanded roles, the PTCB recommended that by 2020, all PTCE candidates be required to complete a training program accredited by the ASHP. Currently, 33 states require training of pharmacy technicians. Eighteen states require national certification to work as a pharmacy technician. Some states require that technicians pass a state-approved certification exam.

BOX 3-5

ASHP Model Curriculum for Pharmacy Technician Education and Training

The ASHP model curriculum goals are categorized into the following areas.

- Personal/Interpersonal Knowledge and Skills
- Foundational Professional Knowledge and Skills
- Processing and Handling of Medications and Medication Orders
- Sterile and Nonsterile Compounding
- Procurement, Billing, Reimbursement, and Inventory Management
- Patient and Medication Safety
- Technology and Informatics
- Regulatory Issues
- Quality Assurance

Personal/Interpersonal Knowledge and Skills
(1) Demonstrate ethical conduct in all job-related activities.
(2) Present an image appropriate for the profession of pharmacy in appearance and behavior.
(3) Communicate clearly when speaking and in writing.
(4) Demonstrate a respectful attitude when interacting with diverse patient populations.
(5) Apply self-management skills, including time management, stress management, and adapting to change.
(6) Apply interpersonal skills, including negotiation skills, conflict resolution, and teamwork.
(7) Apply critical thinking skills, creativity, and innovation to solve problems.

Foundational Professional Knowledge and Skills
(8) Demonstrate understanding of health care occupations and the health care delivery system.
(9) Demonstrate understanding of wellness promotion and disease prevention concepts, such as use of health screenings; health practices and environmental factors that impact health; and adverse effects of alcohol, tobacco, and legal and illegal drugs.

Continued

BOX 3-5

ASHP Model Curriculum for Pharmacy Technician Education and Training—cont'd

(10) Demonstrate commitment to excellence in the pharmacy profession and to continuing education and training.

(11) Demonstrate knowledge and skills in areas of science relevant to the pharmacy technician's role, including anatomy/physiology and pharmacology.

(12) Perform mathematical calculations essential to the duties of pharmacy technicians in a variety of contemporary settings.

(13) Demonstrate understanding of the pharmacy technician's role in the medication-use process.

(14) Demonstrate understanding of major trends, issues, goals, and initiatives taking place in the pharmacy profession.

(15) Demonstrate understanding of nontraditional roles of pharmacy technicians.

(16) Identify and describe emerging therapies.

Processing and Handling of Medications and Medication Orders

(17) Assist pharmacists in collecting, organizing, and recording demographic and clinical information for direct patient care and medication-use review.

(18) Receive and screen prescriptions/medication orders for completeness, accuracy, and authenticity.

(19) Assist pharmacists in the identification of patients who desire/require counseling to optimize the use of medications, equipment, and devices.

(20) Prepare non-patient-specific medications for distribution (e.g., batch, stock medications).

(21) Distribute medications in a manner that follows specified procedures.

(22) Practice effective infection control procedures, including preventing transmission of blood-borne and airborne diseases.

(23) Assist pharmacists in preparing, storing, and distributing medication products requiring special handling and documentation (e.g., controlled substances, immunizations, chemotherapy, investigational drugs, drugs with mandated Risk Evaluation and Mitigation Strategies [REMS]).

(24) Assist pharmacists in the monitoring of medication therapy.

(25) Prepare patient-specific medications for distribution.

(26) Maintain pharmacy facilities and equipment, including automated dispensing equipment.

(27) Use safety data sheets (SDS) to identify, handle, and safely dispose of hazardous materials.

Sterile and Nonsterile Compounding

(28) Prepare medications requiring compounding of sterile products.

(29) Prepare medications requiring compounding of nonsterile products.

(30) Prepare medications requiring compounding of chemotherapy/hazardous products.

Procurement, Billing, Reimbursement, and Inventory Management

(31) Initiate, verify, and assist in the adjudication of billing for pharmacy services and goods, and collect payment for these services.

(32) Apply accepted procedures in purchasing pharmaceuticals, devices, and supplies.

(33) Apply accepted procedures in inventory control of medications, equipment, and devices.

(34) Explain pharmacy reimbursement plans for covering pharmacy services.

Patient and Medication Safety

(35) Apply patient and medication safety practices in all aspects of the pharmacy technician's roles.

(36) Verify measurements, preparation, and/or packaging of medications produced by other health care professionals (e.g., tech-check-tech).

(37) Explain pharmacists' roles when they are responding to emergency situations and how pharmacy technicians can assist pharmacists by being certified as Basic Life Support (BLS) Healthcare Providers.

(38) Demonstrate skills required for effective emergency preparedness.

(39) Assist pharmacists in medication reconciliation.

(40) Assist pharmacists in medication therapy management.

Technology and Informatics

(41) Describe the use of current technology in the health care environment to ensure the safety and accuracy of medication dispensing.

Regulatory Issues

(42) Compare and contrast the roles of pharmacists and pharmacy technicians in ensuring pharmacy department compliance with professional standards and relevant legal, regulatory, formulary, contractual, and safety requirements.

(43) Maintain confidentiality of patient information.

Quality Assurance

(44) Apply quality assurance practices to pharmaceuticals, durable and nondurable medical equipment, devices, and supplies.

(45) Explain procedures and communication channels to use in the event of a product recall or shortage, a medication error, or identification of another problem.

See www.ashp.org for additional information. American Society of Health Systems Pharmacists. The Model Curriculum for Pharmacy Technician Education and Training Programs. (Referenced July 8, 2014). http://www.ashp.org/DocLibrary/Accreditation/Model-Curriculum.pdf

Different Levels of Pharmacy Technicians

There are four levels of pharmacy technicians: pharmacy technicians who have no specialized training or credentials and licensed, registered, and certified technicians. Each level has different qualifications, which may differ from state to state.

Pharmacy Technician

The first level of pharmacy technician requires no specialized training. Some states require pharmacy technicians to attain minimum standards, such as a high school diploma; others do not.

Licensed Pharmacy Technician

A **licensed pharmacy technician** is licensed by the state board of pharmacy. *Licensing* is the process by which an agency of the government grants permission to an individual to engage in a given occupation based on the findings that the applicant has attained the minimum degree of competency necessary to ensure that the public health, safety, and welfare will be reasonably well protected.

Registered Pharmacy Technician

A **registered pharmacy technician** is a pharmacy technician who is registered with the state board of pharmacy. *Registration* is the process of making a list or being enrolled in an existing list; registration should be used to help safeguard the public through tracking of the technician workforce and preventing individuals with documented problems from serving as pharmacy technicians. Registration carries no indication or guarantee of the registrant's knowledge or skills. Each state determines whether continuing education is required of technicians to renew their registration.

Certified Pharmacy Technician

A **certified pharmacy technician** is one who has earned national recognition by a nongovernmental testing agency or association; *certification* indicates that the person has met predetermined qualifications specified by that agency or association (PTCB or NHA). CPhT currently is the main credential available to pharmacy technicians. Certification is an indication of the mastery of a specific core of knowledge. Certified technicians must renew their certification every 2 years and complete at least 20 hours of pharmacy-related continuing education, which must include 1 hour of pharmacy law and 1 hour of medication safety.

National Certification for Technicians

It should be the goal of every pharmacy technician student to become nationally certified. Certification means that you have passed a national exam demonstrating your knowledge of the skills needed to enter the pharmacy technician profession. Many employers prefer certified technicians and often offer them a higher pay scale. Certification, along with education, leads to better job security and additional employment opportunities.

During the infancy of any profession, there is a lack of regular guidelines and standards, or continuity. Currently five types of verification may be required or pursued by technicians: registration, licensing, certification, associate of science (AS) degree in pharmacy technology, or certificate in pharmacy technology. As outlined previously, registration is regulated by the state and requires that the applicant pass a standard background check, in addition to meeting BOP standards. Licensing may also be required by the state, but it is not currently required in all states. A certified pharmacy technician earns a certificate that acknowledges that the technician has a basic understanding of all areas of pharmacy, including federal law. Maintaining certification requires continuing education to keep skills at a minimum level.

Pharmacy technicians work throughout the United States and in all types of pharmacy settings under different rules determined by the individual states, which makes this profession challenging. At some point in the near future, a national minimum standard for the profession must be agreed on across the United States. Although some variations will always exist from state to state, the overall skill level of a pharmacy technician should be a well-known standard. Currently, technicians represent a wide range of skill levels, experience, pay, and belief systems. One of the most basic aspects is the lack of a common title. Pharmacy technicians also are known as pharmacy clerks and pharmacy assistants.

Two national groups certify technicians and are recognized by various states: the Pharmacy Technician Certification Board and the National Healthcareer Association. The **Pharmacy Technician Certification Board (PTCB)** was founded in 1995 by four organizations with the intent of implementing an examination that would certify that a technician has met a basic skill level (Box 3-6). The four organizations that founded the PTCB are the ASHP, the APhA, the Illinois Council of Health-System Pharmacists (ICHP), and the Michigan Pharmacists Association (MPA).

Table 3-1 presents a comparison of two exams, the Pharmacy Technician Certification Exam (PTCE), offered by the PTCB, and the Exam for the Certification of Pharmacy Technicians (ExCPT), offered by the NHA.

As of December 5, 2013, the PTCB offers one sample exam consisting of 90 multiple choice

BOX 3-6

Goals of the PTCE and Eligibility Requirements

Goals
- To work more effectively with pharmacists
- To provide better patient care and service
- To create a minimum standard of knowledge for pharmacy technicians
- To help employers determine the knowledge base of pharmacy technicians

Eligibility Requirements to Take the Exam
To achieve PTCB certification, candidates must satisfy the following eligibility requirements:
- High school diploma or equivalent educational diploma (e.g., a GED or foreign diploma)
- Full disclosure of all criminal and state board of pharmacy registration or licensure actions
- Compliance with all applicable PTCB certification policies
- Passing score on the Pharmacy Technician Certification Exam (PTCE)

A candidate may be disqualified for PTCB certification upon the disclosure or discovery of:
- Criminal conduct involving the candidate
- State board of pharmacy registration or licensure action involving the candidate
- Violation of a PTCB certification policy, including but not limited to the Code of Conduct

The PTCB reserves the right to investigate criminal background, verify candidate eligibility, and deny certification to any individual.

Once certified, Certified Pharmacy Technicians (CPhTs) must report to the PTCB for review any felony conviction, drug or pharmacy-related violations, or state board of pharmacy action taken against their license or registration at the occurrence and at the time of recertification. Disqualification determinations are made on a case-by-case basis.

http://www.nabp.net/programs/cpe-monitor/cpe-monitor-service/technicians#technicians-and-boards-of-pharmacy

questions to be taken within 110 minutes. The new Practice Test is designed to familiarize candidates with the PTCE. The Practice Test is built according to the same content specifications as the PTCE (updated on November 1, 2013), although the Practice Test questions never appear on an actual examination. The cost for this official practice exam is $29. The PTCB expects to add more practice tests in the future. The actual certification exam, administered by the PTCB, is given at a professional testing center and is computerized. Testing can take place once an appointment is made. The PTCE is a computer-based exam administered at PearsonVue test centers nationwide. It is a 2-hour, multiple choice exam that contains 90 questions (80 scored questions and 10 unscored questions). Each question is shown with four possible answers, only one of which is the correct or best answer. Unscored questions are not identified and are randomly distributed throughout the exam. A candidate's exam score is based on the responses to the 80 scored questions. One hour and 50 minutes are allotted for answering the exam questions and 10 minutes for a tutorial and postexam survey. Calculators and scratch pads are provided by the test center. Scoring is done by an independent group that grades the various areas of pharmacy knowledge. The results are immediately calculated at the end of the examination.

The PTCE content was developed by experts in pharmacy technician practice based on a nationwide Job Analysis Study completed in February, 2012. The PTCB's Certification Council and Board of Governors reviewed the 2012 Job Analysis Study and approved a new blueprint for an updated PTCE, which launched on November 1, 2013.

The PTCE assesses knowledge critical to pharmacy technician practice organized into nine knowledge domains, each with a number of knowledge areas (Box 3-7). It is currently the only pharmacy technician certification exam accepted in all 50 states. For more information, visit the PTCB's website at *www.PTCB.org*.

The National Healthcareer Association (NHA)

The **National Healthcareer Association (NHA)** is accredited by boards of the National Community Pharmacists Association (NCPA), the National Commission for Certifying Agencies (NCCA), and the National Association of Chain Drug Stores (NACDS). (For more information about the NHA, visit *www.nhanow.com*.) The exam administered by the NHA is called ExCPT and is given throughout the country at various proctored testing sites. The NHA offers two 50-question sample exams to practice online, at $25 each. One covers just math, whereas the other covers various areas of pharmacy. Currently, ExCPT certification is not recognized in all 50 states. Technicians should check with their individual state boards of pharmacy and employers to determine which certifications are accepted.

Specialty Certifications

One of the recommendations of the 2011 CREST summit involved the creation of specialty pharmacy technician certifications. The PTCB Board of Governors is focused on ensuring that the PTCB program prepares CPhTs for the integral roles they play in supporting pharmacists in all practice settings. Currently, the National Pharmacy Technician

TABLE 3-1

Comparison of Technician Certification Exams

	ExCPT	PTCE
Organization name	National Healthcareer Association (NHA)	Pharmacy Technician Certification Board (PTCB)
Cost	$105	$129
Length of test	2 hours, 110 multiple choice questions	2 hours, 90 multiple choice questions
Frequency of testing	Continuous	Continuous
Testing providers/sites	PSI/Lasergrade	PearsonVue
Results available	Pass/Fail results immediately upon exam completion	Pass/Fail results immediately upon exam completion
Testing requirements	Be at least 18 years of age. Have a high school diploma or GED equivalent Have not been convicted of or pled guilty to a felony Have not had any registration or license revoked, suspended, or subject to any disciplinary action by a state health regulatory board.	High school diploma or equivalent educational diploma (e.g., a GED or foreign diploma). Full disclosure of all criminal and state board of pharmacy registration or licensure actions. Compliance with all applicable PTCB certification policies. Passing score on the Pharmacy Technician Certification Exam (PTCE).
Exam content	Regulations and Technician Duties (approximately 25%): Candidates may expect questions on general technician duties; federal and state law; federal, state and agency rules and regulations; etc. Drugs and Drug Products (approximately 23%): Candidates may expect questions on drug classification, dosage forms, brand and generic drug names, etc. The Dispensing Process (approximately 52%): Candidates may expect questions on prescription information including preparing and dispensing prescriptions, pharmacy calculations, sterile products, repackaging, etc.	1. Pharmacology of technicians; (13.75% of the exam) 2. Pharmacy law and regulations; (12.75% of the exam) 3. Sterile and non-sterile compounding; (8.75% of the exam) 4. Medication safety; (12.5% of the exam) 5. Pharmacy quality assurance; (7.5% of the exam) 6. Medication order entry and fill process; (17.5% of the exam) 7. Pharmacy inventory management; (8.75% of the exam) 8. Pharmacy billing and reimbursement; (8.75% of the exam) 9. Pharmacy information systems usage and application; (10.00% of the exam)
Accredited by the National Commission for Certifying Agencies (NCCA)	Yes	Yes
Website	www.nhanow.com	www.ptcb.org
Recertification requirements	Every 2 years (with a 90-day grace period), 20 hours CE required, including 1 hr of pharmacy law Cost: $40	Every 2 years (no grace period), 20 hours CE requiring 1 hr of pharmacy law and 1 hr of medication safety Cost: $40
Reinstatement requirements	Within 18 months of expiration date Cost: $80	Within 1 year of expiration date Cost: $80
Revocation	For false statements, cheating, conviction of a drug-related felony, revocation of registration/licensure by a state, documented violation of National HealthCareer Association (NHA) Pharmacy Technician Code of Ethics	For false statements, cheating, conviction of a crime or felony of moral turpitude (including but not limited to drug-related crimes), documented gross negligence, intentional misconduct or deficiency in knowledge base
Number of technicians certified	3,000+ (as of December, 2013)	525,365 (as of December 31, 2013)
States that have formally approved test for certification	CT, IA, IN, KA, KY, MD, MA, MN, MT, NV, NH, NJ, NM, OR, RI, TN, UT, WA Seeking approval in many other states	50 states

BOX 3-7

Pharmacy Technician Certification Exam (PTCE) Blueprint

Knowledge Domains and Areas	% of PTCE Content
1.0 Pharmacology for Technicians	13.75%
1.1 Generic and brand names of pharmaceuticals	
1.2 Therapeutic equivalence	
1.3 Drug interactions (e.g., drug-disease, drug-drug, drug–dietary supplement, drug-OTC, drug-laboratory, drug-nutrient)	
1.4 Strengths/dose, dosage forms, physical appearance, routes of administration, and duration of drug therapy*	
1.5 Common and severe side or adverse effects, allergies, and therapeutic contraindications associated with medications	
1.6 Dosage and indication of legend, OTC medications, herbal and dietary supplements	
2.0 Pharmacy Law and Regulations	12.5%*
2.1 Storage, handling, and disposal of hazardous substances and wastes (e.g., SDS)	
2.2 Hazardous substances exposure, prevention, and treatment (e.g., eyewash, spill kit, SDS)	
2.3 Controlled substance transfer regulations (DEA)	
2.4 Controlled substance documentation requirements for receiving, ordering, returning, loss/theft, destruction (DEA)	
2.5 Formula to verify the validity of a prescriber's DEA number (DEA)	
2.6 Record keeping, documentation, and record retention (e.g., length of time prescriptions are maintained on file)	
2.7 Restricted drug programs and related prescription-processing requirements (e.g., thalidomide, isotretinoin, clozapine)	
2.8 Professional standards related to data integrity, security, and confidentiality (e.g., HIPAA, backing up and archiving)	
2.9 Requirement for consultation (e.g., OBRA '90)	
2.10 FDA's recall classification	
2.11 Infection control standards (e.g., laminar air flow, clean room, hand washing, cleaning counting trays, countertop, and equipment) (OSHA, USP 795 and 797)	

Knowledge Domains and Areas	% of PTCE Content
2.12 Record keeping for repackaged and recalled products and supplies (TJC, BOP)	
2.13 Professional standards regarding the roles and responsibilities of pharmacists, pharmacy technicians, and other pharmacy employees (TJC, BOP)	
2.14 Reconciliation between state and federal laws and regulations	
2.15 Facility, equipment, and supply requirements (e.g., space requirements, prescription file storage, cleanliness, reference materials) (TJC, USP, BOP)	
3.0 Sterile and Non–Sterile Compounding	8.75%*
3.1 Infection control (e.g., hand washing, PPE)	
3.2 Handling and disposal requirements (e.g., receptacles, waste streams)	
3.3 Documentation (e.g., batch preparation, compounding record)*	
3.4 Determine product stability (e.g., beyond use dating, signs of incompatibility)*	
3.5 Selection and use of equipment and supplies	
3.6 Sterile compounding processes*	
3.7 Non–sterile compounding processes*	
4.0 Medication Safety	12.5%
4.1 Error prevention strategies for data entry (e.g., prescription or medication order to correct patient)	
4.2 Patient package insert and medication guide requirements (e.g., special directions and precautions)	
4.3 Identify issues that require pharmacist intervention (e.g., DUR, ADE, OTC recommendation, therapeutic substitution, misuse, missed dose)	
4.4 Look-alike, sound-alike medications	
4.5 High-alert/risk medications	
4.6 Common safety strategies (e.g., tall man lettering, separating inventory, leading and trailing zeros, limit use of error-prone abbreviations)	

BOX 3-7

Pharmacy Technician Certification Exam (PTCE) Blueprint

Knowledge Domains and Areas	% of PTCE Content
5.0 Pharmacy Quality Assurance	7.5%
5.1 Quality assurance practices for medication and inventory control systems (e.g., matching NDC number, bar code, data entry)	
5.2 Infection control procedures and documentation (e.g., PPE, needle recapping)	
5.3 Risk management guidelines and regulations (e.g., error prevention strategies)	
5.4 Communication channels necessary to ensure appropriate follow-up and problem resolution (e.g., product recalls, shortages)	
5.5 Productivity, efficiency, and customer satisfaction measures	
6.0 Medication Order Entry and Fill Process	17.5%*
6.1 Order entry process*	
6.2 Intake, interpretation, and data entry*	
6.3 Calculate doses required*	
6.4 Fill process (e.g., select appropriate product, apply special handling requirements, measure, and prepare product for final check)	
6.5 Labeling requirements (e.g., auxiliary and warning labels, expiration date, patient-specific information)	
6.6 Packaging requirements (e.g., type of bags, syringes, glass, PVC, child resistant, light resistant)*	
6.7 Dispensing process (e.g., validation, documentation, and distribution)	

Knowledge Domains and Areas	% of PTCE Content
7.0 Pharmacy Inventory Management	8.75%
7.1 Function and application of NDC, lot numbers, and expiration dates	
7.2 Formulary or approved/preferred product list	
7.3 Ordering and receiving processes (e.g., maintain par levels, rotate stock)*	
7.4 Storage requirements (e.g., refrigeration, freezer, warmer)	
7.5 Removal (e.g., recalls, returns, outdates, reverse distribution)	
8.0 Pharmacy Billing and Reimbursement	8.75%
8.1 Reimbursement policies and plans (e.g., HMOs, PPO, CMS, private plans)	
8.2 Third-party resolution (e.g., prior authorization, rejected claims, plan limitations)*	
8.3 Third-party reimbursement systems (e.g., PBM, medication assistance programs, coupons, and self-pay)	
8.4 Health care reimbursement systems (e.g., home health, long-term care, home infusion)	
8.5 Coordination of benefits	
9.0 Pharmacy Information System Usage and Application	10%
9.1 Pharmacy-related computer applications for documenting the dispensing of prescriptions or medication orders (e.g., maintaining the electronic medical record, patient adherence, risk factors, alcohol drug use, drug allergies, side effects)	
9.2 Databases, pharmacy computer applications, and documentation management (e.g., user access, drug database, interface, inventory report, usage reports, override reports, diversion reports)	

*Denotes content, including calculations.
(Source: Pharmacy Technician Certification Board, www.ptcb.org)
ADE, Adverse Drug Event; *BOP,* board of pharmacy; *CMS,* Centers for Medicare and Medicaid Services; *DEA,* Drug Administration; *DUR,* Drug Utilization Review; *FDA,* U.S. Food and Drug Administration; *HIPAA,* Health Insurance Accountability Act; *HMOs,* health maintenance organizations; *NDC,* National Drug Code; *OSHA,* Occupational Administration; *OTC,* over the counter; *PBM,* pharmacy benefits manager; *PPE,* personal protective equipment organization; *TJC,* the Joint Commission; *USP,* United States Pharmacopeia.

Association (NPTA) offers three specialty certification programs for technicians who want to enhance their skills and marketability: Sterile Products IV certification, Compounding certification, and Chemotherapy certification. To learn more about the PTCB visit the website www.ptcb.org.

Continuing

Technicians w...
certification may
identification tag, i...
pharmacy technician...

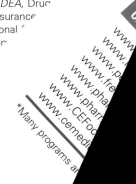

❳ TECHNICIAN PROFILE

Avery is a lead controlled substance pharmacy technician at a Veterans Health Administration hospital. He has worked in the pharmacy for 5 years. Controlled substance distribution is a highly visible and sensitive area for the facility. Avery's position requires an individual who is willing to accept increased responsibility and at the same time pay close attention to details. Most of Avery's duties are performed in the pharmacy vault, setting up controlled substances for dispensing, making appropriate record entries, and reviewing controlled substance administration records. Avery is expected to maintain a high degree of accurate productivity and performance while being extremely sensitive to the contribution to total patient care. He checks in shipments of drugs and supplies, verifies the accuracy of those shipments, and assures the proper storage of all items. All of Avery's activities are supervised by the pharmacy operations manager and the controlled substance pharmacist on duty.

they must earn **continuing education (CE)** credits. All valid CE credits must be approved by the **Accreditation Council for Pharmacy Education (ACPE)**, which is indicated on each CE course. ACPE accredits CE courses for both pharmacists and pharmacy technicians. Although technicians can currently take CE courses meant for pharmacists, the PTCB requires that by 2015, all 20 hours needed for recertification must be pharmacy technician–specific CEs. The letter P indicates that the CE course is designed for pharmacists, whereas a T indicates that the course is for technicians. In addition to the two levels of CE courses (i.e., P and T), current courses may have 05 added to their name; this indicates that the CE course covers a patient safety topic. CEs can be obtained through pharmacy organizations that offer free continuing education to members, journals that include continuing education units, and online webinars or traditional

seminars. Continuing education is less expensive for association members, and many drug companies offer free continuing education units to pharmacists and technicians. Independent pharmacists and other small businesses offer low-cost continuing education credit courses on the Internet (Table 3-2).

Currently, more than one third of jurisdictions have continuing education requirements for technicians to maintain their licensing, certification, or registration. In late 2011, the CPE Monitor was launched as a collaborative effort by the NABP and the ACPE. It provides an electronic system for pharmacists and pharmacy technicians to track their continuing pharmacy education credits. It also offers state boards of pharmacy the opportunity to electronically authenticate the CPE units completed by their licensees, rather than requiring pharmacists and technicians to submit their proof of completion statements upon request or for random audits. Requirements for each state vary; technicians should contact their state boards of pharmacy for information on CPE reporting requirements. In the future, this information may flow from CPE Monitor to the PTCB. The NABP e-profile can be completed by the pharmacist and/or technician at that organization's website (*www.nabp.net*). Once the e-profile has been established, an NABP ID is issued, which is used to register with the CPE Monitor. The pharmacist and/or technician gives the ID to the provider when completing a CPE activity.

 Tech Note!

Many employers may encourage certification and formally recognize achievement. Some pharmacy technicians may receive a raise in pay or expanded career responsibilities after completion of the pharmacy technician certification examination.

TABLE 3-2

Examples of Continuing Education Websites for Technicians

Websites	Online CE	Live/Live Webinar CE	Cost*
.uspharmacist.com	x		Free CE courses available
.rxschool.com	x	x	Free CE courses available
.owerpak.com	x		Free CE courses available
.ece.com	x	x	Free CE courses available
.rmacytechnician.org	x	x	Free CE courses available for members
.macytechce.org	x	x	Free CE courses available members
.usOnline.com	x		Free CE courses available
.cus.com	x		Free CE courses available

*...e available at no charge; occasionally, fee-based programs may also be available, depending on the session provider.

Box 3-8 lists both the qualifications and common duties of pharmacy technicians as established by the PTCB.

According to current statistics, there are more than 484,039 PTCB-certified technicians nationwide. Many states are beginning to recognize the importance of certification to guarantee that the technicians hired are competent in all areas of pharmacy (see Chapter 14, Emily's Act). Employers increasingly are using these credentials as a requirement for hiring technicians.

Opportunities for Technicians

Pharmacies use computers daily; therefore, software must be developed for pharmacy personnel. Some pharmacy-related fields require more education in specific areas, such as computers. With the proper educational training (e.g., an AS degree or a bachelor of science [BS] degree in computer science), the pharmacy technician is well equipped to write software or provide support. Also, because many technicians are given the responsibility of training technicians, their expertise may help them write curriculums, articles, and even books for pharmacy technicians. Many vocational schools hire experienced certified pharmacy technicians to teach students the requirements for becoming competent pharmacy technicians. Completion of such training programs offers different degrees, such as certificates, an associate's degree (associate of arts [AA] or AS), or a bachelor's degree (bachelor of arts [BA] or BS).

Pharmacy technicians also can fill many other, less well known positions, such as the following nontraditional jobs.

- Pharmacy business management operators—Pharmacy business management companies are beginning to realize the importance of knowing not only the trade and generic names of drugs, but also their classifications. They are hiring technicians, rather than registered pharmacists, to help pharmacy customers over the phone, which is a cost savings for the company.
- Computer support technician (PYXIS, SUREMED)—Large companies that supply hospitals, community pharmacies, and other facilities with automated medication dispensing systems are employing technicians as support personnel.
- Software writer—Some pharmacy software writers are using technicians with additional computer background and/or training to prepare software services. Technicians use their terminology and drug knowledge to create new software programs.
- Poison control call center operator—Some poison control centers are using technicians to triage calls coming into the 911 stations. If the call concerns something life-threatening, technicians

BOX 3-8

Common Job Duties and Requirements for Pharmacy Technicians

Job Duties

The following list represents the responsibilities expected of pharmacy technicians, depending on the pharmacy setting and the technician's scope of practice.

- Assist pharmacist in labeling and filling prescriptions
- Assist patients in dropping off and picking up prescriptions
- Enter prescriptions into the computer
- Verify that customer receives the correct prescription or prescriptions
- Compound oral solutions, ointments, and creams
- Schedule and maintain workflow
- Prepackage bulk medications
- Screen calls for pharmacists
- Order medications
- Work with insurance carriers to obtain payment and refilling authority
- Prepare medication inventories
- Prepare chemotherapeutic agents
- Compound total parenteral nutrition solutions
- Compound large volumes of intravenous mixtures
- Assist in outpatient dispensing
- Assist in inpatient dispensing
- Prepare intravenous mixtures
- Assist in purchasing and billing

Knowledge, Skills, Training, and Education

State practice acts and employer policies determine training and education requirements. The following are some commonly desired characteristics.

- Professional attitude
- Strong communication skills
- Ability to work in teams
- Previous customer service experience
- Ability to type 35 words per minute
- Understanding of medical terminology and calculations
- Attention to detail
- Outgoing
- Hard working
- Quick learner
- Pharmacy Technician Certification Board (PTCB) certification (may be desired or mandatory)

(Source: Pharmacy Technician Certification Board. Career Outlook) http://www.ptcb.org/resources/career-outlook#.U7zFiPldVoM (Referenced July 8, 2014)

transfer it to a pharmacist or poison specialist. If the call is less serious, technicians are authorized to take the call.

- Nuclear pharmacy technician—The technician may assist the pharmacist with handling of and preparing physicians' orders for radioactive medications used in diagnosis and treatment.
- Director/instructor—Certified pharmacy technicians can oversee technician training programs and/or serve as instructors in schools around the country. Some programs require a BS degree or vocational education teaching credentials.
- Corporate pharmacy analyst—Working through an independent management service, a technician surveys the efficiency in all areas of the pharmacy and recommends changes to help the pharmacy operate more productively and efficiently. The analyst may travel and even work on the Joint Commission standards to prepare pharmacies for inspection.
- Technician coordinator—Coordinators oversee as many as 50 to 100 technicians in a large hospital pharmacy. They are responsible for training, regulation compliance, and scheduling of all pharmacy technician personnel.
- Home infusion pharmacy technician—Home infusion technicians assist the pharmacist in the preparation of IV solutions, injectable drugs, and enteral nutrition therapy. These medications are dispensed to the patient at home. Technicians process equipment and supply orders and must be knowledgeable about vascular access and infusion devices.

In addition to the positions listed, technicians may continue their education and apply for pharmacy school. Many pharmacists were once technicians. New positions are being developed by different types of pharmacies specifically for technicians. For instance, some hospitals are utilizing pharmacy technicians in the anticoagulant clinic setting to assist the pharmacist in obtaining and assessing information on patient compliance, medication dosages, bleeding symptoms, and a patient's general state of health. Other hospitals are employing pharmacy technicians specializing in pharmacy informatics to provide support for their information and automation systems. Although these positions currently may be nontraditional, their numbers are growing. It would not be surprising if these jobs became commonly held positions for future technicians.

Examples	Setting
Clinical pharmacy technician	Hospital
Anticoagulant pharmacy technician	Hospital
Program director—pharmacy technician	Vocational/technical school

Examples	Setting
Medical billing specialist—pharmacy technician	Health care services
Certified pharmacy technician—loader, driver	Long-term care facility
Implementation pharmacy technician	Pharmacy benefits service
Data entry pharmacy technician	Institutional pharmacy

Incentive Programs

Pharmacies sometimes have an incentive program for employees who want to further their careers in pharmacy. Many pharmacists who began their careers as technicians have used this company benefit to their advantage. Many pharmacy employers provide incentives to their technicians for returning to school and becoming a pharmacist. They may reimburse tuition costs or give pay incentives for agreeing to be employed by the pharmacy a certain number of years upon graduation from pharmacy school. Whether a company supports and partly funds a school program is something a prospective employee should consider when inquiring about a pharmacy position.

As the geriatric age group increases over the next decades, so will the need for qualified medical personnel. Pharmacy technicians are very knowledgeable about the challenges and benefits that pharmacy has to offer. The future of technicians still is being determined, but judging from the advances currently being made by technicians, the only limitations for pharmacy technicians are self-imposed. Many pharmacy companies reimburse their technicians after they pass the PTCB examination. This is more likely to take place in states in which certification is not mandatory but preferred. Attaining higher level skills, including becoming a certified pharmacy technician, opens more doors for technicians in pharmacy.

Professional Technician Associations

There are many pharmacy associations that technicians can join (Table 3-3). Each association has requisite yearly dues, and each has different benefits. These organizations offer continuing education programs and regular conferences or seminars. The following sections give a brief history of each of the national associations. Throughout history it has become clear that professions that form associations provide their participants with an avenue to make changes and advance their careers. It is important that pharmacy technicians not only join pharmacy associations to keep abreast of new information, but

TABLE 3-3

Organizations and Associations for Pharmacy Technicians*

Name of Organization/ Association	Technicians	Pharmacists	Educators	Annual Fees	Special Category/ Technician Student Fees	Journal or Magazine Included	Website
ASHP (has state chapters)	Yes	Yes	N/A	$69 with journal[†]	No/state chapters vary	*AJHP Journal*[‡]	www.ashp.org
APhA (has state chapters)	Yes	Yes	N/A	$67 with journal[†]	No	*JAPhA Journal*[‡]	www.pharmacist.com
AAPT	Yes	Yes	N/A	$40	$10	None	www.pharmacytechnician.com
NPTA	Yes	No	N/A	$69	No	*Today's Technician*	www.pharmacytechnician.org
NCPA	Yes	Yes	N/A	$75	No	None	www.ncpanet.org
PTEC	Yes	Yes	Yes	$86; $55 without journal	No	*Journal of Pharmacy Technology*	www.pharmacytecheducators.com

ASHP, American Society of Health-System Pharmacists; *APhA,* American Pharmacists Association; *AAPT,* American Association of Pharmacy Technicians; *N/A,* not applicable; *NPTA,* National Pharmacy Technician Association; *NCPA,* National Community Pharmacists Association; *PTEC,* Pharmacy Technician Education Council.

*Updated July 15, 2013.

[†]Fees may vary based on state.

[‡]Included for fee.

also that they become active participants. Benefits of association membership include perks such as free CE courses and access to journals; opportunities to attend local, state, and national conventions; and numerous networking possibilities. Association membership is an excellent way for a technician to advance his or her career and form lifelong friendships with pharmacy colleagues.

American Pharmacists Association (APhA)

The APhA, the oldest and largest pharmacist association, was founded in 1852. Members, including pharmacists, technicians, pharmacy students, scientists, and other interested parties, participate in conferences and discussions on pharmacy issues around the world. The association holds annual meetings, which offer opportunities for CE courses and networking. The APhA also participates in the formation of several important government policies, such as Medicare Part D. Technicians can join their local state pharmacists' association in addition to this national organization.

American Society of Health-System Pharmacists (ASHP)

In 1942, 154 members of the APhA separated to form the American Society of Hospital Pharmacists. In 1945 this group established focus areas on minimum standards of pharmaceutical services in the hospital and education about new techniques and medications. The group expanded over time, and in 1950 it published its journal, *Mirror of Hospital Pharmacy.* After the group received feedback from more than 3,000 hospitals, the journal began to publish recommendations to enhance the development of hospital pharmacy. In 1995 it expanded its outreach to areas other than hospital pharmacists. Under its new name, the American Society of Health-System Pharmacists, the association now includes other pharmacy settings, such as home care and ambulatory care; however, most of its members are pharmacists based in hospital settings. The ASHP Commission on Credentialing (COC) is responsible for the accreditation of pharmacy residency programs and pharmacy technician education and training programs. In 2013 the COC finalized a new accreditation standard for pharmacy technician education and training programs that will take effect on January 15, 2015. The new standard was developed to protect the public, to serve as a guide for the development of pharmacy technician education and training programs, and to provide criteria for the evaluation of new and established programs. The ASHP allows technicians to join, and local state chapters also are available.

American Association of Pharmacy Technicians (AAPT)

The **American Association of Pharmacy Technicians (AAPT)**, the first pharmacy technician association, was established in 1979. It has always been managed by volunteer pharmacy technicians and participates in the advancement of pharmacy technicians. Its membership comprises pharmacy technicians, pharmacists, and pharmacy students. The AAPT is a not-for-profit association that serves technicians' interests through the work of the executive board, committees, national office, and local chapters. The AAPT is very involved with the changes occurring in the pharmacy technician field. It offers continuing education programs and a career center to help technicians with their job searches.

National Community Pharmacists Association (NCPA)

The NCPA was founded in 1898 under the National Association of Retail Druggists. Members include pharmacists, pharmacy owners, managers, pharmacy students, and pharmacy technicians. The NCPA represents the professional and proprietary interests of independent community pharmacists. The association is dedicated to the continued growth and prosperity of the independent pharmacies in the United States. The NCPA is governed by elected officers, a chief executive officer, and a board of directors. NCPA committees include technology and communications, compounding, long-term care, national legislation and government affairs, and pharmacy payment programs. The NCPA works on many issues affecting the independent community pharmacy, including health care reform, Medicare Part D, pharmacy benefits manager (PBM) transparency, and stopping legislation promoting mandatory mail-order prescription filling.

National Pharmacy Technician Association (NPTA)

The **National Pharmacy Technician Association (NPTA)** was started in 1999 in Houston. The next year, the association published its magazine, *Today's Technician,* and had its first convention. In 2004 the NPTA gained the approval of the ACPE and began offering its own CE courses. In 2005 the NPTA joined the Committee of European Pharmacy Technicians (CEPT), a European technicians' association. The NPTA also is part of an advocacy group that works to advance education and acknowledgment for technicians. The association's strategic vision includes:

- Mandatory competency-based exams
- Mandatory registration

- Standardized formal education and training requirements
- ACPE-accredited continuing education requirements
- A pharmacy technician representative on each state board of pharmacy

The association is composed of pharmacy technicians from a variety of practice settings, such as retail, nuclear, hospital, independent, formal education, long-term care, and mail-order pharmacies. The NPTA is dedicated to advancing the value of pharmacy technicians in pharmaceutical care.

Professionalism in the Workplace

Pharmacy is an important profession, and pharmacy technician is a great career. As with many things in life, you get out of it what you put into it. If you put 100% effort into your career as a technician, you can achieve a great deal of satisfaction.

A *profession* is a job, occupation, or line of work that becomes a career; a profession is founded on specialized training. **Professionalism** is conforming to the right principles of conduct (work ethics) as accepted by others in the profession. It takes time, hard work, and consistency to be respected as a professional. Because of the increasing depth of education and training that a pharmacy technician needs, today's technicians are the first generation of pharmacy technicians who have been considered professionals. If they do not meet certain responsibilities, they will remain pharmacy assistants and not professionals in the eyes of other health care professionals.

One of the measures of professionalism is projecting the correct behavior; this includes your attitude and interpersonal skills, in addition to your level of competence. Pharmacy technicians work daily with patients, pharmacists, physicians, and nurses (Figure 3-4). How technicians conduct themselves in various situations reveals their professionalism and their personal maturity.

In a 2008 survey of more than 2,000 businesses in the state of Washington, employers said entry-level workers in a variety of professions were lacking in several areas, including problem solving, conflict resolution, and critical observation. These employers came up with a list of six soft skills that every employee needs.

1. Communication skills: These skills include the ability to write a coherent memo, persuade others with a presentation, or simply be able to explain to a co-worker what one needs.
2. Teamwork and collaboration: Employers need people who can work together toward a common goal, who can easily transition from leader to follower, and who can meet assigned deadlines.

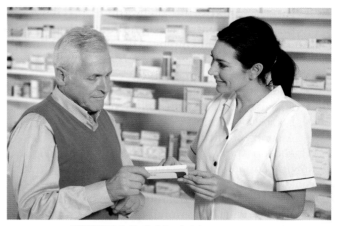

FIGURE 3-4 Technician helping a customer.

3. Adaptability: This skill focuses on the employee's ability to embrace learning and adapt to the changing needs of the organization.
4. Problem solving: Employers expect workers to face problems with a positive attitude. They want people who can explain a dilemma and how it should be approached, involving team members in devising a solution that provides measurable results.
5. Critical observation: This skill involves going beyond the ability to collect and manipulate data; it includes the ability to analyze and interpret it.
6. Conflict resolution: This skill entails being able to negotiate win-win solutions to serve the best interests of the company and the individuals involved.

According to the 2013 Professionalism in the Workplace Study, conducted by the Center for Professional Excellence (CPE) at York College of Pennsylvania, a large portion of the study's participants believed that the professionalism of new employees had decreased over the previous 5 years. Research points to the generation gap between hiring managers and human resources (HR) professionals and the younger entry-level employees as a possible cause. This gap seems to center around the definition of professional standards, which business leaders and managers do not think should change over time. They believe that younger workers should conform to the current standards instead of changing them to match larger societal norms.

The results of the study showed that to be professional in the workplace, an employee should demonstrate the following qualities:

- Appropriate appearance
- Punctuality and regular attendance
- Honesty
- Task completion
- Communication skills

- Interpersonal skills, including civility
- Ability to remain focused and attentive

An unprofessional employee displays the following characteristics:

- Inappropriate appearance
- Poor time management
- Disrespectful or rude behavior
- Poor work ethic
- A sense of entitlement

Based on the research from the CPE study, the following can give a job candidate an edge in getting hired:

1. Learn what it means to be professional.
2. Be committed to doing quality work.
3. Remember, appearance matters.
4. Control your on-the-job use of technology.
5. Be prepared for the interview.

Professional Dress

Statistics from the 2013 Professionalism in the Workplace Study show that 80.6% of the respondents believed that appearance has a high impact on the probability of a candidate being hired. Appearance and attire were also linked with the public's confidence in an employee's ability to perform his or her job requirements. Pharmacy is predominantly a conservative profession. Dressing professionally includes proper clothing, shoes, and hairstyle. Unnatural hair color, facial jewelry, visible tattoos, or any other feature that draws attention away from your personality should be avoided. Medical personnel should appear to be professional, knowledgeable, and competent. It is important that the pharmacy technician show the public that he or she is professional and does not view the vocation as just a job.

Pharmacy technicians must strive to maintain professional behavior when dealing with customers, pharmacists, and fellow health care workers. A professional is honest and dependable and displays integrity in all situations. Job candidates who understand professionalism have a distinct advantage over those who do not.

 Tech Note!

Each year pharmacy technicians celebrate their profession. National Pharmacy Technician Day is observed on the Tuesday of National Pharmacy Week, which is always the third week of October.

The Resume

One of the first encounters you will have with your future employer is through your resume. Recruiters spend only about 10 seconds reviewing each resume. That is why yours should be concise, structured, and

BOX 3-9

Helpful Resume Websites

The following websites can be helpful for the preparation of resumes and letters of interest:

msn.careerbuilder.com
www.1st-writer.com/free_resume_examples.htm
www.collegegrad.com/resume/
    freeresumetemplate.shtml
www.resume-help.org
www.resumeimproved.com
www.resume-now.com

specific. Each resume objective should be tailored to the position for which you are applying. Update it regularly to include recent information pertinent to the current job application. Resumes should be approximately one page long. If possible, list jobs in which you have had customer service experience or those in which you managed yourself or others. These are highly valuable skills that will get you noticed. Because HR managers may not always be familiar with your former employers, it is a good idea to include a hyperlink to the company in the Experience section of your resume. Make sure you can obtain references from your employers at those jobs. Always have references ready on a separate page for your future employer. If you have little or no employment history, focus on your academic qualifications and related skills. Align your achievements with the qualities desired by the hiring organization. Demonstrate your goals and how you will add value to the organization. Seek help in writing your resume and have others look at it to see whether it looks professional (Box 3-9). Larger pharmacy companies may have a standardized format to automate the filing of your resume online. In such cases, it may be helpful to familiarize yourself with the information they request before submitting your application. Don't forget that many hiring managers use social media to search for employees. It is a good idea to include a hyperlink to your LinkedIn profile in the Contact section of your resume.

The Job Search

Job searching has changed drastically over the past several years. Applicants can no longer rely on a generic resume and cover letter to get the job. Now it's about customization and standing out from the crowd. The following are a few suggestions to help you in today's competitive job market.

- Search for specific jobs.
  - Online job listings can be difficult to decipher. Try to stick with sites, such as *US.jobs*, that will

take you directly to the employer website and apply for the position you are most interested in.

- Be prepared for multiple interviews, including some via Skype or Webcam.
  - According to a recent Forbes article, 6 out of 10 recruiters use video interviewing.
- Contact the hiring manager directly.
  - Use sites such as LinkedIn to find specific contact information
- Create and maintain social media profiles.
  - LinkedIn, Twitter, and Facebook can serve as platforms to showcase your accomplishments. Employers are constantly scanning profiles on social media, so be careful what you post. Double-check your spelling and grammar.
- Apply for numerous positions.
  - Interviewing keeps your skills sharp.
- Stay positive.
  - A job search can be stressful, with setbacks and rejections. Remember, you have desirable skills to offer, and you will be an asset to any employer. Hiring managers prefer to hire happy people!

Box 3-10 presents websites that can be helpful in the job search.

Why not start your career while in school? Many student technicians are employed as pharmacy clerks. The benefits are endless; working as a pharmacy clerk not only can strengthen and expand the student's knowledge base about drugs, but also can provide insight into the business of pharmacy and even a possible future job as a technician.

The Future of Pharmacy Technicians Is Bright!

The role of the pharmacy technician is changing! Technicians of the past focused on task-oriented jobs and could be trained by the employer. Today's technician positions are specialized and highly technical in nature. The demand for educated, certified, and

---

> ## BOX 3-10
>
> ### Job Search Engines and Websites
>
> The following websites can be used to search for pharmacy technician jobs:
>
> http://pharmacyjobs.rxcareercenter.com
> www.allpharmacyjobs.com/infusion_pharmacy_jobs.htm
> www.healthjobsusa.com/
> www.careerbuilder.com
> www.indeed.com
> http://linkedin.com
> www.monster.com
> www.pharmacy.org/job.html
> www.pharmacychoice.com/careers/pharmtech.cfm
> http://certified.pharmacy.technician.jobs.com/

skilled pharmacy technicians is great. According to the Bureau of Labor Statistics' *Occupational Outlook Handbook,* the pharmacy technician job market is expected to grow at a rate of 20% through 2022, which is much faster than the average for all occupations. A technician who has graduated from an accredited program and is nationally certified will be the preferred hire. Traditional settings, such as the retail or hospital pharmacy, are not the only places you will find technicians working today. There are many other options for those who do not want to work in the traditional roles. For example, pharmacy technicians can be employed by the federal government (e.g., VA hospitals, prisons, and military pharmacies), quality control offices (repackaging facilities), software companies (pharmacy system software development), and insurance companies (medication consultants). These changes can be positive but challenging as pharmacy technicians take on new and expanded roles. Technicians should be excited about the possibilities the future holds. The outlook for the pharmacy technician is bright!

DO YOU REMEMBER THESE KEY POINTS?

- The common responsibilities and competencies technicians need to function in various pharmacy settings
- Nondiscretionary duties and skills pharmacy technicians can perform
- The ASHP model curriculum and how it relates to technician training
- The levels of pharmacy technician status and the requirements of each
- The process involved in obtaining national certification and the benefits for technicians

- The requirements for maintaining one's national certification after passing the examination
- The advanced pharmacy positions and certifications available to pharmacy technicians
- The types of associations available for pharmacy technicians to join
- The importance of professionalism and networking and how they relate to the job search

Scenario FOLLOW UP

As Olivia continues in her independent pharmacy career, she gradually is gaining more and more responsibilities. She is now able to process prescriptions on the computer. She has learned the inventory ordering system and is involved in processing out-of-date medications. Her communication skills continue to improve, and she is beginning to recognize the customers by name. The pharmacists she works with are very pleased with her progress and professionalism and expect her to continue to excel.

REVIEW QUESTIONS

Multiple Choice Questions

1. The pharmacy association that accredits pharmacy technician education programs is the:
   A. National Pharmacy Technician Association
   B. American Association of Pharmacy Technicians
   C. American Society of Health-System Pharmacists
   D. American Pharmacists Association

2. How often does a nationally certified pharmacy technician have to renew his or her certification?
   A. Yearly
   B. Biannually
   C. Biennially
   D. Every 3 years

3. Which of the following is considered a nondiscretionary duty a pharmacy technician can perform?
   A. Returning expired or damaged stock
   B. Recommending an OTC cold medication
   C. Advising patients about current medications
   D. Changing an order for an IV base

4. Which of the following organizations could revoke a technician's registration?
   A. BOP
   B. ASHP
   C. ACPE
   D. All of the above

5. All pharmacies in their respective states are overseen by:
   A. The National Association of Boards of Pharmacy
   B. Each state's board of pharmacy
   C. Pharmacy managers
   D. Consumer advocacy groups

6. Which of the following would *not* be performed by an inpatient pharmacy technician?
   A. Ordering stock
   B. Accepting payments from patients
   C. Filling medication orders
   D. All of the above would be performed by an inpatient pharmacy technician.

7. Which quality is considered a soft skill preferred by employers?
   A. Honesty
   B. Experience
   C. Personality
   D. Adaptability

8. Once nationally certified by the PTCB, a technician must attain _____ CE units in medication safety every 2 years.
   A. 1
   B. 2
   C. 3
   D. 20

9. Which of the following is an example of a closed door pharmacy?
   A. Children's hospital pharmacy
   B. Nuclear pharmacy
   C. Independent pharmacy
   D. Community pharmacy

10. When preparing a resume, you should:
    A. Have 2 to 3 pages to show all of your accomplishments
    B. Add your LinkedIn profile information to the Contact section
    C. Add your references to the bottom of your resume
    D. All of the above

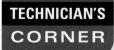

TECHNICIAN'S CORNER Julie is a recent graduate of an accredited pharmacy technician program. She just passed her national certification exam. She has been selected for an interview with a local community pharmacy. Julie has been asked to arrive for the interview with the pharmacist at 1 PM and to bring her resume. Discuss what steps Julie should take to prepare for this interview. How can she demonstrate professionalism and confidence? Julie has a small nose piercing. Should she remove this for the interview? Why or why not?

Bibliography

Harteker LR: *The pharmacy technician companion,* Washington, DC, 1998, American Pharmacists Association.

Manual for pharmacy technicians, ed 3, Bethesda, Md, 2004, American Society of Health-System Pharmacists.

Nordenberg T: Make no mistake: medical errors can be deadly serious. FDA Consumer Sep-Oct 2000. Retrieved March 2, 2003, at www.fda.gov/fdac/features/2000/500_err.html

Phillips J: Generic name confusion. *FDA Safety Page, Drug Topics* 147:90, 2003.

US Food and Drug Administration. Laws. Retrieved July 2, 2013, at www.fda.gov

Western Career College curriculum, Sacramento, Calif, Western Career College.

White paper on pharmacy technicians 2002: Needed changes can no longer wait, *Am J Health-Syst Pharm* 60:37, 2003. Retrieved November 15, 2009, at www.acpe-accredit.org/pdf/whitePaper.pdf

Websites Referenced

A brief history of online pharmacy restrictions. (Referenced January 13, 2014). www.safemedicines.org/online-pharmacy-regulation.html

Accreditation Council for Pharmacy Education. (Referenced July 10, 2013) www.acpe-accredit.org/

American Society of Healthcare Pharmacists. Model curriculum for pharmacy technician training. (Referenced June 29, 2013). www.ashp.org

Center for Drug Evaluation and Research. (Referenced July 10, 2013). www.fda.gov/cder

ExCPT. ICPT creates on-demand testing, the preferred method for certification exams. (Referenced July 3, 2013). www.nationaltechexam.org/documents/On-demand-testing-090908.pdf

Institute for the Certification of Pharmacy Technicians. Code of Ethics for Pharmacy Technicians. (Referenced July 15, 2013). www.nationaltechexam.org/pdf/code-of-ethics.pdf

Koln LT, Corrigan JM, Donaldson MS: To err is human: building a safer health system. Retrieved March 2, 2003, at http://books.nap.edu/books/030906837/html/R1.html

Pharmacy Technician Certification Board. Franco M et al: The National Association of Boards of Pharmacy (NABP) moves to next phase of technician recognition and regulation. May 27, 2009. http://www.ptcb.org/docs/press-releases/the-national-association-of-boards-of-pharmacy-(nabp)-moves-to-next-phase-of-technician-recognition-and-regulation.pdf?sfvrsn=4 (Referenced February 7, 2013).

Pharmacy Technician Career Guide. (Referenced January 13, 2014). V-TECS.org

PTCB announces certification program changes by PTCB staff. (Referenced February 7, 2013). http://ptcb.org/about-ptcb/news-room/news-landing/2013/02/27/ptcb-announces-certification-program-changes#.UeVBkI1QGjk

http://jobsearch.about.com/od/resumetips/fl/best-resume-tips-2014.htm (Referenced February 9, 2104),

http://ptcb.org/docs/get-certified/new_ptce_blueprint.pdf?sfvrsn=6 (Referenced February 8, 2014).

www.aacp.org/governance/COMMITTEES/professionalaffairs/Docs/2014%20PAC%20Charge%201%20Draft%201.13.14.docx (Referenced February 9, 2014).

www.healthcaresource.com/marquis/index.cfm?fuseaction=search.jobDetails&template=dsp_job_details.cfm&cJobId=760506&source=Indeed.com (Referenced February 8, 2014).

www.jobs.net/jobs/rx-relief/en-us/job/united-states/pharmacy-technician-closed-door-facility/J3F45879MSBRMNFVYHP/ (Referenced February 8, 2014).

www.linkedin.com/jobs2/view/9132852 (Referenced February 8, 2014).

www.nabp.net/programs/cpe-monitor/cpe-monitor-service (Referenced January 13, 2014).

www.ncpanet.org/index.php/home/ncpas-mission (Referenced February 9, 2014).

www.ycp.edu/media/york-website/cpe/York-College-Professionalism-in-the-Workplace-Study-2013.pdf (Referenced February 9, 2014).

Communication and Role of the Technician with the Customer/Patient

Bobbi Steelman

OBJECTIVES

Upon completing this chapter, you should be able to do the following:

1. Describe the communication skills needed in the delivery of direct patient care in the pharmacy setting.
2. Explain the communication cycle.
3. Identify various nonverbal and verbal communication skills.
4. Describe ways to improve vocal and verbal communication skills.
5. Use proper telephone and cell phone etiquette and describe its guidelines.
6. Describe the importance of written communication skills in today's workplace.
7. Identify communication skills needed to work with special groups of people, such as the terminally ill, non-English-speaking individuals, and hearing-impaired patients.
8. Explain the significance of working as an effective member of a team.
9. Identify ways to eliminate barriers to effective communication.

TERMS AND DEFINITIONS

Attitude A mental disposition or feeling a technician adopts toward customers, co-workers, or duties at work

Channel A means of communication that can be a written message, spoken words, or body language

Communication The ability to express oneself in such a way that one is understood readily and clearly

Compassion A feeling of wanting to help someone who is sick or in trouble

Diplomacy The skill of dealing with others without causing bad feelings

Etiquette An unwritten guideline or rule of behavior

Perception The way a person thinks about or understands someone or something

Nonverbal communication The act of giving or exchanging information without using spoken words

Tact The ability to do or say things without offending or upsetting other people

Verbal communication The sharing of information by individuals through the use of speech

Introduction

> ### Scenario:
>
> Catherine is a lead technician at a local grocery store pharmacy. She is in charge of training newly hired technicians. Catherine and her supervising pharmacist have developed a 4-week program to help the new trainees integrate successfully into the pharmacy workplace. Currently, Catherine is working with Jackson, preparing for his first day on the job. Module one of the 4-week program is titled "Communication." What topics do you expect Catherine to cover with Jackson in this first section?

Communication

Probably one of the most prevalent concerns of pharmacy managers and pharmacists is the need for pharmacy technicians who are competent in the area of communication. **Communication** is the ability to express oneself in such a way that one is understood readily and clearly. Pharmacy technicians communicate daily with co-workers, health care professionals, and customers (Figure 4-1).

Effective communication skills are critical in achieving optimal patient satisfaction and trust. Virtually all employers consider basic communication abilities a prerequisite to hiring. A competent technician has excellent written and verbal communication skills. In addition, technicians are expected to use skills such as **diplomacy**, **compassion**, sensitivity, responsibility, **tact**, and patience. Good communication is also important for patient safety. A technician who knows exactly what the patient needs and understands how to communicate is able to assist the person with confidence and accuracy.

The Communication Cycle

The communication cycle involves two or more individuals exchanging information. The cycle consists of a sender, a receiver, a message, various channels of communication, and feedback (Figure 4-2). The sender is the person who initiates the communication and sends the message across a **channel**. A channel can be written messages, spoken words, or body language. The receiver decodes the message and provides feedback according to his or her understanding of what is being communicated. To provide optimal patient care, pharmacy technicians must have a clear understanding of the communication cycle.

Listening Skills

Active listening is a communication technique in which listeners confirm understanding by restating or summarizing what they have heard in their own words. This helps both parties make sure the same thing is being discussed. Active listening helps keep the focus on the patient.

Sometimes just listening to a person is all that is required.

If a customer is angry about a medication, regardless of the problem, just listening can ease the person's frustration. Instead of talking over the person or telling the person that he or she is wrong, try to listen until the person is finished and empathize with the dilemma. Most customers know a problem with a medication is not the fault of the pharmacy technician, but they want to be heard. A professional does not allow himself or herself to be directed by another person's inappropriate behavior. Pharmacy technicians must remember to always behave professionally.

Nonverbal Communications

Nonverbal communication, or body language, is the act of giving or exchanging information without using spoken words.

Everyone communicates on a daily basis; however, rarely do we take a step back and evaluate how

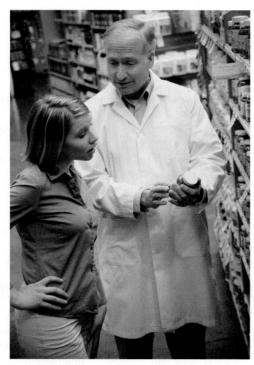

FIGURE 4-1 Communication is very important for pharmacy technicians, especially in daily interactions with customers.

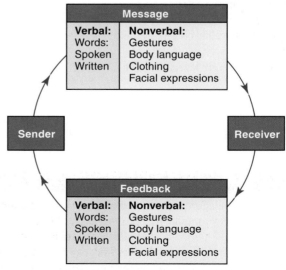

FIGURE 4-2 Communication cycle.

effectively we are communicating. One important aspect of communication is facial expressions. The old phrase "actions speak louder than words" is true. When technicians are working closely with customers in the pharmacy setting or with co-workers, it is important that they maintain a caring but professional attitude at all times.

Most people make a judgment of others within the first 30 seconds of meeting. This is also true in the pharmacy setting. A professional should not bring his or her outside personal problems to work. Stress manifests in various ways, such as frowning, tensing the shoulders, biting one's lip, raising the eyebrows, folding the arms, placing the hands on hips, or other idiosyncrasies. Rolling your eyes or sighing loudly shows impatience and a lack of respect for the customer. If you are counting pills and scowling, the patient may assume you are frustrated. This could keep the person from asking questions or sharing important information. If and when stress begins to transform into this type of body language, it is time to take a step back and maybe a deep breath to help regain focus. If your facial expression is pleasant, the patient will most likely respond in a positive manner. Exhibiting positive body language makes your communication with the patient more effective. The primary goal of pharmacy personnel is to help others, which can be accomplished by being friendly and remaining calm. Facial expressions can show many different emotions, thoughts, and biases. Because you are a pharmacy professional, it is imperative that the only body language you convey is that of a helpful and concerned pharmacy technician.

Box 4-1 presents an example of negative body language. Procedure 4-1 provides an exercise in practicing nonverbal communication.

Verbal Communication

Verbal communication is the sharing of information by individuals through the use of speech.

Verbal communication is an important tool in pharmacy. It is a skill that must be learned and practiced. To be an effective communicator, you must remember that your words and your voice are not always in agreement. Each is a separate entity and can be used to work for or against you. Remember, verbal communication skills have two parts: vocal and verbal.

Vocal Skills: How You Sound

Your voice is a powerful tool that affects the customer or person to whom you are talking. Words alone do not necessarily convey your meaning or feelings; the inflection (pitch), tone, speed, and volume add multitudes of information that is being picked up by the

---

BOX 4-1

Example of Negative Body Language

Ms. Lehman walks up to the counter to have her prescription filled and asks whether it can be done within 5 minutes because her bus will be leaving. John, the pharmacy technician, rolls his eyes and shakes his head in disbelief, wondering why patients think they should never have to wait. He turns and walks away without saying a word.

Alternate response: John shows concern for Ms. Lehman and tells her that her prescription will be filled as soon as possible. John can ask the pharmacist to please fill the prescription as quickly as possible.

PROCEDURE 4-1

Recognizing and Responding to Nonverbal Communications

GOAL: To be able to recognize nonverbal communication and respond to it in a professional manner.

EQUIPMENT AND SUPPLIES
- Various statements that can be communicated in a nonverbal manner

PROCEDURAL STEPS
1. Select a classmate as a partner who will play the role of a patient for this procedure. Use patients of varying cultural backgrounds and ability to communicate in English while practicing the procedure.
   PURPOSE: To practice nonverbal communication with a patient whose responses will not be predictable.
2. Take turns role-playing each nonverbal cue provided.

3. Use appropriate body language and other nonverbal skills in communicating with patients, family, and staff.
   PURPOSE: To make certain that the nonverbal communication sends the same message as the verbal communication.
4. Determine whether the receiver understood the message correctly.
   PURPOSE: To send a nonverbal message that is understood by the receiver.
5. Analyze communications in providing appropriate responses and feedback.
   PURPOSE: To continually improve the communications process between health care professionals, other staff members, and patients.

listener. As an example of the use of inflection, in the following statements, stress the capped word while you say each sentence to a partner, and notice your partner's response to each statement.

- IF you'll wait a moment, I'll get the information you need.
- If you'll WAIT a moment, I'll get the information you need.
- If you'll wait a moment, I'll get the information you need.

As you can see, or hear in this case, the way in which you emphasize a word in a sentence makes a big difference in how it is perceived.

How to Improve Your Vocal Communication Skills

- Try not to talk using the same tone all the time (monotone voice) because it loses the listener's interest and attention.
- Do not talk too rapidly to a customer; the customer may not be able to follow what you are saying.
- Talking very slowly indicates you do not know the answer; if the latter is the case, contact the pharmacist.
- People prefer a lower pitched voice; high, squeaky tones can annoy the listener, and they can result in the listener taking you less seriously.
- A loud or extremely soft voice can annoy and irritate people; speak in a medium tone of voice so you can be heard.
- Articulation is extremely important; mumbling, mispronouncing words, or using slang is one of the fastest ways of sounding unprofessional. Speak in clear, crisp words and sentences.

Verbal Skills: What You Say

Words are also a strong tool that can calm or escalate a situation between you and a customer or patient. Using intimidating words, belittling a person's opinion, or leaving the customer feeling embarrassed, angry, or sad may alienate the patient and result in a loss of business.

 Tech Note!

Remember, customers can choose where they want to fill their prescriptions. Many choices are available to today's consumer. If patients can essentially get the same medication at numerous pharmacies, what is the deciding factor in where they take their business? When all things are equal, such as price and availability, the pharmacy staff is what makes the difference. People want to shop where they receive warm, friendly service and where the staff knows their name. Technicians can be that difference! As author and motivational speaker John C. Maxwell said, "People don't care how much you know, until they know how much you care!"

Be careful of the words you use while addressing a customer. If the customer is definitely wrong, do not tell the person that he or she is wrong. Instead, after carefully listening to the customer, point out the misconception to let the customer know that you understand how this point could be easily confused. Determine which of the scenarios in the following boxes is most appropriate.

Option 1

Customer: When I called earlier, they said the prescriptions would be done by noon; now you tell me they aren't ready. Why do you guys lie like that?
Technician: We don't lie; you probably called in late.
Customer: Oh no; I think I called it in around 10 AM.
Technician: Well, either way, you'll have to wait.
Customer: Let me talk to your manager.

Option 2

Customer: When I called earlier, they said the prescriptions would be done by noon; now you tell me they aren't ready. Why do you guys lie like that?
Technician: I'm sorry; I know the automated system said they would be done by noon, but that's for prescriptions that were called in by a certain time. Did you call in your prescription before 9 AM?
Customer: Oh no; I think I called it in around 10 AM.
Technician: That's okay; let me go take a look to see whether we can get your prescription ready for you as soon as possible.
Customer: Thanks.

How to Improve Your Verbal Skills

- Reading increases your vocabulary.
- Take a course in communication.
- Several types of communication aids are available that you can use to increase your vocabulary, such as CDs, DVDs, and Internet sites.
- Always try to put yourself in the customer's position when talking to him or her. Often the customer is sick or in pain and cannot control his or her emotions; however, you can control yours. Even if the customer is wrong, arguing will not help the situation; instead, it will energize the discussion with negativity. However, if a customer is abusive, the technician should not engage in this type of communication and should notify the pharmacist in charge immediately. If the pharmacist cannot rectify the problem, security is normally called, and the patient is escorted from the premises. Procedure 4-2 provides an exercise for practicing verbal communication skills.

PROCEDURE 4-2

Recognizing and Responding to Verbal Communications

GOAL: To be able to recognize verbal communication and respond to it in a professional manner.

EQUIPMENT AND SUPPLIES
• Various patient scenarios

PROCEDURAL STEPS
1. Select a classmate as a partner who will play the role of a patient for this procedure. Use patients of varying cultural backgrounds and ability to communicate in English while practicing the procedure.
PURPOSE: To practice communication with a patient whose responses will not be predictable.
2. Take turns role-playing each scenario provided.
3. Demonstrate sensitivity appropriate to the message being delivered.

PURPOSE: To send a clearly communicated message.
4. Demonstrate empathy.
PURPOSE: To treat each person fairly and with dignity.
5. Apply active listening skills.
PURPOSE: To make sure your patient understood your message and to allow him or her to communicate a response.
6. Restate the patient's response.
PURPOSE: To ensure that you understood what the patient said.
7. Analyze communications in providing appropriate responses and feedback.
PURPOSE: To continually improve the communications process between health care professionals, other staff members, and patients.

Optimize Your Communication

The following are a few tips to optimize your communication abilities.

1. **Use open-ended questions.** This gets you more than just a "yes" or "no" answer. It shows the patient that the conversation is not just one way and that you care about his or her perspective. If you can get a dialogue going with your customer, you may be able to avoid potential errors. For example, if you ask, "Do you have any allergies?" the customer may just say "No" or shake his head. However, if you say, "What type of medications are you allergic to?" the customer will give you a more detailed answer.

2. **Provide empathetic responses.** This shows the customer that you can see the situation from her point of view. When a patient believes you understand how she feels, she is more inclined to share information that could assist with her care. For example, you might have a patient who had a long wait to see the physician with her sick infant. She is clearly stressed and is now waiting to pick up the baby's medication. She asks you why it is taking so long to get one bottle of medicine. An empathetic response might be, "I know you must be exhausted from all of this waiting. I assure you we are working diligently to get your child's medication ready. Helping her get well is our goal."

3. **Minimize distractions.** The goal for every conversation you have with a patient should be to communicate clearly and make sure your message is understood. If needed, take the patient to a quieter space, such as a designated counseling area, to answer any questions or clarify instructions. For example, you may have a patient who

has received a prescription for Cialis. You ask if he would like to speak with the pharmacist about this new medication. He is hesitant because there are several customers within hearing distance. You should suggest that the patient speak with the pharmacist in the counseling area, which is private and away from the other customers.

 Tech Note!

Always treat customers as you would want to be treated. Remember to be kind, courteous, and respectful at all times.

Scenario CHECK UP 4-1

Catherine has reviewed module one with Jackson, and he is ready to begin interacting with the customers. He will be answering the phone for the first part of his shift. She explains to him that the proper way to greet the customer on the phone is by saying, "Thank you for calling BG pharmacy. This is Jackson, a pharmacy technician. How may I help you?" Is it okay for Jackson to put his own touch on the greeting and change the format, as long as he is friendly? Why is it important for him to identify himself each time he answers the phone?

Telephone Etiquette

Another key area of communication in the pharmacy workplace is telephone interactions. A knowledge of proper phone etiquette is important when dealing with patients. **Etiquette** is an unwritten guideline or rule of behavior. Both traditional phone and cell phone guidelines are discussed.

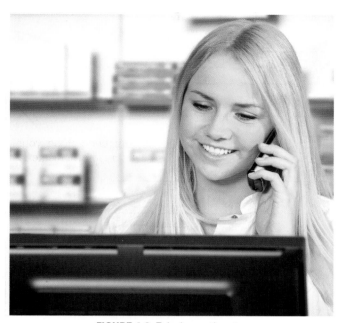

FIGURE 4-3 Telephone etiquette.

BOX 4-2

Example of Unacceptable Phone Etiquette

Patient: Hello, I'm calling because my medication looks different from before, and I need to know if it's the same drug or not.
Pharmacy technician: Would you please hold?
Patient: No, I need to know now because ...
Pharmacy technician: [Places the patient on hold and forgets to get back to the patient.]
  Alternate response: The technician waits to hear the patient's response to the question. When the patient says she cannot wait, the technician waits to hear why and then proceeds to help her.

Answering the phone in a busy pharmacy is traditionally the technician's job. Technicians conduct a great deal of daily business over the telephone. The manner in which they answer the phone can set the tone for the remainder of the conversation. A professional attitude and good judgment should be used at all times. With each call, the technician must decide either to direct the call to the pharmacist or to handle it himself or herself (Figure 4-3).

Sometimes it is necessary to place a customer on hold. If the call must be placed on hold, the technician should check back with the caller at 1- to 2-minute intervals to reassure the patient that he or she has not been forgotten and to verify that the call has not been accidentally disconnected. If the customer raises his or her voice, the technician should let them air the complaint be aired without reacting negatively. The tone of voice used by the technician can either help resolve the problem or escalate a problem into a long, drawn-out argument. It is best to talk in an even tone and always be pleasant and professional. Arguing with the customer can fuel the fire, and the situation may get out of hand, with no resolution (Box 4-2).

Remember the following guidelines when interacting with patients and medical personnel over the phone:

1. Always clearly identify the place of business, your name, and your title when you answer the phone.
2. Carefully listen to the caller to determine the nature of the call.
3. Determine whether the task is within your scope of practice as a technician or whether the call should be forwarded to the pharmacist.
4. If the call can be handled by the technician, make an offer of assistance and restate the purpose of the call before placing the customer on hold or ending the conversation.

🛈 Tech Alert!

Currently, in most states it is not legal for a pharmacy technician to take an oral prescription from a prescriber. As the technician field evolves and more formal education is required, there is reason to believe that technicians may be allowed to perform this function in the future.

Cell Phone Etiquette

According to the Pew Internet Project's research, as of May, 2013:

- 91% of American adults have a cell phone
- 56% of American adults have a smart phone
- 28% of cell phone owners own an Android, 25% of cell phone owners own an iPhone, and 4% own a Blackberry
- 34% of American adults own a tablet computer
- 26% of American adults own an e-reader .

Adult gadget ownership has increased significantly over the past few years; these devices have become a fixture in our daily lives (Figure 4-4).

Good cell phone etiquette is a must for today's pharmacy technicians. There are many ways that cell phones can distract them from delivering excellent customer care. Technicians must be careful not to talk or text on their cell phone while working. Even if you are looking up a drug or medication on your smart phone, it may give the patient the perception that you are focusing on something other than the task at hand. Resist the urge to check your messages or return calls until your break. Technicians have been terminated for inappropriate cell phone use while on the clock. If you have an emergency or an urgent message, ask your supervisor if you can

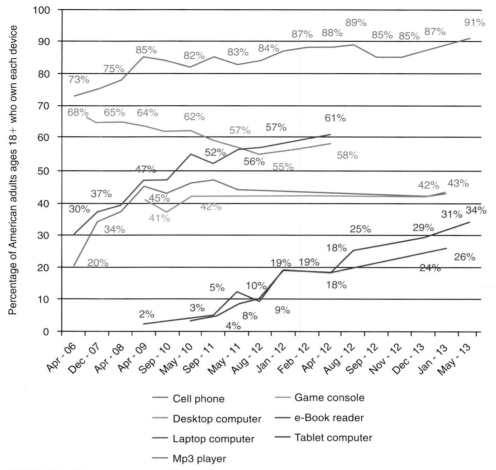

FIGURE 4-4 Adult gadget ownership timeline. Mobile technology fact sheet. Pew Research Center, Washington, D.C. (January 2014). http://www.pewinternet.org/fact-sheets/mobile-technology-fact-sheet (Referenced August 2014).

step out for a moment to check on the call. Excellent patient care should always be your main focus. You cannot afford to be distracted when filling a prescription.

 Tech Note!

Be sure to check with your supervisor about cell phone policies in your workplace. Always err on the side of caution and stay off your phone during work!

Here are a few guidelines for cell phone use in the pharmacy workplace:

1. Always give 100% focus to the customer in front of you. If you are on your phone, your attention is diverted.
2. Keep cell phones out of sight. This could mean in your locker, pocket, handbag, or briefcase.
3. Keep your cell phone on silent or vibrate.
4. Never text or talk on your cell phone while filling a prescription or dealing with a customer.

5. Keep personal calls to a minimum so you do not appear unfocused to the customers or the pharmacy team.

Written Communication Skills

In today's workplace, pharmacy technicians must be proficient in written communication. They must be able to document information, procedures, and actions accurately and clearly. The ability to coordinate written, oral, and electronic communications is vital to a successful pharmacy team. If the technician's writing is inaccurate or illegible, mistakes can be made and poor patient care is the result. Technicians are responsible for written communications such as memos, e-mails, and ordering supplies. Employees with good writing abilities come across as more capable and more credible than their co-workers who make spelling or grammatical errors. In the workplace, remember to proofread all written communications, from e-mails to tweets to company memos.

Message taking is also especially important. Often, technicians take multiple messages for refills or other tasks during a busy pharmacy shift. Sometimes, there may be a delay between the time the message was taken and the time the message is relayed or acted upon. If the message was not written down accurately and legibly, it may be misinterpreted. If a system is not in place on how to record and maintain incoming messages, some may be lost or simply forgotten. The more detailed the message, the less likely the technician is to make a mistake. Illegible handwriting by prescribers can also lead to interpretation problems. Many of the drug errors that have been reported in the news and in medical journals are due to poor handwriting (Box 4-3).

 Tech Note!

Always be sure to get as much information from the caller as possible when taking a message. Be sure to include the date, time, and your initials to avoid confusion. Although a pharmacist needs to check all transcriptions and calculations, it is important that the technician have a good understanding of how to take a message to avoid medication errors.

◢ TECHNICIAN PROFILE

Shelia is an oncology pharmacy technician. She works for a large hospital. Under the direct supervision of the oncology pharmacist, Shelia prepares medication orders for cancer patients. Her duties include compounding or admixing intravenous (IV) drugs, calculating correct dosage volumes by converting between metric and apothecary equivalents, and checking all orders for completeness of information. Record keeping is extremely important. Shelia checks all orders for insurance approval before admixing. This step is crucial because many of these medications are extremely expensive. She maintains current drug inventory and MSDS sheets. All interoffice guidelines and those established by the Occupational Safety and Health Administration (OSHA) must be followed. Shelia's other duties include proper disposal of all materials, both chemotherapy and non-chemotherapy IVs. She must clean the hoods daily or more often as needed. Controlled substances are counted, and weekly logs must be accurate. The requirements for Shelia's position are 2 to 5 years of pharmacy experience in an IV setting, active state registration, CPhT certification, and a clean background check and drug screen. Shelia loves her job because she is able to assist the pharmacist in providing quality medication and care to patients experiencing very difficult challenges. She feels she makes a difference each and every day she goes to work.

Communications with Special Patient Groups

The goal of communication should be to understand and to be clearly understood. The technician should

BOX 4-3

Example of Poor Written Communication Skills

Nurse Johnson calls the pharmacist to ask whether the two drugs she is about to administer are compatible. She is in a hurry. Joe North, CPhT, scribbles down the question but does not get the nurse's name or telephone extension. By the time the nurse calls back to contact the pharmacist, the dose is late and the patient has been in pain while waiting for a response.

Alternate response: The technician, Joe North, tells the nurse he will ask the pharmacist to return her call. Joe then asks for the nurse's name, station, and extension, in addition to the patient's name and medical record number.

Information That Should Be Obtained and Written Down in the Message

- Nurse's or caller's name
- Floor location and extension (hospital setting), the physician's call-back number (community pharmacy), or the patient's preferred call-back number
- The purpose of the call
- The time of the call
- The initials of the technician who took the call
- How soon the information is needed

Only then can a pharmacist quickly and easily relay the correct information to the appropriate person. If your handwriting is illegible, it can cost time and possibly result in a preventable error. There is no excuse for poor handwriting. Poor handwriting is one of the reasons physicians now are transitioning to electronic medication ordering. Thousands of preventable errors can be overcome through the use of computer ordering.

be sensitive to each customer and alert to any special needs the patient might have. This role begins when the technician greets the patient and accepts the prescription.

Terminally Ill Patients

Special consideration should be given to patients who are terminally ill. Remember that they may be feeling overwhelmed. Although each person copes with his or her own mortality differently, there are "normal" progressive steps that people experience. The five stages that terminally ill patients experience are as follows:

Stage	Example
Denial	"This can't be happening …"
Anger	"It isn't fair. I don't deserve this …"
Bargaining	"Please make me better, and I promise …"
Depression	"I will never be able to see you again …"
Acceptance	"I can do this, everyone does …"

Normally the first stage is denial. This is a defense mechanism in which the situation does not seem real. Perhaps the reality is too harsh for the person to accept. The next stage is anger. Sometimes one may have a feeling of unfairness. Bargaining usually follows anger. The person makes promises to himself or herself or to a higher power in the hope of a miracle. Depression may take over at this point, with the realization that nothing is going to change concerning the prognosis. The final phase is acceptance, in which the person concedes his or her own mortality and prepares for eventual death.

Each of these stages can manifest at any time and last for different lengths of time. Therefore, it is important that the technician be compassionate to the patient's situation. Most health care workers do not hesitate to help a dying patient; however, the problem is how to identify these patients. Unfortunately, unless the patient decides to share this information, the pharmacy staff does not necessarily know. Some medications indicate an advancing medical condition. These include pain medications, such as fentanyl patches or morphine; however, these drugs do not definitively identify a fatal condition. Therefore, the pharmacy technician must be objective about each person who enters the pharmacy and realize that he or she does not know what each person is experiencing.

Non-English-Speaking Patients

We live in a culturally diverse society, and technicians often encounter customers who do not speak English as their first language. Technicians who speak multiple languages are in high demand and can play an important role on the pharmacy team. Statistics show that more than 8.6% of the U.S. population speaks English less than "very well." Millions of prescriptions are written for people who have limited English proficiency (LEP) each year. For safety and compliance purposes, it is critical that pharmacy technicians, pharmacists, and LEP patients communicate effectively with each other.

There are many ways pharmacies can help facilitate appropriate communication with the LEP patient. They may employ bilingual staff, provide interpreters, or use software programs that translate the prescription labels and information into various languages. Some pharmacies use pictograms to illustrate a variety of instructions. To view more information on medication pictograms, visit the USP Pictogram Library at *www.usp.org/usp-healthcare-professionals/related -topics-resources/usp-pictograms*

 Tech Note!
Consider learning a foreign language, such a Spanish or Chinese, to increase your employment options.

Hearing-Impaired Patients

Approximately 36 million Americans have hearing loss. An estimated 1 in 3 cases is caused by excessive noise exposure. One in 5 American teens has the same degree of hearing loss found in adults 50 to 60 years old. Considering these statistics, there is a high possibility the pharmacy technician will encounter a hearing-impaired patient. Therefore, it is important to be aware of any special needs the patient might have as the person approaches the pharmacy counter. If you become aware that the patient's hearing is limited or fully impaired, you must determine a plan of action to best interact with that person. First, ask her how she prefers to communicate and note the preference on her patient profile in the computer. Some patients may want to use notes, so the technician should write legibly. However, because many hearing-impaired individuals understand only American Sign Language (ASL), it may be difficult for them to read written English. Others may lip-read, so be sure to look at the patient as you speak. Never yell; instead, use a moderately low voice. If the patient is fully hearing impaired, ask whether anyone knows sign language or if a friend or family member can interpret. Remember to direct your communications to the patient and allow him or her to respond to you through the interpreter. It is considered rude in the deaf community not to keep eye contact when speaking.

 Tech Note!
Consider enrolling in a local American Sign Language class to enhance your ability to communicate with your hearing-impaired customers.

Remember, if the pharmacy technician treats people equally, regardless of their disposition, the technician is behaving appropriately and professionally. The pharmacy technician can influence the development of a positive atmosphere in the pharmacy setting by maintaining an appropriate attitude. **Attitude** is a mental disposition or feeling a technician adopts toward customers, co-workers, or duties at work.

Allowing customers to express frustration, being a good listener, and doing one's best to help others are important components of acting professionally.

Scenario CHECK UP 4-2

Jackson is doing a great job answering the phone. His next call is from a hospice nurse, who begins the conversation by giving Jackson a new prescription for Mr. Jones, a terminally ill cancer patient. What is the problem with this situation? How should Jackson handle this call?

Communication with the Health Care Team

Today, the pharmacy technician is an important member of the health care team. In the retail setting, the team may consist of the technician, the pharmacist, the pharmacy manager, counter personnel, and other store employees. In the institutional setting, the team may include technicians, pharmacists and managers, physicians, nurses, and other departmental personnel. In all pharmacy settings, teams work to provide the best patient care possible. The team leadership establishes clear expectations for each member's responsibilities. Trust and communication are key components of a successful team. Here are a few tips to help you become an effective team player:

1. Make sure you clearly understand your job duties and responsibilities.
2. Take time to discuss the pharmacy's goals with the team.
3. Become a positive part of the decision-making process.
4. Stay informed and know the channels of communication.
5. Be loyal and work to build trust.

Eliminating Communication Barriers

Effective communication is challenging in today's workplace. As discussed earlier, there can be many barriers, such as those involving language differences and hearing impairment. The first step in eliminating these barriers is to recognize that they exist. Then, it is the responsibility of each team member to be knowledgeable about the techniques used to overcome these obstacles. We live in the information age and have access to many devices that help us communicate. However, much of this information exchange lacks real meaning. Real communication occurs when both the speaker and the listener are fully engaged. The best defense against any communication barrier is a strong, cooperative team.

 Tech Note!

Technicians must never assume patients understand medical jargon or pharmacy terminology.

Conclusion

When serving patients, technicians should give each person their undivided attention. They should provide all customers with the opportunity to ask questions. Verification of understanding is needed for optimal compliance and patient safety. Technicians should strive to really hear and understand each individual. Effective communication can increase adherence to treatment and decrease adverse effects, which ultimately leads to improved health and safer patient care.

DO YOU REMEMBER THESE KEY POINTS?

- The terms and definitions covered in this chapter
- The communication skills a competent pharmacy technician must have to successfully relate to both pharmacy team members and customers
- The communication cycle and how it works
- How to incorporate good listening skills into your daily work routine
- The importance of displaying proper body language and how to interpret the body language of others
- The two parts to verbal communication skills: vocal and verbal
- How to use and improve your vocal and verbal communication skills
- Proper telephone and cell phone etiquette
- The importance of good written communication and its role in preventing medication errors
- How to communicate with special groups of people, such as non-English-speaking individuals, those who are hearing impaired, or terminally ill patients
- How to work as an effective pharmacy team member
- Some common communication barriers technicians face when serving patients

Scenario FOLLOW UP

As Jackson completes his training, he thanks Catherine for all the important information she has shared. Her tips for communication both with customers and with medical professionals will serve him well throughout his career. He is now considered a pharmacy tech Level 1, and the pharmacists and other technicians are pleased with his work. What communication challenges do you think Jackson may face as he continues his job as a pharmacy technician?

REVIEW QUESTIONS

Multiple Choice Questions

1. Good communication skills include:
   A. Compassion
   B. Tact
   C. Diplomacy
   D. All of the above
2. Body language should convey an attitude of:
   A. Friendliness and a sense of urgency
   B. Seriousness and professionalism
   C. Helpfulness and concern
   D. Service and dedication
3. This form of communication is judged by others in the first 30 seconds of meeting.
   A. Verbal
   B. Nonverbal
   C. Written
   D. None of the above
4. The primary purpose of having good communication skills is:
   A. To order medications
   B. To relate to pharmacy team members
   C. To relate to customers
   D. All of the above
5. A person's voice can influence how the information is perceived based on:
   A. Inflection
   B. Speed
   C. Volume
   D. All of the above
6. Medication errors have been connected to:
   A. Illegible handwriting
   B. Technician inexperience
   C. Poor phone etiquette
   D. All of the above

7. Which of the following communication tasks is *not* one of the standard technician duties?
   A. Handling angry patients appropriately
   B. Dealing with insurance representatives on the phone
   C. Taking customer refills over the phone
   D. Counseling patients on their medication
8. What is one of the best ways to handle a frustrated customer?
   A. Ask another technician for help
   B. Listen intently
   C. Ask the customer to settle down
   D. All of the above
9. If a technician has tried but is unable to resolve a customer's problem, what step should he or she take next?
   A. Alert the police
   B. Inform the pharmacist
   C. Yell for the technician supervisor
   D. Ask the customer what to do next
10. If any part of a prescription is illegible, technicians should:
    A. Call the prescriber for clarification
    B. Ask another technician for help
    C. See what medication the patient is taking and try to figure it out on their own
    D. None of the above

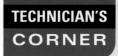 **TECHNICIAN'S CORNER**

Dr. Beth Golden's nurse calls the pharmacy and has the following new prescription for Larry Williams:

    hydrocodone/acetaminophen tablets #50
    Sig: Take 1 tablet q8h prn severe pain
    10 refills

    The pharmacy technician answers the call. Can the technician take the new prescription over the phone? Determine the laws and regulations in your state regarding this call. What other errors do you find in this order?

Bibliography

Ballington DA: *Pharmacy practice for technicians,* ed 4, St Paul, Minn, 2009, EMC/Paradigm.

Gray Morris D: *Calculate with confidence,* ed 6, St Louis, 2013, Elsevier.

National Association of Boards of Pharmacy: *Survey of pharmacy law,* Mount Prospect, Ill, 2013, The Association.

Potter PA, Perry AG: *Fundamentals of nursing,* ed 8, St Louis, 2013, Elsevier.

Proctor DB, Adams AP: *Kinn's the medical assistant,* ed 12, St Louis, 2013, Elsevier.

Websites Referenced

Department of Defense Hearing Center of Excellence. Hearing Loss and Tinnitus in America. (Referenced February 13, 2014.) http://hearing.health.mil/HearingLoss101/StatsandFigures .aspx

Hearing Health Foundation. Hearing Loss and Tinnitus Statistics. (Referenced September 13, 2013.) http://hearinghealthfoundation.org/statistics?gclid=CMbG1dKa1Lk CFY9QOgodMksALw

Learner's Dictionary. (Referenced August 20, 2013.) www.learnersdictionary.com/definition/perception

National Health Law Program. Analysis of State Pharmacy Laws: Impact of Pharmacy Laws on the Provision of Languages Services. (Referenced September 12, 2013.) www.aacp.org/resources/education/documents/pharmacylawbooklet%20final.pdf

Notable Quotes. John C. Maxwell Quotes. (Referenced February 13, 2014.) www.notable-quotes.com/m/maxwell_john_c.html

Pew Research Internet Project. Mobile Technology Fact Sheet. (Referenced September 8, 2013.) http://pewinternet.org/Commentary/2012/February/Pew-Internet-Mobile.aspx

Pharmacy Technician's Letter Online Continuing Education. Effective Communication: A Primer for Technicians. (Referenced February 13, 2014.) http://pharmacytechniciansletter.therapeuticresearch.com/ce/cecourse.aspx?pc=10-402

Rachel Wagner Etiquette and Protocol. Workplace Cell Phone Etiquette—7 Smart Tips. (Referenced September 8, 2013.) www.etiquettetrainer.com/cell-phone-etiquette-workplace/

U.S. Pharmacopeial Convention. USP Pictograms. (Referenced February 13, 2014.) www.usp.org/usp-healthcare-professionals/related-topics-resources/usp-pictograms

WHO Pain and Palliative Care Communications Program. Expanding nurses' role in pain management: international news on nurse prescribing. (Referenced August 16, 2013.) http://whocancerpain.wisc.edu/?q=node/180

Dosage Forms and Routes of Administration

Bobbi Steelman

OBJECTIVES

Upon completing this chapter, you should be able to do the following:

1. List dangerous abbreviations and explain why they are on the "Do Not Use" list.
2. Recognize the general classifications of medications and the related body systems.
3. Identify various dosage formulations and give examples of each.
4. Identify various routes of administration and give examples of each.
5. Explain the difference between pharmacokinetics and pharmacodynamics.
6. List and explain the absorption, distribution, metabolism, elimination, and bioavailability of drugs in the body.
7. Define first-pass metabolism and explain why it is important in drug delivery.

8. Define half-life and describe factors that influence it.
9. Define the bioequivalence of drugs and its relationship to the Orange Book.
10. Describe why excipients (additives) are necessary in the production of medications.
11. List three different common drugs and their storage requirements.
12. List the segments that make up medical terms and provide examples of each.
13. Recognize and interpret common abbreviations as they apply to dosage forms and routes of administration.

TERMS AND DEFINITIONS

Absorption The taking in of nutrients and drugs into the body from food and liquids

Behind-the-counter (BTC) Nonprescription drugs that are kept behind the pharmacy counter; limited amounts may be sold, or the customer may require the permission of a pharmacist to purchase them

Bioavailability The degree to which a drug or other substance becomes available to the target tissue after administration

Bioequivalence The relationship between two drugs that have the same dosage and dosage form and that have similar bioavailability. Generic versions of a medication must show bioequivalence to the original approved brand product as a requirement of drug approval

Distribution The movement of a medication throughout the blood, organs, and tissues after administration

Elimination The final evacuation of a drug or other substance from the body via normal body processes, such as kidney elimination (urine), biliary excretion (bile to stool), sweat, respiration, or saliva

Enteral A route of administration by way of the intestine, such as orally, rectally, or sublingually

First-pass effect A process in which a portion of the drug dose is metabolized before the drug has a chance to be distributed systemically

Half-life 1. The time required for a chemical to be decreased by one half. 2. The time required for half the amount of a substance, such as a drug in a living system, to be eliminated or disintegrated by natural processes. 3. The time required for the concentration of a substance in a body fluid (blood plasma) to decrease by half

Instill To place into; instillation instructions are commonly used for ophthalmic or otic drugs

Legend drugs Drugs that require a prescription; these drugs carry the federal legend: "Federal law prohibits the dispensing of this medication without a prescription"

Metabolism The processes by which the body breaks down or converts medications to active or inactive substances. The primary site of drug metabolism in humans is the liver; however, select drugs are metabolized through other processes

Over-the-counter (OTC) Medications that can be purchased without a prescription

Parenteral A term used to describe a medication that is usually given by injection into a vein, the skin, or muscle that bypasses the gastrointestinal system

Pharmacokinetics The study of the absorption, metabolism, distribution, and elimination of drugs

Pro-drug An inactive substance that is converted to a drug in the body by the action of enzymes or other chemicals

TERMS AND ABBREVIATIONS

Dosage form	Abbreviation/term
Buccal tablet or film	Buccal
Capsule	Cap
Chewable tablet	Chew tab
Diluent	Dil
Elixir	Elix
Enteric-coated tablet	EC tab
Gelatin capsule	Gel cap
Liquid	Liq
Lotion	lot
Lozenge	Loz
Metered dose inhaler	MDI
Mixture	Mix
Ointment	Ung, oint
Patch, transdermal	Patch, TD
Powder	Pdr
Solution	Sol, soln
Suppository	Supp
Suspension	Susp
Syrup	Syr
Tablet	Tab
Tincture	Tinc
Vaginal cream	Vag cr
Vaginal tablet	Vag tab

Main routes of administration (ROA)	Abbreviation
Gastrostomy tube	GT
Inhalant	INH (not to be confused with the abbreviation for isoniazid)
Injection	INJ
Intradermal	ID
Intramuscular	IM
Intrathecal	IT
Intravenous	IV
Intraperitoneal	IP
Intravenous piggyback	IVPB
Nasogastric	NG
Nasogastric tube	NGT
Right ear	AD
Left ear	AS
Both ears	AU
Right eye*	OD
Left eye*	OS
Both eyes*	OU
Orally, by mouth	PO
Rectal, per rectum	PR
Small bowel feeding tube	SBFT
Subcutaneous	SUBCUT, SQ, SC
Vaginal, per vaginal	PV
Sublingual	SL
Topical	TOP

*The Joint Commission (TJC) recommends that the abbreviations OD, OS, and OU be avoided because of possible medication errors due to misinterpretation. TJC suggests that "left ear," "right ear," or "both ears" and "left eye," "right eye," or "both eyes" be written out, for safety purposes.

Introduction

Scenario:

Mary is a new technician at a local compounding pharmacy. She received an associate in applied science (AAS) degree in pharmacy technology and is eager to put her knowledge into practice. After a few days on the job, she realizes that many of the prescriptions are difficult to decipher because of the physician's handwriting. She hesitates to ask for help. What is the best course of action for Mary?

To become proficient in their jobs, pharmacy technicians must be able to interpret orders correctly. Although it may be true that many physicians' handwriting is referred to as "chicken scratch," it is the responsibility of the pharmacy technician and the pharmacist to interpret and clarify orders if necessary. Many of the abbreviations used in prescribing medication look very much alike. For instance, mg (milligram) can look much like mcg (microgram) when written quickly. In this chapter, we explore the common abbreviations seen in pharmacy as they apply to dosage forms and routes of administration. In addition to learning the many different types of dosage forms available and the reasons they are necessary, we will discuss the pharmacokinetics related to the manufacturing of dosage forms. In addition, we will present a brief overview of the segments used to compose medical terms and will cover medical and drug abbreviations.

Where Did Pharmacy Abbreviations Originate?

Much of the terminology in pharmacy and medicine comes from the Latin and Greek languages. Because pharmacy began in Europe, most of the abbreviations have their origins in a foreign language. The use of Latin and Greek has continued into the twenty-first century with little change. Although these abbreviations tend to be confusing at first, they serve an important function. For example, if each pharmacy used its own terminology, it would be virtually impossible for one pharmacy to fill another pharmacy's prescriptions. Therefore, the medical community uses terms in Latin and Greek. These terms serve as a universal language that all medical doctors, nurses, pharmacists, technicians, and other medical personnel can understand. However, the ability to clarify prescribers' orders is still a real dilemma in the United States. The number of errors caused by prescribers' poor handwriting and by inaccurate transcribing of orders by pharmacists and technicians is a great concern (see Chapter 14). Correct interpretation of prescribers' orders by pharmacy staff is obviously extremely important. Interpreting orders can be a time-consuming function of filling prescriptions, and most patients want their medications quickly. This time pressure leaves the pharmacy staff little time to confer or call physicians' offices for every unclear order; however, clarifications must be made if errors are to be avoided. The pharmacy technician must be careful to write the various abbreviations as neatly as possible because other technicians and pharmacists will be reading their writing. Scrolls, stylized, or fancy lettering can easily be misinterpreted. The pharmacy technician must

learn all of the dosage forms and their abbreviations to decipher prescribers' orders.

"Do Not Use" List

Because of the concern over drug errors that have occurred from the misinterpretation of medication orders, both the Institute for Safe Medication Practices (ISMP) and the Joint Commission (TJC) have provided a "Do Not Use List" that outlines the most common misread abbreviations. To reduce the number of mistakes, all practitioners have been informed that these abbreviations should be avoided. In this chapter these specific abbreviations have been included in the Terms and Abbreviations list at the start of the chapter so that student technicians will recognize them when they encounter them. However, these abbreviations should be avoided and instead spelled out in full. The "Do Not Use List" from TJC is provided in Table 5-1, and the list from the ISMP is provided in Table 5-2, which addresses all the areas that influence drug errors.

Dosing Instructions

Dosing times are also abbreviated on prescriptions. Although many abbreviations are listed as "Do Not Use," per the recommendations of both TJC and the ISMP, they will be seen in many orders. In addition, many pharmacy computers are programmed to accept these abbreviations.

Scenario CHECK UP 5-1

Mary continues to enjoy working at the local compounding facility. Her pharmacist gives her a copy of the "Do Not Use" list of abbreviations and asks her to become familiar with it. At first, Mary was skeptical about the value of studying the list. Then one day, as she was compounding a hormone cream, she came across the abbreviation "HS." Did the physician intend for the directions to mean half-strength or at bedtime? At that moment, she realized the significance of the list she had been asked to study. She consulted the pharmacist, who clarified the directions with the physician. What could have been the worst-case scenario in this situation?

Classifications of Medications

Classifications of medications place drugs into groups. Although many medications are used for reasons other than their intended purpose, it is important to know the body system a medication is intended to affect. Each drug can be further broken down into groupings based on pharmacology, intent

TABLE 5-1

The Joint Commission's Official "Do Not Use" List*

Do Not Use	Potential Problem	Use Instead
U, u (unit)	Mistaken for "0" (zero), the number "4" (four) or "cc"	Write "unit"
IU (International Unit)	Mistaken for IV (intravenous) or the number "10" (ten)	Write "International Unit"
Q.D., QD, q.d., qd (daily)	Mistaken for each other	Write "daily"
Q.O.D., QOD, q.o.d, qod (every other day)	Period after the Q mistaken for "i" and the "O" mistaken for "i"	Write "every other day"
Trailing zero (X.0 mg)†	Decimal point is missed	Write X mg
Lack of leading zero (.X mg)		Write 0.X mg
MS	Can mean morphine sulfate or magnesium sulfate	Write "morphine sulfate"
MSO₄ and MgSO₄	Confused for one another	Write "magnesium sulfate"

*Applies to all orders and all medication-related documentation that is handwritten (including free-text computer entry) or on preprinted forms.

†A trailing zero may be used only where required to demonstrate the level of precision of the value being reported, such as for laboratory results, imaging studies that report the size of lesions, or catheter/tube sizes. It may not be used in medication orders or other medication-related documentation.

© The Joint Commission, 2014. Reprinted with permission.

TABLE 5-2

ISMP's List of *Error-Prone Abbreviations, Symbols*, and *Dose Designations*

The abbreviations, symbols, and dose designations found in this table have been reported to ISMP through the ISMP National Medication Errors Reporting Program (ISMP MERP) as being frequently misinterpreted and involved in harmful medication errors. They should **NEVER** be used when communicating medical information. This includes internal communications, telephone/verbal prescriptions, computer-generated labels, labels for drug storage bins, medication administration records, as well as pharmacy and prescriber computer order entry screens.

Abbreviations	Intended Meaning	Misinterpretation	Correction
μg	Microgram	Mistaken as "mg"	Use "mcg"
AD, AS, AU	Right ear, left ear, each ear	Mistaken as OD, OS, OU (right eye, left eye, each eye)	Use "right ear," "left ear," or "each ear"
OD, OS, OU	Right eye, left eye, each eye	Mistaken as AD, AS, AU (right ear, left ear, each ear)	Use "right eye," "left eye," or "each eye"
BT	Bedtime	Mistaken as "BID" (twice daily)	Use "bedtime"
cc	Cubic centimeters	Mistaken as "u" (units)	Use "mL"
D/C	Discharge or discontinue	Premature discontinuation of medications if D/C (intended to mean "discharge") has been misinterpreted as "discontinued" when followed by a list of discharge medications	Use "discharge" and "discontinue"
IJ	Injection	Mistaken as "IV" or "intrajugular"	Use "injection"
IN	Intranasal	Mistaken as "IM" or "IV"	Use "intranasal" or "NAS"
HS	Half-strength	Mistaken as bedtime	Use "half-strength" or "bedtime"
hs	At bedtime, hours of sleep	Mistaken as half-strength	
IU*	International unit	Mistaken as IV (intravenous) or 10 (ten)	Use "units"
o.d. or OD	Once daily	Mistaken as "right eye" (OD–oculus dexter), leading to oral liquid medications administered in the eye	Use "daily"
OJ	Orange juice	Mistaken as OD or OS (right or left eye); drugs meant to be diluted in orange juice may be given in the eye	Use "orange juice"
Per os	By mouth, orally	The "os" can be mistaken as "left eye" (OS–oculus sinister)	Use "PO," "by mouth," or "orally"
q.d. or QD*	Every day	Mistaken as q.i.d., especially if the period after the "q" or the tail of the "q" is misunderstood as an "i"	Use "daily"

Continued

TABLE 5-2

ISMP's List of *Error-Prone Abbreviations, Symbols,* and *Dose Designations*—cont'd

Abbreviations	Intended Meaning	Misinterpretation	Correction
qhs	Nightly at bedtime	Mistaken as "qhr" or every hour	Use "nightly"
qn	Nightly or at bedtime	Mistaken as "qh" (every hour)	Use "nightly" or "at bedtime"
q.o.d. or QOD*	Every other day	Mistaken as "q.d." (daily) or "q.i.d. (four times daily) if the "o" is poorly written	Use "every other day"
q1d	Daily	Mistaken as q.i.d. (four times daily)	Use "daily"
q6PM, etc.	Every evening at 6 PM	Mistaken as every 6 hours	Use "daily at 6 PM" or "6 PM daily"
SC, SQ, sub q	Subcutaneous	SC mistaken as SL (sublingual); SQ mistaken as "5 every;" the "q" in "sub q" has been mistaken as "every" (e.g., a heparin dose ordered "sub q 2 hours before surgery" misunderstood as every 2 hours before surgery)	Use "subcut" or "subcutaneously"
ss	Sliding scale (insulin) or ½ (apothecary)	Mistaken as "55"	Spell out "sliding scale;" use "one-half" or "½"
SSRI	Sliding scale regular insulin	Mistaken as selective-serotonin reuptake inhibitor	Spell out "sliding scale (insulin)"
SSI	Sliding scale insulin	Mistaken as Strong Solution of Iodine (Lugol's)	
i/d	One daily	Mistaken as "tid"	Use "1 daily"
TIW or tiw	3 times a week	Mistaken as "3 times a day" or "twice in a week"	Use "3 times weekly"
U or u*	Unit	Mistaken as the number 0 or 4, causing a 10-fold overdose or greater (e.g., 4U seen as "40" or 4u seen as "44"); mistaken as "cc" so dose given in volume instead of units (e.g., 4u seen as 4 cc)	Use "unit"
UD	As directed ("ut dictum")	Mistaken as unit dose (e.g., diltiazem 125 mg IV infusion "UD" misinterpreted as meaning to give the entire infusion as a unit [bolus] dose)	Use "as directed"

Dose Designations and Other Information	Intended Meaning	Misinterpretation	Correction
Trailing zero after decimal point (e.g., 1.0 mg)*	1 mg	Mistaken as 10 mg if the decimal point is not seen	Do not use trailing zeros for doses expressed in whole numbers
"Naked" decimal point (e.g., .5 mg)*	0.5 mg	Mistaken as 5 mg if the decimal point is not seen	Use zero before a decimal point when the dose is less than a whole unit
Abbreviations such as mg. or mL. with a period following the abbreviation	mg mL	The period is unnecessary and could be mistaken as the number 1 if written poorly	Use mg, mL, etc. without a terminal period
Drug name and dose run together (especially problematic for drug names that end in "l" such as Inderal40 mg; Tegretol300 mg)	Inderal 40 mg Tegretol 300 mg	Mistaken as Inderal 140 mg Mistaken as Tegretol 1300 mg	Place adequate spaces between the drug name, dose, and unit of measure
Numerical dose and unit of measure run together (e.g., 10mg, 100mL)	10 mg 100 mL	The "m" is sometimes mistaken as a zero or two zeros, risking a 10- to 100-fold overdose	Place adequate space between the dose and unit of measure
Large doses without properly placed commas (e.g., 100000 units; 1000000 units)	100,000 units 1,000,000 units	100000 has been mistaken as 10,000 or 1,000,000; 1000000 has been mistaken as 100,000	Use commas for dosing units at or above 1,000, or use words such as 100 "thousand" or 1 "million" to improve readability

TABLE 5-2

ISMP's List of *Error-Prone Abbreviations, Symbols,* and *Dose Designations*—cont'd

Drug Name Abbreviations	Intended Meaning	Misinterpretation	Correction
To avoid confusion, do not abbreviate drug names when communicating medical information. Examples of drug name abbreviations involved in medication errors include:			
APAP	acetaminophen	Not recognized as acetaminophen	Use complete drug name
ARA A	vidarabine	Mistaken as cytarabine (ARA C)	Use complete drug name
AZT	zidovudine (Retrovir)	Mistaken as azathioprine or aztreonam	Use complete drug name
CPZ	Compazine (prochlorperazine)	Mistaken as chlorpromazine	Use complete drug name
DPT	Demerol-Phenergan-Thorazine	Mistaken as diphtheria-pertussis-tetanus (vaccine)	Use complete drug name
DTO	Diluted tincture of opium or deodorized tincture of opium (Paregoric)	Mistaken as tincture of opium	Use complete drug name
HCl	hydrochloric acid or hydrochloride	Mistaken as potassium chloride (The "H" is misinterpreted as "K")	Use complete drug name unless expressed as a salt of a drug
HCT	hydrocortisone	Mistaken as hydrochlorothiazide	Use complete drug name
HCTZ	hydrochlorothiazide	Mistaken as hydrocortisone (seen as HCT250 mg)	Use complete drug name
MgSO4*	magnesium sulfate	Mistaken as morphine sulfate	Use complete drug name
MS, MSO4*	morphine sulfate	Mistaken as magnesium sulfate	Use complete drug name
MTX	methotrexate	Mistaken as mitoxantrone	Use complete drug name
PCA	procainamide	Mistaken as patient controlled analgesia	Use complete drug name
PTU	propylthiouracil	Mistaken as mercaptopurine	Use complete drug name
T3	Tylenol with codeine No. 3	Mistaken as liothyronine	Use complete drug name
TAC	triamcinolone	Mistaken as tetracaine, Adrenalin, cocaine	Use complete drug name
TNK	TNKase	Mistaken as "TPA"	Use complete drug name
ZnSO4	zinc sulfate	Mistaken as morphine sulfate	Use complete drug name

Stemmed Drug Names	Intended Meaning	Misinterpretation	Correction
"Nitro" drip	nitroglycerin infusion	Mistaken as sodium nitroprusside infusion	Use complete drug name
"Norflox"	norfloxacin	Mistaken as Norflex	Use complete drug name
"IV Vanc"	intravenous vancomycin	Mistaken as Invanz	Use complete drug name

Symbols	Intended Meaning	Misinterpretation	Correction
ℨ	Dram	Symbol for dram mistaken as "3"	Use the metric system
ℳ	Minim	Symbol for minim mistaken as "mL"	Use the metric system
×3d	For three days	Mistaken as "3 doses"	Use "for three days"
> and <	Greater than and less than	Mistaken as opposite of intended; mistakenly use incorrect symbol; "< 10" mistaken as "40"	Use "greater than" or "less than"
/ (slash mark)	Separates two doses or indicates "per"	Mistaken as the number 1 (e.g., "25 units/10 units" misread as "25 units and 110" units)	Use "per" rather than a slash mark to separate doses
@	At	Mistaken as "2"	Use "at"
&	And	Mistaken as "2"	Use "and"
+	Plus or and	Mistaken as "4"	Use "and"
°	Hour	Mistaken as a zero (e.g., q2° seen as q 20)	Use "hr," "h," or "hour"
Φ or ∅	zero, null sign	Mistaken as numerals 4, 6, 8, and 9	Use 0 or zero, or describe intent using whole words

*These abbreviations are included on The Joint Commission's "minimum list" of dangerous abbreviations, acronyms, and symbols that must be included on an organization's "Do Not Use" list, effective January 1, 2004. Visit www.jointcommission.org for more information about this Joint Commission requirement.

TABLE 5-3

General Classifications of Medications

Body System	Drug Classification
Gastrointestinal system	Antacids, H_2-antagonists, proton pump inhibitors, antiemetics, laxatives, antidiarrheals
Circulatory system	Anticoagulants, antiplatelets, thrombolytics, antihemorrhagics
Cardiovascular system	Antihypertensives, diuretics, vasodilators, beta-blockers, calcium channel blockers, angiotensin-converting enzyme (ACE) inhibitors, angiotensin II receptor antagonists, antihyperlipidemics
Integumentary system	Emollients, antipruritics, antipsoriatics, medicated dressings
Reproductive system	Hormonal contraceptives, fertility agents, sex hormones
Endocrine system	Hypothalamic-pituitary hormones, corticosteroids, sex hormones, thyroid hormones, antithyroid agents, hypoglycemic agents
Immune system	Antibiotics, antivirals, vaccines, antifungals, antiparasitics
	Anticancer agents
	Immunomodulators
Musculoskeletal system	Anabolic steroids, nonsteroidal antiinflammatory drugs (NSAIDs), antirheumatics, corticosteroids, muscle relaxants, bisphosphonates
Nervous system	Anesthetics, analgesics, anticonvulsants, antidepressants, antiparkinsonian drugs, antipsychotics, stimulants
Respiratory system	Decongestants, bronchodilators, cough medications, H_1-antagonists
Other	Radiopharmaceuticals, contrast media, antidotes

of use, route of administration, or mechanism of action. Various classifications and attributes of drug therapy are discussed later in this chapter. Table 5-3 presents a generalized list so that students can familiarize themselves with the various classifications of available drugs and the body system with which each classification is associated. Each type of medication may have several dosage forms, giving the consumer or physician a choice in how the drug is administered. For consumers, the choice may be based on which dosage form is easier to take, or it may be based on cost. For a physician, the best way to administer medications may be based on how rapidly the medication is needed by the patient.

Classifications of Drug Sales

Currently, three classifications describe drugs' availability to consumers. **Over-the-counter (OTC)** drugs are commonly used and may be purchased without a prescription. **Legend drugs** require a prescription from a prescriber before they can be used and are often denoted as "Rx." **Behind-the-counter (BTC)** drugs do not require a prescription but are kept in the pharmacy; their sales are limited by quantity or may require a pharmacist's approval.

Dosage Forms

Dosage form refers to the means by which a drug is available for use or the vehicle by which the drug is

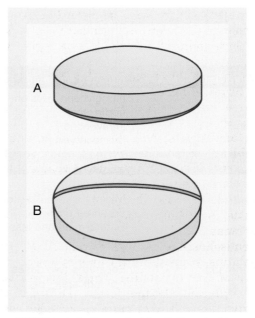

FIGURE 5-1 A, Unscored tablet. **B,** Scored tablet.

delivered. With individual packaging, the dosage form is given on the package. For example, the form may be a tablet or capsule. However, there are many types of tablets and capsules. Tablets are available in a wide variety of shapes and sizes. For example, they may be scored or unscored (Figures 5-1 and 5-2, *B*), or they may be coated or uncoated (Figure 5-2). To a great extent, the dosage form of a

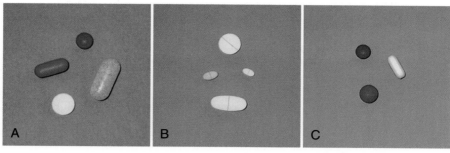

FIGURE 5-2 A, Plain tablets. **B,** Scored tablets. **C,** Enteric-coated tablets.

medication is determined by the drug's pharmacokinetic properties. For instance, heparin (an anticoagulant) is available only in parenteral (intravenous [IV] or subcutaneous [SUBCUT]) form because it becomes ineffective when taken orally as a result of its interaction with stomach acids. Manufacturers prepare certain medications with the ability to release the active ingredient over an extended period. This allows the patient to take the medication less often, which increases compliance. Another consideration is the person taking the drug (e.g., age and health status). If a prescription for sulfamethoxazole/trimethoprim (Bactrim) is intended for a child, that dosage form should be available as a liquid, if at all possible, for ease of administration. The following sections give a brief explanation of the different dosage forms. All the different forms can be divided into three major categories that are composed of subcategories:

- Solids: Tablets, chewable tablets, enteric-coated tablets, extended-release agents, sublingual tablets, capsules, caplets, lozenges, troches, implant capsules, patches
- Liquids: Syrups, elixirs, sprays, inhalant solutions, emulsions, suspensions, solutions, and enemas
- Semisolids: Creams, lotions, ointments, powders, gelatins, suppositories, inhalant powders

Many of the top-selling drugs are available in several different dosage forms. Different dosage forms give the consumer more options; however, the selection of a dosage form also depends on whether the drug will still be effective in a different form. Twenty-five top-selling generic drugs that are available in at least three different dosage forms are shown in Table 5-4. It is always important to know which dosage form is being requested because each form is dosed in different strengths, depending on the drug's reactive properties and the most suitable form for the consumer. For example, if erythromycin tablets are ordered for a young child, the pharmacist may need to call the physician to request either chewable tablets or an oral suspension.

 Tech Note!

Remember that to substitute a different dosage form for the one ordered, the prescriber must give permission. The pharmacist must call the prescriber and explain the reason for the change.

Solids

Solid agents can be contained in various packages and when administered **enterally** can be given orally, rectally, or sublingually. When we think of solids, we normally consider medications given by oral or rectal routes rather than parenteral routes. **Parenteral** is a term used to describe a medication that is usually given by injection into a vein, the skin, or muscle.

Tablets and Caplets

Hundreds of types of tablets are available in a range of sizes, shapes, colors, thickness, and composition. The most common type of tablet contains some type of filler. Fillers are composed of inert substances (no active ingredient) that fill space or cover the tablet (sugar coatings). Sugar coatings improve taste and color or hide unpleasant odors. Certain additives may be used to improve the drug's absorption and/or distribution throughout the body. Some tablets are made to be administered sublingually (under the tongue) or vaginally. Also, some tablets are available in a scored form to allow the dosage to be cut in half if needed. Chewable tablets are convenient for people who have difficulty swallowing tablets and for children who are unable to swallow large tablets. Other tablets are enteric coated to help protect the drug through the acidic environment of the stomach until it reaches the more alkaline intestine. In other cases, the protective covering may delay the release of the drug as it travels through the stomach so that it will not irritate the stomach or become inactive. Orally disintegrating tablets (ODTs) may be dissolved in the mouth without water, easing administration for

TABLE 5-4

25 Examples of Drugs with Multiple Dosage Forms

Examples of Drugs Offered in Multiple Dosage Forms	Tablet	Chewable Tablet	Capsule	Caplet	Solution	Gel Caps	Suspension	Syrup	Elixir	Injectable	Topical patch	Aerosol	Suppositories or Rectal Form	Topical Dosage Forms
Acetaminophen	X	X		X	X	X		X	X				X	
Acetaminophen/codeine	X						X		X				X	
Albuterol	X				X			X				X		
Amoxicillin	X	X	X				X							
Carbamazepine	X	X					X			X				
Clindamycin			X		X					X				X
Diazepam	X				X					X			X	
Digoxin	X		X						X	X				
Diltiazem	X		X							X				
Diphenhydramine	X		X		X		X	X	X	X				X
Erythromycin	X	X	X				X			X				X
Furosemide	X				X					X				
Guaifenesin	X		X		X			X						
Hydrocortisone					X					X			X	X
Hydroxyzine	X		X				X	X		X				
Ibuprofen	X		X		X		X	X		X				
Epinephrine					X					X		X		
Nitroglycerin	X		X							X	X	X		
Phenobarbital	X		X						X	X				
Phenytoin	X		X				X			X				
Potassium chloride	X	X			X					X				
Prednisone	X						X	X						
Promethazine	X							X		X			X	
Ranitidine	X		X		X			X		X				
Risperidone	X				X					X				

individuals who have difficulty swallowing medication. Caplet dosage forms are related closely to tablets but are smooth sided and therefore easier to swallow. The word *caplet* refers to the shape of the tablet. Tablets are often identified by shape, color, and imprint codes, which are determined by the manufacturer.

Many medications have extended-release forms and regular forms. The technician must know which form the physician has ordered. Manufacturers have developed controlled-release formulations to enable the patient to take the medication less often. This improves patient compliance. Abbreviations for agents that release medication over different periods of time and in different quantities are as follows:

CD	Controlled diffusion
CR	Continuous/controlled release
CRT	Controlled-release tablet
IR	Immediate release*
LA	Long acting*
ODT	Orally disintegrating tablet
SA	Sustained action*
SR	Sustained/slow release*
TD	Time delay
TR	Time release
XL	Extra long*
XR	Extended release*

*Also available in capsule forms.

Tech Note!

As a general rule, dosage forms that are specially made to release over time should not be crushed or broken into pieces. This would alter the release process. However, some medications, such as Toprol XL, can be divided if they are scored and approved for such use. Some companies have their own names for extended-release agents. For example, Theo-24 is a theophylline agent that is released over 24 hours, which is why the company named it Theo-24.

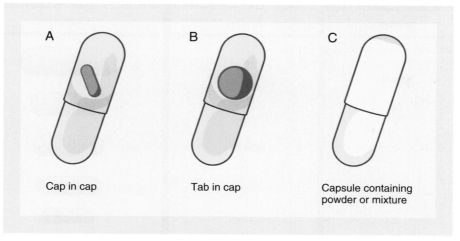

FIGURE 5-3 Different types of capsules.

Capsules

Capsules are composed of a gelatin container. They can have a hard or soft outer shell. The shells of hard capsules are composed of sugar, gelatin, and water. Their color is determined by the manufacturer and is used primarily for identification, along with the capsule imprint coding. Another type of capsule is the pulvule, which is shaped slightly differently for identification purposes. Spansules are capsules that can be pulled apart to sprinkle the medication onto food for children, making it easier to administer. The medication inside a spansule is specially coated to slow the dissolving rate, allowing the medicine to be delivered at a particular time (depending on the coating) after the capsule contents are consumed. The medicine inside a spansule should not be crushed or chewed. Soft-gelatin capsules (gel caps) cannot be pulled apart and often hold medications in liquid form. Because of the many capsule sizes available, capsules can be produced to administer medication in many ways. For example, as seen in Figure 5-3, these capsules can even hold a small capsule or tablet. The reason behind this manufacturing decision is to determine the best absorption and distribution of the medication. Caplets are not capsules; they are simply tablets with a shape similar to a capsule that may ease swallowing. More medications are being prepared as caplets to ensure that they are tamper proof. Figure 5-4 shows more shapes and sizes of capsules.

Capsule Sizes. Capsules are available in different sizes (Figure 5-5). They vary in color, transparency, and identifying marks. The larger half of the capsule is known as the body, and the shorter half is known as the cap. Many companies produce a hard-shelled capsule that cannot be opened, ensuring that it is tamper resistant. Many capsules are designed to be taken orally and swallowed whole. Compounding pharmacies carry empty capsules of varying sizes that can be filled with various amounts of medica-

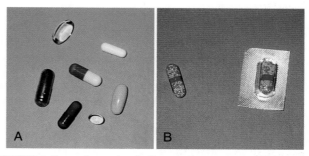

FIGURE 5-4 Types of capsules. **A,** Normal-release capsules. **B,** Extended-release capsules.

tion; a variety of techniques are used to fill them (see Chapter 11 for more information on compounding).

Some capsules are not intended to be swallowed. For example, Topamax Sprinkles are capsules that hold spheres of anticonvulsant medicine inside the capsule. This specific medication can be sprinkled onto a small amount of soft food immediately before dosing for administration; the sprinkles should not be chewed. Pharmacies have capsule dosage forms that hold dry powder medication intended for oral inhalation using inhaler devices; these dosage forms should not be swallowed by the patient.

Examples of Caplets and Capsules. acetaminophen caplets (Tylenol; OTC), hydroxyzine pamoate capsules (Vistaril; Rx)

Lozenges and Troches

Lozenges and troches are other forms of tablets that are not intended to be swallowed; they dissolve in the mouth, which releases the medication more slowly. The medications in lozenges and troches are often aimed at local action in the mouth and/or throat. Many cough drops come in this type of dosage form. Lozenges are similar to hard candy. Troches vary in size. Some are larger than normal-sized tablets and are flat; they usually have a chalky consistency so

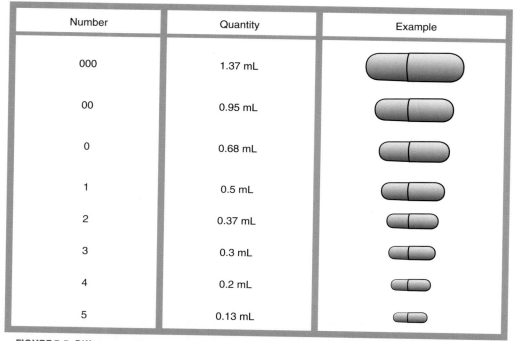

Number	Quantity	Example
000	1.37 mL	
00	0.95 mL	
0	0.68 mL	
1	0.5 mL	
2	0.37 mL	
3	0.3 mL	
4	0.2 mL	
5	0.13 mL	

FIGURE 5-5 Different sizes of capsules. Eight sizes are available; each holds a specific volume, and each holds a specific amount of medication. The size numbers are 5, 4, 3, 2, 1, 0, 00, 000; 5 is the smallest, and 000 is the largest. (From Clayton B, Stock Y: *Basic pharmacology for nurses*, ed 16, St Louis, 2013, Elsevier.)

that they can dissolve in the mouth. Clotrimazole troches are normally administered buccally (in the cheek) and left to dissolve, whereas most lozenges are allowed to dissolve in the mouth.

Examples of Lozenges and Troches. benzocaine and menthol lozenge (Cepacol; OTC); clotrimazole troche (Rx), Numoisyn lozenge (Rx)

Biomaterials

Biomaterials are polymers (long chains of hydrocarbons) that combine with or encapsulate a drug; the drug is then released in a predetermined and predictable way. The dosage form of these drugs can be capsules, tablets, or implants. Both pH and solubility can activate the drug and release its contents over a period of anywhere from 12 hours (e.g., cold medicine) to several years (e.g., Implanon contraceptive implant). These drugs can treat conditions without overdosing or underdosing the patient, and they also promote compliance (patient adherence). These dosage forms help maintain a steady concentration of drug dosing within the accepted therapeutic range or window for the drug. The therapeutic window is essentially a range of concentrations at which a drug is determined to be effective with minimal toxicity to most patients. The top concentration of the range is the maximum concentration for most patients to limit toxicity, and the lowest concentration is the concentration below which the drug is not therapeutically effective for most patients.

Consider two components:
- Water solubility (e.g., ethyl cellulose is water insoluble)
- pH dependency (e.g., sodium alginate is pH dependent, whereas hydroxypropyl methylcellulose is pH independent)

Another consideration with these medications is cost; they are more expensive to manufacture, and that cost is passed along to the consumer.

Implants

Implants are sterile, solid dosage forms that consist of drugs and rate-controlling excipients. They usually are intended for insertion (implantation) into a body cavity or under the skin. Some implants are biosoluble, meaning they degrade in the body over time; others are not and must be removed after a specified time. Many drug-containing implants are actually classified by the U.S. Food and Drug Administration (FDA) as medical devices rather than drugs, such as implantable orthopedic antibiotic beads and various drug-eluting stents for arteries in the heart. Some implants, however, are regulated as prescription drugs. Some popular examples of implants include the Zoladex subcutaneous implant (used for a variety of conditions, including prostate cancer), the Gliadel Wafer (delivers chemotherapy directly to a brain tumor site), and Implanon, a subdermal contraceptive rod (provides birth control that lasts for up to 3 years).

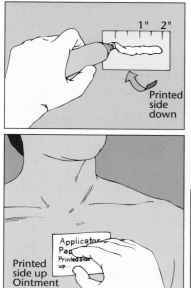
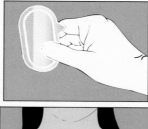
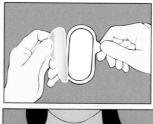
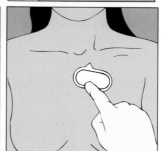

A   B

FIGURE 5-6 **A,** Example of nitroglycerin ointment patch. **B,** Example of a transdermal patch. (From Clayton B, Stock Y: *Basic pharmacology for nurses,* ed 16, St Louis, 2013, Elsevier.)

Transdermal Patches

Transdermal patches are solid pieces of material that hold a specific amount of medication to be released into the skin and absorbed into the bloodstream over time. Patches are convenient dosage forms because they are easily applied and eliminate possible upset stomach. Anginal medication, such as transdermal nitroglycerin patches, can be placed on the chest once daily. Some motion sickness patches (e.g., Transderm Scop) can be applied and left in place for up to 3 days. Fentanyl (Duragesic), a chronic pain medication, is a transdermal patch with a 3-day delivery time (Figure 5-6). Nicotine patches help with smoking cessation, and most are available over the counter. Many estrogen-containing transdermal patches are suited for hormone replacement therapy or prevention of osteoporosis; most are changed once or twice weekly.

Examples of Topical Patches. nitroglycerin patches (Nitro-Dur; Rx), scopolamine transdermal patches (Transderm Scop; Rx), fentanyl patch (Duragesic; Rx)

 Tech Alert!

Never carelessly discard a medication patch in the trash. The medication present on an unprotected, discarded patch may penetrate the skin of a young child or pet. The best approach is to wrap and discard the patch in such a way that a child or pet would not be able to grasp it. One recommendation is to fold the patch onto itself to cover the adhesive area, then place the patch in a pouch or baggie and discard it out of reach of children or pets.

Liquids

Liquids are composed of various mixtures. Traditional names for these dosage forms relate to the types of liquid with which the medication is mixed. Depending on the type of taste, speed of action, or route of administration intended, a physician can choose the best agent for the job. Liquids can be administered by many routes, which makes them a popular choice for drug delivery. For example, enemas are liquid-filled bottles with a dispensing top that can be placed into the rectum to administer the solution into the lower intestine. Other sterile liquids are used in eye and ear products, which are used to treat a variety of conditions. Solutions also can be used topically to treat skin conditions. The following sections discuss the various types of liquids available.

Syrups

Syrups are sugar-based solutions into which medication has been dissolved. The sugar improves the taste of the drug. Syrups tend to be thicker (more viscous) than water.

Examples of Syrups. dextromethorphan syrup (Delsym; OTC), hydrocodone and chlorpheniramine syrup (Tussionex; Rx)

Elixirs

Elixirs are clear, sweetened solutions that contain dissolved medication in a base of water and alcohol (hydroalcoholic base). Drugs that are formulated as elixirs usually require alcohol as a solvent for the drug to be placed into solution. Sweeteners are a

PROCEDURE 5-1

Cleaning Your Nebulizer Equipment

GOAL: To learn the steps for properly cleaning a nebulizer and its tubing to prevent infection.

EQUIPMENT AND SUPPLIES
- Nebulizer kit (tubing and nebulizer chamber)

PROCEDURAL STEPS
1. After each treatment, rinse the nebulizer cup with warm water.

PURPOSE: To wash away any debris or dirt left in the cup.

2. Empty all water from the nebulizer cup and let it air dry.

PURPOSE: To to ensure no moisture is left in the cup, which could allow bacteria to grow.

3. At the end of the day, wash the nebulizer cup, mask, or mouthpiece in warm, soapy water, rinse, and allow to air dry

PURPOSE: To to make sure every part is cleaned thoroughly to avoid and debris or moisture that may be left behind after treatments. All parts should air dry to prevent bacteria growth.

4. Every third day, disinfect the equipment using a vinegar and water solution ($\frac{1}{2}$ cup white vinegar mixed with $1\frac{1}{2}$ cups water).

PURPOSE: White vinegar is a mild disinfectant and is used to kill germs and remove odors.

5. Soak for 20 minutes and rinse well under a steady stream of water.

PURPOSE: Allowing the parts to soak in the vinegar mixture for 20 minutes will ensure the acid has time to kill any germs and remove any odors. Rinsing well will remove any trace of the cleaning mixture and prevent any cross-contamination.

6. Remove excess water and allow to air dry on a paper towel.

PURPOSE: To make sure no moisture is left that might grow bacteria.

7. Make sure all equipment is completely dry before storing it in a plastic resealable bag.

PURPOSE: To avoid any trapped moisture that would be a breeding ground for bacteria.

---

necessary component of elixirs to improve the taste of the alcoholic mixtures. Unlike syrups, elixirs have the same consistency as water.

Examples of Elixirs. brompheniramine/phenylephrine elixir (Dimetapp; OTC), theophylline elixir (Elixophyllin; Rx)

Sprays

Sprays are composed of various bases, such as alcohol or water, in a pump-type dispenser. Sprays are available for use in products such as nasal decongestants and topical sunscreens. A nitroglycerin translingual spray also is available for use under the tongue for relief of anginal pain.

Examples of Sprays. oxymetazoline nasal spray (Afrin; OTC), nitroglycerin sublingual spray (Nitrolingual Pumpspray; Rx)

Inhalants and Aerosols

In certain patients, medications must be delivered directly to the source of inflammation, such as the bronchial tree. Because these areas are so small, the medication particles must be extremely fine to reach them effectively. Inhaler agents are available in a variety of forms, but all must be able to be easily inhaled into the lungs. Common devices of this type, available OTC, are vaporizers that distribute medications when agents are added to a container on the device. In the hospital, respiratory therapists use nebulizers to give breathing treatments to patients;

patients also can use nebulizers at home if they or their caregivers are trained in the use of these devices. Proper daily cleaning and care of the nebulizer equipment helps prevent infection (Procedure 5-1). Inhaled anesthetics are solutions inhaled by a patient undergoing surgery; they are administered during surgery by an anesthesiologist.

Many of the prescribed inhalants contain drugs that treat asthma and allergies. Some devices are called metered dose inhalers (MDIs) and dispense a specific amount of drug with each puff or inhalation (Figure 5-7, *A*); the other common type of medication inhaler is a dry powder inhaler. Some aerosols are used to deliver medication into the nasal passages, whereas others are inhaled orally into the respiratory tract. For orally inhaled agents, although the size of the particles is extremely small, unless the patient uses this device correctly, much of the drug is swallowed rather than inhaled into the lungs where it is needed. Many physicians encourage the use of an AeroChamber or other spacer (Figure 5-7, *B*) along with traditional MDIs. These allow the patient to take a breath of medication without worrying about poor timing and coordination, which could result in loss of medication. The chamber holds the medication until each puff can be inhaled. Dry powder inhalers can be easier to administer because patients prepare the medication before inhalation, allowing them to focus on the proper breathing and administration technique.

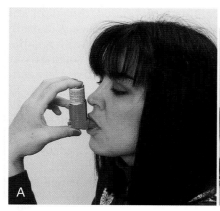
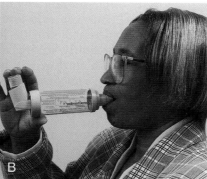

FIGURE 5-7 A, Inhaler. **B,** Inhaler attached to an Aero-Chamber (also known as a spacer). (From Potter PA, Perry AG: *Fundamentals of nursing,* ed 8, St Louis, 2013, Elsevier.)

Examples of Aerosol and MDIs. albuterol (Proventil HFA; Rx), ipratropium bromide and albuterol sulfate metered dose inhaler (Combivent Respimat; Rx)

 Tech Note!

Most inhalants are propelled by the use of various gases. In the past, most propellants contained chlorofluorocarbons (CFCs), which have been found to destroy the ozone layer. As the ozone layer is destroyed, ultraviolet light is allowed to enter the atmosphere at levels that are known to cause skin cancer. Consequently, the FDA ruled that as of January, 2009, inhalers could no longer contain CFCs. Inhalers since then have used a propellant called *hydrofluoroalkane* (HFA). HFA products are more expensive but do not damage the ozone layer.

 Tech Note!

An emulsifier is a substance that binds oil to a water base. An emulsifier binds to both substances and holds them together. For example, take a look at mayonnaise. Mayonnaise is composed of oil and water and uses egg yolks as an emulsifier, which allows the product to form a smooth consistency. Oil can have water as a base; in some cases, water is contained in an oil base. Although most emulsions are used topically, a few parenteral emulsion agents can be given, such as lipids (also known as fat), which are used for nutritional parenteral feedings. Various types of emulsion preparations can be administered topically, orally, and even parenterally.

Emulsions

An emulsion is a mixture of two or more immiscible liquids; in an emulsion, one liquid is dispersed throughout the other. Emulsions are fairly unstable; an emulsifier (a substance that stabilizes an emulsion) is often added to improve stability and dispersion. For example, an emulsifier may be used to bind oil and water into a mixture. Many different types of emulsifiers are used, depending on the medication the manufacturer is preparing. A classic example of an emulsion from your kitchen is simple vinaigrette; vinaigrettes quickly separate unless shaken continually. In the pharmacy, calamine lotion is a classic topical emulsion purchased OTC. Propofol injections and intravenous lipid infusions are prescription medications that are emulsions stabilized with ingredients such as soybean oil and egg lecithin.

Examples of Emulsions. propofol (Diprivan; Rx), cyclosporine ophthalmic emulsion (Restasis; Rx)

Suspensions

Suspensions are liquid dosage forms in which very small solid particles are suspended in the base solution. Certain active ingredients are unstable when dissolved in a solution but stable in a suspension form. Suspensions, such as syrups and other oral solutions, can be used orally by children and older individuals because the patient can take the medication more easily. Oral suspensions should have a "Shake Well" auxiliary label that is easily visible on the front of the bottle and in the directions; if the product is prepared (reconstituted) in the pharmacy, proper adherence to the directions for mixing and placement of the date of expiration ("use by" date) on the label or auxiliary label are very important. Suspension dosage forms are also formulated to be used topically, in the eye or ear, rectally, and even parenterally.

Examples of Suspensions. prednisolone ophthalmic suspension (Pred Forte; Rx), amoxicillin/clavulanate suspension (Augmentin; Rx), ibuprofen suspension (Children's Motrin; OTC)

Enemas

Enemas may be administered for one of two reasons: retention or evacuation. Retention enemas are used to deliver medication to the body in a manner that bypasses the stomach. Conditions such as ulcerative

Tech Note!

It is always important to shake oral suspensions well before using. However, care must be taken with injectable suspensions because some drugs, including many biologic medicines, are inactivated by vigorous shaking. Always follow the manufacturer's directions for handling. For example, some types of insulin suspensions should be rolled, not shaken, to prevent destruction of the proteins that would result from shaking.

Scenario CHECK UP 5-2

Mary begins her day at the compounding pharmacy happy to be putting her education into practice. One of the prescriptions she is to fill is amoxicillin for a baby with otitis media. She knows the drug will need to be reconstituted before it is dispensed. This was a call-in prescription, and the baby's parent will be in around noon to pick it up. What is the proper procedure Mary should follow in this situation? What could happen if Mary prepares the amoxicillin before the parent arrives?

colitis (inflammation of the intestines) can be treated with antiinflammatory agents in this manner. A rectal diazepam gel (Diastat) is available for certain patients for the immediate treatment of seizures. The most common use of enemas, however, is to evacuate the bowel for a variety of reasons, such as preprocedural care (e.g., to prepare for surgeries or examinations involving the intestine) or for women about to give birth. Evacuation enemas can be administered from prefilled squeeze bottles. Some enemas available OTC are used strictly for the relief of constipation. However, because of the dramatic effects of enemas, physicians usually do not recommend them as the first line of treatment for constipation. Enemas are manufactured in a water base, which is faster acting than an oil base. The typical amount of time for an evacuation enema to be effective is less than 10 minutes.

Examples of Enemas. mesalamine enema (Rowasa; Rx), sodium phosphate enema (Fleet enema; OTC)

Semisolids

Semisolid agents are different in their composition from liquids or solids. Although they contain solids and liquids, they normally are intended for topical application. Examples include creams, lotions, ointments, gels, pastes, and suppositories.

Creams

Creams usually have medications in a base that is part oil and part water and is intended for topical or local use. When an emulsifier is added, the water and oil remain combined. Creams are massaged easily into the skin and do not leave a heavy, oily residue. Creams can be formulated to be used vaginally or rectally, taking into account the sensitive tissues to which they will be applied.

Examples of Creams. hydrocortisone cream 1% (Cortaid; OTC), betamethasone cream 0.05% (Diprolene; Rx)

Lotions

Lotions are thinner than creams because their base contains more water. They penetrate well into the skin and do not leave an oily residue after application.

Examples of Lotions. hydrocortisone 1% lotion (Dermarest Eczema Medicated Lotion; OTC), hydrocortisone lotion 2.5% (Rx)

Ointments

Ointments contain medication in a glycol or oil base, such as petrolatum. Ointments can effectively cover the skin's surface while repelling moisture. Ointments can be used rectally or topically and can be formulated and sterilized for use in the eye as an ophthalmic agent.

Examples of Ointments. bacitracin/neomycin/polymyxin ointment (Neosporin; OTC), tacrolimus ointment (Protopic; Rx)

Gels

Gels contain medication in a viscous (thick) liquid that easily penetrates the skin and does not leave a residue. Many sunscreens are available in this dosage form. Medications for various skin conditions also are available in gels.

Examples of Gels. naftifine gel (Naftin; Rx), benzocaine (Orajel; OTC)

Pastes

Pastes contain a lesser amount of liquid base than do solids. They are used for topical application and can absorb secretions, unlike other topical agents.

Example of Pastes. zinc oxide paste 40% (Desitin Maximum Strength; OTC)

Suppositories

Suppositories can be used for rectal, vaginal, or urethral conditions. They can be used for a localized effect (at the site of administration) or a systemic effect (throughout the body). They have several advantages over other dosage forms. Rectal suppositories bypass the stomach, which is important if the patient is experiencing nausea and vomiting. They can relieve these symptoms without the patient having to receive an injection, which is much more invasive. They also are good for relief of constipation.

Rectal antiinflammatory suppositories can be used to help treat inflammatory bowel conditions. Vaginal suppositories are used mostly to treat localized conditions of the vaginal area tissues, including yeast infections and atrophy related to menopause.

Examples of Suppositories. promethazine suppositories (Rx), miconazole vaginal suppositories (Monistat 3; OTC), bisacodyl suppositories (Dulcolax; OTC)

Powders

Powders do not fit neatly into the category of semisolids. Powders are solids, yet they are packaged in some forms that allow them to be sprayed, similar to liquid dosage forms, or inhaled (see inhalants). Therefore, topical powders have been included in the semisolids section. One of the main uses of topical powders is to reduce the wetness in an area. Most antifungal foot agents are available in powdered forms to keep the area as dry as possible, reducing the ability of the fungus to thrive. Powders also can be spread over a wide area if needed.

Examples of Powders. miconazole powder (Desenex spray; OTC), nystatin powder (Mycostatin topical, Rx)

Routes of Administration

Although many other types of dosage forms can be made by manufacturers or compounding pharmacies, the types covered in this chapter are those most commonly seen in the pharmacy. Because medications in the pharmacy are stocked according to their different dosage forms, it is important for student technicians to be familiar with all dosage forms so that they can quickly locate a medication. Table 5-5 lists abbreviations for the most common dosage forms and their routes of administration. The advantages and disadvantages of each type of route of administration determine the physician's final decision on the type of agent the patient should receive. The following sections describe each route of administration and give the pros and cons of each.

By Mouth (Oral)

A positive aspect of taking tablets or capsules or any agent by mouth (PO) is the convenience of the drug for the patient. Most oral medications can be kept readily available throughout the day in a handy bottle. Tablets and capsules do not need to be measured, which increases their ease of use, and most oral forms are much less expensive than other alternatives. Some oral medications are systemic, which means they are absorbed and dispersed throughout the body, while others are not absorbed and act locally in the gastrointestinal tract once swallowed. Oral administration is also one of the safer ways to

give medication because if too much is given, there may be time to react before the drug begins to work. The disadvantage of these drugs is that they do not work as quickly as parenteral medications; they take anywhere from 30 minutes to 1 hour to become active. This can be important, for instance, if the medication is intended for pain relief. Also, some drugs cannot be taken orally because they are not as effective. This complication is due to the acidic pH of the stomach, which breaks down some substances before absorption and makes certain medications of little use orally.

Sublingual and Buccal Agents

Although not many medications are available at this time in the form of sublingual (SL) or buccal (BUC) agents, the few that are commonly used are effective. Nitroglycerin is the most commonly used sublingual tablet (placed under the tongue; Figure 5-8, *A*) that treats anginal attacks. Angina is a common heart ailment that affects millions of people. Its symptoms include shortness of breath and pain in and around the chest cavity. Nitroglycerin sublingual tablets bypass the long passage through the gastrointestinal system and are absorbed readily into the bloodstream. This accelerates the drug's action to a few minutes, compared with the longer time required for oral agents. Buccal agents are another type of uncommon dosage form. Buccal tablets are placed between the gums and cheek (Figure 5-8, *B*), where the medication penetrates the mouth lining and then enters the bloodstream.

Rapidly Disintegrating Oral Tablets

Some drugs are available in a newer dosage form that quickly disintegrates when taken orally and may be administered with or without water. This dosage form allows ease of administration for people who do not take larger sized tablets easily and for those with conditions such as nausea and vomiting, in which taking a tablet may induce vomiting. Examples of ODTs include agents such as ondansetron

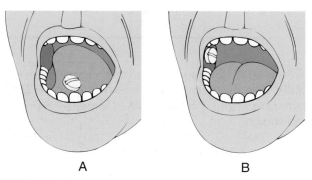

A   B

FIGURE 5-8 A, Sublingual tablet placement. **B,** Buccal tablet placement. (From Clayton B, Stock Y: *Basic pharmacology for nurses,* ed 16, St Louis, 2013, Elsevier.)

TABLE 5-5

Common Abbreviations Used with Dosage Forms

Abbreviation	Route of Administration	Specific Site of Action	Dosage Forms
PO	Oral	Absorbed into bloodstream	Tablet Capsule Solution Syrup Suspension Powder Elixir Tincture Troche
SL	Sublingual	Under the tongue	Tablet Sprays
BUC	Buccal	In the cheek	Lozenge/troche
PR	Per rectum	Rectum	Suppository Solution Enema Ointment
IV	Intravenous	In the vein	Solution/suspension
IM	Intramuscular	In the muscle	Solution/suspension
IT	Intrathecal	In the space surrounding the spinal cord	Solution
IA	Intraarterial	In the artery	Solution
SUBCUT	Subcutaneous	Under the surface of the skin	Solution/suspension

TOP	Epicutaneous or
	    percutaneous
	Transdermal
		On the skin surface
		On the skin surface for delivery through
		    the skin
			Ointment
			Cream
			Paste
			Powder
			Spray
			Solution
			Lotion
			Patch
			Disk

NAS	Intranasal	Nose	Solution Spray Inhalant
INH	Inhalation	Mouth	Solution Aerosol
PV	Per vagina	Vagina	Solution Ointment Foam Gel Suppository Sponge
Urethral	Urethral	Urethra	Solution Suppository

(Zofran ODT) for nausea/vomiting, clonazepam orally ODTs for seizures, donepezil (Aricept ODT) for dementia, and rizatriptan (Maxalt ODT) for migraines.

Rectal Agents

Rectal (PR) agents are used for many different reasons; for example, if a person is vomiting and cannot take oral medications, either suppositories or rectal suspensions can be used to treat the patient's condition. Different preparations are available, depending on the result desired. To reduce inflammation, ointments or creams can be used in addition to suppositories; these types of drugs work locally rather than systemically. However, to treat nausea and vomiting or motion sickness, a systemic-acting suppository can be used. Other agents include rectal solutions that also are used locally for various reasons, usually to clear the intestines of fecal material. The downside is that most people do not feel comfortable using the rectal dosage forms. Also, depending on the drug and the retention time by the patient, the actual amount of drug absorbed may not be as predictable compared with medications taken orally.

Topical Agents

Many different preparations of topical (TOP) treatments are available. The effects of topical preparations range from systemic to localized (e.g., for rashes). The skin is the largest organ of the body because of its large surface area. The skin has many portals through which drugs can pass into the body. Openings include sweat glands, hair follicles, and other small openings in the pores of the skin. Many topical agents fight skin infections, reduce inflammation, and protect the skin from the ultraviolet rays of the sun. Topical agents work at the site of action, which makes them effective for localized use.

In addition, manufacturers have created topical treatments that work systemically, such as medications for angina, blood pressure, hormone replacement, motion sickness, and smoking cessation. These are prepared in a variety of dosage forms, from ointments to patches or small disks that can be applied to the skin. The medication is absorbed through the pores into the bloodstream, where it begins to work.

An advantage of topical agents is the ease of application for the patient. Many topical medications act rapidly at the site of application to relieve itching or inflammation. Patches can be worn all day, which increases patient compliance because the patient does not have to remember to take the medication at various times during the day. In fact, some patches, such as those for motion sickness, can be applied and left in place for days.

The negative aspect of topical drugs is that they may cause skin irritation or may not be adequately absorbed transdermally; therefore, many agents cannot be given by this route of administration. Because patches are generally more expensive to produce than other dosage forms, these medications tend to be more costly than their counterpart oral dosage forms.

Parenteral: Intravenous, Intravenous Piggyback, Intramuscular, and Subcutaneous Agents

The word *parenteral* is Greek in origin and means "side of intestine" or "outside the intestine." A wide range of parenteral dosages and administration sites is available. The most common parenteral medications are given intravenously (IV), into the veins; intramuscularly (IM), into the muscles; or subcuta-

neously (SUBCUT), under the skin. Very small gauge needles are used, and the length depends on the site of injection. Parenteral administration has clear benefits, such as the speed of action and completeness of dosing. Parenteral medications such as insulin have allowed millions of people with diabetes to inject themselves daily, allowing them to lead normal and productive lives. In addition, many parenteral drugs work faster than those given by the oral route. This is important for emergency situations, for patients who are unconscious or combative, and for patients who are unable to swallow. Also, smaller doses may be needed because of the high bioavailability of the agents injected. The disadvantage of parenteral drugs as a group is the increased risk of infection because the techniques for administration are invasive. Any drug injection must be given using as sterile a technique as possible to avoid introducing any microbes into the body. Also, any injection is much more expensive than other routes of administration because of the required preparation and administration by trained personnel. Another disadvantage is that, because injectable drugs work quickly, once the drug has been injected, there is little or no time to alter its availability if an unintended dose is given or if an untoward reaction occurs.

Eye/Ear/Nose (Ophthalmic, Otic, Nasal)

A wide variety of agents is used to treat conditions affecting the eyes, nose, and ears. Pharmacy technicians must remember an important fact when preparing and filling prescriptions for agents that treat the ear or eye: physicians often use eye solutions to treat ear conditions; however, because the eye is sterile, ear solutions cannot be used to treat eye conditions. Therefore, all ophthalmic drugs (eye preparations) are sterile. Otic drugs (ear preparations) are not necessarily always sterile because many otic agents treat the ear canal and do not typically penetrate a sterile environment. The pharmacy technician may prepare ophthalmic drugs in a laminar flow hood using aseptic technique (see Chapter 12). Technicians must remember that all ophthalmic drugs must be kept sterile.

Different dosage forms are used for the eye, ear, and nose, including ointments, solutions, and suspensions. Most treatments for the ear are for fighting an infection or removing earwax buildup. Most nasal sprays are used to treat symptoms of colds and allergies, whereas eye treatments typically are used for infections, inflammation, and conditions such as glaucoma (increased pressure in the eye). These dosage forms are effective at a specific site rather than involving the whole body. They can be administered with ease because of the small package size of the drug. Instructions for eye and ear preparations should use the word **instill** rather than "take" or "put." The main disadvantage of these drugs is that solutions used for the eye, if not kept sterile, can introduce bacteria into the area being treated. Also, ophthalmic drugs do not last as long as other treatments because of blinking of the eye and tearing, which wash the medication away from the site. Therefore, dosing times may be frequent. In addition, most ophthalmic ointments make it difficult to see clearly.

Scenario CHECK UP 5-3

Mary has been extremely busy in the pharmacy today. She only has 1 hour left on her shift, and she is feeling exhausted. She learned that studies show mistakes can occur when technicians are overtired. She receives a prescription for Garamycin drops. Why should Mary read the script extremely carefully? What could occur if Mary interprets the order incorrectly?

Inhalants

Many people suffer from lung diseases and use inhalants (INH) to treat their conditions. As mentioned previously, there are two types of inhalers: those that use a propellant to push the drug to the lungs and those that use dry powder to release the medication as the patient takes a deep, fast breath. The dry powder inhaler may be a dry powder tube inhaler, a powder disk inhaler, or a single-dose dry powder disk inhaler. The choice of inhaler depends on its convenience for the patient and the medication needed. Some agents open the passageways to the lungs (e.g., bronchodilators), and some can be used to reduce inflammation (e.g., corticosteroids).

A positive aspect of inhalants is that most are available in handheld units and are convenient for carrying. The onset of action for short-acting bronchodilators, for example, is quick, which can make an dramatic difference in a person's ability to breathe comfortably. The disadvantage is that if the inhaler is not used properly, little if any of the drug is able to reach the lungs. Breathing in as the inhaler is activated is important, and it may be necessary to shake some inhalers before drug administration. Dry powder inhalants are small and convenient to carry, do not require coordination of breathing at the exact time of medication release, and are not shaken before use, although some models do require cocking the device. Respiratory solutions that are packaged in unit dose ampules or vials are used to deliver a specific amount of drug per treatment with the use of a nebulizer.

Injectables

Injectable medications are normally used to obtain a rapid response. The onset of action of many injectable drugs takes only a few minutes, as opposed to the possible 45 minutes or longer required for oral medications to take effect. People with diabetes may use long-acting insulins along with short-acting insulins. Although people with diabetes are the most common users of injectable drugs outside the hospital setting, other types of injectables used in the home are anticoagulants (e.g., subcutaneous heparins) and certain injectables for patients with multiple sclerosis.

A variety of long-acting parenteral drugs is available that can be used in place of daily dosing. For example, medroxyprogesterone acetate (Depo-Provera, Depo-subQ Provera 104), which can be used for birth control, must be injected every 3 months. Other parenteral long-acting medications include haloperidol decanoate, which is used monthly for the treatment of schizophrenia, and leuprolide acetate injection suspension (e.g., Lupron Depot), which is injected either once monthly or once every 3 months for various hormonal disorders. The technician should note that long-acting depot injectable products are never to be given intravenously.

In the hospital, many oral medications are available in injectable form, and some are *only* available in injectable form. These medications typically are supplied in ampules or vials. Ampules are made of glass (Figure 5-9, *B*) and can range in volume from 0.5 to 50 mL. (Ampules are opened using the techniques outlined in Chapter 12.) Vials can be made of plastic or glass (Figure 5-9, *A*) and range in size from 1 to 100 mL.

A unique type of vial is the ADD-Vantage container, which keeps the medication separate from the diluent until it is time to reconstitute. This saves waste when an expensive drug is used that has a short shelf life after preparation (Figure 5-10 gives instructions on the use of this type of vial). Other medications that are available in intravenous form are premade IV bags and those prepared by the technician. Figure 5-11 presents examples of a large-volume IV and an IV piggyback.

Technicians must pay close attention to the storage requirements for injectable drugs. Some are stored at room temperature, whereas others require refrigeration. For example, phytonadione (vitamin K), must be kept in a light-protected ampule and should be stored at room temperature. Other injectables (e.g., ciprofloxacin) must be stored in light-protected bags after being reconstituted into an IV bag. Glass containers are packaged securely to protect them from breakage.

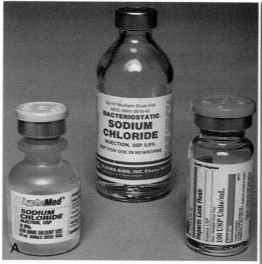
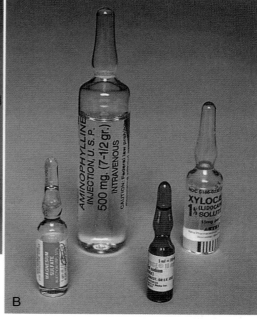

FIGURE 5-9 **A,** Medication in vials. **B,** Medication in ampules.

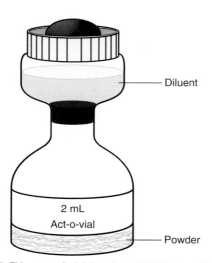

Diluent

2 mL
Act-o-vial

Powder

FIGURE 5-10 This type of vial is called Add-A-Vial or Mix-O-Vial. The advantage of this type of medication dosage form is its longer shelf life. To use this type of vial: 1. Remove the sterile cap. 2. The powder is below, and the sterile diluent is in the top of the vial. The vial is divided by a rubber stopper in the middle. 3. Push the plunger down, forcing the stopper to fall into the bottom of the vial. This allows the diluent to mix with the powder. Shake well. Once dissolved, the medication is ready to be used.

Miscellaneous Routes

Other common routes of administration include vaginal or urethral dosage forms. These forms are suppositories, creams, ointments, foams, gels, and various inserts, such as rings. These types of delivery systems are used for the treatment of infections and inflammation and, in the case of vaginal foams or rings, for local or systemic birth control, respectively.

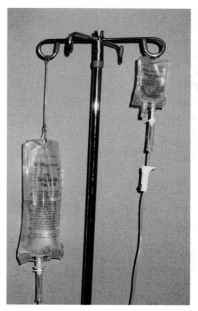

FIGURE 5-11 *Left,* A large-volume IV bag. *Right,* An IV piggyback.

Although there are clear advantages to the use of these agents, such as bypassing a systemic effect for some medications and affecting the specific site only, they are not necessarily applied easily and can be uncomfortable.

Other Considerations: Form and Function

Dosage forms are created based on the results from many clinical trials that investigate the

pharmacokinetics of the medication or the function of the drug in experiments.

Pharmacokinetics and Pharmacodynamics

Pharmacokinetics is an all-inclusive word that represents many different components concerning the actions of the body on a drug, as opposed to *pharmacodynamics* (to be discussed later), which describes the effects the drug has on the body. For example, from the time a person takes a tablet, various considerations are examined, such as the levels of the drug in the blood and tissues, the absorption or movement of the drug into the bloodstream, and the overall distribution of the drug throughout the body, in addition to the metabolism and elimination of the drug. This includes the reaction of the drug with other drugs to determine changes that may occur in the course of the drug's time in the body. As these components are tested and refined, the eventual result is a dosage form that is tailor-made to work at its optimal level, while always keeping patient adherence in mind. Patient adherence is the level at which patients will or will not take their scheduled drugs. If a manufacturer can make a drug that can be taken once daily rather than several times a day, the odds increase that the patient will take the medication as directed.

The following sections describe the overall pharmacokinetics or life of the drug in the body. Absorption, distribution, metabolism, and elimination (ADME) are discussed, as are half-life, bioavailability, and bioequivalence. All information about the pharmacokinetics of a drug and its relation to the proper dosing and use of the drug is listed in several reference books (see Chapter 7) and official drug package inserts.

Absorption

Medications are made specifically to pass through natural body barriers such as the skin, intestines, blood-brain barrier (surrounding the brain), and other membranous tissues. How well the drug passes through these barriers is one factor that determines its ultimate **absorption**, distribution, and effectiveness. Some considerations include whether the barrier is a lipid (fatty) base. Membranes surrounding organs, such as the intestine, have a variety of proteins and other structures implanted in a membranous protective structure that act as carriers for drug transport or as receptor sites. Important chemicals and drugs are able to pass a lock-and-key mechanism by latching onto receptive sites that allow the chemical or drug to pass into the organ to reach the final site of action intended for the drug (Figure 5-12).

Distribution

After systemic absorption, the medication is distributed throughout the body from the bloodstream into the tissues and ultimately organs of the body. **Distribution** is the location of a medication throughout

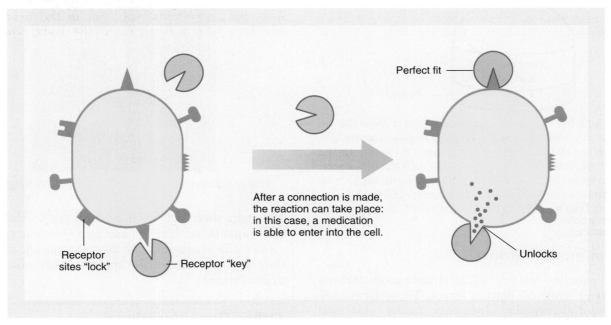

FIGURE 5-12 The "lock-and-key" type mechanism that allows absorption to take place in a cell. These common reactions occur naturally throughout the body. Only after the correct receptor makes a connection with the matching receptor site does the cell allow a reaction to take place. Medications often mimic this natural mechanism.

the blood, organs, and tissues after administration and absorption. For some medications, the distribution of the drug in the blood is measured at certain times throughout the day to keep track of medication concentrations and to ensure therapeutic effectiveness. Clearance (the volume of plasma from which the drug is removed per unit of time) may also be determined from the changes in blood concentrations within the dosing interval. Not all systems are affected equally by the drugs administered; some areas do not allow drugs to infiltrate as rapidly as do other areas. The distribution of a drug, therefore, is not necessarily equal throughout the body. For example, the blood-brain barrier is a built-in system that functions to keep harmful chemicals away from the brain. Certain medications have to be made that can cross this barrier to help treat diseases. Likewise, many medications that may penetrate the blood-brain barrier can cause unwanted side effects, such as confusion. These are just a few of the hurdles drug companies must contend with when creating new medications. Also, most drugs are either weak acids or weak bases, which influences many of their pharmacokinetic characteristics, including their distribution to various body fluids and tissues (Box 5-1).

BOX 5-1

Ionization

Weak acid in weak base is less ionized = Transported more rapidly into lipid membranes
Weak base in weak acid is less ionized = Transported more rapidly into lipid membranes

Protein binding is another important factor related to drug distribution. Most drugs bind to blood proteins to some degree. Warfarin (a "blood thinner," or anticoagulant) and phenytoin (an anticonvulsant) are examples of drugs for which alterations in protein binding can become clinically important to the amount of drug available for distribution and therapeutic effect. If a patient is treated with warfarin along with phenytoin, the drugs compete for protein-binding sites, and free (unbound) warfarin may increase to an unsafe level.

Metabolism

Drug **metabolism** is the biochemical modification or degradation of drugs in the body. As the drug is distributed throughout the body, some of it reenters the bloodstream and ultimately is transferred to the liver, where most drug metabolism takes place. Metabolism changes the chemical structure of the original drug. A **pro-drug** is a drug that is taken in an inactive form and becomes active through the natural metabolic processes. This actually increases the bioavailability of the drug. If a particular drug is poorly absorbed by the body, a pro-drug formulation can increase the amount of drug brought into the circulatory system. This is achieved by reducing the number of polar/ionized particles. Pro-drugs can carry the medication to the specific site before becoming active, which can reduce the side effects (Figure 5-13). Table 5-6 presents examples of pro-drugs and their metabolites.

Some drugs pass initially through the bloodstream from the gastrointestinal tract to the liver before traveling to other organs of the body, where the

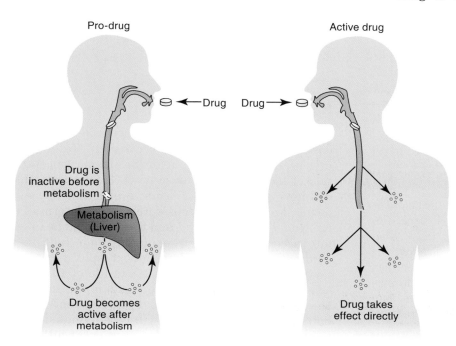

Pro-drug

Active drug

Drug ← Drug   Drug → Drug

Drug is inactive before metabolism

Metabolism (Liver)

Drug becomes active after metabolism

Drug takes effect directly

FIGURE 5-13 The difference between a pro-drug and an active drug.

TABLE 5-6

Examples of Pro-drugs and Their Active Metabolites

Pro-drug	Active Drug
Prontosil	Sulfanilamide
Levodopa	Dopamine
Talampicillin	Ampicillin
Cyclophosphamide	Phosphoramide mustard
Diazepam	Oxazepam
Azathioprine	Mercaptopurine
Cortisone	Hydrocortisone
Dipivefrin	Adrenaline
Prednisone	Prednisolone
Enalapril	Enalaprilat

Data from http://epharmacology.hubpages.com/hub/
Pharmacological-Effects-Prodrugs-Definition-Examples-and-Sources
-of-Drug-Information.

strength of the active ingredient is reduced due to rapid metabolism. This alters the amount of available drug at the site where it is needed.

Many orally administered drugs travel to the liver, and a proportion of the dose is metabolized before the drug has a chance to be distributed; this is called the **first-pass effect**, which lowers the drug's final bioavailability. Drugs that have a first-pass effect are given in higher doses than their injectable counterparts. Certain oral medications do not have this effect and have good bioavailability from oral or injectable routes. Intravenous agents bypass the first-pass phenomenon because they enter the bloodstream directly. Other drugs do not undergo any change at all and are excreted from the body in the same form in which they were introduced. Different influences can alter metabolism, such as age, gender, genetics, diet, and other chemicals ingested.

Most of the final metabolism of a drug takes place in the liver. This is the final processing center of the body; it extracts toxins and unwanted chemicals and forwards them to the sites of the excretion process (e.g., the kidneys). The liver works hard, but the amount it can process in a given time is limited.

Scenario CHECK UP 5-4

As part of Mary's job in the pharmacy, she often helps out with the cashier duties. Mary is waiting on Ms. Black, who is picking up her monthly medications. Ms. Black is an elderly woman who is taking multiple medications for various conditions. Mary notices that today Ms. Black has some OTC cough and cold products she wants to purchase in addition to her regular prescriptions. When Mary offers pharmacist counseling to Ms. Black, she refuses. What should Mary do next?

Individuals with any type of liver damage must be monitored closely when taking various medications to ensure that toxic levels are not present in the liver.

Elimination

Elimination is the last phase of a drug's life in the body. Although elimination usually is associated with urination, it is important to know that there are many ways a drug can be excreted from the body. In addition to elimination via the kidneys, drugs also may be expelled via the feces, exhalation, sweat glands, and even breast milk in women who are lactating. Urination and bowel movements are by far the most common methods of elimination. Remember that drugs that are not eliminated properly may accumulate in the body, which can lead to toxicity. Less common routes of excretion, such as through breast milk, must be considered when a physician prescribes a drug. However, not all drugs are tested by the manufacturer for excretion into breast milk; therefore, the physician must rely on his or her judgment on the use of these agents.

Bioavailability

Bioavailability is the proportion of the drug that is delivered to its destination and is available to the site of action for which it was intended. Different drugs clear in different ways and at different times. This is an important consideration when prescribing drugs and determining drug dosing intervals. Drugs that are intended for certain organs or tissues in the body must pass many different obstacles, such as the destructive actions of stomach acids. By definition, an IV injection has a bioavailability of 100% because the drug does not have to be absorbed; however, bioavailability varies for other routes of administration, such as IM, SUBCUT, topical, and PO.

Half-Life

Half-life refers to the time it takes the body to break down and excrete one half of the drug. To be more precise, it is the time taken for the plasma concentration of the drug to decrease by 50%. Of course, just monitoring the drug's plasma level is not the only factor that should be considered when determining half-life (e.g., muscle, fat, and tissue should be taken into account). After approximately four half-lives, elimination is 94% complete. For example, if a person takes a medication that has a half-life of 10 hours, this means that in 10 hours, one half of the drug will be eliminated, and in another 10 hours, another one half of the remaining drug will be eliminated. This is an important factor in the creation of all drugs because this information tells the manufacturer how long it takes the body to rid itself of the drug; it also helps to determine proper intervals for dosing. If a person takes too much medication or takes doses too close together, the drug can accumulate, which can be dangerous to the patient.

Bioequivalence

Bioequivalence is the comparison of drugs from different manufacturers or from the same manufacturer but different batches (lots). This is an important aspect of a drug because patients assume that every tablet they take is exactly the same as the one before and that all are the exact strength as listed on the label. Generic drug manufacturers strive to achieve equivalence with brand name manufacturers so that they can compete with the original manufacturer. A reference source that can be used to determine whether the generic drug is rated as bioequivalent to the brand name drug is the *Approved Drug Products with Therapeutic Equivalence Evaluations* (the Orange Book).

The Use of Excipients

All medications are prepared with additives (excipients) for many different reasons (Table 5-7). These additives include coloring for better appearance of the product and flavorings to disguise taste and/or smell. Many times fillers are used to increase the size of the medication because the amount of drug may be so small that the medication otherwise would be difficult, if not impossible, to handle. Many different types of preservatives are available; each prevents certain microbes from affecting the drug. These preservatives prolong the shelf life after the patient obtains and opens the drug product. Other types of

additives include those that either increase the dispersal rate of the drug once it reaches the intestines or decreases the rate of distribution of the medication. As mentioned previously, many components involved in the preparation of dosage forms are added to improve the product for the patient's convenience. Patients are more likely to take medication once or twice daily than multiple times per day.

Some patients may be allergic to an ingredient, such as dyes, or may have conditions in which certain ingredients should be avoided. For example, patients with diabetes may be instructed to purchase drug products that are sugar free or alcohol free. Patients with phenylketonuria may need to avoid products containing aspartame as a sweetener. Certain products may be available in the form required, whereas others may not. For patients who need alternative ingredients, a compounding pharmacy may be able to prepare the same drug containing ingredients that are tolerated by the patient.

Manufactured Products

After learning how many different routes of administration there are and the dosage forms used, you may think that that is all there is. However, the ever-changing world of drug manufacturing has made available many different choices and has turned a simple compressed powder, known as a tablet, into an intricate, complicated, and highly structured format. A tablet is not just a tablet, nor a capsule merely a capsule. There are many different types of dosage forms, depending on the desired effect of the drug in question (Table 5-8). All manufactured types of dosage forms must be approved by the FDA (see Chapter 2). Approval of a drug product includes constant testing of the product from batch to batch to ensure continuity of the medication. (Injectable

TABLE 5-7

Description of Additives

Type of Additive	Example of Chemical	Reason
Weak salt acid/base	Hydrochloric acid and sodium hydroxide (base)	Helps dissolve drug more easily once it arrives in the gastrointestinal system
Preservative	Parabens	Increases shelf life
Sweetener	Sucrose	Improves taste
Flavoring	Cherry	Improves taste
Coloring	Yellow dye no. 5	Improves visual appearance
Buffer	Sodium acetate	Adjusts pH
Antifungal	Benzoic acid	Prevents fungal growth
Base	Petrolatum	A common component to which medication is added for ointments and creams
Filler	Starch, powdered cellulose	Increases size of dosage form

TABLE 5-8

Description of Dosage Forms

Dosage Form	Types	Benefits
Oral tablet	Layered	Slow release
	Film-coated	Protects against stomach acid
	Extended-release	Releases medication slowly
	Compressed	Hard dissolves slower; soft dissolves faster
Coated tablet	Sugar added and colored	Protects drug; covers taste
	Caplet	Hard, capsule-shaped tablet
	Colored	Appearance
	Gel	Smaller than a capsule, easier to swallow
	Enteric-coated	Delayed release; easier to swallow
	Oral dissolving	Dissolves in mouth on contact
Sublingual	Soft compressed	Dissolves under the tongue
Buccal		Dissolves in the cheek and the gum
Chewable tablet		Chewed
Capsule	Gelatin cover	Allows for pharmacy-compounded agents; easy to swallow
	Spansule	Capsule holds small pellets or beads
	Pulvule	Manufacturer prepared (bullet shaped)
	Hard gelatin/Dry fill	Filled with powder
	Soft gelatin/Wet fill	Filled with a tablet inside
		Filled with pellets
		Filled with another capsule
		Filled with a liquid
		Filled with a paste
Injectable vial	Multiple-dose vial	May be used more than once
	Single-dose vial	Must be discarded after one use
	ADD-Vantage vial	Rubber stopper is depressed, releasing diluents into powder product

dosage forms are discussed further in Chapter 12.) Pharmacies that provide compounded products must comply with the standards of the United States Pharmacopoeia–National Formulary (USP-NF) monographs.

Packaging and Storage Requirements

Medications are packaged according to manufacturers' specifications to ensure the effectiveness and shelf life of the drug. It is important for technicians to learn the various storage requirements of medications. Medications that have specific storage requirements are clearly marked on the container or box in which they are packaged. Certain medications arrive in dry ice and must be unpacked and stored immediately at the temperature indicated. When the outside of a box is labeled "refrigerate or keep frozen," the contents should never be left at room temperature because this can cause the medication to become unusable. Table 5-9 presents some examples of storage requirements for various drugs, along with special considerations. All medications have a package insert that describes the storage and stability of the drug. Technicians should become familiar with this type of information. In addition

to manufacturer storage requirements, repackaging medications have their own guidelines, which have been instituted by the FDA and can be found in Chapter 11.

Medical Terminology

Another aspect of working with patients is the ability to understand medical terminology. Just as many medication names are derived from the Greek and Latin languages, so are all medical terms. In this section we will cover the basics of medical terminology. The segments of medical terms, along with terms associated with each body system, are described. Medical terms consist of segments, or word parts that, when combined, describe all conditions and anatomy known. Table 5-10 presents a sample of abbreviations used in the medical field.

It is important to know the basics of how medical terminology applies to various conditions. Terms and drugs fit together like hand in glove. There are four segments, or word parts.

1. The prefix
2. The suffix
3. The root word
4. The combining form

TABLE 5-9

Examples of Storage Requirements

Medication	Location	Considerations
Promethazine Suppository	Drug shelf or refrigerator	Intended to melt at body temperature
Latanoprost (Xalatan)	Refrigerator	Stored in refrigerator (2-8°C) until opened; may be kept up to 6 weeks at room temperature after opening
Metronidazole IV	Room temperature	Stored at 15-30°C and protected from light
Vaccines such as Hib, HepA, HepB, human papillomavirus, DTaP, DT, Td, Tdap, influenza, MMR, meningococcal, pneumococcal, rotavirus	Refrigerator	Kept in refrigerator (2-8°C)
Vaccines such as MMR, MMRV, varicella-zoster	Freezer	Kept in freezer (~15°C)
Insulin mixtures containing regular insulin and NPH, including combination formulations (Novolin 70/30, Humulin 70/30)	Room temperature	Stored for 1 month at room temperature Stored for 3 months refrigerated (2-8°C)
Insulin, regular mixed with sterile water or sodium chloride	Room temperature	Must be used within 24 hr
Insulin aspart or combination aspart, NPH (e.g., NovoLog 70/30 FlexPen)	Room temperature	Stored for 14 days (below 30°C)
Penicillin IV	Drug shelf or refrigerator	Must be stored in refrigerator after reconstitution
Mannitol	Room temperature	Mannitol crystallizes at room temperature; do not use crystallized drug; drug must be warmed before using if crystals are present

TABLE 5-10

Additional Abbreviations

Abbreviation	Meaning	Abbreviation	Meaning
ADHD	Attention deficit hyperactivity disorder	HTN	Hypertension
ADR	Adverse drug reaction	ICU	mellitusIntensive care unit
AIDS	Acquired immunodeficiency syndrome	IDDM	Insulin-dependent diabetes
BBB	Blood-brain barrier	KVO	Keep vein open
BUN	Blood urea nitrogen	LBP	Low blood pressure
CABG	Coronary artery bypass graft	LBP	Lower back pain
CAD	Coronary artery disease	LLL	Left lower lobe
CBC	Complete blood count	MI	Myocardial infarction
CCU	Coronary care unit	MRI	Magnetic resonance imaging
CHD	Coronary heart disease	N & V	Nausea and vomiting
CHF	Congestive heart failure	NICU	Neonatal intensive care unit
COPD	Chronic obstructive pulmonary disease	NIDDM	Noninsulin–dependent diabetes mellitus
CVD	Cardiovascular disease	NPO	Nothing by mouth
DNR	Do not resuscitate	OBGYN	Obstetrics and gynecology
DOA	Dead on arrival	OR	Operating room
DOB	Date of birth	PPN	Peripheral parenteral nutrition
DVT	Deep vein thrombosis	PT	Prothrombin time
DX	Diagnosis	RLS	Restless leg syndrome
EEG	Electroencephalogram	SARS	Severe acute respiratory syndrome
EENT	Eye, ear, nose, and throat	SBO	Small bowel obstruction
EKG	Electrocardiogram	SOB	Shortness of breath
ER	Emergency room	TKO	To keep open
FX	Fracture	TPN	Total parenteral nutrition
GERD	Gastroesophageal reflux disease	TX	Treatment
HBP	High blood pressure	UNG	Ointment
HIV	Human immunodeficiency virus	UTI	Urinary tract infection
HPV	Human papillomavirus	WBC	White blood cell count

To combine these word segments, only a few rules must be followed (Box 5-2). A list of common prefixes, suffixes, and root words with their combining forms is shown in Table 5-11.

Although this chapter mentioned many competencies in which a technician must be proficient, you will do most of your learning on the job. However, it is important always to keep learning because this both promotes self-development and enables you to advance in your profession. New dosage forms are always being invented for convenience and to achieve the best results. Technicians can stay current on the new trends through additional reading, continuing education, and on-the-job training.

TECHNICIAN PROFILE

Emory is a pharmacy purchasing agent for a large area hospital. She is a Certified Pharmacy Technician (CPhT) and has worked in the pharmacy department for more than 15 years. The pharmacy buyer's job is a critical component of a well-run facility and requires an individual who is knowledgeable and dedicated to making sure the patients' needs are met. Most of Emory's duties are performed in an office setting. She procures supplies, materials, and pharmaceuticals for the various pharmacies throughout the hospital. She works with vendors to obtain the highest quality products at the optimum price. Emory is responsible for ensuring dependable, expedient delivery of the merchandise. She has a clear understanding of current market fluctuations and drug shortages. She finds her job demanding but very satisfying.

BOX 5-2

Overview of Word Parts of Medical Terminology

Example of how a word is formed:
1. Prefix: placed before each combining form
   Example: peri- (around)
2. Suffix: placed after the combining form
   Example: -itis (inflammation)
3. The root word of the term
   Example: cardia (heart)
4. The combining form
   Example: cardi/o

Read the suffix first, then go back to the beginning and proceed left to right. Put them together: pericarditis (i.e., inflammation around the heart)

Rules
1. Terms can be one to four combinations.
2. Read the suffix first, then go back to the beginning and proceed left to right. Multiple terms can define the same word part.
3. If the combining form has two vowels (e.g., i, o) and the suffix begins with a vowel, drop the "o."

TABLE 5-11

Common Body System Word Segments

Prefixes			
a-	away from, without	-stomy	opening
hyper-	above, elevated	-algia	painful condition
hypo-	below, low	-megaly	enlargement
post-	after, behind	necr/o	tissue death
brady-	slow	scler/o	hardening
tachy-	fast	sten/o	narrowing
poly-	many	-plasty	repair through surgery
sub-	under, less than, below	-gram	picture or record
peri-	around, surrounding	-scopy	use an instrument to examine
pre-	before, in front	-rrhage	excessive flow
dys-	painful or disordered	-rrhea	flow or discharge
		-rrhexis	rupture
		-pnea	breathing
Suffixes			
-al	pertaining to	**Colors**	
-itis	inflammation	cyan/o	blue
-logy	study of	leuk/o	white
-logist	one who studies	rub/o	red
-ectomy	surgical excision	melan/o	black

TABLE 5-11

Common Body System Word Segments—cont'd

Cardiovascular System

cardi/o	heart
angi/o, vas/o	blood vessel
arteri/o	artery
phleb/o	vein
hem/o	blood
capill/o	capillaries

Digestive and Hepatic Systems

gastr/o	stomach
stomat/o	opening
enter/o	relating to the intestine
col/o, colon/o	large intestine
proct/o, rect/o	anus or rectum
hepat/o	liver
cholecyst/o	gallbladder
pancreat/o	pancreas

Eyes

opt/i	eyes
ophthalm/o	eyes
ir/o, irid/o	iris
phac/o, phak/o	lens

Ears

acous/o, ot/o	ears or hearing
pinn/i	external ear, auricle
myring/o	middle ear
tympan/o	membrane of middle ear, eardrum
labyrinth/o	inner ear

Endocrine System

adren/o	adrenal glands
gonad/o	gonads (male, female)
parathyroid/o	parathyroid gland
pineal/o	pineal gland
pituit/o	pituitary glands
thym/o	thymus
thyr/o, thyroid/o	thyroid gland

Integumentary/Skin System

cutane/o	skin
dermat/o, derm/o	skin
seb/o	sebaceous glands
hidr/o	sweat glands

pil/i, pil/o	hair
onych/o	nails

Nervous System

neur/o	nerves
encephal/o	brain
myel/o	spinal cord
mening/o	membranes covering spinal cord and brain

Reproductive System

pen/i, phall/i	penis
orch/o, test/i	testicles
oophor/o	ovaries
salping/o	fallopian tubes
hyster/o	uterus
placent/o	placenta

Respiratory System

nas/o	nose
sinus/o	sinus
rhin/o	nose
pharyng/o	pharynx
laryng/o	larynx
trache/o	trachea
bronchi/o	bronchi
alveol/o	alveoli

Musculoskeletal System

my/o	muscle
oste/o	bones
myel/o	bone marrow
chondr/o	cartilage
arthr/o	joints
ligament/o	ligaments
burs/o	bursa

Urinary System

nephr/o	kidneys
pyel/o	pelvis or kidney
ur/o, urin/o	urine
ureter/o	ureters
cyst/o	bladder
urethr/o	urethra

DO YOU REMEMBER THESE KEY POINTS?

- The abbreviations on the "Do Not Use" list and why they are dangerous
- The general classifications of medications and their associated body systems
- The various dosage forms and routes of administration
- The difference between pharmacokinetics and pharmacodynamics
- How drugs are absorbed, distributed, metabolized, and eliminated from the body
- The bioavailability of drugs in the body
- First-pass metabolism and why it is important in drug delivery

- Half-life and the factors that influence it
- The bioequivalence of drugs and its relationship to the Orange Book
- Types of excipients used in manufacturing dosage forms and the reasons for their use
- Packaging and storage requirements of medications
- Segments of medical terms
- Abbreviations for the routes of administration
- Common medical terms and abbreviations

Scenario FOLLOW UP

As Mary begins to feel more confident in her role as a technician, she finds herself looking forward to the challenges of each new day. Instead of feeling overwhelmed by the sheer number of the different types of drugs and all the various dosage forms she must learn, she understands that with time, she will add to her knowledge base and become a better technician with each passing day.

REVIEW QUESTIONS

Multiple Choice Questions

1. Why are sublingual tablets better for relieving angina attacks than traditional tablets?
   A. They will not cause drowsiness.
   B. They bypass the stomach, entering the bloodstream for quicker relief.
   C. They are administered less frequently than traditional tablets.
   D. They are easier to swallow.

2. Why do manufacturers make dosage forms that are effective over a longer time?
   A. To cut down on the cost of making the drug
   B. To save time preparing each dose
   C. To enable the patient to take the medication less often
   D. To meet Food and Drug Administration standards

3. Parenteral medications are used because:
   A. They work quickly.
   B. They bypass the acidic secretions of the stomach.
   C. The patient is unable to take medication by mouth.
   D. All of the above

4. Which of the following is *not* an example of a semisolid dosage form?
   A. Cream
   B. Gel
   C. Paste
   D. Lozenge

5. Which liquid dosage form has a hydroalcoholic base?
   A. Elixir
   B. Syrup
   C. Enema
   D. Emulsion

6. The organ that performs most of the metabolism of a drug is the:
   A. Kidney
   B. Small intestine
   C. Stomach
   D. Liver

7. If a drug has a half-life of 20 hours, this would mean that:
   A. Half of the drug is eliminated from the body in the first 20 hours, followed by the second half in 20 more hours.
   B. The drug only lasts half as long as needed.
   C. The drug loses half its strength in half of 20 hours.
   D. The drug loses half its strength in 20 hours, followed by half of the remaining strength in the following 20 hours, and so forth.

8. Excipients are used in preparing medications to:
   A. Improve appearance
   B. Disguise taste and/or smell
   C. Increase the size of the medication
   D. All of the above

9. The time taken for the plasma concentration of a drug to decrease by 50% is known as:
   A. Bioavailability
   B. Distribution
   C. Ionization
   D. Half-life

10. Which of the following oral dosage forms should have a "Shake Well" auxiliary label on the bottle?
   A. Suspension
   B. Solution
   C. Syrup
   D. All of the above

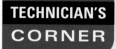

TECHNICIAN'S CORNER

A 30-year-old female was brought into the emergency room experiencing shortness of breath and a rash. She told the nurse she had seafood for dinner. The physician ordered a 0.5 mg dose of epinephrine. Shortly after the IV infusion, the patient complained of chest pain with tingling in her fingers. She was given the *correct* medication but via the *incorrect* route. What should have been the route?

Bibliography

Ansel HC, Allen LV, Popovich NG: *Ansel's pharmaceutical dosage forms and drug delivery systems*, ed 10, Baltimore, 2013, Lippincott Williams & Wilkins.

Brown M, Mulholland J: *Drug calculations*, ed 8, St Louis, 2007, Elsevier.

Drug facts and comparisons, ed 68, St Louis, 2013, Wolters Kluwer Health.

Gray Morris D: *Calculate with confidence*, ed 6, St Louis, 2013, Elsevier.

Potter PA, Perry AG: *Fundamentals of nursing*, ed 8, St Louis, 2013, Elsevier.

Websites Referenced

Approved Drug Products with Therapeutic Equivalence Evaluations (Orange book information). (Referenced September 15, 2013.) www.fda.gov/cder/ob

Cyprotex. ProDrug ADME Services. (Referenced February 19, 2014.) www.cyprotex.com/admepk/prodrug-services/

Difference Between.Net. Difference Between CFC and HFA Inhalers. (Referenced February 20, 2014.) www.differencebetween.net/science/health/disease-health/difference-between-cfc-and-hfa-inhalers/

Epharmacology. Hub Pages. Pharmacological Effects, ProDrugs (Definitions, Examples) and Sources of Drug Information (Referenced June 20, 2014.) http://epharmacology.hubpages.com/hub/Pharmacological-Effects-Prodrugs-Definition-Examples-and-Sources-of-Drug-Information.

Immunization Action Coalition. (Technical reviewed by CDC 2007). Vaccine Handling Tips. (Referenced August 24, 2013.) www.vaccineinformation.org

Institute for Safe Medication Practices. ISMP's List of Error Prone Abbreviations, Symbols, and Dose Designations. (Referenced February 10, 2014.) www.ismp.org/tools/errorproneabbreviations.pdf

Medscape website. Monograph: Insulins General Statement. (Referenced August 24, 2013.) www.medscape.com/druginfo/monoinfobyid?cid=med&drugid=5218&drugname=Humulin+R+Inj&monotype=genstatement&monoid=382933&mononame=Insulins%20General%20Statement&print=1

ProPublica. T. Christian Miller and Jeff Gerth, Dose of confusion. (Referenced September 15, 2013.) www.propublica.org/article/tylenol-mcneil-fda-kids-dose-of-confusion

The Joint Commission. Facts about the official "Do Not Use" list. (Referenced September 29, 2013.) http://www.jointcommission.org/assets/1/18/do_not_use_list.pdf

WebMD. Asthma Health Center. Nebulizers: home and portable. (Referenced September 30, 2013.) www.webmd.com/asthma/guide/home-nebulizer-therapy?page=2

Wisniewski L., RN, Holquist C. The absence of a trade name does not equal a generic drug. (Referenced September 13, 2013.) www.drugtopics.com

Conversions and Calculations

Elaine Simmons Beale, RPh

OBJECTIVES

Upon completing this chapter, you should be able to do the following:

1. Describe the history of the International System of Units.
2. Convert Arabic numbers into Roman numerals.
3. Convert traditional time into international/military time.
4. Convert Fahrenheit to Celsius.
5. Use the following to determine medication dosages:
   - Multiplication and division
   - Fractions
   - Decimals
   - Percentages
   - Ratio and proportion
   - Dimensional analysis
6. Demonstrate the ability to convert between the various systems of measurement used in the practice of pharmacy:
   - Metric system
   - Household measurement

- Apothecary system
- Avoirdupois system

7. Apply the formulas for calculating doses by body weight, body surface area (BSA), Young's Rule, and Clark's Rule.
8. Calculate pediatric and geriatric dosages.
9. Perform calculations involving units and milliequivalents.
10. Calculate infusion rates and drip rates.
11. Understand and apply the calculations involved in dilution.
12. Understand and apply the calculations involved in alligations.

TERMS AND DEFINITIONS

Alligation alternate A mathematical method of solving problems that involves the mixing of two solutions or two solids with different percentage weights to achieve a desired third strength

Apothecary system A system of measurement once used in the practice of pharmacy to measure both volume and weight; this system has been mostly replaced by the metric system

Avoirdupois system A system of measurement previously used in pharmacy for the determination of weight in ounces and pounds; this system has been mostly replaced by the metric system

Conversion factor A fraction with the numerical value of one, which is used to convert one unit to another without changing the value of the number

Diluent/solvent An inert product, either liquid or solid, that is added to a preparation to reduce the strength of the original product

Dilution The process of adding a diluent or solvent to a compound, resulting in a product of increased volume or weight and lower concentration

Dimensional analysis (DA) A method used to solve complicated pharmaceutical calculations that would require numerous sets of ratio and proportion problems; the main benefit of using DA is the ability to keep track of units during the process

Drip rate (DR)/drop rate The number of drops (gtt) administered over a specific time via an intravenous infusion (e.g., gtt/min)

Drop factor The size of drops coming through the tubing; the size is measured in gtt/mL and is found on the tubing package

Flow rate/infusion rate The amount of intravenous (IV) solution administered over a specific period (e.g., mL/min, mL/hr, gtt/min); volume/time

Household system A system of measurement commonly used in the United States; it measures volumes using household utensils

International time A 24-hour method of keeping time; hours are not distinguished as AM or PM, but rather are counted continuously throughout the day

International System of Units (SI) A system of measurement based on seven base units with prefixes that change units by multiples of

10; the prefixes for the modern metric system are taken from the French Système International d'Unités and were adopted to provide a single worldwide system of weights and measures

Markup The amount added to a wholesale price (usually a percentage) to make a profit

Metric system The approved system of measurement for pharmacy in the United States based on multiples of 10; the basic units of measurement are the gram (g) for weight, the liter (L) for volume, and the meter (m) for length

Milliequivalent (mEq) A type of unit used in the United States to express the concentration of electrolytes such as sodium, potassium, magnesium, and calcium

Retail price The wholesale price plus markup

Units A unit of measurement assigned to medications called "biologicals," which have been tested for potency in biological systems; units are specific to each medication, therefore units of one medication cannot be compared to units of a different medication

Volume The amount of liquid enclosed within a container

Wholesale cost The purchase price of a product (in this case, medicine), which is then marked up for resale

Introduction

Scenario:

Victoria is an experienced intravenous (IV) compounding technician. She has worked in her current position at a local hospital pharmacy for 8 years. She is responsible for making IV medications during her shift. Victoria performs many critical calculations on a regular basis. Today she is compounding an antibiotic small volume parenteral for a patient with a staph infection. Why is it important that Victoria's calculations are 100% accurate?

The ability to manipulate conversions and make calculations is a requirement of pharmacy technicians. Unfortunately, in many cases when math is mentioned to new pharmacy technicians, it can trigger instant stress by reminding students of previous bad experiences. However, pharmaceutical calculations are performed on a daily basis and applied to the medications prepared in class and at work. The repetitiveness of these conversions and calculations reinforces the student technician's knowledge and confidence. It is important to learn and feel comfortable with the basic conversions.

 Tech Note!

Although a pharmacist needs to check all transcriptions and calculations, it is important that the technician have a good understanding of these mathematical operations to avoid medication errors.

This chapter describes the types of calculations used throughout history, explains Roman numerals and military time, and presents common math problems involving multiplication, division, fractions, decimals, percentages, and ratios. Other areas of focus include the following:

- Dimensional analysis
- Metric system
- Household system
- Apothecary system
- Avoirdupois system
- Infusion rates, drip rates, and drop factors
- Dilution
- Alligation
- Dosing using mg/kg and body surface area (BSA) in m^2

Special calculations for infants, children, and senior citizens also are discussed; these patients deserve special consideration because of the metabolic differences that exist before adolescence and in old age.

Medication dosing is discussed for the following medications and therapies:

- Insulin
- Heparin
- Chemotherapy
- Parenteral nutrition

Make sure you understand each section before moving on to the next.

History of Pharmacy Calculations

Four different measurement systems have been used throughout the history of pharmacy. Most of the systems involve approximate measurements, so the conversion from one system to another is not precise. The pharmacy technician must have a basic understanding of all systems; however, in the United States, the United States Pharmacopeia (USP) recognizes the **metric system** as the official system of measurement for pharmacy. The metric system (discussed later in the chapter) is based on multiples of 10 and is the most precise of the systems. Technicians in the United States mostly encounter prescriptions expressed in either metric or household systems.

A good way to become familiar with common pharmacy measurements is to start with what you know and build on that knowledge. For example, most people are familiar with the household measurement of a teaspoon. When writing prescriptions, many prescribers prefer to use 5 milliliters (mL) in the metric system rather than 1 teaspoonful (tsp). These two measurements, one in the household system and the other in the metric system, are considered to be equivalent. The pharmacy technician must translate the physician's orders into terms an average person can understand. Always reread what will be printed on the prescription label to consider whether it will make sense to the lay person; never assume that a person understands the meaning of a measurement. This precaution reduces the chance of any misinterpretation of the instructions.

TABLE 6-1

Arabic and Roman Numerals

Arabic Numeral	Roman Numeral	Arabic Numeral	Roman Numeral
1	I	23	XXIII
2	II	24	XXIV
3	III	25	XXV
4	IV	26	XXVI
5	V	27	XXVII
6	VI	28	XXVIII
7	VII	29	XXIX
8	VIII	30	XXX
9	IX	40	XL
10	X	50	L
11	XI	60	LX
12	XII	70	LXX
13	XIII	80	LXXX
14	XIV	90	XC
15	XV	100	C
16	XVI	500	D
17	XVII	600	DC
18	XVIII	700	DCC
19	XIX	800	DCCC
20	XX	900	CM
21	XXI	1000	M
22	XXII		

Roman Numerals

Although Arabic numerals (i.e., 1, 2, 3, and so on) are commonly used in the United States, physicians do not always use this system when ordering medications. Instead, they may use Roman numerals to indicate the quantity of tablets or capsules, the number of fluid ounces, or the number of refills. Roman numerals may be either upper case or lower case letters.

When using Roman numerals, begin with I, II, III (1, 2, 3); then write IV (1 less than 5) to equal 4. Repeat the process at 9 by writing IX (1 less than 10) to equal 9. To write 40, write XL (10 less than 50). However, to write 49, use XLIX (not IL; see rule 9 in the following section). The fraction ½ is written as lower case $\overline{ss}$ (ss with a line over both letters). Table 6-1 presents a comparison of Roman numerals and Arabic numbers.

Rules for Determining Roman Numerals

1. Numbers are represented by combinations of the letters I, V, X, L, C, D, and M, which represent 1, 5, 10, 50, 100, 500, and 1000, respectively.
2. When a numeral is repeated, its value is repeated.
   Examples: II = 2   XXX = 30

3. A numeral may not be repeated more than three times.
   Example: XL = 40, not XXXX
4. V, L, and D are never repeated.
   Example: LL is incorrect for 100 (100 is C)
5. When a smaller numeral is placed after a larger numeral, it is added to the larger numeral.
   Example: CX = 100 + 10 = 110   LXVIII = 50 + 10 + 5 + 3 = 68
6. When a smaller numeral is placed before a larger numeral, it is subtracted from the larger numeral.
   Example: XC = 100 − 10 = 90   XCIX = (100 − 10) + (10 − 1) = 90 + 9 = 99
7. V, L, and D are *never* subtracted. LC is incorrect. (L already is 50)
8. Never subtract more than one numeral!
   Example: 8 = VIII, not IIX
9. When subtracting:
   a. Only subtract powers of 10: I, X, and C (not V or L)
   b. Only use a numeral before the next two higher-value numerals:
      • Use I before V and X, X before L and C, and C before D and M
   Example: 40 = XL, but 49 does not equal IL since I and L are too far apart (49 = XLIX)

EXAMPLE 6-1 WORKING WITH ROMAN NUMERALS

When working with Roman numerals, remember that if a larger number is placed in front of a smaller one, you must add the two to determine the value.

$$XV = X (10) + V (5) = 15$$

However, if a smaller number is placed before a larger number, you must subtract.

$$IX = X (10) - I (1) = 9$$

EXERCISE 6-1 QUICK CHECK

Change the following to Arabic numbers.
1. XIV = _____
2. XC = _____
3. XL = _____
4. VIII = _____
5. IV = _____
6. LX = _____
7. IX = _____
8. XX = _____
9. XXIV = _____
10. LXXV = _____
11. XXXIX = _____
12. CXX = _____

International Time (Military Time)

In a hospital or institutional setting, **international time**, also known as military time, is used exclusively. Orders are written 24 hours a day, and a system is needed to ensure that all medical-related caretakers understand exactly when an order was written and when the medication or treatment is to take place. The system is based on 100. Starting at 0000 (midnight) and continuing with 0100 (1 AM), the clock runs through to 2300 (11 PM) and restarts again at 0000 (midnight) (Figure 6-1). This system is easy for most people to use through 1200 (noon), but then it can become confusing. As the clock hands begin to make their second trip around the face of the clock in the PM hours, the numbers continue. For example, 1300 is 1 PM, and 1400 is 2 PM. Minutes are added to the hours in the last two places through 59. For instance, 1:32 PM is 1332, and 12:01 AM is 0001. When the pharmacy receives orders, the receiver must check the date and time against previous orders to ensure that the most recent order is in effect. Using this system, there is never any question as to when an order was written or which order supersedes another (Box 6-1).

EXERCISE 6-2 QUICK CHECK

Convert each time to either international or standard time.
1. 12:00 AM = _____
2. 4:30 PM = _____
3. 7:00 AM = _____
4. 1:30 AM = _____
5. 11:11 AM = _____
6. 9:15 PM = _____
7. 2:30 PM = _____
8. 2000 = _____
9. 1417 = _____
10. 2101 = _____
11. 2359 = _____
12. 1025 = _____

Temperature Conversion Between Fahrenheit and Celsius

The Fahrenheit temperature scale is most commonly used in the United States. Freezing is 32° F, and boiling is 212° F. The Celsius scale is used in

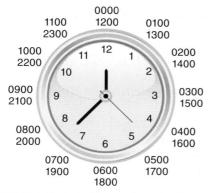

FIGURE 6-1 Clock showing regular and military time.

BOX 6-1

Time Conversions

Midnight (12:00 AM) = 0000 hr	12:00 PM = 1200 hr
1:00 AM = 0100 hr	1:00 PM = 1300 hr
2:00 AM = 0200 hr	2:00 PM = 1400 hr
3:00 AM = 0300 hr	3:00 PM = 1500 hr
4:00 AM = 0400 hr	4:00 PM = 1600 hr
5:00 AM = 0500 hr	5:00 PM = 1700 hr
6:00 AM = 0600 hr	6:00 PM = 1800 hr
7:00 AM = 0700 hr	7:00 PM = 1900 hr
8:00 AM = 0800 hr	8:00 PM = 2000 hr
9:00 AM = 0900 hr	9:00 PM = 2100 hr
10:00 AM = 1000 hr	10:00 PM = 2200 hr
11:00 AM = 1100 hr	11:00 PM = 2300 hr

countries that regularly use the metric system (discussed later in the chapter). The metric system is based on multiples of 10, and the Celsius temperature scale goes from 0° C as the freezing point to 100° C as the boiling point. It is sometimes necessary to convert between these two scales. Formulas for converting can be written with fractions or decimals as follows.

Fahrenheit to Celsius

$$\text{Fraction equation: } °C = (F - 32) \cdot \frac{5}{9}$$

$$\text{Decimal equation: } °C = \frac{(F - 32)}{1.8}$$

EXAMPLE 6-2

Convert 98.6° F to Celsius:

$$°C = (98.6 - 32) \cdot \frac{5}{9} = 37° C \text{ or } °C = \frac{(98.6 - 32)}{1.8} = 37° C$$

Celsius to Fahrenheit

$$\text{Fraction equation: } °F = \left(\frac{9}{5} \cdot C\right) + 32$$
$$\text{Decimal equation: } °F = (1.8 \cdot C) + 32$$

EXAMPLE 6-3

Convert 100° C to Fahrenheit:

$$°F = \frac{9 \cdot 100}{5} + 32 = 212° F \text{ or}$$
$$°F = (1.8 \cdot 100) + 32 = 212° F$$

EXERCISE 6-3 QUICK CHECK

Convert to Fahrenheit or Celsius.
1. 80° C = _____ ° F
2. 72° F = _____ ° C
3. 65° C = _____ ° F
4. 32° F = _____ ° C

Basic Math Skills

It is important for pharmacy technician students to review and be comfortable with basic skills such as adding, subtracting, multiplying, and dividing whole numbers, fractions, and decimals before adding new skills. Multiplication is used repeatedly in pharmacy calculations (Table 6-2). Sometimes it is necessary to increase or reduce a prescription. Multiplication by a number greater than 1 is used to increase a formula. Division, which is the same as multiplying by a proper fraction, is used to determine a part or portion of a prescription.

Review your multiplication and division skills. It is *essential* that you memorize multiplication at least through 12 before continuing. Use flash cards if necessary.

Fractions, Percentages, Ratios, and Proportions

Fractions
A fraction consists of a numerator and a denominator: the numerator is the top number in a fraction, and the denominator is the bottom number. The numerator of a fraction shows the number of equivalent parts in the whole, and the denominator shows how many are being considered as the whole.

TABLE 6-2

Multiplication Chart

	1	2	3	4	5	6	7	8	9	10	11	12
2	2	4	6	8	10	12	14	16	18	20	22	24
3	3	6	9	12	15	18	21	24	27	30	33	36
4	4	8	12	16	20	24	28	32	36	40	44	48
5	5	10	15	20	25	30	35	40	45	50	55	60
6	6	12	18	24	30	36	42	48	54	60	66	72
7	7	14	21	28	35	42	49	56	63	70	77	84
8	8	16	24	32	40	48	56	64	72	80	88	96
9	9	18	27	36	45	54	63	72	81	90	99	108
10	10	20	30	40	50	60	70	80	90	100	110	120
11	11	22	33	44	55	66	77	88	99	110	121	132
12	12	24	36	48	60	72	84	96	108	120	132	144

If an object is divided into four parts, one part can be expressed as ¼, or one part (1) of the whole (4). If we have a 1000-mg tablet:

½ tablet = 500 mg
¼ tablet = 250 mg

Types of Fractions

Proper: The numerator is smaller than the denominator, and the *value* is always less than 1.
Example: ½

Improper: The numerator is greater than or equal to the denominator, and the *value* is always greater than or equal to 1.
Example: ⁵⁄₂

Mixed: A whole number and a proper fraction combined.
Example: 5½

Converting Fractions to Decimals.
When converting fractions to decimals, divide the numerator by the denominator.

1. Converting a proper fraction to a decimal: ½ equals 1 divided by 2, which equals 0.5.
2. Converting an improper fraction to a decimal: ⁵⁄₂ equals 5 divided by 2, which equals 2.5
3. Converting a mixed fraction to a decimal: 3½ equals 3 plus (1 divided by 2 = 0.5), which equals 3.5
   - You can also change 3½ to an improper fraction first:
     - Multiply the denominator by the whole number: 2 times 3 equals 6
     - Add the product to the numerator: 6 plus 1 equals 7
     - Place new numerator over original denominator: ⁷⁄₂
     - ⁷⁄₂ (also written as 7/2) is 7 divided by 2, which equals 3.5

EXERCISE 6-4 QUICK CHECK

Convert the following fractions to decimals.
1. ½ =
2. 4⅝ =
3. ¾ =
4. 2½ =
5. ⁵⁵⁄₂₂ =
6. 1⅛ =
7. ³⁄₂ =
8. ²⁄₁₂ =
9. ⁵⁄₂₀ =
10. ⁹⁄₅ =

Percentages

The term *percent*, and its corresponding sign, %, means "per 100." Percentages represent a portion of a whole. The number 100 is used to represent the whole; therefore, 100% equals the whole.

Converting Decimals and Fractions to Percentages.
To convert a decimal to a percentage, multiply it by 100, which results in the decimal point moving two spaces to the right; then add a percent sign (%).

$$0.75 = 0.75 \times 100 = 75 \quad 75\%$$

To convert a fraction to a percentage, divide the numerator by the denominator and multiply by 100, which results in the decimal point moving two spaces to the right; then add a percent sign (%).

½ is 1 divided by 2, which equals 0.5

$$0.5 \times 100 = 50 \quad 50\%$$

In this chapter, round numbers to the hundredths place, which is two places past the decimal point.

Rounding a Number
1. Determine to what whole number or decimal place the number is to be rounded.
2. Look at the number to the right of the value being rounded.
3. If that number is 5 or greater, round up; if less than 5, round down.
   Examples
   - Round to whole number—use number in tenths place: 3.**4** = 3
   - Round to tenths—use number in hundredths place: 3.4**5** = 3.**5**
   - Round to hundredths—use number in thousandths place: 3.45**7** = 3.4**6**
   - ⅓ is 1 divided by 3, which is 0.333333333... (3 repeats indefinitely)
     - Round to 0.33 (hundredths place); then: 0.33 × 100 = 33%

Converting Percentages to Decimals.
To convert a percentage to a decimal, drop the percent sign and divide by 100. This results in the decimal point moving two spaces to the left.

$$60\% = 60 \text{ divided by } 100 = 0.60$$

Converting Percentages to Fractions.
To convert a percentage to a fraction, drop the percent sign, place the number over 100, and reduce.

$$60\% = \frac{60}{100} = \frac{6}{10} = \frac{3}{5}$$

$$1\% = \frac{1}{100}$$

$$0.5\% = \frac{0.5}{100}$$

This is not an appropriate form, so you must multiply the top and bottom by 10

$$\frac{0.5}{100} \cdot \frac{10}{10} = \frac{5}{1000} = \frac{1}{200}$$

This *does not change the value of the number* because $^{10}\!/_{10} = 1$; however, it removes the decimal from the numerator.

Converting Decimals to Fractions. To convert a decimal to a fraction, place the decimal over 1. Then, as in the previous example, you must multiply the top and bottom of the fraction by a multiple of 10 to remove the decimal point because decimals cannot be part of a fraction.

$$0.02 = \frac{0.02}{1} \cdot \frac{100}{100} = \frac{2}{100} = \frac{1}{50}$$

PRACTICE QUIZ 6-1

1. From 0800 to 1500 hours is _____ hours.
2. A dose given at 0600, 1400, and 2200 hours is _____ hours apart.
3. A dose given at 0005, 1430, and 2045 would be given at _____, _____, and _____ on a 12-hour clock.
4. Write 4:20 PM, 7:15 PM, and 12:00 AM in international time: _____, _____, _____.

Convert international time to 12-hour clock time and vice versa; convert Roman numerals to Arabic numbers and vice versa.

5. 0630 = _____
6. 0230 = _____
7. 0005 = _____
8. 7 PM = _____
9. 5:40 PM = _____
10. 9:20 PM = _____
11. XLV = _____
12. CIX = _____
13. IX = _____
14. XXII = _____
15. XCV = _____
16. 24 = _____
17. 59 = _____
18. 2011 = _____
19. 150 = _____
20. 55 = _____

Convert the following temperatures.

21. 40° C = _____ ° F
22. Insulin is stored in the pharmacy at 36° to 46° F. What is the range in Celsius?

Convert the following percentages to decimals.

23. 50% = _____
24. 12% = _____
25. 175% = _____
26. 2.5% = _____

Convert the following fractions to percentages.

27. $^1\!/_8$ = _____ %
28. $^5\!/_2$ = _____ %
29. $^3\!/_4$ = _____ %
30. $^4\!/_{10}$ = _____ %

Ratios

A ratio expresses a relationship between two quantities or measurements. The following expression is written as a ratio: 1:2, which is read "one is to two." A ratio can also be written as a fraction, in which the first number is the numerator and the second number is the denominator. This ratio can be written either as $^1\!/_2$ or as 1:2. When technicians compound products, they may be required to solve problems using ratios, which can be considered parts or fractions.

Converting Ratios to Percentages. To convert ratios to percentages, first express the ratio as a fraction, then convert it to a decimal, and finally multiply the decimal by 100 and add the percent sign.

$$3:4 = {}^3\!/_4 = 3 \text{ divided by } 4 = 0.75 \quad 0.75 \times 100 = 75 \quad 75\%$$

If two ratios have the same value, they are considered equivalent.

Proportions

A proportion is an equivalent relationship between two ratios.

$^1\!/_2 = {}^2\!/_4$ A proportion may be written as $1:2::2:4$.

This is read "one is to two as two is to four." Most single-step pharmaceutical calculations can be accomplished by using proportions. However, many technicians prefer to use dimensional analysis (discussed later) to make it easier to keep track of units, especially when performing multiple-step calculations.

Solving Proportion Problems. Proportion problems can be solved in two ways. The first method involves cross-multiplying and dividing; the second method is described as "means and extremes." Both methods yield the same answer if set up correctly.

$$\frac{3}{7} = \frac{x}{21} \quad \text{Cross-multiply: } 7x = 3 \cdot 21$$
$$7x = 63$$

Divide both sides by 7 to get the answer: $x = 9$
$3:7::x:21$ means and extremes: 7 times x equals 3 times 21 (same solution as above)

You may reduce a fraction if possible before solving a proportion.

$\dfrac{5}{10} = \dfrac{x}{40}$ may be reduced to $\dfrac{1}{2} = \dfrac{x}{40}$ to simplify the calculations

The ratio and proportion method can also be used to convert ratios to percentages as follows:

Change the ratio $3:4$ to a percentage: $\dfrac{3}{4} = \dfrac{x}{100}$

$x = 75$ 75 out of 100 equal 75%

EXERCISE 6-5 QUICK CHECK

Solve the following proportions.
1. $\frac{2}{10} = \frac{4}{x}$
2. $\frac{4}{40} = \frac{x}{100}$
3. $\frac{55}{82} = \frac{35}{x}$
4. $\frac{250}{500} = \frac{750}{x}$
5. $\frac{1}{25} = \frac{40}{x}$

 Tech Note!

Remember: You must place the proper units (e.g., ml, L, mg, or g) next to the number amount. This cannot be stressed enough, because you may be working with various systems of measurement. Including the units on all numbers helps reduce mistakes.

Working with Word Problems

Many pharmacy technicians have difficulty interpreting word problems. One way you can lessen the confusion of a word problem is by identifying what is known and what is being asked. One of the first things to remember is to dismiss unnecessary information.

In the following ratio and proportion (R&P) examples, identify what strength you have in stock and what strength you need (what the physician is ordering). Next, set up the equation and double-check the calculations. It is important to remember to place the correct units in the correct position. For example, if one side of the equation has milligrams divided by milliliters, then the opposite side of the equation must be expressed as milligrams divided by milliliters.

EXAMPLE 6-4 SINGLE-STEP R&P PROBLEM

You receive an order for Ativan 4 mg. You have 2-mg tablets in stock. How many 2-mg tablets will you need to fill this order?

Note: Most pharmacists will expect you to be able to answer this type of question quickly, without performing written calculations. This example is being used to demonstrate ratio and proportion calculations.

$$\frac{2\text{ mg}}{1\text{ tab}} = \frac{4\text{ mg}}{x} \qquad 2x = 4 \qquad x = 2\text{ tabs}$$

Dimensional Analysis

Dimensional analysis (DA) is a method used to solve more complicated pharmaceutical calculations that would require numerous sets of ratio and proportion problems. The main benefit of using DA is the ability to keep track of units during the process to ensure that the answer has the correct unit and nothing has been overlooked. The steps for DA are as follows:
1. Identify the unit needed in the answer.
2. Write down that unit and an equals sign.
3. Begin the dimensional analysis equation so that the units you want in the *final* answer are in the numerator of the first fraction of the equation; *do not cancel this unit.*
4. Continue with the next fraction in the equation, placed so that the units of its numerator are the same as the units of the denominator of the first fraction, so they will cancel. Continue until all necessary information has been placed in the problem.
5. Cancel your units and multiply the numbers.

EXAMPLE 6-5 DIMENSIONAL ANALYSIS

You receive an order for amoxicillin 250 mg caps qid × 7 d (4 times a day for 7 days).

How many capsules will be needed?

Once again, most pharmacists want their technicians to perform this type of calculation in their head without having to write out a long equation; however, for practice with the concept of DA, the reasoning is as follows:

$$\text{capsules} = \frac{1\text{ cap}}{\text{dose}} \cdot \frac{4\text{ doses}}{\text{day}} \cdot \frac{7\text{ days}}{1} = 28\text{ caps}$$

The unit needed in the answer was placed as the numerator of the first fraction and never canceled. Dose canceled dose and day canceled day, leaving the correct unit as capsules. In this example, the strength of the capsule does not affect the answer and is not used in the calculation.

EXAMPLE 6-6 DIMENSIONAL ANALYSIS

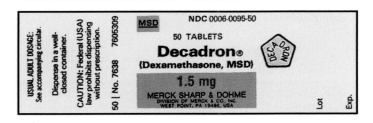

Order: Decadron 3 mg twice a day for 30 days. *How many tablets* are needed to fill this order?

Stock on hand: 1.5-mg tablets

Solve for the total amount of tablets needed for the month.

Set up your equation:

$$\text{tablets} = \frac{1\,\text{tab}}{1.5\,\text{mg}} \cdot \frac{3\,\text{mg}}{1\,\text{dose}} \cdot \frac{2\,\text{doses}}{\text{day}} \cdot \frac{30\,\text{days}}{1} = 120\,\text{tabs}$$

The unit needed in the answer was placed as the numerator of the first fraction and never canceled; mg canceled mg, dose canceled dose, and day canceled day, leaving the correct unit as tablets.

 Tech Note!

Always pay attention to the dosage form. You cannot take one and a half capsules, but you can take one and one half tablets *in some circumstances*. A scored tablet is marked so that it can be split into equal parts. Remember that not all tablets can be split, such as sustained-release or enteric-coated tablets.

EXERCISE 6-6 QUICK CHECK

Use ratio/proportion, DA, or calculate in your head as appropriate.

1. Order: metoprolol tartrate 100 mg tablet twice a day for 30 days.
   Stock: 50 mg tablets. How many tablets will it take to fill this 30-day supply?
2. Order: Augmentin 250 mg four times a day for 7 days.
   Stock: 250 mg capsules. How many capsules are needed to fill this prescription?

Determine 1 Dose

3. Stock: 250-mg tabs; dose 125 mg; give _____ tabs
4. Stock: 10-mg capsules; dose 30 mg; give _____ caps
5. Stock: 4-mg tablets; dose 8 mg; give _____ tabs

Measurement Systems

For a measurement to make sense, it must have a number and a unit. Different measurement systems

TABLE 6-3

Metric Prefixes

Prefix	Meaning
nano-	One-billionth of the basic unit
micro-	One-millionth of the basic unit
milli-	One-thousandth of the basic unit
centi-	One-hundredth of the basic unit
deci-	One-tenth of the basic unit
deca-	10 times the basic unit
hecto-	100 times the basic unit
kilo-	1000 times the basic unit

use different units. For example, the **household system** uses teaspoons and tablespoons for small volumes, whereas the metric system uses milliliters for this size measurement. All answers must have a unit or they are incorrect. Ordering 2 per day makes no sense because it could mean 2 tablets, capsules, teaspoons, milligrams, grams, milliliters, and so on.

Metric System

The USP recognizes the **International System of Units (SI)**, or metric system, as the official system of measurement for pharmacy in the United States. The metric system can be used to measure weight, **volume**, and distance. The basic unit of measurement for weight is the gram (g), for volume is the liter (L), and for length is the meter (m). A pharmacy technician will use the prefixes micro-, milli-, and kilo-, along with the base unit (Table 6-3).

In the metric system, each unit of measurement is a multiple of 10. To convert from a larger unit of measurement to a smaller unit of measurement, multiply by a multiple of 10. To convert from a smaller unit of measurement to a larger unit of measurement, divide by a multiple of 10. A technician must know the difference between the various units used in the metric system. If a prescription for 1 mcg of medication was filled with 1 mg, the patient would receive a 1000-fold overdose; there is a 1000-unit difference between these two measurements. This means that 1000 micrograms (mcg) equals 1 mg. It is extremely important for the technician to know how the units relate to one another.

Metric Measurements

1. The most commonly used metric measurements of weight in pharmacy include, from largest to smallest, the kilogram (kg), the gram (g), the milligram (mg), and the microgram (mcg). There is a 1000-fold difference between kg and g, g and mg, and mg and mcg, as seen in the following:

Metric Measurements of Mass Used in Pharmacy

kg_____g_____mg_____mcg

1 kg = 1000 g   1 g = 1000 mg   1 mg = 1000 mcg

- There is a 1000-unit difference (three decimal places) between kg and g; g and mg; and mg and mcg.
- There is a 1,000,000-unit difference (six decimal places) between kg and mg and between g and mcg.
- There is a 1,000,000,000-unit difference (nine decimal places) between kg and mcg.

2. When measuring volumes, a pharmacy technician uses milliliters (mL) and liters (L).

$$I\,L = 1000\,mL^*$$

3. Meters squared (m²) are used in drug calculations that are based on BSA, which is calculated by a physician or pharmacist using a body surface area calculation chart or a computer program.

 Tech Alert!

One of the most common errors made in pharmacy is the improper use of the decimal point. Physicians who write medication orders without using a leading zero (e.g., .5 g) risk the order being mistaken for 5 g. A leading zero clarifies that the value is less than 1 and helps reduce pharmacy errors (write 0.5 g). The same is true of trailing zeros. An order for 50.0 mg could easily be mistaken for 500 mg. Do not add the decimal point and trailing zero (write 50 mg).

Always seek clarification of an order when it seems that the dose is extremely high or low. When the pharmacy technician performs calculations, he or she must use leading zeros if the number is less than 1. Certain medications given in wrong strengths can harm or even kill the patient (see the following examples). For more information on drug errors, see Chapter 14.

Wrong way: .1 mg could be mistaken for 1 mg
Right way: 0.1 mg is very clear because of the leading zero
Wrong way: 25.0 mg could be mistaken for 250 mg
Right way: 25 mg is very clear because of the lack of decimals and trailing zeros

Converting between Units with DA

Some technicians find it easier to convert between units using DA. DA makes use of a **conversion factor**, a fraction equal to one, which is used

---

*Some prescribers still use cubic centimeter (cc) for volume (1 cc = 1 mL); however this unit is on the official "Do Not Use" List because it is easily confused with 00 when written by hand.

to change the *unit* of a measurement but **not** the *value*.

The following conversion factors are commonly used in the metric system:

$$\frac{1000\,mcg}{1\,mg} \quad \frac{1000\,mg}{1\,g} \quad \frac{1000\,g}{1\,kg} \quad \frac{1000\,mL}{1\,L}$$

Regardless of which value is in the numerator and which value is in the denominator, all of these equal 1 numerically, so multiplying by a conversion factor is like multiplying by 1.

Because 1000 mcg = 1 mg,

both $\dfrac{1000\,mcg}{1\,mg}$ and $\dfrac{1\,mg}{1000\,mcg}$ equals 1

5 g equals how many mg?

$$mg = \frac{1000\,mg}{1\,g} \cdot \frac{5\,g}{1} = 5000\,mg$$

Notice that the decimal moved three places to the *right* because there is a 1000-fold difference between *g* and *mg* and *g is larger than mg.*

250 mcg equals how many mg?

$$mg = \frac{1\,mg}{1000\,mcg} \cdot \frac{250\,mcg}{1} = 0.25\,mg$$

Notice that the decimal moved three places to the *left* because there is a 1000-fold difference between *mcg* and *mg* and *mcg is smaller than mg.*

4.2 g equals how many mcg?

$$mcg = \frac{1000\,mcg}{1\,mg} \cdot \frac{1000\,mg}{1\,g} \cdot \frac{4.2\,g}{1} = 4,200,000\,mcg$$

Notice that the decimal moved six places to the right because there is a 1,000,000-fold difference between *mcg* and *g* and *g is larger than mcg.*

2500 mL equals how many L?

$$L = \frac{1\,L}{1000\,mL} \cdot \frac{2500\,mL}{1} = 2.5\,L$$

The decimal moved three places to the left because *L is larger than mL.*

Metric Rule of Thumb

When converting in the metric system:

- **L**arger unit to **S**maller unit go **R**ight with decimal point (**LSR**)
  Example: Changing kg to g
    6.25 kg = 6250 g
      Moved the decimal three places to the *right* because of the 1000-fold difference between kg and g
      Like multiplying by a multiple of 10, in this case 1000
- **S**maller to **L**arger go **L**eft with decimal point (**SLL**)

Example: Changing mg to g
>   120 mg = 0.120 g
>   Moved the decimal three places to the *left* because of the 1000-fold difference between mg and g
>   Like dividing by a multiple of 10, in this case 1000
>   Remember to place a zero before the decimal point if no other number is there!

Conversions from one metric unit to another become almost automatic once you have practiced them enough. Make sure you know how the units relate to one another.

EXERCISE 6-7 QUICK CHECK

Solve the following problems using the appropriate conversions.
1. You receive a physician's order for 0.88 mcg of drug A. What is the equivalent in milligrams?
2. You receive a physician's order for 5 g of drug B. What is the equivalent in kilograms?
3. You receive an order for 250 mg of drug C. What is the equivalent in micrograms?
4. You receive a physician's order for 250 mg of drug D. What is the equivalent in grams?
5. You receive a physician's order to prepare 0.5 kg of drug E. What is the equivalent in grams?

Household Measurements

The metric system can also be converted into household liquid measurements. The main dry weight measurements in this system are the pound (lb) and the ounce (oz). 1 lb = 16 oz.

Common household measurements of volume are listed in Table 6-4.

The main conversions between household and metric measurements are listed in Table 6-5. Memorize these five conversions. With this information and your knowledge of the household system, you should be able to calculate any volume needed in pharmacy.

The following questions will become easy to answer once you have worked with the measurement systems awhile. They can be performed with ratio and proportion or DA. It is best to use DA if you are performing multistep conversions to keep track of units.

 Tech Note!

Remember that you *only* cross-multiply when there is an equal sign between two ratios indicating that they are equivalent. *Never* cross-multiply with DA.

EXAMPLE 6-7

How many milliliters are in 2 tablespoons? Use 1 Tbsp = 15 mL

R&P: $\dfrac{15\ \text{mL}}{1\ \text{Tbsp}} = \dfrac{x}{2\ \text{Tbsp}}$

>   Cross-multiply and divide to get 30 mL

DA: $\text{mL} = \dfrac{15\ \text{mL}}{1\ \text{Tbsp}} \cdot \dfrac{2\ \text{Tbsp}}{1} = 30\ \text{mL}$

>   (Tbsp units cancel, leaving mL as the answer)

EXAMPLE 6-8

How many mL are in 4 oz?

R&P: $\dfrac{30\ \text{mL}}{1\ \text{oz}} = \dfrac{x}{4\ \text{oz}}$

>   Cross-multiply and divide to get 120 mL

DA: $\text{mL} = \dfrac{30\ \text{mL}}{1\ \text{oz}} \cdot \dfrac{4\ \text{oz}}{1} = 120\ \text{mL}$

>   (oz units cancel, leaving mL as the answer)

 Tech Note!

Compare household kitchen measuring devices to metric measurements in milliliters.

TABLE 6-4

Household Measurements of Volume

	Abbreviations	Equivalents
1 drop	gtt	
1 teaspoon	tsp	60 drops (varies according to dropper size)
1 tablespoon	Tbsp	3 teaspoons
1 ounce	oz	2 Tbsp
1 cup	c	8 oz
1 pint	pt	2 c
1 quart	qt	2 pt
1 gallon	gal	4 qt

TABLE 6-5

Household to Metric Volume Conversions

Household Volume	Metric Volume
1 tsp	5 mL
1 Tbsp	15 mL
1 fl oz	30 mL
1 pt	480 mL
1 gal	3840 mL

EXERCISE 6-8 QUICK CHECK

1. 3 teaspoons = _____ tablespoons = _____ mL
2. 1 ounce = _____ tablespoons = _____ mL
3. 1 cup = _____ ounces = _____ mL
4. 1 pint = _____ tablespoons = _____ mL
5. 1 quart = _____ pints = _____ mL
6. 1 gallon = _____ teaspoons = _____ mL
7. 40 ounces = _____ tablespoons = _____ mL
8. 32 ounces = _____ cups = _____ mL

Apothecary System

The **apothecary system** of measurement, which originated in Europe, is the traditional system of measurement used by physicians and apothecaries. Although it is now largely of historical significance only, components of this system may still be found on some prescriptions.

The apothecary units used in pharmacy include grain (*gr*), dram (℈), ounce (℥), and pound (lb) for dry weight and minim (ℳ), fluid dram (f℥), and fluid ounce (f℥) for volume. When using the apothecary system, place the unit of measurement before the amount and use lower case Roman numerals for the number; for example, 1 grain is written gr i. Historically the most common way to write ½ grain is gr s̄s̄. Now that s̄s̄ is identified as a potentially dangerous abbreviation on the list published by the Institute for Safe Medication Practices (ISMP), you should write gr ½. However, prescribers may still use s̄s̄. Never combine Roman numerals and fractions;

therefore, 3¼ grains would be written gr 3¼ not gr iii ¼.

The following conversion for dry weight is common:

Weight: gr i = 60 mg, 64.8 mg, or 65 mg
(see the following Tech Note!)

 Tech Note!

The weight of a grain in the apothecary system varies between 60 mg, 64.8 mg, and 65 mg. Why? When the grain was used in ancient times to determine weight, real grains of wheat were used, and the weight depended on that year's harvest. If the crop was good, it took fewer grains because each piece weighed more. If the crops were bad that year, it took more grains to equal the same weight. Be aware that some medication labels will state that there are 60 mg/gr, whereas others might have 64.8 mg/gr or 65 mg/gr. For example, 60 mg/gr is used with codeine and nitroglycerin (NTG) tablets, whereas 65 mg/gr is used with aspirin (ASA), acetaminophen (APAP), and iron tablets.

The following conversions for volume are used occasionally:

Volume: 8 fluid drams = 1 fluid ounce
= 30 mL = 2 Tbsp

1 fluid dram = 3.7 mL   This is often considered to be 5 mL or 1 tsp, which is an approximation

Figure 6-2 presents examples of volume conversions between household, metric, and apothecary systems in medication cups. The cups show 8 drams equal to 1 fl oz, 30 mL, and 2 Tbsp.

EXAMPLE 6-9

How many grains are in 325 mg of aspirin (ASA)? Use 65 mg = gr i

$$gr = \frac{gr\ i}{65\ mg} \cdot \frac{325\ mg}{1} = gr\ v$$

Household/metric

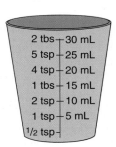

Apothecary/household

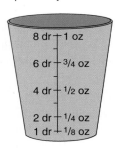

One-ounce medicine cups (30 mL)

FIGURE 6-2 Oral cups show equivalent volumes between household and metric and household and apothecary units. (From Gray Morris D: *Calculate with confidence*, ed 4, St Louis, 2008, Elsevier.)

EXAMPLE 6-10

How many milligrams are in gr $\frac{1}{150}$ of nitroglycerin sublingual (NTG SL) tablets? Use 60 mg = gr i

$$mg = \frac{60 \text{ mg}}{\text{gr i}} \cdot \frac{\text{gr}1/150}{1}$$

$$60 \text{ mg} \cdot \frac{1}{150} = \frac{60 \text{ mg}}{150} = 0.4 \text{ mg}$$

EXERCISE 6-9 QUICK CHECK

Solve the following conversions (refer to tech note for conversion factors).
1. NTG gr $\frac{1}{100}$ = _____ mg
2. NTG gr $\frac{1}{200}$ = _____ mg
3. codeine gr $\frac{1}{2}$ = _____ mg
4. aspirin gr x = _____ mg
5. iron 325 mg = gr _____
6. acetaminophen 130 mg = gr _____
7. 1 oz = _____ fluid drams
8. 1 Tbsp = _____ fluid drams

Avoirdupois System

The **avoirdupois system** is another type of measurement that originated in England. The avoirdupois system is the common system of commerce. It is through this system that items are purchased and sold by the ounce and pound. The avoirdupois system is similar to the apothecary system because it also uses grains, ounces, and pounds for weights. Table 6-6 shows the common avoirdupois weights and volumes.

Avoirdupois Measurements
1. Dry weights use grains (gr), ounces (oz), and pounds (lb).
2. Liquid volumes use fluid ounces (fl oz), pints (pt), and gallons (gal).

TABLE 6-6

Standard Weights and Volumes: Avoirdupois/Metric*

Avoirdupois Weight	Metric Equivalent
Dry Weights	
1 lb	454 g
1 oz	30 g
1 gr	64.8 mg
Liquids	
1 fl oz	30 mL
1 pt	473 mL
1 gal	3785 mL

*Conversions: 60 minims (♏) = 1 fluidrachm or fluid dram (f℥), 8 fluidrachms (480 minims) = 1 fluid ounce (f℥); 16 fl oz = 1 pint (pt); 2 pt (32 fl oz) = 1 quart (qt); 4 qt (8 pt) = 1 gallon (gal).

EXERCISE 6-10 QUICK CHECK

Volume
1. 1 fl dram = _____ mL or approximately _____ mL
2. 8 oz = _____ cup(s) or _____ mL
3. 1 gal = _____ mL
4. 5 mL = _____ tsp
5. 30 mL = _____ tsp or _____ Tbsp

Weight
6. 1 lb = _____ g
7. 1 kg = _____ g or _____ mg
8. acetaminophen gr x = _____ mg
9. 1000 mcg = _____ mg
10. 1 g = _____ mg

PRACTICE QUIZ 6-2

1. 5 mL = _____ tsp
2. 15 mL = _____ Tbsp
3. 30 mL = _____ tsp
4. 1 dram = _____ mL or approximately _____ mL
5. 1 L = _____ mL
6. 454 g = _____ lb
7. 4.4 lb = _____ kg
8. 3000 mcg = _____ mg
9. 450 g = _____ mg
10. 25 kg = _____ mg
11. 1.5 L = _____ mL
12. 3 lb = _____ kg
13. 25 lb = _____ oz
14. 2.25 mcg = _____ mg
15. 240 mL = _____ oz
16. 2 pints = _____ quarts
17. 1 gallon = _____ pints
18. 500 mL = _____ L
19. NTG gr $\frac{1}{100}$ = _____ mg
20. NTG gr $\frac{1}{150}$ = _____ mg
21. ASA 325 mg = gr _____

22. 9000 mg = _____ g
23. 0900 = _____ o'clock (AM or PM)
24. 2110 = _____ o'clock (AM or PM)
25. 1320 = _____ o'clock (AM or PM)
26. 2350 = _____ o'clock (AM or PM)
27. 2:30 PM = _____ (international time)
28. 11:00 AM = _____ (international time)
29. 9:25 PM = _____ (international time)
30. 4:10 AM = _____ (international time)
31. 6 PM = _____ (international time)
32. ix = _____ (Arabic number)
33. viii = _____ (Arabic number)
34. LX = _____ (Arabic number)
35. IV = _____ (Arabic number)
36. XC = _____ (Arabic number)
37. XXX = _____ (Arabic number)

Important Differences Among Systems

You should know how metric system units compare to other units of measure, such as ounces and grains. Most of the time they convert easily, but sometimes there are variances, making conversions between measurement systems approximate in these instances. Because the metric system is the approved system of measurement used in pharmacy, it is the measurement system you should use when preparing a compounded drug. However, you will see differences among manufacturers' products and their weights. For example, some manufacturers consider 473 mL to equal 1 pint, whereas others consider 480 mL to equal 1 pint. The rule is to follow the metric system because it is the approved system of measurement for pharmacy in the United States.

For the following examples, the orders are written in standard abbreviations that indicate how often (frequency) a medication is to be given (Box 6-2).

Calculations with Liquid Medication

Single-step problems with liquid medications can be solved with ratio and proportion.

Order: docusate sodium 20 mg bid
In stock: docusate sodium 4 mg/mL

1. How many milliliters are needed per dose? (Think 4 is to 1 as 20 is to x.)

BOX 6-2

Dosing Schedules (Pharmacy Abbreviations)

bid = 2 times daily	q8h = every 8 hours
q12h = every 12 hours	qid = 4 times daily
tid = 3 times daily	q6h = every 6 hours

$$\frac{4 \text{ mg}}{\text{mL}} = \frac{20 \text{ mg}}{x} \qquad x = 5 \text{ mL}$$

2. How many milliliters are needed per day? 5 mL twice a day equals 10 mL.

Multiple-step problems can be solved with DA to keep track of the units.

1. How many doses can be taken from the 8-oz bottle?

$$\text{doses} = \frac{1 \text{ dose}}{5 \text{ mL}} \cdot \frac{30 \text{ mL}}{1 \text{ oz}} \cdot \frac{8 \text{ oz}}{1} = 48 \text{ doses}$$

EXAMPLE 6-11 SINGLE-STEP PROPORTION PROBLEM

Prepare 240 mg of gentamicin intravenous piggyback (IVPB) using the pharmacy stock concentration of 40 mg/mL (each mL of stock solution contains 40 mg of gentamicin).

How many mL are needed for one dose?

In this case, you need to determine how many *milliliters* of the stock solution are needed to fill the 240 mg order. Write your stock strength or given concentration on the left and the needed amount on the right. Make sure that milligrams are in the numerator and milliliters are in the denominator on both sides. Then cross-multiply and divide; this will give you the necessary milliliters to withdraw from the vial.

$$\frac{40 \text{ mg}}{1 \text{ mL}} = \frac{240 \text{ mg}}{x \text{ mL}} \qquad 40x = 240$$
Divide both sides by 40 $x = 6 \text{ mL}$

EXAMPLE 6-12 SINGLE-STEP PROPORTION PROBLEM

Order: clindamycin 450 mg IVPB q12h
Stock: clindamycin 150 mg/mL

How many mL are needed for one dose?

You are solving for x because you do not know how much clindamycin to draw up into a syringe. To solve for x, you *cross-multiply and divide:*

$$\frac{150 \text{ mg}}{1 \text{ mL}} = \frac{450 \text{ mg}}{x} \qquad 150x = 450 \qquad x = 3 \text{ mL}$$

EXAMPLE 6-13 MULTIPLE-STEP DA PROBLEM

Order: theophylline 45 mg PO
Stock: theophylline 80 mg/Tbsp

How many mL are needed for one dose?

$$\text{mL} = \frac{15 \text{ mL}}{1 \text{ Tbsp}} \cdot \frac{1 \text{ Tbsp}}{80 \text{ mg}} \cdot \frac{45 \text{ mg}}{1} = 8.4 \text{ mL}$$

EXAMPLE 6-14 DIMENSIONAL ANALYSIS

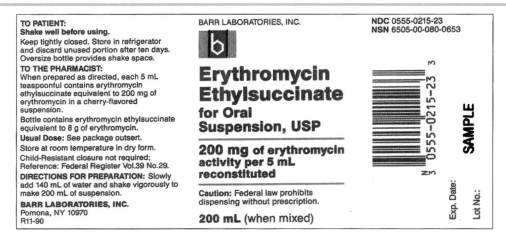

Order: erythromycin suspension 125 mg tid × 10 d. *How many mL* are needed to fill this order? Stock: 200 mg/5 mL. Interpret order: 125 mg to be taken 3 times per day for 10 days.

Set up your equation:

$$mL = \frac{5 \text{ mL}}{200 \text{ mg}} \cdot \frac{125 \text{ mg}}{1 \text{ dose}} \cdot \frac{3 \text{ doses}}{1 \text{ d}} \cdot \frac{10 \text{ d}}{1} = 93.75 \text{ mL}$$

The unit needed in the answer (mL) was placed as the numerator of the first fraction and never canceled (mg canceled mg, dose canceled dose, and day canceled day, leaving the correct unit as mL). On a practical note, this would probably be rounded up to 100 mL.

EXERCISE 6-11 QUICK CHECK

1. Order: 25 mg; stock: 10 mg/mL; give _____ mL
2. Order: 25 mg; stock: 40 mg/mL; give _____ mL
3. Order: 0.6 g; stock: 1.5 g/mL; give _____ mL
4. Order: 500 mg; stock: 25 mg/mL; give _____ mL
5. Order: 250 mg; stock: 500 mg/5mL; give _____ tsp

When preparing intravenous (IV) and other parenteral medications, you may need to calculate the correct dose based on weight, in kg or lb, or BSA, in m²; this is especially true of infants, children, and senior citizens. Chemotherapy medications are often based on the body surface area of the patient. Always check your calculations at least three times before asking a pharmacist to check them. The following sections present examples of the most common methods of performing these calculations.

Calculating the Proper Dose Using Body Weight

All official compendia, drug references, and drug manufacturers provide proper dosing regimens. When these are based on kilograms and the patient's weight is provided in pounds, it is necessary to convert pounds into kilograms. It is important to remember that there are 2.2 lb per kilogram.

$$1 \text{ kg} = 2.2 \text{ lb}$$

What is the weight in kg of a 176-lb person?

$$kg = \frac{1 \text{ kg}}{2.2 \text{ lb}} \cdot \frac{176 \text{ lb}}{1} = 80 \text{ kg}.$$

EXAMPLE 6-15

Dose ordered: 2.5 mg/kg/dose (q8h). Patient weighs 250 lb. How many mg per dose?

$$mg/dose = \frac{2.5 \text{ mg}}{kg / dose} \cdot \frac{1 \text{ kg}}{2.2 \text{ lb}} \cdot \frac{250 \text{ lb}}{1} = 284 \text{ mg/dose}$$

Observe how the units cancel, leaving the correct unit as mg/dose.

If the answer had been required in g, one more conversion would be necessary, as follows:

$$g/dose = \frac{1 \text{ g}}{1000 \text{ mg}} \cdot \frac{2.5 \text{ mg}}{kg / dose} \cdot \frac{1 \text{ kg}}{2.2 \text{ lb}} \cdot \frac{250 \text{ lb}}{1}$$
$$= 0.28 \text{ g/dose}$$

If the question reads: How many g/day, one more conversion would be necessary:

$$g/day = \frac{1\,g}{1000\,mg} \cdot \frac{2.5\,mg}{kg/dose} \cdot \frac{1\,kg}{2.2\,lb} \cdot \frac{250\,lb}{1} \cdot \frac{3\,doses}{day}$$
$$= 0.85\,g/day$$

When working the following exercises, take care to read exactly what the question is asking.

EXERCISE 6-12 QUICK CHECK

1. Dose ordered: 125 mg/kg/dose (q24h). Patient weighs 175 lb. How many *g* per dose?
2. Dose ordered: 55 mg/kg/day (q8h). Patient weighs 48 lb. How many *mg* per dose?
3. Dose ordered: 220 mg/kg/dose (q12h). Patient weighs 141 lb. How many *g* per day?
4. Dose ordered: 1.12 mg/kg/day (q6h). Patient weighs 98 lb. How many *mg* per dose?

 Tech Note!

This is how to remember kilogram conversion: Your weight is more than cut in half when measured in kilograms (2.2 lb = 1 kg). If you weighed 200 lb, you would weigh 91 kg.

Calculating Body Surface Area

The BSA method of calculating a patient's dose results in the most accurate dose because it is based on both the *height* and the *weight* of the patient. BSA calculations are extremely important when determining chemotherapeutic and pediatric doses. A *nomogram* is a table used to determine a patient's body surface area in meters squared (m^2). Most hospitals used computer-based programs to determine BSA.

Solve BSA calculations in the same way you would a dosing problem based on weight.

Patient: length 20 inches; weight 5 lb; BSA 0.18 m^2; dose 75 mg/m^2

How many mg are required per dose?

$$mg = \frac{75\,mg}{m^2} \cdot \frac{0.18\,m^2}{1} = 13.5\,mg$$

EXERCISE 6-13 QUICK CHECK

1. Patient: length 60 inches; weight 85 kg; BSA 1.8 m^2; dose 200 mg/m^2
   How many mg are required per dose?
2. Patient: length 65 inches; weight 150 lb; BSA 1.8 m^2; dose 2.5 g/m^2
   How many g are required per dose?

 Tech Note!

Remember to read the dosage instructions carefully to determine whether the medication is dosed in *kg* or m^2 per dose *or* per day.

Oral and Injectable Syringes

When filling oral liquid prescription orders for pediatric patients and those who cannot take solid dosage forms, you may need to provide an oral syringe with the prescription (Figure 6-3). A needle cannot be attached to an oral syringe, which reduces the possibility of administration errors. In the case of injectable medications, several possible syringe sizes can be selected to withdraw the correct volume of solution. A needle is attached to this type of syringe.

Pediatric and Geriatric Dosing

Liquid medications are used frequently for children and elderly patients. It is important that the parent understand how much medicine to give a child. Using pharmacy-supplied measuring devices, usually marked in household and metric measurements, increases the accuracy of dosing. Very small amounts may be measured with droppers. The pharmacist, not the technician, should show the parent of a patient how to measure the correct amount. Senior citizens must also be careful to take the correct amount of medication. For oral liquids, dosing devices with large, boldface calibrations may help the geriatric patient see the correct amount. Many of these types of dosing devices are sold over the counter.

Calculating Pediatric Dosages

Pediatrics refers to the practice of medicine in children from childbirth until adolescence. This range of ages is subdivided into various groups:

- Neonates: birth to 1 month
- Infant: 1 month to 1 year
- Early childhood: 1 year through 5 years
- Late childhood: 6 years through 12 years
- Adolescence: 13 years through 17 years

Pediatric dosages can be calculated using DA.

EXAMPLE 6-16

The pharmacy receives an order for a baby girl weighing 7 lb.

The order calls for 20 mg/kg/dose.

This means that for every kilogram the child weighs, she should receive 20 mg of medication.

$$mg/dose = \frac{20\,mg}{kg/dose} \cdot \frac{1\,kg}{2.2\,lb} \cdot \frac{7\,lb}{1} = 63.6\,mg/dose$$

Household/metric   Medication Dropper   Syringe

oz/mL

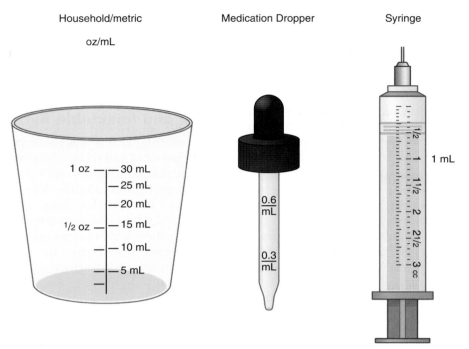

FIGURE 6-3 Common devices used for measuring liquid medications.

Tech Note!

When rounding off numbers, complete all the calculations first and then round off at the end of the calculations if instructed to do so by the pharmacist. If you round off at each step, your answer will not be as accurate.

Other Methods of Calculating Pediatric Doses

Two other methods can be used to calculate pediatric doses. Clark's Rule uses the child's weight in pounds divided by 150 lb (the average weight of an adult) as the basis for calculating the dose from the adult-recommended dose. Young's Rule uses the child's age in years divided by the child's age in years plus 12 as the basis for calculating the child's dose from the adult-recommended dose. Both of these methods are approximations.

Clark's Rule: Child's dose
= Weight of child in lb/150 · Adult dose

Young's Rule: Child's dose = Child's age in
years/(child's age in years + 12) · Adult dose

Clark's Rule is preferred over Young's Rule because it is more accurate to use weight than age.

Geriatric Patients

Geriatric medicine encompasses the management of illness or disability in the elderly. A major consideration in the dosing of elderly patients is reduced kidney function, which may result in reduced drug elimination or increased drug accumulation, leading to toxic drug levels and adverse effects. Renal clearance is extremely important when using specific drugs in elderly patients.

Calculations Involving Units and Milliequivalents (mEq)

Certain parenteral medications, such as insulin, heparin, and penicillin, are measured in units per milliliter. **Units** are assigned to medications called "biologicals," which have been tested for potency in biological systems. To prevent errors, healthcare workers should write out the word "units" rather than abbreviate it as "u." Units are specific to each particular medication because the medication has been tested and shown to produce a specific effect relating to that number of units. Therefore, units of heparin have no relationship to units of insulin.

Heparin is an anticoagulant that is available in many different strengths. Be *very* careful when reading heparin orders and labels because it is a very dangerous medication. It is available in 1000 units/mL, 2000 units/mL, 2500 units/mL, 5000 units/mL,

10,000 units/mL, and 20,000 units/mL. Heparin is also available in 1 unit/mL, 10 units/mL, and 100 units/mL strengths, which are considered heparin lock flushes used to keep a vein open (prevent clotting) so that the IV line remains open for the next dose.

Insulin, a parenteral hypoglycemic medication for lowering the blood glucose level, is also dosed in units. The most common strength used in the United States is U-100, which is 100 units/mL. Regular insulin is the only insulin that can be given intravenously. Other types of insulin, in addition to Regular Insulin, are given subcutaneously.

Some insulin comes in a U-500 strength, which is used only for patients with extreme insulin resistance. This is not a common strength and some pharmacies keep it in a separate location from the U-100 insulins to prevent serious medication errors.

Calculations with units follow the same rules as other calculations.

EXAMPLE 6-17

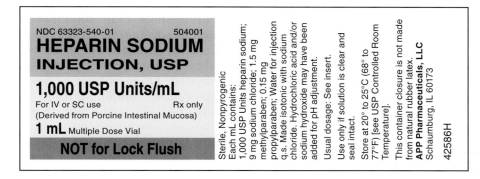

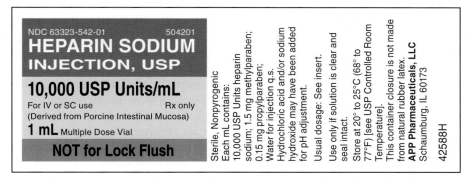

Order: heparin sodium 4000 units subcutaneously (SUBCUT)
Stock choices: heparin sodium 1000 units/mL and heparin sodium 10,000 units/mL

How much of *each* stock volume would be needed for the same dose?

$$\frac{1000 \text{ units}}{1 \text{ mL}} = \frac{4000 \text{ units}}{x} \quad x = 4 \text{ mL} \quad \text{This is too}$$
much volume to inject SUBCUT! (See below)

$$\frac{10,000 \text{ units}}{1 \text{ mL}} = \frac{4000 \text{ units}}{x} \quad x = 0.4 \text{ mL}$$
More appropriate amount for a SUBCUT injection

Choose the 10,000 unit/mL stock solution in this case to keep the dose *volume* smaller.

EXAMPLE 6-18

Order: Regular Insulin 35 units SUBCUT qam
Stock: Regular Insulin 100 units/mL

What volume is needed for this dose?

$$\frac{100 \text{ units}}{1 \text{ mL}} = \frac{35 \text{ units}}{x} \quad \text{Cross-multiply and divide.}$$
$$x = 0.35 \text{ mL}$$

Milliequivalents are a type of unit used in the United States to express the concentration of electrolytes such as sodium, potassium, magnesium, and calcium. With liquid medications, these strengths are expressed as mEq/mL. With solid medications, the strength can be mEq/tablet or mEq/capsule.

Calculations with milliequivalents also follow the same rules as other calculations.

EXAMPLE 6-19

Order: Add 30 mEq of KCl to 1 L normal saline (NS)
Stock: KCl 2 mEq/mL. How many mL should be added to the NS IV?

$$\frac{2 \text{ mEq}}{1 \text{ mL}} = \frac{30 \text{ mEq}}{x} \quad \text{Cross-multiply and divide.}$$
$$x = 15 \text{ mL}$$

EXERCISE 6-14 QUICK CHECK

1. Order: 25 units; stock: 100 units/10 mL; give _____ mL
2. Order: 20,000 units; stock: 25,000 units/2 mL; give _____ mL
3. Order: 40 mEq; stock: 20-mEq tablets; give _____ tablets
4. Order: add 45 mEq of KCl to an IV; stock: KCl 2 mEq/mL; add _____ mL
5. Order: 46 units Regular Insulin; stock: Regular Insulin 100 units/mL; draw up _____ mL

Scenario CHECK UP 6-1

Victoria is nearing the end of a long shift at the hospital. She receives a stat order for 7000 units of heparin subcutaneous to be sent up to the cardiac floor. The supply on hand is heparin 10,000 units per 1 mL. How much will Victoria draw up in the syringe to send to the floor? How quickly must Victoria deliver this medication to the nurse?

Subcutaneous Injections

Subcutaneous (SUBCUT) injections are administered in the subcutaneous or fat layer of the skin. Most subcutaneous doses are less than 1 mL.

Intramuscular Injections

For intramuscular (IM) injections, the needle passes through the cutaneous and subcutaneous layers of the skin, and the injection is given into the muscle. Small volume IM injections are less than 3 mL, and large volume IM injections are 3 to 5 mL. Larger muscles can handle the larger amounts, but 5 mL is the volume limit on IM injections. Therefore, if you calculate an IM dose and your answer is greater than 5 mL, there is probably an error either in the prescribed amount or in your calculations.

Intravenous Medications

Hospital pharmacy technicians prepare and deliver a 24-hour supply of intravenous solutions to nursing stations daily. Large volume parenterals (LVPs) contain more than 250 mL of solution, and small volume parenterals (SVPs) contain 100 mL or less. Most intravenous piggybacks (IVPB) are small volume parenterals that are given over 30 to 60 minutes. Large volume parenterals for continuous intravenous administration are "hung" at the patient's bedside and are allowed to drip slowly into a vein either by gravity or through a pump. They must be given at a slow rate because veins can handle only a small volume over a given time. Both large and small volume parenterals must be infused at a constant rate. In either case, the physician determines the infusion, or flow, rate in terms of milliliters per minute, drops per minute, or amount of drug (milligrams, units, or milliequivalents) per hour. The pharmacy technician must be able to calculate the volume needed to last a certain amount of time to calculate how much longer a currently hanging IV solution will last (Figure 6-4). Depending on the order received, the technician must be able to convert the numbers to determine this information. This ultimately determines the amount of IV solution to be prepared for a 24-hour period.

IV Infusion Rates/Flow Rates

A *rate* is defined as something per unit of time. An **infusion rate** or **flow rate** refers to the amount of IV fluid entering the body over a specific amount of time.

A 1000-mL IV may be ordered to run over 8 hours. The infusion rate would be 1000 mL/8 hr, which reduces to 125 mL/hr.

A 1000-mL IV may be ordered to run at 50 mL/hr.

$$\frac{50 \text{ mL}}{1 \text{ hr}} = \frac{1000 \text{ mL}}{x} \quad x = 20 \text{ hr}$$

The infusion would last for 20 hours.

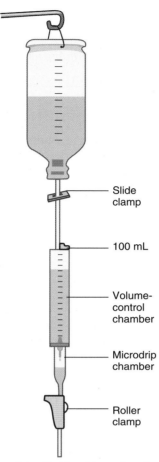

FIGURE 6-4 Large volume IV drip with smaller piggyback attached to tubing on pump.

These calculations involve determining the following:

1. The right amount of medication to be given over time
2. The amount of medication needed to last a certain time
3. The amount of time left until an IV is empty

Basic necessary conversion factors are as follows:

$$1 \text{ hr} = 60 \text{ min} \quad 24 \text{ hr} = 1 \text{ d}$$

EXAMPLE 6-20

Order: Heparin 100 units per 500 mL to run at 10 mL per hour.

How many units will be delivered per hour?

$$\frac{\text{units}}{\text{hr}} = \frac{100 \text{ units}}{500 \text{ mL}} \cdot \frac{10 \text{ mL}}{\text{hr}} = 2 \text{ units/hr}$$

EXERCISE 6-15 QUICK CHECK

When using DA, start by identifying the unit needed in the answer.

1. Order: 2-L TPN to run at 150 mL/hr. How many hours will this solution last?
2. Order: 500-mL solution to run over 24 hr. How many mL per hour?
3. Order: 1 L of NS to run at 100 mL/hr. How many hours will this solution last?

A **drip rate (DR)**, sometimes called a **drop rate**, represents the number of drops (gtt) administered over a specific time via intravenous infusion. It is a specific type of infusion or flow rate usually measured in gtt/min.

Calculations are affected by the size of the tubing used to deliver the medication. A **drop factor** (gtt/mL) is found on the tubing package. Various drop factors are available: 10, 15, and 20 gtt/mL are called *macrodrip,* and 60 gtt/mL is considered a *microdrip.*

 Tech Note!

Remember, the unit abbreviation for drops is *gtt.* Sizes of drops differ between droppers and there are various conversion factors with drops that seem contradictory. When calculating day's supply for insurance company purposes, pharmacists typically use 20 gtt/mL. The household system considers there to be about 60 gtt/tsp, which would convert to 12 gtt/mL.

Also, drops can be intended for drip rates. The number of drops per milliliter in these cases depends on the tubing size of the administration kit.

EXAMPLE 6-21 CALCULATING INFUSION RATES AND DRIP RATES

You receive an order for a 2-L bag to be given over 24 hours. The tubing delivers 15 gtt/mL. What are the drops per minute? To find this out, prepare the problem.

Steps involved in determining drops per minute:
1. Identify the drop factor: 15 gtt/mL
2. How many milliliters will be delivered per hour?

$$2000 \text{ mL/24 hr} = 83.33 \text{ mL/hr}$$

3. How many milliliters per minute?

$$\frac{83.33 \text{ mL}}{1 \text{ hr}} \cdot \frac{1 \text{ hr}}{60 \text{ min}} = 1.38 \text{ mL/min}$$

4. What is the drip rate? You can use DA to go directly from the original question to this final answer because that is how this question will usually be phrased.

$$\frac{gtt}{min} = \frac{15\,gtt}{mL} \cdot \frac{1000\,mL}{1\,L} \cdot \frac{2L}{24\,hr} \cdot \frac{1\,hr}{60\,min} = 20.8\,gtt/min$$

(rounds to 21 gtt/min)

Note: When performing DA calculations with two units in the answer, as above with gtt/min, start your solution with the information that contains the numerator of the answer and continue to add information that will cancel the unwanted units. The above example was begun with gtt/mL because the final answer is needed in gtt/min. Then each consecutive value canceled unwanted units: mL canceled mL, L canceled L, and hr canceled hr, until you were left with gtt/min.

When expressing gtt/min, the number is always rounded *up* to the nearest whole drop. Whether the answer is 20.1 gtt/min or 20.9 gtt/min, it would be rounded up to 21 gtt/min.

EXAMPLE 6-22

A 3-L total parenteral nutrition (TPN) bag is being administered to a patient over 24 hours. The tubing size delivers 15 gtt/mL. How many drops per minute will be delivered?

$$\frac{gtt}{min} = \frac{15\,gtt}{mL} \cdot \frac{1000\,mL}{1\,L} \cdot \frac{3\,L}{24\,hr} \cdot \frac{1\,hr}{60\,min}$$
$$= 31.25\,gtt/min = 32\,gtt/min$$

 Tech Note!

Technicians and pharmacists do not determine the size of the tubing. This is predetermined by the physician's orders to the nurse.

EXERCISE 6-16 QUICK CHECK

1. Aminophylline 500 mg in 1000 mL over 24 hours. The drop factor is 20 gtt/mL.
   a. How many mL would be delivered per hour?
   b. What is the flow rate in drops/min?
2. Heparin 20,000 units in 1 L over 24 hours. The drop factor is 50 gtt/mL.
   a. How many mL would be delivered per hour?
   b. What is the flow rate in drops/min?
3. How many drops per minute would a patient receive at 40 mL/hr using a 20 gtt/mL set?
4. Order: 1500 mL of solution over 12 hr. The tubing size is 20 gtt/mL.
   How many drops per minute will be delivered?
5. Order: 2.5-L solution to run over 20 hr. The tubing size is 15 gtt/mL.
   How many drops per minute will be delivered?

 Tech Note!

A large volume bag can hang for a maximum of 24 hours before it must be changed to prevent microbial growth, according to the USP.

Percentage and Ratio Strengths

In the practice of pharmacy, percentage (%) can be expressed in three ways: weight/weight (g/100 g), weight/volume (g/100 mL), and volume/volume (mL/100 mL). Weight/weight % is the number of grams of solute dissolved in 100 g of final product. Weight/volume % is the number of grams of solute dissolved in 100 mL of solution. Volume/volume % is the number of milliliters of solute dissolved in 100 mL of solution.

EXAMPLE 6-23 USING R&P

How many g of dextrose are in 250 mL of 10% dextrose solution?

$$\frac{10\,g}{100\,mL} = \frac{x}{250\,mL} \qquad 100x = 2500 \qquad x = 25\,g$$

EXAMPLE 6-24

What is the percentage strength of an ointment containing 0.5 g of active ingredient in 50 g?

$$x = 1\,g \qquad 1\,g/100\,g = 1\%$$
$$\frac{0.5\,g}{50\,g} = \frac{x}{100\,g}$$

 Tech Note!

Remember that percent *always* means $x/100$.

A second method of expressing the strength of a substance is by using ratios. Ratio strength is often used to designate the concentration of weak solutions or liquid preparations.

For example, a 1:200 ratio strength is interpreted as the following:
1. Solid in solid (weight to weight, or w/w): 1 g of solute in 200 g of solid preparation
2. Solid in liquid (weight to volume, or w/v): 1 g of solid in 200 mL of solution
3. Liquid in liquid (volume to volume, or v/v): 1 mL of solute in 200 mL of solution

A liquid with a concentration of 1:1000 means there is 1 part active ingredient to 1000 parts total. This could mean 1 gram (g) of drug dissolved in 1000 mL of solution, 1 mL (milliliter) of drug in 1000 mL of solution, or 1 g of drug in 1000 g of product. If you have 25 g of drug dissolved in 100 mL of solution, this can be written as the ratio 25:100, which can be reduced to 1:4.

EXAMPLE 6-25 USING DIMENSIONAL ANALYSIS

How many mg of medication are in 20 mL of a 1:250 solution?

$$mg = \frac{1000 \text{ mg}}{1 \text{ g}} \cdot \frac{1 \text{ g}}{250 \text{ mL}} \cdot \frac{20 \text{ mL}}{1} = 80 \text{ mg}$$

 Tech Note!

Remember that ratio strength is always expressed in the form of 1:*x*.

Converting between percentage and ratio strength is easiest with ratio and proportion as follows.

What is the percentage strength of a 1:1000 solution?

$$\frac{1 \text{ g}}{1000 \text{ mL}} = \frac{x \text{ g}}{100 \text{ mL}} \quad 1000x = 100$$

Divide both sides by 1000 and $x = 0.1$

The answer is 0.1 g over 100 mL, or 0.1%.

The same method can be applied to conversions from percentage strength to ratio strength.

What is the ratio strength of a 5% solution?

$$\frac{5 \text{ g}}{100 \text{ mL}} = \frac{1 \text{ g}}{x \text{ mL}} \quad 5x = 100$$

Divide both sides by 5, so $x = 20$

1 g in 20 mL is a 1:20 ratio strength.

Another method of expressing strength is using fractions such as mg/mL, mEq/mL, and units/mL.

To convert percentage strength to mg/mL with DA, place the unit you want for the answer to the left of the equals sign and line up your known values so that the other units cancel.

Convert 5% (w/v) to mg/mL: 5% means 5 out of 100 and in this case 5 g out of 100 mL.

$$\frac{mg}{mL} = \frac{1000 \text{ mg}}{g} \cdot \frac{5 \text{ g}}{100 \text{ mL}} = \frac{5000 \text{ mg}}{100 \text{ mL}} = \frac{50 \text{ mg}}{mL}$$

To convert ratio strength to mg/mL using DA, place the unit you want for the answer to the left of the equals sign and line up your known values so that the other units cancel.

Convert 1:20,000 (w/v) to mg/mL: 1:20,000 means 1 out of 20,000 and in this case 1 g out of 20,000 mL.

$$\frac{mg}{mL} = \frac{1000 \text{ mg}}{1 \text{ g}} \cdot \frac{1 \text{ g}}{20,000 \text{ mL}} = \frac{1000 \text{ mg}}{20,000 \text{ mL}} = \frac{1 \text{ mg}}{20 \text{ mL}}$$

1 mg/20 mL reduces to 0.05 mg/mL by dividing the top and bottom of the fraction by 20.

EXERCISE 6-17 QUICK CHECK

Calculate the strength in the following problems.
1. How many grams of amino acid are in 500 mL of 8.5% solution?
2. 170 g of medication is dissolved in 1 L of water; what is the percentage strength of the solution formed?
3. How many grams of dextrose are in 250 mL of a 5% solution?
4. What is the ratio strength of a 20% solution?
5. How many mg of drug are in 20 mL of a 1% solution?

Dilution

The pharmacy often receives a prescription for a liquid or solid medication that is not available commercially in the strength prescribed by the physician. Often the commercial strength is greater than the prescribed strength. In this situation, the pharmacist or pharmacy technician must dilute the commercially available product to a lower strength. In this process, called **dilution**, a pharmaceutical preparation is diluted through the addition of a **diluent** or **solvent** to reach the desired strength. The diluent is an inert substance that does not have a concentration; in other words, it has a concentration of 0%. The diluent adds either volume or mass to the preparation. Sterile water is a common diluent for solutions, and petrolatum is a common diluent for solids.

Liquid dilutions involve adding a diluent (e.g., sterile water) with 0% active ingredient to a higher concentration stock solution. During the dilution process, begin with a stock volume (SV) of a particular percentage concentration (SP). Add a diluent to the stock solution to achieve the desired volume (DV) and desired percentage strength (DP). The strengths must always be expressed as percentages, and the volumes must be in the same unit. Usually the volume is requested in mL but occasionally a physician may request L or oz. The process can be expressed mathematically as:

$$SV \cdot SP = DV \cdot DP$$

Three of the four variables are needed to perform this calculation. The amount of diluent needed can be calculated by using the following equation:

$$\text{Amount of diluent needed} = DV - SV$$

The process is the same when diluting weights. Adding a product such as petrolatum to a stock solid dilutes the preparation to a lower strength because petrolatum has 0% active ingredient. Just change the formulas to read:

$$SW \cdot SP = DW \cdot DP \quad \text{Amount of diluent} = DW - SW$$

The technician must remember several important things when using these equations:

1. Convert ratio strengths to percentage strengths before calculating.
2. The stock strength will always be greater than the final strength in a dilution problem.
3. The desired weight or volume will be greater than the initial weight or volume.

EXAMPLE 6-26

How many milliliters of water must be added to 150 mL of a 25% (w/v) stock solution of sodium chloride to prepare a 0.9% (w/v) sodium chloride solution?

Identify the variables: SV = 150 mL, SP = 25%, DV = ?, DP = 0.9%

Place them in the equation and solve for the desired volume:

$$SV \cdot SP = DV \cdot DP$$

$$150\ mL \cdot 25\% = DV \cdot 0.9\%$$

$$3750 = DV \cdot 0.9\% \quad \text{Divide both sides by 0.9}$$

$$4167\ mL = DV$$

Amount of water needed = DV − SV = 4167 mL − 150 mL = 4017 mL

EXAMPLE 6-27

How many milliliters of a 1:50 (w/v) boric acid solution can be prepared from 500 mL of a 10% (w/v) boric acid solution?

First change the ratio strength to a percentage: 1 g/50 mL = x g/100 mL, x = 2 g, so the strength is 2%

Next, identify the variables: SV = 500 mL, SP = 10%, DV = ?, DP = 2%

Place them in the equation and solve for the desired volume:

$$SV \cdot SP = DV \cdot DP$$

$$500\ mL \cdot 10\% = DV \cdot 2\% \quad DV = 2500\ mL$$

 Tech Note!

Remember that the units used for volume must be the same on both sides of the equation.

EXERCISE 6-18 QUICK CHECK

Solve the following dilution problems.

1. If 200 mL of a 20% (w/v) solution is diluted to 1 L, what will be the percentage strength (w/v)?

2. A pharmacist has weighed 3 g of coal tar (100% strength) and given it to the technician to compound a 1% ointment. What will be the final weight of the correctly compounded prescription?
3. An order calls for 120 mL of a 10% magnesium sulfate solution, and you have a 25% magnesium sulfate solution. How many milliliters of the 25% solution will you use?
4. You are to prepare 50 mL of a 1:100 rifampin suspension from a stock 1:20 rifampin suspension. How many milliliters of the 1:20 suspension will you need?
5. The pharmacist receives a prescription for 100 mL of a 30% hydrochloric acid solution. The pharmacy carries a 90% hydrochloric acid solution. How many milliliters of the concentrated solution are needed to fill the prescription?
6. A stock bottle of Lugol's solution contains 4 ounces from the original pint bottle. The technician is able to make four 8-ounce bottles of a more dilute 4% solution. What was the original percentage strength of Lugol's solution?

Total Parenteral Nutrition (TPN)

Total parenteral nutrition is covered thoroughly in Chapter 12: Aseptic Technique and Sterile Compounding. The calculations involve determining amounts of dextrose, amino acids, and lipids, in addition to electrolytes, insulin, and other additives.

EXAMPLE 6-28

Prepare a TPN with 400 mL of 10% Travasol, 500 mL of 70% dextrose, and 100 mL of sterile water. What will be the final strengths of the Travasol and dextrose?

This is actually two dilution questions, so use: SV · SP = DV · DP

DV for both Travasol and dextrose will be 400 mL + 500 mL + 100 mL = 1000 mL

Travasol: $400\ mL \cdot 10\% = 1000\ mL \cdot DP \quad DP = 4\%$

Dextrose: $500\ mL \cdot 70\% = 1000\ mL \cdot DP \quad DP = 35\%$

Electrolytes to be added to TPNs are mostly supplied in mEq/mL strengths.

EXAMPLE 6-29

Add 40 mEq of KCL to the TPN. Stock: KCl 2 mEq/mL.

$$\frac{2\ mEq}{1\ mL} = \frac{40\ mEq}{x} \quad 2x = 40\ mL \quad x = 20\ mL$$

Add 20 mL to the TPN.

Victoria is about halfway through her shift when she receives an order for a total parenteral nutrition (TPN). Her company does not have an automated TPN machine, so she will have to make it by hand, which will take longer. The medication is for a baby in the neonatal unit and has several ingredients. Victoria should calculate the ingredients carefully, recheck them, and then have a pharmacist check them. She needs to be extremely careful when preparing a TPN for a neonate!

Alligation Alternate

Alligation alternate is a method used to calculate the number of parts of two different strengths of medication needed to prepare a third strength that is not in stock. For example, if a physician orders 20% potassium chloride (KCl) and you have only 10% and 50% KCl in stock, you can calculate the amount of each solution needed to attain a 20% solution. You can achieve this only when the strength desired is *between* the two strengths being mixed. This means that you cannot make a 20% solution from a 5% solution and a 10% solution. However, you can make a 20% solution from a 5% and a 70% solution. The alligation process is the same when dealing with weight or volume. If a 0% diluent is used, such as water for volume or petrolatum for weight, you can use the alligation method or the equation from the dilution section.

EXAMPLE 6-30

You have in stock a 70% solution and a 20% solution. How much of each do you need to create 1 L of a 40% solution?

This is as simple as tic-tac-toe; following these basic rules:
1. Draw a tic-tac-toe board.

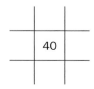

2. Place your desired strength in the middle square.

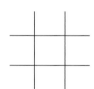

3. Put your higher-strength solution in the top left square.

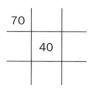

4. Put your lower-strength solution in the bottom left square. If you are using water, you will place a zero in this square because water has a concentration of zero.

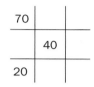

5. Determine the difference between the number in the top left and middle square and place this new number in the bottom right square. Do the same with the bottom left number and middle square and place this result in the top right square. Always use positive numbers as your answers. Both of these numbers are assigned the unit "parts."

70		20	40 – 20 = 20
	40		
20		30	70 – 40 = 30

6. Create a fraction by adding the two new numbers (top and bottom right squares) together for a common denominator. Place the top right number over the denominator and do the same for the bottom right number.

70		20
	40	
20		30

$$\frac{20}{20 + 30} \qquad \frac{30}{20 + 30}$$

7. Divide each fraction, and then multiply by the total volume you need.

70		20
	40	
20		30

$$\frac{20}{50} \times 1000 \text{ mL} = 400 \text{ mL}$$

$$\frac{30}{50} \times 1000 \text{ mL} = 600 \text{ mL}$$

8. Check your answer by adding the two parts. They should equal the total volume.

70		20	400 mL of 70% solution
	40		
20		30	600 mL of 20% solution
			1000 mL of 40% solution

Answer: 400 mL of 70% solution and 600 mL of 20% solution will create a 1-L solution of 40%.

 Tech Note!

Do not read your answer diagonally. Read your answer horizontally!

EXERCISE 6-19 QUICK CHECK

Solve the following alligation problems.
1. Order: Prepare 500 mL of 20% KCl from your stock of 5% and 70% KCl.
   How many mL of each solution are needed?
2. Order: Compound a 2.5% solution from a 10% stock solution and water for a total volume of 8 oz.
   How many mL of each solution do you need? Hint: Change 8 oz to mL first

PRACTICE QUIZ 6-3

1. 2.5 oz = _____ mL
2. 125 lb = _____ kg
3. 2000 mg = _____ g
4. 0900 = _____ o'clock (AM or PM)
5. 1 dram = _____ mL
6. 1.5 L = _____ mL
7. 11:00 AM = _____ (international time)
8. 15 mL = _____ Tbsp
9. 2 pt = _____ qt
10. gr ii = _____ mg (use gr i = 65 mg)
11. 2:30 PM = _____ (international time)
12. 22,500 mcg = _____ g
13. 25,000 units/2 mL = _____ units/mL
14. 30 lb = _____ kg
15. 2350 = _____ o'clock (AM or PM)
16. 240 mL = _____ oz
17. 25 kg = _____ g
18. 10 lb = _____ oz
19. 1.5 g/10 mL = _____ mg/mL
20. 3000 mcg = _____ mg
21. 42 kg = _____ lb
22. 4.4 lb = _____ kg
23. 450 g = _____ mg
24. 908 g = _____ kg
25. 1:1000 = _____ g/_____ mL
26. 6 PM = _____ (international time)

27. 15 mL = _____ tsp
28. 8 Tbsp = _____ mL
29. 50 g/100 mL = _____ mg/mL
30. 2.25 mcg = _____ mg
31. XXX = _____ (Arabic number)
32. 0.02 g = _____ mg
33. You receive an order for gentamicin 90 mg. You have a vial of 40 mg/mL. How many milliliters do you need to fill a one-time dose?
34. How many mL of Prozac 20 mg/5 mL are needed to fill the following prescription: 10 mg once a day for 30 days.
35. You have a pediatric order for amoxicillin 9 mg/kg/dose. The stock strength is 250 mg/5mL. If the child weighs 90 lb, how many milliliters are needed per dose?
36. Order: digoxin 0.25 mg daily. Stock: 125 mcg tabs. How many tablets are needed per dose?
37. Order: 1 L of $D_{10}W$ with 20% KCl to run at 100 mL/hr. How many hours will this bag last?
38. Order: aminophylline drip 500 mL to run over 24 hr with a drop factor of 25 gtt/mL. How many gtt/min will run?
39. Order: make 1-L of a 30% solution. Stock: 10% and 40% KCl. How much of each is needed to prepare 1 L?
40. An order for a baby requires 15 mg/kg/day to be given in three divided doses. If the child weighs 25 lb, how much will each dose be?
41. A pharmacy receives an order for 280 mL of a 5% salicylic acid solution. How much salicylic acid powder is needed to make the solution?
42. The pharmacist has weighed 15 g of coal tar and given it to the technician with instructions to compound a 1% ointment. What will be the final weight of the correctly compounded prescription?
43. The pharmacy has 300 mL of a 50% solution; 200 mL is added to this solution to decrease the concentration. How many grams of active ingredient are in 4 ounces of this diluted solution?
44. If 5 g is dissolved in 100 mL of solution, what is the percentage of the solution?
45. You dilute 100 mL of 5% solution to 500 mL. What is the percentage strength?

Business Calculations

Percentages are used in the pharmacy to identify the strength or concentration of a medication, to perform dilution problems, and to calculate the markup, discounts, net profits, and gross profits in retail pharmacy. Both the Pharmacy Technician Certification Board (PTCB) exam and the Exam for the Certification of Pharmacy Technicians (ExCPT) contain math problems using percentages.

Percentages of Quantities

The easiest method to use for finding percentages of quantities is ratio and proportion because percentage is an amount per 100. Each of the following three questions asks something different, but all can be answered by setting up a ratio and proportion.

What is 50% of 15?

Method 1: Set up a ratio and proportion, cross-multiply, and divide

$$\frac{50}{100} = \frac{x}{15}$$ Reads 50 is to 100 as x is to 15
50 times 15 divided by 100 = 7.5

Method 2: When calculating "what is x percent of" problems, it is also easy to change the percentage to a decimal and then multiply. 50% equals 50 divided by 100 = 0.5

$$0.5 \times 15 = 7.5$$

15 is 60% of what number?
Set up a ratio and proportion, cross-multiply, and divide

$$\frac{60}{100} = \frac{15}{x}$$ Reads 60 is to 100 as 15 is to what?
15 times 100 divided by 60 = 25

You can reduce first:

$$\frac{6}{10} = \frac{15}{x}$$ 15 times 10 divided by 6 = 25

5 is what percent of 20?
Set up a ratio and proportion, cross-multiply, and divide:

$$\frac{x}{100} = \frac{5}{20}$$ Reads x is to 100 as 5 is to 20
5 times 100 divided by 20 = 25

Or reduce first:

$$\frac{x}{100} = \frac{1}{4}$$ 1 times 100 divided by 4 = 25

Most problems in retail pharmacy can be solved with method 2.

EXAMPLE 6-31

An invoice from the supplier states that the pharmacy can receive a 1.5% discount if the invoice is paid within 10 days, but the entire amount is due within 30 days. How is the discount determined? The amount due is $500.

Using Method 2, change 1.5% into a decimal by dividing by 100; 1.5 divided by 100 = 0.015, then multiply 500 by 0.015

$$500 \times 0.015 = 7.50,$$ therefore the discount will be $7.50

The total due within 7 days is $500 − $7.50 = $492.50

EXAMPLE 6-32

Jane, the inventory tech, was calculating the totals for the day after the pharmacy closed. She calculated $3,409.23 as the total income for the day. The pharmacy has an outstanding bill of $8,345 with a drug vendor. The vendor requires a minimum payment of 5% of the outstanding bill each month. How much is owed this month?

Change 5% into a decimal by dividing by 100; 5 divided by 100 = 0.05

$$\$8,345 \times 0.05 = \$417.25$$

If the pharmacy makes this payment from today's total income, what dollar amount will be left outstanding?

$$\$8,345 - \$417.25 = \$7,927.75$$

What will be the pharmacy's required payment next month?

$$\$7,927.75 \times 0.05 = \$396.39$$

The $3,409.23 in income can be ignored because it has nothing to do with the amount due.

EXAMPLE 6-33

The inventory technician is responsible for figuring out how much the pharmacy can save on invoices if they are paid quickly. The total amount of an invoice is $3,500, and the pharmacy is to receive a 2.5% discount.

$$\$3,500 \times 0.025 = \$87.50$$

The discount would be $87.50. It does not sound like a big discount, but remember that this is only one invoice. A pharmacy could save thousands of dollars a year just by paying the invoices quickly.

Another use of percentages is to calculate the **markup** necessary so the pharmacy can make a profit. Remember, the pharmacy has to make a profit so that it can pay you, pay for rent and utilities, and provide the owner with a profit. The pharmacy purchases medications at **wholesale cost** (i.e., the purchase price) and marks them up to the **retail price** (selling price) to make a profit.

EXAMPLE 6-34

The pharmacy must increase the cost of cold medicines by 56% to make a profit. Determine the markup and then calculate the total retail cost of the product.

Tylenol cough and cold liquid:
$5.50 (wholesale price) × 0.56 = $3.08 (markup)

Total retail cost of this medication:
$5.50 + $3.08 = $8.58

Pseudoephedrine tablets:
$2.95 (wholesale price) × 0.56 = $1.65 (markup)

Total retail cost of this medication:
$2.95 + $1.65 = $4.60

Similarly, percentages are used to calculate discounts that pharmacies use as incentives to sell products. Once a product has been marked up, a discount may be advertised on the retail price.

EXAMPLE 6-35

The pharmacy is having a 25% off sale on the medications in Example 6-34. What are the new retail prices?

Tylenol cough and cold liquid:
$8.58 × 0.25 = $2.15 (saving to the customer)

Discounted retail price: $8.58 − $2.15 = $6.43

As you can see, the pharmacy still makes a profit because the wholesale cost was $5.50.

Pseudoephedrine tablets:
$4.60 × 0.25 = $1.15 (savings to the customer)

Discounted retail price: $4.60 − $1.15 = $3.45

Once again, the pharmacy still makes a profit because the wholesale cost was $2.95.

EXERCISE 6-20 QUICK CHECK

Calculate the dollar amount by using the following percentages.
1. $200 = _____ (25%) _____ (50%) _____ (75%)
2. $956 = _____ (15%) _____ (55%) _____ (85%)
3. $2,050 = _____ (20%) _____ (40%) _____ (60%)
4. $10,449 = _____ (2.5%) _____ (5.5%) _____ (7.5%)

5. 6.2% of a $2,100 bill will be given as a discount if the bill is paid before the 15th of the month. What is the savings to the pharmacy if the bill is paid early?
6. These products are on sale for 20% off the regular price. Calculate the total amount of savings to the customer:
Milk of Magnesia 4 oz ($3.25)
Pepcid AC 10-mg tablets ($10.95)
Motrin suspension 120 mL ($6.50)
Vitamin C 250-mg tablets #100 ($2.95)

PRACTICE QUIZ 6-4

1. The pharmacy's drug wholesaler will give a discount of 2% if the bill is paid within 1 week; calculate the final bill if the amount due is $6,544.
2. Your pharmacy is having a big sale on all first aid supplies; take 20% off the following purchase and total the bill.
Tylenol cold and cough, $8.95
Bayer aspirin, $1.95
Pepcid antacid, $18
Vicks Formula 44, $2.95
Imodium chewable tablets, $8.50
3. Your pharmacy received an order of 144 bottles; 25% of the bottles were damaged. How many damaged bottles are being returned?
4. All new prescriptions are being given a 15% discount. What is the dollar amount lost by the pharmacy if all the new prescriptions for the day added up to $2,339?
5. Your pharmacy has Neosporin ointment on sale at 15% off the price of $2.95 per tube. How much will the customer save?

Scenario CHECK UP 6-3

Victoria is cross-trained for many positions in the hospital pharmacy. She often fills in wherever she is needed. On this particular day, the pharmacy buyer is out sick. Victoria is helping out by answering the phones and checking in orders. One of the prime vendors must be paid today in order for the hospital to receive a discount. Victoria looks up the information on the computer and finds the following terms: 3%, net in 30. The balance owed is $3,200. What will the hospital pay if the bill is taken care of today? What will be owed if Victoria waits until the buyer returns to work?

DO YOU REMEMBER THESE KEY POINTS?

- How to convert between Roman numerals and Arabic numbers
- How to convert between the 24-hour clock and the 12-hour clock
- How to convert between fractions, ratios, decimals, and percentages
- The importance of using ratios and proportions in pharmacy calculations
- The importance of using dimensional analysis for tracking units in multistep calculations
- How to convert between units of measurement for weight and volume in the metric system
- The basic measurements of the primary system used in pharmacy—the metric system—in addition to household, avoirdupois, and apothecary units
- The formulas for calculating doses by body weight, body surface area (BSA), Young's Rule, and Clark's Rule

- How to calculate pediatric and geriatric dosages
- Drip rates of intravenous solutions can be expressed either as mL/hr or as gtt/min
- How to determine the duration of an intravenous solution
- Dilution is the process by which an inert substance is added to a preparation so that the final product has a lower concentration than the original product
- Alligation alternate is a method to compound a substance when given two strengths to prepare a third strength in between the two
- All measurements must have units, and it is important to label them correctly while performing calculations and on medication labels to avoid possible errors
- Double-checking calculations is important before preparing medications

Scenario FOLLOW UP

As Victoria continues to excel at the hospital pharmacy, she has learned that it is imperative to check and double-check her calculations. She understands that she can be held accountable for any medication errors she makes. She is diligent in making sure all her work is thoroughly checked by a pharmacist before it reaches the patient.

REVIEW QUESTIONS

Convert the following units to percentages.

1. $\frac{1}{5}$ = _____
2. 0.25 = _____
3. $\frac{10}{25}$ _____
4. 2.275 _____

Convert the following fraction of grains into milligrams.

5. NTG gr $\frac{1}{300}$ = _____ mg

Write the Arabic numbers in Roman numerals and the Roman numerals in Arabic numbers:

6. 20 = _____
7. 50 = _____
8. 59 = _____
9. CXL = _____
10. XC = _____
11. XXXIV = _____

Convert the following temperatures.

12. 37° C = _____ ° F
13. 86° F = _____ ° C

Convert the following metric units into the units indicated.

14. 5 cc = _____ tsp
15. 1 mcg = _____ mg
16. 15 cc = _____ tsp

17. 1000 mg = _____ g
18. 30 mL = _____ tsp
19. 900 mL = _____ oz
20. 1000 mL = _____ L
21. 0.25 L = _____ mL
22. 2 kg = _____ lb
23. 0.25 mg = _____ mcg
24. Order: cimetidine 300 mg tab qid × 30 days. In stock: cimetidine 150 mg tablets
    How many tablets will you need to fill this order?
25. Order: tobramycin IV 60 mg in D₅W 50 mL. In stock: tobramycin 40 mg/mL in 2-mL vials
    How many milliliters are needed to fill the order?
26. Order: vancomycin IV 750 mg bid in D₅W 250 mL. Stock: vancomycin 1 g per 20-mL vial
    How much will you take from the 1-g vial?
27. Order: 10% dextrose solution 1 L. You have 5% and 50% dextrose bags only.
    How much of each solution will it take to make a 1-L bag of 10% dextrose?
28. Order: 0.5 L of a 30% amino acid solution. Stock: 70% amino acids and sterile water
    How much of each solution is required to prepare a 30% solution?

29. Convert the following ratios into grams per milliliter and also to percentage strengths.
    A. 1:10
    B. 2:100
    C. 1:1000
30. Order: dispense ibuprofen liquid 40 mg/kg per day; give qid. You have ibuprofen liquid 100 mg/5 mL in stock.
    How much will this patient receive *per dose* if the patient's weight is 10 lb?
    How much liquid is needed to fill a 7-day supply?
31. 500 mL of heparin is to be given over 20 hours. The tubing size delivers 10 gtt/mL.
    How many drops per minute are being delivered to the patient?
32. What is the percent strength of a 1:25 (w/v) solution?

33. You add 40 g of salicylic acid to white petrolatum to make a total of 800 g.
    What is the percentage strength of the product?
34. What is the initial strength of a solution that is made by adding 200 mL of purified water to make 600 mL of a 25% solution?
35. If you dilute 60 mL of a 30% solution to 480 mL, what is the percentage strength of the new solution?
36. How many milliliters of pure alcohol (w/v) are required to make 480 mL of a solution containing 30% alcohol?
37. You need to mix magic mouthwash that has a ratio of 1:1:1. Using diphenhydramine, Maalox, and lidocaine, how much of each do you need to make 8 oz? Give your answer in milliliters.

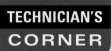

TECHNICIAN'S CORNER   An order comes to the pharmacy with the following directions:
    D$_5$W 250 mL with heparin 10,000 units IV at 500 units/hr
    Calculate the flow rate in mL/hr.

Bibliography

Brown M, Mulholland JM: *Drug calculations: process and problems for clinical practice,* ed 8, St Louis, 2008, Mosby.

Gray Morris D: *Calculate with confidence,* ed 5, St Louis, 2010, Elsevier.

Mizner JJ: *Mosby's review for the Pharmacy Technician Certification Examination,* ed 3, St Louis, 2014, Mosby.

Drug Information References

Bobbi Steelman

OBJECTIVES

Upon completing this chapter, you should be able to do the following:

1. Demonstrate the appropriate way to research drugs and other information from reference books, journals, and electronic resources.
2. Demonstrate the appropriate way to reference drugs and other information from the Internet and other sources.
3. Describe the information contained in the following references:
   - *American Drug Index*
   - *American Hospital Formulary Service Drug Information*
   - *Approved Drug Products with Therapeutic Equivalence Evaluations* (otherwise known as the *"Orange Book"*)
   - *Clinical Pharmacology*
   - *Drug Facts and Comparisons*
   - *Drug Topics Red Book*
   - *Geriatric Dosage Handbook*
   - *Goodman & Gilman's The Pharmacological Basis of Therapeutics*
   - *Handbook of Nonprescription Drugs*

   - *Ident-A-Drug*
   - *Martindale's The Complete Drug Reference*
   - *Micromedex Healthcare Evidence and Clinical Xpert*
   - *Pediatric and Neonatal Dosage Handbook*
   - *Physicians' Desk Reference (PDR)*
   - *Remington's Pharmaceutical Sciences: The Science and Practice of Pharmacy*
   - *Trissel's Handbook on Injectable Drugs*
   - *United States Pharmacist's Pharmacopeia*
   - *United States Pharmacopoeia–National Formulary*
4. Explain the importance of carrying a pocket-sized reference book.
5. List types of electronic reference materials.
6. Explain the importance of journals and newsmagazines as they pertain to pharmacy and continuing education.
7. Describe different considerations when choosing a reference.
8. Identify the benefits of joining a pharmacy association.

TERMS AND DEFINITIONS

Brand/trade name Trademark of a drug or device held by the originating manufacturing company

Chemical structure The makeup of a chemical, including the elements, the shape, the bonding types, the molecular configurations, charges, and so on; the nature of the chemical's structure has much to do with the chemical's stability, reactivity, and physical and chemical properties

Drug classification Categorization based on various characteristics, including the chemical structure of a drug, the action of a drug, and/or the therapeutic or anatomical use of a drug

Drug Facts and Comparisons Reference book found in pharmacies that contains detailed information on more than 22,000 prescription and 6000 over-the-counter medications; drugs are divided into therapeutic groups for easy comparison

Formulary A list of approved drugs to be stocked by the pharmacy; also a list of drugs covered by an insurance company

Generic name Name assigned to a medication or nonproprietary name of a drug

Monograph Comprehensive information on a medication's actions within that class of drugs; also lists generic and trade names, ingredients, dosages, side effects, adverse effects, how the patient should take the medication, and foods or other drugs (e.g., OTC medications, herbals) to avoid while taking the medication

Non-formulary A list of drugs that are not included in the list of preferred medications that a committee of pharmacists and physicians deems to be the safest, most effective, and most economical; they are drugs not included in the drug list approved for reimbursement by the health care plans

Package insert The official prescribing information for a prescription drug; the medication information sheet provided by the manufacturer that includes side effects, dosage forms, indications, and other important information

Trade name The proprietary or brand name given to a drug by the company who developed it; the trade name may be related to the function or main use of the drug

Introduction

Scenario:

Robert is an experienced technician at a busy retail pharmacy. He has been certified with the Pharmacy Technician Certification Board (PTCB) for 6 years. One of his responsibilities is to update the *Drug Facts and Comparisons* loose-leaf binder with the new drug inserts each month. Robert finds this task tedious and time-consuming and often wishes his pharmacist would use an online drug database. Do you think Robert should suggest this change to his supervisors? What would be the best way to approach this subject with the pharmacist? What are the pros and cons of using electronic drug databases in the pharmacy?

Drug information reference books are some of the most important tools used in pharmacy. Physicians, nurses, and other health care professionals call the pharmacy daily to ask questions about various medications. Pharmacists rely on credible, accurate, and up-to-date reference resources to help give the correct information to others. Although a few of the books in pharmacy are highly technical, most give basic information on drugs. Knowing which book to choose for referencing and how to access the information is an important skill for pharmacists and technicians. This chapter covers the references that are more commonly used in a pharmacy. In addition, other types of referencing materials that can be of help specifically to the technician are listed.

Researching a Drug

Before you begin to look for information, take these key points into consideration. First, what exactly is the purpose of your search? What is the question that needs to be answered? Do you need to know the generic drug name only, the drug's interactions and classification, or even perhaps the drug's appearance?

 Tech Alert!

It is important for technicians to be proficient in accessing accurate drug references and materials; however, technicians should not provide patients with information about side effects, dosing, or compatibility. This is out of the technician's scope of practice.

Let's begin with the process of developing, manufacturing, and naming drugs to learn the importance of each one of these components.

 Tech Note!

Technically, all generic drug names are spelled in lower case letters, whereas trade or brand names are capitalized. For example: atenolol (generic) and Tenormin (brand).

When a new drug is in the experimentation phase, the creators or the company give the drug a generic or investigational drug name based on its chemical attributes; the name also prepares the drug for recognition during future marketing after approval. Later, when the drug has been approved by the U.S. Food and Drug Administration (FDA), a **monograph**, or official label, is created to include important findings, such as side effects that were reported during clinical trials.

The **drug classification** is important because it places the drug into proper categories based on its **chemical structure**, mechanism of action, anatomical function, and/or therapeutic use. Many times, drugs in the same class have the same mechanism of action. This information can assist the prescriber and pharmacist in determining the expected therapeutic effect and also possible adverse reactions.

The indications list the main conditions for which the chemical is used. A contraindications list is also an important part of a drug monograph. This list identifies types of individuals who should not be given the medication. Reasons may range from certain serious drug-drug interactions to conditions that conflict with the action of the drug. After all the studies have been done and the data have been analyzed, contraindications may still be discovered in post-market use; these are updated in the drug's

BOX 7-1

Examples of Trade Drug Names That Indicate the Function of the Drug

Lopressor
For hypertension; conveys lowering of blood pressure

Lotensin
For hypertension; conveys lowering of blood pressure

Lipitor
Lowers blood lipids (cholesterol); conveys treatment of lipids

Neurontin
Treats conditions affecting the neurons (nerves); conveys treatment of nerves

Restoril
Treats insomnia; conveys restfulness

Wellbutrin
Treats depression; conveys wellness

Celexa
Treats depression; conveys celebration, wellness

Viagra
Treats erectile dysfunction; conveys vigor, vitality

BOX 7-2

Examples of Similar Endings of Generic Drug Names

Some beta-blockers end in *-olol* (these agents are primarily used to treat high blood pressure [HBP])
atenolol (Tenormin)
nadolol (Corgard)
timolol (Blocadren)
Some angiotensin-converting enzyme (ACE) inhibitors end in *-pril* (these agents are primarily used to treat HBP)
captopril (Capoten)
enalapril (Vasotec)
lisinopril (Prinivil, Zestril)
Some calcium channel blockers end in *-dipine** (these agents are primarily used to treat HBP and heart rhythm disorders)
amlodipine (Norvasc)
nicardipine (Cardene SR)
nifedipine (Procardia XL, Adalat CC)
Penicillins end in *-cillin* (these agents are used to treat infections)
ampicillin (Omnipen)
amoxicillin (Amoxil)
dicloxacillin (Dynapen)
Some antianxiety medications end in *-azepam* (these agents are primarily used to treat anxiety and panic disorders)
diazepam (Valium)
lorazepam (Ativan)
oxazepam (Serax)
Some tricyclic antidepressants end in *-pramine* (these agents are primarily used to treat depression disorders)
desipramine (Norpramin)
imipramine (Tofranil)
clomipramine (Anafranil)
H_2-receptor antagonists end in *-tidine* (these agents are primarily used to treat ulcers and gastro esophageal reflux disorders)
cimetidine (Tagamet)
ranitidine (Zantac)
famotidine (Pepcid)
Proton pump inhibitors end in *-prazole* (these agents are primarily used to treat gastro esophageal reflux disorders)
esomeprazole (Nexium)
lansoprazole (Prevacid)
omeprazole (Prilosec)
Some antifungals end in *-conazole* (these agents are primarily used to treat fungal infections)
ketoconazole (Nizoral)
fluconazole (Diflucan)
miconazole (Monistat)

*Verapamil (Calan) and diltiazem (Cardizem), which are also calcium channel blockers, are exceptions to this pattern.

monograph. It is always helpful to ensure that you are reading the most recent information on a drug. The last date of update is listed directly on the official product labeling.

The founding company assigns the chemical name, **generic name**, and **trade name**, which are found in the product's official label. The chemical name is a scientific name given to a chemical in accordance with the nomenclature system developed by the International Union of Pure & Applied Chemistry, Chemical Abstracts Service, or other authoritative agency. Many times generic names are closely related to the chemical name of the drug, but not always. The trade name (proprietary or brand name) is determined by the company that developed the drug and is therefore the exclusive property of that company. Some trade names may be related to the function or main use of the drug (Box 7-1). Examples of generic names are presented in Box 7-2.

The U.S. Adopted Names Council has established a list of word stems (prefixes, root words. and suffixes) that identify a drug's classification. These word parts reflect a specific drug classification (see Box 7-2). Knowing these word parts makes it easier to learn what a specific drug does.

Tech Note!

Generic drug names do not typically begin with J or W because those letters do not exist in the languages of many countries other than the United States that use generic drugs. Trade names can reflect the drug's primary characteristics or use but cannot imply a cure of a specific part of the body.

References Used in Pharmacy

In addition to being familiar with the official label of a product, technicians should be adept at using basic pharmacy drug references. Most references have a section on how to use the text or online "help" sections to aid the reader in the use of computerized resources. It is helpful for the technician to be familiar with performing a reference search before it is required. Knowing how to use the reference properly allows the technician to find the correct information in a timely manner.

Although many different types of reference materials are available, this chapter describes only the most common types seen in a pharmacy setting.

Many reference materials are available to technicians and pharmacists in a variety of formats, and it should be noted that online interfaces, such as *Micromedex* and *Clinical Pharmacology*, are more and more prevalent in the pharmacy setting. The following examples of commonly used reference materials are normally available in more than one form. All of the books can be found at online booksellers, such as amazon.com. At the end of each description is a list of available product formats.

Drug Facts and Comparisons

Drug Facts and Comparisons is one of the books most frequently used by pharmacists. This reference book was first published in 1946 and was created for quick and accurate reference and drug comparison. Because of its vital information and ease of use, it is a very popular pharmacy reference. *Drug Facts and Comparisons* has five sections (Table 7-1).

At the front of each classification section is extensive information on various aspects of that class of drugs. Included under each drug listing are indications for use. Also, a chart lists all the dosage strengths, dosage forms, sizes, and manufacturers. Most pharmacies carry the unbound book to allow for monthly updates. *Drug Facts and Comparisons* answers many basic questions for the pharmacist. It is available in hardback, loose-leaf hardback, pocket-sized, or electronic subscription (Facts and Comparison eAnswers). An example of how to locate information on either over-the-counter (OTC) or prescription (Rx) drugs is provided in Box 7-3.

TABLE 7-1

Sections in *Drug Facts and Comparisons*

Sections in Order of Reference	Contents of Each Section	Specific Information
Section 1	Index	Generic and trade names
Section 2	Keeping up	Orphan, investigational, and temporary listings
Section 3	Drug monographs	14 chapters of drug descriptions
Section 4	Drug identification	More than 250 drugs shown in color
Section 5	Appendix	Dosage calculations and list of manufacturers

Drug Facts and Comparisons. Facts & Comparisons (database online). St. Louis, 2013, Wolters Kluwer Health, Inc.

Physicians' Desk Reference

The *Physicians' Desk Reference (PDR)* is a popular reference found in most physicians' offices and pharmacies. The *PDR* has been in publication for more than 50 years. It has six sections (Table 7-2).

Each drug referenced in the *PDR* has a complete description, including its chemical structure and study results. This book is a compilation of **package inserts** (official labels) provided by manufacturers who have paid a fee for inclusion in the reference; not all package inserts are available. Package inserts can be difficult to read. Although most pharmacies have a *PDR*, physicians are the primary users, and again, the *PDR* lists only FDA-approved drugs that the manufacturers choose to send for inclusion. This book is not as important in a pharmacy setting as it is in a physician's office. The *PDR* does contain useful drug manufacturer contact information, such as addresses and phone numbers. However, manufacturer information now is available in many other online drug information subscription programs. The *PDR* is available in hardback and electronic formats. Online subscription is free to prescribers.

Drug Topics Red Book

One of the longest published reference guides is the *Drug Topics Red Book*. This book is a good source of information pertaining to average and wholesale drug costs and prices. The *New Red Book* has 10 sections (Table 7-3). Community pharmacies, rather than hospital pharmacies, are more likely to use this book.

BOX 7-3

Example of Information in *Drug Facts and Comparisons*

Omeprazole

OTC	Prilosec OTC	Time-delayed release: 20 mg	14 s, 28 s, 42 s
Rx	Omeprazole (various)	Capsules, delayed release; 10 mg	30 s, 100 s
Rx	Prilosec		1000 s and 30 s

The solid line between drugs indicates that the drugs are of different strength and/or equivalency. A broken line between drugs indicates that the drugs are equivalent; therefore, they can be used interchangeably.

Looking Up Information Under the Trade Name

Prilosec (located in the back of the book under index)

A. Generic name: given next to Prilosec, the trade name
B. Manufacturer: in parentheses under or next to name of drug within the table
C. Dosage forms: given in the middle of the table
D. Strengths: given in the middle of table
E. Package quantities available: given to the right
F. OTC and/or Rx: located to the far left of the drug name
G. Patient information and auxiliary label: located under monograph (see iv)
   i. Under the table are sections on indications, administration, and dosage.
   ii. Overall information on proton pump inhibitors (top of page: classification of drug) is given under the monograph located at the beginning of the section, after the monograph on H_2-antagonists.
   iii. Under the monograph the conditions treated by these types of agents are listed, including pharmacokinetics, contraindications, warnings, precautions, drug interactions, adverse reactions, overdosage, and patient information.
   iv. Under patient information, instructions are provided on the type of auxiliary label that should be used on a prescription bottle.

Looking Up Information Under the Generic Name

Alprazolam

A. Trade name: listed at the heading of the table
B. Classification: at the top of the page
C. Manufacturer: in parentheses under or next to name of drug in the table
D. Dosage forms: given in the middle of the table
E. Strengths: given in the middle of the table
F. Package quantities available: given to the right
G. Schedule: located to the far left of the drug name (Notice that there is no OTC or Rx listed; all scheduled drugs are Rx.)
H. Patient information pertaining to drinking alcohol or taking other central nervous system (CNS) depressants: located under the benzodiazepines monograph

Prilosec oral and Alprazolam oral. *Drug Facts and Comparisons.* Facts & Comparisons (database online). St. Louis, 2013, Wolters Kluwer Health, Inc.

TABLE 7-2

Sections of the *Physicians' Desk Reference*

Sections in Order of Reference	Contents of Each Section	Specific Information
Section 1	Manufacturer indexing	Lists addresses and phone numbers
Section 2	Generic and trade names	Serves as an index for referencing manufacturers
Section 3	Product category index	Lists products by classification or method of action
Section 4	Product identification guide	Drugs shown in color
Section 5	Product information	Most drugs approved by the U.S. Food and Drug Administration (FDA)
Section 6	Diagnostic product information	Information on drug products used as diagnostic agents
Miscellaneous section	Miscellaneous information	List of drug information centers, key to controlled substances, key for FDA pregnancy ratings, FDA telephone directory, and poison control centers

Physicians' Desk Reference Inc. *Red Book: Pharmacy's Fundamental Reference*, Montvale, NJ, 2013, Thomson Reuters.

TABLE 7-3

Sections in the *Drug Topics Red Book*

Sections in Order of Reference	Contents of Each Section	Specific Information
Section 1	Emergency information	Lists addresses and phone numbers
Section 2	Clinical reference guide	Quick guide listings (e.g., sugar-free and alcohol-free products, sulfite-containing drugs, and drugs that cannot be crushed)
Section 3	Practice management and professional development	Disease management programs, listed in alphabetical order with addresses and phone numbers
Section 4	Pharmacy and health care organizations	Lists 25 major organizations, including the ASHP, NABP, and AACP; no technician organizations are listed
Section 5	Drug reimbursement information	Lists State Aid Drug Assistance programs for all states; lists Medicaid upper limit prices and billing rules
Section 6	Manufacturer/wholesaler information	Lists addresses and phone numbers for manufacturers, wholesalers, OBRA '90–participating manufacturers (by identification number), and returned goods policies
Section 7	Product identification	Color photos of limited drugs; also includes list of Look-alike, sound-alike drug names
Section 8	Prescription product listings	Contains *Orange Book,* which lists generic drug, manufacturer, National Drug Code, average wholesale price, direct price, and *Orange Book* code
Section 9	Over-the-counter/nondrug products listing	Lists drugs by generic name or trade name and contains health-related item, universal product code, National Drug Code, average wholesale price, and suggested retail price
Section 10	Complementary/herbal product referencing	Short list of popular herbal remedies, along with a list of those that may be contraindicated, require supervision by medical personnel, and have adverse interactions, followed by a list of both scientific and common herbal names

Drug Facts and Comparisons, ed 66, St Louis, 2012, Wolters Kluwer Health, Inc.
AACP, American Association of Colleges of Pharmacy; *ASHP,* American Society of Health-System Pharmacists; *NABP,* National Association of Boards of Pharmacy; *OBRA '90,* Omnibus Budget Reconciliation Act of 1990.

TABLE 7-4

Abbreviations in the *Drug Topics Red Book*

Abbreviations	Definitions	Information Provided
AWP	Average wholesale price	Average price wholesalers charge pharmacy
NDC	National Drug Code	Identifies each drug by number
OBC	*Orange Book* code	Gives therapeutic equivalence
DP	Direct price	Price for purchasing from manufacturer
NCPDP	National Council for Prescription Drug Programs	Standard billing units (e.g., mL, mg)
HRI	Health-related item	Nonmedication item required to treat patient (e.g., crutches, gauze, tape, lancets)
UPC	Universal product code	Similar to National Drug Code for drug items

Drug Facts and Comparisons, ed 66, St Louis, 2012, Wolters Kluwer Health, Inc.

Red Book contains valuable information, in the form of quick referencing charts, that technicians can use, such as drugs that should not be crushed, drugs that are sugar free and alcohol free, and drugs excreted in breast milk. In addition, *Red Book* includes convenient tables showing pharmacy calculations and dosing instructions translated into Spanish. Although *Red Book* has an extraordinary amount of information, it is not an easy book to reference without knowing the abbreviations for the drug sections (Table 7-4). An added feature of *Red Book* is a listing of all nontraditional doctor of pharmacy

(PharmD) programs, along with requirements and current enrollment numbers. This is information that few, if any other, books contain. This book is available in soft-covered and electronic formats.

Approved Drug Products with Therapeutic Equivalence Evaluations: The *Orange Book*

The *Orange Book* is a comprehensive list of approved drug products with therapeutic equivalence evaluations that is provided by the FDA. This is the book to use for determining whether a generic drug is the same as a brand drug. Other information includes discontinued drug products, orphan product designations, and approval lists. Information searches can be accessed by several different means: active ingredient, patent number, proprietary name, applicant holder, or application number. The *Orange Book* publication is updated annually. Frequent updates are made to the online version, and it can be accessed free of charge.

American Hospital Formulary Service Drug Information

Used mainly by hospitals, the *American Hospital Formulary Service Drug Information (AHFS DI)* provides drug monographs that list drug information, including the following:

- Uses and off-label uses
- Specific dosage and administration information
- Drug interactions
- Adverse reactions
- Acute toxicity
- Preparations, chemistry, and stability
- Mechanism of action
- Spectrum and resistance for antibiotics
- Pharmacology
- Pharmacokinetics
- Laboratory and test references

This information is derived from experts in the fields of medicine, pharmacy, and management, through an independent editorial review process. This book is available in hardback, electronic, and a mobile application version.

United States Pharmacopoeia–National Formulary (USP-NF)

The USP-NF provides access to official standards of the FDA. It is a guide for the specifications—tests, procedures, and acceptance criteria—required for pharmaceutical manufacturing and quality control. This book aids compliance with standards and lists new product development and approvals. It is available in hardback, electronic form, or online with a subscription.

United States Pharmacists' Pharmacopeia

United States Pharmacists' Pharmacopeia is a comprehensive compilation of information on compounding products and ingredients and their safety, in addition to products used to treat specific medical conditions. Also included are the most recent sterile preparation guidelines for USP, the most common **non-formulary** agents, veterinary compounding, dietary supplements, and laws pertaining to compounding. This book is available in hardback or online with a subscription.

Clinical Pharmacology and Other Gold Standard/Elsevier Products

Clinical Pharmacology is an electronic drug compendium commonly encountered in retail and health system pharmacies. Similar to *Drug Facts and Comparisons,* the reference is very popular because of its ease of use and quick access to needed information. The information can be provided to the pharmacy or health system via online, Intranet, electronic, or mobile applications. The reference can be used by physicians, pharmacists, nurses, and other allied health professionals. Similar to the American Society of Health-System Pharmacists (ASHP) and *Micromedex DRUGDEX, Clinical Pharmacology* is an officially recognized compendium by the Centers for Medicare & Medicaid Services (CMS) because of its extensive amount of drug information, including off-label drug uses supported by clinical evidence. Data are continuously updated, making this reference a very timely resource for current drug information. *Gold Standard/Elsevier* also has a complement of other products that can be bundled to the subscription to enhance the base compendia product. The following are examples of the various types of information available:

- Comprehensive drug details, including pharmacology, pharmacokinetics, contraindications, boxed warnings, precautions, pregnancy category, breast-feeding, indications and dosage for all populations, off-label uses, and adverse events
- FDA-approved drugs and "how supplied" data for generic, trade name, prescription, and nonprescription products; drug product images are included
- Drug product comparison reports
- International listing of drugs: Global Drug Name Index
- Drug interactions (available in professional and consumer-friendly reports)

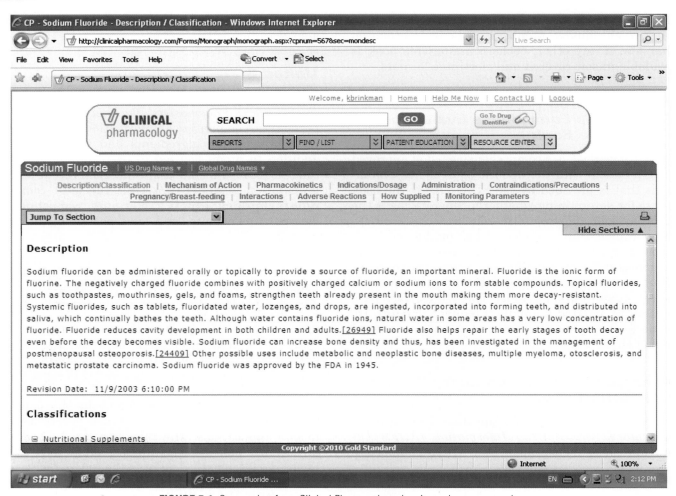

FIGURE 7-1 Screen shot from *Clinical Pharmacology* showing a drug monograph.

- Identification of drug products: Drug IDentifier (includes imprint codes, colors, shapes, scoring, and images)
- Consumer medication information: MedCounselor sheets
- Herbals and dietary supplements, including multivitamin and nutritional product listings
- IV compatibility report
- Integrated drug product data, including clinical decision support and pricing modules:
  - Alchemy
  - Toxicology and poisoning management: ToxED
  - Material safety data sheets: ToxED

Figure 7-1 presents a screen shot of a *Clinical Pharmacology* drug monograph.

Ident-A-Drug

Ident-A-Drug lists tablet and capsule identifications. Most tablets and capsules have a code or number stamped on them by the manufacturer for identification purposes. *Ident-A-Drug* includes more than

38,000 listings. The drugs are not listed by pictures but by identifiable codes, colors, and shapes and also by whether the tablet is available scored. Once these characteristics have been identified, the book provides the name of the manufacturer, generic and brand names, strength, and use of the drug. *Micromedex's* IDENTIDEX and *Clinical Pharmacology's* Drug IDentifier are also useful resources that are currently available in many pharmacies (both hospital and retail). *Micromedex* is an online interface that has pictures to aid in identifying drugs quickly and accurately. This type of referencing is very helpful when patients do not know the name of the drug they are taking but have a capsule or tablet of the drug to use as a reference. Emergency departments often have patients who have overdosed on an unknown drug. If one tablet or capsule is brought in with the patient, the pharmacy probably can identify the drug using the *Ident-A-Drug* book, *Micromedex's* IDENTIDEX, or *Clinical Pharmacology's* Drug IDentifier (Figure 7-2). Although some books, such as *Drug Facts and Comparisons,* have some pictures of tablets and capsules, these are not extensive and are not the

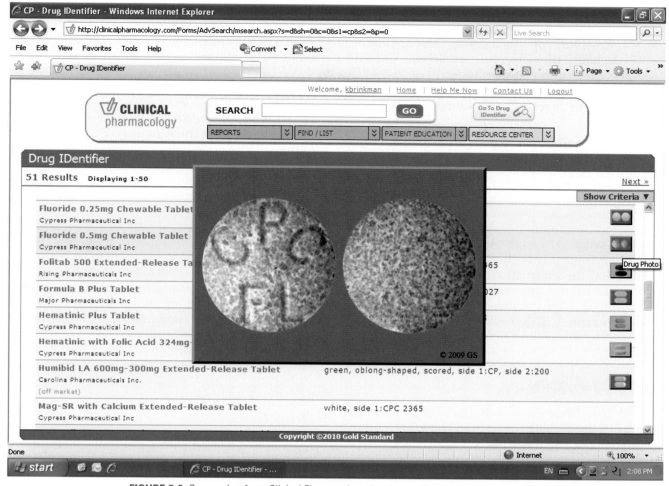

FIGURE 7-2 Screen shot from *Clinical Pharmacology* showing a pill using the Drug IDentifier.

first choice to use in identifying a drug. *Ident-A-Drug* is available as a soft-cover book, mobile application, and online with a subscription.

Micromedex Healthcare Series

Micromedex Healthcare Evidence and Clinical Xpert provides an online and mobile application that can

be used by physicians, pharmacists, and nurses in a health care facility. The information is provided through several different software programs that can be purchased. The following list includes examples of the various types of information available with the specific software programs:

- Comprehensive drug details: DRUGDEX
- FDA-approved drugs: PDR
- International drugs: Index Nominum
- Drug interactions: DRUG-REAX
- Identification of capsules and tablets: IDENTIDEX
- Dosing information and parenteral nutrition solutions for infants: NeoFax
- Pharmacokinetics calculators: KINETIDEX
- Proper drug usage and precautions: DrugNotes
- Drug information for more educated patients: Detailed Drug Information for the Consumer
- Drug pricing: ReadyPrice
- Herbals, supplements, and alternative therapies: AltMedDex
- **Formulary** management for hospitals: Formulary Advisor

- Monographs for pharmacy & therapeutics (P&T) evaluations: P&T QUIK
- Management of medication reconciliation throughout the hospital workflow: Clinical Xpert Medication Reconciliation
- Verification of IV compatibility: IV INDEX
- Safety data sheets: Pharmaceutical SDS

Trissel's Handbook on Injectable Drugs

Mostly used in the hospital setting, the *Handbook on Injectable Drugs* by Lawrence Trissel is a well-known reference used for information on parenteral agents. The monographs discuss products, administration, stability, and compatibility with infusion solutions and other drugs. Although technicians cannot relay information from this book to physicians or nurses, they can find the information and have it ready for the pharmacist. In this way, they can facilitate a rapid response from the pharmacy to the necessary medical personnel. This book is available in hardback, electronic, mobile application, and online formats.*

American Drug Index

The *American Drug Index* contains listings for more than 22,000 drugs, both prescription and OTC. Information includes the following:

- Manufacturers' names
- Pronunciation of drug names
- Active ingredients
- Dosage forms
- Strengths
- Packaging and uses
- Drugs that should not be crushed or chewed
- Look-alike or sound-alike drugs
- Storage requirements for USP drugs
- Trademark glossary
- Normal laboratory values and more

The book is available in hardback or electronic format.

Goodman & Gilman's The Pharmacological Basis of Therapeutics

The following is a list of some of the information provided in *Goodman & Gilman's The Pharmacological Basis of Therapeutics:*

- Pharmacokinetics and pharmacodynamics
- Drug transport/drug transporters
- Drug metabolism pharmacogenomics

- Principles of therapeutics in all areas of the body system

This book is available in hardback format or as an online subscription.

Handbook of Nonprescription Drugs

The *Handbook of Nonprescription Drugs,* a reference published by the American Pharmacists Association (APhA), provides self-care options for the following:

- Nonprescription medications
- Nutritional supplements
- Medical foods
- Complementary and alternative therapies
- Nondrug and preventive measures for self-treatable disorders
- Complementary and alternative medicine
- FDA-approved dosing information and evidence-based research on efficacy and safety considerations of nonprescription, herbal, and homeopathic medications

This book is available in hardback format or as an e-book (textbook is downloaded onto a computer).

Martindale's The Complete Drug Reference

Martindale's The Complete Drug Reference provides information on drugs in clinical use worldwide, in addition to the following:

- Selected investigational and veterinary drugs
- Herbal and complementary medicines
- Pharmaceutical excipients
- Vitamins and nutritional agents
- Vaccines
- Radiopharmaceuticals
- Contrast media and diagnostic agents
- Medicinal gases
- Drugs of abuse and recreational drugs
- Toxic substances
- Disinfectants
- Pesticides

The book is available in hardback or electronic format.

Remington's Pharmaceutical Sciences: The Science and Practice of Pharmacy

Remington's Pharmaceutical Sciences: The Science and Practice of Pharmacy covers the entire scope of pharmacy, from the history of pharmacy and ethics to the specifics of industrial pharmacy and pharmacy practice. The following specific areas are included:

- Manifestations and pathophysiology of diseases
- Immunology

---

*Many online drug compendia, including *Clinical Pharmacology* and *Micromedex*, have incorporated the online Trissel databases into their product offerings.

- Disease state management
- Specialization in pharmacy practice
- Professional communication
- Various aspects of patient care

The book is available in hardback format.

Pediatric and Neonatal Dosage Handbook

The *Pediatric and Neonatal Dosage Handbook,* published by Lexi-Comp, provides information on suggested current dosages for pediatric patients. The twentieth edition features 983 drug monographs. It is alphabetically organized and cross-referenced by U.S. and Canadian brand names. An appendix is provided that contains comparative charts, tables, and other supportive information. A Therapeutic Category and Key Word index also are included. The book is available in hardback format.

Geriatric Dosage Handbook

The *Geriatric Dosage Handbook,* also published by Lexi-Comp, provides information on suggested current dosages for geriatric patients. The brand and generic drug names are alphabetically organized and cross-referenced by page number to the generic drug monograph. Geriatric-sensitive information is provided, along with the latest Beers Criteria (updated 2013). Beers outlines drugs to avoid or to use with caution in older adults. It is available in hardback format.

In addition to these well-known books, many specialty reference books are available, such as those covering information on drugs in pregnancy and breast-feeding, psychotropic medications, and antibiotics. Many pharmacies have a wide range of these types of reference books available (Table 7-5).

TABLE 7-5

Pharmacy Reference Books

Reference Book	Publisher	Available in	Updated
Drug Facts and Comparisons	Wolters Kluwer Health	Hardbound book	Yearly
		Loose-leaf book	Monthly
		Electronic	Current updates
		Mobile application	Current updates
Physicians' Desk Reference	Thomson Healthcare	Hardbound book	Yearly
		Mobile application	Current updates
Drug Topics Red Book	Medical Economics	Softbound book	Yearly and monthly
Orange Book	FDA	Electronic	Current updates
USP-NF	USP	Three-volume hardbound	Monthly
		Online	Current updates
		CD	Monthly
Ident-A-Drug	Therapeutic Research Faculty	Softbound book	Monthly
		Online	Current updates
		Mobile application	Current updates
Goodman & Gilman's The Pharmacological Basis of Therapeutics	McGraw-Hill	Hardbound	Every 5 years
		Electronic	Current updates cut/paste
		Mobile application	With electronic subscription
Remington's Pharmaceutical Sciences: The Science and Practice of Pharmacy	Lippincott Williams & Wilkins	Hardbound	Every 5 years
United States Pharmacopoeia– National Formulary (USP-NF)	USP	Hardbound	Yearly
Drug Information	ASHP	Softbound	Yearly
American Hospital Formulary		Electronic	Current updates
Trissel's Handbook on Injectable Drugs	ASHP	Hardbound	Yearly
Pediatric Dosage Handbook	Lexi-Comp/Wolters Kluwer Health	Hardbound	Yearly
	APhA	Softbound	Yearly
Geriatric Dosage Handbook	Lexi-Comp/Wolters Kluwer Health	Hardbound	Yearly
	APhA	Softbound	Yearly

APhA, American Pharmacists Association; *ASHP,* American Society of Health-System Pharmacists; *USP,* U.S. Pharmacopeial Convention.

Pocket-Sized Reference Books

Technicians traditionally have not carried pocket versions of drug books. However, as roles expand at work, the pharmacy technician needs to have his or her own reference books. Some manufacturers produce small pocket versions of trade/generic name drug books, but the drugs listed often are limited to their drug line only. It is becoming more important for technicians to carry a good pocket guide not only of trade and generic names, but also of drug classifications, indications, and side effects. Before purchasing a pocket guide, technicians should examine a variety of different guides to determine the one that is most pertinent to their jobs. One of the best books to keep is one in which a drug can be looked up by trade or brand name without having to check the index. The cost of these pocket handbooks generally ranges from $5 to $10. The disadvantage is that they are softbound and must be updated yearly to incorporate new drugs or discontinued ones. The advantage is that most of the drugs remain the same over time. You can access a free copy of the Mylan Pharmaceuticals Generic Brand Reference guide at *www.mylan.com/mylan-resources/access-gbr*. You can order by phone, online, or download the app for iPhone, Android, and Blackberry devices.

Scenario CHECK UP 7-2

Robert is a dedicated technician who likes to keep up on the most recent new drugs. His friend Haley suggests he invest in an updated pocket drug guide. Robert tells Haley he would prefer to download one of the new drug apps for his iPhone, but he is not sure if he would be allowed to use it. Employees are not supposed to have their phones out during work. How can Robert solve this dilemma?

Electronic Referencing

Electronic devices, such as smart phones and tablets, are becoming more popular and economical. An assortment of drug databases and other reference materials can be downloaded onto a handheld device for easy access. Several companies offer short-term trial periods for these reference materials before requiring the user to purchase a subscription. Others offer a limited amount of information for free. One example is Epocrates (*www.Epocrates.com*), which offers a basic free drug information package that can be downloaded onto a smart phone or other handheld device. The following information is included:

- Trade and generic name reference
- Classification
- Indications
- Interactions
- Dosing
- Pill identification
- Medication and study updates
- Manufacturer's contact information
- Provider directory
- Resource center

The smart phone with the most drug database options is the iPhone/iTouch/iPad, followed by the Android platform.

The following are several free drug reference apps:

- Medscape Mobile: A combination drug reference and database that includes a drug-drug interaction checker. It is available for iPhone/iTouch/iPad, Android, and Blackberry platforms.
- Micromedex Drug Information (*www.micromedex/products/mobile2*): An extensive drug database with detailed information, including pharmacokinetics, toxicology, and clinical teaching pearls. This currently is available only for iOS, although an Android version is in the works.
- Mobile PDR (*www.skyscape.com/mobilePDR/*): This is an electronic version of the paper book that is published annually. It has a pill search function that includes pictures. This is available to practicing physician assistants (PAs) with a Drug Enforcement Administration (DEA) or National Provider Identifier (NPI) number, and it works on the Skyscape platform for most devices.
- Fingertip Formulary (*www.fingertipformulary.com/*): Provides drug formulary information listed by state. A free version is available for most platforms, and extra drug monograph information is available for licensed providers.

The Internet

Referencing should not be limited to books alone. The Internet has a lot of information; however, it is up to the reader to determine whether the information is reliable and accurate. Finding websites at universities and through publishing companies is a good way to look for information. Accessing personal websites may give you a person's perspective but may not provide medically sound information. A list of reputable websites for news concerning medications is provided at the end of this chapter.

Pharmacy organizations have websites on the Internet, and many have weekly news boards that reference important information concerning pharmacy. Because pharmacy is constantly evolving, much of the information cannot be included in journals. The news links are listed on the website. Many databases have up-to-date information and links (Table 7-6). These are valuable tools for keeping members updated with accurate information. Also,

TABLE 7-6

Websites and Databases Helpful for Pharmacy Technicians

Websites	Name of Organization or Site	Type of Information
www.cdc.gov	Centers for Disease Control and Prevention	Current health issues
www.cms.gov	Centers for Medicare & Medicaid Services	Reimbursement information
www.drugs.com	Online database	Trade/generic names, drug interactions, and pill identifier
drugtopics.modernmedicine.com/	Online information	Up-to-date medical news and pharmacy issues
www.FDA.gov	U.S. Food and Drug Administration (FDA)	Drug, food, and cosmetics safety information
www.fda.gov/drugs/default.htm	FDA drug evaluation and research development	Links to *Orange Book, MedWatch, NDC Directory,* and new drug approvals
www.Health.NIH.gov	National Institutes of Health	Health issues and studies
www.MayoClinic.org	Mayo Clinic	Information on conditions and diseases, lifestyle health issues
www.medicare.gov/part-d/ coverage/part-d-coverage.htm	U.S. Department of Health and Human Services	Information on Medicare Part D, formulary index
www.nlm.nih.gov/medlineplus	National Library of Medicine database	Health and drug information, medical dictionary and encyclopedia
www.medscape.com	Online database	Information on diseases; links to medical journals and continuing education (CE) courses
www.PDRhealth.com	*Physicians' Desktop Reference* online	Interactions database for both legend and over-the-counter (OTC) drugs and also herbs and supplements; information on conditions and diseases
www.Rxlist.com	Online database	Both prescription and OTC drug information
www.webmd.com	Online database	Up-to-date health topics, conditions, and diseases and drug information
www.dailymed.nlm.nih.gov/ dailymed/about.cfm	Online database	Includes package inserts for more than 5000 drugs available in the United States

these association sites have links to other pharmacy sites that may be of interest. Pharmacy associations also may offer Internet links where the user can have questions answered by other members.

Many websites provide continuing education (CE) in the form of online exams and live CE courses. With the online CE courses, the student sometimes can download and study the information before taking the exam online; other online courses require live participation. Once the course has been completed, the certificate is mailed, e-mailed, or provided online to the student. CE certificates should be filed for reference when obtaining recertification. Often these CE courses are offered free of charge, and although a certain number of CE units are required for recertification, there is no limit to the number of CE courses a person may take. Upon completion of the CE exam, you receive notification of your score, and a certificate can be printed and filed in your records as a recertification reference. Beginning in 2015, CE courses appropriate for pharmacy technicians will be identified as such, and technicians will be awarded

CE credit only for pharmacy technician–approved lessons. For more information on continuing education sources, see Chapter 3.

Journals and Newsmagazines

Nearly every pharmacy subscribes to journals and newsmagazines that pertain to pharmacy. They may be paper journals or electronic versions. These can be informative to the pharmacy technician. When a technician becomes nationally certified, he or she must complete continuing education units and may at some point use these journals to complete some if not all the necessary units. Journals offer continuing education at a reasonable cost; in addition, they allow the technician to stay current on the most recent drugs being developed. Journals and newsletters may be published monthly, bimonthly, quarterly, or even weekly. They contain articles on new drugs, technicians, the future of pharmacy, and various legislative changes that may be taking place. The information they can provide about the field of pharmacy

TABLE 7-7

Pharmacy Publications

Publications	Published	Continuing Education Included	Website	Association
AAPT	6 times yearly	Yes	www.pharmacytechnician.com	Yes
Computer Talk	6 times yearly	No	www.computertalk.com	No
Hospital Pharmacy	Monthly	Yes	www.hospitalpharmacyjournal.com	No
Drug Topics	Monthly	Yes	drugtopics.modernmedicine.com	No
Today's Technician	6 times yearly	Yes	www.pharmacytechnician.org	Yes
Pharmacy Times	Monthly	Yes	www.pharmacytimes.com	No
Pharmacy Today (JAPhA)	Monthly	Yes	www.pharmacytoday.org	No
The Script	Monthly	No	www.pharmacy.ca.gov	No
U.S. Pharmacist	Monthly	Yes	www.uspharmacist.com	No
AJHP	Twice monthly	Yes	www.ajhp.org	Yes
Journal of Pharmacy Technology	6 times yearly	Yes	pmt.sagepub.com	No

AAPT, American Association of Pharmacy Technicians; AJHP, American Journal of Health-System Pharmacy; JAPhA, Journal of the American Pharmacists Association.

can be beneficial. Many different journals, newsletters, and magazines are available. Other journals that technicians may not see in the pharmacy setting are those written by pharmacy technician associations. These journals are geared specifically to technician issues. Table 7-7 provides a sample of the types of journals and pharmacy magazines available.

Scenario CHECK UP 7-3

As a certified pharmacy technician, Robert must complete 20 hours of continuing education every 2 years. He has read that the National Pharmacy Technician Association (NPTA) provides free continuing education for its members. He also found that with the yearly membership, he would receive the *Technician Today* magazine. Robert is considering asking his company to pay for his NPTA membership. Do you think this is a good idea? Why or why not?

Additional Types of Information

In addition to large desktop books, pocket handbooks, journals, and the Internet, other sources of information can keep you current and on the cutting edge as a pharmacy technician. For examples of additional references geared to technicians and health care workers, see Table 7-8. Another way to obtain new drug information is to join an association. Membership can be rewarding and can serve as a good source

TABLE 7-8

Additional Reference Books for Pharmacy Technicians*

Name	Useful Information
Gray Morris D: *Calculate with confidence*, ed 6, St Louis, 2014, Elsevier ISBN 978-0-323-08931-9	Math calculations for all types of dosage forms
Potter PA, Perry AG: *Fundamentals of nursing*, ed 8, St Louis, 2013, Elsevier ISBN 978-0-323-07933-4	How nurses approach patients In-depth information on disease states
Mosby's dictionary of medicine, nursing and health professions, ed 9, St Louis, 2013, Elsevier ISBN 978-0-323-07403-2	Anatomical diagrams along with definitions
Gerdin J: *Health careers today*, ed 5, St Louis, 2012, Elsevier ISBN 978-0-323-07504-6	Good description of more than 45 vocations in the medical field Gives technician a better understanding of health fields
Perry AG, Potter PA, Elkin MK: *Nursing interventions & clinical skills*, ed 5, St Louis, 2012, Elsevier ISBN 978-0-323-06968-7	In-depth information on disease states

*Technicians may find these references helpful for understanding various aspects of health care.

divisions are active in supplying continuing education courses to technicians and host various functions for networking and unifying pharmacy technicians from different types of pharmacies. For more information on all associations, refer to Chapter 3.

Seminars and continuing education dinners, provided by pharmacy associations, are sometimes sponsored by drug companies and are another good source of information on drug topics, new drugs, and fulfilling CE requirements. You do not need to be a member of an association to attend, but the cost usually is lower for members. Although seminars normally are held once or twice yearly, depending on the association that is presenting the seminar, continuing education dinners may be hosted monthly by the local chapter of an association. At seminars, many of the technician classes include math, aseptic technique, the future of pharmacy technicians, law updates, and more. Monthly continuing education dinners or events usually have a limited amount of space available; depending on the drug company sponsoring the event, there may be a speaker and a meal for a low cost or (more rarely) no cost. These costs usually are predetermined by the chapter of the association. All of these seminar classes and continuing education dinners can be applied to CE credit for pharmacy technicians.

of information and a way to network. Many associations offer webinars, both live and recorded, for members. CE credits can be earned while learning new material. The associations listed in Box 7-4 currently provide continuing education and information for technicians.

All of these organizations offer a great way to stay current on new drugs, devices, and current and future pharmacy issues. In addition, they usually offer a way to order pharmacy technician certification review books and other reference books, sometimes at a reduced membership rate. These reference books can be found on their websites or at their bookstores (this information may be found at their seminars). The information and support they can provide is limited only by how much they are used. Also, many pharmacist associations, such as the American Society of Health-Systems Pharmacists and American Pharmacists Association and their chapters, have specific divisions for pharmacy technicians, providing technicians with additional sources for learning new information. You must inquire about your local pharmacy associations to determine what they offer. Some technician

Tech Note!

Before you join an association, check out its website for information on the level of involvement of the association with its technician members. Many associations do not have a technician division or offer continuing education classes specifically for technicians. Most, but not all, have yearly seminars and a bimonthly journal containing continuing education and other useful information pertaining specifically to technicians. Becoming familiar with the various conditions of patients and understanding the terminology are essential for becoming a competent pharmacy technician. Table 7-8 lists books that represent various aspects of health care. All health care workers should constantly pursue the acquisition of new information.

TECHNICIAN PROFILE

Ann is a freelance writer for a national pharmacy technician magazine. She is a career hospital technician and has more than 20 years of pharmacy experience. Ann is able to share her knowledge by writing on various topics near and dear to her heart. Many of the duties Ann performed in the hospital pharmacy align well with her freelance job description. Both require attention to detail, love of the technician field, and a willingness to serve. Ann is expected to maintain a high degree of accuracy and to meet all productivity deadlines efficiently. Ann maintains active memberships in her local, state, and national technician associations. These connections allow her to stay current on the issues affecting her peers. She finds being a freelance writer gives her a sense of purpose and accomplishment, and she enjoys the challenge.

Considerations When Choosing a Reference

At times, technicians may need to use a reference for obtaining information on a drug or for billing purposes. Knowing the proper book to reference is important, not only for finding the correct information, but also for saving time and avoiding frustration.

The references listed previously are large reference books that are provided for the staff in the pharmacy. Some online subscription contracts in the pharmacy may have codes that allow you individual access to use the reference at home; check with your employer. If you choose to buy your own reference books or online subscriptions for home use or pocket versions for use at work, you should consider some basics. If your main use of the reference will be to determine generic and trade names, indications, and side effects, a reference such as *Drug Facts and Comparisons* is a good choice. As pharmacies update their reference books, you might be able to obtain a free copy of some print references. Some pharmacies that subscribe to electronic resources also receive complementary access for their employees' use at home; check with your employer. Also, check bookstores on the Internet for the previous year's edition of a desired resource. Older editions can be sold at a reduced price and may contain most of the information you require. However, you should consider the need to have updated information, as drug information changes very quickly. You might check other book companies for similar information. Many reference books contain the same type of information as *Drug Facts and Comparisons*. Another consideration may be the size of the reference book. For instance, although *Drug Facts and Comparisons* is a complete and up-to-date book, it is large and will not fit in your pocket for easy access; however, a pocket version is available. Other publishers also offer pocket versions of their references, including mobile versions for various technical devices.

 Tech Note!

If a technician needs to find a drug price and manufacturer for a drug such as Tenormin and its generic version, a book such as the *PDR* is not helpful because the drugs are listed by manufacturer and the reference does not give prices. *Drug Facts and Comparisons* references drugs by trade or generic name but also does not list prices. *Red Book* is an excellent source to find drug prices using the trade name. It provides prices for the trade name and generic equivalents.

Avoid books that reference drug names in only one way (e.g., only by trade or generic names) because their use can become time-consuming. Most drugs have many names, depending on the drug company that manufactures them. If you are going to keep the book at home or in your office, you might be looking for a larger book. If your space is limited, you may be more interested in a handbook. Remember that smaller books contain less information or have print that is more difficult to read. If you are going to purchase a reference book at a bookstore, take a wide variety of drug names with you to reference in the store. If the book has all the drugs you are looking for and is easy to read, you will use the book more often. Table 7-8 presents additional reference books that are informative for the pharmacy technician. These range from information on various topics in the medical field to resources that can help you practice pharmacy calculations.

DO YOU REMEMBER THESE KEY POINTS?

- The appropriate way to research drugs
- The appropriate way to reference drugs
- The major sources of information a technician most often uses in pharmacy
- The key attributes of each of the reference books explained in this chapter
- The importance of carrying a pocket-sized reference book
- Types of electronic reference materials
- The importance of journals and newsmagazines as they pertain to pharmacy and continuing education
- Different considerations when choosing a reference
- The benefits of joining a pharmacy association

Scenario FOLLOW UP

Robert was thrilled when his company paid for his NPTA membership. He has already learned a great deal from reading the technician journal. He knows that to be the best technician possible, he must have access to the most current and accurate drug information available. He now uses the online *PDR*, the *Clinical Pharmacology* electronic database, and the Epocrates website on a regular basis.

REVIEW QUESTIONS

Multiple Choice Questions

1. Which book provides package inserts from manufacturers?
   A. *Drug Facts and Comparisons*
   B. *Goodman & Gilman's The Pharmacological Basis of Therapeutics*
   C. *Red Book*
   D. *Physicians' Desk Reference*

2. Which book or books is/are the best source for locating manufacturers' addresses?
   A. *Red Book*
   B. *Physicians' Desk Reference*
   C. *Goodman & Gilman's The Pharmacological Basis of Therapeutics*
   D. *Drug Facts and Comparisons*
   E. A, B, and D

3. If you need to find the average wholesale price (AWP) of a drug, the best source to look in is:
   A. *American Drug Index*
   B. *Drug Facts and Comparisons*
   C. *Red Book*
   D. A journal

4. The book that is available both hardbound and loose-leaf to allow for monthly updates is:
   A. *Drug Facts and Comparisons*
   B. *Red Book*
   C. *Goodman & Gilman's The Pharmacological Basis of Therapeutics*
   D. None of the above

5. The most widely used reference book in pharmacy is:
   A. *Goodman & Gilman's The Pharmacological Basis of Therapeutics*
   B. The dictionary
   C. *Remington's Pharmaceutical Sciences: The Science and Practice of Pharmacy*
   D. *Drug Facts and Comparisons*

6. If you need to identify a specific tablet or capsule only by the markings, color, and shape, you would look in:
   A. *Drug Facts and Comparisons;* loose-leaf version
   B. *Ident-A-Drug*
   C. *American Drug Index*
   D. *Red Book*

7. All of the following are updated at least yearly *except:*
   A. *Drug Facts and Comparisons*
   B. *Red Book*
   C. *Goodman & Gilman's The Pharmacological Basis of Therapeutics*
   D. *Physicians' Desk Reference*
   E. All of the above books are updated yearly.

8. All of the following information can be found in the *Drug Facts and Comparisons* (F&C) *except:*
   A. Schedule of a narcotic
   B. Storage and stability
   C. Patient information
   D. All of the above information can be found in the F&C.

9. Information about pharmacy associations can be found:
   A. Online
   B. In journals
   C. In the *Red Book*
   D. A and C

10. All of the following can be found in free downloaded materials from Epocrates *except:*
    A. Contraindications
    B. Herbals
    C. Pill identification
    D. B and C

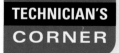 **TECHNICIAN'S CORNER**   A patient arrives at the pharmacy holding a single capsule in her hand and explains that she has lost her prescription bottle. She needs to have the medication refilled. The capsule is white and has the markings "Watson 369" on one side and "5 mg" on the opposite side. What is this drug, and what is its intended use?

Bibliography

Berardi RR et al: *Handbook of nonprescription drugs*, ed 14, Washington, DC, 2004, American Pharmacists Association.

Berardi M et al: *Handbook of nonprescription drugs*, ed 15, Washington, DC, 2006, American Pharmacists Association.

Berardi M et al: *Handbook of nonprescription drugs*, ed 16, Washington, DC, 2009, American Pharmacists Association.

Berardi M et al: *Handbook of nonprescription drugs*, ed 17, Washington, DC, 2011, American Pharmacists Association.

Billups NF, Billups SM: *American drug index 2009*, St Louis, 2008, Wolters Kluwer Health.

Billups N, editor: *American drug index*, Philadelphia, 2008, Lippincott Williams & Wilkins.

Billups N, editor: *American drug index*, Philadelphia, 2012, Lippincott Williams & Wilkins.

Billups N, editor: *American drug index*, Philadelphia, 2013, Lippincott Williams & Wilkins.

Drug facts and comparisons, ed 60, St Louis, 2005, Wolters Kluwer Health.

Drug facts and comparisons, ed 63, St Louis, 2008, Wolters Kluwer Health.

Drug facts and comparisons, ed 66, St Louis, 2012, Wolters Kluwer Health.

Drug topics red book, ed 109, Montvale, NJ, 2005, Thomson.

Drug topics red book, ed 113, Motvale, 2009, Thomson.

Drug topics red book, ed 114, Montvale, NJ, 2010, Thomson.

Gennaro A: *Remington's pharmaceutical sciences: the science and practice of pharmacy*, ed 18, Easton, Pa, 1995, Mack.

Gennaro A: *Remington's pharmaceutical sciences: the science and practice of pharmacy*, ed 21, Philadelphia, 2005, Lippincott Williams & Wilkins.

Hardman JG, Limbird LE, editors: *Goodman & Gilman's the pharmaceutical basis of therapeutics*, ed 11, New York, 2005, McGraw-Hill Professional.

Jellin J, editor: *Ident-a-drug reference: for tablet and capsule identification*, Stockton, Calif, 2008, Therapeutic Research Faculty.

Physicians' Desk Reference.

Physicians' Desk Reference Inc. *Red Book: Pharmacy's Fundamental Reference*. Montvale, NJ: Thomson Reuters; 2013.

Trissel L: *Handbook on injectable drugs*, ed 14, Elk Grove Village, Ill, 2006, American Academy of Pediatrics.

Trissel L: *Handbook on injectable drugs*, ed 15, Elk Grove Village, Ill, 2009, American Society of Health-System Pharmacists.

Trissel, Lawrence: *Handbook on injectable drugs*, ed 17. Elk Grove Village, Ill, 2012, American Society of Health-System Pharmacists.

US pharmacopoeia, ed 30, Rockville, Md, 2006, US Pharmacopeial Convention.

US pharmacopoeia, ed 1, Rockville, Md, 2009, US Pharmacopeial Convention.

US pharmacopoeia, ed 32, Rockville, Md, 2013, US Pharmacopeial Convention.

Websites Referenced

Drug names. (Referenced September 20, 2013.) www.webmd.com/drugs/

Drugs@FDA database. (Referenced October 23, 2013.) www.fda.gov/Drugs/InformationOnDrugs/ucm135821.htm

Gold standard clinical pharmacology. (Referenced October 23, 2013. www.clinicalpharmacology.com/

Ipaktchian S: The name game. (Referenced August 2, 2013.) http://stanmed.stanford.edu/2005summer/name-game.html

Micromedex information. (Referenced October, 2013.) www.micromedex.com/products/hcs/

Orange book: approved drug products with therapeutic equivalence evaluations, ed 33. (Referenced October 23, 2013.) www.fda.gov/cder/ob

Community Pharmacy Practice

James J. Mizner, Jr.

OBJECTIVES

Upon completing this chapter, you should be able to do the following:

1. List and describe the different types of community pharmacies.
2. Explain the pharmacy technician's role in the medication use process.
3. Identify state laws and regulations related to receiving and screening prescription orders.
4. Assess prescription orders for completeness and authenticity when receiving orders via paper or electronic systems.
5. Efficiently obtain information to complete a prescription order.
6. Explain special procedures pharmacy technicians are responsible for in preparing, storing, and distributing controlled substances.
7. Explain the pharmacy technician's role in preparing medications for distribution,
8. Outline the process of creating a new patient profile and entering data into an existing patient profile.
9. Accurately count or measure finished dosage forms as specified by the prescription/medication order.
10. Explain the protocol for assembling appropriate patient information materials.
11. Collect needed information from the patient profile.

12. Identify all situations in which the patient requires the attention of a pharmacist.
13. Identify situations in the screening of refills and renewals in which the technician should notify the pharmacist of potential inappropriateness.
14. Describe the layout of the pharmacy and list the important areas.
15. Discuss effective verbal and written communication skills, including listening skills.
16. Examine strategies for communicating with patients who are non-English speakers or who have other special needs, such as vision or hearing problems, a low reading level, or difficulty understanding instructions.
17. Demonstrate a respectful attitude with diverse groups of people.
18. Recognize effective interpersonal and teamwork skills in working with health care teams.
19. Identify state laws and regulations regarding the technician's role in immunizations.
20. Explain the purpose of monitoring a patient's medication therapy.

TERMS AND DEFINITIONS

Adjudication The process by which a prescription is submitted electronically to a third-party payer for the pharmacy to be reimbursed for the medication dispensed

Aphasia A communication disorder that results from damage or injury to the language parts of the brain; it is more common in older adults, particularly those who have had a stroke

Auxiliary label A label that provides supplementary information about proper and safe administration, use, or storage of a medication

Bank identification number (BIN) A six-digit number on a prescription drug card that is used for routing and identification to process a prescription claim

Behind-the-counter (BTC) medication A class of medications kept behind the pharmacy counter that requires a pharmacist's

intervention before the medication can be sold to a patient; BTC medications are not considered prescription medications

Chain pharmacy A corporate-owned group of pharmacies that share a brand name and central management and usually have standardized business methods and practices

Dispense as Written (DAW) code A numeric set of codes, created by the National Council for Prescription Drug Programs (NCPDP), that is used when filling prescriptions; they can affect reimbursement amounts from insurance companies

Drug Enforcement Administration (DEA) number An alphanumeric number consisting of two letters and seven numbers that is assigned to prescribers authorized by the DEA to prescribe controlled substances

Drug utilization evaluation (DUE) (formerly known as drug utilization review) An authorized, structured, ongoing review of health care provider prescribing, pharmacist dispensing, and patient use of medication

Dysarthria A speech deficiency that interferes with the normal control of the speech mechanism

e-Prescribing The computer-to-computer transfer of prescription data between pharmacies, prescribers, and payers

Federal Legend A statement required on the labeling of all prescription medications: "Federal law prohibits dispensing without a prescription."

Franchise A form of business organization in which a firm that already has a successful product or service (the franchisor) enters into a continuing contractual relationship with other businesses (franchisees) operating under the franchisor's trade name and usually with the franchisor's guidance, in exchange for a fee

Help Desk A toll-free hotline to an insurance company, available 24 hours a day, seven days a week, so that pharmacists can call in specific questions about insurance claims and coverage and pharmacy-specific inquiries

Inscription The name, dosage form, strength, and quantity of the medication prescribed

National Drug Code (NDC) number A unique 10 or 11-digit number, composed of three segments, that is assigned to a medication. The first four digits identify the drug manufacturer, the next four identify specifics about the product, and the last two identify the drug packaging

National Provider Identifier (NPI) A unique 10-digit identification number for covered health care providers that is issued by the Centers for Medicare and Medicaid Services

Nonproprietary (generic) name A short name coined for a drug or chemical that is not subject to proprietary (trademark) rights and is recommended or recognized by an official body

Over-the-counter (OTC) medication A medication that does not require a physician's order or prescription for the patient to purchase

Prescription An order for medication issued by a physician, dentist, or other properly licensed practitioner, such as a physician assistant or nurse practitioner

Proprietary (brand or trade) name A brand name or trademark under which a drug product is marketed

Refill Permission by a prescriber to replenish a prescription

Repackaging The act of reducing the amount of medication taken from a bulk bottle

Signatura (*signa* or *sig*) The directions on a prescription that explain how the patient is to take the prescribed medication; a Latin expression meaning to "write on label"

Sole proprietorship An unincorporated business owned by one person

Subscription The part of the prescription that provides specific instructions to the pharmacist on how to compound the prescription

Superscription The heading of a prescription, represented by the Latin symbol *Rx*, meaning "take thou" or "you take"; the symbol has come to represent prescription or pharmacy

Therapeutic alliance A trust relationship between a health care professional and a patient, incorporating patient perceptions of the acceptability of interventions and mutually agreed upon goals for treatment

Introduction

Scenario:

Andrew is a new pharmacy technician working at a local community pharmacy. During his orientation, he is introduced to the several other pharmacy technicians who are performing various pharmacy activities. He observes one technician accepting new prescriptions from a patient, another pharmacy technician entering information into the pharmacy's computer information system, and one technician checking in a pharmacy order from a drug wholesaler. Andrew is completely overwhelmed by the operations. He asks the pharmacist, "Where do I begin?"

Community pharmacy, also known as *retail* or *ambulatory care pharmacy*, is a vital component of our health care delivery system. There are many types of community pharmacies, including independent, franchise, and chain pharmacies (e.g., CVS and Walgreens).

The independent pharmacy originally was known as the "corner drugstore" in a community. Often these pharmacies were classified as a **sole proprietorship**. A sole proprietor is someone who owns an unincorporated business by himself or herself, according to the Internal Revenue Service. The owner of an independent pharmacy was normally the pharmacist in charge of the pharmacy. The services provided in an independent pharmacy varied based on the pharmacist, the location of the pharmacy, and the patient population. Many independent pharmacies are compounding pharmacies. Independent pharmacies may also sell or rent durable medical equipment. In addition, they now may provide immunizations to the public.

A **franchise** is an authorization, granted to a person or group of people, that allows them to operate under a franchisor's well-established trade name and usually under the franchisor's guidance. A franchise pharmacy is a business organization in which a pharmacy with a successful product or service (the franchisor) enters into a continuing contractual relationship with other pharmacies (franchisees) in exchange for a fee. Examples of franchise pharmacies include Medicine Shoppe, Good Neighbor Pharmacy, and Care Pharmacy.

A **chain pharmacy** is a corporate-owned group of pharmacies that share a brand and central management and usually have standardized business methods and practices. A chain must have at least two locations and have a central headquarters that is overseen by a board of directors. CVS and Walgreens are the two largest pharmacy chains in the United States. According to the National Association of Chain Drugstores (NACDS), in 2012, chain pharmacies filled 2.7 billion prescriptions, or 72% of the total number of prescriptions filled. Chain pharmacies may be classified as mass merchandisers (e.g., Target), discounters (e.g., Wal-Mart and K-Mart), and membership stores (e.g., Costco and BJ's). Many grocery stores have a pharmacy department (e.g., Safeway).

The pharmacy technician plays an instrumental role in our prescription processing system. Pharmacy technicians assist licensed pharmacists, prepare prescription medications, provide customer service, and perform administrative duties in a community pharmacy. They are generally responsible for receiving prescription requests, inputting prescriptions into the pharmacy information system, counting tablets, labeling bottles, maintaining patient profiles, preparing insurance claim forms, and performing administrative functions, such as answering phones, stocking shelves, and operating cash registers. The success of a community pharmacy is very dependent on the knowledge and training of its pharmacy technicians. This chapter focuses on the role of and responsibilities delegated to a pharmacy technician in a community pharmacy.

Role of the Pharmacy Technician

The primary role of the pharmacy technician in a community pharmacy is the same as that in an institutional pharmacy or any other pharmacy setting: *to assist the pharmacist.* A community pharmacy technician may be assigned a specific duty or many different responsibilities in the pharmacy (Figure 8-1). The following are some of the more common duties.

- Provide customer service
- Take the information needed to fill a prescription from customers or health professionals
  - Visually scan new prescriptions to ensure that they contain all of the required information
  - Answer the telephone
  - Obtain refill information from the patient
- Input various types of data into a pharmacy information system
  - Add a prescriber to a database
  - Add a new patient to a database
  - Update a patient's profile or prescriber's information
  - Add insurance plans to a database
  - Add a drug to the database
  - Enter a new prescription
  - Obtain a refill authorization
  - Process a new prescription for prior drug approval
  - Refill, transfer (with a pharmacist's assistance), file, or reverse a prescription
  - Run various productivity reports
- Compound prescriptions
  - Perform necessary calculations before compounding a prescription

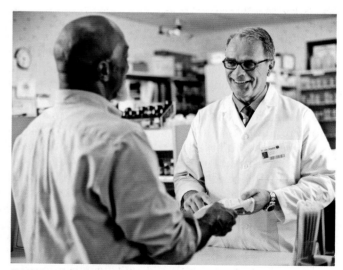

FIGURE 8-1 Pharmacy technicians have a variety of roles in the community pharmacy, including talking with customers, processing and reviewing prescriptions, counting medications, labeling containers, restocking supplies, and other administrative duties. (Copyright © 2014 Fuse, Thinkstock.com. All rights reserved.)

Scenario CHECK UP 8-1

Andrew is manning the prescription drop-off counter at the pharmacy. A patient presents his prescription to Andrew. Andrew collects information from the patient, including the patient's address, contact telephone number, birth date, and prescription drug card coverage. He reads the name of the medication on the prescription, which states that the prescriber wrote for Bayer Aspirin 81 mg. Andrew is bewildered because he has purchased Bayer Aspirin 81 mg in the past for his mother, and he wonders if Bayer Aspirin 81 mg is now a prescription medication. What would you tell him?

- Weigh or measure amounts of medication for prescriptions
- Clean equipment after compounding
- Package and label prescriptions
  - Count the prescribed quantity of medication
  - Select the appropriate container
  - Apply both the prescription and auxiliary label to the container in a professional manner
  - Print the appropriate literature for each prescription to give to the patient
  - Return the medication to the shelf
- Price medications
- Organize inventory and alert pharmacists to any shortages of medications or supplies
  - Reorder medications and pharmacy supplies
  - Check the ordered medication against the packing slip
  - Place ordered medication in its appropriate place on the shelf
  - Check pharmacy stock for medication that may have short dating
- Accept payment for prescriptions and process insurance claims
- Arrange for customers to speak with the pharmacist if customers have questions about medications or health matters
- Perform pharmacy housekeeping tasks

These duties vary, depending on the size of the community pharmacy and the experience of the pharmacy technician.

Prescription

A **prescription** is an order for medication issued by a physician, dentist, or other properly licensed practitioner, such as a physician assistant or nurse practitioner (see Figure 2-9, *A*). In some states, other practitioners have been licensed with a limited scope of practice. A prescription designates a specific medication and dosage to be administered to a particular patient at a specific time. Often the prescribed medication is referred to as a prescription.

There are two broad legal classifications of medications: those that can be obtained only by a prescription, or legend medications, and those that can be obtained without a prescription, or an **over-the-counter (OTC) medication**. A prescription medication is also known as a legend medication because it bears the **Federal Legend**, which states: "Federal law prohibits dispensing without a prescription." OTC medications are deemed safe for an individual to take without being under a physician's supervision. As a result of the Combat Methamphetamine Epidemic Act of 2005, a subclassification of OTC medications has been established; these drugs are

known as **behind-the-counter (BTC)** medications. BTC medications are OTC medications that contain pseudoephedrine, an ingredient used to make methamphetamine, which is a schedule I controlled substance. Individuals who want to purchase products containing pseudoephedrine must buy them at the pharmacy counter under the supervision of a pharmacist and provide proper identification. The purchaser must be at least 16 years of age. An individual may purchase up to 3.6 g in 1 day or no more 9 g within a 30-day period.

A prescription written by a physician may be given to the patient to take to the patient's pharmacy or mailed to a mail-order pharmacy. A physician may designate an employee of his or her practice to telephone a prescription into the pharmacy; in this case, the pharmacist must create a written form of the telephoned order. A physician's office may fax a patient's prescription to the pharmacy. In some states it is legal for a patient to fax his or her prescription to the pharmacy; however, the patient must provide the pharmacy with the original prescription before receiving the medication.

A prescription also may be sent to the pharmacy electronically; this is known as **e-prescribing**. E-prescribing is the computer-to-computer transfer of prescription data between pharmacies, prescribers, and payers. It is not the use of an e-mail or a facsimile transaction. Electronic prescribing functions include messages about new prescriptions, prescription changes, refill requests, prescription fill status notification, prescription cancellation, and medication history. E-prescribing involves a wide range of participants in the health care system: individual practitioners, clinics, hospitals, provider associations, pharmacies, software vendors, trade and professional associations, laboratories and ancillary services, state and federal governments, standards development organizations, terminology and code set organizations, health plans, payers, and processors.

E-prescribing has many advantages, such as:
- Reducing or eliminating errors associated with illegible handwriting
- Enabling prescribers to receive on-screen prompts for drug-specific dosing information
- Linking information from a patient's medical file to a patient's prescription file
- Notifying the prescriber if a drug product is covered by the patient's insurance plan when the order is generated rather than when it is presented at the pharmacy
- Expediting refills
- Facilitating data exchange between the physician and the pharmacist and ultimately their patients

Prescription Information

In most situations it is the pharmacy technician who has the initial contact with the patient when the person drops off a new prescription or requests a **refill** of a prescription. The first thing a pharmacy technician does when receiving a new prescription is determine whether the patient has had prescriptions filled at that pharmacy previously. If the patient has filled prescriptions previously at that pharmacy, the pharmacy technician verifies the accuracy of the information in the patient's profile. If the patient has never had a prescription filled at that pharmacy, the pharmacy technician collects the necessary information, which includes:

- Patient's complete name
- Patient's home address (street, city, state, and zip code)
- Patient's telephone numbers (home, work, and mobile)
- Patient's birth date
- All allergies (drug and food)
- Patient's current physical condition
- Prescription drug card information (group number, member number, and relationship to the cardholder)
- Whether the patient wants to receive generic medications
- A list of any OTC and BTC medications the patient takes
- A list of any herbal supplements the patient takes

This information is used to develop a patient profile for the individual.

A patient profile is a list of the patient's prescriptions and all related information, including the original date of fill, refill dates, and the prescribing practitioner. The Omnibus Budget Reconciliation Act of 1990 (OBRA '90) requires that every ambulatory pharmacy maintain patient profiles. A patient profile is a tool that can help eliminate medication errors. The patient profile is extremely valuable when drug utilization evaluation is performed. During this evaluation, an accurate patient profile can reduce potential drug-food interactions, drug-disease interactions, drug–environmental chemical interactions, and drug-laboratory interactions. In addition, the patient profile can identify multiple pharmacological effects caused by medications being prescribed, distinguish multiple physicians that a patient may be using, detect patient nonadherence to the drug regimen, and disclose possible drug abuse by the patient.

Originally prescriptions were written using Latin abbreviations, and measurements were expressed using the apothecary and avoirdupois systems. Some Latin abbreviations are still used in the practice of pharmacy today (Table 8-1). The metric system (Table 8-2) is the official system of measurement for weights and volumes in the United States; however, some older physicians continue to use the apothecary and avoirdupois systems in writing prescriptions (see Chapter 2).

Prescriber Information

A valid prescription must contain specific information. Every prescription is required to have prescriber information, patient information, a superscription, an inscription, a subscription, and a signa. A prescriber's information includes the prescriber's name, office address, and telephone number. If the prescribed medication is a controlled substance, the physician's **Drug Enforcement Agency (DEA) number** must be included. Some states may require the physician's **National Provider Identifier (NPI) number** and/or medical license to be included on the prescription.

Patient Information

The patient's information includes his or her complete name, home address, and birth date. The patient's birth date is used as an identifier to ensure that the correct patient is receiving the correct medication. At times an illegible prescription will be presented to the pharmacy. The individual who accepts the prescription is responsible for verifying that the information is correct. If the patient's name is not spelled correctly, the patient may question whether he or she is receiving the correct prescription.

Date

The date the prescription was written by the prescriber must appear on the prescription. If there has been a time lapse between the date the prescription was written and when it was received by the pharmacy, the pharmacist may question the intent of the physician and whether the patient's needs are being met. Some medications, such as controlled substances, must be filled or refilled within 6 months of the date the prescription was written. It is the responsibility of the pharmacy technician to be aware of any state regulations regarding the amount of time that may lapse from the date the prescription was written to the date it is presented for filling.

Superscription

The **superscription** (Rx symbol) is a contraction of the Latin verb *recipe*, meaning "take this drug." It is used as the heading on a prescription and usually precedes the inscription. Presently, the Rx symbol represents prescription and the pharmacy.

TABLE 8-1

Pharmacy Abbreviations

Abbreviation	Meaning	Abbreviation	Meaning
aa	of each	mOsm	milliosmole
ac	before meals	N&V	nausea and vomiting
ad	to, up to	noct	at night
ad*	right ear	non rep	do not repeat
ad lib	at pleasure, freely	NS	normal saline
am	morning	OA	osteoarthritis
amp	ampule	OCD	obsessive compulsive disorder
aq	water	od*	right eye
a.s.*	left ear	os*	left eye
a.u.*	each ear	ou*	each eye
bid	twice a day	pc	after meals
BM	bowel movement	pm	afternoon
BP	blood pressure	po	by mouth
BPH	benign prostatic hypertrophy	pr	by rectum
BS	blood sugar	prn	as needed
BSA	body surface area	pulv	powder
c̄	with	PVCs	premature ventricular contractions
Ca	calcium	PVD	peripheral vascular disease
CAD	coronary artery disease	q*	every
cap	capsule	qd	every day
CHF	congestive heart failure	qh	each hour
COPD	chronic obstructive pulmonary disease	qid	four times a day
dil	dilute	qod	every other day
disp	dispense	qs	a sufficient quantity
div	divide	qs ad	a sufficient quantity to prepare
DJD	degenerative joint disease	RA	rheumatoid arthritis
DM	diabetes mellitus	s̄	without
dtd	give of such doses	SC, SQ, SUBCUT, SubQ*	subcutaneous
DW	distilled water	Sig	write on label
Dx	diagnosis	SL	sublingual
elix	elixir	SLE	systemic lupus erythematosus
ft	make	SOB	short of breath
g (gm)	gram	sol	solution
GERD	gastroesophageal reflux disease	s̄s̄	one-half
GI	gastrointestinal	stat	immediately
GU	genitourinary	supp	suppository
gr	grain	susp	suspension
gtt	drop (drops)	Sx	symptom
HA	headache	syr	syrup
HBP	high blood pressure	tab	tablet
HR	heart rate	TB	tuberculosis
hs	at bedtime	Tbsp	teaspoon
HTN	hypertension	TED	thromboembolic disease
ID	intradermal	TIA	transient ischemic attack
inj	injection	tid	three times a day
IV	intravenous	tiw	three times a week
IM	intramuscular	Top	topical
IU*	international units	tsp	tablespoon
JRA	juvenile rheumatoid arthritis	U*	unit
KCl	potassium chloride	UA	uric acid; urinalysis
Kg	kilogram	UC	ulcerative colitis
L	liter	ud	as directed
mcg	microgram	ung	ointment
mEq	milliequivalent	URI	upper respiratory infection
mg	milligram	ut dict	as directed
mg/kg	milligram per kilogram	UTI	urinary tract infection
mg/m²	milligram per square meter	WA	while awake
mL	milliliter	wk	week

*Included in the Institute for Safe Medication Practices (ISMP) "do not use" list of abbreviations; however, physicians still use them in writing prescriptions.

TABLE 8-2

Metric-Household Conversions

Metric (volume)	Household Equivalent
5 mL	1 teaspoon (tsp)
15 mL	1 tablespoon (Tbsp)
30 mL	1 fluid ounce (fl oz)
240 mL	1 cup
480 mL	1 pint (pt)
960 mL	1 quart (qt)
3840 mL	1 gallon (gal)

Inscription

The **inscription** contains the medication name, dosage form, strength, and quantity. Today most medications are already prepared by the pharmaceutical manufacturers. However, the pharmacy may receive a prescription for a nonsterile or sterile compound for which the names and quantities of each ingredient are listed. In this situation the medication or ingredient is listed by its nonproprietary, or generic, name. The quantities should be listed using the metric system; however, some older prescribers may use the apothecary system.

Subscription

The prescription's **subscription** consists of directions to the pharmacist or pharmacy technician on how to compound a prescription. Many of the medications dispensed today do not require compounding and therefore do not contain a subscription.

Signatura (Signa or Sig)

Signatura (*signa* or *sig*) is a Latin expression meaning to "write on label." The *signa* is the directions to the patient on how to take the prescribed medication. These directions are written using English or Latin abbreviations or a combination of the two. They are transcribed by either the pharmacist or the pharmacy technician when this information is entered into the pharmacy's computer system. The *signa* tells the patient how much, when, and how long to take the medication.

Scenario CHECK UP 8-2

A new patient arrives at the pharmacy with a prescription from a local health care provider. The pharmacist asks Andrew to set up a new patient profile in the pharmacy's computer system. What information does Andrew need from the patient to set up a new profile?

Prescription Processing

Intake

A pharmacy may receive a new prescription by a variety of methods. The patient may bring the prescription to the pharmacy; a designated employee from a physician's office may telephone a new prescription into the pharmacy; the physician's office or patient may fax the prescription; or the prescription may be submitted electronically (e-prescribing) from the physician's office. E-prescribing is not the same as a faxed prescription. Pharmacy technicians must be familiar with their state's pharmacy regulations for receiving new prescriptions.

Often the pharmacy technician is the first individual to come in contact with a new prescription brought in by the patient. The pharmacy technician should accept the prescription in a professional manner and review it to ensure that the patient's name, address, and any other required information are on the prescription. If the patient has never had a prescription filled at that pharmacy, the pharmacy technician must collect detailed information from the patient, including medications the patient is currently taking (prescription, nonprescription, vitamins, and herbal supplements), medical conditions, and allergies. Many pharmacies have a form for the patient to complete that requests this information so that a patient profile can be created.

Data Input

Computer systems are standard in pharmacies today because they can provide the following:
- Information to the pharmacist at moment's notice
- Online prescription claim approval
- Speed in processing prescriptions
- Improved efficiency
- Reduction in prescription errors

Patient Information

The pharmacy technician is responsible for inputting the patient's information into the pharmacy's computer information system. Although pharmacy information systems may vary, the system prompts the user for the necessary information. If the information is not entered, the system will not permit the user to continue with the process. Patient information includes the following:
- Full name
- Home address (number, street, city, state, and ZIP code)
- Telephone numbers (home, mobile, and work)
- Birth date
- Gender

Prescription Savings Card

RxBIN: 000000

RxPCN: 0000

Group #: 00000000

ID #:   00000000000

This is NOT insurance - Discount only

FIGURE 8-2 Prescription drug card.

- Allergies
- Generic preference
- Request for non–child-resistant container

A thorough and accurate patient profile can help eliminate possible adverse drug events.

Prescription Drug Benefits

Today many individuals receive prescription drug coverage through medical insurance. Many companies offer prescription drug coverage as an employee benefit. The prescription drug benefit defines the drug coverage that is provided to the member. An individual who is covered under a prescription drug benefit receives a prescription drug card (Figure 8-2). This card contains the necessary information for the pharmacist or pharmacy technician to process the prescription. Information contained on a prescription drug card includes the following:

- A group number, which identifies the coverage for a group of individuals under one contract; normally the group consists of a company's employees.
- A subscriber number, which identifies the individual who pays the premiums
- A person code, which identifies the specific individual covered. Some plans use "01" to identify the card holder, "02" for the card holder's spouse, and "03" for the first child dependent. Person codes may vary according to the plan.
- A **bank identification number (BIN)**, which is a field in the telecommunication standard that is used for the routing and identification of pharmacy claims. The National Council for Prescription Drug Programs (NCPDP) assigns a six-digit BIN to process a prescription claim.
- A Help Desk telephone number, which is a 24-hour service that enables a pharmacy to obtain assistance in processing a prescription claim.

Unfortunately, there is no uniform standard for the information or its format on a prescription drug card.

Prescriber Information

The pharmacy technician must verify that the prescriber's information is accurate in the computer system. The prescriber's information includes his or her name, office address (street number, street, city, state, and ZIP code), office telephone number (including area code), and DEA number for controlled substances only. Depending on state regulations, the NPI number and state medical license number may also be required.

Medication

The pharmacy technician must enter the name of the medication, its strength and quantity, and the number of refills indicated on the prescription. All quantities ordered are to be expressed in metric quantities. For example, 4 fluid ounces would be entered as 120 mL, and 1 pound would be 454 g.

Calculating the Day's Supply

After the quantity has been entered, the pharmacy technician must calculate the day's supply of medication that is being dispensed to the patient. The day's supply can be calculated using the following formula:

$$\text{Day's supply} = \text{Total quantity dispensed} \div \text{Total quantity taken per day}$$

When calculating the day's supply for either ophthalmic or otic drops, the technician should use the conversion of 20 drops per milliliter and calculate according to the following formula:

$$\text{Day's supply} = (20 \text{ gtts/mL} \times \text{Number of mL}) \div \text{Number of drops instilled per day}$$

For inhalation products, use the following formula:

$$\text{Day's supply} = \text{Number of inhalations per container} \div \text{Number of inhalations breathed in each day}$$

In all situations, the day's supply is always rounded to the nearest whole number.

Directions for Use

The directions for use by the patient must be entered into the pharmacy's computer system. Often the prescriber writes the directions using pharmacy abbreviations, and the pharmacy technician must transcribe the directions. Each computer system has developed specific shortcuts that allow the user to use abbreviations that are translated into English when entering the prescription's signa. By becoming familiar with these shortcuts, the user can save time by not having to enter each word. Several hints for inputting the directions for use include:

- Begin with a verb
- Identify the dosage form
- Indicate the route of administration
- Do not use abbreviations
- Use terminology in everyday language so that the patient understands it

If a prescriber writes "as directed" for the directions, the technician should promptly inform the pharmacist of this, and the pharmacist will call the prescriber for explicit directions.

Prescription Refills

The pharmacy technician must enter the approved number of refills from the prescriber into the computer system. The prescriber must provide a specific number of refills for the prescription. Some prescribers may indicate "prn" refills on a prescription. In this situation, the technician must be aware of the state's regulations regarding "prn" refills. The pharmacy technician enters zero refills if a prescriber does not enter any refills on the prescription.

Generic Substitution

If the prescriber authorized a generic drug to be dispensed, the technician will dispense the generic version of the medication. Some states require the prescriber to write "Dispense as Written" or "Brand Name Medically Necessary" in their own handwriting on the prescription; other states may allow the prescriber to check a box on the prescription. The pharmacy technician must be familiar with the state's pharmacy regulations regarding generic substitution.

Dispense as Written (DAW) Codes

Dispense as Written (DAW) codes are a numeric set of codes, created by the NCPDP, that are used when entering prescriptions into the computer (Box 8-1). If a pharmacist or pharmacy technician fails to submit a prescription claim using the correct DAW code, the pharmacy may not be reimbursed properly for the medication that was dispensed. In addition, a pharmacy may be audited by a third-party provider to verify that the DAW code used was correct. If a third-party audit reveals that a pharmacy is improperly using DAW codes, the pharmacy may be held responsible for refunding claims that were submitted incorrectly.

Prescription Adjudication

Prescription **adjudication** is the process by which a prescription is submitted electronically to a third-party payer so that the pharmacy can find out whether it will receive reimbursement for the medication. The pharmacy is notified of the status of the claim within a few seconds of submission. Most of the time, the pharmacy will be reimbursed for the

BOX 8-1

Dispense as Written Codes

0	No product selection indicated
1	Substitution not allowed by provider
2	Substitution allowed—patient requested product dispensed
3	Substitution allowed—pharmacist selected product dispensed
4	Substitution allowed—generic drug not in stock
5	Substitution allowed—brand drug dispensed as generic
6	Override
7	Substitution not allowed—brand drug mandated by law
8	Substitution allowed—generic drug not available in marketplace
9	Other

TABLE 8-3

Prescription Claim Rejection Codes

Rejection Code	Meaning
5	Missing or invalid pharmacy number
6	Missing or invalid group number
7	Missing or invalid cardholder ID number
8	Missing or invalid person code
9	Missing or invalid birth date
11	Missing relationship code
19	Missing days supply
22	Missing or invalid Dispense as Written (DAW)/product selection code
25	Missing or invalid prescriber ID
26	Missing or invalid unit of measure
54	Non-matched National Drug Code (NDC) number
60	Drug not covered for patient
75	Prior authorization required
79	Refill too soon

medication; however, in some situations the prescription claim is rejected. This can occur for a variety of reasons, such as the medication is not covered, the refill was requested too soon, or even the patient is an invalid card holder. If the prescription claim is rejected, the pharmacy is notified of the reason with a one- or two-digit rejection code (Table 8-3).

The prescription claim must be corrected before it is resubmitted. The correct information can be obtained from the patient or the patient's representative or by contacting the Help Desk associated with the third-party provider. The **Help Desk** has a 24/7 toll-free hotline for pharmacists to address specific questions relating to claim rejections, payment status, prior authorization procedures, explanation of drug utilization evaluation messages, and pharmacy-specific inquiries.

Drug Utilization Evaluation

The pharmacist is responsible for reducing medication errors and drug-related illnesses. As a result of OBRA '90, the pharmacist is responsible for obtaining information from Medicaid patients or their caregivers, with the goal of identifying and resolving potential medication-related issues. Patient profiles are created and contain the following information, which the pharmacist uses in reviewing a patient's medication therapy:

- Patient demographic information
- Comprehensive list of medications being taken
- Allergies
- Adverse drug reactions
- Disease states
- Pharmacist's comments regarding a patient's drug therapy.

A prospective drug use review is conducted during **drug utilization evaluation (DUE)**, formerly known as drug utilization review (DUR). This review examines all the patient's medication records before dispensing is conducted. During this review, the following factors are evaluated:

- Drug overutilization
- Drug underutilization
- Therapeutic duplication
- Drug-drug interactions
- Incorrect dosages
- Drug allergy problems
- Incorrect duration of drug treatment
- Clinical abuse or misuse
- Drug-disease contraindications

Pharmacy technicians may be involved with prescription data entry and adjudication, and they should notify the pharmacist immediately of any issues regarding medication. The pharmacist will make a clinical decision based on the information available as to whether the prescription should be processed. It is not within the scope of the pharmacy technician's responsibilities to make judgment decisions regarding medication use.

Scanning the Prescription

Many pharmacies scan the original prescription; therefore, a digital copy of the prescription is available when a prescription is refilled. Also, if the original prescription is misfiled, a digital copy is available for the pharmacist to review. Scanning of prescriptions is a quality assurance tool that can help reduce medication errors.

Prescription Labeling

Every prescription filled should have a visually appealing and professional label (see Figure 2-9, *B*). It is extremely important that the pharmacist or pharmacy technician affix the label neatly to the prescription container. This professional appearance conveys to the patient that care was taken in filling the prescription.

A legal prescription label is required to have several pieces of information:

- Name, address and telephone number of the dispensing pharmacy
- A prescription number (which is used to identify a particular prescription order and to refill the prescription)
- Prescriber's name
- Patient's name
- Date the prescription was dispensed
- Name, strength, and quantity of the medication dispensed
- Directions for use (should be in an easy to understand format for the patient)

Some states may require the name or initials of the individual who dispensed the medication. Often the number of refills may appear on the prescription label. Some pharmacies may list the drug manufacturer's lot number on the label; this makes it easier to identify a medication that has been recalled from the drug manufacturer. In some communities with a large Hispanic population, the prescription label may appear in Spanish.

Auxiliary Labels

Auxiliary labels are normally printed with the pharmacy label (Table 8-4). The auxiliary labels provide patients with additional information about taking their medication. Auxiliary labels may indicate when it is best to take a medication (e.g., before a meal) or a potential side effect ("may cause drowsiness" or "avoid sunlight"), or they may remind the patient to discard the medication after a given time (as with a reconstitutable antibiotic). Auxiliary labels should be affixed to the prescription container so that no important information, such as the **National Drug Code (NDC) number**, lot number, or expiration date, is covered (Figure 8-3).

Patient Product Information

The federal government has required that patient product information (PPI) be provided to the patient when specific medications are dispensed. The purpose

TABLE 8-4

Commonly Used Auxiliary Labels for Side Effects

Classification	Commonly Used Auxiliary Label
Contraceptives	Take as directed
Nonsteroidal antiinflammatory drugs (NSAIDs)	May cause dizziness/drowsiness Take with food
Narcotics	Do not drink alcohol, and/or drinking may increase the effects of the drug
Macrolide antibiotics	Take on an empty stomach Take with plenty of water
All antibiotics	Take until gone
Sulfa antibiotics	May cause sensitivity to light Take on an empty stomach Take with plenty of water
Warfarin	Do not take aspirin unless prescribed

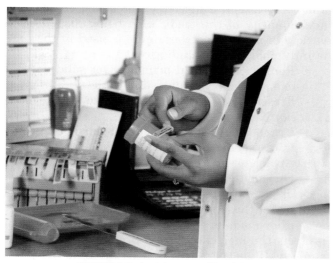

FIGURE 8-3 Applying an auxiliary label.

of the PPI sheet is to ensure that the patient is provided with information on the proper use of the medication. Examples of medications requiring an accompanying PPI include oral contraceptives, estrogens, and NSAIDs. Information contained on a PPI includes:

- **Proprietary (brand or trade) name** and **nonproprietary (generic) name** of the product
- Clinical pharmacology
- Indications and use
- Contraindications
- Warnings
- Precautions
- Adverse reactions
- Drug abuse
- Overdosage

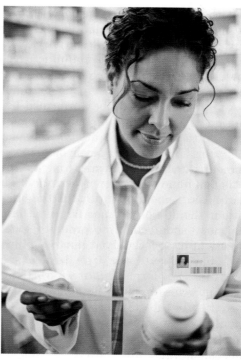

FIGURE 8-4 Technicians should always verify any prescription information with the label on the manufacturer's container. (Copyright © 2014 Fuse, Thinkstock.com. All rights reserved.)

- Dosage and administration
- How supplied

Almost all pharmacies provide supplemental printed instructions to the patient.

Scenario CHECK UP 8-3

Andrew is responsible for inputting the prescription into the pharmacy's computer system and billing the patient's pharmacy benefits manager. During the adjudication process, he receives the following message: #60—Drug Not Covered for Patient. Andrew knows the medication is a prescription drug. What should he do?

Prescription Preparation

After reading and checking the prescription order, the pharmacy technician should decide on the exact procedure to be followed in dispensing or compounding the product. Many of the medications are already prepared for the pharmacy by the drug manufacturers. Pharmacy technicians should take the prescription label with them when they go to the shelf to gather the medication. They should compare the NDC number on the prescription label with the NDC number on the manufacturer's drug label (Figure 8-4; also see Figure 2-4 for a sample label). The technician should pull the medication from the shelf and return it to the dispensing area of the pharmacy. The pharmacy technician must take great care in selecting the prescribed dosage form and strength and the number of dosage units dispensed.

The prescription label should be checked with the original prescription and the manufacturer's label. The prescription should be checked a second time with the prescription and the drug manufacturer's bottle. A final check should be performed before the prescription is bagged for pickup. Any medication that appears to have deteriorated or has passed the manufacturer's date should never be dispensed.

In some instances the pharmacy may not have the medication on hand to fill the prescription. The pharmacy technician should promptly tell the pharmacist. The patient should be informed of the situation, and the pharmacy should offer to order the medication for the patient or to locate it at another pharmacy.

Many pharmacies use a tray with a spatula to count solid dosage forms (Figure 8-5). It is best to count the dosages in multiples of five. To prevent contamination of tablets and capsules, the counting tray should be wiped clean after each use because powder from tablets may remain on the tray. Some pharmacies may use automatic counting machines during dispensing. High-volume community pharmacies may use automatic dispensing equipment (e.g., a Baker Cell) to dispense medications.

Although extemporaneous compounding is still performed in community pharmacies, the percentage of compounded prescriptions is relatively small. However, the pharmacy technician must perform the

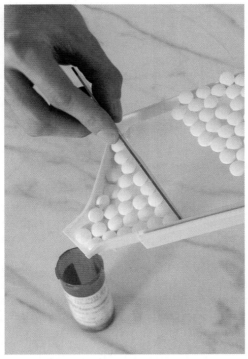

FIGURE 8-5 Counting trays may be used to more easily count and pour tablets into medication vials. (Copyright © 2014 Cornstock Images, Stockbyte, Thinkstock.com. All rights reserved.)

necessary calculations and have them checked before compounding the medication. The pharmacy technician may need to weigh substances or measure liquids before compounding and use the appropriate techniques when adding the ingredients. Extemporaneous compounding is discussed in Chapter 11.

Scanning the Manufacturer's Bottle

Many pharmacies use equipment to scan the bar code on the drug manufacturer's bottle and compare it to the NDC number of the medication selected. If the scanned bar code does not coincide with medication's NDC number, the pharmacist is notified. This process is used as a quality assurance measure to help eliminate medication errors.

Packaging the Prescription

When dispensing a prescription, the pharmacy technician may select a container according to size, color, and composition; the selection is based on the type and quantity of the medication being dispensed. A variety of medication containers is used in the community pharmacy, including:

- Round vials—Used primarily for solid dosages (e.g., tablets, capsules, and caplets)
- Prescription bottles—Used for dispensing liquids
- Dropper bottles—Used for dispensing ophthalmic, otic, nasal, or oral liquid medications
- Applicator bottles—Used for topical medications
- Ointment jars and collapsible tubes—Used to dispense ointments, creams, and gels

Many of these containers are amber in color and are either made of glass or plastic. The amber color protects the medication from breaking down due to sunlight. It is extremely important that the pharmacy technician package the medication in a container that ensures the drug's strength, quality, and purity. Plastic containers have several advantages over glass ones: they are lighter in weight, are more resistant to breakage, and are more adaptable in design.

The Poison Prevention Packaging Act (PPPA) requires the pharmacist to dispense a prescription in a container that has safety closures unless the prescribing physician or patient requests otherwise. This request for a non–child-resistant container may be for a single prescription or for all of a patient's prescriptions. It is the responsibility of the pharmacy staff to obtain a signed waiver from the patient making this request, and this information should be entered into the pharmacy's information system. The PPPA does make exceptions for specific medications not to be dispensed in child-resistant containers. These medications include nitroglycerin (because the patient must have immediate access to the medication in an emergency), oral contraceptives, and various oral and nasal inhalers (because of their unique design and construction). The prescription label should be affixed to the medication container and should convey a professional appearance.

Checking the Prescription

The pharmacist is responsible for checking the final prescription before it is dispensed to the patient to eliminate the possibility of a medication error. The prescription should be checked to verify that the actual medication and strength is being dispensed according to the prescriber's original prescription. The pharmacist should verify the patient's name, the prescription's directions for use, the prescription number, the date, and prescriber's name.

Filing Prescriptions

The pharmacy's information system maintains an electronic record of all filled and refilled prescriptions. The pharmacy is required by law to maintain the actual "hard copy" of the prescription. The Controlled Substance Act provided two options for filing filled prescriptions.

1. Option 1 (three separate files)
   * A file for schedule II controlled substances dispensed
   * A file for schedules III, IV, and V controlled substances dispensed
   * A file for all non-controlled drugs dispensed
2. Option 2 (two separate files):
   * A file for all schedule II controlled substances dispensed
   * A file for all other drugs dispensed (non-controlled and those in schedules III, IV, and V). If this method is used, a prescription for a schedule III, IV, or V drug must be made readily retrievable by use of a red "C" stamp not less than 1 inch high in the lower right hand corner of the prescription. If a pharmacy has an electronic record-keeping system for prescriptions that permits identification by prescription number and retrieval of original documents by prescriber's name, patient's name, drug dispensed, and date filled, the requirement to mark the hard copy with a red "C" is waived.

Electronic Prescription Records

* If a prescription is created, signed, transmitted, and received electronically, all records related to that prescription must be retained electronically.
* Electronic records must be maintained electronically for 2 years from the date of their creation or receipt.

Patient Counseling

OBRA '90 requires that an offer to counsel be made to every Medicaid patient who receives a new prescription. Many states have since adopted this to apply to *all* new prescriptions and refills. Often it is the responsibility of the pharmacy technician to ask a patient whether he or she has any questions for the pharmacist. If a patient has questions about his or her medication, the pharmacy technician should promptly inform the pharmacist. The pharmacist is responsible for identifying and resolving any problems involved with medication use. Only the pharmacist is legally permitted to counsel a patient (Figure 8-6).

Prescription Payment

Often it is the responsibility of the pharmacy technician to collect a patient's payment for the amount due for the prescription. The pharmacy determines the available payment methods. The patient often has the option of paying for the prescription with cash, a check, or a credit card. The person collecting payment for the medication must know how to use the cash register and credit card machine and how to return correct change to the patient if required.

Scenario CHECK UP 8-4

The pharmacy receives a prescription for amoxicillin 250 mg/5 mL 150 mL. The pharmacist asks Andrew to go to the shelf to obtain a bottle. While visually scanning the prescription for completeness, Andrew notes that the prescription calls for 150 mL. Where would he find the amoxicillin in the pharmacy?

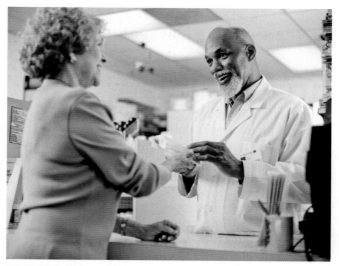

FIGURE 8-6 Patient consultations are performed by the pharmacist, at the agreement or request of the patient. (Copyright © 2014 Fuse, Thinkstock. com. All rights reserved.)

Other Pharmacy Technician Duties

Prescription Refilling

Instructions for refilling a prescription are provided by the prescriber on the original prescription or by verbal communication to the pharmacist. A patient may call the pharmacy or walk in to the pharmacy to request a prescription refill. The pharmacy technician must obtain the following information from the patient:

- Patient's name
- Patient's contact telephone number
- Prescription number
- Medication name and strength
- Physician's name
- Whether the patient will wait or return for the prescription

Many pharmacies use telephone refill trees, which allow the patient to call in 24 hours a day to refill prescriptions. The patient must enter the prescription number and is prompted to verify specific information about the prescription.

Requesting Prescription Refill Authorization

Many states permit a pharmacy technician to contact the prescriber's office for authorization of a refill. Depending on the system used by the pharmacy, the pharmacy technician may submit a refill request electronically, transmit a facsimile of the prescription, or use the telephone to call the prescriber's office. It is important for the technician to be familiar with the schedule category of a medication before requesting a refill authorization. Pharmacies are not permitted to refill schedule II medications; these require a new, handwritten prescription. Also, specific medications, such as isotretinoin, clozapine, and thalidomide, have special processes that must be followed.

Transferring a Prescription

Both federal and state laws govern the transfer of a prescription from one pharmacy to another pharmacy. A pharmacy technician may pull the original prescription from its file or pull it up on the computer system, but the pharmacist is responsible for ensuring that the information transferred is correct. Once the prescription has been transferred from one pharmacy to another pharmacy, the original prescription becomes void. The transferring pharmacist must record the following information from the receiving pharmacist:

- Date of the transfer
- Name, address and telephone number of the receiving pharmacy

- Name of the pharmacist at the receiving pharmacy
- Number of refills transferred
- National Association of Boards of Pharmacy (NABP) number for the receiving pharmacy
- DEA number of the receiving pharmacy (controlled substances only)

This information must appear on the back of the original prescription or in the computer system. The receiving pharmacist must record the following information from the transferring pharmacist:

- Date of the transfer
- Name, address and telephone number of the pharmacy where the prescription was originally filled
- Name of the pharmacist at the original pharmacy
- Number of refills received
- Original date of the written prescription
- NABP number for the originating pharmacy
- DEA number of the originating pharmacy (controlled substances only)

Many states allow a prescription to be transferred only one time.

Scenario CHECK UP 8-5

A patient calls the pharmacy and informs Andrew that she would like to transfer her prescription for hydrochlorothiazide 50 mg, which was originally filled at Ambitious Anthony's Pharmacy, to Andrew's pharmacy. Is it possible for Andrew to transfer the prescription for hydrochlorothiazide 50 mg to his pharmacy? If so, what information would Andrew need to obtain from the patient?

Pharmacy Layout

The state board of pharmacy regulates the practice of pharmacy for that state. Their regulations determine the physical standards for all pharmacies. The standards include the minimum amount of space for the prescription department of the pharmacy. The pharmacy must be well lit and ventilated, and the proper storage temperature must be maintained to meet the specifications of the *U.S. Pharmacopoeia: National Formulary* (USP-NF) for drug storage. The prescription counter should be used only for compounding, dispensing of drugs, and necessary record keeping. The prescription department must have a sink with hot and cold running water. The pharmacy must have adequate refrigeration equipment with a monitoring thermometer for the storage of drugs requiring cold storage temperature if the pharmacy stocks such medications. The pharmacy department must be maintained in a clean, sanitary manner and in good condition. The pharmacy also must have adequate trash receptacles.

The state board requires that each pharmacy maintain a current dispensing information reference source that is consistent with the practice of the pharmacy. Regardless of the state, every pharmacy is required to have a current copy of the Controlled Substance Act, a current copy of the USP-NF, and any other reference mandated by the state board of pharmacy. A pharmacy is required to have a prescription balance that is sensitive to 15 mg and weights or an electronic scale if the pharmacy engages in activities that require weighing of ingredients. The pharmacy must maintain equipment and supplies that are consistent with the pharmacy's practice.

A community pharmacy is required to have a security system that detects attempts to break into the pharmacy. The purpose of the security system is to protect the pharmacy department when it is closed. The security system must meet current alarm industry standards and may be either a sound, microwave, photoelectric, ultrasonic, or any other generally accepted device. The alarm system must have an auxiliary source of power and must be capable of sending an alarm signal to the monitoring company if the main line of communication is not working.

The prescription department of the pharmacy is required to have enclosures that protect the prescription drugs area from unauthorized entry and theft, regardless of whether a pharmacist is on duty. Only authorized personnel, such as pharmacists, pharmacy interns, or pharmacy technicians, are permitted in the pharmacy.

Prescription Intake Window

The prescription intake window is where a patient drops off the prescription to be filled. It is at this location that a pharmacy technician collects the necessary patient information that will be used in developing the patient profile.

Pharmacy Bench

The pharmacy bench is the work area of the pharmacy (Figure 8-7). Numerous tasks are performed at the bench, including:

- Entering patient and prescriber information and prescriptions into the pharmacy's computer information system
- Adjudicating prescription claims
- Scanning prescriptions into the pharmacy's information system
- Pouring and counting medication
- Scanning the manufacturer's drug container for quality assurance purposes
- Packaging and labeling the prescription

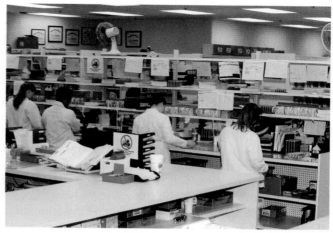

FIGURE 8-7 Technicians filling prescriptions.

- The pharmacist checking the final product against the original prescription order
- Bagging the patient's prescription

A state board of pharmacy may require the pharmacy bench to be a specific length. The pharmacy technician must maintain a clean and clutter-free work area to reduce the possibility of errors. After the pharmacist has checked the pharmacy technician's work and final product, the remaining medication should be returned to its proper location on the shelf.

Pharmacy Stock Area

A community pharmacy stocks many different dosage forms, and the medications are often arranged alphabetically for the various dosage forms. Some pharmacies may arrange the medications on the shelf alphabetically by brand name, whereas other pharmacies may arrange them alphabetically by their generic name. Many pharmacies have a designated area for oral dosage forms (tablets and capsules), oral liquids, reconstituted liquids (antibiotics), oral contraceptives, inhalation products, topical agents, ophthalmic and otic products, vaginal and rectal products, and refrigerated products. Some community pharmacies have an area designated for "fast movers," which are the more commonly dispensed medications for that pharmacy.

A retail pharmacy has a locked safe to ensure that schedule II medications are kept secure at all times. This safe may have a combination lock or a key lock, or it may be opened through biometrics if approved by the state board of pharmacy. Other controlled substances should be dispersed throughout the pharmacy.

If a retail pharmacy stocks drugs that require a cold storage temperature, the pharmacy must have adequate facilities, including a monitoring thermometer, for storage of these drugs in the prescription department. If a pharmacy has controlled substances that must be refrigerated, a separate refrigerator is required for the controlled substances. Pharmacists and pharmacy technicians should *never* place their lunch or a beverage in a refrigerator designated for medications.

Every pharmacy must check its inventory to ensure that all medications are in date. Often the pharmacy's standard operating procedure (SOP) states when this must be performed. If the pharmacy staff identifies medication that has expired, the medication must be removed from the shelf and placed in a designated area in the pharmacy where expired and recalled medications are kept. These medications cannot be dispensed or sold and must be separated from the other stock used for dispensing. These medications should be maintained in this designated area until they are properly discarded.

Non–Sterile Compounding Area

The non–sterile compounding area should be away from other workflow to minimize distractions to the compounder and contamination of the product. The area should be kept clean and free of clutter at all times. It should have a controlled temperature and proper ventilation. All equipment and supplies used in non-sterile compounding should be easily accessible to the compounder. All equipment should be examined for cleanliness before use and washed immediately after use to prevent any cross-contamination between ingredients and the final product. Isopropyl 70% alcohol is often used to clean the compounding area. It is recommended that a log be maintained to show when equipment was cleaned.

A sink with hot and cold running water and proper drainage is required by all state boards of pharmacy. Cleaning products, such as sponges and brushes of various sizes, should be kept next to the sink. Disposable paper towels should be kept adjacent to the sink. Trash receptacles should be kept a distance away from the compounding procedures. All trash should be disposed of safely and properly, including personal protective equipment (PPE) and hazardous waste.

Some of the equipment used in non-sterile compounding includes:
- Balances
- Beakers
- Brushes
- Graduated cylinders
- Evaporating dishes
- Funnels
- Graduates
- Metric weights
- Mortar and pestles
- Pipettes

- Sharps containers
- Spatulas
- Spray bottles
- Stirring rods
- Weighing papers or boats

The pharmacy technician should have a firm understanding of *United States Pharmacopeia Chapter <795>* (USP <795>), the equipment used in non-sterile compounding, and the appropriate techniques.

Sterile Compounding Area

Some retail pharmacies may have a sterile compounding area if the pharmacy administers vaccines or provides intravenous medications to its patients. This area must comply with the *United States Pharmacopeia Chapter <797>* (USP <797>). USP <797> has established specific guidelines for maintaining sterility in compounding and for addressing medication errors. The American Society of Health-System Pharmacists (ASHP) and the National Coordinating Committee on Large Volume Parenterals (NCCLVP) also have released guidelines describing the conditions and practices needed to process compounded sterile preparations (CSPs) so as to prevent harm or even death as a result of cross-contamination.

Pharmacy Order Check-in Area

Many pharmacies have a designated area where warehouse and wholesaler deliveries are received and checked in by the pharmacy technician. The pharmacy technician checks the medication received against the accompanying packaging slip to ensure that everything ordered was received. The pharmacy technician places the medications in their proper places on the pharmacy shelves or in the refrigerator.

Reconstitution Area

All community pharmacies have an area where medication is reconstituted. *Reconstitution* is the process in which a dehydrated product is returned to a liquid state. The most common type of medication that is reconstituted in a retail pharmacy is oral liquid antibiotics. Distilled water is used to reconstitute oral liquid antibiotics. Medications that require reconstitution are not reconstituted until the patient arrives to pick up the prescription because reconstituted medications are good only for a predetermined number of days, as outlined by the drug manufacturer on the bottle. Many reconstituted antibiotics must be refrigerated after mixing with distilled water. Auxiliary labels are affixed to the bottle reminding the patient to shake the bottle before using it and to refrigerate the medication if necessary.

Repackaging Area

Some community pharmacies may repackage medications if they provide pharmacy services to long-term care facilities. These pharmacies may have unit dose packaging equipment to prepare unit dose medications for these facilities. The pharmacy must maintain accurate records for repackaged medications; these records are found in the **repackaging** log. Table 8-5 presents information contained in a repacking log.

A beyond-use date (BUD) is assigned by the pharmacy to replace the drug manufacturer's expiration date. The USP has changed its beyond-use dating method for nonsterile solid and liquid dosage forms that are packaged in single unit and unit dose containers; the BUD is 1 year or less, unless stability data or the manufacturer's labeling indicates otherwise. (See Table 11-4 for examples of manufacturer

abbreviation codes.) Beyond-use dates are nearer than expiration dates to account for the fact that the manufacturer's original container has been opened in the repackaging process, thereby exposing the pharmaceutical article to ambient atmospheric conditions. This exposure, and the fact that containers into which dosage forms are repackaged may not have the integrity of the original package, necessitates a shortening of the expiration period from that originally set by the manufacturer.

Pharmacy Records

All community pharmacies must maintain the original prescription on file for the minimum time required by the state board of pharmacy, including the daily prescription record with the signatures of the filling pharmacists. The pharmacy must maintain all controlled substance invoices for a minimum of 2 years, according to federal regulations. These records include completed DEA Form 222, DEA Form 41, DEA Form 106, biennial inventories, and change of the pharmacist in charge.

Patient Bins

Once a prescription has received its final check from the pharmacist, it is placed in a bin awaiting pickup by the patient (Figure 8-8). These prescriptions may be placed in a secured area outside the prescription

TABLE 8-5

Repackaging Log Information

	Description
Date	Date the drug is repackaged, which includes date, month, and year
Drug	Drug name, usually by generic and then brand name, if indicated on the repackaging log sheet
Dosage form	Examples include tablet, capsule, spansule, troche, suspension, elixir, solution
Drug manufacturer	Drug manufacturer (usually abbreviated)
Drug manufacturer's lot number	Control number located on the side of the label or on the bottom of the bottle
Drug manufacturer's expiration date	Located with the lot number; remember that if the date indicates only the month and year, the medication is good through the end of the month
Assigned pharmacy lot number	Each item repackaged in pharmacy is given a number consecutive to the previous batch prepared
Pharmacy beyond-use date (BUD)	New date assigned to repackaged medications according to *United States Pharmacopeia <795>* guidelines
Pharmacy technician	Must initial logbook entry
Pharmacist	Must check off each item repackaged

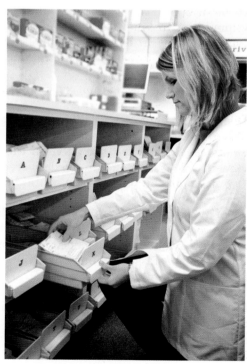

FIGURE 8-8 The patient bins should be in alphabetical order, clearly labeled, and easily accessible to the pharmacy staff.

department, not accessible by the patient, where access to the prescriptions is restricted to individuals designated by the pharmacist. The patient bins are normally arranged in alphabetical order. It is very important that a patient's prescription be placed in the appropriate bin. State pharmacy regulations determine whether a pharmacy technician may provide a patient with his or her medication when the pharmacist is not present.

Prescription Pick-Up Window

Some retail pharmacies have a separate pick-up window for prescriptions. Other pharmacies may have the patient pick up the prescription at the drop-off window. Regardless of the arrangement, there is at least one cash register at this point. Often the pharmacy technician rings up the patient's prescriptions and collects payment. The patient acknowledges receipt of the prescription by signing an electronic device for insurance purposes. When the patient comes to pick up the prescription, the pharmacy technician asks whether he or she has any questions for the pharmacist. If the patient has questions about the medication, the pharmacy technician notifies the pharmacist.

Consultation Area

As the result of changes made through OBRA '90, a pharmacy must have an area designated for patient consultation. Depending on the state board of pharmacy's regulations on counseling, the offer to counsel may be made in any manner the pharmacist feels appropriate, in his or her professional judgment, and may include any one or a combination of the following:

- Face-to-face communication with the pharmacist
- A sign posted so that it can be seen by patients
- A notation affixed to or written on the bag in which the prescription is to be delivered
- A notation on the prescription container
- By telephone

If the offer to counsel is accepted by the patient, the pharmacist counsels the person, presenting the prescription to the extent the pharmacist feels appropriate in his or her professional judgment. Information provided during counseling may include:

- The name and description of the medication
- The dosage form, dosage, route of administration, and duration of drug therapy
- Special directions and precautions for preparation, administration, and use by the patient
- Common adverse or severe side effects or interactions and therapeutic contraindications that

may be encountered, including their avoidance and the action required if they occur
- Techniques for self-monitoring drug therapy
- Proper storage
- Prescription refill information
- Action to be taken in the event of a missed dose

Some pharmacies may have a separate area where the pharmacist can counsel the patient. The consultation area should allow the pharmacist and patient to speak in privacy, away from other patients. Each state board of pharmacy establishes its own criteria.

Drive-Through Window

Within the past two decades, many retail pharmacies have established a drive-through window, where patients can drop off a new prescription, request a refill, or pick up a prescription without leaving their vehicle. The drive-through window is an added customer convenience that saves patients time because they do not have to park their vehicles and walk into the pharmacy. If the pharmacy has a drive-through window, the individual responsible for that area is responsible for collecting all the necessary patient information when a new prescription is presented and payment when it is purchased.

Scenario CHECK UP 8-6

Andrew is working at the pharmacy bench, and he notices one of his co-workers has left random papers and candy wrappers in her work area. Andrew knows it is important to keep the bench clean and organized. How should he handle this situation? What can he do to help his co-worker and the pharmacy maintain the necessary standards of cleanliness?

Communication

Pharmacy technicians have very strong technical skills that are essential in the practice of retail pharmacy. These skills include a strong knowledge base of diseases and their treatment with medication or through behavior modification, solid use of math in performing the necessary pharmacy calculations for compounding, the ability to transcribe a prescriber's order for medications, sound computer skills, and excellent techniques for both sterile and non-sterile compounding. One asset that is just as important as those just mentioned is interpersonal communication skills.

Interpersonal communication skills comprise the process by which messages are generated and transmitted by one individual and subsequently received and translated by another individual. Communication consists of five important components: a sender, the message, receiver, feedback, and barriers. The sender transmits a message to another person. The message is the component that is transmitted from one person to the other person. A message may be a thought, an idea, an emotion, information, or other factors that can be transmitted either verbally or nonverbally. Nonverbal communication includes facial expressions (e.g., smiling, frowning, or grinning) and hand motions. The receiver receives the message from the sender. Feedback is the process whereby the receiver communicates back to the sender his or her understanding of the message. Barriers affect the accuracy of the communication.

Nonverbal communication consists of a complex mix of behaviors, psychological and environmental interactions through which a person consciously and unconsciously relates to another individual. A study by F. Pyothos reported that 55% to 95% of all communication can be attributed to nonverbal communication. Nonverbal communications are distinctive because they mirror an individual's innermost thoughts and feelings. Also, they are difficult to fake during interpersonal communication.

There are numerous barriers in nonverbal communication, including:

- Lack of eye contact
- Facial expressions (e.g., wandering eyes)
- Body position in relation to the patient (e.g., closed or open stance, folded arms, or slouching)
- Tone of voice (e.g., being sarcastic or using a threatening tone)

Although these may be interpreted as barriers in our culture, they may not be a barrier in another culture. Therefore, an understanding of cultural behaviors can be helpful to pharmacy technicians if they have a diverse patient base.

All communication between health professionals and patients has two principal purposes:

- To establish an ongoing rapport between the provider and patient
- To provide the exchange of information necessary to assess a patient's health condition, apply the treatment of a medical problem, and evaluate the effects on a patient's quality of life

Interacting with the Pharmacist

The pharmacist is responsible for communicating with the technician in a clear and concise manner. Using the proper terminology ensures that the pharmacist and pharmacy technician share common definitions associated with the circumstance. Individuals assign meanings to their words based upon their background, values, and experiences. In this situation, the pharmacy technician is responsible for listening intently to the pharmacist. The pharmacist should check with the technician to ensure that he or she understood the communication. It is the pharmacy technician's responsibility to request any clarification of the message. Neither the pharmacist nor the pharmacy technician should ever make assumptions because false assumptions may adversely affect the patient's outcome. Sometimes there is a disconnection between the pharmacist and the pharmacy technician because although the words mean one thing, the nonverbal communication demonstrates something else. Feedback is essential in communications between the pharmacist and the technician. Conversely, when the pharmacy technician is initiating the communication, the pharmacist is responsible for listening and providing feedback to the technician.

Pharmacists play an integral role in making certain their patients obtain the desired outcomes with their medication therapy. The role of the pharmacist has evolved from medication-centered to patient-centered care. To establish a patient-centered care environment, it is essential that the pharmacist develop a trusting relationship with the patient. This allows the pharmacist and patient to be actively involved in the treatment and leads to the desired outcome.

The Institute of Medicine (IOM) defines patient-centered care as "providing care that is respectful of and responsive to individual patient preferences, needs, and values, and ensuring that patient values guide all clinical decisions." To provide patient-centered care, the pharmacist must be able to:

- Understand the patient's illness experience
- Identify the patient's experience as unique
- Foster an unrestricted relationship with the patient
- Build a **therapeutic alliance** with patients to meet mutually understood goals of therapy
- Develop a self-awareness of personal effects on patients

The efforts of the pharmacy technician aid pharmacists in performing their clinical pharmacy activities.

Interacting with the Patient

Often pharmacy communication is delayed due to specific challenges from distinctive obstacles posed by unique groups of patients. Many communication barriers exist within each of these groups of individuals. As a pharmacy technician, it is vital that, if you sense an individual has a specific problem, you check your perception of that individual. If you are dealing with elderly patients, what is your initial perception of them? Are they forgetful? Do you consider them to have visual or auditory issues? Based on your perceptions, you make assumptions about this group of patients.

Elderly Patients

The elderly population is increasing and living longer as a result of advances in the treatment of diseases and disorders with medication and behavioral modification. The elderly experience more chronic conditions than do younger individuals and therefore take a greater number of medications. As individuals age, they may experience a loss in their communication skills (Figure 8-9).

Also, as individuals age, they tend to process information at a slower rate than younger individuals. The rate of speech and the amount of information an elderly patient receives at one time must meet the individual's ability to understand this information. Also, the elderly person's short-term memory, recall, and attention span may be reduced. Elderly patients may perceive things differently from individuals in other age groups and may have specific expectations.

Elderly patients may experience physical changes in their bodies that affect their communication skills. The elderly patient who has experienced a decrease in vision may have difficulty reading the font size of written materials. Therefore, it may be necessary to explain to the individual how to take or store the medications.

An elderly patient may develop hearing impairments. Hearing impairments may occur when something blocks the conduction of sound into the ear's sensory nerve centers, when damage occurs in the sensory center of the inner ear, or when the nerve centers of the brain are affected. A loss of hearing may be due to birth defects, injuries, or chronic exposure to loud noises. The amount of hearing loss varies

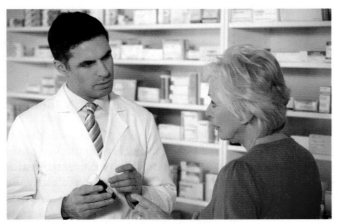

FIGURE 8-9 A technician should be aware of communication issues that may affect elderly patients. (Copyright © 2014 monkeybusinessimages, iStock, Thinkstock.com. All rights reserved.)

among individuals. Some individuals may actually hear words and sounds yet not be able to comprehend the meaning of the words.

Some patients with hearing difficulties depend on speech reading; they watch a person's lips, facial expressions, and gestures to improve their communication skills. As a pharmacy technician, you should position yourself 3 to 6 feet from the hearing-impaired individual. You should never speak directly into the patient's ear because the sound may become distorted. If the patient is experiencing difficulty understanding what you are telling him or her, you should not repeat the sentence, but rather rephrase it in shorter and simpler sentences.

As a pharmacy technician, you may encounter patients with speech impairment. Speech impairments may be caused by a variety of factors, including birth defects, injuries, or other illnesses. **Dysarthria** is a speech impairment involving interference with the normal control of the speech mechanism because of damage to specific facial muscles. Dysarthria can be caused by Parkinson's disease, multiple sclerosis, strokes, and accidents. Often patients with a speech impairment may communicate through the use of notes or sign language. A pharmacy technician should always have a pad of paper at the prescription intake or pick-up station for patients who want to communicate by writing.

Another speech issue that may occur after a patient has experienced a stroke or other adverse event is known as aphasia. **Aphasia** is a complex condition in which an individual has a reduced ability to understand what others are saying and express himself or herself. Depending on the severity of the problem, an individual may have no speech or may have difficulty with names or words. Other individuals may experience difficulty putting words in the proper sequence in a sentence. These patients may encounter problems in understanding oral directions, reading, writing, and the use of numbers. Patients with aphasia may have normal hearing; therefore, speaking loudly to them will not improve the situation. When dealing with a patient who has aphasia, it is best to speak with the patient's caregiver.

Patients with Mental Health Problems

According to a finding in 2012 by the National Institute of Mental Health (NIMH), 43.7 million (18.6%) adults suffered from some form of mental illness. Unfortunately, many pharmacists and pharmacy technicians experience difficulty communicating with patients suffering from mental disease because they do not know what to say to them. There are many stereotypes about patients with mental health problems that some members of the pharmacy team may believe.

Some patients with mental health disorders may be hesitant to speak with members of the pharmacy staff for a variety of reasons. These reasons may include a poor self-image and hesitancy to interact with other people. These patients may believe that they have a condition that may make some individuals feel uncomfortable. Some patients may not feel comfortable interacting with health care professionals.

The pharmacy staff may also have difficulty relating to these individuals. They may feel uncertain about how much information they should provide to the patient. Also, the pharmacy staff may not know what the prescriber has told the patient about his or her condition.

When speaking with patients with mental health issues, it is best to use open-ended questions. Patients suffering from mental illness should not be treated any differently from any other patient who has a condition such as hypertension, chronic obstructive pulmonary disease, diabetes, or thyroid disease. Every patient should be treated with the same dignity and respect.

Terminally Ill Patients

Many individuals find it difficult to interact with terminally ill patients. They may feel uncomfortable discussing the topic of death and experience difficulty finding the correct words to use. Most terminally ill patients need a supportive relationship with family, friends, and health care providers, including both pharmacists and pharmacy technicians. Often the pharmacy team may be the only health care providers in the community that a patient may encounter frequently.

In 1969, Elisabeth Kübler-Ross wrote *On Death and Dying*, which identified five stages of grief: denial, anger, bargaining, depression, and acceptance. By understanding these five stages, a health care professional is better able to understand what a patient is experiencing. In addition to the patient, the person's family also may be experiencing the five stages of grief. Terminally ill patients may be hesitant to discuss various issues, but they may become more receptive as time passes.

Communicating with terminally ill patients and their families is extremely important. You should never avoid talking to them unless you sense they do not want to discuss the illness. Furthermore, not talking to them isolates the individual and may endorse the idea that talking about death is uncomfortable.

Patients with Health Literacy Issues

According to the American Medical Association (AMA), health literacy is defined as the ability to read, understand, and act on health care information. According to the National Patient Safety Foundation (NPSF):

- Ninety million people in the United States may be at risk because of the difficulty some patients experience in understanding and acting upon health information.
- Literacy skills are a stronger predictor of an individual's health status than age, income, employment status, education level, or racial/ethnic group.
- One out of five American adults reads at the fifth grade level or below, and the average American reads at the eighth to ninth grade level; yet most health care materials are written above the tenth grade level.
- Limited health literacy increases the disparity in health care access among exceptionally vulnerable populations (e.g., racial and ethnic minorities and the elderly).
- According to the Center for Health Care Strategies, a disproportionate number of minorities and immigrants are estimated to have literacy problems:
  - 50% of Hispanics
  - 40% of African Americans
  - 33% of Asians
- More than 66% of U.S. adults age 60 or older have either inadequate or marginal literacy skills.
- Annual health care costs for individuals with low literacy skills are four times higher than for those with higher literacy skills.
- Problems with patient compliance and medical errors may be based on poor understanding of health care information. Only about 50% of all patients take medications as directed.
- Patients with low literacy skills were observed to have a 50% increased risk of hospitalization compared with patients who had adequate literacy skills.

Patients with low health literacy are often uncomfortable and fail to inform their pharmacist or pharmacy technician of this situation. Without this knowledge, the pharmacy team is unable to properly assess a patient's understanding of the information they provide. To help these patients, the USP has developed pictographs that illustrate common medication instructions and precautions. (See Figure 14-1 and Chapter 14 for more information on pictographs).

Caregivers

Communication issues develop when information is provided to the caregivers of patients with chronic conditions, parents who take care of children with acute illnesses, family members, or friends. A caregiver must understand a patient's condition and treatment and how to effectively communicate the special instructions to the patient. It is extremely important for the caregiver to understand the importance of refilling the patient's medication. Often it is best to give the caregiver written information so that it can be given to the patient at home.

Patients visit the pharmacy because they need to obtain a medication to treat a current condition or to prevent a condition from occurring. As a pharmacy technician, it is extremely important that you demonstrate empathy toward the patient. By demonstrating to the patient that you understand his or her feelings, you will be able to develop a caring, trusting relationship with the patient. Demonstrating empathy allows patients to understand their own feelings about their conditions and makes it easier for them to solve their own problems. Empathy enables patients to place their trust in the pharmacy team because they have confidence the team will work in their best interest.

A survey conducted in 1997 by the National Harris Survey revealed that many patients do not seek medical attention because of the sensitivity of their condition. A pharmacy technician should be aware that a patient may have difficulty discussing topics such as breast or prostate cancer, contraception, depression, hemorrhoids, incontinence, menopause, and sexual dysfunction. Discreetly approach these sensitive issues, taking the patient's feelings into account to avoid making the person uncomfortable. It is also important to be aware that patients may not adhere to their drug regimens if the situation or the side effects of the medication are difficult for them to discuss.

The pharmacy technician should apply the following techniques when addressing any patient:

- Develop a sense of trustworthiness with the patient by demonstrating friendliness, a sense of ethics, sociability, and fairness
- Avoid using words with more than one meaning
- Avoid using professional jargon
- Use simple ideas and words when obtaining information from the patient
- Recognize that there are differences in cross-cultural styles of speaking

Customer Service

Customer service is defined as the provision of service to customers before, during, and after a purchase. Customer service in health care is different from that in other industries because the customers are recipients of medical services that are critical to their health. The pharmacy provides OTC, BTC, and prescription medications to its customers and patients. In addition, the pharmacist provides information to patients to maximize the therapeutic effects of the medications they are prescribed.

The "five rights" of medication administration used by nurses also apply to pharmacy practice. They are:

- *Right patient:* The patient's identity must be verified against the prescription order to ensure that the correct patient is receiving the medication.
- *Right medication:* It must be verified that the medication written on the prescription order is the same as the medication being prepared for the patient.
- *Right time:* The pharmacist must ensure that the medication is to be taken by the patient at the correct time it was ordered by the physician.
- *Right dose:* The medication dose being prepared must be confirmed against the written medication order before it is dispensed.
- *Right route of administration:* The pharmacist must verify the correct route for delivering the ordered medication to the patient by reading the order and preparing the medication appropriately.

In 2011, J.D. Powers and Associates conducted a National Pharmacy Study of all patients who filled a prescription at a pharmacy over a 2-month period. The study ranked the customer satisfaction of more than 12,300 customers, using a 1000 point scale for their ranking. Customers were asked about their experiences and perceptions as a pharmacy patient, including their satisfaction with the store environment, prescription drop-off and pick-up process, costs, and interactions with pharmacists and other staff. Rick Millard, J.D. Power senior director of the health care practice, said, "Customers are expecting more from their brick-and-mortar pharmacy; not just in terms of wait time, but also in terms of contact with the pharmacist and pharmacy staff."

As a pharmacy technician, you will encounter many unique individuals. Some of these individuals may not fully understand the prescription filling process, the legal requirements of filling a prescription, or their prescription coverage. Table 8-6 presents some complaints that you might hear from your customers.

Given the shrinking margin in prescription profits due to managed care agreements, it is easy to see the importance of customer service in retail pharmacy. Developing excellent customer service skills is important in any job and even more important as a pharmacy technician. Customers that come to your pharmacy will remember if you were rude, uninformative, helpful, or courteous. Your attitude can have a direct effect on whether a pharmacy customer comes back, and it can also alter your image as a technician. Here are some helpful tips you can use on the job.

TABLE 8-6

Common Pharmacy Customer Service Complaints

The wait time to fill a prescription is too long.

I called in my prescription refill 2 days ago; why isn't it ready?

My doctor said they would call the prescription in right away!

My doctor told me that I would be on this medication the rest of my life; what do you mean that there are no refills left on the prescription?

What do you mean my prescription card will not pay for this medication?

What do you mean my prescription coverage will not pay for my medication? I am going on a trip and need to have my prescription refilled before I leave.

What do you mean that if I want the brand name drug, I will have to pay more for it?

Why didn't someone call me to tell me that my doctor wants to see me?

The prescription was for 90 days, and you gave me only a 30-day supply; what do you mean my prescription card will pay only for a 30-day supply?

Why did my doctor prescribe this medication if it is on back order?

- *Appearance.* Individuals who shop and pick up their prescriptions at your pharmacy appreciate a well-groomed pharmacy technician. The way you look has an impact on how others see you.
- *Attitude.* Courtesy and knowledge are important. Be sure to keep up with the pharmacy field and know your subject.
- *Efficiency.* It is imperative to complete your work efficiently and correctly the first time. Mistakes in pharmacy can cause serious illness or even death.
- *Helping out.* Going the extra mile and assisting other co-workers when they are overwhelmed will make you a star worker. Co-workers will also return the favor when you need it.

Box 8-2 shows key customer service statistics that you should keep in mind when serving pharmacy customers.

Scenario CHECK UP 8-7

Andrew is responsible for the prescription drop-off window when a Hispanic customer enters the pharmacy to drop off his prescription. Andrew scans the prescription and notices that there is no address on it. Andrew attempts to ask the patient his address and quickly realizes the patient doesn't speak English. Andrew checks the pharmacy's computer system to see whether the patient has ever filled a prescription at Andrew's pharmacy before and finds that the patient has not. How should Andrew handle the situation?

BOX 8-2

Customer Service Statistics

- The main reason for customer turnover is poor customer service, not price
- 1 negative experience requires 12 positive experiences to change customer opinion
- 96% of dissatisfied customers don't complain
- 91% of dissatisfied customers leave and do not come back
- 70% of customer opinion is based on how customers feel they were treated
- 1 unhappy customer tells between 9 and 15 people about a bad experience
- 13% of unhappy customers will tell more than 20 people
- 1 happy customer will only tell between 4 and 6 people about the good experience
- 55% of customers would pay more if it meant improved service

Data from Digby J: 50 Facts about customer experience. *Return on Behavior Magazine,* October 25, 2010. (Referenced September 23, 2014). http://returnonbehavior.com/2010/10/50-facts-about-customer-experience-for-2011/

Other Pharmacy Services
Immunizations

Many community pharmacies provide immunizations to their patients. These include immunizations for influenza, pneumococcal infection, hepatitis A and B, herpes zoster, and varicella. Currently only pharmacists are permitted to administer immunizations to patients. However, pharmacy technicians can help facilitate immunization programs and reduce some of the barriers to providing superior service. Specific tasks that can be performed by pharmacy technicians include documentation, billing, assisting in the reporting of adverse events, and facilitating communication. Technicians can also take an active role in pharmacy-based immunization programs by obtaining cardiopulmonary resuscitation training and certification. The pharmacy technician is permitted to draw the correct amount of the vaccine into a syringe for the pharmacist.

Medication Therapy Management

Medication therapy management (MTM) is medical care provided by pharmacists whose aim is to optimize drug therapy and improve therapeutic outcomes for patients. Medication therapy management covers a broad range of professional activities, including but not limited to performing a patient assessment and/or a comprehensive medication review, formulating a medication treatment plan, monitoring the efficacy and safety of medication therapy, enhancing medication adherence through patient empowerment and education, and documenting and communicating MTM services to prescribers to maintain comprehensive patient care.

As the pharmacy profession embraces extensive patient counseling in the form of MTM, many aspects of the practice of pharmacy must evolve to ensure the success of the MTM program. Time constraints limit the ability of pharmacists to handle administrative tasks and represent a major barrier to the implementation of MTM programs. Technicians can do some of the work to reduce this barrier. With proper training, technicians can assist pharmacists in the tasks that do not require the professional judgment of a pharmacist, freeing pharmacists to focus on clinical activities and making an MTM program more sustainable. For example, technicians can help in areas such as scheduling and patient reminders through phone calls. Medication histories and health histories can also be documented by technicians, as can chart construction, filing, and the documentation of release forms and health histories. Additional steps can be taken to further increase efficiency in the MTM process, including the creation of a flow map and cross-training of all pharmacy staff.

▶ TECHNICIAN PROFILE

Roberto has been certified as a pharmacy technician by the Pharmacy Technician Certification Board (PTCB) since 1997. He is the lead pharmacy technician at an independent pharmacy in Falls Church, Virginia. Roberto is fluent in Spanish, which is helpful when he is dealing with the pharmacy's Hispanic customers. Recently, the pharmacist has begun providing medication therapy management services to his patients. Roberto understands that he may not counsel patients, but he is able to assist the pharmacist in performing medication therapy management for their patients.

Home Health Care Services

Home health care is defined as health care services and health-related products provided to the patient at home. Pharmacies are able to provide pharmaceutical services and durable medical equipment to patients in their homes. Many community pharmacies provide home health care–related products for their patients for a variety of reasons:

- The number of elderly patients has increased, resulting in a growing need for these products and services.
- Patients prefer to be treated and to convalesce in their homes.

- Services at home are less expensive than staying in a hospital or assisted living facility.
- The patient is able to maintain his or her independence.
- Technology has evolved such that traditional treatments now can be performed in the patient's home.
- Managed care supports the discharge of patients from a hospital to the home.

Most community pharmacies have provided crutches, canes, and walkers for their patients. Within the past several decades, some pharmacies have expanded their inventory of home health care products. These products include:

- Durable medical equipment (e.g., wheelchairs, hospital beds, and commodes)
- Oxygen therapy (e.g., oxygen tanks)
- Wound care and decubitus ulcer (bed sore) products
- Ostomy and incontinence products
- Prosthetic devices
- Orthopedic supplies (e.g., braces)
- Antiembolism stockings (e.g., TED)
- First aid supplies
- Medical instruments (e.g., stethoscopes and blood pressure kits)
- Home diagnostic products (e.g., glucometers and diabetic supplies)
- Prescription medications not for self-administration (e.g., respiratory drugs)
- Nutritional therapy (e.g., Ensure, Sustacal)

Pharmacy technicians who work in community pharmacies that provide home health care products are able to provide excellent customer service if they have received the proper training in the use of these products.

Long-Term Care Services

Some community pharmacies have contracts with long-term care facilities to provide medications for their residents. Long-term care facilities include sub–acute care facilities, correctional facilities, assisted living facilities, and board and care homes. As in a traditional community pharmacy, technicians assist the pharmacist in providing long-term care services. Pharmacy technicians perform many of the dispensing tasks that were previously done by pharmacists. Some of the responsibilities assigned to pharmacy technicians include:

- Entering computer data on prescription drug and nondrug orders
- Repackaging and labeling medications
- Packaging and labeling prescriptions
- Ordering, receiving, and stocking medications and supplies

- Processing returned medications for reuse
- Maintaining repackaging equipment
- Maintaining a drug library
- Maintaining computerized information to include patient profiles and drug information requests
- Billing prescription, over-the-counter, and non-drug services
- Providing the necessary forms to the long-term care facility

- Transporting medications to the facility
- Maintaining delivery records
- Performing general pharmacy housekeeping

As the population continues to age, the need for pharmacy services for long-term care facilities will continue to expand, creating additional employment opportunities for pharmacy technicians in community and retail pharmacy.

DO YOU REMEMBER THESE KEY POINTS?

- The different types of community pharmacies
- The pharmacy technician's role in the medication use process
- State laws and regulations related to receiving and screening prescription orders
- Assessing prescription orders for completeness and authenticity when receiving orders via paper or electronic systems
- Efficiently obtaining information to complete a prescription order
- Special procedures pharmacy technicians are responsible for in preparing, storing, and distributing controlled substances
- The pharmacy technician's role in preparing medications for distribution
- The process of creating a new patient profile or entering data into an existing patient profile
- Accurately counting or measuring finished dosage forms as specified by the prescription/medication order
- The protocol to assemble appropriate patient information materials

- Collecting needed information from the patient profile
- Identifying situations in which the patient requires the attention of the pharmacist
- Applying effective verbal and written communication skills, including listening skills
- Effective strategies for communicating with patients who are non-English speakers or who have other special needs, such as vision or hearing problems, a low reading level, or difficulty understanding instructions.
- Using a respectful attitude with diverse patient groups
- Recognizing effective interpersonal and teamwork skills in working with health care teams
- The pharmacy technician's role in assisting in the administration of immunizations in a community pharmacy
- The purpose of monitoring a patient's medication therapy

REVIEW QUESTIONS

Multiple Choice Questions

1. Which term refers to the name of the prescription?
   A. Inscription
   B. Subscription
   C. Superscription
   D. Signa
2. What Dispense as Written (DAW) code is assigned to a prescription for "No product selection indicated"?
   A. DAW 0
   B. DAW 1
   C. DAW 2
   D. DAW 3

3. Which of the following may be identified during a prospective drug review?
   A. Drug-disease contraindication
   B. Drug duplication
   C. Therapeutic duplication
   D. All of the above
4. Which of the following is *not* one of the patient's rights?
   A. Right patient
   B. Right drug
   C. Right price
   D. Right dosage form

5. Which of the following may a pharmacy technician *not* do regarding immunizations?
   A. Administer the immunization
   B. Bill the patient for the immunization
   C. Collect patient information
   D. Draw the correct amount of vaccine into the syringe

6. What does this signa mean: 1 tsp PO qid ac & hs?
   A. Take 1 teaspoonful by mouth four times a day after meals and at bedtime.
   B. Take 1 teaspoonful by mouth four times a day before meals and at bedtime.
   C. Take 1 tablespoonful by mouth four times a day before meals and at bedtime.
   D. Take 1 tablespoonful by mouth three times a day before meals and at bedtime.

7. Which of the following may a pharmacy technician *not* do in a retail pharmacy?
   A. Accept a new prescription over the telephone from the physician's office
   B. Accept a new prescription from the patient at the intake window
   C. Order medications from a wholesaler
   D. Check medications received from a wholesaler

8. Which of the following should a pharmacy technician *not* demonstrate to a pharmacy patient?
   A. Empathy
   B. Sarcasm
   C. Sensitivity
   D. Understanding

9. Which information may a pharmacist provide to a patient during counseling?
   A. Proper storage
   B. Prescription refill information
   C. Action to be taken in the event of a missed dose
   D. All of the above

10. What is adjudication?
    A. The process by which a prescription is submitted electronically to a third-party payer so that the pharmacy can be reimbursed for the medication dispensed
    B. A number assigned to a medication that indicates the drug manufacturer, drug entity, and drug packaging
    C. A number required to dispense a controlled substance
    D. A number assigned to a health care provider that allows them to be reimbursed by Medicaid or Medicare

TECHNICIAN'S CORNER

One day while you are inputting prescriptions into the pharmacy's computer system, you receive a prescription for ciprofloxacin 500 mg for a Marty Smith who lives at 11608 Happiness Lane in Washington, DC. The pharmacy technician who accepted this prescription failed to obtain the patient's birth date or telephone number. When you search the patient database, you find that you have three Marty Smiths who live at 11608 Happiness Lane in Washington, DC. One of them is 13 years of age, one of them is 45 years old, and the other one is 72 years old.
   How would you handle this situation?
   Is this medication appropriate for all three patients?
   Which of the three patients should not receive ciprofloxacin and why?
   What type of additional training should be provided to the pharmacy technician who accepted the prescription?

Bibliography

Baker DW, Parker RM, Williams MV, Clark WS: Health literacy and the risk of hospital admission, *J Gen Intern Med* 13:791, 1998.

Center for Health Care Strategies: Health literacy and understanding medical information fact sheet. 2013. www.chcs.org/media/CHCS_Health_Literacy_Fact_Sheet.2013.pdf. Accessed 12/10/2013.

Davis K: *Sterile processing for pharmacy technicians*, St Louis, 2014, Elsevier.

Doak CC, Doak LG, Root JH: The literacy problem. In Doak CC, Doak LG, Root JH: *Teaching patients with low literacy skills*, ed 2, Philadelphia, 1996, JB Lippincott.

Harris L: Physician-patient barriers to communication. National Harris Survey. 1997. www.ncbi.nim.nih.gov/PMC/articles/PMC3098184. Accessed 7/7/2014.

Institute of Medicine: Crossing the quality chasm: a new health system for the 21st century, 2001. www.iom.edu/Reports/2001. Accessed 12/02/2013.

Kirsch I, Jungeblut LJ, Kolstad A: A first look at the results of the national adult literacy survey. National Center for Education Statistics, 1993. www.iom.edu/~/media/Files. Accessed March 17, 2014.

Maizes V, Rakel D, Niemiec C: Integrative medicine and patient-centered care. Commissioned for the IOM Summit on Integrative Medicine and the Health of the Public. February 2009. www.nacds.org/pdfs/comm/sfc-statement-on-fy2014-budget-april2013.pdf.

National Association of Chain Drug Stores: Statement of the National Association of Chain Drug Stores for U.S. Senate Committee on Finance. Hearing on the President's Budget for Fiscal Year 2014. April 17, 2013. (Referenced April 17, 2014.) www.nacds.org/pdfs/comm/sfc-statement-on-fy2014-budget-april2013.pdf.

Okeke CC, Bailey L, Medwick T: Revised USP standards for product dating, packaging, and temperature monitoring, *Am J Health Syst Pharm* 57(15), 2000.

Pharmacy management software for pharmacy technicians. DAA Enterprises, 2012. St. Louis, MO.

Pyothos F: *New perspectives in nonverbal communication,* New York, 1983, Pergamon Press.

University of the Sciences in Philadelphia: *Remington: the science and practice of pharmacy,* ed 21, Philadelphia, 2005, Lippincott, Williams & Wilkins.

Weiss BD, editor: *20 common problems in primary care,* New York, 1999, McGraw Hill.

Weiss BD: *Health literacy: a manual for clinicians.* American Medical Association/American Medical Association Foundation, 2003. p. 7, Chicago, IL.

Websites Referenced

An Overview of Aphasia. www.webmd.com/brain/aphasia-causes-symptoms-types-treatments. Accessed July 7, 2014.

Dysarthia. www.nlm.nih.gov/medlineplus/ency/article/007470.htm. Accessed July 7, 2014.

Stats At-a-Glance. www.npsf.org/wp-content/uploads/2011/12/AskMe3. Accessed July 7, 2014.

Statistics. www.nimh.nih.gov/statistics. Accessed July 7, 2014.

Institutional Pharmacy Practice

Bobbi Steelman

OBJECTIVES

Upon completing this chapter, you should be able to do the following:

1. Define the most common tasks performed by hospital pharmacy technicians.
2. Identify different types of hospital pharmacy settings.
3. Discuss different hospital pharmacy standards and procedures.
4. Identify the difference between formulary and non-formulary medication lists.
5. Explain the importance of a good relationship between the pharmacy and the nursing staff.
6. Identify different regulatory agencies that govern the operations of hospitals, including pharmacies in the hospital.
7. List various ways orders are processed by the pharmacy.
8. Identify the difference between stat, ASAP, and standing orders.
9. Describe how POE, CPOE, BPOE, and CADM systems are used in medication ordering.
10. Identify the responsibilities of an institutional pharmacy technician.
11. Describe the technician's role in the IND process.
12. Describe the advantages of using automated dispensing systems (ADS).

13. Explain the importance of counting, dispensing, and tracking controlled substances.
14. Explain what PAR levels are and who is responsible for maintaining them.
15. Identify the difference between hazardous and non-hazardous IV preparation.
16. Explain the importance of aseptic technique for the technician preparing compounded sterile preparations (CSPs).
17. Identify the duties involved in ordering and maintaining the stock levels of the pharmacy.
18. Recognize the differences in floor stock, depending on the area of the hospital.
19. Identify specialty areas of the hospital for which the pharmacy stocks or orders medication.
20. Describe the importance of ongoing technician education and identify professional organizations that institutional technicians can join.

TERMS AND DEFINITIONS

American Society of Health-System Pharmacists (ASHP) An association of pharmacists, pharmacy students, and technicians who practice in hospitals and health care systems, including home health care; ASHP has a long history as an advocate for patient safety and of establishing best practices to improve medication use

ASAP order As soon as possible but not an emergency

Aseptic technique Procedures used in the sterile compounding of hazardous and non-hazardous materials to minimize the introduction of microbes or unwanted debris that could contaminate the preparation

Automated dispensing system(s) (ADS) Computerized cabinets that control inventory on nursing floors, in emergency departments, and in surgical suites and other patient care areas

Computerized physician order entry (CPOE) Computerized order entry

Crash carts Moveable carts containing trays of medications, administration sets, oxygen, and other materials used in life-threatening situations, such as cardiac arrest; also known as *code carts*

Electronic medication administration record (E-MAR) A computer program that automatically documents the administration of medication into certified electronic health record (EHR) systems; the report serves as a legal record of medications administered to a patient at a facility by a health care professional

Floor stock Drugs not labeled for a specific patient and maintained at a nursing station or other department of the institution (excluding the pharmacy) for the purpose of administration to a patient of the facility

Formulary A list of drugs approved for use in hospitals by the pharmacy and therapeutics committee of the institution that have become the standard stock carried by the pharmacy and other departments

Institutional pharmacy A pharmacy in facilities where patients receive care on site (e.g., hospitals, extended-living homes, long-term care, and hospice facilities); institutional pharmacies are also found in government-supported hospitals run by the Department of Veteran Affairs, Indian Health Service, and the Bureau of Prisons

Investigational drug A drug that has not been approved by the U.S. Food and Drug Administration (FDA) for marketing but is in clinical trials; also, an FDA-approved drug seeking a new indication for use

Medication order A prescription written for administration in a hospital or institutional setting

NKA No known allergies

NKDA No known drug allergy

Non-formulary medications Drugs that are not approved for use within an institution unless specific exceptions are filed and accepted by institutional protocols

Parenteral medication Medication that bypasses the digestive system but is intended for systemic action; the term parenteral most commonly describes medications given by injection, such as intravenously or intramuscularly

Periodic automatic replenishment (PAR) A set level of certain medications kept on hospital floors

prn From the Latin term *pro re nata*, meaning "as needed"

Protocol A set of standards and guidelines by which a facility operates

Pyxis An automated dispensing system often used in hospitals

Satellite pharmacy A specialty pharmacy located away from the central pharmacy, such as an operating room (OR), emergency department (ED), or a neonatal pharmacy; satellite pharmacies typically are staffed by a pharmacist and a pharmacy technician

Standing order Written protocols for drugs or treatment that is to be used in a specific situation

Stat order A medication order that must be filled immediately, as quickly as is safely possible to prepare the dose, usually within 5 to 15 minutes

SureMed An automated dispensing system often used in hospitals

The Joint Commission (TJC) An independent, nonprofit organization that accredits hospitals and other health care facilities in the United States; the facility must be accredited to receive Medicare and Medicaid payment

Unit dose (UD) Individualized packaged doses used in institutional practice settings

United States Pharmacopeia <797> (USP <797>) Guidelines enforceable for the safe preparation of sterile products

Introduction

Scenario:

Marcus is employed as a certified pharmacy tech II in a 500-bed hospital. Some of his duties include picking and preparing medications, restocking supplies, delivering supplies and medications to various floors, and refilling the Pyxis machines. During the morning staff meeting the pharmacy manager explains that the Joint Commission (TJC) will be visiting the pharmacy next week. What is TJC, and what will the visit entail?

Probably one of the most challenging settings in which a pharmacy technician can work is a hospital pharmacy, also known as the **institutional pharmacy**. The dynamics of this environment can be exhilarating and exhausting, depending on the circumstances. Because there are fewer hospital pharmacies than community pharmacies, there are fewer job openings for pharmacy technicians in hospitals. However, as a result of the current changes in the pharmacist's role in hospitals, the number of highly skilled technicians needed has increased. Pharmacists once prepared all intravenous antibiotics, chemotherapy drugs, and large volume parenteral medications, in addition to other inpatient tasks. Because of the increase in patient volume and the need for pharmacy interventions and evaluations as they pertain to patient profiles, today's pharmacists do not have time to perform many of the important tasks they did in the past. Technicians have

assumed control of these tasks, which include preparing intravenous medications, loading patient medication drawers or **Pyxis** machines, and entering patient data into the pharmacy computer systems. This chapter outlines the daily tasks of a pharmacy technician, lists the various areas or departments of a hospital that require medication supply from the pharmacy, and describes **the Joint Commission (TJC)** standards relevant to pharmacy and medication use. As the health care industry changes and improves, so will the vital roles required of pharmacy technicians as they strive to provide improved health care services.

Types of Hospitals

Depending on the function of the hospital (facility), patient populations vary. The size of a hospital may be thought of in terms of the number of beds available for patient use. Many small cities or towns may have small facilities, with a capacity of 50 beds or fewer. Larger urban areas have facilities that can range from 50 beds to more than 250 beds. There are nonprofit and for-profit hospitals. A nonprofit hospital is a facility that does not pay either state or local property taxes or federal income taxes because it is considered a charity. Nonprofit organizations must meet certain criteria established by state and federal guidelines. A for-profit, or investor-owned, hospital is a facility owned by private investors or owned publicly by shareholders. For-profit hospitals issue shares of stock to raise funds to expand the hospital activities.

Other factors that differentiate hospitals from one another are their capabilities for diagnosis, surgery, and outpatient services. For instance, many hospitals do not have the funds to house computed tomography (CT) scanners. CT scanners use a computer that takes data from several radiographic images of structures inside the body. The multiple views create a cross-sectional image of the bones and soft tissue on the computer screen. If a facility does not have a CT scanner, patients who need such scans must be sent to another hospital to have procedures or diagnostic examinations performed.

Another important difference between hospitals is the organization of their pharmacies. Many older hospitals may have one central inpatient pharmacy that is responsible for supplying the entire hospital

and all clinics. Larger hospitals and those with specialized areas may have a central pharmacy and, in addition, smaller **satellite pharmacies** at various points throughout the facility. For instance, a large teaching facility may have specialized areas of treatment, such as pediatrics, burn units, intensive care units, and cancer units. Because of the large volume and specialty of the medications needed for these areas, these units may have small pharmacies that stock specific medications. This practice can accelerate the distribution of commonly used medications and allow the pharmacist to work directly with physicians, nurses, and patients on an individualized basis to address specific medical problems.

Hospitals are funded by various entities. Health insurance companies and Medicare pay for services in many institutions; others are funded by donation. An example of donation-funded institutions are Shriners Hospitals for Children, which treat children who cannot afford treatment in mainstream hospitals. Other institutions are managed completely by the government (e.g., Veterans Affairs hospitals). Table 9-1 lists hospital facilities and types of pharmacy arrangements.

Hospital Pharmacy Settings

As mentioned, in addition to the typical inpatient pharmacy, hospitals may have additional types of pharmacies that are more specialized. For instance,

TABLE 9-1

Examples of Various Sizes and Types of Hospitals

Type	Bed Capacity	Usually One Pharmacy	Central Pharmacy and Satellites	Pharmacies Independent from One Another	Type of Care Given
Small	25-50	X			Limited, minor surgeries; critical care is temporary
Medium	50-100	X			Most surgeries, a coronary care unit, and an intensive care unit
Large	100	X	X	X	Treats most conditions; physical therapy, intensive care unit, coronary care unit; may have specialty areas, such as burn or pediatric unit
Teaching	100	X	X	X	Covers all conditions and has specialty areas for teaching purposes; trains medical physicians and other health care providers
Institutional	10-100	X		X	Care ranges from treating severe emergencies to continuing treatment but also may include triage to a larger facility that specializes in a particular area; found in institutions such as prisons and mental facilities
Convalescent or long-term care	100	X			Depending on type of convalescent home, level of care may vary; some patients are sent to a hospital for surgery and recovery and then are sent back to their main resident home

more hospitals are incorporating satellite pharmacies to expedite order preparation and delivery. Specialty medications can be stocked in these pharmacies, as is the case for units such as oncology, pediatrics, and intensive care. Certain hospitals interconnect inpatient and discharge pharmacies; this is an area where a technician may work with both inpatients and outpatients concurrently.

Satellite Pharmacies

Satellites are small specialty pharmacies that supply a clinic, such as the emergency department, or an entire floor of a hospital. Larger hospitals, such as teaching institutions, use satellite pharmacies because obtaining the medication from one centralized pharmacy can be too time-consuming. The number of satellites varies, depending on the size of the facility, but most are small and minimally staffed. The satellites fill most of the daily medications for patients on their floors. They may be equipped with an intravenous (IV) hood for parenteral product preparation if necessary, and they also are used to replace any missing medications in the automated systems or in the patient's cassette drawers. Most of the **floor stock** used by the satellites is supplied by the large central pharmacy of the hospital. The pharmacist's role is to monitor regulatory compliance and oversee all medications dispensed from the particular satellite to ensure optimum patient care. A pharmacist working in a satellite facility must have a thorough knowledge of all medications used in that specialty setting. Technicians who work in the satellites are responsible for filling all medication orders and delivering them to the nurses' stations. Other duties include answering phones, keeping satellites stocked, filling stat orders, preparing IV medications, replacing missing doses, and replenishing pharmacy stock.

Discharge Pharmacies

Many hospitals have a discharge and/or outpatient pharmacy that fills prescriptions in the same manner as a community pharmacy except that it is located in the institution. Physicians' orders are written on special discharge order forms that are sent to the pharmacy with other orders via the fax machine or pneumatic tube, or are delivered by staff. Other hospitals have designated pharmacies where patients can pick up their discharge medications. The discharge orders may be sent via the hospital computer to the outpatient pharmacy for filling. Once a discharge order has been sent, the pharmacy fills the order by the same process used in any community pharmacy. This includes determining the patient's address, phone number, and insurance coverage.

Pharmacy technicians normally process the prescription just as they would an outpatient pharmacy prescription. After the patient information has been entered into the computer system, the order is filled. All auxiliary labels are attached, if required, and the medications must have a final check by the pharmacist. Once these orders are complete, the medication can be sent back to the floor for the nurse to give to the patient; alternatively, if the drug is a controlled substance or a new medication for the patient, the nurse can transport the patient directly to the pharmacy to receive the medication and consult the pharmacist if necessary. If the orders are sent to an outpatient pharmacy, they are filled in the same manner but then placed in a holding bag for pickup. These are kept in alphabetical order according to the patient's last name. Depending on the protocol of the hospital and the location of the pharmacy, filled prescriptions may remain in the pharmacy from 3 to several days before they are returned to stock. A large hospital may have an adjacent pharmacy that functions both as a discharge pharmacy and as a community pharmacy.

Hospital Pharmacy Standards and Procedures

Policies and Standard Operating Procedures

All pharmacies have a policies and procedures (P&P) manual (also known as *standard operating procedures* [SOPs]). This manual contains the policies that outline the rules of the facility and the procedures that explain how, when, and/or why the policies are to be executed; in other words, the **protocol** of the facility. These rules apply to all pharmacy employees. Adherence to these policies and procedures keeps patients safe and comprises the department's quality assurance and quality control plans. For example, information contained in the P&P manual concerns daily work routines and responsibilities, benefits, protocols for emergency situations, mandatory training, and other important and useful information. Technicians should be familiar with the P&P manuals of their facilities.

 Tech Note!

All pharmacy employees are responsible for knowing the policies and procedures (P&P) and the standard operating procedures (SOPs) of the pharmacy where they are employed. During your externship, be sure to familiarize yourself with the specific rules and regulations of the pharmacy by reading the P&P manual.

Hospital Protocol

Protocol also defines the guidelines within the hospital, such as the **formulary** medications (those that are approved for use) and **non-formulary** medications (those not approved). Formularies are developed by a group of physicians and pharmacists from a variety of medical specialties who do not work for the entity requiring the formulary. These group members review new and current medications to evaluate selections based on cost, effectiveness, and safety of the drugs, and patient demographics. If the recommended criteria are not met, the drug is considered non-formulary and is not included on the approved list.

These rules must be enforced and updated constantly. The Pharmacy and Therapeutics Committee, composed of pharmacists, physicians, nurses, other health care workers, and administrators, meets on a routine basis to discuss appropriate changes to the protocol. The purpose of the committee is to choose the best medicine for patients at the best cost. A drug education coordinator is a pharmacist who helps educate the health care providers about the changes in protocol concerning drug coverage and who also assists the hospital pharmacy in implementing these changes. Not all hospitals have the extra help needed to perform these duties; sometimes the tasks of the drug education coordinator may be part of the job description of staff pharmacists or the pharmacy manager.

 Tech Note!

The abbreviation **NKA** means "no known allergies"; the abbreviation **NKDA** indicates "no known drug allergies." Both of these abbreviations are used in pharmacy and by hospital personnel. Allergy information and any other previous history of a serious adverse drug event must be entered into the computer system before any medications can be released to the nursing floors; this information includes any specific allergies to foods, dyes, preservatives, or inactive ingredients because these allergies may also pertain to medications. Proper recording of this information in the patient's computer profile helps ensure that the patient does not experience any preventable allergic or untoward reactions. All pharmacy staff members are responsible for making sure the patient information is maintained and updated on a regular basis.

Pharmacy and Nursing Staff Relationship

The pharmacy staff probably works more with nurses than with anyone else in the hospital. Nurses are the pharmacy's primary customers and should be provided with the highest level of support. They depend on the pharmacy for all their medications; they generally are responsible for more than 80% of the total calls or electronic contacts with the inpatient

pharmacy. The subjects of these inquiries include the status of their patients' medications and requests for information about drug interactions, dosing ranges, and pharmacy calculations. By far the most common question asked of the pharmacy is, "Where are the medications I ordered?" Any pharmacy technician can answer this question by simply accessing the computer system to see whether the medication was sent or by checking the orders that have not yet been entered. The technician can also check the automated dispensing system (ADS) to see whether the stock is empty; this can be done from the main pharmacy ADS machine. All other questions should be referred to the pharmacist.

As a result of the newer technology, many facilities receive fewer phone calls and more computerized communications about missing medications. The technician can look into the ADS machine to see whether the stock is empty and fill the missing medication. The technician then can notify the nurse (via computer) that the order is being processed.

Remember, collaboration between nurses and pharmacy teams is important to ensure that medication errors are prevented. Teamwork opens channels of communication and improves patient care.

 Tech Note!

Clearly identify yourself as a technician when answering the phone. Immediately let callers know whether you can help them. This information prevents the caller from having to repeat a possibly lengthy question.

Regulatory Agencies

All hospitals must meet federal and state guidelines if they are to be reimbursed for patients who have Medicare or Medicaid insurance coverage. Various agencies, such as the U.S. Department of Health and Human Services, ensure that hospitals meet all standards of safe operation. Each state's board of pharmacy may inspect pharmacies to guarantee that all personnel are working within legal guidelines. The board has the authority to fine, and even close, any pharmacy that is noncompliant with current laws.

The following are some of the agencies that govern the operations of hospitals.

- *The Joint Commission (TJC).* Hospitals pay a fee for TJC accreditation. Joint Commission surveyors visit accredited health care organizations a minimum of once every 39 months (2 years for laboratories) to evaluate standards compliance. This visit is called a survey, and all Joint Commission accreditation surveys are unannounced. The Joint Commission can require compliance with applicable local rules and regulations, so it can indirectly enforce *United States Pharmacopeia*

<797> (**USP <797>**) in states that have adopted USP <797> in their pharmacy rules and regulations.

- *Centers for Medicare and Medicaid Services (CMS).* This agency was formerly known as the Health Care Financing Administration (HCFA). It regulates and administers Medicare, Medicaid, the Children's Health Insurance Program (CHIP), the Health Insurance Portability and Accountability Act (HIPAA) standards, and several other health-related programs. The CMS inspects facilities and must give approval for hospitals to provide care and receive reimbursement for patients covered by Medicaid and Medicare.
- *Department of Health and Human Services (HHS).* This department is the primary agency that protects the health of the American people and provides essential human services. It includes more than 300 agencies, covering areas such as infection and disease, preventive care, and disaster preparedness.
- *Department of Public Health (DPH).* Each state's department of public health inspects hospitals and hospital pharmacies to ensure that they are in compliance with DPH regulations.
- *State board of pharmacy (BOP).* Each state's BOP develops, implements, and enforces pharmacy practice standards in that state for the purpose of protecting the public. State BOPs regulate the pharmacists and pharmacy technicians that work in each hospital facility.

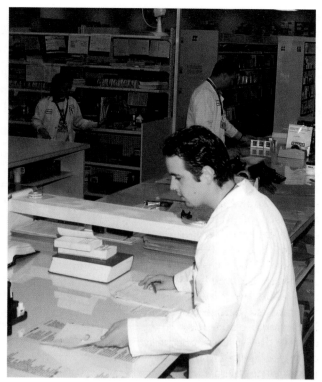

FIGURE 9-1 The flow of orders. As orders arrive, they are entered into the computer. If an order is unclear or if there is a question, the pharmacist contacts the physician.

Scenario CHECK UP 9-1

Marcus and the entire pharmacy staff are continually preparing for a possible Joint Commission visit. The hospital's goal is to meet or exceed the standards outlined by TJC and to provide the highest level of patient care possible. Marcus is assigned to verify the refrigerator temperature logs. What does this duty involve and why is it important?*

*For information about the Joint Commission's standards for medication management, see the commission's website at *www.jointcommission.org/standards_information/jcfaq.aspx? ProgramId=39*

Hospital Orders

Flow of Orders

When a physician visits a patient in the hospital, he or she may write a medication order for the patient. A **medication order** is a prescription written for administration in a hospital or institutional setting. Figure 9-1 shows a visual representation of the flow of orders. The order is written on a physician's order

sheet and is placed in the patient's chart (Figure 9-2). The chart is a record that contains all the medical orders written by medical staff, along with nursing assessments and notes, medication administration records, laboratory results, and other vital information about the patient's admission. The chart remains in the patient care area where the patient is admitted. The unit clerk or nurse periodically checks all records for new orders that must be sent to various areas of the hospital. These include dietary restrictions to be sent to the dietary department, laboratory test requests to be sent to the laboratory, and orders for medications to be sent to the pharmacy. Pharmacists review the patient profiles, their histories, progress, and laboratory values to monitor the effectiveness of the prescribed medications. The physician, nurse, or unit clerk must include all the necessary information on the patient's admitting record and subsequent medication orders to ensure that the orders are filled correctly. This includes the patient's full name, date of birth, medical record number, room number, diagnosis, weight, and, of course, drug allergies.

Some hospital pharmacies are not open 24 hours a day or on weekends or holidays, whereas others are open all day, 365 days of the year. For those that are not staffed by pharmacy personnel at all times, contingent policies and regulations allow specific nursing

---

UNIVERSITY HOSPITAL AND MEDICAL CENTER

PHYSICIAN ORDER SHEET

Patient name: *Jonathan Simmons*
Medical Record Number: *88454959 - 2*
Physician: *Dr. Cynthia Gardella*

Medication or Patient Treatment

- Press firmly using a ball point pen
- White copy remains in patient record. Fax copy to pharmacy
- Do not enter antibiotics or TPN orders on this sheet

Date	Time	
6/23/2014	10²⁰ A	V.O. Dr. Gardella → C. Kipton, RN
		Percocet 5mg. TABS
		ii po Q4 HRS for pain
		C. Kipton, RN 10²⁰ A

FIGURE 9-2 Example of a physician's order. Note the medical record number in place of a prescription number. Also, the patient's room number and allergies should be listed (not shown). (Modified from Perry AG, Potter PA, Elkin MK: *Nursing interventions and clinical skills,* ed 5, St Louis, 2012, Elsevier.)

personnel to have limited inpatient pharmacy access to obtain needed medications. In other facilities, an "on-call" pharmacist may provide the necessary services in times of less than full operation. Still other pharmacies may have off-site pharmacies that provide courier services to deliver needed orders.

Various methods are used to send orders to the pharmacy. **Computerized physician order entry (CPOE)** is a new technology by which the medication order is sent electronically to the pharmacy. (More detailed information on CPOE systems can be found in Chapter 14.) Another method is a pneumatic tube system, which allows a person to send orders and other small items by way of an air-propelled tube. In this system, cylindrical canisters can carry IV bags and other medications to the hospital floor (Figure 9-3). A disadvantage of this system is that the carrier can get jammed, or the item can accidentally be sent to the incorrect department. Also, fragile items (e.g., those encased in glass), controlled substances, expensive medications, and protein-derived medications require special packaging to be sent safely via the pneumatic tube system because they can break during the rough ride. Some pharmacies may receive orders via a fax machine. Although the fax machine is an effective way to send orders to the pharmacy quickly, it is being replaced by computerized order entry.

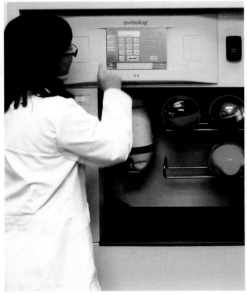

FIGURE 9-3 Pneumatic tube system. A pneumatic tube system is used to transport orders to the pharmacy and medications to hospital floors. (Courtesy Swisslog Healthcare Solutions, Buchs/Aarau, Switzerland.)

Another method of transmitting physicians' orders is to have a staff member deliver the order to the pharmacy. This normally is done when a system (e.g., the pneumatic tube system) breaks down or if the facility is extremely small.

Once the orders have been received in the pharmacy, they must be processed in the same way a regular prescription is processed. However, instead of using the name, address, and phone number for identification, the pharmacy uses the patient's medical record number. Even though this method is the primary way patients are identified, all information, including name and room number, should always be verified against the order. In this way, errors are reduced, especially when two patients with the same last name are on the same floor. When two patients have the same last name and are on the same floor, the pharmacy uses name alert stickers, which are placed on the patient's drawer and medication. Many computer systems also have name alert functions to help distinguish between patients with similar identifying characteristics.

Most computer systems allow pharmacy technicians to enter the patient's medical record number and drug orders. In many hospitals, the pharmacist enters the order because if the information is entered by the technician, it must be checked by the pharmacist to ensure accuracy before a label is released. Many pharmacists believe that the work is doubled if the technician enters an order and then the pharmacist must reread and approve the order. After an order is signed off, a printer produces a label that has the patient's name, medical record number, and room number, along with the medication information. The name of the drug, strength, dosage form, route of administration, dose, quantity, and dosing interval are included on printed label. Because the labels are produced continually, the technician usually pulls them off the printer and fills the order from the unit dose pick station. A variety of medication and dosage forms is always kept in stock for starter doses and for medications not stocked in automated dispensing systems.

To make sure the technician retrieves the correct medication, a bar coding system may be used. The technician uses a handheld device to scan the medication's National Drug Code (NDC) to verify that the correct item has been selected. If it is correct, the label will print and the medication can be given to the pharmacist for final verification. (For additional information on bar coding technology and regulations, see Chapter 14.) Patient drug labels should be placed so that medications can be checked visibly against the label by the pharmacist before they are placed in a pneumatic tube or taken to the patient's floor.

Stat, ASAP, and Standing Orders

Medication orders that need to be filled within minutes are referred to as **stat orders**. When the pharmacy receives a stat order, it should take precedence over all other orders. Normally, a stat order can be filled in 5 to 15 minutes, depending on the preparation time required for the medication. Some stat orders can be filled quickly using stock off the shelf, whereas others may require special preparation, such as the mixing of an IV preparation. In such cases, the medication is made as quickly as possible using proper aseptic technique. Stat orders can mean the difference between life and death; they must be taken seriously. If possible, a stat order should be hand delivered to ensure that it arrives at the correct destination safely and quickly.

An **ASAP order** is not normally as urgent as a stat order. However, these orders should be put in front of the new orders to ensure fast processing by the pharmacist. If the order has any discrepancies, it is the pharmacist's responsibility to contact either the nurse or the physician caring for the patient. Once the orders have been cleared, they are entered, verified, and sent.

Standing orders are written protocols for drugs or treatment that are to be used in a specific situation. For example, if a procedure is to be performed, a preprinted order with the list of medications to be administered is on file for the physician to use. This saves the physician from having to write the same order each time he or she performs the procedure. This includes orders for **prn** (as needed) drugs that can be given in case the patient needs additional medication. A standing order may have a variety of prn medications with dosage forms, routes of administration, and dosing times that require only the physician's checkmark and signature.

Point of Entry (POE) Systems

Published reports from many drug error prevention studies are responsible for a complete revamping of order entry. According to the 2006 Institute of Medicine report, "Preventing Medication Errors," it was estimated that 1.5 million preventable medication errors occur annually in the United States alone. One major change that can counteract errors is the implementation of electronic systems that can quickly and clearly transfer patient information to and from the pharmacy. POE systems provide electronic access to medical information and drug information data and allow physicians, nurses, and pharmacists to directly communicate with one another, limiting errors of transcription. Systems used include CPOE, IV smart pumps for infusible medications, computerized adverse drug event monitoring (CADM), and bar code point of entry (BPOE) medication systems. These systems are a technological step above the previous systems, called computers on wheels (COWs), which are computers on stands located at the bedside of the patient. These new COW systems are used mainly in specialty units such as intensive care units

(ICUs), where it is important that the nurse stay in close proximity to the patient. However, their usefulness is limited because they do not have bar code reading abilities and are much larger than handheld devices.

Computerized Physician Order Entry

Although CPOE technology is still new and is not used in every hospital, it is becoming more popular because it eliminates the need to decipher physicians' handwriting, and the order is sent safely to the pharmacy for processing via computer entry. The Health Information Technology for Economic and Clinical Health (HITECH) Act, enacted as part of the American Recovery and Reinvestment Act of 2009, was signed into law in February, 2009. It promotes the adoption and meaningful use of health information technology. Health care providers are offered financial incentives for demonstrating meaningful use of electronic health records (EHRs). Incentives are offered until 2015. After that, penalties will be assessed for noncompliance. Midway through 2012, it was estimated that approximately 20% of hospitals attested to stage 1 meaningful use of CPOE.

With CPOE, medication orders can be clearly identified, and the computer systems check new medications against current medications for interactions or contraindications. If an interaction is possible, the computer shows an alert icon on the screen, and the order cannot proceed until the problem is resolved. The systems may also check for proper dosage selection based on patient parameters and diagnoses. Physicians can enter all laboratory results, dietary requirements, medications, and special notes in the computer, which makes all the patients' information accessible to them at one time. Medication orders are sent directly to the pharmacy, eliminating the possibility of a lost order.

Bar Code Point of Entry

Nurses are now electronically connected to the pharmacy through the use of bar codes. The nurse can ensure accuracy of medication dosages at the patient's bedside before any medications are given. Each unit dosed medication is bar coded and can be scanned with a handheld device. Information is linked to pharmacy and to **electronic medication administration record (E-MAR)** systems. The nurse is alerted to any special notes or warnings as each dose is verified for the patient. If there is any discrepancy between the current orders and the medications sent for the patient, it is detected by the scanner and the nurse is alerted to the specific problem. For example, a medication is sent to the floor for administration; the nurse scans the tablet's bar code; and the BPOE system informs the nurse that the order has been discontinued. An error has been averted.

Orders are sent to the nurse in "real time" on the nurse's handheld device, along with any notes. Once the order has been sent to the nurse, it must be verified before administration. If there is a discrepancy, the nurse can send a note to the pharmacy for clarification. This constant communication between nurses and the pharmacy staff ultimately benefits patient care. The interaction between the nurse and the E-MAR is useful because the patient's vital signs and other chart notes can be entered from the bedside directly onto the E-MAR. For example, the patient's blood pressure, respiration rate, and pain levels can be entered. The nurse's ability to check on dosages at the patient's bedside helps ensure that the five rights of medication safety are followed, reduces the time required for charting, and creates less paperwork, so the nurse can spend more time attending to the patient. The five rights include: the right person, the right dose, the right time, the right drug, and the right route.

Computerized Adverse Drug Event Monitoring

CADM systems detect and monitor adverse drug events. Although pharmacy has used this type of system for years, it is now being integrated into the CPOE and EHR systems. This allows for a more comprehensive health care practice.

The overall change with the use of these new systems is not without problems. Pharmacy must make sure all medications are bar coded for identification, and the information in the computer must accurately reflect how the dosage form is to be given. The usual workflow of personnel is often affected and must be adjusted to accommodate the new technologies. Training pharmacists, physicians, and nurses to use these electronic systems is a significant task and must be analyzed continually for accuracy and interactions between systems already in place. Most people find major changes in their daily routine very difficult to accept; therefore, it is important to implement a system that is not too difficult to use. More hospitals are implementing these systems as new versions are developed for ease of use and accuracy.

Institutional Pharmacy Technicians

Pharmacy technicians must have many skills in today's pharmacy; because the roles of pharmacists are continually expanding, so must the roles of the pharmacy technician. Because pharmacists now have more interaction with the proper dosing of medications and implementation of formularies, the pharmacy technician completes many of the daily tasks that were previously delegated to the pharmacist. The institutional pharmacy has many different functions that depend mostly on the size of the hospital and number of pharmacies in operation. Many hospitals have 24-hour pharmacies. Technicians need to be flexible to work all shifts, including holidays. They also need to be multifunctional because there are usually half as many technicians and pharmacists employed during night and weekend shifts in most hospital pharmacies. However, the patient load may remain the same or even increase during these times. Therefore, it is essential that the technician be able to perform all the functions necessary for all shifts.

Table 9-2 outlines a variety of institutional pharmacy technician jobs and their descriptions. Because institutional pharmacies need to be staffed around the clock, it is important to have employees who can function in all areas. Technicians who are cross-trained in a variety of institutional settings become more valuable employees.

Specialty Tasks

In addition to the previously outlined tasks that technicians commonly perform, there are additional duties that require the skills of a technician. These duties include assisting with clinical duties and anticoagulant therapy tasks. Some hospitals that have nuclear medication pharmacies are using technicians to prepare these medications. These agents may be used in diagnostic procedures. Some hospitals employ investigational drug technicians. An **investigational drug** is an agent not yet approved by the U.S. Food and Drug Administration (FDA) for use. After a drug has finished prehuman testing, and if the results are positive, the next phase involves testing with human volunteers. The drug company must apply for permission through the FDA. The application is referred to as an Investigational New Drug (IND) application. The FDA must approve the use (through

TABLE 9-2

Job Descriptions for Institutional Pharmacy Technicians

Technician Responsibilities	Description
IV room	Prepares all parenteral intravenous preparations, including large volume drips and parenteral nutrition; prepares drugs that are under investigational trial and logs these special medications in appropriate manner as required by law
Chemotherapy	Prepares cytotoxic agents and other medications that may accompany these agents
Controlled substances	Gathers all controlled substance inventory sheets from all areas of the hospital; technician also may fill and deliver all controlled substances; pharmacist is required to verify pharmacy inventory daily
Patient medication	Fills medication drawers on a pharmacy cart that will deliver filling medications to all hospital patients; also may deliver carts to all patient areas and restock any floor stock medications; if hospital uses an automated medication dispensing system instead, technician must fill this unit on all floors; fills prescriptions for patients who will be discharged on an as-needed basis
Preparation of medication	Fills unit dosing bulk medications; compounds drugs such as for ointments, creams, and solutions
Filling requisitions	Fills all requisitions sent to pharmacy; stocks inventory; orders pharmacy stock; controls narcotics inventory and audits narcotics if required; transports medications throughout hospital facility
Inventory	Orders all medications and supplies for the pharmacy; also may order specialty items for other areas of the hospital; handles all returns and recalled items that must be sent back to the manufacturer; responsible for handling all invoices and for putting all stock in appropriate bins; rotates stock, performs nursing floor inspections, and inspects other pharmacy supply areas for outdated drugs and inventory levels; restocks these areas if necessary; this may include the operating room, postoperative area, preoperative area, and other sterile areas
Discharge pharmacy	Fills prescription orders as patients are discharged from the hospital; medications are sent to the floor for patients, or patients may come to the pharmacy window to pick up medications
Satellite pharmacy	May be responsible for all tasks related to a small, isolated pharmacy, such as answering phones, ordering and putting away stock, preparing parenteral medications, transcribing and pulling all medication orders, and making deliveries to nursing stations
Medication reconciliation	Reviews and documents patient's arrival medication (for pharmacist review), assuring appropriate dose, route, frequency, and duration of therapy; may review records for drug-drug interactions, duplication, and drug-allergy interactions; assists with arrival medication order entry; participates in hospital committees relevant to practice area
Miscellaneous duties	Able to work in all areas of the pharmacy as needed; answers phones, trains new technicians and pharmacist interns; works on a team with other technicians, clerks, and pharmacists

clinical trials) of an investigational drug to ensure that the patient would not be exposed to high risks. If the drug is approved, patients can apply to participate in a clinical trial. Under certain circumstances the clinical trial may be performed in the hospital.

People want to participate in a clinical trial for many reasons. Common reasons include they have exhausted all other currently approved treatments, and they believe the investigational drug will be more effective than what they are currently using. Others may want to participate in the study to promote the future development of medicine.

Hospitals frequently treat patients with investigational drugs. Depending on the hospital, this practice may be more or less common. The Joint Commission regulations must be met, and strict protocols regulate the ordering, storing, inventory, and final disposal of the drug or drugs. All investigational drugs are delivered to the central pharmacy, where they are signed in by the pharmacist and stored separately from other drugs. Each drug has a logbook that must contain the following information:

- Drug name
- Drug strength
- Unit size
- Protocol title and numbers
- Principal investigator
- Manufacturer's lot number
- Identification
- Date dispensed
- Units and/or doses dispensed
- Stock balance
- Pharmacist's initials

The investigational drug technician assists in preparing, maintaining, monitoring, and auditing investigational drug study agents and related pharmacy documentation.

Once the study is complete, the remaining drugs are returned to the sponsor. along with the log records. Copies of the records are kept by the pharmacy under "closed studies."

Tech Note!

Institutional technicians can join the American Society of Health-System Pharmacists (ASHP). This national organization has more than 40,000 members, including pharmacists, pharmacy technicians, and pharmacy students, who serve patients in hospitals, health systems, and ambulatory clinics. For more information on membership, visit the society's website at *www.ashp.org*.

Patient Cassette Drawers and/or Pyxis Machines

A long-standing daily task of pharmacy technicians is loading the patient cassette drawer from a pick

Scenario CHECK UP 9-2

Today Marcus is busy supervising the Pyxis refills. Marcus works in a state that allows certified technicians to check the work of fellow technicians. He begins to check the cassette drawers of his co-worker, Janet. Janet is normally a very hardworking and responsible technician. Today she seems distracted. Marcus finds several errors in the drawers Janet has completed. How should he handle this situation? Do you think technicians should be allowed to check other technicians' work? Explain your answer.

station. These stations in the pharmacy can be quite extensive, depending on the hospital's needs. All unit dose medications are arranged in order by generic name and are located in sections that separate solid oral dosage forms, liquids, suppositories, and other miscellaneous types of medication containers. Even though pick stations can hold many medications, some patients may require medications that must be taken from the normal stock area, such as injectable dosage forms.

After a new order is received, a starter dose is sent to the floor. The medications that will be needed for the next day are loaded in the patient cassette drawer. The technician reads the daily medication record printed each morning and fills the necessary medications into the cassettes. Normally, routine medications are placed in these drawers in the front, and as-needed (prn) doses are put in the back, separated by a divider. Routine medications are taken on a schedule every day, whereas prn medications are taken only if needed. For example, most acetaminophen (Tylenol) is ordered as needed for headache or fever.

The patient cassette drawers are held in large push carts so they can be delivered to the floor each day. All medications are delivered to the patient floors using two carts that are rotated daily. Before the patients' drawers are loaded with the next 24-hour supply, all previous medications should be emptied from the drawer. This is to reduce the possibility of errors. Many hospitals use a combination of patient cassette drawers and automated dispensing systems (discussed in the next section). Commonly used medications are stocked in the automated machines, whereas specialty or uncommon medication dosages are loaded in the cassettes.

One type of automated system used by large hospital pharmacies is the robot dispensing machine. This machine uses mechanical arms to scan bar codes on each unit dosed medication to identify the correct dose. (Dose information is fed into the machine by computer input from the pharmacist or technician.) The machine fills each patient's medication cassette with 99% accuracy as the cassette moves along a conveyer belt. Once the medication has been filled, the cassette is delivered by the technician, who returns the previous day's cassette for the next day's filling.

Although some hospitals still use solely the patient cassette system, most facilities use automated dispensing systems and robotics. These systems accelerate delivery of medication to the patient and also help to ensure accuracy. Automated floor dispensing systems used in hospital settings include Pyxis and **SureMed**. Both Pyxis and SureMed are machines on the nursing floor that are preloaded with a variety of commonly used medications. The pharmacist need only enter the order and verify it; the nurse then can retrieve the medication on the patient's floor by using a thermal fingerprint for access. These dispensing systems require continual filling and updating, which are duties of properly trained technicians.

Automated Dispensing Systems

An example of an **automated dispensing system (ADS)** is the Pyxis MedStation 4000 system. This automated system uses a biometric user identification security system. This means the user's fingerprint is scanned and verified before the system grants the user access. Many automated systems similar to the Pyxis MedStation system rely on passwords or identification swipe cards to control access. This approach puts security at risk because the card could be given to or stolen by unauthorized personnel. The advantage of the Pyxis MedStation 4000 system is that it helps ensure the security of the system and ultimate control over access to medications. Once the fingerprint scanner verifies the user, the user can access the drawers in the station for filling or dispensing purposes, according to the privileges the user is assigned.

After obtaining access to the station, the nurse selects the patient for whom he or she wants to remove medication by touching the name of the patient and the name of the medication on the display screen. The appropriate drawer with the medication opens. When the drawer is closed, the amount of medication removed is recorded for inventory tracking purposes. The pharmacy can generate reports that identify who accessed the station, when the station was accessed, which medication was removed, and how much of each medication was supposedly removed. This information is valuable in solving discrepancies and managing inventory.

Other products offered by the Pyxis Products division of Cardinal Health include the Pyxis CII Safe system and the Pyxis Oral Solid Packager. The Pyxis CII Safe system is a controlled substance management system that creates detailed tracking and reporting for each transaction to improve inventory

management. This system is separate from the Pyxis MedStation 4000 system, but the inventory management functions between the two systems can be integrated. The Pyxis Oral Solid Packager is an automated packager and bar code labeling system.

Most hospitals have incorporated automated dispensing machines to hold all types of stock. These containers are available in many different sizes, from countertop models to 6-foot-tall cabinets that hold tubing, large volume IVs, and dressings. The three main advantages of this type of cabinet are as follows:

- Inventory control: Inventory sheets can be generated in the pharmacy. Also, the patient can be charged exactly as each item is dispensed from the ADS machine.
- Reduced wait time: Nurses can directly access the patient's drugs from the ADS. No starter dose needs to be sent to the floor from the pharmacy.
- Accuracy: Nurses who access the ADS machines are allowed to take only the specific medication or medications ordered for their patients. In this way, an incorrect medication is less likely to be dispensed.

Several companies supply ADS machines, but all the machines operate on the same premise. The central unit is located in the pharmacy, where stock levels can be generated for any department at any time. Depending on the size and activity of the hospital, stock levels may have to be replenished once daily to several times a day. Periodic automatic replenishment (PAR) levels are predetermined for each drug. When the count is lower than the PAR level, the technician can pull the amount needed to restore the original count. All orders must be checked against the pull list before delivery by either a qualified technician or a pharmacist. All narcotics are kept in drawers that are physically separated from other medication, although all medications are open for removal when the main drawer opens. Box 9-1 lists various manufacturers of ADS machines and their websites.

Larger facilities may receive daily stock from an electronically produced inventory sheet that is sent to the distributor, such as Cardinal Health. For example, Cardinal Health pulls all the unit dose ADS medication, identifies the intended location on each bag, and sends it to the hospital each day at a specific time. The pharmacist checks the order, and the technician merely needs to fill the ADS machines. This saves time for the technician because only a fraction of the drawers needs to be filled.

Unit Dose Medications

Another important daily task technicians perform is the preparation of **unit dose (UD)** medications that

BOX 9-1

Manufacturers of Automated Dispensing Systems

Pyxis Stations by Cardinal Health	www.cardinalhealth.com
medDISPENSE Cabinets by Metro Healthcare	www.metro.com/ healthcare/automated-dispensing
Medselect Flex, Supplyselect, Centrack by Amerisourcebergen	www .amerisourcebergendrug .com
OmniRX, Singlepointe by Omnicell	www.omnicell.com
Compact Robotic System (CRS), SP200, SP Unit Dispenser (SPUD), SP Automation Center (SPace) by Scriptpro	www.scriptpro.com
MedRover, MedTower, ATP system, PillPick, BoxPicker. UniPick 2 by Swisslog Inspired Solutions	www.swisslog.com

are not available from the manufacturer or stocked by the pharmacy. Although many premade unit dose containers are available from manufacturers, not all drugs are available in UD form. In other cases, the hospital may prefer to make its own unit dose packaging because it can be less expensive and the hospital can make specific amounts to reduce waste.

Technicians are responsible for determining which medications need to be made based on the use of stock by patients, documenting all necessary information per protocol, and preparing the doses. The final check is done by the pharmacist. Bulk bottles of medication are pulled from stock shelves and made into UD oral syringes and other dosage forms. Many different types of methods and machines can aid in the preparation of UD medications (see Chapter 11). Only medications used on a regular basis are made into UDs. For uncommon medication orders or dosage strengths, the technician must prepare individual dosages as patient needs arise.

Unit Dose Liquids

In the past, bulk liquid items were sent to the floor for several days' use. For example, if a physician ordered Mylanta 15 mL 5 times daily, the pharmacy would send an 8-oz bottle that would stay on the patient's floor until empty. This minimized the need to place several UD cups in a small cassette drawer. As a result of new standards implemented to reduce drug errors (see Chapter 14), the Joint Commission now requires hospitals to make all medications patient-dose specific. This means that every liquid

dose must be prepared in a unit dose package and labeled before it is sent to the patient's room. A hospital may have a separate room dedicated to the preparation of all oral liquid medications and may use oral syringes to prepare each dose. Other pharmacies may make all their own unit dose cups from their bulk stock; this would be done by a technician following repackaging guidelines outlined in Chapter 11.

Controlled Substances

The task of counting, dispensing, and tracking controlled substances is a critical job that requires perfection. Many hospitals use pharmacy technicians to restock and fill narcotics for the entire hospital. In each hospital unit that stocks controlled substances, two nurses must conduct an actual count before the beginning of each shift. Therefore, all controlled substances are counted two or three times daily, depending on the length of a nursing shift. One nurse counts the controlled substances while the other nurse confirms the count on the controlled substance sheet or on the ADS record. If the narcotics are documented on paper, the count is transferred to a new inventory sheet each morning, and the last day's sheet is sent to the pharmacy for filing. **Periodic automatic replenishment (PAR)** levels are written at the top of the controlled substance sheets identifying the amounts of medications that should be kept on the floor at all times. Often the technician is responsible for retrieving these sheets daily from all units and beginning assessment of how many controlled substances of various sizes and strengths must be provided to keep the unit at its PAR level. If ADS machines are used, a PAR list is generated daily that records the current count of narcotics. Narcotics that are not being used may be returned to the pharmacy at the time of delivery.

In the pharmacy, controlled substances are normally kept in a locked room or vault, which may be under surveillance. All written records must be in pen. A registered pharmacist must verify all inventories.

Each hospital has its own system for delivering controlled substances, but one of the most important aspects is to keep the controlled substances nonidentifiable. For example, hospitals without ADS units might place controlled substances in brown paper bags that are stapled shut; most people would never know that controlled substances were being delivered in this type of package. Even so, the pharmacy technician should never let these controlled substances out of sight when delivering them throughout the hospital. Other hospitals may have lockboxes for narcotics delivery.

After the technician has confirmed the pharmacy's controlled substances count for the day, he or she must sign out each drug onto a dispensing sheet that is used to deliver the controlled substances. A pharmacist must check all narcotics before they leave the pharmacy. A pharmacist must also verify all final counts. Monthly or bimonthly inventories are taken, depending on state regulations.

All controlled substances are signed into the nursing department by adding them to the department's controlled substances sheet. A technician and nurse must observe the addition or return of stock. Only registered nurses (RNs), not licensed practical nurses, can sign in controlled substances. All controlled substances then must be countersigned onto or off of the pharmacy inventory sheet by both the technician and the nurse. The nurse and pharmacy technician should perform an actual count of the current levels of controlled substances to verify all existing controlled substances before adding additional ones into stock. In addition to delivering controlled substances, the technician may be asked by the nurse to return certain substances to the pharmacy. The same validation system is used to enter onto the pharmacy inventory sheet any drugs that are to be returned to the pharmacy.

An ADS machine verifies the count as the technician enters the narcotic to be added. An electronic record is maintained that includes the time the drawer was accessed, the name of the person accessing the drawer, the count before opening the drawer, the amount added or deleted, and the final count. In many hospitals, an RN is still required to countersign on the delivery sheet to verify that it is the correct drug and the correct beginning and ending inventory, in addition to the correct ADS station. All additions and deletions are documented by the ADS machine, which shows who opened the cabinet, when the cabinet was opened, and in which drawer the additions or deletions were made. The technician must count first, then add or remove items, and then recount afterward. Only one type of narcotic dosage form is allowed per drawer container. The stock is put into the ADS, and a receipt is printed. This verification receipt is taken to the pharmacy and kept in the narcotic count area.

Upon return to the pharmacy, all controlled substances must be signed back into the pharmacy stock, along with the receipt from the ADS machine if one has been used. This normally is done by a technician and verified and countersigned by a pharmacist. One of the most important parts of this job is to verify that all numbers are correct. The pharmacist must never sign in controlled substances without first visually counting the existing and returned stock.

Narcotics are normally filed in stock under their generic name and by their schedule. All controlled substances are confined in the same area. Binders may be used to keep inventory of each drug. As stock is removed, the amount is taken off the inventory sheet, and the remainder must be counted and correct. Certain scheduled drugs are also stored in a refrigerator, and in the pharmacy a small refrigerator is often kept in the locked room or vault for this purpose. Nursing units have a lockbox in their medication refrigerator for scheduled drugs.

⏺ *Scenario* CHECK UP 9-3

Marcus continues preparing for the Joint Commission visit. His pharmacist has asked him to look over the controlled substance logs to check for any errors or irregularities. He also MUST do a count of the current controlled substance inventory along with the supervising pharmacist. During the review, Marcus finds that one particular technician had an unusually high number of accesses to the controlled substance drawer. What could this mean? What precautions SHOULD Marcus take during this review?

Intravenous Preparations

At certain intervals throughout the day, IV labels representing all current orders are printed from the computer system. All changes in IV medication information are kept updated by the technician and the pharmacist who work in the intravenous room. Only specially trained and properly garbed pharmacy personnel are allowed into the clean room.

Normally, while the technician labels all premade IV antibiotics and other IV medications, the pharmacist answers the phones and enters new and changed orders. Pharmacists are also responsible for contacting the nurse or physician if a problem arises with an order. For example, if an order is sent to the pharmacy for ampicillin/sulbactam (Unasyn) and the patient is allergic to penicillin, the pharmacist contacts the physician and asks the physician to replace this antibiotic with one that will not cause an allergic reaction in the patient.

Orders in an inpatient pharmacy are affected by the time of day. For example, in the early morning several preoperative (preop) medications may be ordered, and later in the morning postoperative (postop) medications may be ordered for surgical patients. Also, more diagnostic exams are performed in the morning or afternoon hours than in the evening. Medications that are required for these diagnostic tests usually must be sent by the pharmacy.

The pharmacy technician is responsible for stocking the IV room with all the supplies needed for the day. The technician also must make sure the work area stays clean. Usually the same technician prepares all IV medications, and at the end of the shift, he or she delivers them to the nursing floors. When the IV medications are delivered to the nursing stations, the unused IV medications are returned to the pharmacy. If they have not expired, they are placed in the refrigerator or back into stock for future use; otherwise, they are logged and discarded properly according to pharmacy policy. Because each IV preparation must be registered and justified, most pharmacies keep a binder or book in which information about all wasted IV preparations is written. Technicians must remember that it is important to complete all tasks before the end of the shift and to replace all stock items as best they can for the next shift.

Aseptic Technique

Aseptic technique is a set of procedures used to prevent the contamination of an object by microorganisms. Use of this technique is important in the preparation of all IV medications, IV nutrition solutions, chemotherapy products, and compounded ophthalmic medications. All personnel preparing sterile preparations must be tested periodically on the proper guidelines of aseptic technique; this usually is done by management at the yearly evaluation. Samples normally are taken from a newly prepared parenteral medication and are sent to the laboratory for testing, or media fill kits may be used to test on site. This testing is performed to ensure that microbial contamination is not present in medications that must be sterile. Aseptic technique is discussed in detail in Chapter 12.

Non-Hazardous IV Preparation

An IV tech is responsible for the preparation of various **parenteral medications**. Parenteral medications bypass the digestive system and are intended for quick systemic action. Parenteral medications are given by injection via the intramuscular or IV route. This includes piggyback antibiotics, large volume IV solutions (e.g., sodium chloride, dextrose, and amino acid infusions), and other parenteral medication orders. Some hospital pharmacies are responsible only for the large volumes of IV medications that must be prepared with special additives; the nurses on the floor maintain a floor stock of premade, large volume bags that can be supplied by central supply or by the pharmacy. Typical antibiotics and other IV admixtures can be prepared in a horizontal laminar flow hood after the proper personnel cleansing procedures and garbing order have been followed (Procedure 9-1).

PROCEDURE 9-1

Personnel Cleansing and Garbing Order for Sterile Compounding

GOAL: To learn the steps required to cleanse and garb up to properly prepare compounded sterile preparations.

EQUIPMENT AND SUPPLIES
- Antiseptic hand cleanser
- Surgical scrub
- Shoe cover
- Head and facial hair cover
- Face mask or eye shield
- Non-shedding gown
- Sterile, powder-free gloves

PROCEDURAL STEPS
- Remove all personal outer garments.

PURPOSE: Outer garments such as jackets or coats may have shedding fibers or hairs that could contaminate the compounding area.
- Remove all cosmetics and jewelry (no artificial nails are allowed).

PURPOSE: Cosmetics can flake off and jewelry and artificial nails can have dirt and other debris on and under the surface. These contaminants can be carried into the compounding area if not removed.
- Put on personal protective equipment (PPE) in the following order:
  - Shoe covers
  - Head and facial hair covers
  - Face masks/eye shields

PURPOSE: Shoe covers help prevent any germs that may be on your shoes from entering the compounding area. Head and facial hair covers are used to keep any hairs from falling into the compounding area. Face masks and eye shields are used to protect the technician from exposure to medications that may splash or may accidentally spill during the compounding process.
- Perform aseptic hand cleansing procedures with a surgical scrub.

PURPOSE: Proper hand washing with a surgical scrub helps to lessen the bacteria found on the hands before beginning the compounding process.
- Put on a non-shedding gown.

PURPOSE: Donning a non-shedding gown serves to prevent any contaminants that may be on the technician's clothes from getting into the compounding area. Most gowns are resistant to penetration by moisture, which helps protect the technician if a spill occurs.
- Put on the sterile, powder-free gloves.

PURPOSE: Gloves protect the compounding area from skin that is constantly shedding from our hands. They also protect the technician from exposure to medications that may be used in the compounding process. Double gloving is recommended when compounding hazardous drugs or chemicals.

IV preparation areas are required to have a clean room outside the compounding area that meets federal standards. These clean rooms buffer the IV admixture room and allow preparation of IV labels and stock to be maintained in a clean yet separate area. They also must meet USP <797> standards. Only the necessary supplies should be carried into the buffer room, and the room must be cleaned with specific cleaning solutions and devices.

Many hospitals cannot convert their compounding areas to USP <797> standards; therefore, they have begun to contract out the bulk of their IV preparations to USP <797>–certified compounding pharmacies. The policies vary from hospital to hospital.

Horizontal laminar flow hoods are cabinets that direct filtered air horizontally toward the opening of the cabinet, which provides a sterile environment for preparing parenteral medications (Figure 9-4). There are other types of hoods, such as partially covered vertical hoods and biological safety cabinets (BSCs). Each type meets specific environmental requirements. For more information on flow hoods and their uses, see Chapter 12.

A horizontal flow hood or laminar airflow workbench (LAFW) is used for preparing non-hazardous IV medications. A high-efficiency particulate air (HEPA) filter is located at the back of the hood. When the technician is working inside the horizontal flow hood, the orientation of the hands must not block the flow of first-air. First-air is the air issuing directly from the HEPA filter. This means that hands cannot be moved between the vial, needle, or IV bag and the first-air. Blocking the flow of first-air can allow contamination of the preparation. Technicians must practice and master proper aseptic technique. Nonhazardous IV preparations can also be made by robotic systems.

The hospital technician may be responsible for preparing chemotherapeutic medications. The same aseptic techniques are used in preventing contamination when preparing any parenteral medication. However a few differences between the intravenous and chemotherapy environments should be noted. All chemo compounds are prepared within a vertical flow hood BSC, glove box, or a compounding aseptic containment isolator (CACI).

USP <797> regulations state that compounding should take place in an International Standards Organization (ISO) Class 8 or better clean room. There are different levels of clean rooms. The ISO ranks clean rooms as ISO Class 1 (the cleanest) through ISO Class 9. The lower the ISO rating, the cleaner the environment. Contamination is measured by particle count. HEPA filters capture the contaminated particles. An ISO Class 8 environment means that the filter captures 3,520,000 parts per cubic meter that measure greater than 0.5 mcg.

There must also be an anteroom for gowning and degowning and movement of personnel into and out of the clean room. Additionally, a hood known as the primary engineering control (PEC) providing an ISO Class 5 or better environment must be used to perform compounding activities.

Building and operating a clean room can be expensive and may not be in the budget for smaller hospitals. Fortunately, glove box isolators (or barrier isolators) can now be added to comply with USP <797> requirements.

There are different classes of glove boxes, but they are all based on the same premise, that all medication preparation is performed in a closed, sterile environment (Figure 9-5). Glove boxes have been found to reduce the possibility of contamination, which is a major concern in error prevention. All materials are placed in a side cabinet attached to the main cabinet and then transferred into the main cabinet for preparation. The hood must be cleaned both before and after each use with special cleaning cloths and 70% isopropyl alcohol. Guidelines for proper use and cleaning are provided by the manufacturer.

Glove boxes can be used for higher risk IV admixtures per USP <797> regulations. Air is filtered through a HEPA filter and then through a final HEPA filter before it is exhausted to the outside of the facility (not into the work area). The technician never

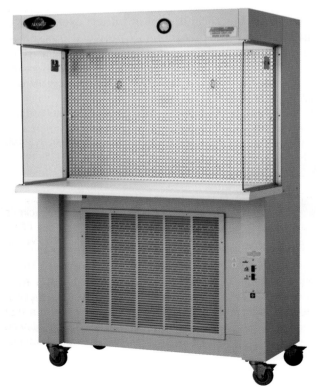

FIGURE 9-4 Horizontal laminar flow hood clean bench (Airegard 301). (Courtesy NuAire, Plymouth, Minn.)

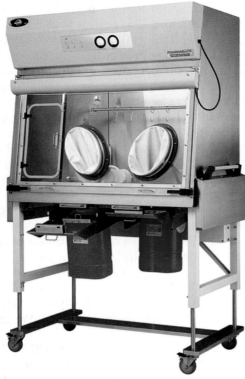

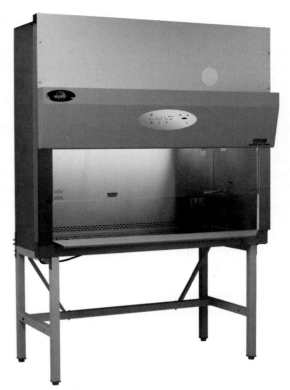

FIGURE 9-5 Glove box for IV admixture (Pharmagard 797). (Courtesy NuAire, Plymouth, Minn.)

FIGURE 9-6 Biological safety cabinet with vertical flow hood (Labgard 437). (Courtesy NuAire, Plymouth, Minn.)

directly contacts the medication while manipulating it in the hood. This is a closed system, unlike the partially shielded vertical flow hood or horizontal flow hood. In a glove box the airflow is also vertical; therefore, hands must not move over the top of any vial, needle, or IV bag. If the hands do move into these areas, aseptic technique has been broken. Regardless of which hood is used, it is most important that aseptic technique is always practiced (see Chapter 12).

BSCs are partially open front vertical airflow hoods used to prepare chemotherapeutic agents (Figure 9-6). The air is pulled down toward the tabletop filter from the ceiling of the hood, which contains the first HEPA filter. The chemotherapy hood does not allow the air to leave the container compartment; instead, the air is recycled through a second HEPA filter that removes any particulate matter before the air is recirculated into the work environment. The flow of air vertically helps protect the person preparing the agents from unwanted exposure. To maintain sufficient airflow, hands should not move over or above the items in the vertical flow hood. Technicians must follow the standard personnel cleansing and garbing regulations, with a few extra precautions. For safety, a special impervious chemotherapy gown must be worn, along with eye protection and double gloves (latex or non-latex) or special chemical safety

gloves (nitrile or neoprene rubber and polyurethane). The first pair is worn under the wrist cuff of the gown, and the second pair is pulled over the wrist cuff of the gown. Hazardous IV preparations can also be made by robotic systems such as CYTOCARE.

 Tech Alert!
Safe practices recommend that gloves used to prepare chemotherapeutic agents should not be worn longer than 30 minutes. Hands must always be washed before and after removal of gloves.

Scenario CHECK UP 9-4

Today Marcus is working in the IV compounding area. He receives an order for IVIG for Ms. Wallace, who comes in once a month to the outpatient care unit. Marcus knows that this is a very expensive medication, and he has never compounded it before. How should he approach this challenge? What makes this IV preparation different from most compounded sterile preparations?

Labeling

The proper placement of labels is important to ensure visibility of the parenteral solution and contents

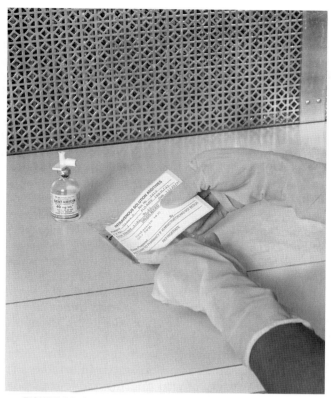

FIGURE 9-7 Proper placement of labels on parenteral solutions.

(Figure 9-7). All labels must be placed squarely onto the medication and should be clear and easy to read.

The technician must initial all medications, even if the label is placed on a premade bag. Before IV piggybacks and drips are delivered to the appropriate floors, the pharmacist must check each medication and countersign with his or her initials. Labels usually contain the same type of information, regardless of the facility. In addition to labeling parenteral medications, the technician must be aware of additional information, such as medications that need to be placed in light-protected bags and those requiring refrigeration. The technician must know the storage requirements and the stability of the medications he or she prepares.

Tech Alert!

Gloves must be surface cleaned before you wipe down the final preparation, place the label on the preparation, and move the preparation to the pass-through area for removal from the sterile parenteral preparation room. The inner pair of gloves (used when preparing chemotherapeutic agents) is used to affix labels and place the agent in a sealable containment bag for transport; this must be done within the BSC. You must put on a new pair of gloves before handling the completed preparation to avoid any exposure to the agent by yourself or others.

All drugs must be labeled before they leave the pharmacy. The required parts of a label include the patient's name, patient's medical record number and room number, name of the drug, strength of the medication, name of the solution with which the medication was mixed, and the rate of infusion. The pharmacy technician must check this information several times before he or she applies the label to the medication. Additional information on a label includes the time the dose should be given, the date, and the expiration date. Expiration dates are important because many IV preparations are returned to stock if not expired.

Several references can provide stability information:

- *Trissel's Stability of Compounded Formulations*
- *Trissel's Handbook of Injectable Drugs*
- *USP Dispensing Information*
- *Journal of Pharmaceutical Sciences*
- *American Journal of Health-System Pharmacy*
- *Remington: The Science and Practice of Pharmacy*

Beyond-use dating is described in USP <797> as consisting of two components, chemical stability and microbial sterility. Storing a compounded sterile preparation for an extended period before use creates the potential for microbial growth and pyrogen formation. Therefore, the risk level is based on the duration of storage.

When IVs are delivered to the floor, the technician checks the remaining IVs for unused medications. If the IV was not used, it is picked up by the pharmacy at the time of the daily IV delivery and returned to stock for later use. IVs that have expired are logged into a logbook. The IV is emptied (normally into the sink), and the Viaflex bag is disposed of in the garbage. Viaflex bags are made of flexible polyvinyl chloride (PVC). If the drug removed from the IV bag is a potential environmental hazard or biohazard, it must be disposed of according to certain regulations. These regulations vary by state and local requirements and also by rules established by federal agencies, including the FDA, Environmental Protection Agency (EPA), Department of Transportation (DOT), and Occupational Safety and Health Administration (OSHA). The technician should always be familiar with the disposal regulations of the facility before emptying any medications into sewage systems.

Maintaining Stock and Supplying Specialty Areas

In several areas of a hospital the pharmacy must maintain a PAR level of medications. Technicians must recognize each of the abbreviations representing the units and clinics that require medication from the pharmacy (Box 9-2). The supplies kept on hand in these units are referred to as *floor stock*. The

BOX 9-2

Examples of Primary Units and Areas That Require Medication from the Pharmacy

CCU	Coronary care unit
Clinics	Patients may visit a clinic to be seen by a physician, physician's assistant, or nurse practitioner
ED or ER	Emergency department; area of hospital where patients can receive emergency care; physicians and nurses are on staff 24 hours a day
ICU	Intensive care unit
L&D	Labor and delivery; unit where a woman goes through labor and delivers a baby
MED-SURG	Medical unit for patients who have undergone surgery or who may be under observation
NICU	Neonatal intensive care unit; can also stand for neurological intensive care unit
NSY	Nursery; unit where babies are taken for care and observation by nurses
OB/GYN	Obstetrics/gynecology; unit that takes care of expectant mothers or those who have just given birth
ONCOLOGY	Unit that takes care of patients with cancer
OR	Operating room
ORTHO	Orthopedics unit; takes care of patients who may need treatment or surgery on bones or joints
PACU	Postanesthesia care unit
PED	Pediatrics; unit for children younger than age 14 years
POSTOP	Unit where patient is kept after an operation or procedure
PREOP	Unit where patient is kept before an operation or procedure
UROLOGY	Unit that takes care of patients who may need treatment, surgery, or procedures on the urinary system

technician must be fully aware of the types of medications used in each of these areas because each unit, ward, or clinic has its own special stock. Because of the special needs of each area, many pharmacies have special forms that are preprinted with complete descriptions of commonly used drugs. This helps reduce the incidence of stock being sent to the wrong areas in the hospital. The pharmacy normally receives the supply ordering forms from the specialty areas daily. Although they are not a high-priority task, these orders should be filled before the end of the day. In addition, the technician may need to deliver the medications and check various areas of the hospital for any outdated medications. This task

should be done monthly, preferably before the end of the month. Outdated medications normally can be returned to the pharmacy if they will expire within 3 months. Expired medications may be returned to the manufacturer for credit (most manufacturers accept returned expired medications in batches of 100), or they may be taken by an independent company and destroyed in a proper manner. This depends on the contract between the hospital and the manufacturer. Some hospitals contract with an outside company that specializes in drug inventory to visit the pharmacy periodically and document all expired medications before they are destroyed.

Each department (e.g., preop, postop, operating room, wards, and clinics) is stocked with specific medications, depending on the type of services it provides. Because of the many different areas throughout a hospital, the pharmacy must stock a wide variety of medications in different dosage forms. Therefore, the pharmacy technician must have a good understanding of which medications are appropriate for each department. Departments such as the emergency department, operating room, and intensive care unit stock many drugs in injectable form and a wide variety of oral and injectable controlled substances. Pediatrics uses many of the same medications that are used in the other departments, except in lower doses, in addition to medications in special pediatric dosage forms. The labor and delivery department stocks injectables and other drugs used for labor, contractions, and cesarean births. The tasks of collecting and filling all floor stock medications are part of the daily routine of a technician. As always, it is necessary that all orders be verified and initialed by a pharmacist before they can be delivered to the correct departments unless the tech-check-tech process has been approved under hospital protocol.

⚠ *Tech Alert!*

When refilling a crash cart, *never* assume that the unused drugs left inside the tray are correct. A prime example is the common error of failing to differentiate between pediatric and adult strengths of lidocaine. As another example, epinephrine is always stocked on a crash cart. Both adult and pediatric strengths are packaged in prefilled syringes, and they have a similar appearance. *Note the dosages of pediatric-strength epinephrine (1:1000 [1 mg/mL]) and adult-strength epinephrine (1:10,000 [0.1 mg/mL]). Placing adult-dose epinephrine in pediatric trays is a common error.* However, if an adult dose of the medication is filled into a pediatric tray, this could result in death rather than save a life. Always remove all medications and start anew. Following the prepared list, check all the strengths of the medications and the expiration dates.

BOX 9-3

Examples of Hospital Codes*

- Code red: Fire
- Code blue: Medical emergency—adult
- Code white: Medical emergency—pediatric
- Code pink: Infant abduction
- Code purple: Child abduction
- Code yellow: Bomb threat
- Code gray: Combative person
- Code silver: Person with a weapon and/or hostage situation
- Code orange: Hazardous material spill/release
- Code triage internal: An internal disaster
- Code triage external: An external disaster

*Codes vary among hospitals.

Crash Carts

Another important pharmacy task is the refilling of **crash carts**. These are trays used by all areas of the hospital. They contain injectable medications used for a code situation (e.g., cardiopulmonary distress). Each hospital has a set of codes (Box 9-3). It is the responsibility of each employee to know the hospital's code names. The naming of the code varies from hospital to hospital. Table 9-3 lists examples of the types of injectable drugs commonly used on crash carts. The pharmacy stocks extra trays in case of a stat call for another tray. The three types of trays are adult, pediatric, and neonatal. Each type of tray contains a different strength of drug. When a tray has been used, the pharmacy technician takes a new tray, retrieves the used tray, and refills the missing contents. Also at this time the technician checks expiration dates on all medications. These dates are listed on a preprinted form. All crash cart medications should always be placed in the tray in the same order. The familiar order enhances the ability of nurses and physicians to quickly grab a needed medication. If all crash carts were in a different order, the nurse would have to search for the life-saving medication. As always, it is necessary that all orders be verified and initialed by a pharmacist before they can be delivered to the correct departments. All crash carts are wrapped in a disposable cover and assigned a lock, which is broken at the time of use. Each lock is imprinted with a number controlled by the pharmacy, and the location of every crash cart is documented.

Supplying Nonclinical Areas

Nonclinical areas of a hospital can include areas that a patient never sees or areas that are used as temporary patient care areas. Some examples of these special areas of the hospital, along with the types of

TABLE 9-3

Commonly Used Crash Cart Medications and Their Classification

Medication	Classification	Common Dosage Forms Stored on Cart
Adenosine	Antiarrhythmic	Vial
Amiodarone	Antiarrhythmic	Ampule, vial
Atropine sulfate	Anticholinergic	PFS
Calcium chloride	Electrolyte	PFS
Dextrose	Carbohydrate	IV solution bags*
Dextrose 50%	Carbohydrate	PFS
Digoxin	Cardiac glycoside	Ampule
Dobutamine	Vasopressor	Vial
Dopamine	Vasopressor	Vial, IV bag*
Enalapril	ACE inhibitor	Vial
Epinephrine	Vasopressor	PFS
Furosemide	Loop diuretic	Vial
Glucagon	Glucose-elevating agent	Vial
Heparin	Anticoagulant	IV bag,* vial
Lidocaine	Antiarrhythmic	PFS, IV bag*
Magnesium sulfate	Electrolyte	Vial
Mannitol	Osmotic diuretic	Vial, IV bag*
Metoprolol	Beta-blocker	Ampule
Naloxone	Narcotic antagonist	Ampule
Nitroglycerin	Antianginal	Vial
Nitroprusside	Antihypertensive	Vial
Norepinephrine	Vasopressor	Ampule
Procainamide	Antiarrhythmic	Vial
Propranolol	Beta-blocker	Vial
Sodium bicarbonate	Alkalinizing agent	PFS
Sodium chloride	Electrolyte	Vial, IV solution bags*
Vasopressin	Vasopressor	Vial
Verapamil	Calcium channel blocker	Vial

ACE, Angiotensin-converting enzyme; *IV,* intravenous; *PFS,* prefilled syringe.
*Bags of medications may be kept in a drawer different from the medication tray.

Scenario CHECK UP 9-5

Today Marcus and Janet are preparing to update all the crash carts. The Joint Commission will be checking for accuracy and any outdated medications. While filling the crash cart Marcus notices that Janet has the correct medication, but she is putting it into the tray in a different order than usual. When he discusses this with Janet, she becomes defensive and insists her order is correct. What should Marcus do next? What are the dangers associated with this situation?

BOX 9-4

Special Departments Stocked by the Pharmacy

Anesthesia	Physicians or nurse anesthesiologists administer medications used before and throughout surgery
Respiratory	Therapists administer breathing treatments to hospitalized or clinic patients
Injection clinic	Nurses administer adult and pediatric immunizations and also may perform allergy skin tests
Radiology or imaging department	Technicians and physicians may administer dyes for imaging and may need to use a medication cart (known as a *crash cart*) for adverse reactions or incidents

medications the pharmacy may be responsible for ordering and stocking, are presented in Box 9-4.

Central Supply

Another area that stocks supplies for the hospital is central supply. Usually boxes of large volume IVs and mixtures are kept here, in addition to dressings, tubing, and instruments used by various departments. The pharmacy orders stock normally on a daily basis from central supply. The type of stock ordered includes sterile water and various strengths of solutions, such as premade potassium chloride (KCl) bags or lactated Ringer's solution. These are supplied in case-size boxes that can weigh almost 15 pounds each. They are ordered early in the morning and are delivered within a few hours. It is the responsibility of the stock person to ensure that all stock was delivered. The IV tech normally obtains his or her order from the stock delivered and restocks the pharmacy IV room. At the end of the day, the stock for the following day must be ordered by contacting the order clerk. Drugs are not stocked in central supply; they must be ordered directly from the manufacturer or distributor.

The Future for Institutional Pharmacy Technicians

The **American Society of Health-System Pharmacists (ASHP)** Pharmacy Practice Model Initiative (*www.ashpmedia.org/ppmi/*) recognizes pharmacy technicians as a cornerstone of the future of pharmacy practice. This initiative recommends increased educational requirements for technicians to prepare them for expanded roles and increased responsibilities. The benefits of technician education are numerous. Technicians play an integral role in the institutional pharmacy practice. With continuing education, they become more engaged in their work, which leads to better accountability and greater job satisfaction. The technician who has experience in many different settings and a broad knowledge of pharmacy practices will be in high demand.

> **TECHNICIAN** PROFILE

Dana is a pharmacy technician manager and recruiter for a large teaching hospital. She is certified with the Pharmacy Technician Certification Board (PTCB) and has 10 years' experience as a technician. She holds a bachelor's degree in health care administration and an associate's degree in pharmacy technology. Her job is to provide operations management and support to specialized areas. In this position, she worked to develop a career ladder for technicians that allowed for increased pay for advanced education and training. Dana supervises the new-hire orientation process and is responsible for overseeing the technician schedules for 10 different pharmacies in the hospital complex. She works side by side with many dedicated pharmacists who support and encourage advanced roles for technicians. Dana believes that broadening the responsibilities of pharmacy technicians is a critical component to improving patient care and safety.

DO YOU REMEMBER THESE KEY POINTS?

- Different types of hospital pharmacies, what differentiates them from one another, and how that affects the overall service they may provide
- What an SOP and a P&P include
- The difference between formulary and nonformulary medication lists
- The importance of a good relationship between the pharmacy and the nursing staff
- Which agencies monitor hospitals, including pharmacies in the hospital
- The various ways orders are processed by the pharmacy

- The difference between stat, ASAP, and standing orders
- How POE, CPOE, BPOE, and CADM systems are used to reduce drug errors
- The various duties of an institutional pharmacy technician, including the areas described in this chapter
- The technician's role in the IND process
- How ADS machines function in the hospital setting and how they are stocked
- The steps in and frequency of filling automated medication dispensing systems

- The importance of counting, dispensing, and tracking controlled substances
- What PAR levels are and who is responsible for maintaining them
- How often medications are supplied to nursing units using a cart-filling method
- The difference between hazardous and non-hazardous IV preparation
- The importance of aseptic technique for the technician preparing compounded sterile preparations (CSPs)

- Duties involved in ordering and maintaining the stock levels of the pharmacy
- Hospital areas that the pharmacy stocks
- Specialty areas of the hospital for which the pharmacy stocks or orders medication
- Why technician education is important and the name of a professional organization that institutional technicians can join

Scenario FOLLOW UP

The Joint Commission visit is over, and Marcus is proud to report that the pharmacy received only one finding. The commission found an outdated flu vaccine in the back of the pharmacy refrigerator. Several technicians and pharmacists had checked for out-of-date medications, but somehow one was missed. Everyone understood the danger of possibly administering an outdated vaccine and determined to be more diligent in the future to prevent the same mistake. Overall, the visit was a success, and the pharmacy staff was proud of their efforts to ensure quality patient care.

REVIEW QUESTIONS

Multiple Choice Questions

1. P&P manuals contain information pertaining to all of the following *except*:
   A. Employees' weekly schedule
   B. Emergency situations
   C. Training
   D. Daily work routines
2. The Joint Commission does *not* inspect or accredit:
   A. Long-term care pharmacies
   B. Hospital pharmacies
   C. Retail pharmacists
   D. All of the above are inspected and accredited by the Joint Commission.
3. Hospital orders contain which information?
   A. Drug interactions
   B. Dietary restrictions
   C. Medication orders
   D. All of the above
4. What is the meaning of the acronym CPOE?
   A. Computerized pharmacy operating element
   B. Counseling program offering education
   C. Counseling pharmacy operations elective
   D. Computerized prescriber order entry
5. Hospital technicians must be available to:
   A. Work various shifts
   B. Work weekends
   C. Fill different jobs per operational needs
   D. All of the above

6. Technicians have all of the following responsibilities *except*:
   A. Printing labels for IV medications before filling the container
   B. Preparing antibiotics
   C. Discontinuing intravenous medications per physician's orders
   D. Contacting the physician for order clarification
7. Which statement about investigational drugs is false?
   A. An IND application must be filed with the FDA before the clinical study.
   B. All investigational drugs must be disposed of on site at the hospital where the study has taken place.
   C. A logbook containing all required information on the investigational drug must be maintained by the pharmacy.
   D. A clinical trial with investigational drugs is the last phase before a drug is approved by the FDA.
8. Stat orders should be filled within:
   A. 15 minutes
   B. 20 minutes
   C. 25 minutes
   D. 30 minutes

9. Which of the following provides guidelines and regulations for the compounding of sterile preparations?
   A. HHS
   B. USP <797>
   C. USP <795>
   D. DPH

10. Which is *not* an ADS?
    A. Pyxis
    B. Glove box
    C. SureMed
    D. SmartCart

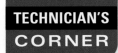

TECHNICIAN'S CORNER

You receive an order for Ms. Jeni Gilbert. Only her name and her room number are written on the order. The order is for ceftriaxone 1 g q4h.
Is this an appropriate dosing regimen for this medication?
What information must you have before you can process this order?
What actions should you take concerning the dosing regimen for this medication?

Bibliography

Ansel H, Allen L, Popovich N: *Pharmaceutical dosage forms and drug delivery systems*, ed 9, Baltimore, 2011, Lippincott Williams & Wilkins.

Elkin M, Perry A, Potter P: *Nursing interventions and clinical skills*, ed 5, St Louis, 2011, Elsevier.

United States Pharmacopeia <797>: Pharmaceutical compounding: sterile preparations. Rockville, MD. United States Pharmacopeial Convention. Revision Bulletin, 2013.

Websites Referenced

American Society of Health-System Pharmacists. Discussion Guide for Compounding Sterile Preparations. (Referenced January 23, 2014.) www.ashp.org/s_ashp/docs/files/HACC_797 guide.pdf.

American Society of Health-System Pharmacists. Medication Reconciliation and Pharmacy Technicians. (Referenced March 5, 2014). http://www.ashp.org/DocLibrary/MemberCenter/Webinars/Webinar20081023.aspx.

eHow. What is the Meaning of Non-Formulary Drugs. (Referenced February 24, 2014.) www.ehow.com/about_6749588_meaning-non_formulary-drugs_.html?ref=Track2&utm_source=ask.

Healthcare IT News. Is CPOE Getting better—or just bigger? (Referenced December 20, 2013.) www.healthcareitnews.com/news/cpoe-getting-better-%E2%80%93-or-just-bigger.

Lionheart Publishing. Patient safety and quality healthcare. Healthcare-Associated Infection Reports. (Referenced November 10, 2013.) http://www.psqh.com/magazine-top/1796-health care-associated-infection-reports?highlight=WyJub3ZlbWJlc iIsMjAxMywibm92ZW1iZXIgMjAxMyJd.

Society of Nuclear Medicine and Molecular Imaging. Frequently Asked Questions about USP <797>. (Referenced February 24, 2014.) http://interactive.snm.org/index.cfm?PageID=7897.

UNC Eshelman School of Pharmacy. The Pharmaceutics and Compounding Laboratory. Assigning Beyond Use Dates. (Referenced March 4, 2014.) http://pharmlabs.unc.edu/labs/prescriptions/beyond.htm.

University of Kentucky Hospital Chandler Medical Center. Department of Pharmacy Policy. (Referenced November 10, 2013.) www.ashp.org/DocLibrary/Policy/IDS/Receiptand Control.aspx.

Wyoming State Board of Pharmacy. Wyoming Pharmacy Act, Rules and Regulations. Institutional Pharmacy Practice Regulations. (Referenced March 5, 2014.) http://pharmacyboard.state.wy.us/laws/Chapter_12_Pharmacy_Act.pdf.

Additional Pharmacy Practice Settings

Julie Beccarelli

OBJECTIVES

Upon completing this chapter, you should be able to do the following:

1. List and describe the roles and responsibilities of a pharmacy purchasing agent.
2. Identify and explain the requirements for becoming a pharmacy purchasing agent.
3. List and describe the roles and responsibilities of a managed care pharmacy technician.
4. Identify and explain the requirements for becoming a managed care pharmacy technician.
5. List and describe the roles and responsibilities of a pharmacy technician educator or trainer.
6. Identify and explain the requirements for becoming a pharmacy technician educator or trainer.
7. List and describe the roles and responsibilities of a pharmaceutical sales representative.
8. Identify and explain the requirements for becoming a pharmaceutical sales representative.
9. List and describe the roles and responsibilities of a nuclear pharmacy technician.

10. Identify and explain the requirements for becoming a nuclear pharmacy technician.
11. List and describe the roles and responsibilities of a telepharmacy/remote pharmacy technician.
12. Identify and explain the requirements for becoming a telepharmacy/remote pharmacy technician.
13. List and describe the roles and responsibilities of a medication reconciliation pharmacy technician.
14. Identify and explain the requirements for becoming a medication reconciliation pharmacy technician.
15. List and describe the roles and responsibilities of a pharmacy informatics pharmacy technician.
16. Identify and explain the requirements for becoming a pharmacy informatics pharmacy technician.
17. Evaluate how each additional role of the pharmacy technician plays a part in patient safety.

TERMS AND DEFINITIONS

Managed care An organized health care delivery system designed to improve both the quality and accessibility of health care, including pharmaceutical care, while containing costs

Medication reconciliation The process of comparing a patient's medication orders with all the medications the patient was taking before admission to the hospital

Pharmacy benefit management (PBM) The development and management of broad and cost-efficient prescription drug benefits for a large group of patient populations

Telepharmacy The provision of pharmaceutical care to patients at a distance through the use of telecommunications and information technologies

Introduction

Scenario:

John is a certified pharmacy technician at a local hospital. Recently, the department added a new technician role, medication management tech. John is very interested in this position and wants to apply for it. He has the required 2 years of experience in the pharmacy and a good understanding of brand and generic medication names. What other attributes would make him successful in this position?

As the field of pharmacy evolves, so do the responsibilities of and opportunities for the pharmacy technician. The expected employment growth rate for pharmacy technician careers between 2010 and 2020 is 32%. There are several reasons for this increase in the need for technicians with advanced qualifications, such as medication safety regulations, the increasing development of new medications, and the rapid growth of the elderly population, who have polypharmacy (the simultaneous use of multiple drugs to treat a single ailment or condition) concerns.

The role of the pharmacy technician was once considered a clerk-type position—stocking shelves and running the register. However, the technician's role has grown into a position with important responsibilities, and most states require the pharmacy technician to be licensed or registered with the state board of pharmacy. In some cases national certification is required to obtain a position as a pharmacy technician. More than 50% of pharmacy technicians work in the traditional settings, such as community pharmacies and hospitals. However, with the increase in qualified, experienced, and well-trained technicians, many other opportunities, at an advanced level, have become available to pharmacy technicians. Previous chapters have discussed the job responsibilities and requirements for an entry-level position. This chapter discusses advanced-level opportunities and the requirements for obtaining these positions.

Advanced-Level Pharmacy Technician Opportunities

Employers hiring pharmacy technicians in an advanced-level pharmacy setting often look for individuals who have had previous formal training and often certification. Technicians applying for the types of positions discussed in the following sections should keep in mind that the more entry-level experience they have, the more competitive their resume will be.

 Tech Note!
Of the fastest growing jobs overall in the United States, the career of pharmacy technician ranks no. 60. It ranks no. 10 for workers age 16 to 24, and no. 22 for women.

Pharmacy Purchasing Agent

With the increasing number of medications being prescribed, pharmacies need at least one employee to do the purchasing for the department. Most commonly found in an institutional setting, pharmacy purchasing agents also can work in retail, nuclear, or mail-order settings (Figure 10-1). Also known as the pharmacy procurement specialist or pharmacy buyer, the pharmacy purchasing agent has several responsibilities, including the following:

- Placing daily orders to keep the department stocked so that patients' needs can be met
- Meeting with pharmaceutical sales representatives to discuss new and alternative medications
- Negotiating prices and contracts
- Planning ahead for the demand for certain products
- Establishing cost-effective practices
- Working closely with pharmacy management to take advantage of cost-saving opportunities

In most facilities the requirements for the position of pharmacy purchasing agent usually include up to 2 years of experience as a pharmacy technician and related on-the-job training. Additional requirements

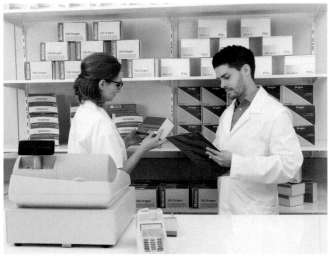

FIGURE 10-1 Placing orders is an important responsibility of the pharmacy purchasing agent. (Copyright © 2014 AndreyPopov, iStock, Thinkstock.com. All rights reserved.)

may include one or more pharmacy technician certifications. Also, an associate's or bachelor's degree, although not required, is often preferred. A person interested in this type of position should have general clerical and computer knowledge and excellent communication skills.

Medication Reconciliation Technician

Pharmacy Times has defined medication reconciliation as "the process of comparing a patient's medication orders with all of the medications that the patient has been taking prior to admission to the hospital."

The pharmacy medication reconciliation technician is an essential factor in patient safety. The goal of this position is to prevent medication errors. Performing **medication reconciliation** (or med recon) can prevent drug omissions, duplications, errors in dosing, and drug-drug interactions (Figure 10-2). Since 2009, the process of medication reconciliation has reduced medication errors (e.g., prescribing, dispensing, and administering) to less than 5%.

The step-by-step med recon process is as follows:
1. Developing a list of current medications.
2. Developing a list of medications to be ordered/ prescribed.
3. Comparing the information on the two lists.
4. Making clinical decisions.
5. Communicating the new list to appropriate individuals.

The technician's responsibilities begin with interviewing patients about their at-home medications, including prescription and over-the-counter medications, vitamins, and herbal supplements. The list

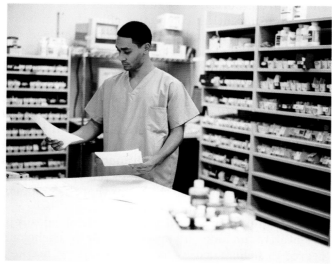

FIGURE 10-2 A medication reconciliation technician must be sure to compare information for all of the patient's prescriptions, to ensure that everything is correct and there are no conflicts or interactions. (Copyright © 2014 Jupiterimages, Photos.com, Thinkstock.com. All rights reserved.)

should include the drug name, dosage, frequency, and any notes included with the medication. The technician may have to call different sources to get all the information required to complete each patient's list. Calls are frequently made to pharmacies, prescriber's offices, long-term care facilities (e.g., assisted living facilities and nursing homes), and other health care settings. Once a patient's list is complete, the technician is responsible for entering the information into the computer system, being careful to avoid any errors, so that it is available to the health care provider. This information helps the provider make informed decisions about the patient's medication regimen.

Although additional education is not required for the position of medication reconciliation technician, the pharmacy technician is always at an advantage if he or she is certified. Medication reconciliation technicians must be familiar with medications and possible side effects and/or drug-drug interactions or food-drug interactions. As a result, the technician must have significant experience in the pharmacy field. Medication reconciliation technicians also must have good communication skills and a strong sense of professionalism because they communicate with the patient in person.

Managed Care Pharmacy Technician

The definition of **managed care** is "an organized health care delivery system designed to improve both the quality and the accessibility of healthcare, including pharmaceutical care, while containing costs." Congress passed the Health Maintenance Organization Act in 1973, creating health maintenance organizations, or HMOs. When HMOs started up, the cost of prescription medications accounted for only about 5% of health care costs. However, because of improved health care and the discovery of more effective treatments for medical conditions and diseases, the number of elderly patients has increased. Most elderly patients take multiple medications, increasing the need for the management of prescription drug use. As a result, **pharmacy benefit management (PBM)** companies were created (e.g., ClearScript). The purpose of PBMs is to develop and manage broad and cost-efficient prescription drug benefits for a large group of patient populations.

The responsibilities of a pharmacist in a PBM setting include building formularies, creating drug benefit plans, and negotiating contracts with community pharmacies. The role of the pharmacy technician in this setting varies even more broadly. Managed care pharmacy technicians work mainly in an office, and their responsibilities include the following:
- Providing benefit information to the patient or client

- Determining the proper use of benefits
- Receiving and entering clinical data
- Processing claims for members according to their benefits
- Troubleshooting rejected claims
- Entering and preparing mail-order prescriptions

Although no additional formal education is required for the position of managed care pharmacy technician, companies usually require experience in the pharmacy field and prefer call center experience. The training required for this position is most commonly company-based training.

Scenario CHECK UP 10-1

John was given the new position of medication reconciliation tech in his department. He really enjoys his new role and wants to stay current with all the new medications coming out. What is the best way for him to stay current with new drugs on the market?

Pharmacy Technician Educator or Trainer

Another specialty area for a pharmacy technician is education or training. An experienced pharmacy technician can take on a role as an educator at an accredited school or lead training for new pharmacy employees.

As a pharmacy technician trainer, a technician must have adequate experience in the practice area he or she is teaching. A trainer's responsibility is to provide on-the-job training for new employees or for technicians in new roles. The training usually continues until the trainer and the new employee both feel confident that the new employee can perform the task with minimal supervision. In some instances, the trainee may have to take a test to prove that he or she understands some tasks and can competently complete the work.

The pharmacy technician educator is most commonly found working for an accredited college or university, either on campus or online. Some community pharmacies (e.g., Walgreens and CVS) offer a training course that is certified by the American Society of Health-System Pharmacists (ASHP) and differs from on-the-job training. The responsibilities of a pharmacy technician educator include teaching pharmacy technician students the knowledge and skills they need to pass an ASHP-approved national certification exam and become certified pharmacy technicians. Subjects taught by pharmacy technician educators include:

- Personal/interpersonal knowledge and skills
- Foundational professional knowledge and skills
- Processing and handling of medications and medication orders

- Sterile and non-sterile compounding
- Procurement, billing, reimbursement and inventory management
- Patient and medication safety
- Technology and informatics
- Regulatory issues
- Quality assurance

Most schools with campuses provide a hands-on laboratory where students learn and demonstrate compounding techniques, intravenous (IV) solution admixture, prescription processing, and the correct way to handle products in the pharmacy setting. All pharmacy technician programs are moving toward becoming ASHP approved, which requires the programs to teach the 45 goals and objectives of an accredited program found on the ASHP website (*www.ashp.org*).

Technicians interested in a rewarding career as a pharmacy technician educator must have national certification, meet their state's regulations for practice, and have a minimum of 3 years of experience in the pharmacy setting. Most employers look for candidates with retail and hospital pharmacy experience, and individuals with an associate's or a bachelor's degree tend to be more competitive.

Pharmaceutical Sales Representative

Although a pharmaceutical sales representative career is a more nontraditional setting for a pharmacy technician, it has its advantages. The pay for a pharmaceutical sales representative is significantly higher than that for a pharmacy technician in a traditional setting. According to the Bureau Labor of Statistics, as of 2012, the median salary for a pharmacy technician is about $29,320; the median salary for a pharmaceutical sales representative is $57,870. Most pharmaceutical companies offer their employees a company car and a great benefits package.

The responsibilities of pharmaceutical sales representatives include traveling to the clients' sites and promoting their assigned medications (Figure 10-3). The representative should have on hand important information on the medication he or she is trying to sell, including up-to-date reports on clinical studies and side effects, in addition to a pharmacological knowledge of the drug. The ultimate goal of a sales rep is to do everything possible to sell specific products, often by persuading the buyer that the products are the best on the market.

The requirements for a pharmaceutical sales representative include an associate's or a bachelor's degree in fields such as biology, chemistry, marketing, business, or a related field. The candidate also must have excellent communication skills. Other qualifications for a candidate in the pharmacy sales industry include self-motivation and self-confidence. Experience in business relations is preferred. This

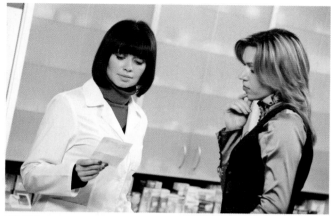

FIGURE 10-3 A pharmacy technician may have the opportunity to become a pharmaceutical sales representative or may be in communication with various sales reps as part of a job in a community pharmacy. (Copyright © 2014 kadmy, iStock, Thinkstock.com. All rights reserved.)

area of pharmacy does not require national certification; however, a candidate who is knowledgeable about the policies and procedures of pharmacy is at an advantage.

Nuclear Pharmacy

As defined by the Department of Pharmacy Practice at Purdue University, nuclear pharmacy is a "a specialty area of pharmacy practice dedicated to compounding and dispensing of radioactive materials for use in nuclear medicine procedures." Nuclear pharmacy developed after the specialty of nuclear medicine was recognized by the American Medical Association (AMA). With the increase in the use of nuclear products, it became evident that individuals were needed to prepare these products. Larger hospitals were able to accommodate this activity. However, many smaller hospitals did not have the staff or capability to handle the radioactive materials, resulting in the concept of centralized, freestanding nuclear pharmacies.

When an order or prescription is written and presented for a particular radioactive product, it is entered by the pharmacist, just as it would be in a traditional setting. The pharmacy technician, taking specific safety precautions, prepares the product as ordered. The final product is checked by the pharmacist and dispensed or shipped to its destination using proper procedures to reduce the risk of exposure.

Radiopharmaceuticals are a special class of drugs used in the nuclear pharmacy. The Mayo Clinic defines radiopharmaceuticals as "agents used to diagnose certain medical problems or to treat certain diseases [that] may be given by mouth, by injection, or placed into the eye or into the bladder." Examples of these types of medications are fluorodeoxyglucose,

diethylenetriamine penta-acetic acid, and pertechnetate, to name a few. The technician must be aware of special risks, such as exposure to radioactive material, when preparing and handling these materials, and specialized training is required for everyone handling these products, including the pharmacist and pharmacy technician. The University of Arkansas for Medical Sciences, along with the University of New Mexico, Purdue University, and Ohio State University, currently are the only schools that offer an approved training program for nuclear pharmacy technicians.

Because of the strict guidelines required to perform the duties of a nuclear technician, many nuclear pharmacies send new employees to attend these programs to complete their training. Some very important competencies required of the nuclear pharmacy technician include:

- A thorough knowledge of the terms, abbreviations, and symbols often used in the prescription of radiopharmaceuticals
- The ability to differentiate between therapeutic and diagnostic use of radiopharmaceuticals
- A knowledge of procedures related to the reconstitution, packaging, labeling, aseptic compounding, and validation of parenteral admixture techniques
- The ability to perform the calculations required to compound the preparation
- A knowledge of the record-keeping procedures for the compounding and dispensing of radiopharmaceuticals, including those involving quality control and testing

Because of the risks associated with the nuclear pharmacy setting, the pay in this area of pharmacy is most often higher than in a traditional pharmacy setting. Furthermore, because of the specialized nature of this practice, opportunities in the nuclear pharmacy setting are very limited.

> **❯ TECHNICIAN** PROFILE
>
> Justin is a nuclear pharmacy technician for a large company. He graduated from a program accredited by the ASHP and obtained his certification from the Pharmacy Technician Certification Board (PTCB) during the program. He had 5 years' experience before obtaining this position, and after he was hired, he went to the University of Arkansas for additional training in nuclear practice. Justin's job includes working with radiopharmaceutical drugs and preparing sterile preparations every day for delivery. He takes orders over the phone and uses his knowledge of pharmacology and aseptic technique to prepare products for techniques such as magnetic resonance imaging (MRI) and other diagnostic procedures. Justin is a very detail-oriented technician who finds his job challenging and rewarding.

John recently had a patient encounter with an individual who was taking more than 15 medications. As a result of his reading and knowledge of some recently released medications, John notices that one of the medications the patient has been taking for a long time is very similar to a new medication she recently started. He is concerned about the duplication. What should he do to help the patient?

Pharmacy Technician Positions of the Future

With changes and improvements in technology come changes and improvements in the practice of medicine, focusing mainly on patient safety.

Remote/Telepharmacy

Since the early 2000s, the National Association of Boards of Pharmacy (NABP) has included **telepharmacy** in its Model Pharmacy Act defining pharmacy practices. The Model Pharmacy Act, updated every August, provides the boards of pharmacy with model language that may be used when developing state laws or board rules. The NABP defines telepharmacy as "the provision of pharmaceutical care through the use of telecommunications and information technologies to patients at a distance."

Telepharmacy has expanded nationwide since its start in rural areas of North Dakota. This system has had positive results serving communities that have been without pharmacies for years. Within the past decade, a total of 16 states have written rules and regulations that allow this practice. Other states are considering moving forward with rules and regulations to begin the telepharmacy practice, and no state laws prohibit the practice of telepharmacy.

As the practice of telepharmacy grows, it is no longer restricted to rural areas. Veterans Affairs health care organizations across the country are using the technology of telepharmacy in their community-based clinics.

A telepharmacy consists of a centralized pharmacy, where the pharmacist is located, and a community pharmacy, where the technician is located. The centralized pharmacy is connected to the community pharmacy via audio and/or visual technology, allowing the pharmacist to communicate with the pharmacy technician while remaining in the community pharmacy (Figure 10-4). The technology also allows the pharmacist to communicate with the patient and to check and verify the prescriptions being dispensed.

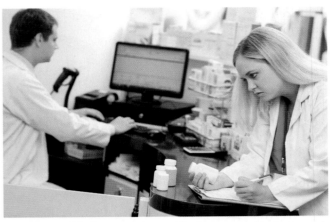

FIGURE 10-4 Telepharmacy helps provide pharmacy services to communities through the use of technology to link pharmacists in a central location with technicians at local pharmacies. (Copyright © 2014 DragonImages, iStock, Thinkstock.com. All rights reserved.)

The job responsibilities of a pharmacy technician in a telepharmacy setting are much like those of the technician in a community or hospital pharmacy. However, because the pharmacist is not physically on site with the technician, a candidate for this position must have experience, self-motivation, and self-confidence. In some states, a "tech-check-tech" procedure is an approved practice when the pharmacist is not available; one technician can check another technician's work. No extra formal education is required for a telepharmacy technician position, although a candidate who is certified is preferable.

Pharmacy Informatics

Pharmacy informatics is a specialty practice of pharmacy that focuses on the use of information technology and drug information to optimize medication use. With the requirements set forth by the government to help reduce medication errors through the use of technology, informatics has become an increasingly important field.

The main responsibility of a pharmacy informatics technician is to provide support for pharmacy information in clinical systems. The technician assists in building new systems to be used by the pharmacy staff and must also be available to help troubleshoot if anything needs to be fixed. In this setting, the technician should build in relevant pharmacy information (e.g., pharmaceutical, formulary, financial, and operational information) into informatics materials.

No additional education is required for the position of pharmacy informatics technician; however, most employers look for candidates with a bachelor's degree, preferably in computer science, and a knowledge of pharmacology. A minimum of 2 years' experience in a community or hospital pharmacy is required for a prospective candidate in pharmacy informatics.

Future Opportunities for the Pharmacy Technician

Advances in technology are making new medical treatments ever more available; a growing population of elderly requires more medications; and the health care industry in general is rapidly expanding. As a result of all these factors, pharmacy technician employment is expected to continue to grow. As new treatments are discovered and new technology is created, the role of the pharmacy technician also will evolve. Education and experience are common requirements for the current and future practice settings of pharmacy, but professionalism is the most important characteristic of a candidate seeking any health care position.

 Tech Note!
The current job growth rate for pharmacy technician is 28.8%.

DO YOU REMEMBER THESE KEY POINTS?

- The roles and responsibilities of a pharmacy purchasing agent
- The requirements for becoming a pharmacy purchasing agent
- The roles and responsibilities of a medication reconciliation pharmacy technician
- The requirements for becoming a medication reconciliation pharmacy technician
- The roles and responsibilities of a managed care pharmacy technician
- The requirements for becoming a managed care pharmacy technician
- The roles and responsibilities of a pharmacy technician educator
- The requirements for becoming a pharmacy technician educator
- The roles and responsibilities of a pharmaceutical sales representative

- The requirements for becoming a pharmaceutical sales representative
- The roles and responsibilities of a nuclear pharmacy technician
- The requirements for becoming a nuclear pharmacy technician
- The roles and responsibilities of a telepharmacy/remote pharmacy technician
- The requirements for becoming a telepharmacy/remote pharmacy technician
- The roles and responsibilities of a pharmacy informatics pharmacy technician
- The requirements for becoming a pharmacy informatics pharmacy technician
- How each additional role of the pharmacy technician plays a part in patient safety

 ## *Scenario* FOLLOW UP

John has been working as a medication reconciliation technician now for 1 year and doing a great job. He has learned so much and has helped many patients with their medications and compliance. Staying current with the medications has really made a difference, and the future is bright.

REVIEW QUESTIONS

Multiple Choice Questions

1. Which pharmacy setting does not have a pharmacist on site?
   A. Pharmacy informatics
   B. Telepharmacy
   C. Nuclear pharmacy
   D. Managed care pharmacy
2. The expected growth rate for the pharmacy technician profession is _____ between 2010 and 2020.
   A. 28%
   B. 30%
   C. 32%
   D. 34%

3. Providing benefit information to the patient is a responsibility of which pharmacy technician practice?
   A. Pharmaceutical sales representative
   B. Managed care pharmacy technician
   C. Pharmacy technician educator
   D. Telepharmacy pharmacy technician
4. Which professional works closely with the pharmacy management in implementing cost-saving opportunities?
   A. Pharmaceutical sales representative
   B. Managed care pharmacy technician
   C. Pharmacy purchasing agent
   D. Nuclear pharmacy technician

5. When health maintenance organizations were created in 1973, the cost of prescription medications was about ____ of health care costs.
   A. 2%
   B. 32%
   C. 10%
   D. 5%

6. A specialty area of pharmacy practice dedicated to compounding and dispensing of radioactive materials is _____.
   A. pharmacy informatics
   B. nuclear pharmacy
   C. managed care pharmacy
   D. none of the above

7. Telepharmacy began in rural areas of:
   A. South Dakota
   B. North Dakota
   C. Maine
   D. Montana

8. Which pharmacy technician position requires the technician to interview patients about their medications?
   A. Pharmaceutical sales representative
   B. Telepharmacy technician
   C. Medication reconciliation technician
   D. Pharmacy informatics technician

9. A pharmacy technician may be employed by the IT department of a health care organization in which type of pharmacy practice?
   A. Telepharmacy
   B. Pharmacy informatics
   C. Pharmacy purchasing agent
   D. Pharmacy technician educator

10. The pharmacy field highly prefers a candidate to have experience in business and business relations for the position of _____.
    A. pharmacy purchasing agent
    B. pharmacy informatics
    C. pharmaceutical sales representatives
    D. pharmacy technician trainer

TECHNICIAN'S CORNER

Pamela is a pharmacy technician in a telepharmacy setting. There has been a power outage in the area. Mr. Jones, a patient, has a very important question for the pharmacist about his medication. Pamela can't get through to the pharmacist, and Mr. Jones is anxious. What can Pamela do to make sure Mr. Jones' question is answered?

Bibliography

Hamlett K: Schools that offer nuclear pharmacy technician programs. (Referenced September 17, 2013.) www.ehow.com/list_7230135_schools-nuclear-pharmacy-tech-programs.html

Levitz MD: Med recon: the role of the pharmacy technician. *Pharmacy Times* (online). (Referenced August 9, 2013.) www.pharmacytimes.com/publications/Directions-in-Pharmacy/2013/August2013/Medication-Recon-The-Role-of-the-Pharmacy-Technician

Mayo Clinic: Radiopharmaceuticals. July 13, 2013. (Referenced September 17, 2013.) www.mayoclinic.com/health/drug-information/DR602307

North Dakota State University: Telepharmacy. June 28, 2013. (Referenced September 17, 2013.) www.ndsu.edu/telepharmacy/

Purdue University, Nuclear Pharmacy Program: What is nuclear pharmacy? (Referenced September 17, 2013.) nuclear.pharmacy.purdue.edu/what.php

U.S. Department of Labor, Bureau of Labor Statistics: Occupational outlook handbook, 2012-2013. (Referenced September 17, 2013.) www.bls.gov/ooh/healthcare/pharmacy-technicians.html

Websites Referenced

www.ashp.org
www.bpsweb.org/specialties/nuclear.cfm
www.himss.org/library/pharmacy-informatics
www.nabp.net
www.pharmacypurchasing.com/
www.ptcb.org
www.thesepht.org

Bulk Repackaging and Non-Sterile Compounding

Karen Davis

OBJECTIVES

Upon completing this chapter, you should be able to do the following:

1. Explain the need for packaging products in the appropriate type and size of container.
2. List the steps in the bulk repackaging of medications.
3. List five reasons pharmacies often repackage bulk medications into unit dose packages.
4. Describe the proper handling of medications during bulk repackaging.
5. Demonstrate how to complete a repacking logbook with the necessary information.
6. Explain the importance of the accurate labeling of pharmaceuticals.
7. Explain the calculations used to determine the beyond-use date when repackaging.
8. List the common reasons for using unit dose medications.
9. Describe the types of containers used for repackaged and compounded medications.
10. Name three advantages of blister card packaging.
11. Define non-sterile compounding.
12. List the common reasons patients need compounded medications.
13. Explain the important considerations in the storage and stability of compounded products.
14. Describe the equipment used in compounding drugs.
15. Differentiate between the types of scales used to weigh compounds.
16. Demonstrate how to complete a compounding sheet with the necessary information.
17. Demonstrate compounding procedures.
18. Describe the types of dosage forms compounded for animal use.

TERMS AND DEFINITIONS

Bubble pack (blister card) A preformed card with 28-, 30-, and 31-day depressions that can hold medications; the medication is sealed into the pack with a foil card backboard; this type of packaging usually is used for long-term care medications

Bulk repackaging The process by which the pharmacy transfers a medication manually or by means of an automated system from a manufacturer's original container to another type of container

Calibration The markings on a measuring device

Compounding The act of mixing, reconstituting, and packaging a drug

Compounding record (CR) The form that documents a non–sterile compounding process

Cream A hydrophilic base

Elixir A base solution that is a mixture of alcohol and water

Emulsion A mixture of two or more liquids that do not usually blend using a stabilizing agent; the process of making an emulsion is called emulsification

Excipient An inert substance added to a drug to form a suitable consistency for dosing

FDA Acronym for the U.S. Food and Drug Administration

Formulation record (FR) A document similar to a recipe that is used in the preparation of non-sterile compounds

Good Manufacturing Practices (GMP) Federal guidelines that must be followed by all entities that prepare and package medication or medical devices

Hydrophilic Having a strong affinity for water; any substance that easily mixes in water

Hydrophobic Lacking an affinity for water; any substance that does not mix or dissolve in water

Mortar and pestle A bowl and tool with a rounded knob used to grind substances into fine powder or to mix liquids

Non–sterile compounding The compounding of two or more medications in a non-sterile environment (no clean room or hood is required)

Ointment A hydrophobic product, such as petroleum jelly

Oleaginous base An ingredient used in compounding that does not dissolve in water

Periodic automatic replacement (PAR) level A minimum set amount of stock that must be kept on hand

Punch method Manual filling of capsules with powdered medication that has been premixed

Reconstitution The mixing of a liquid and a powder to form a suspension or solution

Solute The ingredient that is dissolved into a solution

Solution A water base in which one or more ingredients are dissolved completely

Solvent The greater part of a solution that dissolves a solute

Strip pack (unit dose pack) A strip of heat-sealed packets, each holding one tablet or capsule; used in the bulk repackaging process

Suspension A solution in which the powder does not dissolve into the base; the solution must be shaken before use

Syrup A sugar-based liquid

Triturate To grind or crush powder, such as a tablet, into fine particles

Troche A flat, disklike tablet that dissolves between the gum and cheek

Unit dose A single dose of a drug

Introduction

Scenario:

Judy recently began her career as a technician at a long-term care pharmacy. She graduated from a technician training program accredited by the American Society of Health-System Pharmacists (ASHP). She is cross-trained in many different areas, including order entry, repackaging, extemporaneous compounding, and intravenous (IV) admixture. During her training, she compounded many different dosage forms, such as troches, ointments, creams, and suspensions, in an actual laboratory setting. What are the advantages of this type of hands-on training?

There are several different pharmacy settings, and each stocks specific types of medications and dosage forms that best suit its functions. This chapter discusses methods of providing single or unit doses for patients in institutional settings such as hospitals, nursing homes, or long-term care facilities.

Repackaging medications into single doses, known as **bulk repackaging**, and preparing patient-specific medication doses or formulas, known as **non–sterile compounding**, are two common tasks performed in modern pharmacies. **Compounding** may be done in a specialty or compounding pharmacy or in a community or retail pharmacy that provides this service. These pharmacies are equipped to prepare a wide assortment of solutions, ointments, creams, suppositories, and other drug delivery systems. Compounding pharmacies also prepare medications in various dosage forms and strengths for animals. Although the types of products compounded may differ, many of the same rules apply for medications compounded for both humans and animals. This chapter covers the skills, formulas, equipment, procedures, and documentation necessary for repackaging and compounding nonsterile products.

Bulk Repackaging

Institutional pharmacies often purchase medication in bulk quantities. These are large-count bottles, containing up to 1000 doses each, that are sold at a much lower cost because of their size. For example, a bottle of 100-count aspirin 81-mg tablets can be packaged into 100 individual containers. The department employs technicians to repackage these medications into single doses, or what is commonly referred to as "unit dose medication," to save a substantial amount of money and to create an inventory of medications for the automated dispensing machines. These unit doses are dispensed to specific patients one dose at a time when they are needed per the physician's order. Even liquids can be divided into single 15- to 30-mL dose cups to allow the nurse to dispense just the correct amount for a single dose. This process is called bulk repackaging, and it can be done manually or by means of an automated system, transferring medications from a manufacturer's original container to another type of container before the need arises to dispense a prescriber's order. Prepackaged medications may be in unit dose, single dose, bubble or blister pack, or in a container used in a traditional dispensing system.

One dose is referred to as a **unit dose**. Hospitals use unit dose containers; they order them from the manufacturer and make their own when necessary. These include **unit dose packs** or **strip packs** and liquid cups that contain one medication for one dose. Nursing and home health care facilities may use a **blister card** or **bubble pack** (i.e., punch cards), which may contain one to several tablets or capsules for dosing several days of medication.

Only one drug product at a time should be prepackaged in a specific work area. All federal and state laws and regulations must be followed. Label requirements include the proprietary and nonproprietary names, dosage form, strength, strength of an individual dose, total contents delivered, beyond-use date, and lot number. Proper procedures must be followed in the repackaging of medications; these require accuracy, technique, and documentation.

The following are five possible reasons a pharmacy may repackage bulk medication:

1. Certain medications are not available unit dosed.
2. The cost of repackaging bulk medication may be less than purchasing it unit dosed.
3. Repackaging may allow the pharmacy to provide a patient with a new medication more quickly, rather than having to order the drug and wait for it to be delivered.
4. Labeling each individual dose reduces the chance of errors.
5. If unit dose medication is not used, it can be returned to stock and used for another patient at a later time.

Although packaging guidelines are not exactly the same between pharmacies and manufacturers, both entities must use good manufacturing practices. **Good Manufacturing Practices (GMP)** are guidelines established by the U.S. Food and Drug Administration (**FDA**) to guarantee safe and effective products for consumers. Examples of GMP guidelines that the technician and pharmacist should follow when preparing unit dose medications are listed in Table 11-1. GMP guidelines that should be followed when repackaging include the type of packaging used. Some medications degrade upon exposure to sunlight. These products must be packaged in amber-colored bottles or vials. Examples of the types of containers used in repackaging are listed in Table 11-2. Each type of container holds specific amounts and types of medications (Figure 11-1). Liquids normally are placed in glass or plastic bottles or plastic or foil cups. Tablets and capsules usually are placed in individual or strip packs (Figure 11-2).

 Tech Note!

It is common practice to use only amber-colored containers to avoid possible degradation of medication, although clear unit dose packs are available.

Bulk Repackaging Equipment

Types of unit dosing equipment vary, depending on the amount of drugs to be repackaged. Large

TABLE 11-1

Examples of Good Manufacturing Practice Guidelines for Repackaging

Item	Guidelines
Drugs and labels	All medications must be checked by a registered pharmacist
Equipment	In good condition and clean
Beyond-use date	One year from the date repackaged or the expiration date on the manufacturer's container, whichever is earlier (unless stated otherwise in the manufacturer's literature)
Package	Appropriate for the drug
Preparation	Not more than one item prepared at a time
Records	All items repackaged are logged for reference

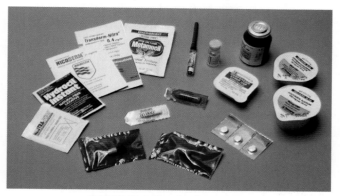

FIGURE 11-1 Sample of containers.

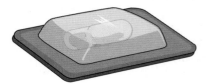

FIGURE 11-2 Sample of a blister pack container for one unit dose.

pharmacies that supply many patient medications may use automated packaging machines. These machines not only fill the unit dose containers, but also may generate bar coded labels for the drugs and apply them to the containers as they pass through the machine (Figure 11-3). Other types of equipment are much less high-tech. A technician can manually place each tablet or capsule into the individual blister pack and then apply the label. Although this type of repackaging is considered nonsterile, the technician should carefully use appropriate aseptic techniques to keep the process of preparing medications as clean as possible.

TABLE 11-2

Unit Dose Containers

Type of Container	Medication Types	Volume/Size
Plastic cups	Liquids, suspensions	5, 10, 15, 30 mL
Syringes	Parenterals, oral liquids, transdermal gels	0.5, 1, 3, 5, 10, 15, 20, 30, 60 mL
Oral syringes	Liquids	1, 3, 5, 10 mL
Heat-sealed strip packs	Tablets, capsules, troches	1 unit dose
Amber blister packs	Tablets, capsules	1 unit dose
Various sizes of bubble packs	Tablets, capsules, troches	1 to 3 medications
Amber glass	Liquids	5, 10, 25, 30 mL
Applicators	Suppositories, creams, ointments	1 application
Foil cups	Liquids, suspensions	5, 10, 30 mL
Plastic suppository shells	Suppositories	1- to 5-g sizes in different colors

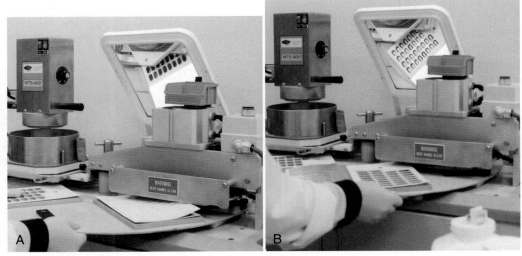

FIGURE 11-3 A technician is responsible for the proper preparation and labeling of all repackaged medications. **A,** The empty medication card is rotated under the hopper, where the medication is placed into the card. The medication card is then rotated to the heating element, where the seal is made to enclose each tablet. **B,** The technician uses a mirror to verify that each sheet is filled completely.

Bulk Repackaging Techniques

Sterile technique is not required for repackaging. However, technicians must observe the following rules for garments, techniques, and equipment to ensure that the environment is as clean as possible:

- Wear a lab coat.
- Pull the hair back.
- Wash the hands.
- Wear a face mask when appropriate.
- Wear gloves if the tablets or capsules will be touched.
- Use a pill counting tray and spatula if the tablets will be dispensed from the tray.

All equipment should be kept clean and in good condition at all times. The process of repackaging should take place in a designated area of the pharmacy, away from high-traffic areas. This reduces airflow over the medication, which may cause contamination. If the technician is using manual methods to load medications into blister packs, it is important that he or she wear gloves after washing the hands. If a pill tray is used to guide tablets or capsules into their containers, the tray should be washed with alcohol after each use. If tablets or capsules are to be unit dosed, it is important to have enough packages and labels ready for use. In addition to having these supplies, keeping medications separate from one another is important. Only one item at a time should be prepared because leaving multiple drugs on a countertop leads to errors. Keeping the area clean and well organized not only helps avoid contamination of drugs, but also reduces the chance of errors.

Tech Note!

To reduce cross-contamination of patients' prescriptions, pill counting trays should be cleaned after each use. If residue is left behind on the pill counter and the next patient is allergic to the previously counted medication, that patient may have an allergic reaction. When chemotherapy medication is counted, a tray marked specifically for counting chemotherapeutic drugs should be used to avoid cross-contamination. All trays are cleaned with alcohol prep pads.

Documentation

Keeping track of the products you are repackaging is a major step that must not be overlooked. Just as manufacturers must document all drugs they have packaged, so must the pharmacy. If a manufacturer recalls a drug that has been repackaged, it is essential to have an accurate count of how many unit doses were made with the recalled product and to be able to identify them by the lot number on each. Therefore, documentation for repackaged drugs must include the information shown in Table 11-3. Table 11-4 provides examples of how the drug manufacturers' names normally are abbreviated. It is important to enter as much information as possible on the unit dose log record, which is usually a separate binder used for record keeping. Figure 11-4 shows an example of a unit dose log record.

Scenario CHECK UP 11-1

Today Judy is assigned to work in the repackaging station. As she gets ready to begin her shift, she notices that her co-worker is filling blister packs by hand without wearing gloves. Judy knows that even though repackaging is considered non-sterile, gloves should be worn to limit contamination possibilities. Should Judy discuss this with her co-worker? What is the best way to handle this situation?

Labeling and Checking Bulk Repackaged Medications

Common dosage forms of drugs that normally are repackaged in a pharmacy include oral medications such as tablets, capsules, and liquids. Tablets may be cut in half and repackaged per facility protocol.

Many different types of computer labeling programs are used to generate unit dose labels in the pharmacy. The pharmacy technician is responsible for determining which drugs are needed to replenish the pharmacy stock according to **periodic automatic replacement (PAR) levels** and then preparing the necessary medications. Technicians must calculate the correct beyond-use date, document the

TABLE 11-3

Example of Unit Dose Record Log Sheet Information*

Item	Description
Date	Date the drug is repackaged, which includes day, month, and year
Drug	Drug name, usually by generic and then brand name if indicated on log sheet
Dosage form	Tablet, capsule, spansule, troche, suspension, elixir, solution
Manufacturer	Manufacturer of drug, usually abbreviated
Manufacturer's lot number	Control number located on side of label or on bottom of bottle
Manufacturer's expiration date	Located with lot number; remember that if the date indicates only the month and year, the drug is good through the end of the month
Pharmacy lot number	Each item repackaged in the pharmacy is given a number consecutive to the previous batch prepared
Pharmacy beyond-use date	One year from the date packaged or the expiration date on the manufacturer's container, whichever is earlier
Technician	Must initial logbook entry
Pharmacist	Each item repackaged must be checked off by a pharmacist

*Much less information is required on the label of the unit dose item than in the logbook, but it is just as important. The components necessary on a typical unit dose label include the name of the drug, generic name, trade name (the trade name commonly given for easy identification of the proper medication), strength, dosage form, lot number, and beyond-use date.

essential information, generate the labels, fill the medication, and apply the label neatly on the container. Finally, the pharmacist checks the completed work to ensure that the label, drug, and logging of the medication are correct.

In specific situations, a technician who has received specialized training may check another technician's work; this is referred to as tech-check-tech. Certain states allow pharmacy technicians to check the work of other technicians. This is limited to checking repackaged unit doses, floor stock, and patient medication drawers. Even if your state has approved the use of the tech-check-tech process, each pharmacy can choose whether to adopt the process and provide the necessary training (see Chapter 3).

Storage and Stability

Medications in a solid form (e.g., tablets) usually have a longer shelf life than liquid forms because it

TABLE 11-4

Examples of Manufacturer Abbreviation Codes

Manufacturer	Code	Manufacturer	Code
3M Pharmaceuticals	3MP	Johnson & Johnson	JJ
Abbott Laboratories	ABB	Lederle	LED
A H Robins	ROB	Marion Merrell Dow	MMD
AstraZeneca	AZN	Mead Johnson Nutritionals	M/J
Barr Laboratories	BRR	Merck & Co	MSD
Bausch & Lomb	B-L	Novartis Pharmaceuticals	NVR
Bayer Pharmaceuticals Corp	BYR	Novo Nordisk	NNP
Boehringer Ingelheim	B-I	Novopharm	NOV
Burroughs Wellcome	BW	Parke-Davis	P-D
Ciba Pharmaceuticals	CIB	Pfizer Pharmaceuticals	FD
Colgate Oral Pharmaceuticals	COP	Pharmacia & Upjohn	UPJ
Dey LP	DEY	Procter & Gamble	PG
DuPont Pharmaceuticals	DUP	Purdue Pharma	PUR
Econo Med Pharmaceuticals	ECO	Roche Laboratories	ORC
Eli Lilly and Company	LY	Roxane Laboratories	ROX
Endo Pharmaceuticals	END	Rugby Laboratories	RUG
Eon Laboratories	EON	Sandoz	SAN
Fujisawa Pharmaceutical	FUJ	SmithKline Beecham Pharmaceuticals	SKF
G & W Laboratories	G&W	Taro Pharmaceuticals	TRO
Geigy Pharmaceuticals	GEI	Teva Pharmaceuticals	TEV
Geneva Pharmaceuticals	GG	Upsher Smith Laboratories	UPS
GlaxoWellcome	GLX	Wyeth-Ayerst	WY
Hoechst Marion Roussel	HMR	Zenith Goldline Pharmaceuticals	Z/G
ICN Pharmaceuticals	ICN		

	Date	Drug (generic)	Strength	Dosage form	Amount	MFG	MFG lot#	MFG exp date	Pharmacy expiration date	Pharmacy lot #	Tech	RPH
1	2/11/2015	aspirin	81 mg	tab	100	Bayer	JGH405	7/15/2012	Jun-16	A1001	LP	TG
2	2/12/2015	perphenazine	2 mg	tab	100	Schering	XYZ124	12/1/2012	Jul-16	A1002	TK	DS
3												
4												
5												
6												
7												
8												
9												

FIGURE 11-4 Example of a unit dose log record.

 Tech Alert!

PAR levels are set amounts of drugs or equipment that must be kept in stock at all times. All departments have PAR levels. Stock is normally ordered on preprinted sheets that list the PAR level and have a space for entering the amount of medication needed to replenish the PAR level.

is easier for a liquid product to degrade or for its components to separate. The FDA is responsible for providing guidelines for all manufacturers that package medications. Expiration dates are determined on the basis of tests conducted by manufactur-ers and the FDA; however, these rules do not apply to medications repackaged in a hospital setting for individual patient use. *Once the medication is removed from its original packaging, the expiration date changes.* The beyond-use dates assigned to repackaged products are established according to the guidelines in *United States Pharmacopeia <795>,* "Pharmaceutical Compounding—Nonsterile Preparations" (USP <795>). Items repackaged for use in a hospital or for a specific patient's use cannot be mass produced. Only drug manufacturing companies following FDA guidelines may mass produce medications.

Expiration Dates and Beyond-Use Dating

There is an important distinction between "expiration" dates and "beyond-use" dates. Expiration dates are assigned by the manufacturer. When reading a manufacturer's expiration date, such as 9/15, it means that the drug is effective through the last day of the month, in this case September 2015. Beyond-use dates are calculated by the pharmacy when repackaging or compounding medications. Assigning beyond-use dates is an important process. Once a bulk bottle is opened and the medication is repackaged, the manufacturer's expiration date may no longer be valid.

Determining Beyond-Use Date

The beyond-use date (BUD) of a repackaged nonsterile solid or liquid dose is one year from the date repackaged or the expiration date on the manufactuer's container, whichever is earlier (unless otherwise stated in the manufacturer's literature). The manufacturer's expiration date is the exact amount of time the drug is usable. Once repackaged, this may be different. This applies to unit dosing as well as filling prescriptions in a retail pharmacy. Example 11-1 shows this calculation for proper dating.

EXAMPLE 11-1: BEYOND-USE DATING

Acetaminophen 500-mg tablets
Today's date: August 15, 2015
Per the manufacturer, the medication expires in December 2018

Because the manufacturer's expiration date is more than 1 year away, you may give this drug a 1-year beyond-use date of August 15, 2016.

 Tech Alert!

Proper repacking techniques are paramount during the preparation of unit dose medications. Gloves must be worn, and the pill counting tray or device should be cleaned between uses to avoid cross-contamination.

Scenario CHECK UP 11-2

Judy continues her work at the long-term care pharmacy. She is busy finishing up the repackaging for the day. It is her responsibility to check her partner's work before it goes to the pharmacist for final approval. Judy notices that the beyond-use dates have been calculated incorrectly. What steps should she take to correct this error? What if the mistake had been overlooked entirely?

Long-Term Care Packaging

Often patients need their medications packaged in 28- to 31-day cards for ease of individual administration and accuracy in dosing. The method is often referred to as "blister packing" or "bubble packaging." The medications prescribed by a physician are put into individual pockets in a card that holds a month's worth of medication. Morning doses and the night doses can be placed in different cards, and each dose is put in an individual pocket. This method has many advantages for patients and health care providers. For example, it makes compliance easier for patients in taking their medication correctly, and it allows timely monitoring by health care team members. Also, the unsteady hands of an elderly patient can get one tablet from the card without spilling the entire contents of a bottle or touching the other tablets in the card. If a dose is changed (and with long-term care patients this is often the case due to their chronic or multiple disease states), the remaining uncontaminated medications in the card can be returned and reused. The card is a visible way to easily identify missed doses and to aid the patient in medication compliance.

Non–Sterile Compounding

History

The art of compounding dates back more than 4000 years, beginning with medicinal mixtures using plants, animals, and minerals. Historians have found recipes for various treatments written on scrolls from 1500 BC, and **mortars and pestles** have been unearthed that were used in the early Egyptian and Roman societies. Even throughout recent civilization, pharmacists compounded each prescription individually. In the United States the first pharmacopoeia was published in 1820 and listed more than 80% of the prescriptions that were made; all were compounded products at that time. As the pharmaceutical business grew, more drugs were manufactured in common dosages by drug companies, which reduced the number of products that needed to be compounded by the pharmacy. It was not until the late 1990s that compounding once again became popular.

Premade dosages are not always appropriate for everyone; each person is different because of other concurrent conditions or physiological factors that affect the drug prescribed. This is evident in pediatrics, where dosages must be calculated and provided based on the weight of the child because the metabolic rate of children is quite different from that of adults. Dosages that are much easier for a child to take also are needed. Examples of these dosage forms

BOX 11-1

Why Compound Medications?

Medications may need to be compounded by a pharmacy for several reasons, including the following:

- The medication is no longer manufactured by the drug company.
- The patient is allergic to a preservative, dye, or other additive in the normal drug.
- A specialized dosage or strength is needed for a patient with unique needs (e.g., an infant or a patient with diabetes).
- Combining several medications will increase patient compliance.
- The patient cannot ingest the normal dosage form.
- The medication requires flavorings and/or additives to make it more palatable for patients, most often children.

BOX 11-2

Examples of Dosage Forms That Can Be Compounded

Topicals
- Creams
- Gels, jellies
- Ointments
- Pastes
- Sticks

Oral Liquids
- Elixirs
- Solutions
- Suspensions
- Syrups
- Tinctures

Oral Solids
- Capsules
- Lollipops
- Lozenges
- Popsicles
- Tablets
- Troches
- Effervescent tablets

Suppositories
- Rectal
- Urethral
- Vaginal

include popsicles and lozenges that deliver medications. Hospice patients, who may not be able to swallow oral medications or have injections, require a different dosage form that is not available by a manufacturer. A list of reasons for compounding medications is given in Box 11-1. People who would benefit from a combination drug that is not already packaged can have a combination drug made specifically for them. For example, women who are menopausal can have compounded medications made specifically for their hormone supplementation needs.

Use of Non–Sterile Compounding

Non–sterile compounding consists of compounding two or more medications in a nonsterile environment. Aseptic technique (sterile compounding) is discussed in depth in Chapter 12. Most community pharmacies do not have the staff, the wide variety of supplies, or the time to compound various dosage forms and medication strengths. This type of task is performed by specialized compounding pharmacies. However, the average technician will perform some basic types of nonsterile compounding when working in institutional settings or community pharmacies. Compounding standards, common preparations prepared in most pharmacies, and types of items prepared in specialized compounding pharmacies are discussed.

The FDA requires that nonsterile compounded products meet the *United States Pharmacopoeia: National Formulary (USP-NF)* <795> standards, although they do not specifically regulate compounding. Compounding pharmacies must follow each state's board of pharmacy regulations, in addition to USP-NF <795> standards. Other standards that must be followed involve the quality and stability of ingredients, assigning BUDs, the policies and procedures used during preparation, the equipment required, and the quality control and documentation guidelines that must be followed (per the board of pharmacy). Box 11-2 lists the types of dosage forms that can be compounded under USP-NF <795>.

Determining Beyond-Use Dating for Nonsterile Compounds

Unless there is specific information available in the literature for a particular nonsterile compounded drug preparation, USP <795> provides general guidelines to follow. The USP <795> guidelines for determining beyond-use dating for non–sterile compounding are shown in Table 11-13; however, more stringent specific state requirements may dictate the method used. This information should be outlined in each facility's policies and procedures manual. According to USP <795>, a nonsterile compound has three main parts: the active ingredient, medication, or active pharmaceutical ingredient (API); the inactive ingredient; and the diluent or vehicle. When the shelf life or BUD of a compound is determined, the expiration dates for these three parts are taken into consideration. Nonaqueous formulations should be assigned a beyond-use date that is the sooner of 6 months or the earliest expiration date of any of the ingredients. Beyond-use dating should be no more than 14 days (refrigerated) for formulations that contain water. All other formulations have a recommended beyond-use dating of 30 days or until the end of therapy, whichever comes first.

Compounding Area

Certain criteria established by USP <795> must be met in setting up a compounding area. Although the compounding area and its supplies can be located in a pharmacy, the compounding area should be away from areas where normal prescription processing, chemicals, dust, or open boxes are located. The compounding surface area should be nonporous, smooth, and in good condition, and provide good lighting. Overhanging shelves or ledges should not be located over the workspace because dust can accumulate in these spaces. There should be a sink located close to the compounding site for hand washing and cleaning. When in use, all surfaces should be cleaned on a routine basis, between compounding procedures and at the beginning and the end of the day, to avoid cross-contamination. The temperature and humidity should be monitored to avoid decomposition of chemicals.

Equipment

Types of compounding equipment include personal protective equipment, measuring and weighing devices, an assortment of containers, and labels. The minimum required equipment list is provided by each state board of pharmacy (see your state's requirements), although pharmacies may want to stock additional types of equipment for preparing products (Table 11-5). This determination normally is made on the basis of the amounts and types of nonsterile products the pharmacy provides. The maintenance, calibration, and cleaning of each piece of equipment is required according to the manufacturer's specifications, and documentation, in the form of logs, is required by USP <795> (Figure 11-5). Various types of compounding equipment that are required for specific uses are discussed in the following sections.

Personal Protective Equipment

Personal protective equipment is used to ensure the sterility of the product and to protect the technician from spills while working. The following are considered necessary personal protective equipment:

- Gloves
- Goggles
- Gown
- Hair cover
- Lab coat
- Mask
- Shoe covers

Measuring Devices

Graduated cylinders (Figure 11-6) are available in various sizes (from 1 mL to 1 L), types (e.g., glass and plastic), and shapes (e.g., conical and cylindrical) to measure liquids (Table 11-6). Other types of measuring instruments can range from syringes (for small volumes) and pipettes (for minute volumes) to large automated measuring machines. These electronic machines, ointment mills, and capsule-filling machines are used in compounding pharmacies to prepare large amounts of medications. Capsule-filling machines normally fill anywhere from 100 to 300 capsules at a time.

Mixing Equipment

Various sizes of glass and porcelain mortars and pestles are necessary, depending on the types of ingredients to be prepared (Figure 11-7). Various spatula types include metal and plastic (Table 11-7). Automated mortars and pestles, used for ointments and creams, have settings for mixing times and speed (Figure 11-8). These allow the preparer to set up the machine for a time to mix according to a formulation compound or recipe. An automated ointment mill also is available for mixing creams and ointments (Figure 11-9).

Weighing Equipment

One of the most expensive pieces of compounding equipment is the balance or scale used to weigh powders. Scales differ in their range of weight and style. A Class III balance, also called a Class A balance (Figure 11-10, *A*), is a torsion balance. This type of scale uses a counterbalance (weights) to determine the weight of the substance being measured, and is referred to as a mechanical scale (required by most state boards of pharmacy). This type of scale has special weights that are labeled in a range of milligrams and grams (Figure 11-10, *B*). The minimum weighable quantity for a Class A balance is 120 mg. Weights used on this type of scale should be stored in a hard-shelled container and should be handled only with the accompanying tweezers.

Another style of balance is the analytical electronic balance (Class II) (Figure 11-10, *C*), which provides a digital readout of the weight. No weights are used with this balance; instead, the calibrations are electronic. Digital balances are more commonly used than two-pan torsion balances. They can weigh heavier substances than the Class III balance, as shown in the following comparisons:

- Digital balance/Class II: Capacity 100 g; readable to 0.0001 g (e.g., Sartoris GD503)
- Digital balance/Class II: Capacity 200 g; readable to 0.01 g (e.g., PCE-LSM200)
- Class III balance: Capacity 60 to 120 g; sensitivity of 6 mg or less (e.g., DRX-3 Torbal)

Appropriate calibration, care, and cleaning of these sensitive instruments are the responsibility of

TABLE 11-5

Examples of Compounding Equipment

Equipment	Use/Description
Autoclave	For sterilization
Balance	Class A balance, torsion digital balance
Beakers	1, 5, 10, 20, 50, 100, 500, 1000 mL
Blender	Electric
Capsule molds	For making multiple capsules
Containers	Spray bottles, ointment tubes, plastic jars, vials, bottles, stick containers, ophthalmic containers
Crimpers	For sealing tubes and glass bottles
Disposable weighing devices	Papers (glycerin), boats (plastic)
Droppers	Sterile and nonsterile
Filters	0.5 and 0.2 micrometers
Foil wraps	For wrapping suppositories
Funnels	For transferring liquids
Glass stirring rods	For stirring/mixing liquids
Glass tile	For mixing ingredients
Graduated cylinders	For performing various measurements
Heat gun	For sealing packages
Hot plate	For melting ingredients
Magnetic stir plate	Automatically stirs for long periods
Magnetic stirrers	Used in beaker to stir contents
Metal measuring scoop	For transferring powders to scale
Molds	Capsules, tablets, lozenges, troches, suppositories, popsicles, lollipops
Mortar and pestle	Glass, porcelain
Ointment mill	For increasing the overall surface area of the active substance, thereby maximizing the benefit to the patient; produces very smooth and elegant ointments
Paper sheets 12 × 12	For levigation and mixing ingredients
Pipettes	For adding minute amounts of liquids: 50 micrograms (mcg) to 1 mL
Refrigerator	For storage
Rubber grippers	For removing glass from hot plates
Sieves	For removing particles
Sink	For washing all equipment
Solvents	For cleaning surface area of compounding room
Spatulas	For moving and mixing ingredients
Thermometers	For ingredients that must be prepared at a certain temperature
Tongs	For removing hot contents
Wash bottle	For rinsing
Weights	Brass weights used on Class A balance

the person using them and should be performed before, during, and after use.

 Tech Alert!
Always place and use a scale outside of direct airflow to obtain the most accurate reading.

Additional Supplies

Mold Forms

Various suppository molds can be used to prepare suppositories. These include the traditional metal molds, in which cavity openings range from 1 to 2.5 g. Different mold sizes (6 to 100) allow for different numbers of suppositories to be prepared. The molds are held together by nuts and screws while the ingredients solidify. Another option is hard rubber molds, which are similar to the metal molds. Hard rubber molds are held together by screws that are loosened when the suppositories are solid. Flexible rubber molds in strips that can be placed in the refrigerator, if necessary, are also available. When strips of molds are used, the exact number of suppositories can be removed to fill a prescription, and the remainder can be left in the refrigerator for the next order.

Excipients

Excipients are inert (not medicinally active) ingredients that are added to preparations to achieve the required consistency, effectiveness, and functional

Title of SOP: Room Cleaning Procedures—Compounding Room

SOP No. 5.008

Original: ☐ Yes ☐ No   Revision: ☐ Yes ☐ No   Revision No.: _____

Responsibility:

The pharmacist-in-charge and the support staff or contract labor are responsible for this procedure.

Purpose:

The purpose of this standard operating procedure is to establish appropriate guidelines and documentation for the maintenance of the compounding room.

Equipment/Supplies Required:

- Cleaning items designated for compounding room cleaning only—mop, bucket, floor soap, proper cleaning attire
- Cleaning Maintenance Log

Procedure:

General

A. Use cleaning items that are designated for compounding room cleaning only. ***WARNING:*** *Do not use cleaning items that are designated for clean room cleaning only. Do not perform cleaning procedures during a compounding process.*

B. Clean areas immediately following any repairs or spills.

Preparation of Cleaning Solutions

A. Prepare cleaning solutions on the day of use. ***WARNING:*** *Do not combine cleaning solutions or use in concentrations other than those outlined in the appropriate SOPs and/or the manufacturer's instructions.*

B. Discard any unused cleaning solutions immediately after the cleaning has been completed.

Cleaning Schedule

A. Document all cleanings on the Cleaning Maintenance Log.

B. Perform the following daily cleaning duties:

    1. Empty all waste receptacles.

    2. Sweep the floors.

    3. Clean the counter tops as needed.

    4. Wash dishes, utensils, and drain items.

C. Perform the following weekly cleaning duties:

    1. Damp mop the floor.

D. Perform the following monthly cleaning duties:

    1. Clean the shelving and items stored on the shelving.

Approved by _____ Date _____

Implemented by _____ Date _____

FIGURE 11-5 Log for cleaning of the compounding room. (Courtesy Karen Davis.)

Continued

Cleaning Maintenance Log								
Room Description: (Check one)	☐ IV room ☐ Compounding laboratory ☐ Anteroom			☐ Ancillary room ☐ IV infusion room				
Check activity as completed								
Month				Year				
	Daily				Weekly	Monthly		
Date	Waste removal	Sweep floors	Clean counter tops	Wash dishes, utensils	Mop floor	Check out-of-date drugs	Clean and disinfect shelves of bulk drug	Signature
1								
2								
3								
4								
5								
6								
7								
8								
9								
10								
11								
12								
13								
14								
15								
16								
17								
18								
19								
20								
21								
22								
23								
24								
25								
26								
27								
28								
29								
30								
31								

Approved by _____ Date _____

Implemented by _____ Date _____

FIGURE 11-5, cont'd

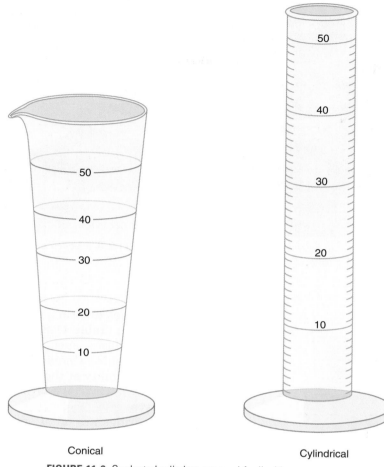

Conical   Cylindrical

FIGURE 11-6 Graduated cylinders are used for liquid measurement.

TABLE 11-6

Types of Graduated Cylinders

Type	Use
Glass	Used for hot liquids or liquids not compatible with plastic devices
Plastic	Used for cold liquids
Cylindrical	Used to measure liquids more accurately
Conical	Wider platform is more stable when measuring viscous liquids and makes it easier to mix solutions; however, because sides flare outward, reading meniscus is more difficult, which affects accuracy of measurement

TABLE 11-7

Types of Compounding Mixing Equipment

Mortars and Pestles

Glass	Used for preparing liquids such as solutions and suspensions and for mixing oily or staining materials
Porcelain	Used for blending powders and pulverizing soft aggregates or crystals

Spatulas

Plastic	Used for mixtures that may react with metal
Metal	Used for mixing ointments or creams and handling dry chemicals
Long (>6 inches)	Used for ointments or creams and powder blends for capsules
Short (≤6 inches)	Used in handling dry chemicals

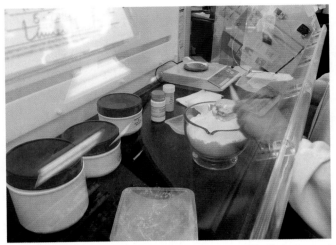

FIGURE 11-7 Mortars and pestles are used to crush solids. Both glass and porcelain types are used in compounding. (Courtesy Karen Davis.)

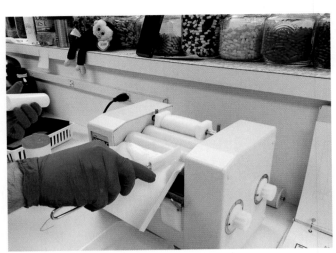

FIGURE 11-9 A three-roll ointment mill in operation. (Courtesy Karen Davis.)

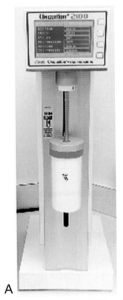

A

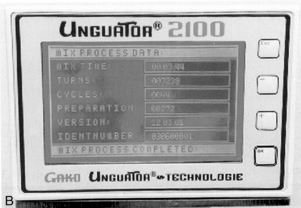

B

FIGURE 11-8 A, Electronic mortar and pestle. **B,** The screen shows a variety of settings for preparing different compounds. (Courtesy Karen Davis.)

properties to form a suitable dosage form for administration (Table 11-8). They are used in a variety of dosage forms, such as liquids, suspensions, tablets, and capsules. Chemicals may be used to alter the pH and solubility of the active medication as needed.

Taste

Flavorings are often added to medications to mask the bad taste of the ingredients. The tongue recognizes four basic tastes: sweet, sour, salty, and bitter. Masking the taste becomes more difficult as the distaste increases. Flavorings such as saccharin impart a bitter taste followed by a sweet taste, whereas sucrose gives an immediate sweet taste. Sucrose flavorings are the most commonly used because of this property. Preservatives can alter the properties of flavorings, causing different results in taste. Many of the flavorings have a color additive; for those that do not, dyes can be used, although they are not absolutely necessary. Colors should match the flavor; for example, cherry flavor should be colored red. Each recipe indicates which flavorings and/or colors can be mixed into the compounded product. Examples of the types of agents used as flavorings when compounding antibiotics, antihistamines, barbiturates, decongestants, and electrolytes are shown in Table 11-9. Considerations must always be given to the stability and solubility of the additives. Also, the patient's record must be checked for any allergies before preparation. Children's medications are often flavored with types of flavors similar to those found in candy and drinks.

Personal Preparation

Before beginning the compounding process, the technician should tie back long hair and put on a lab coat

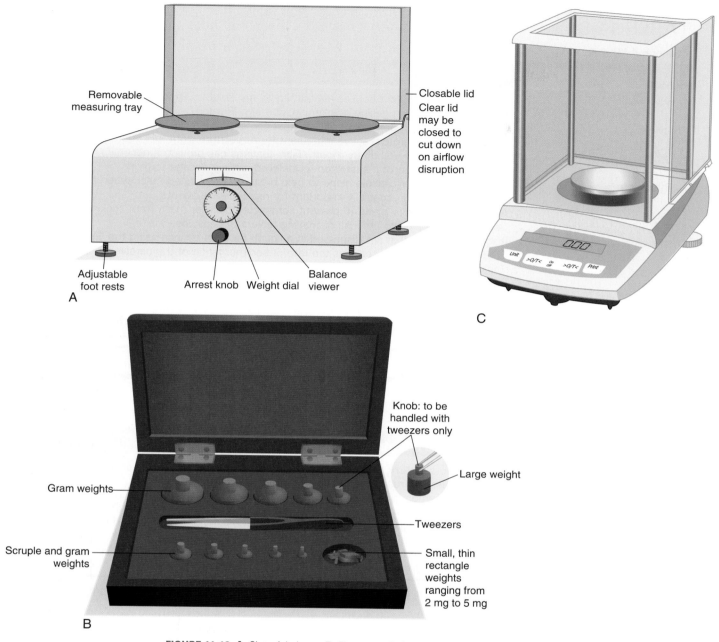

FIGURE 11-10 A, Class A balance. **B,** Pharmaceutical weights. **C,** Analytical balance.

and gloves to reduce contamination of the product. In addition to these personal considerations, a technician who is sick or has any open wounds should not compound any products. For commonly compounded items, pharmacists and technicians use a recipe book or formula cards listing compounds, their weights, and step-by-step instructions. The pharmacy technician should be competent in several skills to reduce the possibility of errors when compounding (Box 11-3).

Weighing Techniques

When using a Class A balance, begin by gathering the necessary ingredients and supplies, such as glycerin paper or weighing boats and weights. The balance has adjustable legs for leveling it on the compounding surface, if necessary. Each balance also has an arrest knob that is used to lock the scale in place, which reduces the possibility of damage to the balance. The proper setup of a balance involves six steps (Procedure 11-1), and each step is critical to

TABLE 11-8

Common Additives

Additive	Description
Gums	Naturally occurring plant derivatives that are water soluble. They provide a variety of properties, including gelling, thickening, and film forming.
Coatings	Surrounding layer of polymeric material that coats a tablet, capsule, or pellet. This is done to change color; protect active ingredient from moisture, light, pH of stomach; hide bad taste or odor when taken by mouth. Film coatings can provide functional properties that enable the creation of a sustained- or delayed-release dosage form.
Disintegrants	Added to a tablet or capsule blend to help break up compacted mass when put into a fluid environment; especially important for rapid-release agents.
Lubricants	Additive for a powder blend to prevent compacted powder mass from sticking to equipment during the process of making tablets or capsules.
Suspending agents	Insoluble particles that are dispersed in a liquid; they act by increasing the viscosity of the liquid vehicle. This reduces the rate of sedimentation of the particles in a suspension.
Plasticizers	Blend of plasticizers in acrylic emulsion coatings. They have a wide variety of functional properties (e.g., retarding drug release) and allow for flexibility in coating.
Emulsifying agents	Maintain dispersion of finely divided liquid droplets in a liquid vehicle; made from two or more immiscible liquids (e.g., water and oil) and can be a liquid or semisolid (creams and lotions).

TABLE 11-9

Common Flavoring Additives for Taste*

Drug Class	Most Suitable Flavorings
Antibiotics	Citrus flavors, cherry, pineapple, orange, berry, banana, strawberry-vanilla, banana-vanilla, lemon custard, fruit cinnamon
Antihistamines	Cherry, cinnamon, grape, lime, peach-orange, raspberry, root beer, wild cherry, apricot
Barbiturates	Lime, orange, banana-vanilla, banana-pineapple, peach-orange, root beer
Decongestants and expectorants	Cherry, lemon, loganberry, gooseberry, orange-peach, apricot, strawberry, pineapple, raspberry, tangerine, custard-mint-strawberry
Electrolytes	Cherry, grape, lemon-lime, raspberry, wild cherry
Geriatrics	Black currant, grenadine-strawberry, lime, root beer, wild strawberry

*Additional flavorings include menthol, monosodium glutamate (flavor enhancer), peppermint oil, spearmint oil, and wintergreen.

obtaining the proper weight of a substance. Inside the container that holds the weights is a pair of tweezers for grasping the brass or metal weights. Use of these tweezers prevents hand oils from being transferred to the surface of the metal. Oils can corrode the metal, altering the exact weight.

Pharmacy balances are very sensitive. Regardless of the substance you are weighing, it is important to keep airflow around the balance to a minimum. Even the motion of a person walking by can set the balance into a rocking motion, making calibration difficult. Pharmacy balances have a glass lid that can be used to impede air currents while compounds are weighed. As the balance levels, it is important to add less and less substance to it. One way of doing this is to use a spatula and pick up a small amount of substance, then lightly tap the side of the spatula (from behind

the substance) to flick on a few granules at a time. This technique is easier with powders than with other substances. Compounding is time-consuming. It is important to always strive for accuracy. Thus, you must take your time.

 Tech Note!

Always place the weights on the right side of the balance using a weighing boat or paper. This is done to ensure continuity of measurement.

Measuring Liquids

Measuring liquids requires a few simple steps to ensure the proper volume. Because water molecules cling to the sides of a container (called *capillary*

BOX 11-3

Technician Competencies for Compounding

To reduce the likelihood of errors and to maximize the quality of the compounded preparation, the pharmacy technician should follow several steps, including the following:

1. Identify the equipment needed to prepare the medication.
2. Wear the proper gear.
3. Wash hands appropriately.
4. Clean the compounding area and necessary equipment with antibacterial solvent.
5. Assemble all necessary materials before beginning the compounding process.
6. Perform all necessary calculations to determine the amounts of ingredients necessary.
7. Determine the intended use, safety, and legal limitations of the prescription to be compounded.
8. Compound only one preparation at a time.
9. Compound the preparation according to the prescription or formula (recipe).
10. Assess the weight variation, consistency of mixture, and the color, odor, clarity, and pH of preparation.
11. Determine the beyond-use dating for the product prepared.
12. Complete the log sheet and add a notation to describe the appearance of the formulation.
13. Label the prescription container, making sure to include all required information.
14. Immediately clean and store all equipment used.
15. Thoroughly clean surface areas.

Before compounding, ensure that you know your state's laws for compounding. If you have any questions on how to prepare a product, ask the pharmacist before you begin the compounding process, not in the middle of it.

PROCEDURE 11-1

Instructions for Using a Class A Balance

GOAL: To learn the steps involved in using a Class A balance.

EQUIPMENT AND SUPPLIES
- Class A balance
- Material to be weighed
- Log to record weight
- Lightweight papers
- Weighing boats
- Weights

PROCEDURAL STEPS

1. Turn the arrest knob to arrest the balance. Make sure the balance is steady on the counter.
2. Level the balance from front to back using the adjustable legs.
PURPOSE: The balance must be level to ensure accuracy.
3. Turn the calibrated dial to zero to set the internal weights.
PURPOSE: The weights must start at zero to ensure accuracy.
4. Level the balance from left to right using the adjustable legs.
PURPOSE: The balance must be level to ensure accuracy.
5. Add lightweight papers or weighing boats to both sides of the balance.
PURPOSE: Papers or weighing boats protect the weighing plates and hold the substance being weighed.
6. "Zero out" the balance.
PURPOSE: This prevents the paper from being included in the weight of the drug.
7. Place weights on the right side of the balance and set the balance to reflect the proper weight.
PURPOSE: The balance should indicate the correct amount of the weights; if it does not, make the necessary adjustments before weighing the material.
8. Place the substance to be measured on the left side of the balance and view the pointer. Add and/or remove material until the pointer is in the center.
PURPOSE: The pointer is in the center if the right side and the left side of the balance contain exactly the same weight.

For more details and to watch a video of this procedure, visit the following website: http://pharmlabs.unc.edu/labs/measurements/balance_operate.htm.

action), the amount of liquid appears to be more than the actual amount. When reading the calibrations of a beaker or graduated cylinder, you must have the liquid at eye level. You must read the graduated cylinder at the bottom of the liquid line, also known as the *meniscus* (Figure 11-11).

When choosing a container in which to measure your liquids, remember that it is best to choose the size closest to the volume required because the calibrations are more accurate than in larger containers. For maximum accuracy in measuring liquids, use the 20% rule: measure no less than 20% of the capacity

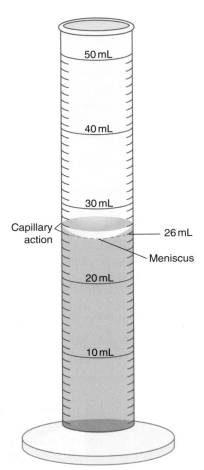

FIGURE 11-11 The meniscus is the level at which liquids are measured and recorded. For accuracy always have the container at eye level when determining the volume.

ingredient or agent dissolved in the solvent; and the **solution** is the result, the final mixture of the solute and solvent. Most solutions are compounded by adding the solute to the solvent in portions for proper mixing or by adding two solutions together. Two of the most important techniques of mixing solutions are to measure carefully and mix thoroughly. Solutions are prepared in all types of pharmacy settings. Always check the final solution for any precipitation or discoloration.

Solubility

A drug's solubility dictates the type of dosage form that must be prepared. For example, if the drug is water soluble, a **syrup** or solution can be prepared; however, if it is insoluble, an **elixir**, a **suspension**, or possibly an **emulsion** can be made. The pH also affects the solubility of a drug; in such cases buffers may be used to maintain the correct solubility characteristics. Buffers are solutions that resist pH changes when either acids or bases are added to the solution. Factors that affect solubility characteristics are listed in Box 11-4.

 Tech Note!

When orders indicate a solution to be a specific strength with instruction to "qs" to a final volume, this means that the solution is to yield a final volume and final strength exactly as ordered by the physician. The "qs" (quantity sufficient) means to add a sufficient quantity of liquid to reach that final required volume.

Reconstituting Premade Suspensions

The only type of compounding that may be done away from the compounding area is the **reconstitution** of premade oral suspensions. Reconstituting involves mixing a diluent (liquid) into a powder to form a solution or suspension. These products are simple to prepare and do not need to be logged or labeled in the same manner as compounded products.

When prepackaged drugs are reconstituted (e.g., an amoxicillin suspension), the label is already

of any graduate. For example, a 100-mL graduated cylinder should be used to measure no less than 20 mL (20% of 100) of liquid. Likewise, a 250-mL cylinder should be used to measure no less than 50 mL (20% of 250). In the case of small or extremely small amounts, a syringe or micropipette is used. It would not be accurate to measure 1 mL of liquid in a 10-mL graduated cylinder because 20% of 10 mL is 2 mL. This amount is much more accurately measured with a 3-mL syringe.

Depending on the type of product being prepared, different techniques are required. Each type of compounded product requires specific steps that must be carefully followed, including appropriate labeling. Pharmacy technicians often prepare compounded products and should be familiar with the behavior of each type of additive and of the final product.

Preparing Solutions

When preparing solutions, you must understand the major parts of the liquid: the **solvent** is the vehicle used to dissolve something; the **solute** is the

TABLE 11-10

Common Auxiliary Labels Placed on Medication Containers

Dosage Form	Auxiliary Label
Suspensions	SHAKE WELL
Ophthalmic preparations	FOR THE EYE
Otic preparations	FOR THE EAR
Ointments, creams, lotions	FOR TOPICAL USE; FOR EXTERNAL USE ONLY
Suppositories	FOR RECTAL USE; FOR VAGINAL USE
Patches	APPLY TO SKIN

BOX 11-5

Tablet Additives

- Diluent bases: These can be combined to increase the firmness of the tablet.
  - Dextrose
  - Lactose
  - Mannitol
  - Sucrose
- For drugs that react chemically with sugars, the following can be added:
  - Bentonite
  - Calcium carbonate
  - Calcium phosphate
  - Kaolin
- Liquids can be added to moisten and mold powder:
  - Mixture of alcohol and water in different percentages (50% to 80% alcohol): Alcohol accelerates drying, and water causes sugar to dissolve and bind the tablet. If the ingredients dissolve in water quickly, adding water can be omitted.

attached to the product. All the technician must do is read the side panel and follow the directions indicating the proper amount of sterile water (SW) to be mixed with the powder. The beyond-use date that must be applied to the product after reconstitution is marked clearly on the side of the medication, which is active as soon as the suspension is mixed. Therefore, after mixing the drug, the technician should write the beyond-use date on the front of the label. In addition, the patient information and any necessary auxiliary labels must be attached (Table 11-10).

Suspensions are different from solutions because they mix a **hydrophobic** (not water soluble) ingredient into a **hydrophilic** (water soluble) solution. When you reconstitute a suspension, if the manufacturer suggests 110 mL of distilled water to be mixed with the powder in the bottle, you should at first add only part of the water, as the manufacturer directs. This allows the powder to mix with the water in enough free space in the bottle; this lower volume in the bottle makes it easier to mix in the remaining amount. The powdered ingredient is suspended in sterile water after mixing. Therefore, all suspensions must be shaken well before each use to mix the powder evenly, allowing delivery of the proper amount of medication. Many antibiotics, but not all, must be refrigerated after mixing.

Solids: Tablets, Capsules, and Lozenges

Tablets, capsules, and lozenges can be compounded by pharmacy technicians. These preparations have the advantage of providing a custom-made medication for each patient's specific needs. Molds are used to make these oral dosage forms. A product can be made accurately using careful measuring, weighing, and mixing procedures. Technicians must have great skill and experience to prepare these dosage forms.

Pharmacies can provide individualized strengths and dosage forms to meet the needs of the patient. Molded tablets can be prepared using a tablet **triturate** mold. Compressed tablets are made using a pellet press or single-punch tablet-making machine. Tablets by far are the most common dosage form used because of their ease of administration; they can be taken orally, sublingually, or as a buccal dose, or they can be prepared similar to troches and wafers.

Molded Tablets

Molded tablets disintegrate quickly when they are exposed to moisture. Because molded tablets are small, they are limited to substances that require a smaller dose. Ingredients used in the preparation of molded tablets include a base and additives (Box 11-5), as well as the active drug.

Tablet Molds. Tablet molds are made of metal and consist of a top plate (i.e., cavity plate) with holes and a bottom plate (i.e., peg plate) with pegs. Capacities for tablet molds can range from 60 to 100 mg.

Steps Necessary for Preparation of Molded Tablets. Because molds have a fixed volume, they must be **calibrated** (Procedure 11-2). This is because each base used in preparing a molded tablet has a different density, which changes the capacity of each hole in the mold plate. Procedure 11-3 presents the process used to compound molded tablets.

Compressed Tablets and Lozenges

To prepare tablets or lozenges, a single-punch tablet press can be used to make one dose at a time, or a

PROCEDURE 11-2

Calibrating the Mold

GOAL: To be able to calibrate the mold before making molded tablets.

EQUIPMENT AND SUPPLIES
- Mold
- Calculator
- Pencil/pen

PROCEDURAL STEPS

1. Make tablets that contain only a powder base first. Weigh the entire batch and then average the weight per tablet.

PURPOSE: It is important to know what each tablet will weigh once it is molded to confirm that it has been properly made.

2. Determine the average weight of only the active drug; fill a few cavities in the mold and average the weight per tablet.

PURPOSE: Knowing the average weight of the active drug can help determine the proper weight of the molded tablet.

3. The quantity of the total prescription is divided by the average weight of each tablet's active ingredient.

PURPOSE: This gives the percentage of the cavity volume required by the active drug, which affects the amount of other material used in the molded tablet.

4. Subtract the percentage in step 3 from 100%; this equals the volume (%) available for the base.

PURPOSE: Knowing the volume is necessary to determine the correct amount of base to include in the molded tablet.

5. Use percentages of both the active drug in the cavity and the base in the cavity to calculate the amount of base and drug to weigh. (For example, if the mold holds 10 cavities, each holding 100 mg, then 1000 mg of mixture is needed to fill the entire mold.) From this calculation, calculate the base and drug to weigh. (For example, multiply 1000 by the two different percentages from steps 3 and 4.)

PURPOSE: This calculation provides the amount of active drug and the amount of base need for the entire batch. Once those amounts have been determined, the mixture can be prepared and placed in the mold (see Procedure 11-3).

6. Prepare 5% to 10% excess mixture .

PURPOSE: Creating excess mixture allows for powder loss and any variance in the capacity of the molds.

For more details and to watch a video of this procedure, visit the following website: http://pharmlabs.unc.edu/labs/tablets/molded.htm.

PROCEDURE 11-3

Compounding Procedure for Molded Tablets

GOAL: To be able to accurately compound pharmaceutically elegant tablets with a mold.

EQUIPMENT AND SUPPLIES
- 80- to 100-mesh sieve
- Tablet mold
- Ointment tile or glass plate
- Hard rubber spatula
- Powder mixture
- Water
- Alcohol

PROCEDURAL STEPS

1. Prepare the powder mixture using proper techniques for that specific recipe; then sift the mixture through the 80- to 100-mesh sieve.

PURPOSE: The sieve is used to reduce the particle size. A good powder formulation has a uniform particle size distribution. If the particle size distribution is not uniform, the powder can segregate according to the different particle sizes, which may result in inaccurate dosing or inconsistent performance.

2. Moisten the mix (alcohol/water) until it adheres to the pestle.

PURPOSE: To make sure the mixture sets up properly.

3. Place the cavity plate on either an ointment tile or a glass plate.

PURPOSE: To make sure the cavity plate is on an even surface before filling.

4. Take the molded form and press the mixture into the cavity plate using a hard rubber spatula. The choice of material for the spatula depends on any reaction with the ingredients.

PURPOSE: To evenly distribute the tablet material throughout the cavity plate.

5. Apply sufficient pressure to each cavity to make sure all cavities are entirely filled.

PURPOSE: To ensure uniformity of all the tablets.

6. Inspect the cavity plate to ensure that all cavities are filled to capacity (there should be very little mixture left unused).

PURPOSE: To visually check for consistency and accuracy.

7. Align the cavity plate onto the peg plate and then slowly press down evenly on the peg plate.

PURPOSE: To use the mold to form tablets.

8. The cavity plate will fall, having pushed out the tablets onto the pegs.

PURPOSE: To use the tablet mold to form individual, uniform tablets.

9. Leave the tablets on the pegs until dried. This typically takes 1 to 2 hours.

PURPOSE: To allow the tablets to dry so that they can be easily removed.

10. Invert the plate and press the tablets off.

To watch a video of this procedure, visit the following website: http://pharmlabs.unc.edu/labs/tablets/videos.htm.

metal punch press can be used to make multiple doses. These presses are available in a variety of sizes to make various strengths of tablets or lozenges. Types of lozenges include hard or soft, and tablets can be chewable, effervescent, or disintegrating. The metal punch press is composed of two parts: the bottom has a small cavity in one end of the tube; the top has a rod that pushes through the cavity. The rod does not extend totally through the cavity; instead, it leaves a small gap. The punch fits into the press. As the handle is depressed and then released, the rod moves in and out of the bottom piece.

Making a Tablet. The following steps are used to make a compressed tablet:

1. Place the powder in the bottom piece.
2. Depress the handle and then release. The powders are compressed and will occupy the gap left in the press.
3. Let the tablets harden; then remove them from the punch press.

Compounding Capsules. Various sizes of capsules are kept in stock for the compounding of encapsulated drugs. Advantages of capsules include masking of ingredients' taste and ease of swallowing compared with tablets. After the proper proportions have been prepared, the powder is then blocked. With a steel spatula, the powder is gathered and compressed onto a flat surface, making it easier to fill the capsule using the **punch method**. The body (i.e., the longer and thinner part of the capsule) is punched, attached to the cap (i.e., the shorter and wider part of the capsule), and then weighed to make sure each capsule is filled with the same amount of drug. The error rate is calculated by recording each capsule's weight and determining the average weight. According to quality control measures from USP <795>, capsules, powders, lozenges, and tablets must not weigh less than 90% or more than 110% of the calculated weight for each unit.

In larger pharmacies, automated capsule-filling machines can quickly and accurately fill various capsule sizes, saving the pharmacy staff hours of compounding and allowing them to fill other orders or prepare more difficult mixtures. The punch method is used when smaller quantities of capsules are prepared. Capsules are composed of vegetable-based or gelatinous materials. Great care must be taken to load the capsule accurately. Table 11-11 shows the sizes of capsules and the quantity of medication each one holds.

Other solids include mini-tabs (mostly used for pediatric patients), troches, and lozenges. **Troches** and lozenges are larger than tablets and are intended to dissolve slowly in the mouth. Troches often are placed in the cheek (buccal) for administration.

Lozenges. **Lozenges** are made by molding or compression and have several advantages. They are

TABLE 11-11

Capsule Sizes

Number	Contains Approximate Amount (mg)	Example
000	1000	
00	750	
0	500	
1	400	
2	300	
3	200	
4	150	
5	100	

normally made with flavors to enhance their taste. They also can be used as buccal tablets that are absorbed through the buccal lining of the mouth when the appropriate ingredients are used. Children have a much easier time taking gummy-type lozenges than other dosage forms because they look like candy. Lozenges either dissolve or disintegrate slowly in the mouth.

The following traditional ingredients are used to make lozenges:

- Phenol
- Sodium phenolate
- Benzocaine
- Cetylpyridinium chloride
- May also contain anesthetics, antimicrobials, antitussives, antiemetics, and decongestants

Molding mixtures are used to prepare different types of lozenges and may contain the following ingredients:

- Sugars to form a hard lozenge
- Polyethylene glycol (PEG) to form a soft lozenge
- Gelatin to form a chewable lozenge

Hard Lozenges. Hard lozenges can be made into the traditional round shape or manufactured to look like a lollipop or sucker. A combination of sugars is mixed with other ingredients and the medication, and the mixture is poured into a mold and allowed to cool before removal. When the various ingredients are heated together, great care must be taken in monitoring the temperature, moisture content, and pH of the final product.

Considerations in preparing hard lozenges include the following:

- Drugs that may degrade in high heat cannot be made into hard lozenges.
- The dosage form needs a low moisture content, between 0.5% and 1.5%.
- Certain syrups cannot be stirred until a specific temperature is reached.
- Between 55% and 65% sucrose and between 35% and 45% corn syrup must be used to avoid a grainy consistency.
- The use of acidic flavorings lowers the pH; calcium carbonate, sodium bicarbonate, or magnesium hydroxide must be used to raise the pH to 5 or 6.

EXAMPLE 11-2: HARD LOZENGE FORMULA

1. Drug: 2 g
2. Powdered sugar: 70 g
3. Corn syrup: 46 g
4. Water: 48 mL
5. Mint extract: 2 mL

Use food coloring to confirm adequate mixing in the laboratory.

Soft Lozenges. Soft lozenges can be made relatively quickly and then colored and flavored. They can be chewed or dissolved in the mouth. Ingredients include PEG 1000 or 1450, chocolate, or a sugar/acacia base. Lozenges can be hand rolled and cut into pieces or poured while warm into a plastic troche mold. After the mold cools, a spatula is used to level the excess solution; using a hair blow-dryer gives a smooth appearance.

Softeners are mixed and heated to 50° C; mixtures may include the following ingredients:

- Acacia gel: Used to add texture and smoothness
- Silica gel: Used as a suspending agent to keep materials from settling to the bottom of the mold
- Flavoring
- Food extracts
- Syrup flavor concentrates
- Volatile oils
- Sweeteners
- 9 parts NutraSweet and 1 part saccharin

EXAMPLE 11-3: SOFT LOZENGE FORMULA

1. Drug: 1 g
2. PEG: 10 g
3. Aspartame: 20 packets
4. Mint extract: 1 mL
5. Color: qs

Chewable Lozenges. Gummy-type lozenges are made primarily for children. The formulations consist of glycerinated gelatin and water. Fruit flavoring is used to sweeten the ingredients and disguise the taste of glycerin, which is very acidic. After the ingredients have been combined, they are heated at a low heat until a fluid forms; the fluid is then poured into preshaped gummy molds and cooled.

EXAMPLE 11-4: CHEWABLE LOZENGE FORMULA

1. Drug: 0.5 g
2. Glycerin: 70 mL
3. Gelatin: 18 g
4. Water: 12 mL
5. Methylparabenzamide: 0.4 g
6. Flavoring oil: 3 to 4 gtt
7. Color: qs

Semisolids

Ointments (Box 11-6), pastes, and creams each have different consistencies, depending on the amount of solids used. Pastes have more solids than ointments and creams. **Creams** are semisolid emulsions that are similar to ointments, but they are opaque (cloudy) instead of translucent. All three final forms have smooth consistencies.

Semisolids are prepared in all types of pharmacy settings. It is important to mix all ingredients in the right order, following the recipe exactly for uniformity.

Medication Sticks

Medication sticks provide another way of administering medication. Agents such as antibiotics, local anesthetics, sunscreens, antivirals, and oncological drugs can be manufactured as medication sticks and applied directly to the site on the body that needs treatment. They can also be applied to certain epidermal sites for a systemic effect (i.e., affecting the whole body).

Various waxes are used to make either hard or soft sticks; specific blends and temperatures are used to achieve the desired consistency. Additional ingredients, such as resins, polymers, oils, and gels, determine the texture and appearance (i.e., clear or opaque) of the finished product.

When combining two or more ingredients that have different ranges of melting points, melt the ingredients sequentially from highest to lowest melting point. Reducing the temperature on the hot plate prevents overheating.

Filling Ointment Jars

An appropriately sized container should be selected for an ointment preparation. Containers range in

BOX 11-6

Classifications of Ointment Bases

Absorption Bases

Properties: Absorb water; highly compatible with medications; increased stability to heat; greasy; most not washable. Examples include:
- Hydrophilic (water-loving) petrolatum bases (USP)
- Petrolatum-based ointment (Aquaphor)

Emulsion Bases

Properties: Insoluble in water; not washable unless mixed with water-in-oil (w/o) base; subject to water loss; washable and nongreasy when in an oil-in-water (o/w) base; more prone to mold growth unless a preservative is added. Examples include:
- Lanolin
- cold cream for w/o and dermabase for o/w
- Hydrophilic ointment
- USP (o/w)
- Vanishing creams (o/w)

Oleaginous Bases

Properties: Insoluble in water; good compatibility with a variety of medications; difficult to remove from clothing and skin; difficult to determine the amount of medication released upon application. The following are types of oleaginous bases.
- Petrolatum (Vaseline)
  - Consistency can be altered by adding mineral oil or white wax
  - Will not absorb much water unless mixed with cholesterol

- Stable bases that mix well with most substances
- All bases are greasy
- Melting point between 38° and 60°C
- Jelene (Plastibase)
  - Mixture of hydrocarbons in both liquid and wax types
  - Jellylike consistency
  - Able to withstand a wider range of temperatures before melting
  - Releases medication faster than petrolatum base
- Silicones
  - Polymers of silicon and oxygen
  - Protect skin from moisture

Water-Soluble Bases

Properties: Both absorb and dissolve in water; nongreasy and therefore washable; not susceptible to mold or microbial growth; color of the base can change in the presence of certain drugs unless cetyl alcohol is added. Example includes:
- Polyethylene glycols (also called carbowaxes): Consistency dependent on molecular weight, which is noted by a number; the increasing number relates to the solidity of the agent. Carbowax 300 is a liquid at room temperature, whereas 1540 is a solid.

---

size from $\frac{1}{4}$ ounce to 1 pound. Using a small spatula, pack the ointment carefully into the bottom and sides of the container and then fill the center. The jar can be tapped to release any trapped bubbles. As the final step, top off the jar, smoothing the ointment level at the top. For melted ointments, pour the ointment into the jar while still warm, let the ointment solidify, and then smooth off the top using a heated metal spatula.

Filling Ointment Tubes

Ointment tubes are available in different sizes. First roll the ointment (on glassine paper) into a cylinder slightly smaller than the circumference and length of the appropriately sized tube. Before placing the roll into the back of the tube, take off the cap to release the displaced air when the ointment is inserted. Place both the ointment and the rolling paper into the tube; then cover the end of the tube with a spatula and carefully pull out the paper, leaving the ointment inside the tube. Fold the end of the tube over twice, use crimpers to seal the end of the tube, and label the product.

Soft Sticks

Soft sticks can be clear or opaque; they spread the medication evenly when applied, soften at body temperature, and do not leave a residue on the skin after application.

Ingredients used in soft sticks include:
- Waxes
- Polymers
- Oils
- Gels
- Petrolatum
- Cocoa butter
- PEG

EXAMPLE 11-5: SOFT OPAQUE STICK FORMULATION

1. White beeswax: 30 g
2. Cetyl alcohol: 8 g
3. Cocoa butter: 6 g
4. Carnauba wax: 1 g
5. Castor oil (tasteless): 2 mL
6. Aquabase T: 20 g

7. Petrolatum: 13.5 g
8. Perfume: 0.9 mL
9. Preservative: 0.1 g
10. Butyl stearate: 5 mg
11. Active drug: qs

EXAMPLE 11-6: SOFT CLEAR STICK FORMULATION

The example given here is an analgesic stick; methyl salicylate is the active ingredient for topical pain relief.
1. Sodium stearate: 13%
2. Methyl salicylate: 35%
3. Menthol: 15%
4. Propylene glycol: 25%
5. Water: 12%

Hard Sticks

Hard sticks contain crystalline powders that are held together either by heat or by a binding agent. This type of stick must be moistened before it becomes active, and it leaves a white residue when applied.

EXAMPLE 11-7: HARD STICK FORMULATION

The example given here is a styptic stick, which stops bleeding from minor cuts, such as razor cuts.
1. Ammonium chloride: 7 g
2. Aluminum sulfate: 27 g
3. Ferric sulfate: 40 g
4. Copper sulfate: 26 g

The following are additional types of ingredients that can be used in sticks:
- Lubricants
  - Paraffin
  - Castor oil
  - Corn oil
  - Cottonseed oil
  - Oleic oil
  - Peanut oil
  - Soybean oil
  - PEG 300 or 400
- Skin care additives
  - Vitamin A
  - Vitamin E
- Sun protection agents
  - Zinc oxide
  - *p*-Aminobenzoic acid (PABA)

Sizes and styles of applicators differ, depending on their intended use. Lip balms are prepared in small, cylindrical-shaped plastic applicators. To fill the applicators without leaving an indentation in the top (caused by the cooling process), follow these steps:
1. Turn the base of the applicator two full turns to raise the bale (the bottom platform).
2. Slightly overfill the tube with the base. Do this when the mixture has cooled as much as possible to avoid shrinkage.
3. Top the base by pressing a warm spatula on the top of the base to cover any hole that may have appeared during the cooling process.
4. Turn the base of the applicator downward and place the cap on top.

Suppositories

Several sizes and shapes of suppositories are used to administer medications to vaginal, rectal, and urethral areas; suppositories are made with either solutions or ointments. Suppositories can be prepared in three ways: hand rolling, compression, and fusion molding. The various bases used in suppositories serve two purposes: they provide a medium that can carry the medication to the site of absorption, and they allow the medication to be released over different lengths of time. Common bases used are listed in the following sections.

Oleaginous Bases. **Oleaginous bases**, such as cocoa butter or synthetic triglycerides, can be used because they remain solid at room and body temperatures and melt at warm temperatures. However, care must be taken when heating suppositories made with cocoa butter. If a suppository is heated above 35° C (95° F), its properties change and it will not keep a solid form when the temperatures rise to 30° C (77° F). The synthetic triglycerides are more stable, although they are more expensive. Stepan (Northfield, Illinois), the manufacturer of Wecobee, makes several bases from coconut oil with a temperature range of 33.9° C up to 40.5° C, depending on which formula is used. Other triglyceride products by different manufacturers include Dehydag, Hydro-Kote, Suppocire, and Witepsol. Because of the temperature range at which suppositories melt, they should be stored in a cool place or in the refrigerator.

Water-Soluble Bases. PEG polymers or glycerinated gelatins can be used in the manufacturing of suppositories. These types of ingredients dissolve in body fluids and are not as dependent on temperature; therefore, they can be stored at room temperature. PEG polymers are a popular choice because of their properties: they are nonirritating, they can be used to make suppositories either by molding or by compression, and they have a wide melting point range. Different weights of PEG bases are normally mixed together or with another base to form different levels of solidity and dissolving lengths. The combinations include the following:
- PEG 1450 (30%) and PEG 8000 (70%)
- PEG 1000 (75%) and PEG 3350 (25%)
- PEG 1450 (2.3 g) and silica gel (25 mg)
- PEG 300 (60%) and PEG 8000 (40%)

Glycerinated Gelatins. These are often used for vaginal suppositories and have a wide range of additives, such as zinc oxide and boric acid. Their properties include an ability to disperse slowly in mucous secretions; they are translucent and gelatinous solids. They must be kept in a cool, dry place because they decompose in humid environments. If they are to be kept for an extended period, preservatives are added, such as methylparaben, propylparaben, or a combination of the two. They should be dipped in water before administration to activate the gelatin.

Preparing Suppositories

Using Molds. If suppository molds are used, they must be kept at room temperature because the rapid cooling of refrigeration can cause the suppositories to break. The formulation should be poured into each mold cavity in a steady and consistent manner to prevent a layered appearance. Also, pouring the ingredients just before they reach their congealing point allows for a solid suppository. Pouring the mixture too soon (after heating) can produce a hole in the top of the suppository; this is due to contraction. Hard molds, such as metal or rubber, require a lubricant, which aids in removal of the suppositories. For this purpose, a light coat of vegetable oil spray can be applied to the mold before the mixture is poured.

When filling molds, pour to the top of each one; filling slightly over the mold is also permissible because the excess can be removed with a heated metal spatula. A black light (to improve visualization) is used to fill suppository shells (unit dose) to ensure that the ingredients are filled to the proper line. These shells may be filled either by pouring or by using a syringe, which limits spillage and allows better control over the volume filled. It is important to be very careful when removing suppositories; the two halves should not be pried apart; instead, they should be pushed away from one another by placing the top of the screws on the table and pushing down on the mold (Figure 11-12).

Hand-Rolling Method. Another way of preparing only a few suppositories is to roll them by hand. For this method cocoa butter is used as a base because it does not have to be melted. Triturate the grated cocoa butter, along with the active ingredient, in a mortar. Form a ball-like shape using the palm of your hands; then roll the suppository into a cylinder using a large spatula or a small flat board on a pill tile. The cylinder is cut into suppository segments, which are then rolled on one end to form a conical shape.

Packaging Suppositories. If plastic shells are not used, each suppository must be wrapped separately, using foil wrappers that are available in different sizes and colors.

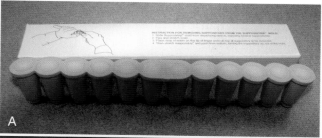
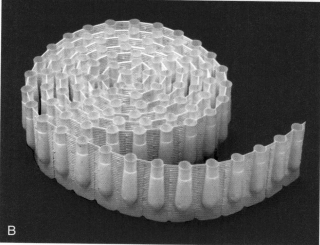

FIGURE 11-12 Suppository molds can be used in addition to the hand-rolled method. **A,** Suppository molds prepared in the pharmacy. **B,** Suppository packaging. (Courtesy Total Pharmacy Supply, Inc., Arlington, TX)

👤 *Scenario* CHECK UP 11-3

Judy is looking forward to her day because she has been assigned to the compounding station. She loves to prepare medications by following the formula! It is always a challenge to make the most pharmaceutically elegant (the special use of a finishing technique to give the final product a professional look) product possible. Her first task is to measure a liquid in a graduated cylinder. What should Julie remember about measuring liquid in a cylinder? What process should she follow to determine the proper amount of liquid?

Nasal Preparations: Ointments, Suspensions, Gels, and Solutions

Nasal preparations can be compounded as jellies, gels, ointments, solutions, or suspensions. They can be used for topical application (e.g., ointments, gels, jellies), as sprays, as inhalers, or as drops. Excipients used include buffers, preservatives, tonicity-adjusting agents, gelling agents, and antioxidants, all of which must be nonirritating. These are the same types of agents that are used in ophthalmic formulations. They are quickly absorbed into the bloodstream for rapid onset of activity.

Common preservatives used in nasal products include the following:

- Benzalkonium chloride
- Benzethonium chloride

- Phenylmercuric acetate
- Phenylmercuric nitrate
- Thimerosal
- *p*-Hydroxybenzoates

The preparation method for each type of dosage form begins with accurate measuring and weighing of each ingredient.

Preparing Solutions

1. Dissolve ingredients into three fourths of the total amount of sterile water for the injection to be used; mix well.
2. qs with SW to the total volume required.
3. Determine the pH, clarity, and other quality control factors from a sample of the solution.
4. Filter through a sterile 0.2-micrometer filter into a sterile nasal container.
5. Package and label.

Preparing Suspensions

1. Repeat steps 1 through 3 under Preparing Solutions.
2. Package in an appropriate container for autoclaving.
3. Autoclave, cool, and then label (this step is optional, depending on the recipe).
4. Choose a random sample to check for quality of product (e.g., sterility, pH).
5. Package and label; shake well before using.

Preparing Ointments

1. Repeat step 1 under Preparing Solutions.
2. Sterilize each ingredient using an appropriate method.
3. Mix each of the ingredients with the sterile vehicle.
4. Perform quality control on a sample of the mixture.
5. Package and label; for topical use only.

Preparing Gels

1. Repeat step 1 under Preparing Solutions.
2. Filter through a 0.2-micrometer filter into a sterile container.
3. Add the (sterilized) gelling agent and mix well.
4. Add SW for injection to volume/weight and mix well.
5. Perform quality assurance (QA) on sample.
6. Package and label; for topical use only.

> ### Tech Alert!
> Ophthalmic, inhalant, otic, and nasal preparations carry a high risk of cross-contamination if used by more than one patient. Patients should be advised never to share these agents because they are considered sterile.

Packaging

The types of containers used for compounded products must be appropriate. The container must protect the contents and have a child-resistant cap (if applicable), the appropriate label, and any auxiliary labels required. Once mixed to the proper concentration, all products are filled into the appropriately sized container. This should be done neatly to avoid waste. Containers vary in size and in manufactured materials, depending on the circumstances in which the drug is used (Table 11-12). Containers used to package compounded products include glass and plastic bottles, syringes, dropper bottles, and jars of various sizes. Containers in a variety of sizes are used to hold medications and suppository molds for rectal preparations.

Syringes sometimes are used to prepare oral, vaginal, or parenteral compounds. Once the drug has been loaded into the barrel of the syringe, a cap is placed over the top to keep the contents inside. For items that should not be injected, an oral syringe or other syringe to which a needle cannot be attached should be used; using an oral/nonparenteral syringe reduces dosage administration errors.

Certain containers do not have childproof caps or lids; therefore, the patient must be instructed by the pharmacist to keep these types of containers out of the reach of children. The following are some examples of these types of containers:

- Syringes
- Cream or ointment jars
- Dropper bottles
- Ointment tubes

> ### Tech Note!
> Read all instructions before beginning to compound materials. Make sure that all the ingredients are available to avoid a delay in product preparation. Also, it is important to reorder stock after ingredients have been depleted so that the ingredients are available for the next prescription.

TABLE 11-12

Containers and Sealants and Associated Dosage Forms

Container/Sealant	Dosage Forms
Foil paper	Suppositories
Polystyrene	Solids in bottles and jars
Metal tubes	Ointments and semisolids
Amber bottles	Tablets, capsules, liquids
Heat-sealed strips*	Tablets, capsules
Amber blister packs*	Tablets, capsules

*For institutional use only.

Stability

Several factors affect the stability of a drug. The amount of light and air, the temperature, and even the pH alter the longevity of a drug. Legally, the date given to a pharmacy-prepared product cannot be longer than that for any of the ingredients in the product. The pharmacist or the pharmacy technician must find the appropriate beyond-use date in the manufacturer's literature if it is not already provided. In addition to this reference, many compounding books contain calculations that determine appropriate beyond-use dates. Prepared recipes contain all necessary information. The beyond-use date of a preparation is set from the time of compounding, not from the time when the medication is dispensed. If no literature is available to determine the beyond-use date, USP <795> provides guidelines that can be used to set the appropriate date (Table 11-13).

Documentation

As in the case of repackaging, documentation of compounded medications is important. Keeping accurate records ensures the integrity of the product dispensed and meets FDA guidelines for quality assurance. Although protocols vary between pharmacy settings, most compounding ingredients and steps are put into a recipe format known as the **formulation record (FR)** for the person preparing the medication. The FR includes a list of ingredients, the preparation methods, safety requirements, BUD information, and references for the preparer. This documentation ensures that the procedures are consistent and can be reproduced (Figure 11-13). In addition to the FR, pharmacies are required to have a **compounding record (CR)**, or log sheet that is

a record of finished compounds and includes all ingredients in the mix, the BUD assigned, the preparer, and assigned lot numbers (Box 11-7). Also required are Safety Data Sheets (SDSs) for all chemicals and drug substances, either in hard copy or as electronically accessible forms. However, if commercial products are used in preparing the medication, the package insert may be used.

Once the label has been affixed to the container, all necessary auxiliary labels are chosen. Many auxiliary labels not only instruct the patient in the intended use of the product, but also indicate the appropriate storage requirements. In addition, some labels allow for beyond-use dates to be added.

Scenario CHECK UP 11-4

Judy is in the middle of her shift in the compounding area. She is documenting her completed prescription in the compounding log. She notices that the technician who worked the previous shift forgot to list the lot numbers on her last two medications. Why are the lot numbers so important? What should Judy do next?

BOX 11-7

Information Necessary on Compounding Log Sheets and Medication Labels

Log Sheet Information
- Date prepared
- Names of ingredients
- Manufacturer of each ingredient
- Lot number and expiration date of each ingredient (includes sterile water container, if used)
- Amount or weight of each ingredient
- Dosage form of each ingredient
- Pharmacy lot number assigned
- Pharmacy beyond-use date assigned
- Technician's initials
- Pharmacist's initials
- Date dispensed
- Patient's name and medical record number
Documents are kept on the pharmacy premises for no less than 3 years from the time the medication was prepared.

Medication Label Information
- Name of patient and medical record number
- Date
- Drug name
- Drug strength
- Physician
- Sig: directions
- Pharmacy lot number and beyond-use date
- Initials of both technician and pharmacist

TABLE 11-13

USP <795> Guidelines for Beyond-Use Dating with Nonsterile Compounding*

Medication Forms	Guidelines
Nonaqueous formulations	The sooner of 6 months or the expiration date of any of the ingredients
Water-containing oral formulations	No later than 14 days when stored in refrigerator
Water-containing topical/ dermal and mucosal liquid and semisolid formulations	No later than 30 days or the intended duration of therapy, whichever comes first

*These guidelines are used if there is no stability information available for the particular medication or formulation.

Safety

All chemicals should be safely stored inside cabinets or behind shelf brackets to avoid spillage. Several additives can be harmful if they are inhaled or come in contact with the eyes or skin. Every pharmacy has an SDS binder with information about all chemical products and how to handle spillage or contact. It is important to know where the SDS binder is kept in the pharmacy department.

Cleaning up excess ingredients appropriately is important; the method of cleaning up and disposing of agents or any equipment used depends on the type of agents used. Hazardous chemicals must be discarded properly according to pharmacy protocol. Nonhazardous chemicals normally can be discarded

---

Progesterone 100 mg SR Capsules Size #0 (LoxOral™)

SUGGESTED FORMULA FOR

Progesterone 100 mg SR Capsules Size #0 (LoxOral™)

Version: 1.0

100 Capsules

PROGESTERONE USP, PCCA SPECIAL MICRONIZED	10 g
METHOCEL® E4M PREMIUM CR [HYPROMELLOSE USP]	14 g
BASE, PCCA LOXORAL™	14.857 g

SUGGESTED COMPOUNDING PROCEDURE

Note: It is recommended that you follow USP <795> recommendations for potency testing which states "... each preparation shall contain not less than 90.0% and not more than 110.0% of the theoretically calculated and labeled quantity of active ingredient...". In order to provide some guidance in this area, please contact Eagle Analytical Services regarding the use of Skip Lot testing.

Note: This is a theoretical formula and has not been tested in the PCCA lab.

Note: This formula was calculated using the following capsule packing statistics:

        Progesterone USP, PCCA Special Micronized:

                Lot #C151637, 327 milligrams in a size #0 capsule

        Methocel ® E4M Premium CR (Hypromellose USP):

                Lot #C104616. 350 milligrams in a size #0 capsule

        Base, PCCA LoxOral™:

                Lot #PILOT, 505 milligrams in a size #0 capsule

Pack stats will vary from lot to lot so it is recommended that you perform your own packing statistics before proceeding with this formulation. Please contact PCCA's Pharmacy Consulting Department for further assistance.

1. Using the Principles of Geometric Dilution, mix Progesterone, Methacel E4M and PCCA LoxOral Base together with trituration in a mortar and pestle.
2. Capsule formulations should have powders where the particle size is the same throughout. Once powders are thoroughly mixed, sieve through an 80 mesh sieve (PCCA #35-3125) to ensure even particle size. Do not force large particles through the sieve as this destroys the integrity of the sieve. Instead, any particles remaining in the sieve should be triturated in a mortar and pestle to reduce particle size, and ALL powders should be sieved again.
3. Encapsulate in size #0 capsules.

Progesterone 100 mg SR Capsules Size #0 (LoxOral™) (10802)

Page 1/2

FIGURE 11-13 Formulation record.

Principles of Geometric Dilution:

This procedure should be followed when mixing an ingredient of a larger quantity (L) with a second ingredient of a smaller quantity (S). L is to be mixed into S in small proportions.

First, add a portion of L which has the same volume of that of S followed by thorough mixing. You will get a mixture (M1).

Then, add another portion of L which has the same volume of that of M1 followed by thorough mixing. Do the mixing based on the above principle until L is mixed into S completely.

Under no circumstance should the entire quantity of L be added at once to S in the expectation that uniform dispersion of the latter will be more expeditiously achieved on brief trituration of the mixture.

WARNING!

SAFETY WHEN COMPOUNDING:

Precautions should be taken when compounding hormone and other steroids, as they can be absorbed through skin, mucous membranes and lungs. Wear appropriate lab apparel, eye protection and respirator. Use an appropriate filter system to reduce the amount of airborne chemical particles in your lab. Monitor to ensure there is no direct exposure to the compounder. Consider using Flow Sciences Vented Balance Safety Enclosures - PCCA #35-3310 or PCCA #35-3311. Pregnant women and compounders with hormone related cancer should not compound hormone therapy.

See PCCA #35-3020, Pharmacy Safety Kit in catalog, and review "Safety in the Compounding Pharmacy" Video PCCA #35-3025, CD-ROM PCCA #35-3120. (These two are available at no charge or they may be viewed on the PCCA Members Only Website.) Call PCCA Pharmacy Consulting Department with questions.

Note: No claims are made as to the safety or efficacy of this preparation. This formulation is provided solely at the unsolicited request of the pharmacist.

Note: Beyond Use Dates of preparations are conservative estimates by the formulator using reference books, peer reviewed literature, intended duration of therapy, formulation from commercially available products, organoleptic stability observations and current USP guidelines. Compounders may have stability tests performed by a reputable laboratory if they wish to extend the Beyond Use Date.

Note: Beyond Use Date after compounding is estimated to be <u>180 days.</u>

10802
Revised: Fri Oct 18, 2013

Progesterone 100 mg SR Capsules Size #0 (LoOral™) (10802)

Page 2/2

FIGURE 11-13, cont'd

in a regular trash container. Any glass or needles must be placed in a sharps container.

Compounding Professionalism

Pharmaceutical elegance is the special use of a finishing technique to give the final product a professional look. Great care must be taken when topping off jars of creams and ointments. By holding the spatula very straight across the top of the ingredients and slowly turning the container, the top achieves a smooth appearance. Then slowly lift the spatula, as you are turning, to leave a small curl in the center of the cream or ointment.

Regulatory and Quality Control

The repackaging and compounding of pharmaceutical products are subject to regulatory control. The manner in which the medication is packaged affects both the product inside the package and the user's compliance with the physician's orders for taking the medication. Many medications can degrade with ultraviolet (UV) light exposure; therefore, they must be placed in amber-colored containers to protect the medication. Storage is another consideration for a prepared product in a specific type of container. All labeling requirements must be followed, or the prescription is considered misbranded. Under the FDA Modernization Act of 1997, the following restrictions were placed on pharmacies:

- Compounded drugs may be made in limited quantities.
- Compounded products must be made from approved ingredients that meet manufacturing and safety standards.
- The drug product must not be identified by the FDA as a product that presents demonstrable difficulties for compounding in terms of safety or effectiveness.

Veterinary Medications

Many pet owners must medicate their animals. Administering oral medications to a pet can be difficult. Many delivery systems have been developed to avoid forcing a tablet down the throat of an animal. For example, dog treats can be made that have the medication mixed into the treat; other forms of dosing include liquids and transdermal routes of administration. Sticks can be prepared to administer antibiotics to the inside of the ear; liquids poured onto a pet's food reduce the stress on both the animal and the owner. Labeling requirements for compounded veterinary products are listed in Box 11-8.

Compounding pharmacies provide many more choices for patients to administer their medications in the appropriate strength and dosage form to their pets (Table 11-14).

Personnel Training

Pharmacy programs must include supportive personnel (technicians) with adequate training to perform the necessary functions of compounding. To enable technicians to build and maintain a high skill level, training programs should be offered periodically. Instructions on compounding should include the following:

- Calculations
- Compounding equipment
- Dosage forms
- Interpretation of symbols
- Literature
- Safety
- Techniques

BOX 11-8

Labeling Requirements for Animal Prescriptions

1. Name and address of veterinarian
2. Active ingredient or ingredients
3. Date dispensed and beyond-use date
4. Name of pet
5. Directions for use specified by practitioner and the class/species or identification of the animal
6. Dosage
7. Frequency
8. Route of administration
9. Duration of therapy
10. Any warnings and information on side effects must be given by the veterinarian and/or the pharmacist to ensure safety
11. Name and address of the dispenser (pharmacy/pharmacist)
12. Prescription number
13. Date filled

TABLE 11-14

Pet Dosage Forms and Uses

Dosage Form	Uses
Treats	Chewable flavored tablets (beef, chicken, turkey) for oral doses
Sticks	Transdermal gel applicators used for topical administration
Miniature tablets	Extremely small tablets; easy to put into food
Beads and pellets	Biodegradable dosage forms used in chemotherapeutic and other compounded agents

---

❭ TECHNICIAN PROFILE

Shevala is a certified compounding technician at an independently owned pharmacy. She has worked in this position for 7 years. Her responsibilities include using a computerized compounding system, weighing and recording chemicals, combining chemicals into appropriate dosage forms per formula instructions, and properly using and calibrating all lab equipment, including scales, electronic meters, and IV pumps. Shevala is also responsible for following all safety and USP guidelines, recording daily refrigerator and freezer temperatures, and ordering medication and supplies as needed. She has the strong math skills and basic knowledge of compounding laws and regulations that are essential to this position. She enjoys her job and the opportunity to help individualize medications to optimize the patient's health.

These programs may include watching instructional videos or observation and dialog between instructor and personnel. The instruction should also include either a written test or a quality control test of finished preparations. The highest level of competency in compounding procedures is ensured if pharmacies provide initial training followed by recurrent training in methods, regulations, and techniques of compounding. In this way, the pharmacy can provide the customer with the highest product quality.

Compounding Calculations

Many formulas are already documented in a compounding recipe book; however, in some situations the final product may have to be prepared in a strength or volume different from that listed in the recipe, or products of different strengths may need to be used to prepare a final percentage solution. In such cases the pharmacist or technician must perform calculations to attain the correct weights and/or volumes for the final product. The following sections discuss calculation procedures for reducing or increasing formulas, determining partial dosage units, changing stock solutions, mixing products of different strengths, performing solubility expressions, and converting units to weights.

Increasing or Decreasing a Formulation's Quantity

EXAMPLE 11-8: INCREASING A FORMULATION'S QUANTITY

Recipe is for 100 mL of 2% ibuprofen gel.
By definition a 2% gel means 2 g per 100 mL of gel, so set up a ratio and proportion to determine how much ibuprofen powder is required to prepare 240 mL of gel.

$$\frac{2\,g}{100\,mL} = \frac{x}{240\,mL}$$

$$(x)(100\,mL) = (2\,g)(240\,mL)$$

$$x = (2\,g)(240\,mL)/(100\,mL)$$

$$x = 4.8\,g \text{ of ibuprofen powder needed}$$

EXAMPLE 11-9: REDUCING A FORMULATION'S QUANTITY

Recipe is for 100 mL of 2% ibuprofen gel.
How much ibuprofen powder is required to prepare 40 mL of gel?

$$\frac{2\,g}{100\,mL} = \frac{x}{40\,mL}$$

$$(x)(100\,mL) = (2\,g)(40\,mL)$$

$$x = (2\,g)(40\,mL)/(100\,mL)$$

$$x = 0.8\,g \text{ of ibuprofen powder needed}$$

EXAMPLE 11-10: REDUCING A FORMULATION'S QUANTITY

Recipe is for 100 mL of 5 mg/mL of drug D.
Ingredients:
- Drug D: 50-mg tablets #10
- Sterile water for injection: 4 mL
- Artificial banana flavoring: 3 mL
- Simple syrup (with suspending agent) mixture: qs to 100 mL

Reduce this recipe to 35 mL of drug D, 5 mg/mL suspension.

The new volume ordered (35 mL) divided by the amount in the recipe in the original (100 mL) gives the final percentage to alter the formula. Reduce the entire formula to 35% of the original by multiplying each ingredient by 0.35.

$$\frac{35}{100} = 0.35$$

Drug D: 10 tablets $\times$ 0.35 = 3.5 tablets

Sterile water: 4 mL $\times$ 0.35 = 1.4 mL

Banana flavoring: 3 mL $\times$ 0.35 = 1.05 mL

Sterile water for injection: qs to 35 mL

EXAMPLE 11-11: DETERMINING PARTIAL DOSAGE UNITS

Recipe: Mixture M, the original formula, calls for 125 mg of active ingredient M.
Active ingredient M: 125 mg (need 5 capsules at 25 mg each)
Ora-Plus: 60 mL
Ora-Sweet: qs 120 mL
Using 25-mg capsules, determine the amount needed to make only 120 mg:

$$\frac{25\,mg}{1\,cap} = \frac{120\,mg}{x}$$

$$(x)(25\,mg) = (1\,cap)(120\,mg)$$

$$x = (1\,cap)(120\,mg)/(25\,mg)$$

$$x = 4.8\,caps$$

Then:
1. Empty 5 capsules onto a weighing boat or paper and weigh.

2. Determine how many grams you need to remove. If the weight of 5 capsules of active ingredient and filler is 1600 mg:

$$\frac{1600 \text{ mg}}{5 \text{ caps}} = \frac{x}{4.8 \text{ caps}}$$

$$(x)(5 \text{ caps}) = (1600 \text{ mg})(4.8 \text{ caps})$$

$$x = (1600 \text{ mg})(4.8 \text{ caps})/(5 \text{ caps})$$

$$x = 1536 \text{ mg needed}$$

3. Remove 64 mg from the balance to retain the necessary 1536 mg.

EXAMPLE 11-12: CHANGING STOCK SOLUTIONS

Order: Prepare three 15-mL bottles of medicated solution with 0.01% ingredient A.
In stock: 17% ingredient A solution
How much of the 17% ingredient A solution is needed?
Note: 0.01% final strength needed = 0.01 g/100 mL; ingredient A 17% = 17 g/100 mL.

$$15 \text{ mL} \cdot 3 = 45 \text{ mL}$$

$$\frac{0.01 \text{ g}}{100 \text{ mL}} = \frac{x}{45 \text{ mL}}$$

$$100 \text{ mL} \cdot x = 0.01 \text{ g} \cdot 45 \text{ mL}$$

$$x = 0.0045 \text{ g of ingredient A needed}$$

$$\frac{17 \text{ g}}{100 \text{ mL}} = \frac{0.0045 \text{ g}}{x}$$

$$17 \text{ g} \cdot x = 0.0045 \text{ g} \cdot 100 \text{ mL}$$

$$x = 0.026 \text{ mL of 17% solution needed}$$

Use 0.026 mL of 17% solution and qs with appropriate liquid to 45 mL.
An easier way to approach this question is to use the equation from Chapter 6 for diluting stock solutions: SV · SP = DV · DP

Identify the variables: SV = ?
SP = 17%   DV = 45 mL   DP = 0.01%

SV · 17% = 45 mL · 0.01%   SV = 0.026 mL

EXAMPLE 11-13: MIXING PRODUCTS OF DIFFERENT STRENGTHS

Order: 120 g of 0.1% ointment B
In stock: 1 oz of 0.1% ointment B base
0.5 oz of 0.15% ointment B base
2.5 oz of 0.005% ointment B base

If these three ingredients are mixed together, how much of ointment powder drug B must be added to prepare the prescription to attain 120 g of 0.1% ointment B?
Note: This cannot be done using the SV · SP = DV · DP equation or the alligation alternate method because three strengths are being combined.
Use dimensional analysis to determine how many mg of ingredient B are in each amount. Remember from Chapter 6 to begin with the conversion that has the unit of your desired answer (mg) in the numerator and add information in order to cancel unwanted units with each subsequent fraction.

$$\frac{1000 \text{ mg}}{1 \text{ g}} \cdot \frac{0.1 \text{ g}}{100 \text{ mL}} \cdot \frac{30 \text{ mL}}{1 \text{ oz}} \cdot \frac{1 \text{ oz}}{1} = 30 \text{ mg}$$

$$\frac{1000 \text{ mg}}{1 \text{ g}} \cdot \frac{0.15 \text{ g}}{100 \text{ mL}} \cdot \frac{30 \text{ mL}}{1 \text{ oz}} \cdot \frac{0.5 \text{ oz}}{1} = 22.5 \text{ mg}$$

$$\frac{1000 \text{ mg}}{1 \text{ g}} \cdot \frac{0.005 \text{ g}}{100 \text{ mL}} \cdot \frac{30 \text{ mL}}{1 \text{ oz}} \cdot \frac{2.5 \text{ oz}}{1} = 3.75 \text{ mg}$$

Total amount = 56.25 mg

120 mg – 56.25 mg = 63.75 mg additional ingredient B powder needed

EXAMPLE 11-14: PERFORMING SOLUBILITY EXPRESSIONS

Order: Prepare 150 mL of a 1:15 strength solution of drug X.
How much of drug X is required to fill this order?
This is a single-step problem that is easy to solve with ratio and proportion.

$$\frac{1 \text{ g}}{15 \text{ mL}} = \frac{x}{150 \text{ mL}} \quad x = 10 \text{ g}$$

EXAMPLE 11-15: CONVERTING UNITS TO WEIGHTS

Order: 150,000 units of drug N per gram of ointment; quantity: 60 g to be dispensed.
How much of drug N should be weighed (based on 4400 [USP] units/mg)?
This is a multistep problem so use dimensional analysis to keep track of units.

$$\frac{1 \text{ g}}{1000 \text{ mg}} \cdot \frac{1 \text{ mg}}{4,400 \text{ units}} \cdot \frac{150,000 \text{ units}}{1 \text{ g}} \cdot \frac{60 \text{ g}}{1} = 2.045 \text{ g}$$

DO YOU REMEMBER THESE KEY POINTS?

- The need for packaging products in the appropriate type and size container
- The proper steps to follow in the bulk repackaging medication
- Five reasons pharmacies often repackage bulk medications into unit dose packages
- The proper handling of medications during bulk repackaging
- The documentation necessary for repackaged and compounded products
- Information required on labels
- Common auxiliary labels used on compounded products
- How expiration and beyond-use dates are determined when repackaging
- Common reasons for using unit dose medications
- The various types of containers used in repackaged and compounded products
- Definition of non–sterile compounding

- Common reasons patients need compounded medications
- The various types of equipment used in compounded medications
- The various types of scales used in compounding
- How to complete a compounding sheet with necessary information
- The proper steps to follow when compounding a product
- Types of additives that are used to improve the taste and appearance of oral solutions
- The sizes of capsules used in compounding
- How ointments, suppositories, nasal sprays, and other dosage forms are prepared
- GMP used when preparing compounded products
- Regulations pertaining to compounding pharmacies on limits of quantities
- The use of compounded products for animals

REVIEW QUESTIONS

Multiple Choice Questions

1. The guideline for assigning a beyond-use date to a bulk repackaged solid or liquid is:
   A. Half of the manufacturer's expiration date
   B. Less than the manufacturer's date
   C. No sooner than 6 months from the date the medication was repackaged
   D. One year from the date repackaged or the expiration date on the manufacturer's container, whichever is earlier

2. To grind or crush powders into fine particles using a mortar and pestle best describes:
   A. Trituration
   B. Levigation
   C. Mixing
   D. Stirring

3. Determine the beyond-use date of a drug to be repackaged into unit doses that has a manufacturer's expiration date of 7/14. If today's date is 6/13, the BUD is:
   A. 9/13
   B. 7/13
   C. 6/14
   D. 3/14

4. The type of balance(s) that can weigh 10 g of powder accurately is(are):
   A. Class A
   B. Class B
   C. Both A and B
   D. None of the above

5. A meniscus is best described as:
   A. A beaker filled with a small amount of water
   B. Water molecules attaching to the sides of a container
   C. A container used to measure very small amounts of liquid
   D. The lowest level of liquid, which is the point that should be used to assign a measurement

6. The arrest knob on a balance is used to:
   A. Measure the weight of a compound
   B. Balance the feet of the balance
   C. Adjust the balance's weights
   D. Lock the balance

7. Emulsion bases are:
   A. absorbent
   B. insoluble in water
   C. greasy
   D. not susceptible to mold growth

8. Which type of medication can be compounded for animal use?
   A. Tiny tablets
   B. Transdermal sticks
   C. Transdermal patches
   D. All of the above

9. According to FDA regulatory guidelines, compounding pharmacies are *not* allowed to:
   A. Advertise their compounding products
   B. Prepare large quantities of compounded product
   C. Prepare transdermal medications
   D. None of the above

10. Beyond-use dating differs from expiration dates because:
   A. Beyond-use dating is used only when compounding, and expiration dates are used for repackaging
   B. Beyond-use dating is used when repackaging or compounding products, whereas only manufacturers use expiration dates
   C. Expiration dates are used only for medications, whereas beyond-use dating applies to all additives
   D. None of the above

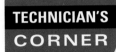

TECHNICIAN'S CORNER

You receive an order for 50 g of 2.5% hydrocortisone cream. You have hydrocortisone powder and Dermabase in stock.
How many grams of hydrocortisone powder are needed?
How much Dermabase do you need to qs to 50 g?
What documentation is required for these items?
What information would you place on the label (include auxiliary labels needed)?

Bibliography

Allen L: *The art, science, and technology of pharmaceutical compounding*, Washington, 2002, American Pharmaceutical Association.

Allen L: USP <795> Pharmaceutical Compounding—Nonsterile Preparations. *Secundum Artem* Current and Practical Compounding Information for the Pharmacist. Volume 13, Number 4 (ACPE No. 748-000-05-001-H01).

Ansel H, Allen L, Popovich N: *Pharmaceutical dosage forms and drug delivery systems*, ed 8, Baltimore, 2004, Lippincott Williams & Wilkins.

Leon S et al: *Comprehensive pharmacy review*, ed 7, Baltimore, 2009, Lippincott Williams & Wilkins.

USP Bulletin: Compounding pharmacies at the forefront of personalized medicine, 96:6, 2007,

Websites Referenced

Allen L Jr: Compounding oral liquids. *Secundum Artem* vol 5 no 1. (Referenced August 22, 2013.) www.paddocklabs.com/forms/secundum/volume_3_1.pdf

American Society for Health-System Pharmacists (ASHP): Technical assistance bulletin on compounding nonsterile products in pharmacies, 1994, p 73. (Referenced August 22, 2013.) www.ashp.org/DocLibrary/BestPractices/CompoundingNonsterile.aspx

American Society of Consultant Pharmacists (ASCP): Guidelines for prepackaging of medications. (Referenced November 15, 2013.) www.ascp.com/resources/policy/upload/Gui98-Prepackaging%20meds.pdf

Compounding nasal preparations. *Secundum Artem* vol 7, no 1. (Referenced November 15, 2013.) www.paddocklabs.com/images/PadSec7-1.pdf

Compounding rectal dosage forms. II. *Secundem Artem* vol 14, no 1. (Referenced August 22, 2013.) www.paddocklabs.com/forms/secundum/Volume14.4.pdf

Excipients category list. (Referenced October 19, 2013.) www.pformulate.com/labclass/categories.htm

Limited FDA survey of compounding drug products. (Referenced August 22, 2013.) www.fda.gov/Drugs/GuidanceComplianceRegulatoryInformation/PharmacyCompounding/ucm155725.htm

Pharmaceutics and Compounding Laboratory: Pharmaceutical solutions. III. Ophthalmic solutions. (Referenced November 15, 2013.) http://pharmlabs.unc.edu/labs/ophthalmics/objectives.htm

UNC School of Pharmacy, Pharmaceutics and Compounding Laboratory: Compounding lab exercises. (Referenced November 15, 2013.) http://pharmlabs.unc.edu/index.htm

USP & Compounding: Compounding pharmacy resources. (Referenced August 12, 2009.) www.usp.org/pdf/EN/distributors/compounding.pdf

Wedgewood Pharmacy: Veterinary dosage forms. 2009. (Referenced November 15, 2013.) www.wedgewoodpharmacy.com/dosage forms Veterinary Dosage Forms

Aseptic Technique and Sterile Compounding

Bobbi Steelman

OBJECTIVES

Upon completing this chapter, you should be able to do the following:

1. Explain why certain medications must be sterile.
2. Define common terms used in sterile compounding.
3. Describe Standard Precautions necessary when preparing compounded sterile preparations.
4. Describe standard supplies and equipment used to prepare compounded sterile preparations.
5. Explain the anatomy of a syringe and needle.
6. List the sizes of syringes and needles used in the pharmacy setting.
7. Explain when and why filters are used in sterile compounding.
8. List the types of stock used within a clean room.
9. Describe various medication delivery systems.
10. Explain the history of USP <797>.
11. List the main components of USP <797> regulations.
12. List the three risk levels of drug preparation determined by USP <797>.
13. Explain the differences between the various types of hoods.
14. Describe how often hoods must be inspected.
15. Describe how to properly clean various types of hoods and prepare them for use.
16. Describe proper aseptic technique.
17. Demonstrate the steps in drawing up medication from an ampule.
18. Demonstrate the steps in drawing up medication from a vial.
19. Describe different types of intravenous (IV) parenteral medications.
20. Describe how to properly dispose of needles, vials, and cytotoxic supplies.

TERMS AND DEFINITIONS

Anteroom The room adjacent to the "clean room" used for donning all personnel protective equipment (PPE) and wiping down all supplies that will be used in the compounding area

Aseptic technique The procedures used to eliminate the possibility of a drug becoming contaminated with microbes or particles

Beyond-use date (BUD) Defined by USP <797> as the date or time after which a compounded sterile preparation (CSP) shall not be administered, stored, or transported; it is determined from the date the preparation is compounded

Biological safety cabinet (BSC) A hood that should be used for making hazardous sterile preparations in the clean room

Clean room In pharmacy, a contained and controlled environment in the pharmacy that has a low level of environmental pollutants (e.g., dust, airborne microbes, aerosol particles, and chemical vapors); the clean room is used for preparing sterile medication products

Compounded sterile preparations (CSPs) Preparations prepared in a sterile environment using nonsterile ingredients or devices that must be sterilized before administration

Gauge The size of the needle opening

Hazardous drug Any drug that has been proven to have dangerous effects during animal or human testing; it may cause cancer or may harm certain organs or pregnant women

Hazardous waste Any waste that meets the Resource Conservation and Recovery Act (RCRA) criteria of ignitability, corrosiveness, reactivity, or toxicity

Health care–associated infection (HAI) An infection that patients acquire during the course of receiving treatments for other conditions in an institutional setting

Horizontal laminar flow hood An environment for the preparation of compounded sterile preparations in which air originating from the back of the hood moves forward across the hood and into the room

Hyperalimentation Parenteral nutrition for individuals who are unable to eat solids or liquids

Infection control Policies and procedures put in place to minimize the risk of spreading infections in hospitals or other health care facilities

Laminar flow hood An environment for the preparation of sterile products

Parenteral medication Medication that bypasses the digestive system but is intended for systemic action; the term *parenteral* most commonly describes medications given by injection, such as intravenously or intramuscularly

Peripheral parenteral Injection of a medication into the veins on the periphery of the body instead of into a central vein or artery

Peripheral parenteral nutrition (PPN) Intravenous nutrition administered through veins on the periphery of the body rather than through a central vein or artery

Precipitate To separate from solution or suspension; a solid that emerges from a liquid solution

Reconstitute To add a diluent (e.g., saline or sterile water) to a powder

Standard operating procedures (SOPs) Written guidelines and criteria that list specific steps for various competencies

Standard Precautions (i.e., Universal Precautions) A set of standards that reduces the possibility of contamination and the risk of transmission of infectious disease; these standards are used throughout a health care facility, including to prepare medications

Sterile preparation A preparation that contains no living microorganisms

Total parenteral nutrition (TPN) Large volume intravenous nutrition administered through a central vein (e.g., subclavian vein), which allows for a higher concentration of solutions

United States Pharmacopeia <797> (USP <797>) Chapter 797, "Pharmaceutical Compounding—Sterile Preparations," of the *USP National Formulary*. It contains a set of enforceable sterile compounding standards; describes the guidelines, procedures, and compliance requirements for compounding sterile preparations; and sets the standards that apply to all settings in which sterile preparations are compounded.

Vertical laminar flow hood An environment for the preparation of chemotherapeutic and hazardous agents in which air originating from the roof of the hood moves downward (over the agent) and is captured in a vent on the floor of the hood

Introduction

Scenario:

Ken is a total parenteral nutrition (TPN) technician specialist at a prominent hospital pharmacy. He received his training on the job and has more than 20 years of experience. Ken is nationally certified with the Pharmacy Technician Certification Board (PTCB) and is an active member of the American Society of Health-System Pharmacists (ASHP). He works rotating shifts, in which he is scheduled one weekend per month in addition to his normal work week. Ken has seen many changes in the hospital pharmacy over the years. He remembers when the TPN medications were made by hand, which was very time-consuming and labor intensive. He enjoys his job and believes that his department plays an important role in providing quality patient care. Why is it important that all parenteral medications be prepared by well-trained pharmacy technicians?

Proper preparation of **parenteral medications** is one of the most crucial responsibilities of the hospital pharmacy technician. Preparation of all parenteral medications in a manner that reduces the chance of contamination is important. This is possible only through the proper manipulation of materials used within the appropriate hood. Various sizes and types of hoods are available; all are capable of excluding bacteria and other unwanted particulates if the technician uses proper aseptic technique. **Aseptic technique** involves procedures used to eliminate the possibility of a drug becoming contaminated with microbes or other unwanted particles.

The pharmacy technician may prepare **compounded sterile preparations (CSPs)** in pharmacy settings such as home health services and long-term care facilities. This chapter predominantly focuses on the technician working in a hospital pharmacy. The regulations of *United States Pharmacopeia <797> (USP <797>)*, "Pharmaceutical Compounding—Sterile Preparations," are explored, as are policies established by other organizations to monitor compliance in the **sterile preparation** of compounded products.

Wider varieties of parenteral medications are used in the hospital than in any other setting. In the hospital, the pharmacy technician may be responsible for many daily tasks related to compounding sterile preparations. Each skill has its own set of guidelines, which are outlined in the three risk levels of USP <797> (discussed later).

This chapter explores several types of parenteral medications, including the terminology and equipment commonly associated with medications and the various methods used in their preparation. The student technician must understand many important aspects of sterile preparation of medications before filling an order, including the type of drug to be prepared, equipment used, sterilization steps per USP <797>, expiration dates, storage, and proper disposal of equipment. These are the technician's

BOX 12-1

Abbreviations and Descriptions of Pharmacy Stock

Types of Containers Used for Preparing Parenteral Medications

Amp	Ampule; 1- to 50-mL glass container
Vial	0.5- to 100-mL glass or plastic container with a stopper
MDV	Multidose vial; holds multiple doses of medication
SDV	Single dose vial; holds one dose of medication
Flexible bag	Plastic container (empty or filled with various fluids ranging from 50 to 3000 mL)

Common Types of Solutions Used/Ordered for Parenteral Agents

Diluent	Agent used to dilute medications; can be sterile water, normal saline (NS), or others
D_5NS	5% dextrose in normal saline
$D_{10}NS$	10% dextrose in normal saline
NS	Normal saline; has a concentration of 0.9% sodium chloride
0.45 NaCl	One-half normal saline; has a concentration 0.45% sodium chloride
LR	Lactated Ringer's solution; isotonic solution containing sodium, potassium, calcium, acetate, and chloride
$\frac{1}{4}NS$	One-fourth normal saline (concentration 0.225% sodium chloride)
$D_5\frac{1}{2}NS$	5% dextrose and 0.45% normal saline contained in the same bag of solution
SWFI	Sterile water for injection; usually used to reconstitute other medications
D_5W	5% dextrose in water
$D_{10}W$	10% dextrose in water

Routes of Administration for Parenteral Agents

IV	Intravenous; into the vein
IV push	Into the vein directly from a syringe
IM	Intramuscular; into the muscle
ID	Intradermal injection up to 1 mL into the upper layers of the skin
SUBCUT	Subcutaneous; under the skin
IT	Intrathecal; into a sheath (hollow tube), such as the lumbar sheath located at the base of the spine

Miscellaneous Terms Used with Parenteral Medications

On call	Physician wants dose to be ready when he or she decides to give the medication; most anesthesiologists order on-call preoperative medications
NPO	Nothing by mouth
Preop	Medication to be given before surgery (e.g., sedative or antiemetic)
Postop	Medication to be given after surgery (e.g., pain control or antiemetic)
prn	Medication to be given as needed
qs	Quantity sufficient; adding enough diluent or medication to attain the correct amount needed
Drip or infusion	An intravenous bag medication that is infused over a specified amount of time but is not given IV push

responsibilities in producing a compounded sterile preparation; in addition, technicians must be competent in using drug abbreviations and performing calculations that may be required to prepare medications. These are all important skills of a pharmacy technician.

Terminology Used in Pharmacy

Solutions, medications, and supplies may be required when preparing sterile products. The terms used to identify these items often are abbreviated in prescribers' orders and on supply lists. Pharmacy technicians need to understand these terms and abbreviations to interpret orders and fill stock levels

in the intravenous (IV) room. Box 12-1 lists some of the most common terms and abbreviations used for IV supplies.

Standard Precautions for a Health Care Worker

When working in a hospital setting all employees must comply with the policies of **Standard Precautions (i.e., Universal Precautions)**. To prevent the dissemination of highly contagious diseases, hospitals usually require an employee to receive both tuberculosis (TB) testing and an immunization against influenza annually. Standard Precautions are practices followed to prevent the transmission of infection and contamination; they are based on the principle that all blood, body fluids, secretions, excretions (except sweat), nonintact skin, and mucous membranes may contain infectious agents. Based on the anticipated exposure to potentially infectious substances, each area in the hospital has specific **infection control** guidelines (which can be found in the facility's policies and procedures manual); employees are expected to meet these requirements, including hand washing, orderliness, and cleanliness. The pharmacy does not supply blood or blood products. However, pharmacy personnel must participate in training sessions on blood-borne pathogens so that they not only understand various aspects of contamination, but also are aware of ways to prevent exposure and transmission of infections. For example, training includes the interpretation of room signs that indicate patient isolation (e.g., droplet or contact isolation) and the precautions and procedures that should be followed if access to these rooms is necessary.

Other hospital-wide standards include the following:

- Employees are not to use patient restrooms; they should use only employee restrooms.
- Medication refrigerators and freezers may hold only medications; they should not be used to store food or drink.
- Eating is prohibited in any drug preparation or patient care areas.

The following are examples of procedures specific to the pharmacy:

- All injectable drugs and other compounded sterile preparations must be made in a "clean room" under laminar flow hoods.
- All flow hoods are recertified every 6 months by an independent contractor or anytime the hood is moved.
- Routine maintenance of the hoods includes cleaning all work surfaces and prefilters.
- Records of all inspections are to be kept on file in the pharmacy department.

Scenario CHECK UP 12-1

Ken begins his shift by donning the proper personal protective equipment (PPE) and preparing to clean the hood. He cleans all work surfaces with sterile 70% isopropyl alcohol and checks the prefilters. He notices that the hood certification expires in 30 days. What should Ken do before the end of the month? Why must hoods be inspected every 6 months?

Supplies

Before discussing the actual techniques required to prepare injections, IV drips, chemotherapeutic drugs,

and other compounded sterile preparations, the types of supplies and equipment necessary for these processes should be explained. Different types of equipment are available for IV preparation, depending on the amount or volumes to be prepared. For instance, many different types of automated pumps automatically fill IV bags and other sterile containers. These pumps range in complexity and cost. For example, if large multiadditive automated machines are rented by the pharmacy, only the tubing required for that specific pump needs to be purchased. Small pumps, such as Baxa's Repeater pump, are used to administer smaller reconstituted volumes into single dose vials (SDVs) or larger volumes into multidose vials (MDVs). In addition, a wide variety of supplies used in the **clean room** must be kept in stock for daily use (Table 12-1). For this reason, the technician must inventory these supplies and reorder stock daily, anticipating the stock needed for the next day.

Syringes

Syringes used in the pharmacy are available in eight basic sizes: 0.5, 1, 3, 5, 10, 20, 30, and 60 mL. As the size of the syringe increases, the accuracy decreases (Figure 12-1). For parenteral products, the exact amount of drug ordered must be obtained. Syringe tips are available in two types. A tension-type syringe has a 1-mL volume. In this case the needle is attached by friction only (Figure 12-2, *A*). This type of syringe can be used for withdrawing insulin and other medications that require volumes equal to or less than 1 mL. However, tension-type tips cannot be used when preparing doses of chemotherapeutic drugs because of the risk of the needle detaching from the syringe and causing a spill or a possible needle stick to the technician. On all other sizes of syringes, the needle is held in place by a locking mechanism, commonly referred to as a Luer-Lok (Figure 12-2, *B*). This ensures a safe seal for withdrawal of the medication.

Most syringes are made of plastic and must be discarded after one use. Glass syringes rarely are used in the pharmacy, although they can be used when a patient is allergic to plastics. Glass syringes, unlike plastic syringes, can be sterilized and reused.

Another type of syringe is a Tubex or Carpuject (Figure 12-3). These cartridge systems can hold a variety of medications and are available in volumes from 0.5 mL up to 3 mL. The bottom of the cartridge is screwed into the system's syringe holder. The syringe cartridge holders for these systems are reusable and normally are dispensed to the nursing units by the pharmacy upon request. The Tubex or Carpuject cartridge is discarded after use; if desired, the holders may be autoclaved for sterility.

TABLE 12-1

Commonly Used Intravenous Room Supplies

Supplies	Common Description
70% isopropyl alcohol	Antiseptic for cleaning the hood
Ampule breaker	Plastic device on which one end is smaller for small ampules, the other end is used for larger ampules; helps to prevent crushing of the glass or cutting oneself when opening ampules
Filter needles	Needle that includes a filter; it prevents glass from entering the final solution when drawing from an ampule
Filter straws	Used for withdrawing medication from ampules
Filters	Used for specific medications to trap particles 0.22 to 5.0 μm from entering IV fluids
Male/female adapter	Universal size; fits a syringe on each end for mixing two contents
Sterile 70% alcohol pads	Alcohol on pads for convenience
Syringe needles	Most common bore sizes used in pharmacy are 16 to 20 gauge
Syringe caps	A sterile cap used to prevent contamination of syringes during transportation out of pharmacy
Syringes	Instrument that holds 0.5-60 mL for administration of medications
Transfer needles	A needle on both ends used to transfer a vial to a bottle
Tubing for pumps	Tubing is specific to manufacturer's machine
Tubing transfer sets	Blood transfer sets; used to transfer the contents of large containers into empty containers
Mini-spike	Large-bore spike that is pushed into vial with a syringe attachment at the other end
Forceps	Instruments that lock; used to obstruct tubing while transferring medications

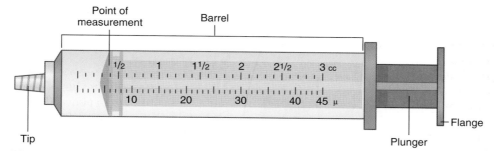

FIGURE 12-1 Anatomy of a syringe. As the syringe decreases in size, the calibrations (volume markers) become larger, allowing a more accurate dosage.

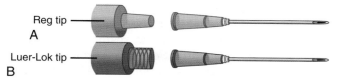

FIGURE 12-2 Two types of syringes. **A,** Regular tip syringe. The regular tip is held in place by pressure, as seen in the 1-mL syringe. **B,** The Luer-Lok syringe has spirals to secure the needle, as seen on a larger 3-mL syringe. (From Potter PA, Perry AG: *Fundamentals of nursing,* ed 8, St Louis, 2013, Mosby.)

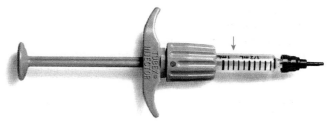

FIGURE 12-3 Tubex holders are intended to be reused. They hold the disposable Tubex or Carpuject cartridges. Each cartridge is prelabeled with the medication name, strength, volume, and concentration. The pharmacy stocks holders and cartridges.

Needles

Needles are made of aluminum or stainless steel and are available in many different **gauges** (sizes) and lengths. Higher gauge needles (e.g., 20 to 25 gauge) are used by nurses to administer injections. The nurse determines which gauge and needle length to use according to the injection site. In the pharmacy, needles are used to draw solutions into a syringe, not to administer medications to patients. A limited number of needle gauges are available in the pharmacy, and the lower gauge needles make drawing medications easier. The most common needle sizes used for preparing IV medications are 19, 18, and 16 gauge, which are used to draw solutions from vials or other containers (Figure 12-4). These needles are normally 1 to 1.5 inches long. The gauge (size) number of a needle is inversely proportional to the

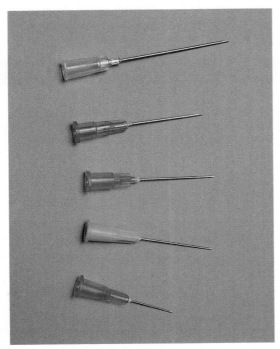

FIGURE 12-4 *Top to bottom,* Needle sizes 19, 20, 21, 23, and 25 gauge. Technicians may use a 19-gauge needle for small volumes, such as 1 mL or less. Larger gauges (not shown) include 18 and 16 gauge for larger volumes. (From Potter PA, Perry AG: *Fundamentals of nursing,* ed 8, St Louis, 2013, Mosby.)

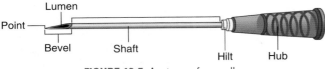

FIGURE 12-5 Anatomy of a needle.

bore (opening) size of the needle. This means that as the bore size increases, the gauge decreases. For example, a 25-gauge needle has a much smaller opening than a 19-gauge needle. The *bore size* refers to the circumference of the needle opening; as this increases, so does the probability of coring or cutting out a piece of rubber from the vial's rubber stopper. When a vial is cored, a chunk of rubber is dislodged and may fall into the vial. To avoid coring, the bevel edge should face upward. If coring does occur, a filter needle must be used to prevent the piece of cored rubber from entering the parenteral solution. No part of a needle below the hub should be touched (Figure 12-5). The point and shaft must remain sterile.

 Tech Note!

You should not wipe needles with sterile 70% alcohol. If you touch the needle with alcohol or something unintended (e.g., the outside of a vial), the needle must be discarded and replaced with a new one.

Filters

Different types and sizes of filters can be used when preparing parenteral medications. Filters are located within the hub of the needle, depending on the type used. Typical filter sizes are 10, 5, 1, and 0.45 micrometer (μm); the smallest filter is 0.22 micrometer, which removes all unwanted particles from the solution. If use of a filter needle is necessary, the technician must follow the manufacturer's guidelines regarding filter needles suggested for the specific medication. Some medications should never be filtered because filtering would remove active drug from the solution. Filter needles are for single direction use only and cannot be used to both withdraw and inject a solution.

Another type of filter is the filter straw. This strawlike needle can withdraw a larger amount of solution quickly, sifting it through a filter in the hub of the needle. The filter straw often is used to remove any fine particles of glass from an ampule. The filter straw must be replaced with a normal needle before the medication is pushed into the final container. Figure 12-6 shows the types of filters and other materials used in the IV room.

Stock Levels

All the items stored in the IV room of the pharmacy must be kept in stock above their minimum levels at all times. Current USP <797> standards (revised in 2008) require that a minimum number of supply items be kept in the clean room. Only items that will be used immediately for direct compounding should be in the clean room. Supply items must be wiped down with an appropriate cleaning solution before they are brought into the clean room.

Before and after each shift, the IV technician is responsible for reordering and restocking the clean room for the next shift. Some IV supplies may be ordered from the central supply area of the hospital and arrive by the next shift. However, most supplies are ordered directly from the pharmacy wholesaler, and delivery can take 2 days to 1 week. Therefore, to ensure that required pharmacy stock is always on hand, the technician must be knowledgeable about delivery options.

Many IV antibiotics are available in premade bulk packs; for example, 12 or 24 packs are frozen in boxes. Although these are convenient, they are more expensive than those prepared by technicians. Most of the time, technicians prepare the IVs needed throughout the week. Certain IV medications can be frozen in either IV solutions or syringes, but each bag must be marked with the date of reconstitution, the **beyond-use date (BUD)**, the concentration/strength, and the preparer's initials.

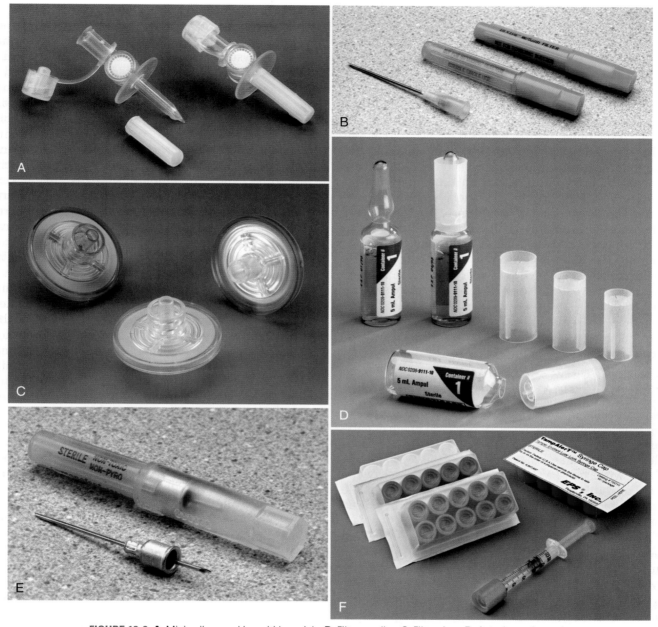

FIGURE 12-6 A, Mini-spikes used in multidose vials. **B,** Filter needles. **C,** Filter sizes. **D,** Ampules and ampule breakers. **E,** Transfer needle. **F,** Syringe and caps. (Courtesy Medi-Dose/EPS.)

The expiration dates for frozen, refrigerated, or room temperature products are determined by using the manufacturer's information, the known stability data, and other pharmaceutical specialty publications and research. Large, temperature-controlled refrigerators may be used to store thawed IV medications. Antibiotics and other medications in multidose vials can be stored in the refrigerator after opening, sometimes for days, and used as determined by USP guidelines for MDVs. All these items should be visually checked each day for stock levels and out-of-date medications.

Routes of Administration

Because prepared solutions differ in their volumes and/or concentrations, understanding the routes of administration (ROA) is important. For example, if a dose of ceftriaxone 1 g is to be given intramuscularly (IM), it is normally divided into two syringes for the nurse to inject into each side of the hip area. Injections can be given on several areas of the body. The route of administration of each type of medication must be stated on the label (this is discussed later in the chapter).

Medication Delivery Systems

Many different types of containers are used to deliver medications. Such containers are developed to be stable and easy to use. In addition, because many medications are not premade for final use by the manufacturer and must be prepared in the pharmacy, it is important to determine whether the medication must be discarded (i.e., wasted) if not administered to the patient in a timely manner. For example, once a medication has been **reconstituted**, it must be used within a certain time or it expires, resulting in lost revenue for the pharmacy. Sometimes the drug may not be given to the patient for whom it was prepared; the physician may have decided to use a medication of a different dose, type, volume, and solution. This type of waste only adds to the high costs of health care. Systems can be used to eliminate waste, such as the ADD-Vantage system. Although these systems are expensive, they can be beneficial by reducing waste and ultimately adding cost efficiency. These systems, and others, are discussed later.

Piggyback Containers

Flexible bags and bottles are the two main types of piggyback containers. Most IV bags are made of polyvinyl chloride (PVC), which consists of several flexible layers of plastics. Other types of IV bags are made with non-PVC materials, such as ethylene vinyl acetate (EVA). The EVA bags are not as flexible as PVC bags. Piggyback IVs are intended to be placed on top of a primary IV using tubing connection sets (Figure 12-7). Containers can be purchased prefilled with solutions or may be empty and filled with a custom-made IV solution. The sizes and types of piggyback containers and solutions range from 50 to

250 mL. Examples of specialized containers used for medication dispensing include large and small volume drips, syringe pumps, and miscellaneous dispensing systems. Many controlled substances also are prepared in such systems and are dispensed to the nursing floor after they have been documented according to established procedures for controlled substances.

Large and Small Volume Drips

Large volume drips include Viaflex bags in 500-mL and 1-, 2-, and 3-L volumes. Volumes greater than 1 L are often reserved for use with parenteral nutritional formulas. Bottles are also available in various sizes, ranging from 500 mL to 1 L. These can deliver a variety of fluids, including parenteral nutrition. Parenteral nutrition is a combination of essential nutrients that is administered through a drip system for several hours or up to 24 hours. (Parenteral nutrition solutions are discussed later in the chapter.) Small volume piggyback containers and solutions are available in 50-, 100-, 150-, and 250-mL volumes. Small volume drips can be piggybacked onto large volume drips. All Viaflex bags have a 10% overfill of solution. To attain an accurate final concentration of drug, some mixtures require that a volume of base solution equal to the volume of medication being added, plus the solution overfill, be removed during the mixing process. This type of procedure usually occurs with critical care medication drips, in which small changes in drug concentration may greatly influence the dosage given to the patient and the subsequent patient response.

 Tech Note!

All dosage forms of controlled substances that are delivered to nursing floors must be signed out of the pharmacy stock and into the floor stock of the receiving station. Documents registering controlled substances should be kept up to date, and all controlled substances should be counted at the end of every shift to account for all narcotic use or waste.

Continuous Analgesic Delivery Systems

Patients who require analgesics after major surgery and individuals who are in hospice normally have their medications prepared in the pharmacy. In the hospital setting, nursing stations stock various strengths of controlled substances intended to relieve extreme pain. Depending on the physician's order, the nurse can prepare intramuscular or IV push doses from the controlled substances cabinet.

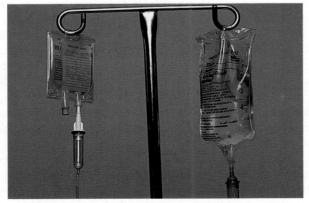

FIGURE 12-7 This gravity pump system intravenous piggyback setup shows a 100-mL Viaflex container *(left)* piggybacked to a large volume 1-L IV *(right)*. (From Potter PA, Perry AG: *Fundamentals of nursing*, ed 8, St Louis, 2013, Mosby.)

When a patient is in severe pain, physicians often order analgesic medications such as morphine or fentanyl (both schedule II [C-II] drugs) on a schedule (e.g., every 6 or 8 hours). When this strength of analgesic is given in larger doses to patients who have no history of opioid use, the initial effects of the medication may be extreme, causing side effects such as nausea, vomiting, and in some cases difficulty breathing. Toward the end of the 6 or 8 hours, some patients are once again suffering from pain and waiting for the next dose to be administered. To provide a more constant degree of comfort and to limit unwanted side effects, some patients may be given either an implantable port or a catheter system attached to a portable electronic pump system, which administers a steady flow of analgesics that controls the patient's pain more effectively. These pumps are used to dispense controlled substances at a specific rate of infusion. Two types of portable electronic pumps can be used to deliver controlled substances: a syringe system or a cassette system. Technicians may prepare either syringes or cassettes that are placed into a pump that automatically delivers the medication over a predetermined time. These pumps can be programmed for short or long durations to deliver medication, not to exceed a 24-hour period. These devices are especially effective for patients who require constant pain control and those discharged home with this type of medication. Another type of dispensing system that uses syringes relies on gravity for delivering the solution. The syringes are placed in a freestanding IV pump system on wheels; these are used only in the hospital.

Patient-Controlled Analgesia Syringe System

Patient-controlled analgesia (PCA) is a method of administration that allows the patient to control the rate at which the drug is delivered for the relief of pain. The PCA pump holds a syringe of pain medication that is attached to the IV line and is regulated by a computerized device that automatically dispenses the medication. The pump may be programmed to deliver a small, constant dose of pain medicine, and the patient has the option of receiving additional doses (bolus) if necessary. This is done by depressing a button attached to a line on the machine. The boluses are preset for amount and frequency; even if the patient presses the button many times, he or she receives only the predetermined amount of drug. For example, if the dose is set at 1 mg/mL with dosing intervals every 6 minutes and a 1-hour lockout dose of 10 mg, regardless of how many times the patient presses the button within 6 minutes, he or she receives only 1 dose. The 1-hour lockout limits medication administration to a total dose of 10 mg

in 1 hour. This safeguards the patient from overdosing. The PCA syringe device is normally used in a hospital setting for acute postoperative pain control. Children ages 7 years and older can typically use this pump device independently once they are familiar with it. Young or debilitated patients need assistance from a nurse or caregiver to receive their dosing. Many manufacturers provide prefilled PCA syringes that may be used directly from the packaging in these pumps. Alternatively, pharmacy technicians (using aseptic technique in a **horizontal laminar flow hood**) can prepare the syringes for PCA pumps. Each syringe must be labeled, capped, and checked by the pharmacist before delivery. When the pharmacy technician is ready to have a prepared medication inspected by the pharmacist, he or she should include the finished product, along with the syringe, the opioid analgesic container, and the diluent used in its preparation.

PCA Syringe Systems
The following are some manufacturers of PCA syringe systems:
- Smiths/Medical (Medfusion): *www.smiths-medical.com*
- B Braun: *www.bbraunusa.com*
- Aitecs: *www.aitecs.com*

Patient-Controlled Analgesia Cassette System

Cassette pumps are another type of PCA system that can be used at home. The programmed pumps work similarly to the syringe pumps in that they are preset for dosage administration. Additional boluses may be programmed into the pump per the physician's orders and cannot be altered by the patient. A *bolus* is a predetermined amount of drug that can be administered by the patient at one time when pain intensifies. The cassettes are available in various sizes, such as 50- or 100-mL volumes. The pharmacy may prepare the cassettes. A short piece of tubing with a Luer-Lok can be connected to a 60-mL syringe that is used to load the proper amount of solution. After the cassette has been filled, the line (tubing) must be primed. To prime a line, the tubing is allowed to fill with solution so that there is no air in the tubing; the tubing then is secured with a twist cap. This is usually done by the pharmacy at the time the medication is prepared. Figure 12-8 shows an example of a PCA device.

PCA Cassette Systems
The following are some manufacturers of PCA cassette systems:
- CADD pumps: *www.smiths-medical.com*
- LMA e-PainCare System: *www.lmana.com*

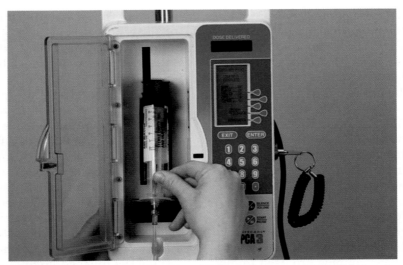

FIGURE 12-8 PCA device with cartridge. (From Perry AG, Potter PA, Ostendorf WR: *Clinical nursing skills and techniques*, ed 8, St Louis, 2014, Elsevier.)

United States Pharmacopeia (USP) <797>

History of USP <797>

The *United States Pharmacopeia (USP)* is responsible for providing safety guidelines for the preparation of parenteral and other sterile medications. In the 1970s, because of the dramatic increase in nosocomial infections, the National Coordinating Committee on Large Volume Parenterals (NCCLVP) provided guidelines for the preparation of parenterals. Nosocomial infections, or **health care–associated infections (HAIs)**, are infections that originate in a hospital. Later, in the 1980s, the efforts of the NCCLVP were replaced by several other organizations as they began to establish standards for pharmacists and technicians in the safe preparation of parenterals. These organizations included the American Society of Health-System Pharmacists (ASHP), the National Association of Boards of Pharmacy (NABP), and the United States Pharmacopeial Convention (USP). Through the 1990s these organizations wrote both recommendations and guidelines for safe standards, but they were not monitored or enforced. In the mid-1990s it was determined through health system surveys that very few pharmacies followed these standards explicitly. For example, most pharmacies did not perform quality assurance checks or solution tests on a regular basis for prepared parenterals, and many did not provide education and training for personnel on a periodic basis. In addition, various IV medications were reported contaminated with bacteria because of poor aseptic technique. The reports of patient harm from improper preparation of medications by pharmacies continued through the 1990s.

In 2004 the USP <797> regulations were written with the intent that they would constitute an enforceable standard. The USP <797> standards must be met in all practice settings where sterile products are compounded. The USP, ASHP, and the Joint Commission (TJC) outlined a timeline for total compliance, realizing that it would take time for pharmacies to implement all the changes mandated. Pharmacies and other areas that prepare compounded sterile preparations must research, create, and document their **standard operating procedures (SOPs)** for meeting USP <797> regulations.

In 2008 the USP <797> regulations were updated, effective June 1, 2008. A number of changes were made, including clarification regarding the use of alternative technologies when preparing a compounded sterile product (CSP). A comprehensive list of definitions, including the terms used in this chapter, was provided. The risk categories of CSPs were revised, and a new low-risk, 12-hour BUD category was added. The **hazardous drug** section was updated to match the guidelines of the National Institute for Occupational Safety and Health (NIOSH). New guidelines were provided on the use of single use and multiuse vials, and specifics were outlined on the minimum frequency for cleaning and disinfecting the clean room (Table 12-2). Appendix 1 of the revised chapter outlines competencies, procedures, and quality assurance practices that are required and those that are recommended (more information on the revisions can be found at the USP website, *www.usp.org*). In 2013, as a result of the fungal meningitis tragedy at the New England Compounding Center, a group of executives from the sterile compounding industry formed the Specialty Sterile Pharmaceutical Society (SSPS). It was founded to support more stringent standards of practice

TABLE 12-2

Environmental Cleaning Schedule

Site	Minimum Frequency
Laminar airflow hood, biologic safety cabinet, compounding aseptic isolator, compounding aseptic containment isolator	Start of each shift, start of each batch, at least every 30 minutes, and after spills or when surface is contaminated
Counters and work surfaces	Daily
Floors	Daily
Walls, ceilings, and storage shelves	Monthly

regarding quality control and to ensure the safety and welfare of individuals receiving CSPs. (For more information about SSPS standards and activities, visit the website *www.sterilepharma.net*.)

Sections of USP <797>

USP <797> has three major sections:

1. Responsibilities of personnel: The risk levels of classification of compounded sterile preparations
2. Verification: Accuracy and sterility of compounded sterile preparations
3. Training: Individual training and continued evaluation of personnel with respect to compounded products, including both quality and control of the preparation environment

Furthermore, USP <797> requires SOPs that include automated systems used in compounding procedures, storing compounded sterile preparations, and assigning expiration dates, to maintain both quality and control even after the parenteral medication leaves the pharmacy. Other areas under USP <797> include any medication prepared by nurses, physicians, or other practitioners intended for patient use, regardless of the setting. The types of products include diagnostics, nutrients, irrigations, radiopharmaceuticals, and otic and ophthalmic solutions. Additionally, patient or caregiver training, patient monitoring, and adverse event reporting (see Chapter 14) must be maintained. Table 12-3 presents many of the terms and abbreviations used in describing areas of the pharmacy where aseptic technique is used.

Risk Levels

USP <797> has identified three risk levels (low, medium, high), which are based on various criteria

(Table 12-4). Additional requirements include the amount of space between the hood areas and sink and the storage location of products. (For more information on the standards of USP <797>, visit the USP website, *www.usp.org*.)

Low Risk: Level 1

Risk level 1 encompasses medications and procedures used to prepare compounded sterile preparations, including sterile medications, needles, and syringes; sterile technique; and use of an International Organization for Standardization (ISO) Class 5 hood. The technique must require only minimal manipulations within the hood. This is the most common type of IV preparation performed. Technicians must wear gown, gloves, cap, and mask during manipulation; these items of clothing are typically referred to as personal protective equipment and must be provided by the facility. The technician must verify all ingredients and instructions and visually inspect the solution after preparation. Each person's knowledge of aseptic technique and proper manipulations must be monitored and verified annually. An annual media-fill test must be done for each person compounding products in the hood. Safety measures include proper testing and certification of the hood.

Medium Risk: Level 2

Risk level 2 encompasses bulk compounding; this includes multiple IVs prepared for several patients or multiple compounded products to be used for one patient over several days. This includes preparing a **hyperalimentation** to be used over 1 week. A hyperalimentation is an IV nutritional product prepared for individuals who are unable to take in food through the alimentary tract. Many manipulations must be performed while in the hood. The requirements include all those listed for level 1 plus additional guidelines. A more in-depth evaluation must be performed, including a more stringent media-fill test to be conducted annually. This is done by performing a systematic evaluation of manipulations to determine that a compounded sterile preparation has been prepared.

High Risk: Level 3

Risk level 3 includes all the requirements of levels 1 and 2 plus additional guidelines. The types of products that this level encompasses are those that are susceptible to contamination because of the preparation of nonsterile products and/or delayed sterilization. An example is the preparation of a morphine and bupivacaine solution from a bulk powder (nonsterile) for use in an intrathecal pump. The requirements for this level include semiannual certification of aseptic compounding. Technicians must demonstrate that they can prepare such a product and

TABLE 12-3

Terms and Abbreviations Used in Pharmacy

Terms	Definition
Ante area	An area in which all preparations for IV admixture are gathered, including labels, gowning, and drug materials
Beyond-use date (BUD)	The date or time a drug or material can no longer be used; the drug is ineffective after this date
Biological safety cabinet (BSC)	A cabinet with a high-efficiency particulate air (HEPA) filter for laminar airflow
Buffer area	An area in which hoods are kept and IV preparation takes place
Clean room	A space where microbial containment is kept at a specific level of safety to ensure a certain level of cleanliness
Compounding aseptic isolator (CAI)	An isolator cabinet designed to contain all contaminants; prevents contaminants from escaping IVs and being transferred to the surrounding area
Critical site	An area exposed to air or touch, such as a vial, a needle, or an ampule
Direct compounding area (DCA)	A critical area within the hood (International Standards Organization [ISO] Class 5) where compounding materials are exposed to filtered air; also known as *first-air*
First-air	The air from the HEPA filter that passes over materials; this air is contaminant free
Hazardous drugs	Drugs that have been proven to have dangerous effects during animal or human testing; they may cause cancer or harm to certain organs or to pregnant women
Media-fill test	A test performed on compounded products to ensure that no contamination has taken place during preparation phase
Multiple dose container/vial (MDV)	A vial or container that can be used for more than one admixture; MDVs normally contain preservatives; the maximum dating is 28 days unless specified by the manufacturer
Negative pressure room	A room that has lower pressure than the adjacent rooms; net airflow is into the room.
Positive pressure room	A room that has a higher pressure than the adjacent rooms; net airflow is out of the room.
Primary engineering control (PEC)	A practice in which an ISO Class 5 system is in place that provides safety for admixtures; this includes laminar flow hood, glove boxes, vertical flow hoods, or compounding aseptic isolators
Single dose container/vial (SDV)	A vial or container that can be used only once

TABLE 12-4

USP <797> Risk Levels

Low Risk	Medium Risk	High Risk
Prepared in an ISO Class 5 (Class 100) laminar flow hood; located in an ISO Class 8 (Class 100,000) buffer room (clean room) with an ante area; sterile ingredients/devices; only syringe transfer used for measuring/mixing no more than three products	Prepared in an ISO Class 5 (Class 100) laminar flow hood; located in an ISO Class 8 (Class 100,000) buffer room (clean room) with an ante area; all low risk plus no broad-spectrum antibiotic present even over "x" days; complex aseptic technique manipulations; multiple doses in one container for multiple patients or multiple doses for one patient	Prepared in an ISO Class 5 (Class 100) laminar flow hood; located in an ISO Class 8 (Class 100,000) buffer room (clean room) with a separate ante area; all low/medium risk plus sterile products compounded from nonsterile ingredients; use of nonsterile device before terminal sterilization; sterile ingredients, components, or devices exposed to air quality; open system transfers
Batch doses with preservatives	Batch doses; no preservatives	Preparation of CSPs from bulk, nonsterile components, or final containers that are nonsterile and must be terminally sterilized (e.g., nuclear pharmaceuticals)
	Reconstituted doses; no preservatives	95% purity of ingredients
Ampule extraction using filter needles	Preparation of IVs that contain more than one additive and evacuate air; kept at room temperature over several days	IV preparations reconstituted from nonsterile powder that will be terminally sterilized
		Compounded bladder irrigations
Manually prepared TPN with only three ingredients	TPN prepared by an automated compounder.	Parenteral nutrition

CSPs, Compounded sterile products; *ISO,* International Standards Organization; *TPN,* total parenteral nutrition.

ensure its sterility. In addition, any batches over 25 units require pyrogen testing to verify that the batch is free of any contamination.

Storage and Stability

As the length of time a compounded IV is exposed to room temperature increases, so does the risk of bacterial growth. In addition, refrigeration temperatures must be monitored at least once daily to ensure constant conditions. As required by risk level, guidelines are provided for both temperature ranges and expiration dates of compounded medications (Table 12-5). The limits are for products that are aseptically prepared but have not passed a sterility test. The limits do not apply to batches that have been tested. Products that have been tested for sterility may be given longer expiration dates. Storage requirements also include training the patient and/or caretaker in the proper use and storage of compounded products. Monitoring of any adverse events and reporting them through the proper channels must be performed consistently and documented.

Requirements for Compounding

All personnel who prepare parenteral medications are required to be trained and monitored for compliance with techniques on a periodic basis. This includes ensuring that the drug ingredients, containers, labeling, and equipment are correct. Products must be stored according to manufacturer guidelines or other scientific findings (to be discussed later). In addition, pharmacists must determine the risk level of each type of preparation. Although USP <797> outlines risk, the standards do not rate every type of manipulation; the standards outline basic guidelines. The determination of which level applies to additional types of manipulations must be made by the pharmacist on an individual basis. The hoods and clean room, in addition to the pharmacy rooms adjacent to these rooms, must be within the guidelines of USP <797>. It is essential that any contamination be kept away from these areas. The guidelines for air standards in IV areas and individual hoods are listed in Table 12-6.

IV Environment

Most pharmacies can easily meet the educational and training aspects of USP <797>; however, this is not true of the new regulations related to the areas where these products are prepared. Each type of environment in the pharmacy is required to meet minimum standards pertaining to particle size and quantity. According to studies conducted by USP, using a **laminar flow hood** in an open room is no safer than preparing products on a countertop. This has been one of the most significant changes in pharmacy. As a result of the enormous expense required to create these new areas, many hospitals now contract out to specialized pharmacies to prepare their compounded sterile preparations. Facilities that have been able to meet USP standards must

TABLE 12-5

Storage Risk Levels: Temperature Ranges and Expiration Dates of Compounded Medications

Level of Risk	Room Temperature (20°-25° C [68°-77° F])	Refrigeration (2°-8° C [36°-46° F])	Freezer (5°-10° C [13°-14° F])
Low	12 hours or less	12 hours or less	N/A
Low	48 hours	14 days	45 days
Medium	30 hours	9 days	45 days
High	24 hours	3 days	45 days

TABLE 12-6

USP <797> Air Standards Based on 0.5-μm Particle Size

BSC or Room	Description	Number of Particles/m^3	Area in Pharmacy	Required Testing for Compliance
ISO Class 8	Class 100,000	3,520,000	Nonhazardous room	Checked every 12 months
ISO Class 7	Class 10,000	352,000	Clean room (i.e., buffer room and anteroom)	Checked every 12 months
ISO Class 6	Class 1000	35,200	Anteroom	Checked every 6 months
ISO Class 5	Class 100	3,520	IV hood	Checked every 6 months

BSC, Biological safety cabinet; *ISO,* International Standards Organization.

BOX 12-2

Environment Terminology

Clean or buffer room: Space adjacent to the primary engineering control (PEC) room where sterile preparation takes place

Anteroom: Space adjacent to the clean or buffer room

Primary engineering control (PEC): Space or hood where sterile preparation takes place

Biological safety cabinet (BSC): A hood that should be used for hazardous sterile preparation in the clean room

Laminar airflow hood (LAFH): A hood that should be used for nonhazardous sterile preparation in the clean room

Compounding aseptic isolator (CAI): A Class III glove box that can have either negative or positive air pressure

Compounding aseptic containment isolator (CACI): Another type of Class III CAI glove box that exhausts 100% of the air through a high-efficiency particulate air (HEPA) filter; to be used for preparation of hazardous medications; may also have either negative or positive air pressure

Air lock: A space of separation between two different air pressures; may be a pass-through chamber or room; a door must be present to prevent loss of pressure in the higher pressured room

Air pressure: Can be either positive or negative; positive air pressure environments may be used only for nonhazardous sterile preparation; negative air pressure environments can be used to prepare both nonhazardous and hazardous sterile preparations

---

positive or negative airflow; these are known as a glove box or barrier isolator hood (see Figure 9-5). All types of hoods have high-efficiency particulate air (HEPA) filters, although the way in which they expel the air differs. Proper use of these hoods requires additional training. The hoods must be verified and certified every 6 months or whenever moved to ensure their ability to filter contaminants. Both anterooms and clean rooms must be within standards. Assessments must be completed annually; any movement of the equipment requires additional inspection.

Pharmacies must use special equipment and chemicals to sterilize the anteroom and clean room; specialty knowledge about the proper way to clean each room is also required. For example, hoods and surface areas must be cleaned and sterilized daily, the walls and floor weekly. SOPs must be written and studied, and all who work in these areas must take evaluation exams.

Hood Cleaning and Maintenance

Airflow

Three types of hoods are used, depending on the sterile product being prepared: horizontal flow hoods, **vertical laminar flow hoods**, and glove boxes (i.e., BSCs). Laminar airflow workbenches (LAFWs) (i.e., hoods) are used for many types of parenteral or sterile product preparations. Horizontal hoods provide positive air pressure, moving the filtered air outward toward the preparer. For chemotherapeutic agents, a vertical flow hood can be used because of the direction of the airflow and the specifications of the hood. A vertical flow hood provides negative air pressure, circulating the air through an additional HEPA filter and then through a vent away from the preparer. A vertical flow hood can be used to mix non–chemotherapeutic agents if needed; however, chemotherapeutic agents should never be mixed in a horizontal flow hood. Glove boxes are closed systems that use a HEPA filter and a sophisticated venting system. These provide the greatest amount of safety to the preparer because of the containment ability. With all systems, strict aseptic technique and care must be used because spillage can still occur on the surface of the IV bag or container and can cause contamination or unwanted exposure on removal from the hood.

In a horizontal flow hood, the outside airflow starts in the back of the hood, passes through a special filter, and circulates out toward the opening. This special filter is a HEPA filter that traps all particles larger than 0.2 micrometers. The sides of the hood and items within the hood create a disruption of airflow. For this reason, the technician must work at least 6 inches from the sides and front of the hood.

also test the air periodically to ensure that guidelines are met. The terms and definitions used to describe types of environments are listed in Box 12-2.

The **anteroom** is adjacent to the buffer room (or clean room) and is sometimes called the gowning/degowning area. The minimum size of air particles allowed in the anteroom is 0.5 micrometers. All donning of the personnel protective equipment (PPE) occurs in the anteroom The clean room, where the technician actually prepares compounded sterile preparations, must meet more stringent requirements for air particulate size (Figure 12-9).

USP <797> also requires specific types of hoods to be used for compounding specific sterile products. Laminar flow hoods that have only positive (horizontal) airflow may be used to prepare nonhazardous medications (see Figure 9-4), whereas a negative (vertical) airflow environment may be used to prepare hazardous products per USP guidelines (see Figure 9-6). **Biological safety cabinets (BSCs)** are totally enclosed environments that are available in either

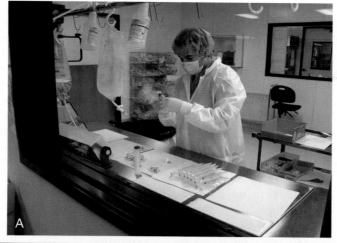

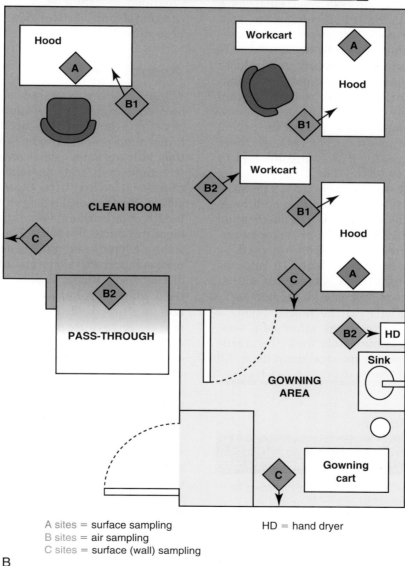

A sites = surface sampling   HD = hand dryer
B sites = air sampling
C sites = surface (wall) sampling

FIGURE 12-9 Clean room. **A,** Technician working in a clean room. **B,** The layout of a clean room. (**B** from Davis K: *Sterile processing for pharmacy technicians*, St Louis, 2014, Elsevier.)

In addition, movement within the hood should be kept to a minimum to reduce disruption of airflow.

The concept is similar for a vertical flow hood, although air cannot be released back into the room. For this reason, vertical hoods have a Plexiglas shield that separates the technician from the inside work surface. The air passes into the HEPA filter and then into the workspace area. The technician must not block the downward flow of air while working. A grid at the front of the tabletop draws in the air and filters it once again through a HEPA filter before it is released into the workspace area or is vented to the outside, depending on the type of venting system used. Both horizontal and vertical flow hoods must be turned on at least 30 minutes before use.

As mentioned, the BSC is also referred to as a glove box or barrier isolator. It is becoming the most popular type of hood for sterile preparation. It reduces the risk of contamination caused by accidental mishandling of drugs during compounding and reduces the number of environmental microbial contaminants, thus increasing the sterility of the prepared product. This ultimately protects patients from possibly harmful medications. It also protects the person preparing a chemotherapeutic agent because these medications can be harmful if they are inhaled or come in contact with the skin. The HEPA filtering system standards are listed in Table 12-7. The air is redirected through a HEPA filter, and an additional airflow system helps decontaminate the medication preparation. Daily monitoring of the pressure gauge, flow indicators, or alarms should be documented.

A BSC must be turned on at least 10 minutes before use. After the technician washes his or her hands and cleans the hood properly, all the necessary materials and medications can be placed inside a sterile holding chamber. Using the attached gloves, the technician takes the materials from the sterile chamber and transfers them into the main hood. All

products and supplies should be placed at least 4 inches inside the sash. At this point, the technician may prepare the medication. Any high-risk medication can be prepared in this type of hood. Inspections should be performed every 6 months. In an effort to comply with USP <797> guidelines, more pharmacies are using these types of hoods.

Cleaning and Maintaining Hoods

All hoods in the pharmacy must be thoroughly cleaned using the appropriate solvent and cleaning methods (see Table 12-2 for the cleaning schedule). Procedure 12-1 lists systematic instructions for cleaning a horizontal flow hood, and Procedure 12-2 lists the instructions for cleaning a vertical flow hood. Cleaning of BSCs differs from the cleaning of horizontal and vertical flow hoods, as described in Procedure 12-3.

Aseptic Technique

When CSPs are prepared, aseptic techniques must be used. Normally nurses do not have the advantage of using a laminar flow hood; however, they sometimes must prepare products for immediate use, and they still must use strict aseptic technique. Aseptic technique is directly associated with Universal Precautions (also known as Standard Precautions). Universal Precautions are guidelines followed by all health care workers when exposure to body fluids or blood products is likely. These precautions involve washing hands and putting on gloves and gowns (i.e., personal protective equipment) when in the presence of any body fluids. Similarly, aseptic technique is used when both hazardous and nonhazardous products are prepared. Products that have been tested and shown to cause adverse or toxic effects in humans are classified as hazardous. Examples of these types of medications include chemotherapeutic agents, radioactive compounds, and various hazardous chemicals, such as phenol and glacial acetic acid. These precautions are used to prevent contamination by a product or to a product.

For pharmacy technicians, the importance of using aseptic technique cannot be stressed enough. A medication that contains any microbes or unwanted debris can cause a dangerous infection, or even death, when administered to a patient. The steps used in aseptic technique begin with hand hygiene (Procedure 12-4), followed by proper donning of gloves and gown, cleaning of the flow hood, and, finally, preparation of the parenteral medication. Procedure 12-5 lists the preparation required for aseptic technique; except for putting on the surgical face mask immediately before entering the hood, all these steps should be completed outside the clean room. On leaving the IV area, the technician must remove the hair cover,

TABLE 12-7

HEPA Filtering System Standards

Class	Risk Levels	Safety Level	Filtering System
Class I	Low- to moderate-risk biologicals	Biosafety level I	HEPA filters air before it is exhausted.
Class II	Low- to moderate-risk biologicals	Biosafety level II	HEPA filters exhaust air to room or to a facility exhaust system.
Class III	High-risk biologicals	Biosafety level III	Containment of hazardous materials

PROCEDURE 12-1

Cleaning a Horizontal Laminar Airflow Hood

GOAL: To learn to properly clean a horizontal laminar airflow hood.

EQUIPMENT AND SUPPLIES
- Horizontal laminar airflow hood
- Sterile water
- Lint-free wipes or gauze
- Sterile 70% alcohol

REMEMBER
- Procedures for cleaning and disinfecting the hood should be developed, implemented, and practiced by trained compounding personnel. These procedures must follow USP <797> guidelines and should be written in the facility's standard operating procedures (SOPs).
- Cleaning and disinfecting are to be completed before any compounding is performed.
- The hood should be turned on and running at least 30 minutes before cleaning.
- Follow proper hand washing procedure and technique.
- Put on appropriate apparel, following proper garbing technique.

PROCEDURAL STEPS
1. Remove any items from within the hood.
PURPOSE: The hood should be completely empty so that all surfaces can be cleaned. Unnecessary items clutter the workspace and may contaminate the area.
2. Clean all surfaces inside the hood with a lint-free wipe and sterile water.
PURPOSE: To make certain all surfaces are clean and free from any loose material or residue.
3. Inspect all surfaces for any crystallized solutions. Clean these with sterile water before continuing.
PURPOSE: To make certain nothing is left on the surface that may contaminate the compounded sterile preparations (CSPs).
4. Moisten a 4 × 4-inch gauze or other lint-free cloth with sterile 70% alcohol.

PURPOSE: To prepare to disinfect the surfaces in the hood. If used properly, sterile 70% alcohol reduces the probability of contamination.

Remember to use a new wipe moistened with sterile 70% alcohol on each section of the hood cleaned.*
5. Wipe the top of the hood first. Clean in a side-to-side motion from left to right, working from back to front.
PURPOSE: To ensure uniformity of the cleaning procedure from shift to shift and person to person. This also follows the method of cleaning from top to bottom to ensure nothing falls from a higher surface to contaminate a lower surface.
6. Wipe the horizontal IV pole and any hooks or brackets using a smooth motion from left to right.
PURPOSE: To ensure that the IV pole is disinfected and ready to use if any items need to be attached during the compounding process.
7. Wipe from top to bottom on each side of the hood. Always work from the back to the front.
PURPOSE: To disinfect the sides of the hood to prepare for the compounding process.
8. Wipe the rear wall of the hood using a side-to-side motion from left to right, beginning at the top and working down to the bottom.
PURPOSE: To disinfect the rear wall of the hood to prepare for the compounding process. Remember, the HEPA filter is delicate and easily damaged. Never put too much pressure on the filter cover when cleaning. This could drive one of the aluminum separators into the filter, causing damage that can be detected only through testing.
9. Finally, wipe the flat work surface area using a side-to-side motion from left to right, working from back to front.
PURPOSE: To disinfect the work surface area of the hood to prepare for the compounding process.
10. Allow the sterile 70% alcohol to remain on surfaces to be disinfected for at least 30 seconds before such surfaces are used to prepare CSPs.
PURPOSE: To kill organisms that may contaminate the CSPs. If the alcohol is not allowed to dry completely, it may itself act as a vehicle for the transfer of contaminants.

*Never attempt to clean the HEPA filter or spray any solutions toward the HEPA filter. Also, discard alcohol bottles when empty and be sure to disinfect the spray head if transferring it to a new bottle to avoid contamination.

gloves, and face mask. Another consideration is the preparation of the rooms and equipment used in preparing CSPs. Accuracy in performing calculations and measuring medications is paramount; all calculations and measurements should be double-checked and must be verified by a pharmacist.

Hand Placement

Regardless of the type of hood used, the placement of the hands is one of the most important aspects to consider when preparing sterile medications. The technician should practice some simple yet important techniques that reduce the possibility of contamination and errors when preparing CSPs. Figure 12-10 outlines the necessary steps for withdrawing a liquid from a vial while working in the hood. When working in a horizontal hood, you must not block the airflow at any time; to prevent this, grasp the vial or ampule by the front; avoid placing the hands or fingers right behind the top of the container. When holding up the vial or ampule, keep the fingers from

PROCEDURE 12-2

Cleaning a Vertical Airflow Hood

GOAL: To learn to properly clean a vertical laminar airflow hood.

EQUIPMENT AND SUPPLIES
- Vertical airflow hood
- Sterile water
- Lint-free wipes or gauze
- Sterile 70% alcohol

REMEMBER
- Procedures for cleaning and disinfecting the hood should be developed, implemented, and practiced by trained compounding personnel. These procedures must follow USP <797> guidelines and should be written in the facility's standard operating procedures (SOPs).
- Cleaning and disinfecting are to be completed before any compounding is performed.
- The hood should be turned on and running at least 30 minutes before cleaning.
- Follow proper hand washing procedure and technique.
- Put on appropriate apparel, following proper garbing technique.

PROCEDURAL STEPS
1. Remove any items from within the hood.
PURPOSE: The hood should be completely empty so that all surfaces can be cleaned. Unnecessary items clutter the workspace and may contaminate the area.
2. Clean all surfaces inside the hood with a lint-free wipe and sterile water.
PURPOSE: To make certain all surfaces are clean and free from any loose material or residue.
3. Inspect all surfaces for any crystallized solutions. Clean these with sterile water before continuing.

PURPOSE: To make certain nothing is left on the surface that may contaminate the compounded sterile preparations (CSPs).
4. Moisten a 4 × 4-inch gauze or other lint-free cloth with sterile 70% alcohol.
PURPOSE: To prepare to disinfect the surfaces in the hood. If used properly, sterile 70% alcohol reduces the probability of contamination.
   *Remember to use a new wipe moistened with sterile 70% alcohol on each section of the hood cleaned.**
5. Wipe the horizontal IV pole and any hooks or brackets using a smooth motion from left to right.
PURPOSE: To ensure that the IV pole is disinfected and ready to use if any items need to be attached during the compounding process.
6. Wipe from top to bottom on each side of the hood. Work side to side with overlapping strokes.
PURPOSE: To disinfect the sides of the hood to prepare for the compounding process.
7. Wipe the rear wall of the hood and inside the front shield using a side-to-side motion from left to right, beginning at the top and working down to the bottom.
PURPOSE: To disinfect the rear wall and front shield of the hood to prepare for the compounding process.
8. Finally, wipe the flat work surface area using a side-to-side motion from left to right, working from back to front.
PURPOSE: To disinfect the work surface area of the hood to prepare for the compounding process.
9. Allow the sterile 70% alcohol to remain on surfaces to be disinfected for at least 30 seconds before such surfaces are used to prepare CSPs.
PURPOSE: To kill organisms that may contaminate the CSPs. If the alcohol is not allowed to dry completely, it may itself act as a vehicle for the transfer of contaminants.

*Never attempt to clean the HEPA filter or spray any solutions toward the HEPA filter. Also, discard alcohol bottles when empty and be sure to disinfect the spray head if transferring it to a new bottle to avoid contamination. Treat cleaning supplies as hazardous waste for disposal purposes.

blocking airflow. This technique takes time to perfect and should be practiced constantly until it becomes second nature. When working in a vertical flow hood, avoid placing the hands and fingers over the container because this would break airflow. It is also important not to overload the hood with drugs and supplies, which can lead to a break in aseptic technique and increases the likelihood of drug errors. When using a BSC, you must follow strict protocol in handling and transferring solutions.

Use of Ampules to Prepare Medications

Intravenous push or intramuscular medications can be prepared by the nurse at the nursing station or at the patient's bedside; however, the pharmacy does

prepare some IV push and IM medications. These agents are placed in a syringe and sealed with a syringe cap until it is time to administer the medication. The technician must follow the five steps outlined in the following sections and Figure 12-11 when preparing these syringes from ampules; the procedures differ from those followed when using a vial.

Technique

When solution is pulled from an ampule, there is no positive or negative pressure because this is an open system; that is, the container is open and able to allow air to enter it, replacing the missing volume of solution. However, it is important to remember to use a filter needle when transferring drug from an

PROCEDURE 12-3

Cleaning a Biological Safety Cabinet

GOAL: To learn to properly clean a biological safety cabinet.

EQUIPMENT AND SUPPLIES
- Biological safety cabinet
- Sterile water
- Lint-free wipes or gauze
- Sterile 70% alcohol

REMEMBER
- Procedures for cleaning and disinfecting the biological safety cabinet should be developed, implemented, and practiced by trained compounding personnel. These procedures must follow USP <797> guidelines and should be written in the facility's standard operating procedures (SOPs).
- Cleaning and disinfecting are to be completed before any compounding is performed.
- Biological safety cabinets are intended to operate 24 hours a day. They must be cleaned every 30 minutes while continuous compounding is taking place.
- Follow proper hand washing procedure and technique.
- Put on appropriate apparel, following proper garbing technique.

PROCEDURAL STEPS

1. Remove any items from within the biological safety cabinet.
PURPOSE: The biological safety cabinet should be completely empty so that all surfaces can be cleaned. Unnecessary items clutter the workspace and may contaminate the area.
2. Clean all surfaces inside the biological safety cabinet with a lint-free wipe and sterile water.
PURPOSE: To make certain all surfaces are clean and free from any loose material or residue.
3. Inspect all surfaces for any crystallized solutions. Clean these with sterile water before continuing.
PURPOSE: To make certain nothing is left on the surface that may contaminate the compounded sterile preparations (CSPs).

4. Moisten a 4 × 4-inch gauze or other lint-free cloth with sterile 70% alcohol.
PURPOSE: To prepare to disinfect the surfaces in the biological safety cabinet. If used properly, sterile 70% alcohol reduces the probability of contamination.
   *Remember to use a new wipe moistened with sterile 70% alcohol on each section of the biological safety cabinet cleaned.**
5. Wipe the horizontal IV pole and any hooks or brackets using a smooth motion from left to right.
PURPOSE: To ensure that the IV pole is disinfected and ready to use if any items need to be attached during the compounding process.
6. Wipe from top to bottom on each side of the biological safety cabinet. Work side to side with overlapping strokes.
PURPOSE: To disinfect the sides of the biological safety cabinet to prepare for the compounding process.
7. Wipe the rear wall of the biological safety cabinet and inside the front shield using a side-to-side motion from left to right, beginning at the top and working down to the bottom.
PURPOSE: To disinfect the rear wall and front shield of the biological safety cabinet to prepare for the compounding process.
8. Finally, wipe the flat work surface area using a side-to-side motion from left to right, working from back to front.
PURPOSE: To disinfect the work surface area of the biological safety cabinet to prepare for the compounding process.
9. Allow the sterile 70% alcohol to remain on surfaces to be disinfected for at least 30 seconds before such surfaces are used to prepare CSPs.
PURPOSE: To kill organisms that may contaminate the CSPs. If the alcohol is not allowed to dry completely, it may itself act as a vehicle for the transfer of contaminants.

*Never attempt to clean the HEPA filter or spray any solutions toward the HEPA filter. Also, discard alcohol bottles when empty and be sure to disinfect the spray head if transferring it to a new bottle to avoid contamination. Treat cleaning supplies as hazardous waste for disposal purposes.

ampule because small pieces of the ampule may detach and fall into the solution when the ampule is broken. A filter needle may be used only for one draw (push or pull); either it can be replaced by a regular needle before the drug is pushed into a piggyback. or a regular needle can be used to withdraw the solution and then a filter needle can be used to push the filtered solution into the piggyback. Otherwise, the glass trapped in the filter needle is pushed into the final solution.

Scenario CHECK UP 12-2

After cleaning the hood and the Automix compounder, Ken gathers his orders and supplies to begin his TPN compounding. It is extremely important that all TPN medications be prepared in a manner that reduces the possibility of contamination. The first order calls for magnesium chloride as one of the additives; this is supplied in a 10-mL ampule. In addition to the syringe, what will Ken need to draw up this additive? Why is this extra step critical?

PROCEDURE 12-4

Proper Hand Hygiene

GOAL: To learn to follow proper hand washing procedures to prevent the spread of infection.

EQUIPMENT AND SUPPLIES
- Warm water
- Facility-approved hand cleanser
- Nail brush or scrub sponge
- Waterless alcohol-based hand rub
- Non-shedding disposable towels or an electronic hand dryer

REMEMBER
- Personal electronic devices, such as cell phones or iPods and any associated attachments, must be removed before hand washing and should not be used in the sterile compounding area.

PROCEDURAL STEPS

1. Remove all visible jewelry and cosmetics before beginning the hand washing process.
   PURPOSE: To minimize the risk of bacterial contamination by minimizing the number of particles introduced into the sterile compounding area.
2. Wash the hands, nails, wrists, and forearms up to the elbows for at least 30 seconds with a brush and/or sponge, warm water, and a facility-approved cleansing agent.
   PURPOSE: To make certain all surfaces are clean and free from any residue. The cleansing agent should remain in contact with the skin for at least 30 seconds to complete the bactericidal activity.
3. Rinse thoroughly with the hands and forearms in an upright position, beginning with the fingertips down to the elbows.
   PURPOSE: To make certain contaminants flow away from the hands and all cleansing residue is removed.

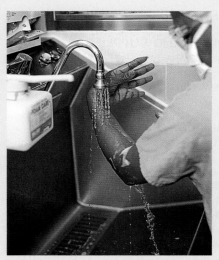

(From Potter PA, Perry AG: *Fundamentals of nursing,* ed 8, St Louis, 2013, Mosby.)

4. Dry the hands and arms with a non-shedding or lint-free cloth or with an electronic hand dryer.
   PURPOSE: To ensure that no contaminants are transferred from the towel to the clean hands.
   *Remember to leave the water running while you dry your hands and arms and do not touch any part of the sink or dryer surfaces.**
5. After the hands and arms are completely dry, throw away damp towels and use a new towel to turn off the running water.
   PURPOSE: To ensure that clean hands and arms are not contaminated by touching any unclean surfaces.
6. Sanitize the hands by applying a waterless, alcohol-based hand rub and allow it to dry completely before putting on sterile gloves.
   PURPOSE: To prohibit regrowth of bacteria after hand washing.

*Touch is the most common source of contamination. Hands and gloves remain sterile only until they touch something.

Vials

The two types of vials are those intended for immediate use (single dose vials [SDVs]) and those that can be used more than once (multidose vials [MDVs]). Because they are not discarded after one use, MDVs contain preservatives. Volumes for SDVs and MDVs range from 1 mL up to 100 mL, and vials may contain either solution for withdrawal or powder for reconstitution. When an MDV solution is used, the date the vial was opened must be written on the label, along with the initials of the person who opened the vial.

 Tech Note!

Never use an unmarked reconstituted vial because the amount of diluent is unknown. Instead, discard unmarked reconstituted vials. Frozen parenteral products must be thawed slowly, using either a cool bath or a thawing platform. They should never be placed in hot water or in a microwave oven. Once such medications have been thawed, they must be marked with the new expiration date per literature or the manufacturer's guidelines.

PROCEDURE 12-5

Personnel Cleansing and Garbing Order

GOAL: To learn the steps required to cleanse and garb up to properly prepare compounded sterile preparations

EQUIPMENT AND SUPPLIES

- Antiseptic hand cleanser
- Surgical scrub
- Shoe covers
- Head and facial hair cover
- Face mask or eye shield
- Non-shedding gown
- Sterile powder-free gloves

PROCEDURAL STEPS

1. Remove all personal outer garments.

PURPOSE: Outer garments such as jackets or coats may have shedding fibers or hairs that could contaminate the compounding area.

2. Remove all cosmetics and jewelry (no artificial nails are allowed).

PURPOSE: Cosmetics can flake off and jewelry and artificial nails can have dirt and other debris on and under the surface. These contaminants can be carried into the compounding area if not removed.

3. Put on personal protective equipment (PPE) in the following order:

Shoe covers

Head and facial hair covers

Face masks/eye shields

PURPOSE: Shoe covers help prevent any germs that may be on your shoes from entering the compounding area. Head and facial hair covers are used to keep any hairs from falling into the compounding area. Face masks and eye shields are used to protect the technician from exposure to medications that may splash or may accidentally spill during the compounding process.

4. Perform aseptic hand cleansing procedures with a surgical scrub.

PURPOSE: Proper hand washing with a surgical scrub helps to lessen the bacteria found on the hands before beginning the compounding process.

5. Put on a non-shedding gown.

PURPOSE: Donning a non-shedding gown serves to prevent any contaminants that may be on the technician's clothes from getting into the compounding area. Most gowns are resistant to penetration by moisture, which helps protect the technician if a spill occurs.

6. Put on the sterile, powder-free gloves.

PURPOSE: Gloves protect the compounding area from skin that is constantly shedding from our hands. They also protect the technician from exposure to medications that may be used in the compounding process. Double gloving is recommended when compounding hazardous drugs or chemicals.

Reconstituting a medication is the addition of a diluent, such as sterile water, to convert the medication into solution form. If an antibiotic MDV portion has been used, the following information must be indicated on the vial: the date the vial was opened, the date the vial expires, the diluent used (if applicable), the concentration (e.g., mg/mL), and the technician's initials. Bulk vials can be reconstituted in varying concentrations per the manufacturer's instructions to provide multiple IV bags for future use. For example, a cefazolin 10 g bulk vial can be reconstituted with 45 mL of sterile water, which provides a final concentration of 1 g per 5 mL. This supplies 10, 1-g bags of cefazolin that can be used immediately or can be refrigerated or frozen for later

use. Beyond-use dates differ between frozen and refrigerated medications. Many antibiotics are available in bulk containers.

Specialized types of vials, such as the ADD-Vantage system (Figure 12-12), can be placed on a small piggyback solution via an adapter; these are not mixed with the solution until immediately before administration. The pharmacy technician is responsible for proper attachment of the vial to the proper solution, but the nurse is responsible for breaking the adapter seal between the vial and the piggyback and mixing the powdered drug with the solution. Because the medication does not mix with the solution until the seal is broken, the IV can be returned to the pharmacy if it is not used. This greatly reduces the amount of wasted medication.

A controlled-release infusion system (CRIS) is another type of delivery system in which the vial is reconstituted (mixed) but is not added to the piggyback. At the time of administration, the vial is attached to a special port on the side of the tubing set that allows the medication to enter the piggyback, from which it then is delivered through the IV tubing.

Scenario *CHECK UP 12-3*

Ken is preparing to inject the next additive into the TPN mixture. He notices that the additive is from a multidose vial, which has been opened. The date the vial was opened is missing. What should Ken do in this situation? What could be the result if he uses the vial without proper documentation?

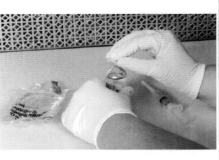

1

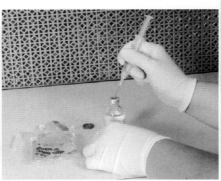

2

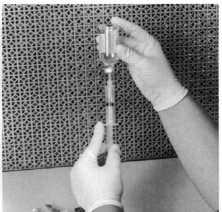

3

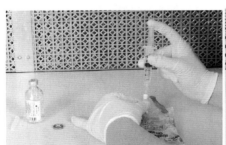

4

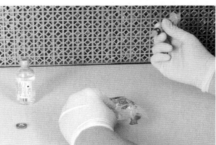

5

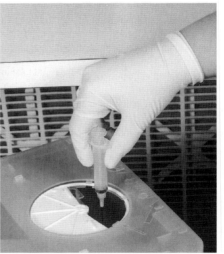

6

FIGURE 12-10 The six-step process for drawing medication from a vial. (1) Using sterile 70% alcohol, wipe the tops of the vials and the ports on the intravenous (IV) bags from back to front (wipe around the vial and bag rather than over or behind). (2) Place the needle bevel side up and push it into the rubber stopper of the vial. Preload the syringe with the necessary amount of air to replace solution. (3) Invert the vial and syringe 180 degrees. Push in the air from the syringe and pull out the solution. (4) After removing the syringe from the vial, insert the needle into the IV bag and inject the medication using a steady hand. (5) After injecting the IV bag with the medication, immediately flip the bag over. This reduces the likelihood of forgetting which bags have been injected and which have not. (6) Never recap the used needles; instead, discard each syringe in a sharps container, along with the uncapped needle, after use. Syringes cannot be reused when changing from one drug to another. This reduces the chance of drug-to-drug contamination.

 Tech Note!

When a diluent is added to a powder, it is important to read the instructions on the vial for reconstitution volumes. The final concentrations of many medications depend on both the volume of the diluent and the volume of the powder. For example, cefazolin 10 g powder and 45 mL of sterile water yield 10 g/50 mL; the cefazolin powder is responsible for the additional 5 mL of volume. Each manufacturer indicates how much diluent to use, along with the final concentration.

Parenteral Antibiotics and Solutions

Manufacturers have suggested guidelines for dosing regimens and volumes of solutions that most physicians follow (Table 12-8). The manufacturer's guidelines are determined by which microbe is targeted. Pharmacies have a chart that instructs the person preparing the medication as to the type and amount of diluent needed, the normal dosing times, and expiration dates. Antibiotics also differ in how they should be prepared and how long it takes the powder to dissolve in the diluent. Once the drug has been

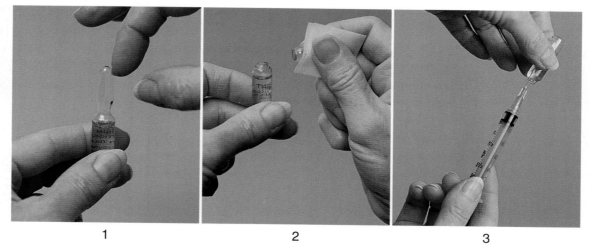

FIGURE 12-11 Proper manipulation of an ampule. Ampules are glass containers that range in size from 1 to 50 mL. For larger ampules, an ampule breaker is suggested. For smaller ampules, follow these steps: (1) Tap the top of the ampule to empty the top of the container. (2) Using a sterile 70% alcohol swab, wipe the neck of the ampule and snap it open (away from you). (3) Tilt the ampule at an angle (the solution will not spill) and withdraw the required amount of drug using a filter needle. (4) Replace the filter needle with a regular needle and inject the drug into the IV solution; however, if the drug is to be transported in the syringe, remove the needle and cap the end of the syringe. (5) Label the container and place it in the proper location for the pharmacist's inspection. (From Potter PA, Perry AG: *Fundamentals of nursing,* ed 8, St Louis, 2013, Mosby.)

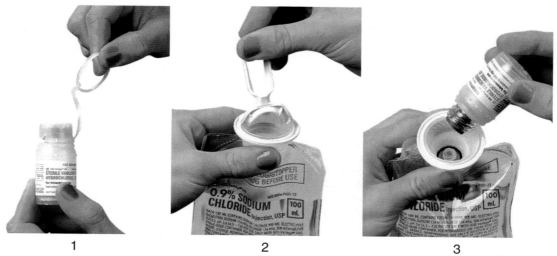

FIGURE 12-12 ADD-Vantage system. To prepare an IV medication, follow these three steps: (1) Remove the top of the vial. (2) Pull up the flange, removing the seal on the IV bag. (3) Screw the vial into the port. Do not break the seal between the vial and the bag.

reconstituted, the solution should be checked for color and clarity.

Technique

When a diluent is added to a powder, an equal amount of air must be removed from the vial or positive pressure is created, which causes pressure resistance in the syringe. For example, if you are adding 10 mL of diluent to a powder, push on the syringe until you feel a very slight resistance and then stop and withdraw an equal amount of air from the vial to relieve the positive pressure. Repeat this until all

the diluent has been added. To work with negative pressure, first withdraw air from the vial until you feel resistance and then allow the vial to pull diluent out of the syringe. Never let go of a syringe. This type of technique works well because there is less chance of a spill.

Hyperalimentation

Hyperalimentation (also known as hyperals) is a term for large volumes of parenteral nutrition solutions normally prepared for individuals who cannot

TABLE 12-8

Examples of Suggested Dosing Times, Solutions, and Appropriate Volumes for Antibiotics

Generic Name	Trade Name	Common Dosing Regimens (hr)	Common Solutions	Common Volumes
Ampicillin	Omnipen	q6-q8	NS	Less than 1.5 g (50 mL), more than 1.5 g (100 mL)
Cefazolin	Ancef, Kefzol	q6-q8	D₅W or NS	Less than 2 g (50 mL), more than 2 g (100 mL)
Cefotaxime	Claforan	q6-q12	D₅W or NS	Less than 2 g (50 mL), more than 2 g (100 mL)
Ceftazidime	Fortaz	q6-q8	D₅W or NS	Less than 2 g (50 mL), more than 2 g (100 mL)
Ceftriaxone	Rocephin	q8-q24	D₅W or NS	Less than 2 g (50 mL), more than 2 g (100 mL)
Doxycycline	Vibramycin	q12	D₅W or NS	250 mL
Erythromycin	E-Mycin	q6-q24	NS	250 mL* (10 mg) or 500 mL (20 mg) lidocaine
Gentamicin	Garamycin	q8-q18† based on glycoside levels	D₅W or NS	Less than 100 mg (50 mL), more than 100 mg (100 mL)
Imipenem-cilastatin	Primaxin	q6-q12	NS	Less than 500 mg (100 mL), more than 500 mg (250 mL)

D₅W, 5% dextrose in water; *NS*, normal saline.

*Erythromycin stings when given intravenously; therefore it is commonly mixed with lidocaine to relieve the pain.

†See Chapter 25 for more information on antibiotics.

TECHICIAN PROFILE

Rita is an IV technician specialist at a local medical center. Her position requires completion of an ASHP-accredited pharmacy technician program and PTCB certification. Six months experience in a hospital setting is mandatory before hire. Rita's duties are performed under the supervision of the pharmacist. She is responsible for accurately preparing IV admixtures, parenteral nutrition, and other injectable preparations using aseptic technique. She is skilled in the operation and maintenance of the automated systems used in the IV compounding area. It is Rita's job to be knowledgeable about the USP <797> guidelines and their implementation. Rita maintains active memberships in her state and national ASHP associations. These memberships allow her to keep abreast of important information related to IV compounding. She finds her position both challenging and rewarding and prepares each IV with the utmost care, always keeping the end user in mind.

---

orally consume nutrition (i.e., they cannot eat). Some reasons for this inability to eat include:

- Recent stomach or intestinal surgery
- Unconsciousness (coma)
- Various conditions that may adversely affect the gastrointestinal system.

Two main types of hyperalimentation are prepared in the pharmacy: **total parenteral nutrition (TPN)** and **peripheral parenteral nutrition (PPN)**. A **peripheral parenteral injection** is administered into the veins on the periphery of the body (arms, hands, or feet) instead of into a central vein or artery.

In a hospital setting, after the initial hyperalimentation (hyperal) has been prepared and hung, daily laboratory tests of electrolyte levels are drawn from the patient to determine necessary changes. For example, if a patient's potassium levels begin to drop, the next hyperal is altered to compensate for this decrease. In this way, the patient receives exactly the nutrients needed each day. Home health clinics and some hospitals prepare hyperalimentation solutions that last 1 week. If this is done, the vitamin additive must be added daily to the hyperal because this is one limiting factor for the bag's 24-hour expiration. Electrolyte levels are tested weekly instead of daily. Some patients may receive this type of nutrition for many months. Figure 12-13 shows a TPN preparation connected to an automatic infusion pump system.

Many different protocols are used to prepare parenteral nutrition. The following is a list of typical solutions prepared in a hospital pharmacy. The large volume components (e.g., protein, carbohydrates, and fats) are premixed and ordered in cases from the manufacturer. Added to these solutions are the various electrolytes and other compatible medications requested by the patient's attending physician:

- TPN normally contains 50% dextrose, 10% amino acids, and 20% fat.
- PPN normally contains 25% dextrose, 10% amino acids, and 10% fat.
- Hyperals are prepared for neonates, children, and adults.

Because of the regulations established by USP <797>, many pharmacies contract out their TPN/PPN orders to specialized compounding companies. Bags can range in volumes from 50 mL for neonates up to 3 L for adults. It is important to note that neonatal and pediatric additives differ in concentration from adult formulas; therefore, great care must be taken when pulling the correct medication for preparation if your facility prepares these products.

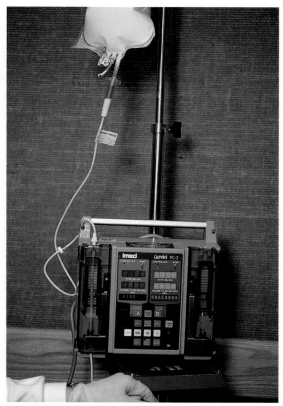

FIGURE 12-13 Total parenteral nutrition preparation connected to an infusion set. (From Perry AG, Potter PA, Elkin MK: *Nursing interventions and clinical skills,* ed 5, St Louis, 2012, Elsevier.)

 Scenario CHECK UP 12-4

Ken is now compounding a TPN for a baby in the intensive care unit. The physician's TPN order included directions to add zinc in a concentration of 200 mcg/100 mL. The automated compounder requires entry of zinc in a mcg/kg dose. What will happen if the pharmacist enters the zinc dose into the pharmacy computer as mg instead of mcg? What should Ken do if he discovers the error? A scenario similar to this one actually happened. For more information on the story, visit the website *www.ncbi.nlm.nih.gov/pmc/ articles/PMC3171817/.*

Tech Note!

Some chemicals can **precipitate** other chemicals, creating solid flakes in the intravenous solution. Always check your IV bag for clarity after you finish preparing the solution.

Because of their range of concentrations, PPN solutions are administered differently from the higher concentration TPN solutions. TPN is administered intravenously via the subclavian vein and superior vena cava because of the higher concentra-tion of nutrients. Patients must have a catheter surgically inserted for this procedure. PPN is administered via a peripheral vein, either in the back of the hand or in another peripheral area in the upper extremity, and therefore is a less complicated procedure. Most facilities have a standard order to initiate patient hyperalimentation. The volume of hyperalimentation typically ranges from 2 to 3 L. The physician determines the rate of infusion over the course of 24 hours. Regardless of how many milliliters run per hour, the hyperalimentation must be changed at least every 24 hours to ensure the sterility of the solution. A standard rate of infusion is 100 mL/hour; therefore, 2400 mL may be used over the course of a day. Most hyperalimentation preparations are tailor-made for each patient. Figure 12-14 gives an example of a protocol order.

Tech Note!

The final product must always be checked for color, clarity, and evidence of precipitation.

Electrolytes and Additives

All TPN preparations contain dextrose and amino acids; both ingredients help nourish the body. The metabolism of dextrose (i.e., sugar) provides calories and a quick energy source for the body, whereas amino acids are the essential components the body uses to synthesize protein, needed enzymes, and other important molecules. Lipids commonly are added to give the body the fat needed for synthesis of important cell components, such as cell membranes. The rest of the additives are additional electrolytes (Table 12-9). These components can be determined daily if the patient is in a hospital. Other medications, such as ranitidine, cimetidine, or famotidine (all histamine$_2$-antagonists), which help patients with stomach problems, also can be added to hyperalimentation. Besides stomach medications, insulin often is added in quantities up to 100 units per bag. Only regular insulin is added to hyperalimentation preparations because it is the only insulin product that may be given intravenously.

Compatibility Considerations of Parenteral Medications

Many different types of medications are prepared in a clean room. Some medications must be protected from light, whereas others must be kept in bottles (as discussed previously). Table 12-10 presents additional considerations in the preparation of parenteral drugs. Special instructions for the preparation of many types of parenteral medications can be found

TPN ORDER SHEET

HOME HEALTH	DATE
PATIENT	ADDRESS

TPN FORMULA:

AMINO ACIDS: ☐ 5.5% ☐ 8.5% ☑ 10% ☐ WITH STANDARD ELECTROLYTES	425 mL
DEXTROSE: ☐ 10% ☐ 20% ☐ 40% ☐ 50% ☑ 70% (check one)	357 mL
LIPIDS: ☐ 10% ☑ 20% FOR ALL-IN-ONE FORMULA	125 mL

FINAL VOLUME qsad STERILE WATER FOR INJECTION	400mL	1307 mL

Calcium Gluconate	0.465m Eq/mL	5	mEq
Magnesium Sulfate	4m Eq/mL	5	mEq
Potassium Acetate	2m Eq/mL		mEq
Potassium Chloride	2m Eq/mL		mEq
Potassium Phosphate	3m M/mL	22	mM
Sodium Acetate	2m Eq/mL		mEq
Sodium Chloride	4m Eq/mL	35	mEq
Sodium Phosphate	3m M/mL		mM
TRACE ELEMENTS CONCENTRATE	☐ 4 ☐ 5 ☐ 6		mL

Patient Additives:

☐ MVC 9 + 3 10 mL Daily

☐ HUMULIN-R __10__ u Daily

☐ FOLIC ACID _____ mg
_____ times weekly

☐ VITAMIN K _____ mg
_____ times weekly

☐ OTHER: __MVI 12 1.5mL/daily__

☐ OTHER: _____

Directions:

INFUSE: ☑ DAILY
☐ ____ TIMES WEEKLY

OTHER DIRECTIONS:

_____

_____

_____

_____

Rate: ☐ CYCLIC INFUSION: OVER ____ HOURS (TAPER UP AND DOWN)	" " "	☐ CONTINUOUS INFUSION: AT ____ mL PER HOUR	" " "	☑ STANDARD RATE: AT __110__ mL PER HOUR FOR __12__ HOURS

LAB ORDERS:

☐ STANDARD LAB ORDERS
SMAC-20, CO2, Mg+2 TWICE WEEKLY
CBC WITH AUTO DIFF WEEKLY
UNTIL STABLE, THEN:
SMAC-20, CO2, Mg+2 WEEKLY
CBC WITH AUTO DIFF MONTHLY

☐ OTHER: _____

_____

_____

VALIDATION:

_____
DOCTOR'S SIGNATURE

Print Name: _____

Office Address: _____

_____

Phone: _____

WHITE: Home Health   CANARY: Physician

FIGURE 12-14 Total parenteral nutrition order.

TABLE 12-9

Types of Parenteral Additives

Abbreviation	Meaning	Concentration	Notes
KCl	Potassium chloride	2 mEq/mL	
KPO$_4$	Potassium phosphate	Potassium 2 mEq/mL; phosphate 3 mEq/mL	Always determine phosphate concentration first
CaGluconate	Calcium gluconate	0.465 mEq/mL	
MgSO$_4$	Magnesium sulfate	1 mg/mL	
KAc	Potassium acetate	2 mEq/mL	Used to balance*
NaAcetate	Sodium acetate	2 mEq/mL	Used to balance*
NaPO$_4$	Sodium phosphate	2 mEq/mL	
NaCl	Sodium chloride	2 mEq/mL	Used to balance*
Miscellaneous Additives			
MVI	Multivitamin		Both adult and pediatric dosing
MTE	Multiple trace elements		Both adult and pediatric dosing
Zn	Zinc		
Se	Selenium		
Regular insulin	Insulin		Can be added to TPN and PPN

Other Nonsupplements Added to TPN or PPN Solutions		
Generic Name	**Trade Name**	**Concentration**
Ranitidine	Zantac	40 mg/mL
Famotidine	Pepcid	20 mg/mL
Cimetidine	Tagamet	150 mg/mL

PPN, Peripheral parenteral nutrition; *TPN,* total parenteral nutrition.
To balance means the pharmacist determines the amount to be added.

TABLE 12-10

Additional Considerations for the Preparation of Drugs

Medication	Special Instructions
Insulin	NS or ½NS; must be placed in glass container
Amiodarone	D$_5$W
Nitroglycerin	D$_5$NS or NS; must be placed in glass container
Ciprofloxacin	Protect from light
Lorazepam	Protect from light; stable longer in glass than in plastic

D$_5$NS, 5% dextrose in normal saline; *D$_5$W,* 5% dextrose in water; *NS,* normal saline.

in reference books in IV rooms. The IV technician must become familiar with the idiosyncrasies of medications to ensure that all solutions he or she makes are effective and safe.

Components of a Label for Intravenous Medication

The final step in preparing parenteral medications is the application of the label. First, check the label against the medication and the physician's orders to

 Tech Note!

Each type of medication has its own unique properties. For example, ceftazidime produces gas when reconstituted. Therefore, to prevent the solution from shooting out of the vial, the gas must be released first. This can be done by puncturing the vial membrane with a needle to allow venting of the gas. Erythromycin powder is difficult to dissolve into the diluent; therefore, it is important to allow additional time when reconstituting erythromycin. Allow the vial to sit in the hood (and shake it occasionally) until the powder turns into a solution.

ensure that the right medication is being given to the right patient. Although each pharmacy prepares its own label, all labels require the same minimum information (Figure 12-15).

All labels produced for parenteral medications must be initialed by the technician who prepares them. A registered pharmacist is responsible for the final label inspection. If the medication is not used, perhaps because of a discontinued order, it is recycled for use with another patient.

After the labels have been applied, the IV preparations are left for the pharmacist to check, along with the vial or container of medication used to make the

HOME INFUSION PHARMACY

Patient A   Date: 03/26/2012
RX#37856

Amino*Acids 10%=425 mL Dextrose*70%=357 mL
Ster*Water=400 mL Lipids*20%=125 mL
MVI=10 ml/day *Additives per liter*
Sod*Chlor=35 mEq Pot*Phos=15 mM Calcium=
5 mEq Magnesium=5 mEq

Qty#   TPN 40–51GM Protein+Lipids
Infuse nightly 8pm to 8am thru IV PICC line via sigma
pump. *****Add 10 units Humulin-R to each bag just
prior to infusion***** **Note: contains TPN soln+lipids:
rate adjusted** Settings: rate=104 mL/hr
volume=1248 mL

REFRIGERATE

Expiration date: 04/01/07

FIGURE 12-15 IV medication label.

IV preparation. When this check has been completed, the IV preparations are loaded onto a cart or delivery vehicle that delivers them to their destinations. In a home health setting, a delivery service may be used to transport the medications to the patient's home. In a hospital, this task normally is done by the technician. When the IV preparations are placed in the correct nursing unit, all unused IV preparations are collected and returned to the pharmacy for recycling. As long as the IV preparations are within their expiration dates and are kept at proper temperature, they can be used to fill new orders.

Disposal

Once the technician has finished using the hood area, he or she should clean all unused materials and discard any used products. To clean a horizontal flow hood, wipe down the surface with a sterile 70% isopropyl alcohol swab and then allow the surface to air dry. Dispose of all paper products in a trash bin; dispose of needles, syringes, and vials in a sharps container. Most sharps containers are made of heavy-duty plastic; they have a separate lid that can be locked into place on top of the container and a one-way opening in the lid for the disposal of needles and other sharps. Normally a 7-gallon size is used and is located outside the hood. When cleaning a vertical flow hood, discard needles, syringes, and vials in a small sharps container placed inside the hood area. Wrap all other materials to be discarded into the spill-proof pad and place inside a chemotherapeutic protective bag. This may be discarded in a special hazardous materials bin located outside the hood. All materials used in the BSC, including

disposable needles and syringes, must be placed in appropriate sharps disposal containers and discarded as infectious waste. This is located inside the hood area.

For all hoods, the last step is to clean the entire area with the proper sterile 70% alcohol solution as appropriate for the type of cabinet involved. Sharps containers are to be replaced when two-thirds full and must be picked up or delivered to an approved "red bag" or medical waste treatment site.

Tech Note!

Always check the pharmacy protocol for the disposal of sharps containers. This information can be found in the policies and procedures handbook. Never insert your hand into a sharps or hazardous waste container! This could result in a needle stick or exposure to a hazardous chemical.

Chemotherapeutic Agents

Special considerations apply in the preparation of chemotherapeutic agents. Because of the risks involved in handling chemotherapy drugs, technicians must be thoroughly trained in chemotherapy admixture technique to reduce the chances of exposure. Hazardous medications should be prepared only in a safe environment, such as a vertical flow barrier hood or a BSC. Pharmacy technicians should always follow chemo guidelines and should be trained in proper disposal of hazardous substances. Special chemo gowns are worn to repel any substances that might spill or drip onto the technician during the compounding process. Double gloves are worn for extra protection. Face and eye shields help the technician avoid contamination of the eyes. Masks are worn to prevent inhalation of any dangerous chemicals. When chemotherapeutic agents are compounded, preparation and cleanup must be done slowly and carefully, and the proper documentation should be completed.

Spills

If a spill occurs in a horizontal flow hood, it may be cleaned using a gauze pad and sterile 70% isopropyl alcohol. The gauze can be discarded in a regular trash bin. Always wear the proper protective equipment for the type of spill to be handled. If a small spill occurs in a vertical flow hood, it should be cleaned with sterile gauze and 70% isopropyl alcohol and discarded inside a chemotherapeutic protective bag. If a small spill occurs in a BSC, wipe up the spill with a disinfectant-soaked paper towel and then clean the surface with 70% isopropyl alcohol. The outer pair of gloves must be replaced after cleaning up a spill. Dispose of the materials in the appropriate container. For specific information on spill size and cleaning techniques, see the policies and procedures binder.

 Tech Note!

Always know the location of the cleanup kit for **hazardous waste** spills. In addition, take time to review the policies and procedures in case of a chemotherapeutic drug spill.

Scenario CHECK UP 12-5

Ken is required to complete an aseptic validation certification each year to maintain his position. He must complete a media-fill simulation test that demonstrates his ability to use aseptic procedures to compound sterile pharmacy products. He must meet the verification and sterility testing requirements as detailed in USP <797>. What should be his margin of error? Should he be allowed more than one attempt? What should be the consequence of failing this simulation test?

Education and Training

Both pharmacists and technicians must be able to show competency in compounding. Before compounding is permitted, the pharmacist and technician must complete video and written and practical instruction, followed by a media-fill test and a written exam. Training and testing must be repeated annually for low- and medium-risk levels and semiannually for the high-risk level.

Although individuals who prepare sterile products must receive training on standards of sterile compounding, those instructions differ, depending on the number and type of manipulations performed. Normally physicians, nurses, and emergency medical technicians (EMTs) prepare only low-risk products. Pharmacy technicians and pharmacists must be instructed on all standards if they are to prepare all types of compounded sterile preparations. For example, an IV technician may need only risk level 2 training, whereas technicians who prepare chemotherapeutic agents or hyperalimentation need training for risk level 3 preparations.

Several steps must be accomplished to complete the proper training. By viewing instructional videos from the ASHP, technicians can learn safe handling of compounded sterile preparations. In addition, aseptic technique verification services, such as Valiteq Products, provide training packets for various risk levels. Both ASHP and Valiteq have

---

BOX 12-3

Media-Fill Tests

What is a media-fill test?
For a media-fill test, a microbial growth medium (e.g., trypticase soy broth [TSB]) solution is substituted for the actual drug to simulate the admixture compounding technique. After the TSB is injected into the compounded sterile product, the final container is incubated at 20° to 35° C for 14 days and then checked for turbidity. A positive test result confirms the presence of microbial contaminants.

How often are media-fill tests performed?
Per USP <797> regulations, a media-fill test must be completed at the time of hire. Thereafter, it must be performed at least yearly for low- and medium-risk compounding levels and twice a year for high-risk compounding levels.

Under what conditions is a media-fill test performed?
It is suggested that the test be performed in a manner to mimic a real case scenario; for example, at the end of the day when the preparer is tired or at stressful work times during the day.

What happens if the test results are positive?
The written policies for the pharmacy include steps that should be taken for positive test results; they include retraining in aseptic techniques with a mentor and then repeating the media-fill test. If the test results are positive after the retest, it is suggested that the clean room and hoods be tested for any contamination. All results should be documented.

---

compounding manuals that can be used throughout the training period. Valiteq includes media-fill tests (Box 12-3) and a written exam, in addition to a visual check-off list for observation of the preparer. Once the preparation is complete, the growth medium is incubated according to set requirements and tested at various times for any abnormal growth. No growth is acceptable for a passing score. A 90% passing score is required on the written test and practical observation in the hood. These check-offs must be completed and passed before the technician is permitted to prepare compounded sterile preparations. Personnel who fail any of the tests must repeat instruction and reevaluation. Check-lists are often made by pharmacies to document the evaluation of the person compounding. A sample form (Figure 12-16) lists the standards required of personnel who prepare CSPs. To ensure compliance, an observer must rate each standard while preparations are being compounded.

COMPOUNDING EVALUATION CHECKLIST
(circle answer)

No jewelry	YES	NO	N/A
Hair tied back	YES	NO	N/A
All calculations done prior	YES	NO	N/A
All products gathered prior	YES	NO	N/A
Washes hands appropriately	YES	NO	N/A
Gowns appropriately	YES	NO	N/A
Cleans hood 70% isopropyl alcohol	YES	NO	N/A
Cleans hood appropriately	YES	NO	N/A
Puts all items into the hood properly	YES	NO	N/A
Uses aseptic manipulation in the hood	YES	NO	N/A
Works within 6" radius of hood	YES	NO	N/A
If left the hood, sterilizes gloves prior to re-entering	YES	NO	N/A
Checked label 3 times	YES	NO	N/A
Uses proper equipment while in the hood	YES	NO	N/A
Uses foil cover on port after adding medication	YES	NO	N/A
Checks final product for color, clarity	YES	NO	N/A
Places label properly on product	YES	NO	N/A
Label is correct	YES	NO	N/A
Calculations are correct	YES	NO	N/A
Expiration date given	YES	NO	N/A
Signature of preparer signed	YES	NO	N/A
Disposes of vial and used packages appropriately	YES	NO	N/A
Cleans hood after use	YES	NO	N/A
Did not spill any contents	YES	NO	N/A
Did not break airflow	YES	NO	N/A
Checked for any particulates in diluted solution	YES	NO	N/A

Name _____   Date_____Time _____

Evaluator _____

Comments:_____

FIGURE 12-16 Compounding evaluation checklist.

DO YOU REMEMBER THESE KEY POINTS?

- Why certain medication must be sterile
- Common terms used in sterile compounding
- The Standard Precautions necessary when preparing compounded sterile preparations
- The standard supplies and equipment used to prepare compounded sterile preparations
- The anatomy of a syringe and needle
- The sizes of syringes and needles used in the pharmacy setting
- When and why filters are used in sterile compounding
- Types of stock used in a clean room
- The various medication delivery systems
- The history of USP <797>

- The main components of USP <797> regulations
- The three risk levels of drug preparation determined by USP <797>
- The various types of hoods
- How often hoods must be inspected
- How to properly clean various types of hoods and prepare them for use
- The proper aseptic technique
- The steps in drawing up medication from an ampule
- The steps in drawing up medication from a vial
- Different types of IV parenteral medications
- How to properly dispose of needles, vials, and cytotoxic supplies

Scenario FOLLOW UP

Ken completes his yearly aseptic validation certification and receives his results. He is delighted to see that his compounded parenteral products were 98% particulate free. He knows the only way to ensure product quality is to continually demonstrate proper procedure. His goal is to produce 100% contaminant-free TPN and IV admixtures. Do you think this is an attainable goal? Why or why not?

REVIEW QUESTIONS

Multiple Choice Questions

1. The smallest filter that can be used is a:
   A. Filter straw
   B. Filter needle
   C. 5-μm filter
   D. 0.22-μm filter

2. Laminar flow hoods should be cleaned:
   A. With 70% isopropyl alcohol
   B. At least 30 minutes before using
   C. After any spill
   D. All of the above

3. Chemotherapeutic agents should be disposed of:
   A. In a plastic chemotherapy bag
   B. In a sharps container
   C. Only at the end of a shift
   D. By a biohazard team of professionals

4. HEPA stands for _____, which traps particles larger than _____:
   A. heated environmental parenteral air filter; 2 μm
   B. high-environmental particulate air filter; 0.2 μm
   C. horizontal-efficiency particulate air filter; 0.2 μm
   D. high-efficiency particulate air filter; 0.2 μm

5. How far should you be working in the hood when compounding?
   A. At least 12 inches
   B. At least 6 inches
   C. Just past the front grill
   D. At least halfway between the front grill and the HEPA filter

6. A room adjacent to the clean room must meet standards classified as:
   A. ISO Class 5
   B. ISO Class 6
   C. ISO Class 8
   D. ISO Class 10

7. First-air refers to:
   A. The air from the HEPA filter that passes over the materials
   B. The first air that you breathe in the clean room
   C. The air contained inside a vial
   D. The air contained inside a syringe

8. Low-risk IVs kept at refrigerated temperatures expire within:
   A. 7 days
   B. 14 days
   C. 21 days
   D. 30 days

9. Horizontal flow hoods should be inspected every:
   A. Month
   B. 3 months
   C. 6 months
   D. 12 months

10. SOP means:
    A. Safe operating protocol
    B. Safe operations policy
    C. Standard operating policy
    D. Standard operating procedure

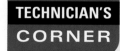
TECHNICIAN'S CORNER

Laura recently moved to a new city and was hired as an IV technician for the local hospital. She has 5 years of IV room experience and is a certified pharmacy technician with the PTCB. During her first week at her new job, she notices that some of her co-workers do not always follow proper aseptic technique. A few wear makeup and jewelry into the compounding area on a regular basis. Laura knows that these behaviors put the patients at risk. How should she handle this dilemma?

Bibliography

Bachenheimer BS: *Manual for pharmacy technicians,* ed 4, Bethesda, Md, 2010, American Society of Health-Systems Pharmacists.

Ballington D: *Pharmacy practice for technicians,* ed 5, St Paul, 2014, EMC/Paradigm.

Baxa Corporation: Englewood, Colorado, USP <797> training requirements: 2011 course schedule.

Holmes CJ, Ausman RK, Kundsin RB, Walter CW: Effect of freezing and microwave thawing on the stability of six antibiotic admixtures in plastic bags, *Am J Hosp Pharm* 39:104, 1982. (Referenced December 9, 2013.) www.ncbi.nlm.nih.gov/pubmed/6798865

Perry A, Potter P, Elkin M: *Nursing interventions and clinical skills,* ed 5, St Louis, 2012, Elsevier.

Potter P, Perry A: *Fundamentals of nursing,* ed 8, St Louis, 2013, Mosby.

Simmons H: Best practices for aseptic media-fill testing. *Pharmacy Purchasing & Products.* (Referenced December 8, 2013.) www.pppmag.com/documents/V4N8/p2_4_5.pdf

Websites Referenced

Centers for Disease Control and Prevention: 2014 Biosafety and Operations Management. (Referenced December 15, 2013.) www.cdc.gov/OD/OHS/biosfty/bsc/BSC2000sec5.htm

Controlled Environments: What Do the New Sterile Compounding Pharmacy Regulations Mean to You? (Referenced March 25, 2014.) http://www.cemag.us/articles/2014/02/what-do-new-sterile-compounding-pharmacy-regulations-mean-you

Device Link: (Referenced December 15, 2013.) www.devicelink.com/pmpn/archive/02/04/005.html

Micro-Clean, Inc: Sample Cleaning and Sanitizing Procedure. (Referenced December 8, 2013.) www.microcln.com/PDF/CleaningandSanitizingProcedure.pdf

University of Illinois at Chicago College of Pharmacy, Drug Information Group: What Are the New Changes for USP <797> for 2008? (Referenced December 3, 2013.) www.uic.edu/pharmacy/services/di/faq/usp797.php

Pharmacy Billing and Inventory Management

Bobbi Steelman

OBJECTIVES

Upon completing this chapter, you should be able to do the following:

1. Discuss the importance of pharmacy billing and inventory management to the pharmacy practice.
2. Explain the function of a drug formulary in insurance plans.
3. Describe the role of the pharmacy technician in the drug utilization evaluation.
4. Discuss how a drug formulary or an approved/preferred product list affects pharmacy billing and inventory control.
5. Assess the differences between generic and trade name (proprietary) drugs in pharmacy billing.
6. List the primary types of private and group medical insurance plans.
7. Describe how each type of private and group insurance manages drug coverage.
8. Differentiate between Medicare, Medicaid, and Medigap programs.
9. List the four parts of Medicare coverage.
10. Differentiate between TRICARE and CHAMPVA benefits.
11. Describe workers' compensation coverage.
12. Explain the purpose of third-party billing.
13. Describe the purpose of point of sale billing.
14. Describe the role of prior authorization in claims processing.
15. List the information found on a prescription card.
16. Determine the information needed to complete a patient profile for a pharmacy database.
17. Discuss online adjudication.
18. Identify the information needed to complete a universal claim form.
19. List and discuss reasons for claim rejections.
20. Describe the process of resubmitting rejected claims.
21. Discuss the types of plan limitations common in managed care.
22. Explain the various prescription payment methods, including self-pay, discount programs or coupons, private plans, and health savings accounts/flexible spending accounts.
23. Explain the importance of inventory management.
24. Define the periodic automatic replenishment level and describe how it affects inventory management.
25. Describe the role of an inventory control technician.
26. Discuss the purpose of the National Drug Code (NDC) numbers, lot numbers, and expiration and beyond-use dates.
27. Explain the inventory ordering and receiving processes, including special orders, bar coding, manual ordering, and new stock.
28. List the types of automated dispensing systems used in pharmacy.
29. Describe storage requirements for various types of inventory.
30. Outline the steps for handling recalled, returned, or expired medications.
31. List the types of suppliers of pharmacy stock.
32. Identify any special considerations related to drug ordering and storage.

TERMS AND DEFINITIONS

Adjudication Electronic insurance billing for medication payment

Average wholesale price (AWP) The average price at which a drug is sold; the data are compiled from information provided by manufacturers, distributors, and pharmacies; the AWP is often used in calculations related to medication reimbursement

Civilian Health and Medical Program of the Department of Veterans Affairs (CHAMPVA) A program for veterans with permanent service-related disabilities and their dependents and for the spouses and children of veterans who died from service-connected disability; also known as the Veterans Health Administration (VHA)

Closed formulary Tight restriction of medication use to the medications included on the formulary list; medications that are not listed as preapproved drugs per the health plan provider or pharmacy benefits manager are not reimbursed except under extenuating circumstances and with proper documentation

Coinsurance A type of insurance in which the policyholder pays a share of the payment made against a claim

Copayment The portion of the prescription bill that the patient is responsible for paying

Deductible The amount paid by a policyholder out of pocket before the insurance company pays a claim

Direct manufacturer ordering Pharmacies may join a group purchasing organization (GPO) and contract directly with the manufacturer to obtain better pricing.

Drug Topics Red Book A reference book listing National Drug Code (NDC) numbers, manufacturers, and average wholesale pricing of drug products; note that pharmacies often include this type of product and pricing information in their online database systems, which are provided by companies such as First DataBank and Gold Standard

Drug utilization evaluation (DUE) or review (DUR) An ongoing review by a pharmacist of the prescribing, dispensing, and use of medications, based on predetermined criteria, to decide whether changes need to be made in a patient's drug therapy

Formulary A list of preapproved medications that are covered under a prescription plan or within an institution

Health Insurance Portability and Accountability Act (HIPAA) Federal guidelines for the protection of a patient's personal health information

Health Maintenance Organization (HMO) An insurance plan that that allows coverage for in-network only physicians and services and uses the primary care physician (or provider) as the "gatekeeper" for the patient's health care; patients often have copays to defray the costs of medical care and prescription drugs

Inventory The amount of product a pharmacy has for sale

Just-in-time ordering A system that orders a product just before it is used

Medicaid A government-managed insurance program that provides health care services to low-income children, the elderly, blind, and those with disabilities

Medicare A government-managed insurance program composed of several coverage plans for health care services and supplies; it is funded by both federal and state entities, and individuals must meet specific requirements to be eligible; individuals must be 65 years or older, be younger than 65 with long-term disabilities, or suffer from end-stage renal disease

Medicare Modernization Act (MMA) The enactment of prescription drug coverage provided for individuals covered under Medicare

Medigap plan Supplemental insurance provided through private insurance companies to help cover costs not reimbursed by the Medicare plan, such as coinsurance, copays, and deductibles

National Drug Code (NDC) A 10-digit number given to all drugs for identification purposes; in health and drug databases, the NDC is represented as an 11-digit number, in which placeholder zeros are inserted in the proper order in the code for the purpose of standardizing data transmissions

National Provider Identifier (NPI) A number assigned to any health care provider that is used for the purpose of standardizing health data transmissions

Open formulary A formulary list that is essentially unrestricted in the types of drug choices offered or that can be prescribed and reimbursed under the health provider plan or pharmacy benefit plan

Patient profile A document listing necessary patient personal and health information, including comprehensive information on the medications the patient is taking, disease states, and any food or drug allergies the person might have

Periodic automatic replenishment (PAR) The periodic automatic replenishment of stock levels to a certain number of allowed units

Pharmacy and therapeutics committee (P&T committee) Medical staff composed of physicians, pharmacists, pharmacy technicians, nurses, and dieticians who provide necessary information and advice to the institution or insurer on whether a drug should be added to a formulary

Point of sale (POS) A system that allows inventory to be tracked as it is used

Preferred provider organization (PPO) An insurance plan in which patients choose a provider from a specified list, resulting in reduced costs for medical services

Prime vendor A large distributor of medications and retail products that contracts with the pharmacy to deliver the bulk of their medications in exchange for lower prices; examples of prime vendors are McKesson, Cardinal Health, and AmerisourceBergen

Prior authorization Insurance-required approval for a restricted, nonformulary, or noncovered medication before a prescription medication can be filled

Safety Data Sheets (SDS) Information sheets supplied to the pharmacy from the manufacturer of chemical products; the SDS lists the hazards of the product and procedures to follow if a person is exposed to that product

Trade, brand, or proprietary drug name The name a company assigns for marketing and identification purposes to a commercial drug product; most brand names are trademarked and belong to originator products; the named products are often protected for a time by patents

Treatment authorization request (TAR) The process used by Medicare and Medicaid for authorization of assistive technology devices costing more than $100; durable medical equipment (e.g., wheelchairs and walkers) also require a TAR; similar to a preauthorization form

TRICARE (formerly CHAMPUS) A health benefit program for active duty and retired personnel in all seven uniformed services; it also covers dependents of military personnel who were killed while on active duty

Wholesalers Companies that stock a variety of drug manufacturers' medications and normally have a "just-in-time" turnaround for ordered drugs; this means that drugs ordered today arrive the next day

Workers' compensation Government-required and government-enforced medical coverage for workers injured on the job, paid for by the employer; the programs are managed by each state in accordance with the state's workers' compensation laws

Introduction

Everyone working in the pharmacy is responsible for maintaining the **inventory** stock. This is an essential part of the daily tasks of pharmacy staff. As stock is depleted, it is important to order replacement inventory. Although many different systems are available for ordering stock, the task of ordering may be delegated to a specific person in the pharmacy. It is then the responsibility of the staff to inform the inventory control person of decreasing stock levels. One method of replenishing the stock is "just-in-time" ordering. This is an inventory strategy in which medications are ordered and received only as they are used.

Along with ordering stock, pharmacy technicians help manage the third-party billing process. Knowledge of proper billing procedures is a skill that normally is learned by experience over time as a technician works in the pharmacy. Because each pharmacy contracts to accept different insurance companies, the technician must become acquainted with the normal billing procedures of that particular pharmacy and its associated insurance companies. Common types of billing practices are covered in this chapter to help you understand the proper information needed to file a claim for reimbursement.

In addition, the chapter introduces the pharmacy technician to basic information about the major types of insurance coverage. A firm knowledge of terminology and guidelines must be in place for proper ordering and billing practices. This chapter begins with a discussion of formularies and the knowledge needed about insurance companies. Also discussed are pharmacy inventory, some major types of devices used to keep track of inventory, and ways to handle special obstacles as they occur.

Formulary and Drug Utilization

A formulary is analogous to a backbone. The **formulary** is a list that describes all the medications covered under a specific insurance plan approved for use in an institution, such as a hospital. It may also offer alternative medications if the first choice is not covered. For medications to become part of a formulary, they must meet certain requirements, such as effectiveness and cost. These are determined by pharmacists, pharmacy technicians, physicians, nurses, and administrators who are members of the **pharmacy and therapeutics committee (P&T committee)**. Formularies are not the same at all institutional pharmacies or for all health plans. An institution can have an **open formulary**, which means any drug can be ordered and stocked for patient use; a **closed formulary** places certain restrictions on the drugs ordered.

Often retail pharmacies stock a variety of medications to accommodate both their patients and the many different insurance companies for which they are contracted providers. Each insurance company has its own formulary, with recommendations for therapeutic alternatives when a drug is not covered under a particular plan. A therapeutic alternative is a drug that may differ chemically from the one prescribed but provides the same effect when administered to the patient. Many insurance companies have a variety of prescription plans and formularies that coincide with the many different types of health plans they provide. Specific formulary information can usually be found on insurance company websites. A hospital or home health care pharmacy is more likely to have a closed formulary, or a specific list of drugs to be kept on hand and dispensed to the patients and health plans served by the pharmacy.

Drug utilization evaluation (DUE), formerly known as **drug utilization review (DUR)**, is an important process in ensuring that the correct drug is prescribed for a condition. Pharmacists must perform this function, but pharmacy technicians play an important role in the DUE process. When technicians are inputting prescriptions, DUE alerts interrupt the process if a drug interaction or duplicate therapy is found. Technicians must *never* override these warnings on the computer! They must notify the pharmacist immediately so he or she can screen the medication order for potential problems, such as drug-drug interactions, duplicate therapy, or other possible errors. This is done before the drug is dispensed, which reduces the risk of the patient receiving the wrong treatment.

Many formulary drugs are generic versions of proprietary (brand name) products. These drugs are as effective as the brand name drugs. They meet the same bioequivalence requirements but are less expensive. A health plan or prescription plan committee composed of pharmacists, physicians, and other health care administrators reviews drugs that have been approved by the U.S. Food and Drug Administration (FDA) to ensure that they are cost-effective. In addition, consideration may be given to drug companies that bid or give rebates when their drug is chosen for a formulary. This decrease in price to the pharmacy ultimately saves money for both the insurance company and the patient. Although most insurance companies cover most of the cost of a generic drug, some do allow the patient to choose the brand name drug. However, if the patient selects the brand name drug, he or she is responsible for the amount due based on calculation of the copay as outlined in the third-party agreement. For example, if the normal **copayment** is $5 per prescription and the patient chooses a brand name medication that costs $10 more than the generic equivalent, the patient must pay $15. The dollar amount of a prescription also depends on orders such as dispense as written (DAW) drugs that require specialty codes. The three DAW codes that are most often used in the pharmacy setting are 0, 1, and 2.

- DAW 0 indicates that the physician authorizes a therapeutic alternative and the pharmacy can dispense the generic drug to the patient. If a generic is not available. the trade name product must be given; however, the DAW code must still be zero because this indicates that if a generic becomes available at a later date, the physician has given permission to the pharmacy to make the substitution. The pharmacist can find the therapeutic equivalent in the *Orange Book*.
- DAW 1 indicates dispense as written and is usually used by the physician to indicate that the trade or brand name medication is in some way medically necessary for the successful treatment of the patient. Often patients must have proof that other therapies have been tried but failed. Sometimes, such as in the case of the drug Celebrex, a patient must be age 50 or older. Physicians must write either "Brand Name Medically Necessary" or "Dispense as Written" in their own handwriting.
- DAW 2 indicates that the physician has approved the generic substitution of the medication prescribed; however, the patient has insisted on receiving the brand name medication.

 Tech Note!
Technicians must be aware of and understand the proper use of DAW codes for accurate insurance billing.

Other DAW codes are assigned very infrequently and should be used only under the direction of the pharmacist. It is important to pay attention to the DAW codes and to use the correct one.

Insurance companies audit pharmacies; they specifically verify whether DAW 1 claims sent by the pharmacy have prescriptions in which the physician specifically indicates a brand name drug be dispensed. The selection of proper DAW codes is easy to overlook and can cause seemingly simple mistakes. If these mistakes are found in an audit, however, they can cause the reversal and repayment of the inaccurate claims and may result in the insurance company terminating its contract with a pharmacy.

Formularies are constantly changing. If and when new generic drugs are introduced, cost and other factors are reviewed again. Typically, the types of drugs not included on a formulary are new drugs, uncommon drugs, and extremely expensive drugs. However, if a non-formulary drug can be justified as a medically necessary substitution by the physician, it may be approved for reimbursement under the insurance plan.

Generic Versus Trade Name Drugs

The terms **trade**, **brand**, and **proprietary** are used interchangeably to refer to the name of a drug product that was first patented and marketed by the owner or manufacturer. Another name for such a product is *innovator product*. After a certain time passes, the patent expires. Eventually other drug companies can apply for the right to produce the same drug product, although not all drugs will be available in generic form. For example, it is usually not advantageous to drug companies to make generic medications that are used by a small percentage of the population. Brand name drugs that are produced by nonproprietary companies as an alternative to the proprietary product are considered "generic." A common example in pharmacy is the many different generic brands of birth control pills. Although the FDA approves generic drugs as equivalent to the trade name drug, the drugs often have different appearances because of different manufacturing procedures. Brand name drugs generally are protected for 17 to 20 years (depending on a drug company's petition to the FDA) before patents expire (CDER). Once generic competition is introduced, prices can drop 50% to 80%. Drug price competition and patent term restoration expedite the availability of less costly generic drugs by permitting the FDA to approve applications to market generic versions without repeating the research needed to prove them safe and effective. At the same time, the brand name companies can apply for up to 5 years of additional patent protection for the new medicines they developed or for a new indication of a medication to compensate for the time lost while their products were undergoing the FDA approval process.

Types of Private and Group Medical Insurance Plans

Many different types of medical insurance plans are available. Understanding the policies and procedures of these plans is challenging, especially because their guidelines change regularly. Therefore, this chapter covers the most basic information applied to the major types of insurance. Technicians must be able to differentiate between the different types of insurance, obtain the necessary information from the insurance card, determine whether the patient has prescription (Rx) coverage and who should be billed, and transmit the claim correctly. The types of medical insurance plans and cards in use today include the following:

- Pharmacy benefits card (has "Rx Yes" printed on it)
- Medical insurance ID card
- Drug discount card
- Prescription coupon card provided by drug manufacturers to patients: Coupon cards are provided either as an incentive for the patient to try the drug or as an aid to patients who meet certain income requirements
- Medicare card
- Medicaid card
- Medicare Advantage card
- Medigap card
- CHAMPVA card
- TRICARE card
- Workers' compensation (no card is required)

Health Maintenance Organization

A **health maintenance organization (HMO)** has specific features that distinguish it from traditional insurance programs. An HMO is an effective method of controlling health care costs. Aetna, Anthem, United Healthcare, and Kaiser are just a few examples of the many insurance companies that offer HMO coverage. HMOs include the following:

1. Primary care physician (PCP): The insurance company requires the patient to choose a primary physician to coordinate all of the patient's medical needs.
2. Independent physician association (IPA): The provider offers a discounted rate to the patient through the contract made with the insurance company. In return, the physician accepts a lower payment than normally is charged for the procedure performed. These are contracted providers; examples of contracted providers are certain hospitals, clinics, and medical groups.
3. Copay: The insurance company requires the patient to pay a predetermined amount for office visits, emergency department visits, and drugs, regardless of the final cost. The rate varies, depending on the patient's coverage plan. The insurance company is responsible for the remainder of the cost.
4. Capitation: Some physicians are independent and see both HMO policyholders and nonmembers in their practice. In this situation the HMO pays the physician a fixed amount for each member patient regardless of how many times the patient visits the physician. This method of payment is known as capitation.

What If Your Patient Has HMO Insurance?

If a patient has HMO insurance, the technician must obtain information from the patient such as address, date of birth, insurance number, and full name. The technician also must obtain the patient's prescription insurance card and verify that the pharmacy is a contracted provider for that particular insurance company and group. The pharmacy bills the insurance company first, through online adjudication, and receives an authorization number and copay information for the patient. **Adjudication** is the processing of claims over a computerized system. If the insurance claim is rejected, the pharmacy either must troubleshoot the issues or have the patient pay full price for the medication. It is then the patient's responsibility to contact the insurance company and attempt to obtain reimbursement. The patient is responsible for the entire cost only if the insurance company denies coverage based on eligibility or authorization not received before service. HMOs may require **prior authorization** on certain medications per their formulary guidelines. State regulations regarding the types of forms used to approve such medications may vary. The prescriber must justify the therapeutic basis for the prescribed medication. This prior authorization must be entered into the system before payment is approved. One example is Botox. Botox is used to treat muscular disorders but can also be used cosmetically. If a patient's plan does not cover cosmetic services but the drug is prescribed to treat a muscular disorder, a prior authorization is required. Technicians are crucial personnel in securing the prior authorization for the patient. They may call the physician's office and/or the insurance companies to ensure that the patient's needs are met.

There are opportunities to specialize and work specifically as a prior authorization technician. These technicians are considered experts in prior authorization and provide customer service support to members, customers, and/or providers. They take incoming requests for prior authorizations for both formulary and non-formulary medications. Requests can be received via fax or telephone, from providers' offices, and from pharmacists. The position provides clinical review for authorizations in keeping with legal and contractual requirements, including but not limited to turn around times (TATs) and service level agreements (SLAs). The technician must provide the information clearly, accurately, and in a professional manner. Interactions with callers must be documented per contractual and various regulatory and legal requirements.

Scenario CHECK UP 13-1

Brian has begun working on the tech 3 learning materials. He has passed the first three chapters with flying colors, and his pharmacist is impressed with his work. A co-worker is also vying for the tech 3 spot. While contemplating how he can improve his productivity, Brian decides to develop a plan that will reduce time spent dealing with securing prior authorizations. What are some ideas Brian might implement?

Preferred Provider Organization

A **preferred provider organization (PPO)** provides health care for members for a discounted fee. The benefit is that the patient can choose a physician from the insurance plan's list of contracted providers or may choose to consult any specialty physician without primary care physician referrals. There are no requirements to choose a specific primary care physician.

Aetna, Anthem, United Healthcare, State Farm Insurance, and others offer PPO plans. Patients choosing a PPO may have a higher copay for their office visits than an HMO copay. Members of a PPO may have to meet a yearly **deductible** (the amount that the patient must pay before the insurance company pays). The insurance then pays a certain percentage of the medical expenses and medication bills if the patient's claims meet the criteria (i.e., charges were incurred by a contracted provider and the service provided was within the allowed amount of the PPO). This helps control the cost to the insurance company because the patient pays everything the insurance company does not pay.

What If Your Patient Has PPO Insurance?
You must determine whether the patient has medication coverage through the PPO plan. In addition, you must establish whether the patient pays the complete cost for the medication and then files for direct reimbursement, has a deductible, or has a copay. This is determined from the information on the patient's health insurance card and through the online billing process. An example of a health insurance card is shown in Figure 13-1. After the information is transmitted to the insurance provider, an approval code is sent to the pharmacy. If the patient has a copay or deductible, the insurance company should monitor the patient's obligation. If the patient must self-bill the insurance company for reimbursement, the patient needs the receipt to submit to the insurance company.

From the pharmacy perspective, the billing processes for an HMO and a PPO are similar. The

---

HOPPER HEALTH

HOSPITAL ADMISSIONS REQUIRE PRIOR APPROVAL

JOHN A DOE
YBC999999999 99

GROUP: 272550000001

75.00 EMER ROOM
20.00 OFFICE VISIT

BCBSKC RX   1-800-228-1436

BC PLAN: 240   BS PLAN: 740

CUST SERV: 816-232-8396/800-822-2583

FIGURE 13-1 Example of a health insurance card.

difference is that if the patient has a PPO, he or she may have a deductible to meet before the cost share (such as a percentage) or copay becomes activated. Most HMO and PPO insurance plans have separate deductibles for medical and prescription services. Often patients forget they have a deductible to meet, or they do not realize it resets at the beginning of the year. In addition, they may not realize that each family member may be required to meet his or her own deductible before the insurance pays that individual's portion. For example, for a family of four with a $1,000 individual deductible, if one family member receives $1,000 of medical services, the insurance pays a portion of that family member's medication for the remainder of the year. However, if another family member then needs medication, the second family member's $1,000 deductible must be met before the insurance pays a portion of the second family member's medication.

Government-Managed Insurance Programs

Programs such as Medicare and Medicaid are examples of state-managed and federal-managed medical insurance plans. Each employee in the United States pays the government a percentage of his or her income toward Medicare. A percentage of each state budget is applied toward Medicaid. Each plan has specific guidelines that must be followed precisely for patients to qualify for reimbursement.

History of Medicare and Medicaid

Both Medicaid and Medicare were implemented in 1965. **Medicaid** provided health care services to low-income children, the elderly, the blind, and people with disabilities. Until 1977, Medicaid was associated with the Social Security Administration. Later, in 1986, coverage was expanded to infants of pregnant women with low incomes and became state regulated. Through the following years, many revisions were made, including increasing the eligibility age of children and covering certain individuals who were disabled or unable to return to work. Medicaid is funded by both federal and state governments, and the benefits vary widely. Each state is responsible for payment to health care providers. Participants must prove that their income and financial resources are at or below national poverty levels. Although each state may vary in its scope of coverage, the state must provide a minimum level of benefits according to federal guidelines. The following benefits are included:

- Hospital inpatient services
- Outpatient services

BOX 13-1

Types of Medicare Coverage

Part A: Covers institutional costs if the participant meets the criteria established by federal and state regulations.

Part B: Covers physician and other outpatient services, including diabetes testing, physical therapy, and other preventive costs.

Part C: Also known as Medicare Advantage; this is an optional plan to Parts A and B. It is a private plan that uses Medicare and must be equivalent to coverage provided by Parts A and B. Some Part C plans cover certain prescription drugs. A person should have either Part C or Medigap, because the two are not cumulative in coverage.

Part D: Specifically covers prescription drugs. The coverage is provided by individual private insurance plans that are overseen by Medicare. A monthly premium is paid, and the plan chosen by the patient may have an annual deductible. Once the deductible has been paid, the insurance plan pays either all or some of the remaining costs, After the maximum benefit has been reached, there is a gap in the coverage of drug costs, and the patient must pay for prescriptions out-of-pocket.

- Physician services
- Skilled nursing care
- Home health care
- Laboratory services
- Radiology services

In 1966, more than 19 million people enrolled into the newly formed **Medicare** program. Coverage consisted of several parts (Box 13-1). As of 1972 Medicare eligibility was extended to include people older than age 65, those younger than 65 with long-term disabilities, and individuals suffering from end-stage renal disease (ESRD).

In 1987, both Medicare and Medicaid required health care providers to include patient privacy provisions if they were to participate in the government-sponsored programs. Medicare revised its coverage in 1988, implementing prescription drug benefits, along with a cap on patient liability. In 1996 the **Health Insurance Portability and Accountability Act (HIPAA)** (linked to the Employee Retirement Income Security Act of 1974) provided new rules for improving portability (continuity) of coverage and simplified standards for electronic transactions, among other changes.

In 1997, Medicare implemented additional changes, including the following:

- Expanded education; new information helped participants make a more informed choice about their health care.

- Five new payment systems for services, including:
  - Inpatient rehabilitation hospital or unit services
  - Skilled nursing facility services
  - Home health services
  - Hospital outpatient services and rehabilitation
  - Expanded preventive benefits

A significant change was made in 2003 with the **Medicare Modernization Act (MMA)** and the creation of prescription drug discount cards, which allowed competition between health plans, benefiting participants. In 2006 Medicare Part D was enacted; this requires the federal government to provide subsidies to participants whose income is less than 150% of the federal poverty limit. Those with higher incomes would pay a greater share of drug costs as of 2007. Certain individuals may be covered under both Medicaid and Medicare and are known as "dual eligible"; Medicaid supplements Medicare coverage. In 2010 the Affordable Care Act (ACA) was signed into law and has had a significant impact on Medicare and Medicaid services. According to the *Washington Post,* as of December 31, 2013, about 4.4 million Americans had signed up for Medicaid coverage via the health care exchanges (see Chapter 2 for more information on the Affordable Care Act [ACA]).

Many savings programs assist low-income participants with out-of-pocket health care costs. Each state has its own programs for assistance and may or may not include services such as home-delivered personal care and other community-based services for the disabled. Table 13-1 presents a timeline that explains various changes in the coverage and events in both Medicare and Medicaid programs.

 Tech Note!

In 1997, both Medicaid and Medicare were reorganized and became subsidiaries of the Health Care Financing Administration (HCFA), now called the Centers for Medicare and Medicaid Services (CMS). In 2010, the Affordable Care Act was signed into law. It will be implemented in phases, and changes related to the practice of pharmacy will begin to occur. Technicians should familiarize themselves with the language of the ACA, in particular changes dealing with medication management and Medicare Part D.

Current Use of Medicare/Medicaid Insurance

Medicare

Medicare is a federally sponsored program for seniors, the disabled, and dialysis patients. It functions much like an HMO and a PPO. The patient must see a provider who accepts Medicare, but the patient has a yearly deductible and a percentage share of the cost. The share of the cost is similar to a deductible and copay combined. The patient is responsible for paying a deductible up to a certain amount in a hospital setting. Medicare has four parts: Parts A, B, C, and D.

- **Medicare Part A** (Hospital Insurance): Part A helps cover inpatient care in hospitals, skilled nursing facilities, and critical care hospitals. It also helps cover hospice and some home health care. Patients who are eligible for Social Security benefits are automatically enrolled in Medicare Part A. Most people do not pay a premium, but those who are 65 or older who do not qualify for Social Security benefits may enroll with the understanding that they will be required to pay a premium to obtain benefits.
- **Medicare Part B** (Medical Insurance): Part B helps pay for physicians' services and outpatient care. It helps pay for services that Part A does not cover, such as durable medical equipment and even physical and occupational therapists when deemed medically necessary. This coverage is optional, and most people pay a monthly premium.

 Tech Note!

If a patient has Medicare Part B, the technician should ask the patient for the most current card at each visit. Some states require Part B to be renewed monthly, so it is important to verify that it has not expired. Medicare Part B also includes coverage for durable medical equipment (DME).

- **Medicare Part C** (Medicare Advantage): Part C allows participants in Medicare Parts A and B to obtain additional insurance through private HMOs or PPOs. The MMA changed the rules for contracting with these private health insurance companies to provide participants with better benefits and lower costs.
- **Medicare Part D** (Prescription Drug Plan): Part D provides people who are eligible for Medicare a voluntary prescription drug plan. This plan covers medications, insulin, vaccines, and certain medical supplies. Most enrollees pay a monthly premium for the discounted prices, and not all medications are covered. Technicians, along with the pharmacist, can assist patients in choosing the best prescription drug plan based on their particular medications. Most Medicare prescription plans have a coverage gap known as the "donut hole." This means that there is a limit to how much a particular plan covers for drugs. In 2014, once you and your plan had spent $2,850 on covered medications, which included your deductible, you

TABLE 13-1

Chronological Changes in Medicare/Medicaid Coverage

Year	Description
1965	Medicaid and Medicare were signed into law.
1966	Nineteen million people requested Medicare benefits.
1972	Medicare expanded coverage to include individuals younger than age 65 with low income and those with end-stage renal failure.
1977	Medicaid and Medicare were placed under the control of the Social Security Administration.
1980	Medigap was introduced to fill a gap in Medicare coverage; patients could choose among 12 different Medigap plans.
1986	Medicaid expanded coverage to include infants and pregnant women of low income.
1987	Medicare and Medicaid payment was linked to the Omnibus Budget Reconciliation Act of 1987 (OBRA '87) and specifically addressed poor conditions of nursing homes.
1988	Medicare introduced a prescription drug benefit plan.
1990	OBRA '90 required that all health care personnel participating in Medicare and Medicaid programs protect patient privacy; it also required patient consultation with pharmacists.
1996	The Health Insurance Portability and Accountability Act (HIPAA) implemented patient privacy rules for Medicare payment and provided electronic payment methods.
1997	Medicare made several important changes that expanded coverage and developed five new payment systems.
1997	Both Medicare and Medicaid were placed under the control of the Health Care Financing Administration.
2003	The Medicare Modernization Act (MMA) provided drug discount cards to eligible individuals.
2003	Medicare Part D was introduced under MMA; it provided subsidies for eligible people, to be implemented by 2006.
2004	A temporary Medicare-approved drug discount card program began, along with a transitional assistance program to provide a $600 annual credit to low-income Medicare beneficiaries without prescription drug coverage in 2004 and 2005.
2005	Medicare begins covering a "Welcome to Medicare" physical, along with other preventive services, such as cardiovascular screening blood tests and diabetes screening tests. Medicare begins education and outreach activities to implement the 2006 prescription drug benefit.
2006	Medicare Part D was enacted, requiring the federal government to provide subsidies to participants whose income was less than 150% of the federal poverty limit.
2010	Medicare spending was reduced; Medicaid enrollment and spending were increased; and new payment and reimbursement guidelines for Medicare and Medicaid services were introduced. These changes were associated with the Health Care and Education Affordability Reconciliation Act (HCERA) of 2010.
2011	Medicare began covering preventative care services, such as mammograms and colonoscopies, without charging Part B **coinsurance** or deductibles. Yearly "wellness" visits were also covered.
2011	Effective July 1, 2011, federal payments were prohibited to states for Medicaid services related to certain health care–acquired conditions.
2012	States received 2 more years of funding for the Children's Health Insurance Program (CHIP) to continue coverage for children not eligible for Medicaid.
2013	Effective January 1, 2013, to December 31, 2014, the Affordable Care Act (ACA) requires an increase in Medicaid payments for primary care physician services. This increase is fully funded by the federal government.
2014	Creation and implementation of Affordable Insurance Exchanges. Individuals and small businesses can sign up and buy affordable health benefit plans. The new system will determine eligibility and coordinate enrollment for Medicaid and the CHIP.
2015	Effective October, 2015, federal matching funds for CHIP will increase by 23 percentage points, with a cap of 100%, to help states pay for coverage of uninsured children.

were in the coverage gap. This amount varies from year to year. For 2014, once you had reached the coverage gap, you had to pay out of pocket 47.5% of the price for brand name drugs and 72% of the price for generic drugs. The portion you pay for generic drugs decreases each year until it reaches 25% in 2020.

Medicare services were expanded in 1980 with the creation of the **Medigap plan**, which is also regulated by the federal government. The last significant update to Medigap plans was in June 2010, when Medicare SELECT was introduced in some states. This required participants to use specific hospitals and specific providers for full coverage.

BOX 13-2

Medigap Coverage

A patient has Medicare Part D prescription coverage. This sample plan shows that the patient typically pays for generic medications or brand name drugs with a yearly maximum payout of $1,200. If the patient purchases $1,200 in medication in the first 3 months of the year, the patient's insurance will not pay for any medication prescribed during the remainder of the year. At this point, the patient can apply for coverage for this "gap." This coverage can help pay the deductible or co-pay on Medicare Parts A, B, and D. The patient must determine whether Medigap would be beneficial.

BOX 13-3

Various Supplies Covered by Medicare

Typical supplies or prescriptions that may be covered under specific parts of Medicare insurance include:
- Blood glucose testing strips (Part B)
- Lasix (generic only, Part D)
- Hospital stay (Part A)
- Heparin for home dialysis (Part B)
- Lancets (Part B)
- Insulin (Part D)

The traditional Medigap plan offers optional insurance policies that can be purchased through privately owned insurance companies. The plans are intended to fill the gap in the Medicare program coverage. However, if you have Medicare Part C, Medigap cannot be used. There are 12 different Medigap policies, labeled A through L. Most of the insurer plans do not differ significantly in their policies. Each person must purchase his or her own policy. Medicare is the primary payer, and the Medigap carrier is secondary. There is also a 6-month open enrollment for Medigap coverage (Box 13-2).

What If Your Patient Has Medicare Insurance? Any changes in Medicare drug coverage increase the number of consultations by the pharmacist, because pharmacists must explain different issues caused by a change in medications. In addition, people may need to have their prescriptions filled at a different pharmacy. This is because of the time it takes to register the patient in the Medicare database. Pharmacies must apply for a **National Provider Identifier (NPI)** from the Centers for Medicare and Medicaid Services (CMS). All providers who bill electronically must use an NPI, which is required by HIPAA. Any pharmacist who provides services such as consultation and does not bill for this time under a pharmacy with an NPI must have his or her own NPI. The NPI number may be assigned either per person or per pharmacy, depending on each state's laws. For example, in Nevada, individual pharmacists must apply for an NPI number to process prescriptions covered by Medicare, whereas in California, this number is assigned for each pharmacy. If a patient is not in the system yet and the physician has ordered a drug that is not covered, the pharmacist may call the physician for a substitute if possible, or the patient may pay out of pocket for the medication and try to obtain reimbursement when he or she is in the system.

An important "bottom line" approach to consider is this:

The patient will be encouraged to receive generic drugs. Brand name drugs are often covered at a much higher cost if a generic is available, and this cost may be prohibitive enough to force many people into using the generic versions. Typically, brand name drugs are covered at the generic price and the patient is responsible for paying the difference. For a drug such as Zocor (generic name, simvastatin), this difference in cost can be as much as $100. The overall use of generic drugs has increased greatly under Medicare Part D.

In the past, open enrollment for Medicare plans ran from November 15 to December 31. This period was changed in 2011 to ensure that Medicare has enough time to process plan choices so that coverage begins at the beginning of the New Year. Currently, the election period begins on October 15 and ends on December 7 each year. This is when a patient can change plans.

Because different items are covered under different parts of the plan, it is important for the technician to obtain not only the Medicare Part D card (Figure 13-2) for pharmacy billing, but also a copy of the Part A and Part B cards, in case other items are needed (Box 13-3).

Scenario CHECK UP 13-2

Brian has completed approximately one half of the required lessons for tech 3 status. He is in the middle of a busy work day when he encounters an elderly customer who wants to pick up her prescription. Brian rings up the medication on the register and explains to the patient that her portion of the cost is $50. She explains that she now has Medigap insurance and should not have to pay any money out of pocket. How should Brian handle this situation?

Medicaid

Medicaid is a federal assistance program based on income and other circumstances. Individuals earning

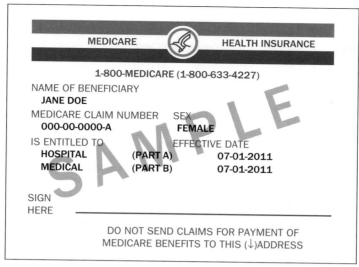

FIGURE 13-2 Example of a Medicare Part D card.

below the national poverty level are eligible for health care services. Each state has its own Medicaid program for low-income residents. This also includes uninsured pregnant women and those with certain disabilities. Medicaid is funded by both the state and the federal government. Depending on a state's level of unemployment and poverty, it may receive matching funds from the federal government. Medicaid can be used with Medicare if the person qualifies. In addition, each state may have many different programs that help defer the cost of health care and medication. The following are the three major levels of coverage in the Medicaid system:

1. The patient may not be responsible for any cost.
2. Share of cost: The patient's plan requires that the patient pay a deductible (i.e., a specific dollar amount must be met before the insurance company pays). For instance, the patient may be responsible for the first $1,000, but any remaining amount is paid by Medicaid.
3. Geographical managed care program: A geographical managed care plan allows patients to belong to a medical group with which Medicaid has a contractual agreement. This includes HMOs, thus allowing patients to have Medicaid benefits similar to benefits offered by HMOs. The regulations may vary from state to state.

Effective January 1, 2014, Medicaid benefits were expanded to include individuals age 19 to 65 with incomes up to 138% of the federal poverty level. For a single person, that translates into an annual income of $15, 856. This change opened up Medicaid for many childless adults who were not previously eligible.

States must provide certain mandatory benefits for Medicaid participants, such as:

- Inpatient hospital services
- Outpatient hospital services
- Physician services
- Laboratory and x-ray services
- Family planning services
- Home health services
- Smoking cessation for pregnant women
- Prenatal and nurse midwife services

States can also choose to provide optional benefits for Medicaid participants, such as:

- Prescription drugs
- Physical therapy
- Dentures
- Eyeglasses
- Respiratory care
- Chiropractic services

What If Your Patient Has Medicaid Insurance? You must know whether the patient has Medicaid benefits. If the patient is covered under Medicaid, you need a copy of the patient's insurance card. This card identifies the program under which the patient is covered. Because different states authorize coverage at varying durations, it is important for the technician to verify eligibility each time the patient has a prescription filled. Many states use the Electronic Medicaid Eligibility Verification System (EMEVS), which verifies coverage by electronic transmission or by telephone.

Other Government Medical Insurance Plans: TRICARE and CHAMPVA

TRICARE

TRICARE is a health care program for military personnel and their families. This includes approximately 9.6 million active duty service members, National Guard and Reserve members, and retirees. TRICARE is managed by the Defense Health Agency and covers beneficiaries in the Army, Navy, Marines, Air Force, and the Coast Guard. TRICARE eligibility

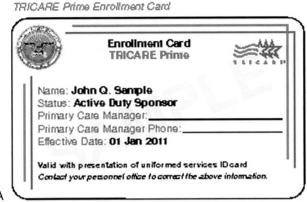

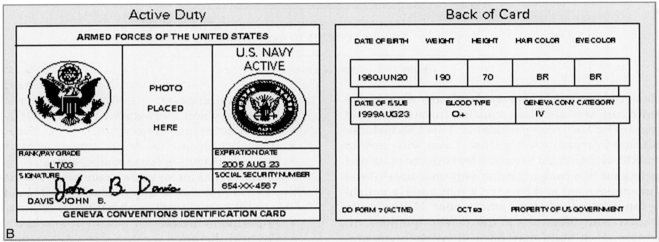

FIGURE 13-3 **A,** Example of a TRICARE Prime card. All TRICARE cards are valid only when accompanied by a uniformed services ID card **(B).** (From Fordney M: *Insurance handbook for the medical office,* ed 13, St Louis, 2014, Elsevier.)

is tracked through a worldwide database known as the Defense Enrollment Eligibility Reporting System (DEERS). Active duty and retired service members are automatically entered into DEERS, but family members must be registered separately. This system helps eliminate fraudulent claims. Figure 13-3, *A* shows an example of a TRICARE Prime card; Figure 13-3, *B* shows an example of a uniformed services ID card, which must be presented with the TRICARE card.

CHAMPVA

The **Civilian Health and Medical Program of the Department of Veteran Affairs (CHAMPVA)** (also known as the Veterans Health Administration) is a health benefits program in which the VA shares the cost of certain health care services with eligible participants. This includes families of veterans who are totally or permanently disabled due to service-related injuries. To be eligible for CHAMPVA, an individual cannot be eligible for TRICARE. In most cases, CHAMPVA pays comparable to Medicare/TRICARE rates. Drugs and medications are covered under CHAMPVA when the following conditions are met:

- The medication has a valid National Drug Code (NDC).
- The drug has been approved by the FDA for the condition being treated.
- The drug is medically necessary.
- The drug is prescribed by an authorized prescriber and dispensed lawfully.

Figure 13-4 shows an example of a CHAMPVA card.

Workers' Compensation

Workers' compensation is a type of insurance paid by employers to entirely cover injuries suffered by employees while on the job. Federal law requires employers with a certain number of employees to offer workers' compensation. Insurance coverage is provided by private insurance carriers.

Anyone who works for a company that pays into workers' compensation may be eligible to use this insurance if he or she has a work-related injury. The patient does not have to pay anything. Instead, claims are filed electronically or on hard copy to the insurance companies. If the patient arrives at the

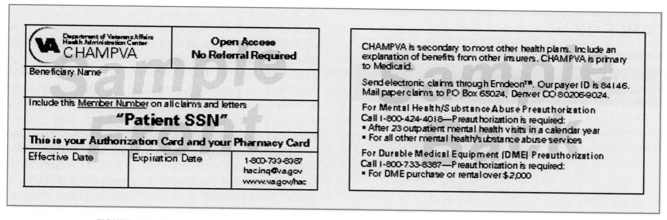

FIGURE 13-4 Example of a CHAMPVA card. (From Fordney M: *Insurance handbook for the medical office,* ed 13, St Louis, 2014, Elsevier.)

pharmacy with a workers' compensation claim, it is important to obtain billing information before dispensing medication, if possible. This may involve contacting the patient's employer, obtaining the billing information over the phone from the human resources department, and then calling the workers' compensation insurance company for further information. To avoid any billing errors, it is important to keep detailed notes regarding communication when processing workers' compensation claims. Be sure to include the name of the person who was consulted, the date of the consultation, and detailed notes about your conversation. It is also important to follow HIPAA guidelines. The only people who need to know that the patient is injured or ill are those in the human resources department. They do not need to be given a specific diagnosis from the pharmacy; they just need to provide the billing information.

Tech Note!
Regardless of the patient's type of insurance, you should always treat people with respect. Take care to ensure that the patient is treated with respect and receives superior service when handling prescription billing.

Third-Party Billing

The term *third-party billing* refers to the portion of payment reimbursed by insurance companies. The three entities that are responsible for payment include the patient, the pharmacy, and the insurance company. It is customary for the pharmacy to bill the insurance company on behalf of the patient. The patient is often responsible for meeting the copayment or deductible at the time the medication is dispensed, and the pharmacy must collect the rest of the drug cost from the insurance based on contracted rates and dispensing fees. A copay is a predetermined

amount the patient always pays when a medication is dispensed, whereas a deductible is the amount of out-of-pocket cost the patient must pay before his or her insurance coverage is activated. Copays can be a fixed dollar amount or a fixed percentage. Because there are so many different insurance companies, each with different billing requirements, it often takes more than 1 year for a technician to become proficient in third-party adjudication, or claim billing.

The information needed by insurance companies to process a claim from the pharmacy or to reimburse the patient is the same as the information required on a pharmacy label, plus date of birth, insurance group number, and identification number. All information must be verified before the medication is dispensed. Once the patient's information has been entered into the pharmacy computer system, it is important to keep that information updated both for the pharmacy and for the insurance company (Table 13-2).

Point of Sale Billing

Pharmacies that send claims electronically to an insurance company participate in **point of sale (POS)** billing. Electronic billing is performed via a secure data and transactional network to ensure patient confidentiality. The insurance company verifies eligibility, identifies covered drugs, prices a claim, and returns a response to submitting pharmacies within seconds during the prescription processing functions.

Tech Note!
Authorization forms can be submitted electronically, along with any supporting documentation. This is due to the development of electronic prior authorization (ePA) modules, in addition to the ability to send these documents through secure, HIPAA-compliant electronic channels.

TABLE 13-2

Minimum Information Required by Insurance Companies

Required by Insurance Company	Reason
Patient's name	To verify insurance coverage
Date medication is filled	To process claim for reimbursement purposes; must be done within a specific period determined by provider
Pharmacy name and address	To pay pharmacy
Medication prescribed	To verify whether drug is on the formulary and is covered
Dosage	To determine cost of medication
Date of birth	To verify medication is dispensed to correct patient
Identification number	To provide authorization of coverage

Prior Authorization

Often an insurance company pays for a medication only if a prior authorization is first received. Prior authorization is needed for a variety of reasons; for example, the drug of choice may not be included in the formulary, or the insurance company may have determined that less costly methods of treatment are available and the patient must use those first. Two types of forms are used: a prior authorization form (or **treatment authorization request [TAR]**) or an eTAR, which is a web-based, paperless process for submitting an electronic TAR for payment. Most insurance companies require a prior authorization form. The pharmacy typically does not contact the insurance company about prior authorization. If a third-party claim is rejected as "prior authorization required," then either the pharmacy contacts the patient's physician or the pharmacy directly notifies the physician's office. The physician's office then contacts the insurance company to request the prior authorization. Policies may vary, depending on the insurance provider and the medication prescribed. For Medicare and Medicaid the TAR form is used, which requires the same information as forms used for standard insurance companies (Figure 13-5).

The physician often must produce documentation explaining why a specific course of therapy is needed, such as "The patient tried the other therapies, and they were ineffective"; "The patient has allergies to certain medications"; or "The patient must undergo diagnostic tests that require the requested therapy." All of this information must be provided by the

physician because the pharmacy does not have access to the patient's records. The insurance company either approves or denies the authorization in 24 to 48 hours. Rarely does the insurance company or the physician alert the pharmacy when authorization has been approved; therefore, the pharmacy should attempt to rebill the claim in 48 to 72 hours. If the claim is still denied, the pharmacy may need to contact the physician's office or the insurance company to determine whether the authorization was submitted and whether a special override code is needed to bill the claim. Regardless of whether the claim is approved or denied, the patient should be contacted within 3 days so he or she is not waiting for a medication that has been denied.

Each plan has its own formulary, limitations, and exclusions. In addition to these variances, each pharmacy has certain insurance types that it accepts or rejects. This means that if the pharmacy accepts the copayment as payment in full, the pharmacy bills the insurance company for the cost of the medication. Otherwise, the pharmacy may not accept the insurance based on the limits of payment. Insurance cards have all the information necessary to perform the billing process. An explanation of the information contained on an insurance prescription card is presented in Box 13-4.

 Tech Note!

Identify each insurance card as a prescription discount card, prescription coupon card, or insurance card. For each card, identify the payer and the Pharmacy Benefit International Identification Number (RxBIN), the Pharmacy Benefit Processor Control Number (RxPCN), and the group and ID numbers.

Scenario CHECK UP 13-3

Brian is working with Ms. Jones, a new patient at the pharmacy. He begins by explaining to Ms. Jones that he will need to get some important information from her before he can begin filling her prescription. Brian brings up a new patient profile on the computer. What questions do you think he will ask Ms. Jones?

Patient Profiles

Each pharmacy has its own specific computer system, which details each **patient profile**. Figure 13-6 shows an example of a pharmacy patient profile database. This profile must be kept updated for proper billing. Basic information that can be viewed on this computer system includes the following:

- Name
- Date of birth

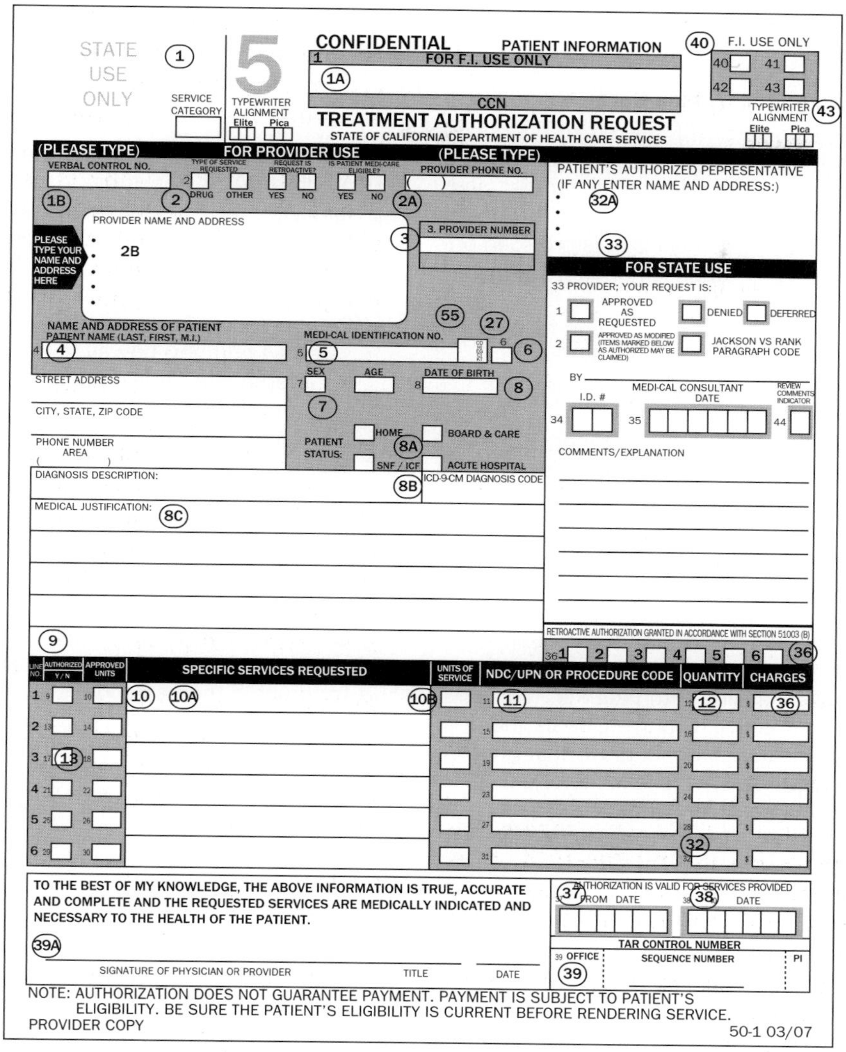

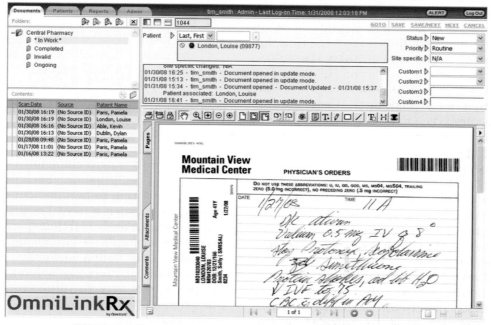

FIGURE 13-5 Treatment authorization request (TAR) form.

FIGURE 13-6 Computer patient profile using OmniLinkRx. (Courtesy Omnicell.)

BOX 13-4

Information Included on a Prescription Card

Each insurance card contains information about the coverage plan, the patient's name and identification number, and the phone number of the insurance company. The basic information needed to bill a third-party claim is provided on the card. If any additional information is needed, the insurance company or provider should be contacted.

- Pharmacy Benefit International Identification number (RxBIN)—Used much like an IP address to direct the claim to the correct third-party provider. All network pharmacy payers have an RxBIN.
- Pharmacy Benefit Processor Control Number (PCN)—Some, but not all, network pharmacy payers use this number, labeled RxPCN, for network pharmacy benefit routing, along with the RxBIN. If used, this number is required for specialized health care coverage plans, such as those that begin with the letter U, W, X, or Y. For example, dental coverage plans are identified by a PCN identifier with the letter "W." This has been used increasingly in the past few years because of the greater number of plans available to patients.
- Prescription group number (Rx Grp #)—Directs the claim to the specific insurance benefits for that group. Groups are usually organized by collections of people who work for the same company or have similar benefits packages.

- Identification number (ID #)—A unique identification number that is specific to each member or member family group. Some insurance companies, such as Kaiser, issue an ID number to each person in the plan. Some issue one to the cardholder and each member of the family has the same ID number.
- Person code—Each member of the family has the same ID number; however, an individual code is used to differentiate family members from one another. Often the cardholder, or the primary person on the insurance, is person 00 or 01. The spouse or other insured adult is person 01 or 02. The children covered under the plan are listed in numeric order according to their birth order.
- Date of birth (DOB)—Must match the date the insurance company has on file for each patient.
- Sex code—Must match gender filed by insurance company. The insurance company also rejects claims for drugs if the sex code is incorrect. For instance, if the technician submits a claim stating that Mary Clein is a male and attempts to bill her insurance for Ortho Tri-Cyclen, the claim may be rejected by the insurance company because males typically are not prescribed birth control pills.

- Address
- Phone number
- Gender
- Allergies (both drug and food)
- Insurance provider's information: provider's phone number and insurance number (per hospital or institution policies)
- Over-the-counter (OTC) medications
- Diagnoses or disease states

If the information contains a mistake, the insurance claim may be rejected.

If the patient does not have insurance, he or she must pay full price for prescriptions. The cost of a prescription can vary greatly. Many pharmacies offer certain generics at a lower cost, $4 for a 30-day supply or $10 for a 90-day supply. The use of generic drugs can reduce the medication cost greatly.

If the patient has insurance, determining the guidelines of the program is of primary importance if the pharmacy is to receive reimbursement. The process by which all claims are processed over a computerized system is referred to as adjudication. The insurance determines the amount of coverage per medication based on various criteria, such as the following:

- Average wholesale price (AWP): The average wholesale price can be found in *Drug Topics*

Red Book, or this information may be contained in a portion of the pharmacy database. Use the *Red Book* to determine the price of a medication based on the listed price. The *Red Book* is available electronically, and the online databases supply real-time updates to medication price changes.

- Copay: A relatively small fixed fee required by the health insurer to be paid by the patient at the time of each office visit, outpatient service, or filling of a prescription.

Processing Claims

When handling a patient's medication claim, the pharmacy technician may be responsible for using the insurance company claim form to relay the necessary patient information. Because each company requires its forms to be filled out entirely and correctly, the technician must know the specific needs of the company. Universal claim forms (UCFs) (Figure 13-7) are used in certain circumstances. For instance, because a compounded medication does not have an NDC number, it cannot be submitted in the normal manner, as are manufactured products. However, it can be submitted using a UCF. Sometimes patients arrive at the pharmacy with a claim form that the

NCPDP UNIVERSAL CLAIM FORM (UCF)

1A4

TYPE OR PRINT ALL INFORMATION NEATLY AND COMPLETELY IN APPROPRIATE SPACES

I.D. ____ GROUP I.D. ____

NAME ____ PLAN NAME ____

PATIENT NAME ____ OTHER COVERAGE CODE (1) ____ PERSON CODE (2) ____

PATIENT DATE OF BIRTH __ __ __ (MM DD CCYY) PATIENT (3) GENDER CODE ____ PATIENT (4) RELATIONSHIP CODE ____

PHARMACY NAME ____

ADDRESS ____ SERVICE PROVIDER I.D. ____ QUAL (5) ____

CITY ____ PHONE NO. ( )

STATE & ZIP CODE ____ FAX NO. ( )

FOR OFFICE USE ONLY

WORKERS COMP. INFORMATION

EMPLOYER NAME ____

ADDRESS ____

CITY ____ STATE ____ ZIP CODE ____

CARRIER I.D. (6) ____ EMPLOYER PHONE NO. ____

DATE OF INJURY __ __ __ (MM DD CCYY) CLAIM (7) REFERENCE I.D. ____

I have hereby read the Certification Statement on the reverse side. I hereby certify to and accept the terms thereof. I also certify that I have received 1 or 2 (please circle number) prescription(s) listed below.

PATIENT/ AUTHORIZED REPRESENTATIVE ____

ATTENTION RECIPIENT PLEASE READ CERTIFICATION STATEMENT ON REVERSE SIDE

1

PRESCRIPTION/SERV. REF. #	QUAL (8)	DATE WRITTEN MM DD CCYY	DATE OF SERVICE MM DD CCYY	FILL#	QTY DISPENSED (9)	DAYS SUPPLY

PRODUCT/SERVICE I.D.	QUAL (10)	DAW CODE	PRIOR AUTH # SUBMITTED	PA TYPE (11)	PRESCRIBER I.D.	QUAL (12)

DUR/PPS CODES (13)	BASS COST (14)	PROVIDER I.D.	QUAL (15)	DIAGNOSIS CODE	QUAL (16)
A B C					

OTHER PAYER DATE MM DD CCYY	OTHER PAYER I.D.	QUAL (17)	OTHER PAYER REJECT CODES	USUAL & CUST. CHARGE

	INGREDIENT COST SUBMITTED
	DISPENSING FEE SUBMITTED
	INCENTIVE AMOUNT SUBMITTED
	OTHER AMOUNT SUBMITTED
	SALES TAX SUBMITTED
	GROSS AMOUNT DUE SUBMITTED
	PATIENT PAID AMOUNT
	OTHER PAYER AMOUNT PAID
	NET AMOUNT DUE

2

PRESCRIPTION/SERV. REF. #	QUAL (8)	DATE WRITTEN MM DD CCYY	DATE OF SERVICE MM DD CCYY	FILL#	QTY DISPENSED (9)	DAYS SUPPLY

PRODUCT/SERVICE I.D.	QUAL (10)	DAW CODE	PRIOR AUTH # SUBMITTED	PA TYPE (11)	PRESCRIBER I.D.	QUAL (12)

DUR/PPS CODES (13)	BASS COST (14)	PROVIDER I.D.	QUAL (15)	DIAGNOSIS CODE	QUAL (16)
A B C					

OTHER PAYER DATE MM DD CCYY	OTHER PAYER I.D.	QUAL (17)	OTHER PAYER REJECT CODES	USUAL & CUST. CHARGE

	INGREDIENT COST SUBMITTED
	DISPENSING FEE SUBMITTED
	INCENTIVE AMOUNT SUBMITTED
	OTHER AMOUNT SUBMITTED
	SALES TAX SUBMITTED
	GROSS AMOUNT DUE SUBMITTED
	PATIENT PAID AMOUNT
	OTHER PAYER AMOUNT PAID
	NET AMOUNT DUE

FIGURE 13-7 Universal claim form.

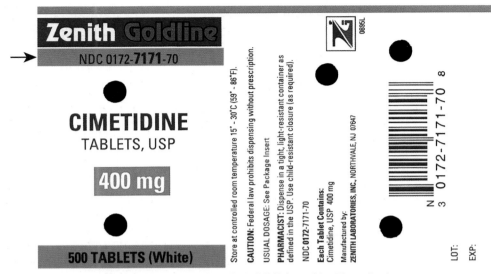

Store at controlled room temperature 15°-30°C (59°-86°F).

CAUTION: Federal law prohibits dispensing without prescription.

USUAL DOSAGE: See Package Insert

PHARMACIST: Dispense in a tight, light-resistant container as defined in the USP. Use child-resistant closure (as required).

NDC 0172-7171-70

Each Tablet Contains:
Cimetidine, USP 400 mg

Manufactured by:
ZENITH LABORATORIES, INC., NORTHVALE, NJ 07647

LOT:

EXP:

Zenith Goldline

NDC 0172-**7171**-70

CIMETIDINE
TABLETS, USP

400 mg

500 TABLETS (White)

N 3 0172-7171-70 8

FIGURE 13-8 National Drug Code (NDC) *(arrow)* for this medication.

pharmacy needs to complete for reimbursement. Claims are filed electronically. The general types of information required may include the following:

- Processor: Typically the insurance company
- Member's identification number: Can be either the assigned number specific to that patient or the Social Security number; however, fewer insurance companies are using Social Security numbers because of the potential for identity theft
- Group number (if applicable)
- Plan code (if applicable)
- Insurance carrier

Claim Problems

A prescription may not be covered for the insured patient for many reasons. For example, the **National Drug Code (NDC)** may not be covered. The NDC number is organized into three sections: the labeler code, the product code, and the package code (Figure 13-8). All medications have an NDC number. When a prescription is not covered, it can be frustrating for both the patient and the technician, and even for the insurance company representative. Other common reasons that a prescription may not be covered are as follows:

- Coverage has expired.
- Coverage limits have been exceeded.
- Patient is trying to refill a prescription too early.
- The cardholder's information does not match the processor's information.
- The physician who wrote the prescription is not the patient's primary care physician.
- The prescription is written for an invalid amount of medication; most insurance companies cover only a 30-day supply unless it is

mail-order, which covers a 90-day supply. Many insurance companies are now requiring patients to use mail-order for certain maintenance medications.

Coverage Expiration Policy for Drugs

If the patient has lost his or her coverage, the claim is rejected. Following HIPAA regulations, the pharmacy does not have access to information about the reason for rejection, and only a termination date is disclosed. Patients often are unaware of why coverage has been discontinued and may want the pharmacy to investigate. Pharmacy personnel are not permitted to call the patient's insurance carrier about these types of inquiries. Patient confidentiality would be breached, and legal action could result. The only recourse is to explain to the patient that he or she must contact the insurance company to resolve the issue. In the interim, the patient must pay full price for the medications. If there has been an error, reimbursement is made after the insurance company corrects the problem.

Limitation of Plan Exceeded

The phrase *limitation of plan exceeded* refers to a patient who has exhausted his or her pharmacy benefits for the specified time period or quantity limitation on a drug.

If a prescription requests a greater quantity of the drug than is allowed by the insurance plan, the plan limits are exceeded. For example, some government insurance plans limit the number of prescriptions that can be filled per month or per year. If the prescription is written for a specific quantity of medication that exceeds the maximum amount to be filled per day, the prescription is rejected and the patient must contact the insurance company for special permission to obtain the drug. "Limit exceeded" could also mean that the patient has met a yearly or lifetime benefit amount.

Some patients are exempt from these types of limitations because of their illness. These include individuals who suffer from diabetes and those who have been diagnosed with human immunodeficiency virus (HIV) infection or acquired immunodeficiency syndrome (AIDS). People with diabetes mellitus require a continuous refill of lancets and blood-testing strips to monitor their blood glucose levels. In addition, they must refill their insulin syringes monthly. In the case of patients treated for HIV infection or AIDS, the medication is expensive, and these patients usually have to take many medications simultaneously. When a claim is rejected because the maximum limits of the insurance are exceeded, the technician must explain the problem to the patient. The patient is ultimately responsible for contacting the insurance company to dispute the problem.

 Tech Note!

Only a pharmacist can contact the physician to request a change in medication.

Handling Non-Formulary Drugs or Noncovered National Drug Codes

Formularies tend to be specific. This includes the decision on which drugs are included in the member's plan. These drugs are identified by their NDC, a code assigned to every drug in the United States. If the code submitted is not in the formulary, the claim is rejected by the insurance company. In pharmacy, these types of medications are referred to as *non-formulary drugs*. In this case, two options can be explored. First, the pharmacist can contact the physician and request that the prescription be changed to a drug that is covered under the patient's insurance plan. Second, the physician can submit a prior authorization form to the insurance company indicating why the patient must take the non-formulary drug. The type of prior authorization form varies, depending on insurance company guidelines. Physicians normally complete and submit the prior authorization form for approval. This approval process can take up to 2 weeks. Therefore, the patient can either purchase the medication for immediate use or wait to have the prescription filled after approval or rejection is given by the insurance company. If the patient pays upfront and the medication is approved, the patient is reimbursed by the insurance company after the pharmacist completes a reimbursement form for the patient. The form is sent to the insurance company to reimburse the patient for the covered drug cost.

Filling a Prescription Too Soon

Patients attempt to have their prescriptions refilled when they still have medication remaining for several reasons. Most of the time it is not a problem to obtain a refill 1 week before the prescription's refill date; however, there are instances in which the patient may request a refill as early as 1 week after having the prescription filled. For example, the patient may be leaving the country for an extended time and wants to ensure that sufficient medication is available until he or she returns. Most insurance plans allow extra refills in circumstances such as vacations or the occurrence of devastating events. For example, when Hurricane Sandy devastated the East Coast of the United States, many insurance companies allowed early refills and replacement fills on prescriptions, and even permitted patients to be treated by physicians outside their medical plan.

If the patient's insurance will not pay, the patient is responsible for the cost of the medication. Prescriptions normally are written for a 30-, 60-, or 90-day supply, depending on the condition treated. Mail-order companies usually fill up to a 90-day supply for certain maintenance drugs, such as diabetic or heart medications. Sometimes the amount of medication prescribed is limited because of safety or legal issues regarding the dispensing of a specific medication. Because certain medications are dangerous, they may not be prescribed for more than 30 days. Examples include Drug Enforcement Agency (DEA) schedule II controlled substances and a specific drug, isotretinoin (an acne medication), which has been linked to teratogenicity if given to pregnant women. Many insurance plans allow additional savings if refills are ordered via mail-order pharmacies that are on their list of participating pharmacies.

Sometimes a physician instructs the patient to increase the dosage, thus forcing the refill process before its allotted time. In this case a new prescription order must be submitted to the insurance company. In some cases the technician must contact the insurance company "help desk" to explain the circumstances of the prescription change. However, some insurance companies may require a direct response from the patient's physician before granting approval.

Non-Identification Match

Probably one of the most common problems arises when the cardholder's information does not match the processor's information, thus resulting in a claim rejection. To determine whether this is the case, the technician should always recheck the information submitted to the insurance company. Items to double-check include the following:

- Health plan card number, identification number, and insurance number
- Patient's name, date of birth, and relationship to the insured person

The relationship of the patient to the cardholder is important because he or she may be a new spouse or adopted child, or other significant changes may have occurred. In this case the technician may be able to ask for a new insurance card for the member through the insurance help desk.

Scenario CHECK UP 13-4

Brian is learning a great deal from the training materials he has been studying. He just completed a lesson on how to effectively resolve rejected insurance claims. Today at work, a new technician asks if Brian can help her with a billing problem. It seems that when she sends the prescription to the insurance company for adjudication, it comes back with a "non-identification match" rejection code. When Brian double-checks the patient's name, date of birth, and relationship to the insured person, he finds that the information entered is correct. Upon further investigation, he learns that the patient is one of a set of identical twins who have the same birth date and same first name but different middle names. What can Brian do to help the new technician get this prescription processed?

Resubmitting Rejected Claims

Sometimes an insurance company mistakenly rejects a valid claim. When this happens, the pharmacy technician can resubmit the claim a second time. Special attention should be paid to the rejection codes provided by the payer in the remittance information. Next, the insurance company determines whether the issue has been resolved and the claim can be processed and paid. It is the responsibility of the pharmacy to keep records of claims that are submitted until they are processed or denied. Follow-up is the key to ensuring that payment is received.

Plan Limitations

Often insurance carriers enact plan limitations to control drug use and reduce drug costs. Some examples include:

- Maximum amounts on medication that can be dispensed at one time
- Days' supply restrictions: 30 days for retail and 90 days for mail-order supplies
- Refill limits

- Requiring prior authorization for certain medications
- Step therapy: One or more cheaper medications must be demonstrated to be ineffective before more expensive medications may be used.

These limits are sometimes called "cost utilization measures" and are designed to reduce health care costs.

 Tech Note!

Fraud involving pharmacy insurance claims is a serious issue and should not be taken lightly. Falsely billing charges for medication that was not dispensed is a crime.

Other Methods of Payment

Self-Pay

Some patients do not have insurance coverage and are solely responsible for their prescription cost. These patients can pay with cash, check, or credit or debit card.

Drug Discount Cards or Drug Coupon Cards

Patients can obtain drug discount cards from a variety of sources. These do not offer insurance benefits, but instead allow the patient to obtain medications at the contracted provider rate. For example, if a drug discount card contracts with a pharmacy to pay the **average wholesale price (AWP)** −10% plus a $2 dispensing fee for a drug that would normally be sold at retail for AWP +15% plus a $5 dispensing fee, the patient can obtain the medicine at the less expensive rate through a prescription discount card.

Drug manufacturers provide drug coupon cards to patients either as an incentive for the patient to take the drug or as an aid to patients who meet certain income requirements. Both types of cards are billed as a third-party claim for the pharmacy to receive reimbursement and the patient to receive his or her discount.

Private Plans

With a private plan, the patient obtains a prescription drug card from a pharmacy benefits manager. Usually these plans are very expensive.

Health Savings Account/Flexible Spending Account

Health savings accounts and flexible spending accounts are something like a savings account that can be used to pay medical bills before a deductible has been met, along with copays for prescriptions and office visits. The government has put limits on the amounts that can be put into these accounts per calendar year. There is also a "use it or lose it" component. Some employers contribute to these accounts and some do not. Restrictions are placed on what is covered. Participants must be knowledgeable about the regulations affecting these types of accounts.

Many times pharmacists must explain the various types of benefits to patients. Technicians play an important role in helping patients understand their coverage. They should keep themselves updated on any changes in the system to ensure that the billing process goes smoothly. Technicians must have patience and good communications skills to explain technical issues or terms, such as *coverage, formulary, generic availability,* and so on, in language the patient can understand.

Inventory Management

Proper inventory management is the key to an efficiently run pharmacy. Having the needed medications and supplies on hand to serve the patients' needs is a top priority. Minimizing the carrying cost of the pharmacy's inventory investment enhances the pharmacy's ability to earn a profit. Inventory management focuses on ordering stock, proper storage of medication and supplies, repackaging, disposal of used and unused pharmaceutical products, and distribution systems.

Pharmacy Stock

Everyone working in the pharmacy is responsible for maintaining the inventory stock. This is an essential part of the daily tasks of pharmacy staff. As stocks are depleted, it is important to order replacement inventories. Although many different systems are available for ordering stock, the task of ordering can be delegated to a specific person in the pharmacy. It is then the responsibility of staff to inform the inventory control person of decreasing stock levels.

Each pharmacy orders drugs that include formulary drugs and a limited amount of non-formulary or less commonly used drugs. The established level of medication stock kept on hand at any given time is referred to as the **periodic automatic replenishment (PAR)** level. This is the minimum amount of medication that should be maintained in the pharmacy at any given time. Just as insurance billing has become a common task of pharmacy technicians, so has the responsibility of ordering medications. Different systems are available that can keep an updated inventory of medications and alert the technician when new stock must be ordered. This can be done

in several ways, such as at the point of sale, by order cards, or by handheld inventory computers. Because so many different types of systems are in use today, this section of the chapter explores the main characteristics of various systems and explains when and how stock arrives at the pharmacy. Proper storage of all drugs is also discussed. In addition, this chapter discusses how recalls are addressed and how returns are processed.

Although some pharmacies may contract out the job of processing returns and sending them to the manufacturer, this function is usually assigned to a pharmacy technician who is an employee of the pharmacy. Typically, an inventory technician is in charge of all aspects of ordering, restocking, and returning stock in the pharmacy.

Inventory Control Technician

Most hospitals have a technician who is in charge of maintaining stock levels and completing the special ordering of medications. The technician who orders the stock is responsible for the actual ordering, billing, and restocking of the pharmacy shelves; however, it takes a group effort in the pharmacy to maintain stock levels and avoid having to borrow items from another hospital or special-order them at a higher cost.

Many methods of keeping stock at necessary levels are available. Before today's electronic stocking methods became available, a hospital pharmacy used ordering cards to reorder stock when it was low. Each person was responsible for pulling the card (normally kept with the medications) and placing it in a designated area where the inventory technician could place the order. When the order arrived, the card was put back into the box along with the new stock. For the electronic stocking method typically used today, a handheld device that reads bar codes is used for electronic ordering. In this case, the inventory technician must check visually to see which medications need to be ordered.

A third method of stocking requires each item to be tagged with a manufacturer's sticker as it arrives in the pharmacy. Stickers are provided by the manufacturer and must be affixed to each item before it is placed on the shelf. This sticker lists the stock number of the medication along with the price. When an item needs to be reordered, the sticker is taken off the container and placed on an ordering sheet, also known as a "want book." It is then entered into an electronic device for transmission by phone or by online ordering.

Duties

Every day the pharmacy depletes some of its stock of drugs and supplies. Although pharmacies have different systems of ordering the medications, most orders normally are placed using a computer. Depending on the location of the warehouse or manufacturer, the turnaround time for the shipment may vary. For example, if a supplier is thousands of miles away, that medication must be ordered earlier than a medication from the pharmacy's warehouse (which usually takes less than 24 hours). Knowing the right time to order medications is a skill that pharmacy technicians must acquire; it is crucial to keep the pharmacy completely stocked with necessary medications.

When the shipment arrives, all included medications and supplies must be verified against the inventory list; initialing and writing "received" on each invoice are important. Some medications are backordered; these items are currently not in stock from the manufacturer but will be sent as soon as they are available. If the medication is one that cannot be left out of stock for any length of time, it may be necessary to borrow from another pharmacy. This can be done by calling a pharmacist at a neighboring hospital and asking whether that pharmacy has enough to share. A loan/borrow sheet is filled out, and either a taxi or a hospital courier normally is sent to carry the medication from one location to the other. After the original ordered stock arrives, replacements for the borrowed items are returned to the lending pharmacy.

Placing stock on the shelves is another important duty of the pharmacy technician; it is the point at which the stock is rotated (Figure 13-9). Placing medications with later expiration dates farthest back on

the shelf ensures that the medications with the earliest expiration dates are used first. The inventory technician is also responsible for returning damaged items and expired agents and handling recall items according to the manufacturer's guidelines.

Timing is probably one of the most important aspects of keeping inventory at a constant level. The technician can order appropriately if he or she learns the pharmacy protocol for ordering, compensates for items that take longer to ship, and considers upcoming holidays. Patient load also directly relates to the types of medications to be ordered. It is a well-known fact that during the winter months, hospitals have more patients because more people become ill at this time of year. The elderly are especially at risk. Also, certain hospitals have primary functions, such as burn centers, rehabilitation, or specific surgeries, and their specialties influence the overall increase in the use of medications specific to those patients' needs.

Ordering Process

Maintaining a PAR level in the pharmacy is important for several reasons. Many manufacturers do not fill orders on weekends or holidays. Thus if the pharmacy depletes its stock during this time, it may have to wait until the following delivery day to receive the necessary stock. It is serious if a patient cannot obtain an essential medication because the pharmacy is out of stock. Patients visiting a community pharmacy may be able to go elsewhere to have prescriptions filled, but hospitalized patients rely on the hospital pharmacy to stock medications.

If stock will not arrive until the following Monday or Tuesday, the only recourse is to use an express delivery company contracted by the pharmacy or to borrow the medication from another pharmacy. Express delivery can range from delivery of a medication by courier to air delivery of the medication. In some cases pharmacies even contact other stores in the area to "borrow" stock for patients. Of course this is done only in case of an emergency, when all other options have been exhausted. Express delivery also is expensive and in many cases unnecessary if the pharmacy staff understands when to reorder a specific drug. Shipping time varies, depending on the type of drug ordered. This is when pharmacy personnel must demonstrate their teamwork. It is improper and inappropriate to assume that medication ordering is another team member's responsibility.

Special Orders

When a pharmacy does not carry a medication (perhaps it is new or uncommon), it may be ordered from a drug wholesaler. It is important to know the length of time needed for the wholesaler to deliver a

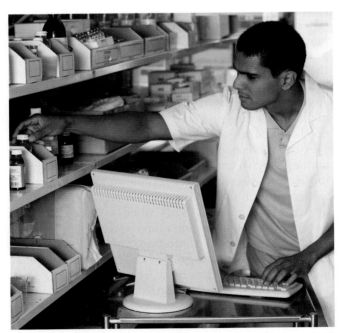

FIGURE 13-9 Inventory control technicians help maintain pharmacy stock by ordering drugs, stocking shelves, and managing returns. (Copyright © 2014 Fuse, Thinkstock.com. All rights reserved.)

medication and to follow the order's progress. Special order prescriptions should be filed in a specific location in the pharmacy. The technician must check for special orders each time stock arrives. This ensures that the patient is not waiting for a medication that was received by the pharmacy a week ago. In addition, if medication has not been delivered by the expected date, the wholesaler should be contacted to determine whether there is a back-order, ordering problem, or other issue. Notification of any ordering issues as soon as possible means that patients will not have their therapy delayed any longer than necessary.

More pharmacies rely on computerized systems that are programmed to order medications. This is by far one of the best ways to maintain appropriate stock levels, although not all pharmacies have this system. Three main systems are discussed in this chapter, although there are many more types. All systems are similar to those discussed in the following sections.

Bar Coding

Most manufacturers identify their products with bar codes that can be scanned. This process accelerates the input of information because one pass of the bar code device identifies the drug, strength, dosage form, quantity, cost, package size, and any other information necessary to fill the medication or device. Pharmacies also can use these bar codes. The medication is scanned at the register, known as the point of sale, and electronically deleted from the computerized inventory list. When the in-stock quantity drops below the PAR level, it is reordered automatically. Other devices used to scan drugs are handheld components that identify the necessary drug information. The technician needs to enter only the quantity to be ordered. The information from this handheld set then is transferred to the main computer ordering system.

Automated Dispensing Systems

Automated dispensing systems (ADSs) involve technology designed to reduce labor and increase patient safety. ADSs store medications and control electronic dispensing.

ADSs are used in community pharmacies to monitor the inventory as tablets and capsules are dispensed into a drug vial from a bulk bin. As the pills pass a beam of light, they automatically are removed from the inventory. An example of this type of system is a Baker Cell system. Technicians are responsible for filling, cleaning, and troubleshooting these systems when a problem occurs. In the hospital, the pharmacy is responsible for stocking the various clinics and nursing units. To avoid a stock shortage, dispensing systems that link the nursing units to the pharmacy computer system allow the stock levels to be viewed at any time. Each time the nurse indicates the type and amount of drug taken from these drug cabinets, it is deducted from the current stock levels in the cabinet and this information is transferred electronically to the pharmacy unit. Various reports can be generated from this centralized unit, which can provide an overall stock inventory for a specific drug. In addition to the inventory status, such units also monitor controlled substance use and inventory. All individuals adding drugs to or taking drugs from the unit are identified, and a log is kept of all users. This also ensures the proper use of controlled substances and detects any discrepancies. Examples of these types of ADS are hospital units such as Pyxis (see Chapter 9), OmniRx (Figure 13-10), or Baker Cell systems. Again, technicians are responsible for the maintenance of these systems, including filling, cleaning, and troubleshooting when necessary. Technicians also run various reports needed for filling the medication drawers and other reconciliation procedures.

✎ *Tech Note!*

Automated systems in hospitals are being transitioned from personal codes entered by nurses and pharmacy personnel to biometric identification, making it more difficult to misuse the system.

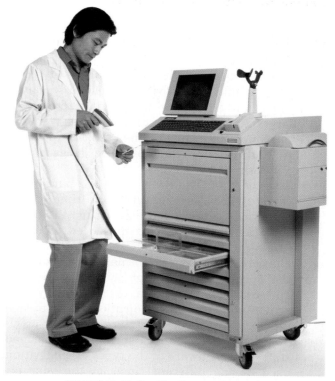

FIGURE 13-10 OmniRx. (Courtesy Omnicell.)

Manual Ordering

Although manual ordering is being eliminated slowly as the primary ordering technique, it is still important in the continued monitoring of stock levels. Some pharmacies still visually note that stock is getting low or use ordering cards that stay inside the medication box. These cards list the drug information, including the ordering number and the necessary PAR levels, to aid the technician in ordering the proper amount. Using the card system or simply writing down the right amount of stock to be ordered depends on the PAR levels or special orders.

More commonly, orders are processed electronically via the computer or handheld computers that transmit the order. The following list categorizes the drugs stocked by many pharmacies:

- *Formulary:* In a hospital pharmacy, these drugs, normally stocked by the pharmacy, are approved by a pharmacy and therapeutics (P&T) committee. In a retail pharmacy, a specific formulary indicates which drugs are on the approved list of a patient's insurance company. Because there are many different insurance companies and thus many different formularies, retail pharmacies stock a wide range of products.
- *Fast mover:* These drugs typically are kept in a separate area from the normal stock because of the high volume of use. These must be ordered in larger quantities, keeping the overstock in close proximity, or must be ordered more often.
- *Slow mover:* These drugs are prescribed regularly by a few physicians but are not commonly prescribed. They must be checked before ordering and periodically to ensure that the drugs are not close to expiring.
- *Special orders:* These are drugs typically used by only a few patients, but they may be important for proper treatment. It is easy to forget to order these drugs because of their infrequent use. Usually they are ordered at the time of use, and some of these drugs may be non-formulary.
- *Time of year:* The drugs that are part of this category vary, depending on the time of year. Many medications that are fast movers during a particular time of year may need their PAR levels raised during that period. For example, albuterol inhalers are normally fast movers in the spring, when allergy symptoms increase and consequent asthma or respiratory tract symptoms. Antiviral medications used to treat influenza are prescribed more often during the flu season, from fall to spring. All pharmacy staff must be aware of the types of medications used during different times of the year and understand how levels fluctuate.

 Tech Note!

When stock begins to become depleted, it is everyone's responsibility to make sure that the stock is ordered.

New Stock

Stock normally arrives daily at the pharmacy (excluding weekends and holidays) from different sources (except for central supply in a hospital setting, which functions 7 days a week). For billing purposes, it is important that all stock be checked completely against the packing list when first received. Procedure 13-1 presents a step-by-step approach that should be used when receiving stock.

▶ TECHNICIAN PROFILE

Melissa works in a large hospital as an inventory control technician. She has been in the pharmacy for 15 years and works under the supervision of the pharmacy director. Her position requires an individual who is skilled in data entry, mathematics, and computer software applications, and who can type at least 30 words per minute. She is nationally certified and is an active member of the American Society of Health-System Pharmacists (ASHP). Melissa's duties include maintaining adequate levels of drug inventory, purchasing drugs according to contract and cost, and alerting the director to any drug shortages. She also tracks the controlled substance ordering and delivery and receipt of all medications for the entire hospital. Although her job is very demanding, she works as a part of a very effective team. Each member plays a key role in ensuring that all patients have the needed medication available. Melissa is considered a specialty technician.

Proper Storage

As stock arrives, it is important to follow the manufacturer's requirements for storage. Certain medications must be frozen at temperatures between −20° and −10° C, refrigerated at temperatures between 2° and 8° C, or stored at room temperature (23° C). Light or humidity can also affect the stability of the medication; therefore, care must be taken to protect stock from either light sources or excessive humidity. If these guidelines are not followed, the medication is compromised, rendering it unusable. Just as it is important to return unused stock to its proper location when it is returned from the nursing floors (in hospital pharmacy), it likewise is essential that the pharmacy technician place new stock items in their respective areas of storage as soon as possible. Chemicals such as phenol and other toxic materials are usually kept behind cabinet doors and low to the ground. It is not wise to leave these types of materials exposed to the public, because they are toxic. Read the packaging on all medications and follow the

---

PROCEDURE 13-1

Receiving Stock in the Pharmacy

GOAL: To learn the steps involved in properly receiving and checking in pharmacy stock.

EQUIPMENT AND SUPPLIES
- Manufacturer or warehouse invoice
- Medication to be checked in
- Clipboard and pen

PROCEDURAL STEPS
1. Retrieve the manufacturer or warehouse invoice.
PURPOSE: You must have the appropriate invoice to accurately check in the order.
2. Account for all boxes.
PURPOSE: To make certain that if the invoice indicates there are five boxes, you verify that there are indeed five boxes.
3. Inspect all boxes for storage requirements.
PURPOSE: To make certain that if any box is marked "Refrigerate" or "Freeze," you immediately comply with the instructions to avoid product damage.
4. Check all information against the invoice, which includes the drug name, strength, dosage form, and quantity. Also check that the expiration date is not too soon.
PURPOSE: To confirm that all information on the invoice matches the product you are checking in.
5. Compare the invoice with the order form to ensure that only the items requested were received.
PURPOSE: To ensure that no drugs are missing or shorted and that you have no extra items you did not order.

6. Sign and date the invoice and forward it for processing per pharmacy protocol.
PURPOSE: To ensure that the invoice is forwarded and stored appropriately for future reference and accounting purposes.
7. Place the stock in the correct location per pharmacy protocol, placing new stock behind existing stock, with the most current expiration dates in the front.
PURPOSE: To rotate stock appropriately to avoid accumulation of expired drugs that may be used accidentally.
8. Return inventory cards to the medication box for future use.
PURPOSE: To prevent medication inventory from becoming depleted due to failure to properly reorder out-of-stock items.

NOTE!
- Proper inventory control is very important. Marking stock shelves clearly reduces the probability of drug errors. For example, if a drug is accidentally placed in a box intended for a different drug with a similar sounding name, it may be used to fill a prescription for the sound-alike drug and ultimately affect the patient's health and well-being.
- Checking the expiration date is important. Drugs that are used rarely and have short expiration dates may stay on the shelf and expire before use.

---

manufacturer's requirements for storage. Storing medications in the proper location is the responsibility of everyone working in pharmacy.

Returns

Medication is returned to the warehouse or manufacturer for four main reasons:
1. Drug recalls
   - Class I: Recalls for drugs that may pose a serious threat to users' health or even death
   - Class II: Recalls for drugs that may cause a temporary health problem and have a low risk of creating a serious problem
   - Class III: Recalls for drugs that violate FDA regulations concerning container defects or have a strange taste or color
2. Damaged stock
3. Expired stock
4. Medication is about to expire; the pharmacy may return the drug to the wholesaler for credit or full price if the drug has at least a 9-month expiration date later than the date of return.

Depending on the reason, certain documentation must accompany the medication. Pharmacy policies and procedures should list the steps involved for returns. Except for scheduled drugs that fall under the jurisdiction of the DEA (see Chapter 2), most medications can be returned by the technician without a pharmacist's signature.

Drug Recalls
Manufacturers are required by law to recall any product that has been found to violate any of the following guidelines:
- Labeling is wrong.
- Product was not packaged or produced properly.
- Drug batch was contaminated.
- The FDA has required removal of the drug from the market as a result of safety risks.
- Any other change occurs that causes the drug to fall outside the FDA or manufacturer's guidelines.

Recall notices may arrive at the pharmacy by mail, e-mail, or fax. Notices should identify the necessary information about the drug or device in question and describe the necessary steps to follow the recall procedure. This information includes the drug name and the reason it is being recalled. One of the most important pieces of information provided is the *lot number* of the drug. Lot numbers are assigned by the drug manufacturer to identify a specific batch of medication. This is the key to identifying the recalled medication. Retail pharmacy corporations and hospitals often have detailed procedures and teams of people who ensure the documentation, implementation, and completion of recall procedures, including final notification to the manufacturer and the FDA of the completion of removal of the recalled product. Upon receipt of the recall notification, pharmacy staff should immediately inspect and remove all stock from shelves, refrigerators, and freezers. If a pharmacy finds recalled medication on its shelves, a report is normally generated identifying the patients who may have received the medication within the past 30 days, and the patient is notified. The prescriber should be notified if a patient has received any of a recalled medication.

The pharmacy should place the recalled medication in a designated area or container for return to the manufacturer or disposal in accordance with the recall notice. Technicians are responsible for checking all the drug stock throughout the pharmacy and facility to ensure that the recalled drug is not in stock. If this is the case, the recall form is initialed to indicate that the item is not in stock. If pharmacy stock does include a drug with the recalled lot number, the pharmacist must be notified in case a patient has been issued one of these products. Prescribers also are notified by manufacturers and the FDA in the same manner as the pharmacy. It is the responsibility of the prescriber to notify patients currently using a recalled medication or device if treatment is to be discontinued or altered. The pharmacy can help facilitate the patient's return or disposal of a recalled medication. Although the FDA can issue mandatory drug recalls, most are voluntary recalls issued by the manufacturers. All recalls monitored by the FDA are included in a weekly Enforcement Report and are classified as to the level of hazard involved. These Enforcement Reports are available on the FDA website (*www.fda.gov*). You can sign up to receive the reports via e-mail. Box 13-5 presents an example of a recall notification.

BOX 13-5

Recall Notification

Recall—Firm Press Release
The U.S. Food and Drug Administration (FDA) posts press releases and other notices of recalls and market withdrawals from the firms involved as a service to consumers, the media, and other interested parties. The FDA does not endorse either the product or the company.

Alexion Provides Update on Previously Communicated November 2013 Voluntary Nationwide Recall of Two Lots of Soliris® (eculizumab) Concentrated Solution for Intravenous Infusion

Contact
Consumer
Irving Adler
203-271-8210

Media
Kim Diamond
203-439-9600

FOR IMMEDIATE RELEASE—December 13, 2013—Cheshire, Conn.,—Alexion Pharmaceuticals, Inc. (NASDAQ: ALXN) today is providing further information regarding a previously communicated voluntary recall of two lots of Soliris® (eculizumab) Concentrated Solution for Intrave-

nous Infusion. As stated on Nov. 12, 2013, the two lots were found to contain visible particles. At that time, Alexion provided instructions to return any unused vials of Soliris from these two lots at the distributor level. Alexion is now providing the same instructions at the hospital/ user level.

The administration of particulate, if present in a parenteral drug, poses a potential safety risk to patients in two general areas: immunogenicity and thromboembolic events. Particulates could cause blockage of flow of blood in vessels, which could be life-threatening. To date, there have been no product complaints of particulates or identifiable safety concerns attributed to the product consumed from the affected lots. As previously stated, Alexion does not anticipate any interruption to patient supply of Soliris.

The product is approved as a treatment for patients with paroxysmal nocturnal hemoglobinuria and atypical hemolytic uremic syndrome, two ultra-rare disorders. Alexion and its distributors typically ship Soliris to health care providers in small quantities, which are timed to individual patient infusions, with the product being consumed before more is shipped. As product was last shipped on Nov. 1, 2013, Alexion believes there is little, if any, inventory currently being held at the hospital or user level.

BOX 13-5

Recall Notification—cont'd

The following table lists the two affected lots, which were distributed nationwide.

Product	Lot	Expiration Date	First Ship Date	Last Ship Date
Soliris® (eculizumab) 300 mg/30 mL	10010A	Oct. 31, 2015	Oct. 11, 2013	Nov. 1, 2013
Concentrated solution for intravenous infusion only NDC 25682-001-01	10001-1	July 31, 2014	June 4, 2012	May 8, 2013

As previously disclosed, Alexion believes that it has identified the filling process step that resulted in the presence of the visible particles and implemented the change necessary to correct the issue. To date, visible particles have not been observed in other lots of Soliris distributed in the United States.

Any person in possession of vials of Soliris from these lots should stop use and arrange for return of the product to Alexion immediately by calling 1-888-SOLIRIS (888-765-4747).

Alexion will replace any recalled vials of Soliris. Unaffected lot numbers can continue to be used according to the instructions for use.

Health care professionals and pharmacists with questions about this recall can contact Alexion at 1-888-765-4747. Patients should contact their physician or health care provider if they have experienced any problems that may be related to taking or using this drug product.

Adverse reactions or quality problems experienced with the use of this product may be reported to the FDA's MedWatch Adverse Event Reporting program either online, by regular mail, or by fax.

- Online: www.fda.gov/MedWatch/report.htm
- Regular mail: Use postage-paid, preaddressed Form FDA 3500 available at: www.fda.gov/MedWatch/getforms.htm. Mail to address on the preaddressed form.
- Fax: 1-800-FDA-0178

This recall is being conducted with the knowledge of the U.S. Food and Drug Administration.

About Alexion

Alexion Pharmaceuticals, Inc. is a biopharmaceutical company focused on serving patients with severe and ultra-rare disorders through the innovation, development, and commercialization of life-transforming therapeutic products. Alexion is the global leader in complement inhibition and has developed and markets Soliris® (eculizumab) as a treatment for patients with PNH and aHUS, two debilitating, ultra-rare and life-threatening disorders caused by chronic uncontrolled complement activation. Soliris is currently approved in nearly 50 countries for the treatment of PNH, and in the United States, European Union, Japan and other countries for the treatment of aHUS. Alexion is evaluating other potential indications for Soliris in additional severe and ultra-rare disorders beyond PNH and aHUS, and is developing other highly innovative biotechnology product candidates across multiple therapeutic areas. This press release and further information about Alexion Pharmaceuticals, Inc. can be found at: *www.alexionpharma.com*.

Safe Harbor Statement

This news release includes forward-looking statements relating to continued adequacy of the supply of Soliris and identification and correction of the cause of the visible particles. These statements are subject to risks, uncertainties, and other factors, including risks related to continuous product inventory and supply, the uncertainties involved in manufacturing of biologic products, and whether the FDA, EMA or other international regulatory authorities decide to take corrective or disciplinary actions against Alexion, as well as the risks that are described in detail in Alexion's Quarterly Report on Form 10-Q for the quarter ended Sept. 30, 2013, as filed with the U.S. Securities and Exchange Commission. These risks, uncertainties, and other factors could cause actual results to differ materially from those referred to in the forward-looking statements. The reader is cautioned not to place undue reliance on these forward-looking statements. All forward-looking statements are based on information currently available to Alexion, and Alexion assumes no duty or obligation to update or revise any such forward-looking statements or any other statement in this report. See: *www.fda.gov/Safety/Recalls/ucm378614.htm*

Damaged Stock

If you notice that some drugs were damaged en route to the pharmacy but you were not aware of damage at the time of delivery, it is not too late to return the damaged stock to the manufacturer. It may be necessary to first contact the manufacturer and obtain an authorization before the damaged goods are returned. The patient may also notice damaged stock. Sometimes EpiPen or Imitrex injections have bent needles, broken plungers, or other issues. In these cases the patient returns the medications, and the pharmacy replaces the item. The pharmacy must then contact the manufacturer, who sends a replacement to the pharmacy directly and may or may not collect the damaged merchandise.

Expired Stock

Some pharmacies have a policy to pull any medication that expires in 3 months or sooner. This ensures that no drugs on the shelves are close to their expiration date. Depending on the contract between the pharmacy and the manufacturer, it may be acceptable to return items as long as they can be bundled into a minimum package size rather than as partials. For instance, if the stock of cimetidine expires within 3 months, the manufacturer may allow it to be returned for full or partial credit if a box of 100 tablets can be returned at one time. Following manufacturers' guidelines for returns is important. Hazardous chemicals, including cytotoxic agents, must be repackaged carefully to avoid breakage during transport.

Pharmacy personnel can also pull and return slow-moving stock that has 9 to 12 months before expiration; the pharmacy can receive credit from the wholesaler, who in turn may be able to resell the drug to another pharmacy. This applies only to unopened bottles, and regulations vary according to the wholesaler's or manufacturer's specific operating policies.

Many pharmacies have a service that processes returns to drug companies for a percentage of the credits obtained. These companies visit the pharmacy at various times, ranging from once every 3 months to once a year, and complete all the paperwork and documentation for returning expired inventory.

Tech Note!
Patients should be instructed in the proper disposal of unused medications. For many drugs, it is advisable to mix them with either coffee grounds or kitty litter and then place them in the garbage. Used transdermal patches and other novel dosage forms will need special care for disposal to prevent accidental exposures. Certain pharmacies allow patients to return to the pharmacy any expired or unused prescriptions found in their medicine cabinets. Check with your pharmacy supervisor to see whether your pharmacy offers this service. Medications should never be emptied into a toilet or a drain because the drugs can infiltrate the water supply. The Drug Enforcement Agency (DEA) initiated a National Prescription Drug Take-Back Day in 2010 and has been holding take-back days twice a year ever since. The program provides a safe, convenient, and responsible means of disposing of prescription drugs while educating the public about the potential for medication abuse. For more information about this program in your state, visit the website *www.deadiversion.usdoj.gov/drug_disposal/takeback/*.

Automated Return Companies
Some companies' sole job is to process returns for hospitals, wholesalers, pharmacy chain stores, and independent retailers. They are responsible for all records and recalled items and for disposal of hazardous waste. Pharmacies contract with these companies for regular pickups; it is the pharmacy's responsibility to choose a licensed, qualified business to perform these services. Some examples of automated return companies are Return Solutions, Guaranteed Returns, and PharmaLink.

Tech Alert!
No medications taken out of the pharmacy by a patient can be returned to stock!

Nonreturnable Drugs and Their Disposal
Many items cannot be returned to manufacturers. Some examples of nonreturnable drugs are any drug that is reconstituted or compounded in the pharmacy; partially used bottles of medication; and any drugs that have been repackaged by the pharmacy. These drugs, including most reconstituted agents (e.g., amoxicillin suspension), can be discarded in the pharmacy garbage. They should not be allowed to infiltrate the water supply. In most cases, especially in chain pharmacies, the drugs are sent to a central location for destruction or returned to the manufacturer for credit.

Many agents must be disposed of carefully. Cytotoxic agents must be discarded in a specialized sharps container marked "hazardous waste." Nontoxic intravenous agents should be discarded in a standard sharps container marked for proper disposal. Controlled substances must be counted and cosigned by a pharmacist before they are destroyed. Before any scheduled medications are destroyed, the DEA must be contacted for specific instructions concerning their destruction. A pharmacist must always be present to cosign for the disposal of controlled substances and must return required information about the disposal to the DEA. The DEA issues a receipt for schedule II merchandise destroyed. This receipt must be kept for 2 years from the date of receipt or disposal with the schedule II inventory.

Suppliers
When ordering stock for the pharmacy, the technician orders from a centralized warehouse the pharmacy owns, from a wholesaler, or directly from the manufacturer. Medications, devices, and other pharmacy supplies are available from various sources.

- **Prime vendors** are large distributors of various medications and retail products to pharmacies. A contract outlining the cost, delivery dates, return policies, and payment schedule is made between the pharmacy and the distributor, usually requiring the pharmacy to order medications through their specific company. Even with the percentage

TABLE 13-3

Difference in Ordering from Manufacturers, Wholesalers, and Warehouse Repackaging Plants

Factors to Consider	Manufacturer	Wholesaler/Vendor Repackaging Plant	Warehouse
Supplier cost	No shipping fees	Lower per contract	Lowest cost
Supplier has electronic inventory control mechanism	No	Yes	Yes
Supplier can stock large supplies when ordering	Yes	No	Yes
Supplier provides special delivery service	Varies by manufacturer	Yes	Yes
Supplier handles special orders	Yes	Some special orders must be made through manufacturer	Some special orders must be made through manufacturer

fee that is added for this type of supplier, there can be a substantial savings to the pharmacy. Examples of prime vendors include Amerisource-Bergen, McKesson, Total Pharmacy Supply, and Cardinal Health. Advantages of the prime vendor agreement are lower costs and emergency delivery services.

- **Wholesalers** are companies that stock a variety of drug manufacturers' medications and normally have a "just-in-time" turnaround for ordered drugs. This means that drugs ordered today will arrive tomorrow. This type of ordering is very useful in pharmacies where space is limited for overstock items or the medication is needed by the next day. A percentage fee is added onto the shipments, but the additional fees can be offset by ordering in bulk, resulting in a substantial savings overall. Examples of wholesalers include HD Smith, Anda, and Cardinal Health.
- **Direct manufacturer ordering** may be used under certain circumstances. For example, a group of pharmacies may join a group purchasing organization (GPO) that contracts with the manufacturer for better pricing. The contract is usually based on the quantity ordered and includes specific return policies and conditions. Other reasons might arise for directly ordering from manufacturers; for example, the wholesaler and/or prime vendor may not stock the drug; the drug may not be available from the normal source at the time of ordering; or the medication may be available only to select patients who meet certain treatment parameters (e.g., FDA regulations or investigational protocols). In such cases, the manufacturer records and verifies the information before sending the medication for the specific patient. Examples of drug manufacturers include Abbott Laboratories, Bristol-Myers Squibb, Janssen Pharmaceuticals, and Upsher-Smith Laboratories.

Each of these types of suppliers has pros and cons. As seen in Table 13-3, the benefits of using wholesalers as opposed to dealing directly with the manufacturer differ mostly in the amount of stock that must be ordered and kept as overstock and the difference in cost. The fourth column of Table 13-3 describes factors to consider when ordering medications from a warehouse; in this situation, the pharmaceutical company orders high volumes of drugs from the manufacturer and may repackage the medications into more suitable sizes for the ordering physician. This serves several purposes, such as easier handling, increased productivity, and lower cost. However, large-quantity bottles are hard to handle. They are more likely to be dropped, spilling the contents. Medications may be prepackaged in smaller, easy-to-handle containers to eliminate the bulkiness of the larger bottles. If the pharmacy warehouse prepackages common dosages, the labeling process is faster. For example, sulfamethoxazole/trimethoprim (Septra, Bactrim) normally is taken twice daily for 10 days or twice daily for 15 days. These tablets are prepackaged in bottles of 20 and 30, eliminating the time it takes to count out the proper amount at the pharmacy counter. The technician must check the label against the prescription to determine the appropriate drug and quantity, then the prescription is ready to be inspected by the pharmacist and dispensed. Finally, because the volume of drugs is much higher than what a typical pharmacy can stock, pharmacies have contracts with these warehouses that save the pharmacy a substantial amount of money. This ultimately keeps the cost lower for the consumer.

Special Considerations

Special considerations apply to a host of drugs ordered by pharmacy, such as controlled substances, investigational drugs, cytotoxic drugs, and hazardous substances. Each of these types of medications requires special ordering, inventory, storage, handling, and return documentation. The DEA requires special forms to be completed for ordering, transferring, and returning schedule II controlled substances.

Investigational drugs typically have documentation that must be completed and returned to the manufacturer each time a medication is dispensed. These drugs are stored and inventoried separately. Cytotoxic drugs do not need special documentation, but they should be handled with great care and placed in a safety cabinet according to the manufacturer's guidelines. Certain cytotoxic agents must be refrigerated and should be clearly marked to separate them from other agents. Most pharmacies stock certain chemicals that are considered hazardous. You must know where the **Safety Data Sheets (SDS)** of your pharmacy are located in case of a spill. Agents such as phenol should be stored behind cabinet doors to protect individuals from accidentally knocking the bottle off a shelf and inhaling the toxic fumes or coming in contact with the agent.

Although many of the guidelines can be found in each pharmacy's policies and procedures manual, it is the responsibility of the pharmacy technician to be aware of these guidelines and of federal and state regulations. This requires continuous effort to ensure that the regulations that apply to your pharmacy are updated to reflect the current requirements. Patients rely on the knowledge of the pharmacy technician, which is why competencies in the area of billing and inventory are extremely important in the daily functions of pharmacy.

DO YOU REMEMBER THESE KEY POINTS?

- Why pharmacy formularies are important
- The major types of insurance and the differences between them
- The differences between government-managed insurance programs
- The parts of a health insurance card
- The necessary information patients must provide to the pharmacy for billing prescriptions to third parties
- The steps involved in billing insurance companies
- The types of problems that often arise when processing insurance claims
- The importance of the National Drug Code and how to decipher it

- The responsibilities of a pharmacy technician concerning stock levels and ordering stock for the pharmacy
- Common types of automated dispensing systems and pharmacy settings in which they are used
- The steps that should be followed when receiving stock
- Reasons for returning stock to the manufacturer or supplier
- Who issues recalls and how they are addressed
- How to return expired or recalled stock
- The importance of storing stock at the appropriate temperature

Scenario FOLLOW UP

Brian is now the new level 3 technician. He is proud of this accomplishment and plans to continue to look for ways to improve his working environment. He understands that this new position includes more responsibility, and he welcomes the challenge. With his positive attitude and willingness to step up as a leader, Brian has a bright and exciting future in the pharmacy technician field.

REVIEW QUESTIONS

Multiple Choice Questions

1. Which of the following is responsible for developing the formulary used by an institution?
   - **A.** State board of pharmacy
   - **B.** Pharmacy and therapeutics committee
   - **C.** Food and Drug Administration
   - **D.** All of the above.

2. Medicare is a government-managed insurance program that covers all of the following *except:*
   - **A.** Senior citizens
   - **B.** Patients using dialysis
   - **C.** Children
   - **D.** People who are disabled

3. Medicaid covers all of the following *except:*
   A. People who are disabled
   B. People with a low income
   C. Women who are pregnant
   D. Single working people with above-average income

4. Which health plan covers in-network provider visits only?
   A. A medical group that is covered under Medicare
   B. Preferred provider organization (PPO)
   C. Health maintenance organization (HMO)
   D. Point of service plan (POS)

5. Which regulatory body can issue a drug recall?
   A. FDA
   B. TJC
   C. DEA
   D. BOP

6. Insurance claims that are transmitted electronically to the insurance provider are called:
   A. E-mail claims
   B. NDC claims
   C. Adjudicated claims
   D. Co-pay claims

7. Various types of agents ordered for a pharmacy may include:
   A. Formulary drugs
   B. Hazardous substances
   C. Cytotoxic drugs
   D. All of the above

8. Which program makes prescription drugs available through private insurance plans?
   A. Medicare Part A
   B. Medicare Part B
   C. Medicare Part C
   D. Medicare Part D

9. An inventory system that automatically orders stock as it is used is called:
   A. Pyxis
   B. POS
   C. Omnicell
   D. Baker Cell

10. When a workers' compensation claim arrives at the pharmacy, the technician must:
    A. Obtain permission from a government agency at a later time
    B. Obtain information from the patient's human resources department
    C. Collect payment from the patient, who then will be reimbursed by the insurance company
    D. Wait until payment is made by the insurance company before releasing the medication

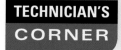
TECHNICIAN'S CORNER

Amber is working as a pharmacy technician in a busy retail pharmacy. A patient brings in a prescription for Pegasys, a drug used to treat hepatitis C. When Amber tries to process the medication using the customer's third-party billing information, she gets the rejection code for "prior authorization required." How should Amber handle this situation? What should she do first?

Bibliography

CBS News: U.S. prescription drug spending drops for first time in 58 years. May 9, 2013. (Referenced June 10, 2014). www.cbsnews.com/news/us-prescription-drug-spending-drops-for-first-time-in-58-years/

Kaiser Family Foundation: Medicare: a timeline of key developments. [blog post]. (Referenced July 17, 2014.) http://kaiserfamilyfoundation.files.wordpress.com/2005/06/5-02-13-medicare-timeline.pdf

Klein E: Obamacare really signed up 10 million people? January 6, 2014. *Wonk Blog, The Washington Post.* (Referenced May 20, 2014.) www.washingtonpost.com/blogs/wonkblog/wp/2014/01/06/has-obamacare-really-signed-up-10-million-people/

Medical plans offer more help to quit smoking: February 1, 2008. *Purdue Today.* (Referenced May 20, 2014.) www.purdue.edu/uns/insidepurdue/2008/080201_Cessation.html

Medicare: 8 Things to consider when choosing or changing your coverage. (Referenced June 10, 2014.) www.medicare.gov/sign-up-change-plans/decide-how-to-get-medicare/things-to-consider/8-things-to-consider.html

US Department of Justice. Drug Enforcement Administration. Office of Diversion Control: *Pharmacist's manual.* Section IX.

The Drug Enforcement Agency: Valid prescription requirements. (Referenced May 20, 2014.) www.deadiversion.usdoj.gov/pubs/manuals/pharm2/pharm_content.htm

Websites Referenced

(Referenced December 2013.) www.medicare.gov
(Referenced December 2013.) www.ConsumerReports.org
(Referenced December 2013.) www.Webmd.com
(Referenced December 2013.) www.drugtopics.com
(Referenced December 2013.) www.accesstobenefits.org
(Referenced December 2013.) www.nlm.nih.gov
(Referenced December 2013.) www.fda.gov
(Referenced December 2013.) www.texmed.org
(Referenced December 2013.) www.prescriptiondrugrecall.com/
(Referenced December 2013.) www.purdue.edu/uns/insidepurdue/2008/080201_Cessation.html

Centers for Medicare and Medicaid Services: Medicare Program General Information. (Referenced January 2014.) www.cms.gov/Medicare/Medicare-General-nformation/MedicareGenInfo/index.html

Department of Veteran Affairs: CHAMPVA. Pharmacy Benefits Fact Sheet. (Referenced January 2014.) www.va.gov/hac/factsheets/champva/factsheet01-24.pdf

Medicaid.Gov: Keeping America Healthy. Affordable Care Act Timeline. (Referenced January 2014.) www.medicaid.gov/AffordableCareAct/Timeline/Timeline.html

Medicaid.Gov: Keeping America Healthy. Medicaid Benefits. (Referenced January 2014.) www.medicaid.gov/Medicaid-CHIP-Program-Information/By-Topics/Benefits/Medicaid-Benefits.html

Medicare.Gov: State Pharmaceutical Assistance Programs. (Referenced April 2014.) www.medicare.gov/pharmaceutical-assistance-program/state-programs.aspx

Military.Com Benefits: TRICARE Eligibility. (Referenced January 2014.). www.military.com/benefits/tricare/tricare-eligibility.html?comp=7000022779075&rank=1

TRICARE: Tricare Welcome Information. (Referenced January 2014.) www.tricare.mil/Welcome.aspx

U.S. Department of Justice. Drug Enforcement Administration: Office of Diversion Control. National Take-Back Initiative. (Referenced January 2014.) www.deadiversion.usdoj.gov/drug_disposal/takeback/

U.S. Department of Veteran Affairs: CHAMPVA Frequently Asked Questions. (Referenced January 2014.) www.va.gov/hac/forbeneficiaries/champva/faqs.asp

U.S. Food and Drug Administration: About the Center for Drug Evaluation and Research. (Referenced April 2014.) www.fda.gov/AboutFDA/CentersOffices/OfficeofMedicalProductsandTobacco/CDER/default.htm

U.S. Food and Drug Administration: Enforcement Reports. (Referenced January 2014.) www.fda.gov/Safety/Recalls/EnforcementReports/default.htm

U.S. Food and Drug Administration: National Drug Code Directory. (Referenced January 2014.) www.fda.gov/Drugs/InformationOnDrugs/ucm142438.htm

Medication Safety and Error Prevention

Bobbi Steelman

OBJECTIVES

Upon completing this chapter, you should be able to do the following:

1. List the five patient rights and give an example of each.
2. Describe what constitutes an error.
3. Differentiate between the various types of medication errors.
4. Explain the various causes of medication errors.
5. Explain the necessity of reporting medication errors.
6. List the organizations or groups that track and report medication errors.
7. Identify safety strategies pharmacies, pharmacists, and pharmacy technicians can use to reduce medication errors.
8. List and describe four automated systems and explain how they prevent errors.
9. Explain how electronic prescribing is used to reduce errors.
10. Describe the role training and education plays in the reduction of medication errors.

TERMS AND DEFINITIONS

American Society of Health-System Pharmacists (ASHP) An association of pharmacists, pharmacy students, and technicians practicing in hospitals and health care systems, including home health care; ASHP has a long history of advocating for patient safety and establishing best practices to improve medication use

Automated dispensing system (ADS) Electronic system used to dispense medications

Institute for Healthcare Improvement (IHI) A nonprofit organization committed to the improvement of health care by promoting promising concepts through safety, efficiency, and other patient-centered goals

Institute of Medicine (IOM) Established under the National Academies and a part of the National Academy of Sciences, this nonprofit organization provides scientifically informed analysis and guidance regarding health and health policy; projects include studies of drug safety systems in the United States and recommendations for patient safety

Institute for Safe Medication Practices (ISMP) A nonprofit organization devoted entirely to promoting safe medication use and preventing medication errors; it gathers information on drug errors and suggests new, safer standards to avoid such errors

Medication error Any preventable event that may cause or lead to inappropriate medication use or patient harm

Medication error prevention Methods used by pharmacy, medicine, nursing, and other allied health professionals to prevent medication errors

MedMARx A national Internet-accessible database that hospitals and health care systems use to track adverse drug reactions and medication errors

MedWatch A program established by the U.S. Food and Drug Administration (FDA) for reporting drug and medical product safety alerts and label changes; the program also provides a voluntary adverse event reporting system for medications, medical products, and devices

National Coordinating Council for Medication Error Reporting and Prevention (NCCMERP) Founded by the United States Pharmacopeia, this is an independent council of more than 25 organizations gathered to address interdisciplinary causes of medication errors and strategies for prevention

Pharmacy Technician Certification Board (PTCB) An organization that offers national certification for pharmacy technicians in the United States

Pharmacy Technician Educators Council (PTEC) A U.S. organization that promotes teachers' strategies and instructions for pharmacy technician education

Risk evaluation and mitigation strategy (REMS) A strategy for managing a known or potential serious risk associated with a drug or biological product

Society for the Education of Pharmacy Technicians (SEPhT) A national pharmacy technician organization that promotes the education and training of pharmacy technicians; it provides links to medication safety and quality practices for technicians

United States Pharmacopeial Convention (USP) An independent organization that strives to ensure the quality, safety, and benefit of medicines and dietary supplements by setting standards and certification processes

Introduction

Scenario:

Jonathan is an experienced technician at a large municipal hospital pharmacy. He began his career after graduating from a 2-year technician training program. He is certified by the Pharmacy Technician Certification Board (PTCB) and works full-time as an inpatient technician. He has been asked by the pharmacy director to participate on a committee looking into medication errors. What types of issues do you think the committee will address? How can Jonathan prepare for this new assignment?

Drug errors are unacceptable in any situation involving medical treatment or medications, but the reality is that they will never disappear. It is a human trait that people make mistakes. At times, errors may not be realized before they cause harm. When discussing drug errors, it is important to note that not all errors are harmful and not all are caused by the pharmacy. In this chapter, the types and incidence of errors are discussed, and specific cases that unfortunately caused harm are presented. An attempt is made to identify the common causes of many drug errors and ultimately the ways in which they can be avoided. Other topics discussed in this chapter include the process of drug error reporting (i.e., when errors should be reported and who should be contacted) and the importance of helping patients learn to take responsibility for their own medical treatment, including their medications.

Pharmacy technicians are at the forefront in the effort to prevent drug errors; ironically, they also can cause errors relatively easily. Many technicians have relied on the pharmacist to catch their mistakes, but this is not the correct approach to preventing medication errors. Anyone can make a mistake, including pharmacists, physicians, and nurses.

It takes a team working together to prevent medication errors. The knowledge requirements for technicians are increasing, along with their additional responsibilities. Today's pharmacy techs must understand their scope of practice and strive to meet the highest standard.

Overview

In 2010 the Office of the Inspector General for Health and Human Services reported that bad hospital care contributed to the deaths of 180,000 Medicare patients. A study in the *Journal of Patient Safety,* published in September, 2013, estimated that from 210,000 to more than 400,000 patients per year suffer some type of preventable adverse event while in the hospital that contributes to their death; this was a much higher estimate than the estimate in a 1999 study completed by the **Institute of Medicine (IOM)**. The higher estimate was developed by John T. James, PhD, a toxicologist at NASA's space center in Houston. Mr. James became involved in patient safety issues after his 19-year-old son died as a result of insufficient hospital care. The **Institute for Safe Medication Practices (ISMP)** estimates that about 7000 deaths per year are linked to actual medication errors. High-alert medications are drugs with a heightened risk of causing significant patient harm when used in error. According to the ISMP, some medications considered "highest alert" in connection with errors are insulin, narcotics and opiates, methotrexate, warfarin, and potassium chloride injections (Box 14-1).

Five Rights of Medication Safety

There are five basic rights involving medication safety. Pharmacy personnel and other health care professionals are expected to adhere to these guidelines to avoid medication errors.

Effective patient care results from the concentrated efforts of the entire pharmacy team. Every patient is entitled to expect the highest standard of accuracy with regard to his or her medication. This accuracy standard is expressed as the following rights and examples.

1. The right patient
   - Always make certain the patient identification information is correct.

BOX 14-1

High-Alert Medications

Acute Care Settings
Epinephrine, subcutaneous
- epoprostenol (Flolan), IV
- insulin U-500 (special emphasis)*
- magnesium sulfate injection
- methotrexate, oral, nononcologic use
- opium tincture
- oxytocin, IV
- nitroprusside sodium for injection
- potassium chloride for injection concentrate
- potassium phosphates injection
- promethazine, IV
- vasopressin, IV or intraosseous

Community and Ambulatory Healthcare Settings
- carbamazepine
- chloral hydrate liquid, for sedation of children
- heparin, including unfractionated and low molecular weight heparin
- metformin
- methotrexate, non-oncologic use
- midazolam liquid, for sedation of children
- propylthiouracil
- warfarin

*All forms of insulin, subcutaneous and IV, are considered a class of high-alert medications. Insulin U500 has been singled out for special emphasis to bring attention to the need for distinct strategies to prevent the types of errors that occur with this concentrated form of insulin.
From the Institute for Safe Medication Practices. ISMP List of High-Alert Medications in Acute Care Settings and ISMP List of High-Alert Medications in Community/Ambulatory Healthcare. https://www.ismp.org/tools/highalertmedicationLists.asp Accessed September 30, 2014.

2. The right medication
   - Verify that the medication is exactly what the physician ordered.
   - Is it brand name or generic?
3. The right dose
   - Verify how many doses or tablets are to be taken per day.
   - How long is the patient to continue on the medication?
4. The right route
   - Should it be swallowed or chewed?
   - Can it be crushed or broken in half?
   - Is it for injection or to be taken orally?
5. The right time
   - What time of day should the medication be taken?
   - Is it taken after or before meals?
   - Is it given at bedtime?

Each pharmacy should incorporate checking these rights into the procedural guidelines of their organization as one of the safety goals of the medication process.

What Constitutes an Error?

An error is any type of preventable event that may cause or lead to inappropriate medication use or patient harm. Patients themselves cause many drug errors when taking their own medications at home. They may take their medications at the wrong time, in the wrong amount, in the wrong combination, or with an improper administration technique. It is difficult to know how many drug errors occur at home because they typically are not reported to anyone and may continue to occur unless recognized by the physician or pharmacist or, even worse, manifested by an adverse drug event or reaction (ADE or ADR). These types of situations are part of the drug error dilemma and are taken very seriously by all involved in patient care. An error can involve prescription or over-the-counter (OTC) medications and can be committed by both experienced and inexperienced staff. The **American Society of Health-System Pharmacists (ASHP)** and the **National Coordinating Council for Medication Error Reporting and Prevention (NCCMERP)**, frequently referred to simply as MERP, outline the most common types of errors that may occur (Tables 14-1 and 14-2).

Types of Medication Errors

Medication errors can be broken down into three main categories: prescribing errors, dispensing errors, and administration errors.

Examples of prescribing errors may include:
- Incorrect strength of a medication
- Quantity and refill information omitted
- Route of administration not specified
- Illegible handwriting

Examples of dispensing errors may include:
- Incorrect prescription interpretation
- Incorrect calculations
- Incorrect drug utilization evaluation

Sound-alike or look-alike drug errors may include:
- Incorrect prescription interpretation
- Incorrect calculations
- Incorrect drug utilization evaluation

Examples of administration errors may include:
- Ear medications being placed in the eye
- Oral medications given intravenously
- Intravenous syringes used to measure oral medications
- Failure to document medication administration records accurately

Physicians' handwriting has long been known for its illegibility, which means that reading drug names, strengths, and dosages can be very problematic.

TABLE 14-1

Types of Medication Errors (ASHP)

Error	Description
Prescribing error	Prescriber orders a medication that is incorrect (e.g., incorrect usage, dosage form, route, concentration, rate of infusion) or is selected incorrectly based on indications or contraindications (allergies, existing condition); medication reaches patient
Omission error	Failure to administer an ordered dose to a patient before next dose is due, without an apparent reason for omission or appropriate documentation (e.g., nurse forgets to give a dose to patient)
Wrong time error	Medication administered outside scheduled time frame; if facility allows plus or minus 30 minutes, dose is given outside of this variance (each facility sets an acceptable time frame for variances)
Unauthorized drug error	Medication administered to a patient from an unauthorized prescriber; physician not licensed in that state or not an authorized prescriber
Improper dose error	Patient administered a dose that is greater or less than prescribed amount (e.g., aspirin 325 mg is given instead of 500 mg)
Wrong dosage form	Medication administered in a dosage form other than what was ordered (e.g., capsule for tablet, ointment for cream)
Wrong drug preparation	Drug is incorrectly formulated (e.g., wrong calculations or wrong solution used for reconstitution) or manipulated (e.g., break in aseptic technique), and medication is administered to patient
Wrong administration	Drug is given using wrong procedure or technique (e.g., giving an intramuscular [IM] dose as an intravenous [IV] dose or placing an ophthalmic solution in wrong eye)
Deteriorated drug error	Medication is administered that has expired or the integrity of ingredients has been compromised (e.g., storing a drug at room temperature when it should be refrigerated)
Monitoring error	Failure to review a prescribed medication for proper regimen, appropriateness (e.g., not monitoring patient's response to prescribed medication), detection of problems in dosage (e.g., not recognizing side effects from drugs), or failure in using laboratory results to correctly adjust dose
Compliance error	Patient does not adhere to prescribed medication regimen (e.g., taking a q8h dose every 6 hr or stopping a medication before scheduled)

Medication Misadventures—Guidelines. ASHP Guidelines for Preventing Medication Errors in Hospitals. Types of Medication Errors. (Referenced July 2, 2014.) http://www.ashp.org/s_ashp/docs/files/medmis_gdl_hosp.pdf

TABLE 14-2

Medication Error Reporting and Prevention Categories

Category	Definition	Type of Resulting Error
A	Circumstances that have potential for causing errors	No error
B	Error occurred but did not reach patient	Error, No harm
C	Error reached patient but did not cause harm	Error, No harm
D	Error reached patient, did not cause harm, but needed monitoring or intervention to prove no harm resulted	Error, No harm
E	Error occurred that may have contributed to or resulted in temporary harm to patient and patient required intervention	Error, Harm
F	Error occurred that may have contributed to or resulted in temporary harm to patient and resulted in monitoring or hospitalization	Error, Harm
G	Error occurred that may have contributed to or resulted in temporary or permanent harm to patient	Error, Harm
H	Error occurred that may have contributed to or resulted in harm to patient and required hospitalization to sustain life	Error, Harm
I	Error occurred that may have contributed to or resulted in patient's death	Error, Death

Institute for Safe Medication Practices. Medication Error Index for Categorizing Errors. (Referenced June 10, 2014.) https://www.ismp.org/Newsletters/acutecare/articles/19960911.asp

An alternative to a handwritten prescription is a new technology called *e-prescribing*. Prescriptions can be sent by computer or mobile device directly to the pharmacy, where they can be easily and quickly interpreted. Several software programs facilitate e-prescribing. Although e-prescribing has been implemented in various medical institutions and physicians' offices, many physicians still write their orders by hand on prescription pads or order sheets. It is the responsibility of the pharmacy and nurses to interpret these prescriptions correctly.

Case scenario examples show the possible progression of an ultimate drug error.

Scenario 1: Misinterpretation of Physician's Orders

A prescription arrives in the pharmacy for digoxin 0.125 mg; because of the illegibility of the physician's handwriting, it is transcribed inaccurately as 0.25 mg. The wrong medication strength is sent to the floor, where the nurse gives the patient the wrong dose.

Scenario 2: Missed Dose

A medication order arrives in the pharmacy and is processed correctly and sent to the patient. The nurse pulls the correct drug and dose but forgets to give it to the patient; therefore, the patient misses a dose. Whether the nurse forgets to give the dose or the patient (at home) forgets to take the medication, this constitutes a medication error.

Scenario 3: Wrong Patient

A medication order arrives in the pharmacy and is processed and sent to the floor correctly, but the nurse gives the drug to the wrong patient.

Scenario 4: Adverse Effect

A patient takes an OTC drug along with a prescription drug, which results in an adverse or toxic effect because of a drug-drug interaction.

Scenario 5: Noncompliance

A patient obtains his or her prescription at the local pharmacy and begins to take the medication; the prescription instructs the patient to take daily for 30 days. After 1 week the patient feels much better and stops taking the medication.

Responsibility for Errors

Unfortunately, the first response to an error is normally to blame rather than to explain the reasons behind such an occurrence. All health care workers are at risk of being found guilty of errors that are considered negligence according to federal and state laws. The case of a medical error reported in Colorado (Case Study 1) identifies the complexity of a drug error. Two cases that were highly publicized across the country (Case Studies 2 and 3) clearly illustrate the need for well-educated and trained technicians.

Case Study 1

Police charged three nurses with negligent homicide after an infant's death from a fatal overdose of potassium chloride. A subsequent analysis uncovered a chain of numerous errors from the time of prescription to the time of injection. The police did not charge the physician who wrote the cryptic prescription or the pharmacist who misread the dosage.

Case Study 2

The Ohio State Board of Pharmacy revoked the license of a staff pharmacist at Rainbow Baby's and Children's Hospital in Cleveland after Emily, a 2-year-old patient, died as a result of a sodium overdose in a chemotherapy solution. The board concluded that the pharmacist did not follow proper hospital procedures for the supervision of a pharmacy technician who prepared the solution. No disciplinary action was taken against the technician because Ohio does not license or register pharmacy technicians. The technician resigned in the aftermath of the incident. William Winsley, RPh, MS, executive director of the board, stated that both the pharmacist and the technician were experienced and had prepared intravenous and chemotherapy solutions many times. However, he said, "The pharmacist failed to adequately check the technician's work." The supervising pharmacist who failed to notice the technician's mistake lost his state license and pleaded no contest to involuntary manslaughter; he was sentenced to 6 months in jail and 6 months of house arrest. In 2009 Emily's Law was signed by the governor of Ohio. This act requires all pharmacy technicians in the state to be of legal age, to have a high school diploma or equivalent, to pass a state and federal background check, and to pass a certifying competency examination approved by the board of pharmacy before being awarded technician status. The National Pharmacy Technician Association (NPTA) supports the legislation as a model for national and state standards. U.S. Representative Steve LaTourette proposed Emily's Act for congressional approval on March 1, 2009, but it was rejected.

Case Study 3

In March, 2010, ABC News reported that a Florida appeals court had ordered Walgreens to pay a $25.8

BOX 14-2

ASHP Common Causes of Medication Errors

1. Ambiguous strength designation on labels or in packaging
2. Drug product nomenclature (look-alike or sound-alike names, use of lettered or numbered prefixes and suffixes in drug names)
3. Equipment failure or malfunction
4. Illegible handwriting
5. Improper transcription
6. Inaccurate dosage calculation
7. Inadequately trained personnel
8. Inappropriate abbreviations used in prescribing
9. Labeling errors
10. Excessive workload
11. Lapses in individual performance
12. Medication unavailable

Medication Misadventures—Guidelines. ASHP Guidelines for Preventing Medication Errors in Hospitals. (Referenced July 2, 2014.) http://www.ashp.org/s_ashp/docs/files/medmis_gdl_hosp.pdf

million judgment for an error made by Janelle Banks.* Ms. Banks was a teenage pharmacy technician who had no formal training and had previously worked at a movie theater popping popcorn. In court, she testified that she typed in "ten milligrams" on the prescription when it should have been "one milligram." As a result of this error, Beth Hippely received a dosage of her blood thinner medication that was 10 times too much. She suffered a massive stroke.

Where Errors Are Made

Medication errors can occur in many different settings, including hospitals, clinics, pharmacies, physicians' offices, and even patients' homes. These errors may be intentional or unintentional and often go undetected. Box 14-2 presents a list of common causes of medication errors compiled by the ASHP.

Although errors are made in many different settings, they most often are reported in community and institutional pharmacies, such as hospitals. MERP tracks errors and their causes and has created a list of five recommendations for avoiding errors specifically in nonhospital settings.

*Florida no longer allows on-the-job training. Effective January 1, 2011, any individual who wanted to work as a pharmacy technician in the state of Florida had to register with the Florida Board of Pharmacy. To register with the Florida Board of Pharmacy, an applicant had to submit a Pharmacy Technician Registration Application and proof of completion of a board-approved pharmacy technician training program.

Why Errors Occur

It is human nature to make errors; humans are not perfect. A person can look at the name and strength of a drug yet fail to register the correct information, substituting unintended information in its place. Errors can result from focusing on more than one task at a time. People tend to filter out information even under normal circumstances. Think about the examples below of errors in everyday life and note whether any have ever happened to you:

- You pick up the phone to call a specific person, and you call someone else instead.
- You leave to drive to school, and you start to drive to work.
- You read the words on a page of a textbook, and although you read each word correctly, you do not remember what you have just read.
- You reach for the correct spice on the kitchen shelf, and you grab the wrong one because it was similar in size, shape, color, or labeling.

Even the most highly skilled person occasionally makes errors. You know what you want to do, but your mind changes its focus, and you follow the wrong information. This type of "automatic behavior" plays a role in the occurrence of errors. In addition, when repetitive actions are carried out daily, it is easy to become complacent and lose focus on the task at hand.

Both treating patients and supplying medications accurately are critical responsibilities, and it is expected that errors will be avoided. All health care workers strive to avoid errors on a daily basis. However, various situations and circumstances often hinder this effort. The following are some examples of the daily obstructions encountered by pharmacy personnel:

- Stress, because of the fast-paced environment and the increase in the number of prescriptions processed daily
- Stress related to difficulties encountered during the insurance online adjudication process
- Noise in the workplace that distracts focus from the medication ordered
- Multitasking; doing two or more things at once (e.g., answering the phone and checking medications at the same time) can distract attention from the order
- Medication names that sound alike
- Medications that look similar (e.g., colors, shapes, sizes, or a similar area where they are stored)
- Labels that look similar because of the same color and/or lettering
- Labels that are difficult to read because of small print
- Prescriptions with illegible handwriting
- Excessive workload

Stress

Many studies have shown that over the past few decades, Americans' stress levels have been on the rise. Job stress has been identified as a major source of stress for adults. Excessive pressure and demands placed on individuals at work can cause them to feel overwhelmed and unable to perform at their best. This is when errors can occur.

In pharmacies, shortages in personnel and an increasing demand for services contribute to workplace stress. Eventually, this stress can translate into higher occurrences of errors and lower job satisfaction. Some stressors include dealing with angry patients or customers, rude health care personnel, high prescription volumes, employees calling in sick, inadequate supplies or stock, and insurance processing complications. Stress affects everyone, including the pharmacist, pharmacy technician, and other pharmacy personnel. Stress reduction goals should be addressed on a regular basis. Open and honest communication should be used when discussing workplace stressors. Placing blame should be avoided.

Noise

A typical pharmacy environment is full of many types of noise. Sounds such as telephones, machines, intercoms, cell phones, and voices are considered normal. However, an overly noisy workplace can cause distractions, affecting concentration on the task at hand, which could result in medication errors.

Talking or laughing among employees during the prescription filling process can be disruptive and may seem uncaring or unprofessional to the customers or patients. The noise or vibration of a text message can be equally distracting. Most organizations have restrictions on cell phone use and texting at work. We are all very aware of how dangerous texting and driving can be. However, sending and receiving text messages at work can be just as dangerous. Anything that takes the focus away from accurately filling a patient's prescription should be avoided. Every pharmacy employee should be aware of the company policy regarding cell phone use. Patient and staff safety is always the goal. Standards governing the appropriate sound environment should be reviewed with new employees and updated regularly.

Case Study

Hanna worked at a pharmaceutical plant as a packaging technician. She was responsible for making sure the pills were distributed into the correct bottles using the appropriate machines. During her lunch she was texting her boyfriend about their upcoming trip. After lunch she brought her cell phone back into the production area in case her boyfriend needed to text her about the trip. She knew this was against policy, but everyone broke the rule occasionally.

About an hour into her shift, her phone vibrated. When she went to answer it, she dropped it on the conveyor belt. She knew it would jam up the machine and halt the production line, so she reached to stop it. Her hand got caught, and she lost two fingers.

Case Study Follow-Up

How could Hanna have avoided this accident? Is there ever an excuse to break the safety rules?

Texting distracts from the job at hand. It is the responsibility of each pharmacy professional to respect the safety guidelines and adhere to company policy.

Multitasking

An article published in 2012 by *Harvard Health* states that multitasking can increase the chance of making mistakes and hinder problem solving and creativity. With more and more health care professionals using electronic devices at work, the temptation to multitask is great. Often errors occur when one task is interrupted by some other device. Everyone needs to be aware of the distractions that come with the use of new technologies. Focusing on one task at a time, giving your full attention before moving on, helps ensure patient safety.

Case Study

An older man suffering from dementia was admitted to the hospital. One of his physicians decided to increase the dose of warfarin he was taking. The next day, the physician decided to reevaluate the warfarin regimen to see whether it was even necessary. He gave the order to temporarily stop the blood thinner to a resident to submit. As the resident was completing the new order via the computerized order entry system, she was interrupted by a text message from a friend and failed to complete the temporary stop on the warfarin. As a result, the man's blood became so thin, he needed open heart surgery to save his life.

Case Study Follow-Up

Remember to always finish one task before going on to the next task. Text messages can wait. Numerous distractions may arise during any particular work shift. It is the technician's responsibility to be 100% focused on patient safety and accuracy.

Look-Alike, Sound-Alike (LASA) Drugs

Each year, in an effort to reduce confusion between drug names that look alike or sound alike, the U.S. Food and Drug Administration (FDA) reviews approximately 300 drug names before they are

Scenario CHECK UP 14-1

Jonathan is training a newly hired technician today. He is very excited to share his knowledge with his co-worker. Their first task is to scan and put up the medications that arrived from the wholesaler. Jonathan takes time to explain the hospital policy on look-alike, sound-alike drugs. He shows her the posted list of commonly confused drug names and describes how the tall man lettering works. Why does a new employee need this information if the pharmacist has the last check to verify accuracy?

allowed to enter the market. Approximately one third of the names that companies propose are rejected. To test these drug names, the FDA enlists the help of about 120 FDA health professionals. This group simulates real-life drug order situations. In addition, the FDA has created a computer program to detect similar names.

Risk Evaluation and Mitigation Strategies (REMS)

The decision to approve a new drug always includes the question, "Do the benefits outweigh the risks for the patient?" Manufacturers and the FDA are continually evaluating these risks and benefits throughout the entire life cycle of a drug. Traditionally, these risks have been communicated via the manufacturer's package insert. However, in some cases the FDA and/or the manufacturer determine that the risks are significant enough to require additional product labeling to ensure patient safety. In these cases, a **risk evaluation and mitigation strategy (REMS)** is recommended to ensure that benefits outweigh the risks.

The implementation of REMS in the pharmacy workplace is unique to each practice setting. Pharmacists provide education to patients on the benefits and risks of REM medications. Pharmacy technicians are involved with keeping a list of REM medications requiring MedGuides for dispensing and any medications that require REM components, in addition to a MedGuide. Medication Guides are paper handouts that address issues specific to particular drugs and drug classes. They contain FDA-approved information designed to help patients avoid serious adverse events. The list can be found at: *www.fda.gov.*

Pharmacy technicians can identify medications requiring MedGuides by looking for the indication in bold lettering on the stock bottle or box or by looking for a red or yellow symbol. Some pharmacies have a special symbol that prints out with the label for REMS medications. MedGuides can be printed directly from the FDA website.

Look-Alike Drug Names and Tall Man Lettering

The ISMP and the Joint Commission (TJC) promote the use of tall man lettering as one means of reducing confusion between similar drug names. Tall man lettering uses mixed case letters to draw attention to the dissimilarities in look-alike drug names, as in the following examples:

buPROPion—busPIRone
clomiPHENE—clomiPRAMINE
cycloSPORINE—cycloSERINE
DAUNOrubicin—DOXOrubicin
glipiZIDE—glyBURIDE
hydrALAZINE—hydrOXYzine
medroxyPROGESTERone—methylPREDNISolone—
    methylTESTOSTERone
niCARdipine—NIFEdipine
predniSONE—prednisoLONE
sulfADIAZINE—sulfiSOXAZOLE

A complete list of look-alike drug names is available on the ISMP website.

Case Study

An elderly male patient was operated on for a coronary arterial bypass and was recovering from anesthesia in the cardiac intensive care unit (ICU). He showed mild metabolic acidosis (condition in which there is too much acid in the body fluids) due to hypothermia. Sodium bicarbonate was to be given intravenously slowly. A few seconds after injection, the patient's heart stopped. Cardiac resuscitation was initiated, and the patient was revived successfully with an intravenous bolus injection of adrenaline, calcium, and sodium bicarbonate.

Upon analysis of the event, five broken ampules of potassium chloride were found lying on the patient's medication table. The staff attending the patient had given 50 mL (100 mEq) of potassium chloride (KCl) instead of 50 mL (50 mEq) of sodium bicarbonate. It was determined that the error occurred because of the similar color of the labels of sodium bicarbonate and KCl. The ampules for both drugs were from the same pharmaceutical company; they were both packaged in 10-mL ampules with a red label, and the two medications were kept on the same shelf, side by side. Use of different-sized ampules kept in different places could have prevented this type of look-alike medication error.

Drug Labeling

Drug companies are urged to make changes in the labeling of any type of medication that can be confusing or misinterpreted. The use of color coding, tall man lettering, and boldface lettering can help make drug selection errors less likely. For example, using tall man lettering helps differentiate the drug hydrOXYzine from the drug hydrALAzine. Changes to drug stocking include placing "Name Alert" stickers on the bins containing problematic sound-alike or look-alike drugs or placing the bins in different areas of the pharmacy to reduce the possibility of pulling the wrong drug. Drug companies have been encouraged to name their new drugs differently from other medications to help reduce confusion.

Case Study

A woman undergoing a radiology procedure was mistakenly given an injection of chlorhexidine, a skin cleansing agent. She was supposed to have received an injection of contrast dye. The two solutions were in similar, unlabeled containers. The mistake was irreversible, and the patient died.

Case Study Follow-Up

The pharmacy could have implemented procedures to clearly label all containers and train the personnel to never use an unlabeled bottle.

Excessive Workload

Many pharmacists and pharmacy technicians believe that their excessive workloads are a threat to the public's safety. The demands of processing hundreds of prescriptions in a 10- to 12-hour shift are increasing the risks of error. Many pharmacy employees complain of few or no breaks, no time to eat lunch or dinner, and very little time to go to the bathroom when needed. Several state boards of pharmacy (BOP), such as the Iowa BOP and the Oregon BOP, are beginning to address this issue and develop strategies to combat these problems. In March, 2013, the Iowa BOP received the following recommendations from its patient safety task force:

- Require the pharmacy to provide sufficient personnel to prevent fatigue, distractions, or conditions that interfere with a pharmacist's ability to practice safely
- Require the pharmacy to provide opportunities for rest periods and meal breaks
- Require the pharmacy to provide adequate time for a pharmacist to complete professional duties and responsibilities
- Prohibit introduction of external factors (e.g., productivity quotas or programs such as time limits) that interfere with the pharmacist's ability to provide appropriate professional services

More information on this issue is available at the website *www.nodakpharmacy.com.*

Case Study

A part-time pharmacy technician at Walgreens in Florida mistakenly filled a prescription for methadone with the instruction to take "as needed." The instruction was supposed to read "Take four 10 mg tablets twice daily." The patient took 22 pills over the course of a day and a half, nearly twice as many as prescribed. His wife found him dead, his body curled on the shower floor. The pharmacy filled 380 prescriptions that day. No one had offered the patient any counseling.

Case Study Follow-Up

It is important to offer counseling to each patient so that he or she has the opportunity to discuss the medication regimen with the pharmacist. Patient safety is of the utmost importance, and we should never be too busy to ask patients whether they have any questions. If the technician would have made sure the patient understood the instruction by discussing it with the pharmacist, this tragedy might have been prevented.

Drug Interactions as a Source of Error

Drug interactions are another source of errors in the pharmacy. The probability of drug-drug interactions is increased in seniors and severely ill patients because of the multiple medications they often receive. Seniors may have multiple conditions that are treated concurrently. In addition to the changes in metabolism that occur with aging, taking similar drugs that have the same side effects may increase the risk and/or severity of adverse effects. Table 14-3

TABLE 14-3

Examples of Drug-Drug Interactions

Drug	Drug	Result of Drug Interaction
Angiotensin-converting enzyme (ACE) inhibitors	Spironolactone	Increased serum potassium levels
Ciprofloxacin	Multivitamin with minerals	Decreased effect of ciprofloxacin because minerals in multivitamins can decrease antibiotic absorption if taken at the same time
Digoxin	Verapamil and amiodarone	Digoxin toxicity
Theophylline	Quinolones	Theophylline toxicity

lists examples of drugs that should not be given concurrently.

Warfarin (Coumadin) Interactions

Coumadin anticoagulants, such as warfarin, have the potential for many interactions with drugs, food, and dietary or herbal supplements. Certain warfarin interactions can be deadly. Warfarin is given to prevent clots that can cause strokes or heart attacks; the prothrombin time (PT) and the international normalized ratio (INR) must be maintained at a specific level to ensure that blood clots do not form and that the patient does not bleed internally. Regular blood tests are performed to check the PT/INR level of patients taking warfarin. Examples of common warfarin interactions are shown in Table 14-4. Although warfarin has several drug-drug and drug-food interactions, many other drugs also have the potential to cause severe interactions.

Errors in the Pharmacy

No one wants to make an error, but when it does happen, negative feelings and assumptions may emerge. For example, it may seem that the person who made the mistake is careless, lazy, or untrained. Suspension or termination is a frightening event to consider; the reality that a patient suffered as a result of an error is horrible. Additional fears are the

legal ramifications of lawsuits and possible public humiliation. All of these fears are in the back of the technician's mind, along with the constant need to maintain the workflow.

In fact, a pharmacy can fill 1000 prescriptions correctly, but if one error occurs, the pharmacy management will likely counsel the technician and pharmacist to "be more careful," thus placing the blame on these employees specifically. This fear of being reprimanded adds to the stress on the pharmacy staff. Many times no action is taken to review the overall process of how the mistake occurred.

Many pharmacy organizations and entities, such as MedWatch, TJC, ISMP, MERP, and others, have recognized the need to study errors in a much different light. First, the need for open error reporting without fear of retaliation is essential if the root causes of errors are to be revealed. Pharmacy staff members need to know that they will not be punished; instead, the error will be examined, and new strategies may be established that make it more difficult for errors to occur. It is important to have tools that can be used for error prevention. Even then, human factor errors will occur, but the goal is to reduce them as much as possible through the knowledge of how they occur. MedWatch and other error-reporting agencies encourage reporting of all types of errors by both health care workers and the public. A MedWatch report can be accessed via the Internet, which makes it a simple way to report an error.

TABLE 14-4

Examples of Warfarin Interactions with Drugs, Supplements, and Foods

Drugs		
Warfarin	Aspirin	Possible increased risk of bleeding
Warfarin	Phenytoin	Increased phenytoin or warfarin levels
Warfarin	Quinolones	Increased chance of bleeding
Warfarin	Sulfa drugs	Increased chance of bleeding
Warfarin	Cimetidine	Increased chance of bleeding
Warfarin	Heparin	Increased chance of bleeding
Warfarin	Amiodarone	Increased chance of bleeding
Warfarin	Nonsteroidal antiinflammatory drugs (NSAIDs)	Increased chance of bleeding
Supplements		
Warfarin	Gingko biloba	Increased chance of bleeding
Warfarin	Vitamin K	Decreased activity of warfarin
Warfarin	Garlic	Increased chance of bleeding
Warfarin	Ginseng	Decreased activity of warfarin
Warfarin	St. John's wort	Decreased activity of warfarin
Foods		
Warfarin	Broccoli and other green vegetables or foods high in vitamin K	Decreased effect of warfarin
Warfarin	Soybean and canola oils	Altered effect of warfarin
Warfarin	Cranberry juice	Altered effect of warfarin

(Figure 2-3 presents an example of a MedWatch form.)

Although drug errors do not necessarily cause dire consequences for all patients, in many instances they do. In these cases the only adequate outcome is to identify the causes of the error and establish safeguards that prevent the error from recurring. For grieving family and friends, this is of little help, and for the person or persons responsible, this is a life-changing event that can result in loss of license, penalty fines, and, in certain instances, incarceration. Examples of various errors are listed in the following sections.

Errors Related to Patient Care

Health Care–Associated Infections

Health care–associated infections (HAIs) have plagued hospitals for decades. It is estimated that at any given time, 1 in 20 inpatients has an infection related to hospital care. Most HAIs involve urinary tract infections, surgical site infections, bloodstream infections, and pneumonia. All hospitals and other institutions have infection control specialists who are responsible for training both staff members and patients as part of the investigation of all cases of HAI. However, the training from institution to institution varies widely. Using Universal Precautions (e.g., hand washing) is a necessity in all institutions.

Home Health Care Errors

Many patients are discharged home with instructions for self-administration of medications or with the help of visiting nurses. This is due to rising costs associated with hospital stays. According to the 2011 IMS National Health Perspectives, home health represented a $2.8 billion retail channel for pharmaceuticals. In 2010, the Medicare Payment Advisory Commission (MedPAC) reported payments for home health totaled $19.4 billion. The home infusion industry has grown over the past few years and accounts for somewhere between $9 billion and $11 billion annually.

Receiving care in the home carries the risk of improper dosing and contamination of intravenous (IV) sets that may ultimately cause infections. Many elderly and disabled patients do not have coverage for infusion sets and supplies because Medicare covers only the cost of medication. Self-dosing errors can increase the risk of an adverse effect. Patients may try to use medical supplies intended for single use more than once to try to save money; poor aseptic technique may increase the risk of infection.

Age-Related Errors

Medication Errors and the Elderly

More people are living into their 80s and beyond. Life expectancy in the United States has risen from 49 years (1900) to 79 years in the past century. By 2050 approximately one third of the United States population will be over age 55, and 20% will be over age 65. Individuals over age 80 will be the fastest growing segment of the population for the next 40 years. This is due to several reasons, including increased activity, better diets, and improved health care. Medication plays an important role in the longevity of people suffering from various conditions, such as osteoporosis, cardiovascular disease, and diabetes. It is estimated that nearly half of all Americans age 55 or older take some type of prescription drugs, and about 40% take OTC medications. Many seniors mix medications on a daily basis, and as the number of medications increases, so does the possibility of drug-drug interactions. People tend to believe that any medication purchased over the counter is safe. This is a misconception, especially when these agents are mixed with prescription medications. Consideration also must be given to drug-food interactions.

Medical Errors and Pediatric Patients

Most emergency department (ED) cases relating to pediatric patients and medication (more than 66%) are due to overdosing of prescription and OTC medications. Most overdoses are primarily a result of failure to store medications in a secure area out of reach of children. In the United States alone, more than 71,000 children under age 19 are taken to the ED for unintentional overdoses of drugs kept at home. Toddlers (2-year-olds) were most likely to experience poisoning.

Pictograms and the use of plain language have been shown to reduce the possibility of parents dosing their children inappropriately. Pictograms are standardized graphics (pictures) that depict such things as how to take medication, how to store medication, and when to take medication (Figure 14-1). Many parents in the United States have problems reading and understanding dosage instructions because of low reading levels or lack of understanding of the English language. This is more prevalent in multicultural areas where English is a second language. In a study conducted in an urban public hospital ED, a control group (standard labeling information) and an intervention group (using pictograms and plain language) were studied. Both were given standard instructions by the medical staff. Results showed that parent nonadherence was lower in the intervention group (9.3%) than in the control group (38%).

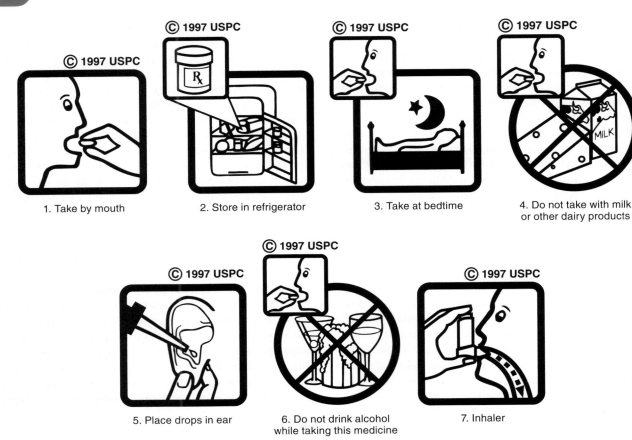

© 1997 USPC

1. Take by mouth

© 1997 USPC

2. Store in refrigerator

© 1997 USPC

3. Take at bedtime

© 1997 USPC

4. Do not take with milk or other dairy products

© 1997 USPC

5. Place drops in ear

© 1997 USPC

6. Do not drink alcohol while taking this medicine

© 1997 USPC

7. Inhaler

FIGURE 14-1 Medication pictograms. (Courtesy U.S. Pharmacopeial Convention.)

FDA committees have also suggested the use of new labeling on certain OTC medications to ensure that parents receive proper advice before administering medications to young children. New labels read, "Do not dose children under the age of 4 years." In addition, the new labels state that a physician should be consulted for children ages 4 to 6 years. This has changed from the previous guidelines of not dosing children under 2 years of age. Hopefully, these changes in labeling (voluntarily made by manufacturers) will reduce the number of parents who administer incorrect doses or dose their children at the wrong time. In some cases parents do not use the medication for its intended purpose.

Children and infants are also at risk of drug errors in the hospital; incorrect dosing is the most commonly reported error. Dosing errors include computation errors in dosage and dosing intervals. Children vary in weight, body surface area, and organ system maturity; all of these factors affect their ability both to metabolize and to excrete medication. In addition, not many standardized dosing regimens are available for children, which increases the probability of drug errors. Various causes have been identified for errors in the hospital; for example, the procedure or protocol was not followed, miscommunication, inaccurate or omitted transcription, improper

documentation, incorrect calculations, drug distribution system error, computer entry error, and lack of system safeguards.

Scenario CHECK UP 14-2

Jonathan is continuing to train Jennifer, the new employee. He explains to her the process for reporting medication errors in the pharmacy. Jennifer has recently read about several cases in which the technician was involved in a fatal medication error. What are some of the reasons technicians fail to report their mistakes? What are the possible consequences if errors go unreported?

Medication Errors That Involve Allergies

Although many people are aware of the medications to which they are allergic, many allergic reactions cannot be avoided before drug administration.

Allergic reactions are not always medication errors; however, many people can have an allergic reaction as a result of the physician failing to document or review the patient's allergies before prescribing medications. In one study of more than 50 patients hospitalized because of allergic reactions to medications, contributing factors to the allergic events were reported and included the following:

- Physician was not aware of allergy (41%).
- Physician did not believe allergy was real (5%).
- Physician was aware of allergy but felt the benefit outweighed the risk (4%).
- Physician was not aware that the agent was in the same class of drugs (3%).

The primary reasons for allergy-related prescribing errors included workload and failure to review the patient's drug history and profile. However, on most occasions the physician was alerted about the allergies by a nurse or a pharmacist; most errors were prevented by pharmacists.

Parenteral Errors

The most frightening errors are those that take effect quickly and may not be easily reversed. This is the case with parenteral medications. Several cases of heparin and insulin overdoses have occurred. Heparin is of great concern because it is common to flush IV lines with Hep-Lock solutions, which may be confused with similarly sized and labeled vials of much more concentrated heparin solutions. In the hospital, many floors keep several different concentrations of heparin, and the labels can be confusing because they are similar in appearance. Potassium chloride (KCl) solutions are also problematic. In several cases patients have died from the administration of concentrated KCl injections by personnel who misunderstood the labeling; concentrated KCl should *never* be given undiluted. As a result of these errors, concentrated KCl has been pulled from nursing floors and is strictly regulated by the pharmacy, yet errors can still occur.

Other considerations are important when administering parenterals. Pharmacy technicians need to be aware of the range of normal dosages, and if an ordered dose is suspect, they must alert the pharmacist immediately. For example, if a patient with diabetes has orders for several IVs, which are normally prepared in dextrose, this order should be suspect because of the patient's diabetic condition. The physician may not want the medication prepared in dextrose but instead may wish to use normal saline.

Sustained-Released Dosage Form Errors

The clear advantage of sustained-released (SR) medications is the ability of the patient to take his or her medication once daily rather than several times a day. This improves patient compliance and can ultimately result in better health. Directions that the dosage is in sustained-release form are usually printed below the drug name on the manufacturer's label. If an SR medication is given in place of a regular dose, adverse effects can occur, including death. In addition, if a patient is receiving nourishment through a feeding tube and an SR dose is crushed, it becomes an immediate release (IR) dose that is much higher in strength and can result in an adverse reaction. Many errors occur because of suffixes on drug products that are not clearly understood. According to a report from the ISMP, suffixes such as LA, CR, CD, ER, XL, and SR on drug products do not provide a clear meaning to indicate release properties or dosing frequency. The *United States Pharmacopeia* defines two categories of modified release formulations: delayed release and extended release. Delayed release denotes a formulation that has a coating to delay release of the drug until the product has passed through the stomach. Extended release denotes any formulation designed to deliver the dose over a longer interval than an IR product of the same drug. Because of the confusion of suffixes (i.e., the choice of a wrong suffix, the use of an unclear suffix, or the omission of a proper suffix during prescribing or dispensing), one form of drug may be given in place of the proper drug product.

Necessity of Reporting Errors

Pharmacist's Daily Routine

Most pharmacies are located in the retail setting, and most pharmacists are overworked on a daily basis. Many pharmacies fill as many as 300 to 400 prescriptions a day; the workload also includes addressing discrepancies in orders and counseling patients. In addition, pharmacists must check the work of technicians.

The limited time that a rushed pharmacist has to check technicians' work adds to the potential for errors. Another potentially dangerous situation arises when the same pharmacists and technicians work together for a long time. After pharmacists have worked many years with the same technicians, a bond of trust may develop, and pharmacists may become complacent about checking the technicians' work, either not checking it at all or just quickly scanning the completed order.

Computerized Prescription Order Entry

Many new systems are available that can help reduce errors. Many physicians use e-prescribing from the physician's office to the pharmacy or computerized physician order entry (CPOE) by the prescriber in institutional settings. The idea behind this type of ordering (i.e., electronic ordering) is that it circumvents having to decipher poor handwriting because orders are sent by computer directly to the pharmacy. However, many physicians and institutions have not yet accepted this type of ordering. It should be noted that even when the CPOE system is used, errors can still be made; selecting the wrong drug or dose from drop-down menus is still possible. In addition, introducing new technology often results in the introduction of new types of possible errors. More insurance companies and government-funded plans are pressuring physicians to use e-prescribing to be eligible for bonus payments. However, adoption of the technology can be costly, and in some cases state or federal laws have not allowed for full adoption of e-prescribing in all circumstances (e.g., allowing the prescription of controlled substances). Data transmission standards must be agreed upon and adhered to by all technologies to ensure proper communication between devices and computer databases.

In hospitals and other inpatient institutions, the use of CPOE is becoming more popular, along with bar coding methods (see Figure 14-2). Bar codes provide the following three forms of identification of a drug:

- National Drug Code
- Lot number of the drug
- Expiration date of the drug

Although the overall risk of errors is reduced by the use of CPOE, these systems are not 100% error free. Concerns have arisen about the lack of evaluation of their effectiveness because many different types are marketed. Potential dangers in certain CPOE systems include the facts that the computerized software does not recognize discrepancies in prescribing between the outpatient medication regimen and the hospital treatment plan, and many systems do not require prescribers to address computer alerts.

Other concerns pertaining to CPOE systems include ordering and administration problems (e.g., misidentification of patients and patient variables, such as height and weight) and mismatching of drug orders to chemotherapy protocols or miscalculations.

The problems with these systems are due to the newness of the technology. It takes time to address the flaws, which may be why many hospitals are slow to implement these systems. It is very time-consuming to electronically connect all the necessary personnel and still ensure that patient confidentiality is maintained. In addition, it takes time to understand new steps introduced into the health care professional's workflow. For example, after seeing their patients, physicians can sit at a computer or use a handheld device to enter new or changed orders and send them directly to the pharmacy. Nurses may also enter additional nursing notes that are documented in the system.

> ### Tech Note!
> Pharmacy employees need to know they will not be punished; instead, the error will be examined and new strategies will be established to ensure that errors are reduced in the future. It is important to have an error prevention plan in place. The goal is to reduce mistakes as much as possible using the knowledge of how they occur.

Reporting Errors

The most important aspect of dealing with errors is the reporting process. In years past, the most common response to an error was to place blame on the person who caused it and then tell the person to be more careful. This type of response was found to be nonproductive because most people will not report errors if they know they will be reprimanded. Also, "trying to be more careful" does not give the person the tools necessary to avoid further errors. Therefore, an emphasis on finding the causes of mistakes and ways to reduce errors has been found to be more productive. For this reason, the tracking systems in place do not target blame, but rather focus more on how the error occurred. Thus the reasons an error occurred can be examined, and constructive changes can be made and tracked. Examples of organizations that track medication errors in this way are listed in Box 14-3.

The ISMP tracks drug errors and works toward reducing them through MERP. MERP can be accessed via the Internet, *https://www.ismp.org/orderforms/reporterrortoismp.asp*, where health care workers can report incidences of errors, near-errors, or hazardous conditions in the workplace. When reporting incidents, questions concerning how the error was discovered and recommendations for preventing recurrence of the error are included in the report (follow this link to view an error report form: *http://www.consumermedsafety.org/report-a-medication-error*).

BOX 14-3

Organizations That Track Medication Errors

- U.S. Food and Drug Administration (FDA) and Centers for Disease Control and Prevention (CDC)
- FDA MedWatch
- FDA Adverse Event Reporting System (FAERS)
- Institute of Medicine (IOM)
- Institute for Safe Medication Practices (ISMP)
- National Coordinating Council for Medication Error Reporting and Prevention (NCCMERP)
- *United States Pharmacopeia (USP)* Medication Errors Reporting Program and MEDMARX
- The Joint Commission (TJC)

Specific incidents include the following:
- Administering the wrong:
  - Drug, dose, strength, or dosage form or using the wrong route of administration
- Errors in:
  - Prescribing medications
  - Transcribing medications
  - Dispensing medications
  - Monitoring medications
  - Performing calculations
  - Preparing medications

MERP recommendations include the following:
- **Medication error understanding:** Improves the collection, classification, and analysis of data linked to types, causes, and sources of error and the impact of errors on patients. Tracking medication errors in a systematic manner and prioritizing reduction activities are also included.
- **Medication error reporting:** Increases awareness of reporting systems available, such as MERP, **MedMARx**, and **MedWatch** (FDA). These programs maintain a classification system that identifies types of errors; the data obtained can then be used to analyze and report error statistics.
- **Medication error prevention:** With continuous research and reporting, areas can be identified where changes can be made to prevent future errors. This includes distinctive packaging, labeling, and nomenclature for drugs that are at high risk of errors.

Reporting can be done anonymously and voluntarily without fear of retribution. The MERP institute reviews all medication error reports, attempts to understand the reason or reasons for errors, and works toward producing initiatives to educate health care workers and improve medication safety. The following five guidelines are used to share information with health care professionals about potentially dangerous events:
1. Knowledge
2. Analysis (the evaluation of data)
3. Education
   - Providing confidential consulting services to health care systems to proactively evaluate medication systems
   - Educational programs that include:
     - Teleconferences on medications and issues
     - Patient resources (e.g., posters, pamphlets, videos, books)
   - High alert drugs (newsletter) and potentially dangerous abbreviations
4. Cooperation
   - Working with other entities:
     - Legislative and regulatory bodies
     - Health care practitioners
     - Health care institutions
     - Regulatory and accrediting agencies
     - Pharmaceutical industry
5. Communication
   - Bringing information to:
     - Consumers
     - Employers
     - Health care providers
   - Providing a voluntary reporting program

In 2012, the ISMP launched the National Vaccine Error Reporting Program (ISMP VERP) to capture the unique causes and consequences of vaccine-related errors. Health care practitioners from all areas can report a vaccine error by logging onto the website *http://verp.ismp.org*. All reports submitted to this website are shared with the FDA. Errors in vaccine administration are common, but little data are available as to why they occur. Hopefully, this new reporting system will produce valuable data in the fight to reduce errors.

 Tech Note!
One area of concern is the use of abbreviations. Many have been misinterpreted, which has resulted in drug errors. The ISMP has provided a list of terms to be avoided (see Table 5-2); they recommend that the term be spelled out completely.

The Joint Commission is another organization that helps institutions implement safety standards to reduce errors. TJC's five areas (each having 10 criteria) for ensuring patient safety are summarized as follows:
1. **Leadership process and accountability:** The leadership structure, individual accountability, policies and procedures (in all areas), and the managing of daily operations are identified. The institution is compliant with all laws and regulations. Leaders are educated about quality and are actively involved in setting quality and safety priorities. Both leaders and managers collaborate on quality and patient safety activities (e.g., patient assessments, medication use systems). The organization provides a mechanism based on the safety of the patient, as it relates to any type of drug research and/or organ transplantation that may take place, through data collection, analysis, and improvement.
2. **Competent and capable workforce:** Personnel files contain the credentials of all employees (e.g., education, training, licensure, work history, and copies of evaluations). Personnel job descriptions match the worker's credentials. Proper training is given in areas including cardiopulmonary

resuscitation (CPR), basic life support (BLS), infection prevention, and safety. Staff health and safety standards are met, and accurate patient records are reviewed and transferred to the appropriate unit or nurse. The credentials, licensure, education, training, and competence of physicians are reviewed. Nurses' ability to provide appropriate patient services, based on their competence, licensure, training, and education, is reviewed. The credentials of other health professionals are reviewed. Health care students in the institution are adequately monitored, supervised, and oriented to patient safety.

3. **Safe environment for staff and patients:** The institution has regular safety inspections of the building's environment (e.g., broken furniture, faulty equipment, and missing signs) and ensures fire safety measures (i.e., must work properly, exits not blocked). Water quality and electrical sources required 24 hours a day, 7 days a week work properly; alternate source plans are in place to ensure the safety of patients. All biomedical equipment and biohazardous materials are properly used and maintained. Education, training, and certification (if applicable) of employees in infection prevention and control is ensured, including proper disposal of needles and infectious wastes. A hand hygiene program with documented guidelines is followed. Reduction of health care–associated infections is achieved through proper implementation of a hand hygiene program and barrier techniques (e.g., gloves, masks, eye protection).

4. **Clinical care of patients:** The patient's identification is checked before medication, blood products, treatments, or procedures are administered. Patients understand the risks, treatments, and procedures before giving consent. Medical and nursing assessments are documented in the patient's record in a reasonable time frame so that treatment can take place as soon as possible. Laboratory and diagnostic services are available, reliable, and safe. Consent forms are completed for all treatments and/or procedures. Patient education and training are provided so that patients can participate in their own care (e.g., granting consent during hospitalization and learning proper medication use after discharge). All services (e.g., surgery, anesthesia, postsurgical unit) are appropriate to the patient's needs.

5. **Improving quality and safety:** An adverse event reporting system is in place, and the system is analyzed. Changes are made to increase patient safety based on causes of adverse events; these include medication errors, unanticipated death of a patient, surgery on the wrong patient or body part, and patient falls. High-risk patients are

monitored (e.g., immunosuppressed, comatose, emergency care patients). Patient and staff satisfaction is monitored in the facility for improvement purposes. A complaint process is in place for both patients and family members. Staff members understand how to improve processes by participating in improvement activities. Clinical outcomes are monitored and improved if necessary. Quality and safety information is communicated to staff members (e.g., through newsletters, reports, and posters) to improve patient safety.

A primary responsibility of TJC is to review documentation that tracks progress in each of these areas. For a comprehensive outline of the five safety standards, visit the website *www.jointcommission.org*.

Strategies for Reducing Errors

As we have learned, many factors contribute to medication errors. Each pharmacy should develop a system designed to strengthen its medication management practices and help reduce the number of preventable medication errors. The ISMP has launched the 2014-15 Targeted Medication Safety Best Practices for Hospitals to help identify and reduce medication errors that recur despite repeated warnings. These best practices provide strategies for error prevention and target a group of six key safety issues.

ISMP's 2014-2015 targeted medication safety best practices for hospitals are:

BEST PRACTICE 1
Dispense vincristine (and other vinca alkaloids) in a minibag of a compatible solution and not in a syringe.

BEST PRACTICE 2
a. Use a weekly dosage regimen default for oral methotrexate. If overrode to daily, require a hard stop verification of an appropriate oncologic indication.

b. Provide patient education by a pharmacist for all weekly oral methotrexate discharge orders.

BEST PRACTICE 3
Measure and express patient weights in metric units only. Ensure that scales used for weighing patients are set and measure only in metric units.

BEST PRACTICE 4
Ensure that all oral liquids that are not commercially available as unit dose are dispensed by the pharmacy in an oral syringe.

BEST PRACTICE 5
Purchase oral liquid dosing devices (oral syringes/cups/droppers) that display only the metric scale.

BEST PRACTICE 6
Eliminate glacial acetic acid from all areas of the hospital.

Common Pharmacy Technology

Bar Codes

Another part of the medication safety plan for hospitals involves the use of bar coding technology (Figure 14-2). Bar codes provide the following three forms of identification of a drug:

- National Drug Code (NDC)
- Lot number of the drug
- Expiration date of the drug

Although electronic communication between physician, pharmacy, and nursing reduces the number of errors, the system does have some problems. For example, if the nurse scans an alternative dose strength (e.g., two 5-mg tablets are substituted for one 10-mg tablet), the system reads this as an error. The nurse must then override the computer to administer the medication.

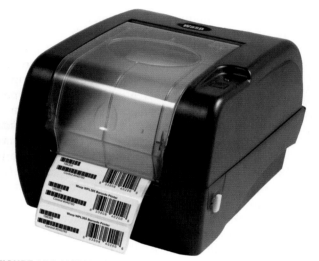

FIGURE 14-2 WPL305 desktop bar code printer. (Courtesy Wasp Barcode Technologies.)

Scenario CHECK UP 14-3

Today Jonathan is restocking the Robot-Rx. The regular robot filler is out sick. Jonathan has been cross-trained in many positions. His supervisors consider him a very valuable employee. Jennifer is still shadowing Jonathan during her orientation process. She has heard that sometimes these automated machines take the place of technicians, eliminating certain jobs. Is this a true statement? What are the advantages and disadvantages of automation in the pharmacy?

Robot-Rx Machines

Large robotic machines have been used for many years in some hospitals. Patient medication records are read by the machine through the use of bar coding; the appropriate medication's bar code is scanned from the package and then matched to the electronic medication administration record (E-MAR). Once the bar code has been verified, the machine (Figure 14-3) pulls from a rack of prepackaged unit dose medications stored in the unit. The medications are placed in a patient envelope, from which they can be delivered to the appropriate floor. These large

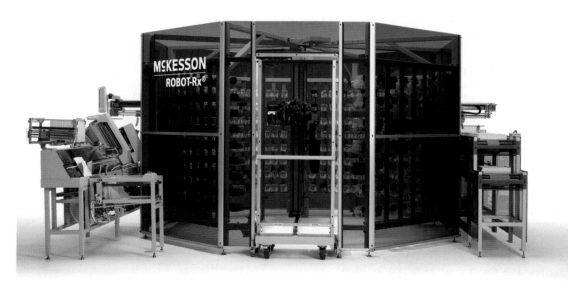

FIGURE 14-3 Robot-Rx machine. (Courtesy McKesson Corp.)

fillers are expensive and require a large area to function.

Hospital Pharmacy Automated Dispensing System Machines

Automated dispensing system (ADS) machines have been used for years in hospitals and institutions. ADS machines store unit dosed medications and nursing supplies to be accessed by nurses on patient floors. The pharmacy receives an order and enters it into the ADS computer, which then allows the nurse to access the medication using the patient's name. These systems work effectively if the medication in the drawer is correct; if the wrong medication is loaded into the drawer and the nurse fails to catch the mistake, an error can occur. However, coupling this system with bar coding greatly reduces the risk of errors. Each cubicle has an attached bar code that identifies the medication; when the technician attempts to fill the cubicle, he or she must match the bar code on the cubicle to the bar code on the medication. The nurse then can use the bar code to match the drug to the patient.

Another type of automated dispensing machine is the MedCarousel. The MedCarousel is a vertical, automated storage and retrieval system for medications in hospital pharmacies. MedCarousel automates medication dispensing and inventory control with its rotating shelves, pick-to-light technology, and forced compliance bar code scanning process (Figure 14-4).

Community Pharmacy Automated Dispensing Systems

For many years ADS machines have been used in community pharmacies. They are available in many different sizes to accommodate the prescription load. Bar coding is used to verify that the correct dosage is dispensed to the correct patient. The following three main types of ADS are used in community pharmacies:

- Tabletop automatic pill counters (e.g., model KL20 by Kirby Lester [Figure 14-5]): These devices are used for counting and verifying every order. The device instructs the technician first to scan the patient's prescription label and then to scan the bottle of medication to ensure a match (of medication, dosage, and quantity to be dispensed). The device's touch screen displays a picture of the medication and specific information about the drug. The tablets or capsules are poured into a hopper and are counted electronically. The device estimates the correct vial size (in drams) to use. The medication is then dispensed into a tray, and the technician pours its contents into a vial. A technician can fill a typical prescription with a KL20 device in 3 to 6 seconds.
- Large wall units that use cassettes, such as Baker Cell systems: The number of cassettes is limited only by the wall space available, and each cassette holds an assortment of preloaded medications. Again, the bar code on the

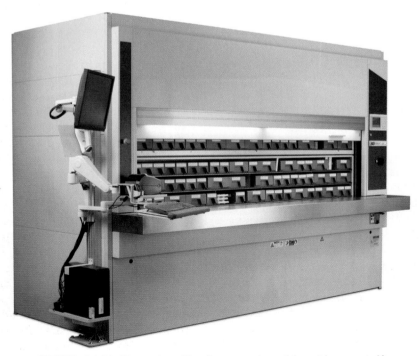

FIGURE 14-4 MedCarousel machine. (Image courtesy of Aesynt Incorporated.)

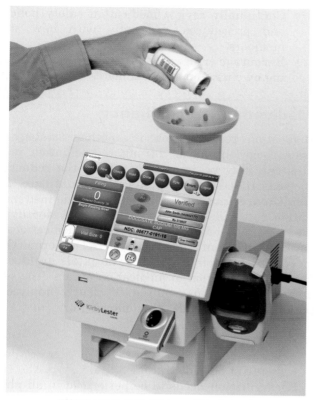

FIGURE 14-5 KL20. (Courtesy Kirby Lester.)

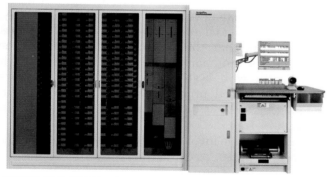

FIGURE 14-6 SP 200 robotic prescription dispensing system. (Courtesy ScriptPro.)

prescription label is scanned, and the appropriate amount is then dispensed. The pharmacist then scans the bottle for a final check. A screen displays the correct appearance of the medication, along with specific information on the drug.

- Robot technology (e.g., the SP 200 System by ScriptPro [Figure 14-6]): This system is a fully automated robotic prescription dispensing system. It accepts prescription dispensing instructions from pharmacy computers and delivers filled and labeled vials at a rate of up to 100 prescriptions per hour.

Many types of community pharmacy ADS and software programs are available, although they are very expensive and require training to use. More pharmacies use these systems so that they can fill more prescriptions in less time and concurrently reduce errors.

Mark is a level 2 technician at a large hospital. He has worked in the pharmacy for 8 years. When the pharmacy management began installing robots to help fill patient medications, he was among the first to apply for the new position of robot filler. Mark received extensive training on how to load these million-dollar machines and how to keep them running smoothly. The automated systems allowed the pharmacy to fill more orders in less time and reduce errors. Mark's position requires an individual who is technologically savvy, has an eye for detail, and is a problem solver. Machines break down, and glitches occur on a regular basis. It is the filler's job to know how to get the operation back on track. Mark reports directly to the pharmacy manager and works with each department to maintain adequate supplies and timely delivery of medications.

Patient Dose-Specific Orders

In the past, when patients required a large amount of liquids over a 24-hour period, a bulk bottle was placed in the patient's drawer. Also, if the liquid was not available in unit dose form, it would be sent in bulk form. The nurse would pour the proper amount per the medication administration record (MAR) and use the liquid until the bottle was empty. The nurse would then send a refill request to the pharmacy. The bottles sometimes would be labeled with just the patient's name and room number. Because specific dosing instructions were not denoted on the bottle, there was an increased likelihood that the nurse might dose the liquid medication inappropriately. Also, opening and closing lids can increase the risk of contamination of a medication. The pharmacy must have control over each dose to ensure accuracy. TJC requires hospitals and institutions to prepackage all liquid doses in oral syringes or containers. Each dose is prepared by the technician and is labeled with the patient's name, medical record number, and room number. In addition, the name of the drug, dose, strength, and time of administration are indicated on each dose. In this way, each dose is strictly controlled by the pharmacy. Automated robots can also fill and label doses, reducing the time needed by a technician to fill daily doses.

United States Pharmacopeia <797> Regulations

One of the regulations established by *United States Pharmacopeia* (USP) <797> addresses the problem of contamination of any type of sterile product. The adoption of USP <797> has been one of the most dramatic changes for any pharmacy that prepares sterile products, such as IVs and other parenterals. Because of the new regulations, many pharmacies are contracting their sterile preparations to companies that specialize in this area and have met all guidelines of USP <797>. Chapter 12 lists specifics of USP <797> regulations.

Medication safety is the responsibility of all pharmacy personnel. For any safety system to succeed, there must be an effective leader at the helm. ASHP has identified this role as the medication safety leader. This person is most often a pharmacist and is looked to as an expert on safe medication use. The medication safety leader usually reports to the risk management department or senior administrator; these individuals lead the team in developing strategies for reducing errors.

To reduce errors, pharmacists can:
- Check prescriptions carefully and thoroughly
- Initial checked prescriptions
- Document all clarifications made to any orders
- Visually check the product in the bottle
- Counsel all patients with new prescriptions
- Report all errors or adverse events

To reduce errors, pharmacy technicians can:
- Refer any questions regarding illegible handwriting or ambiguous orders to the pharmacist immediately
- Triple-count controlled substances
- Double-check dosage calculations with the pharmacist
- Keep the work area free of clutter
- Always keep the prescription and the label together during the filling process
- Check the drug three times: when removing the medication from the stock, after placing the medication in the prescription bottle, and before returning the medication bottle to the stock
- Observe and report to the pharmacist any pertinent OTC purchases made by patients

To reduce errors, pharmacies can:
- Use automated filling systems
- Scan the original prescription
- Use electronic prescribing
- Keep high-alert medications in a separate location in the pharmacy
- Maintain accurate, up-to-date patient profiles that include OTC and herbal medications
- Designate a medication safety leader

- Continually review medication safety policies and procedures, especially with new staff members
- Encourage error reporting by employees, focusing on change not punishment

Medication Reconciliation

Medication reconciliation is another strategy to prevent patient harm. Strong reconciliation practices can play an important role in the reduction of medication-related events. The **Institute for Healthcare Improvement (IHI)** has defined medication reconciliation as the process of identifying the most up-to-date list of all the medications a patient is currently taking. The IHI reported that more than 50% of all errors in hospitals are due to poor communication of medication orders. The necessary information required to clearly analyze a patient's needs includes the following:
- Name of drug
- Dosage
- Frequency
- Route of administration

Reconciliation needs to be performed in all pharmacy settings, although each type of pharmacy must develop its own specific strategies. In institutional settings it is important to compare the current list of medications with the list shown at the time of admission, at the time of any transfer within the facility, after surgeries, and at the time of discharge. The goal is to ensure that the patient is given the proper medications at all points as he or she moves through the health care system. In this way any errors can be identified promptly. The steps involved in completing a medication reconciliation are shown in Procedure 14-1.

Reconciliation involves several parties: the patient, physician, nurse, and pharmacist. Orders must be rewritten each time the patient is transferred to or from the intensive care unit (ICU) or returns from surgery. In the past, physicians would sometimes write "resume previous medications." This allowed misinterpretation of the medications being dosed. It was much easier to lose track of the medications the patient was taking. This resulted in adverse drug reactions and possible harm to the patient. TJC has since prohibited the use of these "blanket orders." At each point throughout the course of treatment, the previous medications must be compared with the current orders. Normally, facilities use a reconciliation form (Figure 14-7) that can be viewed by the physician, nurse, and pharmacist. In addition, at the time of discharge, the community pharmacy must perform reconciliation. Finally, the patient must be informed about the current instructions compared with any previous instructions. Many resources are

PROCEDURE 14-1

Medication Reconciliation

GOAL: To understand the steps required to complete a medication reconciliation form (the goal is to ensure that the patient is given the correct medication at all points as he or she moves through the health care system).

EQUIPMENT AND SUPPLIES
• Medication Reconciliation Form

PROCEDURAL STEPS*
• Verification: Obtain the patient's medication history and other medical information. This includes all medications, over-the-counter (OTC) drugs, and herbal remedies.
PURPOSE: It is critical to have the patient medication history to prevent any drug interactions, contraindications, or therapeutic duplications.

• Clarification: Make sure the medications and dosages are appropriate for the patient. The current physician's orders are compared with the patient's medication list.
PURPOSE: It is important to clarify the medications are within the acceptable dosage range for the patient, otherwise the patient may be harmed.
• Reconciliation: Clinical decisions are made based on the comparison between the two drug lists. Resolving any observed discrepancies or errors through documentation and direct communication is the final step.
PURPOSE: This is done to ensure the patient receives the optimum care and no drug interactions or therapeutic duplications of medications are overlooked.

*These steps are usually performed by a nurse and may be reviewed by the physician, another nurse, pharmacist, or trained pharmacy technician.

available to help pharmacies develop a strong medication reconciliation program. Some examples are given in the website list at the end of the chapter.

Other Considerations

Other conditions that can help reduce errors when filling prescriptions include using good lighting to clearly read the label and checking the drug against the prescription. Also, filling protocol systems must be reviewed and altered if they potentially can cause an error. Reducing the fear and anxiety of reporting errors should be implemented in all medical settings. Each prescription should be checked several times to ensure that it is correct. Physicians should use the metric system when writing doses. In the future, all prescriptions should be electronic rather than written, because this greatly improves clarity. Software systems must be improved to aid the pharmacy in identifying potential problems with dosing regimens.

Training and Education

One of the best ways to reduce errors is through training and education. Many states do not have standardized exams or use the national exam to pretest technicians. Some states do not even fingerprint or conduct a background check on pharmacy technicians. Many schools with pharmacy technician programs are not accredited and do not have standards of learning. Many large pharmacies train

their own employees to become technicians. The **Pharmacy Technician Certification Board (PTCB)** and ASHP have worked toward implementing training standards, and organizations such as the **Society for the Education of Pharmacy Technicians (SEPhT)** promote education and training before and after certification. In addition to obtaining certification, it is important for the technician to consistently self-educate through staff meetings, continuing education, and journal reports.

Beyond certification and continuous training, technicians should always check each prescription three times throughout the filling process. If anything about the prescription seems unclear or confusing, the pharmacist should be notified immediately.

The **Pharmacy Technician Educator's Council (PTEC)** is an organization of instructors whose goals are to improve teaching techniques and competencies of students. Members include both Canadian and U.S. instructors. As technicians' initial training improves, they are more able to address probable errors and to recognize questionable doses.

Conclusion

There are no simple solutions for preventing medication mistakes. However, through consistent monitoring and evaluation, the number of errors can be greatly reduced. The technician must approach each action taken in the pharmacy and other medication settings as requiring 100% commitment to the goal of perfection. Accurate interpretation of drugs and

Patient Name
MRN

MEDICATION RECONCILIATION FORM

ADMISSION / POINT OF ENTRY RECONCILIATION

- The first nurse to interview the patient should initiate completion of this form. Additional nurses and clinicians may continue to use the same form for the same patient.
- **Circle all sources of information:**   Patient   Caregiver   Rx bottle   EMS   Primary provider   Other:_____

ALLERGIES AND ADVERSE DRUG REACTIONS : _____

ACTIVE MEDICATION LIST				Date of Admission / Point of Entry:			RECONCILIATION
List below all medications patient was taking at time of admission. (Dosing information REQUIRED, if available.)							Continue on Admission?
Medication Name	Dose	Route	Frequency	Last Dose (Date/Time)	Date	Initials	Circle **Y** (yes) or **N** (no)*
1.							Y N
2.							Y N
3.							Y N
4.							Y N
5.							Y N
6.							Y N
7.							Y N
8.							Y N
9.							Y N
10.							Y N
11.							Y N
12.							Y N
13.							Y N
14.							Y N
15.							Y N
OTC Medications, Herbals, etc.							
							Y N
							Y N
							Y N
							Y N

*If order to be discontinued, see Admitting Note for comments.

Medication list recorded by RN/MD/PA/NP/LPN/RPh							
Initials	Print Name/Stamp	Signature	Date	Initials	Print Name/Stamp	Signature	Date

Reconciling Prescriber (MD/PA/NP/CNM)			
Print Name/Stamp	Signature	Title	Date

TRANSFER RECONCILIATION	DISCHARGE RECONCILIATION
- See Physician Orders for active medication orders upon transfer. - See Medication Administration Record for last dose given.	- See Patient Discharge Plan for list of medications patient should continue after discharge. - Discharge plan should include stopped medications.
Reconciling Prescriber (**Provide name, date, signature.**)	Reconciling Prescriber (**Provide name, date, signature.**)

☐   Check here if multiple pages needed. Please indicate: Page ____ of ____

Pilot Number 2/06

FIGURE 14-7 Example of a reconciliation form.

drug orders can mean the difference between life and death to a patient. Reporting drug errors can help instigate a change in the current protocol of a pharmacy that can prevent further errors of the same type. Technicians play an integral part in helping to identify and prevent errors.

It is true that many of the electronic software and hardware systems being implemented in pharmacies, institutions, physicians' offices, and clinics are helping to reduce errors, but these systems can malfunction. The ability to catch mistakes before they occur will always be the responsibility of the personnel involved in the prescribing, filling, and dosing of medications. For this reason, it is imperative that every health care worker view drug error prevention as a priority. Only through continuous education and training can errors be controlled, now and in the future. A summary of practices that can be used to reduce the occurrence of medication errors is presented in Box 14-4.

BOX 14-4

Methods for Avoiding Errors in the Pharmacy

- Medication name alerts
- Computerized physician order entry (CPOE) systems
- Bar coding
- Automatic dispensing system (ADS) machines
- Software systems used for identification
- Pharmacy robots
- Tall man lettering
- Color coding
- Education
- Training
- Altering system factors (e.g., clutter, lighting, workflow, distractions, interruptions, poorly designed procedures, stress, fear of reporting errors)
- Patient dose-specific repackaging
- Medication reconciliation

DO YOU REMEMBER THESE KEY POINTS?

- The five patient rights
- What constitutes an error
- Different types of medication errors
- The main causes of drug errors
- Where to report an adverse drug event
- The organization or groups that track and report medication errors
- The safety strategies that pharmacies, pharmacists, and pharmacy technicians can use to reduce medication errors

- The types of automated systems used to reduce drug errors
- How CPOE can reduce the number of confusing drug orders
- The role of training and education in reducing medication errors

---

Scenario FOLLOW UP

Jonathan finishes training Jennifer and congratulates her on a job well done. He feels confident she will work to prevent errors and promote patient safety. He understands the importance of education and knowledge in the quest to eliminate medication misadventures. Since the implementation of the tech-check-tech system, he has come to realize that he plays an important role in maintaining high standards for order accuracy and patient care. He is proud of the trust his pharmacists have in his abilities, and he is determined to do his best at all times.

REVIEW QUESTIONS

Multiple Choice Questions

1. Which of the following is *not* an example of a medication error?
   A. Giving the patient a medication intended for someone else
   B. Giving a chewable tablet instead of a liquid at the patient's request
   C. Giving a generic medication when the physician had prescribed a brand name medication and had signed "no substitutions"
   D. Giving a nitroglycerin patch when the intended route was nitroglycerin sublingual

2. What is the first step a pharmacy technician should take upon detecting a medication error?
   A. Notify the patient.
   B. Notify the physician.
   C. Alert the pharmacist.
   D. Alert the lead pharmacy technician.

3. REMS is a strategy used to manage known and potential serious risks of a drug or biological product. The FDA requires REMS to ensure that the benefits of a drug outweigh its risks. What does the acronym REMS stand for?
   A. Registered emergency medication system
   B. Risk evaluation and mitigation strategy
   C. Risk event monitoring strategy
   D. Registered emergency monitoring system

4. Which of the following does the ISMP consider to be a high-alert medication?
   A. IV oxytocin
   B. IM oxytocin
   C. Oral OxyContin
   D. All of the above

5. When dispensing medication, it is critical to remember the five rights of medication safety. What are the five rights?
   A. Right name, right date of birth, right address, right medication, right route
   B. Right quantity, right refills, right time, right date, right patient
   C. Right patient, right route, right time, right quantity, right dose
   D. Right patient, right time, right route, right dose, right medication

6. Which strategy to reduce errors would label bupropion and buspirone as buPROPion and bus-PIRone on the pharmacy shelf?
   A. Strategic inventory management (SIM)
   B. Tall man lettering
   C. Risk evaluation and mitigation strategy (REMS)
   D. Inventory bar coding strategy (IBS)

7. Which of the following are used in error reporting?
   A. MERP
   B. REMS
   C. ADS
   D. All of the above

8. The organization that accredits pharmacy technician programs is:
   A. PTCB
   B. ASHP
   C. PTEC
   D. TJC

9. Which of the following is *not* an ADS?
   A. Kirby Lester
   B. Robot-Rx
   C. CPOE
   D. MedCarousel

10. Which organization oversees MedWatch?
    A. ISMP
    B. IOM
    C. TJC
    D. FDA

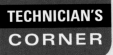

TECHNICIAN'S CORNER   What is your opinion on the criminalization of medication errors? Read the article by Jesse Vivian, "Criminalization of Medication Errors," at the website *www.uspharmacist.com/content/d/pharmacy%20law/c/16572/*. Discuss with your classmates and instructor what you believe is the proper punishment for technicians and pharmacists who are involved in medication errors. Research your state laws on this topic and any cases that have been recently brought before your state board of pharmacy.

Bibliography

Aesynt: MedCarousel: Increases Accuracy and efficiency of medication dispensing and inventory management. (Referenced April 20, 2014.) http://aesynt.com/medcarousel

American Society of Hospital Pharmacies: Guidelines on preventing medication errors in hospitals. (Referenced May 25, 2013.) www.ashp.org/DocLibrary/BestPractices/MedMisGdlHosp.aspx

Anthony L: Home infusion enhances specialty pharmaceutical distribution. *Pharmaceutical Commerce.* July 12, 2012. (Referenced January 12, 2014.) http://pharmaceuticalcommerce.com/special_report?articleid=26575

Arthur D, Cacchione J, Farrell B et al: Health forum: hospital-acquired infections—leadership challenges. Panel discussion. *Hosp Health Netw* 82:56, 2008. (Referenced January 12, 2014.)

Ballantyne C: Mystery solved: polo ponies probably died of selenium overdose. *Scientific American* (blog post). April 30, 2009. (Referenced December 9, 2013.) www.scientificamerican.com/blog/post.cfm?id=mystery-solved-polo-ponies-probably-2009-04-30

Bates DW: Sustained-release preparations and medication errors, *J Gen Intern Med* 17:657, 2002. (Referenced December 9, 2013.) www.ncbi.nlm.nih.gov/pmc/articles/PMC1495086/

Binder L: The shocking truth about medication errors. *Forbes* (blog post). September 3, 2013. (Referenced December 9, 2013.) www.forbes.com/sites/leahbinder/2013/09/03/the-shocking-truth-about-medication-errors/

Centers for Disease Control and Prevention: Get Smart for Healthcare (website). (Referenced April 2, 2014.) www.cdc.gov/getsmart/healthcare/

Fox News: Mom sues pharmacy alleging morphine overdose killed her daughter (online), August 22, 2013. (Referenced December 9, 2013.) www.foxnews.com/health/2013/08/22/mom-sues-pharmacy-alleging-morphine-overdose-killed-her-daughter/

Hendrick B: Sleep apnea, daytime sleepiness: risky combo. *WebMD Health News* (online), April 1, 2011. (Referenced December 9, 2013.) www.medicinenet.com/script/main/art.asp?articlekey=142618

Hodes RJ: Fiscal year 2014 budget request: statement for the record. Senate Subcommittee on Labor–HHS–Education Appropriations. Department of Health and Human Services and National Institutes of Health. (Referenced November 25, 2013.) http://olpa.od.nih.gov/PDFs%20Files/Congressional%20Hearings%20page/Congress%20113th/Hodes-Senate%20LHHS%20NIA%20FY%202014%20Opening%20Statement%20-%20FINAL.pdf

Institute of Medicine: To err is human: building a safer health system. November 1999. (Referenced December 10, 2013.) www.iom.edu/~/media/Files/Report%20Files/1999/To-Err-is-Human/To%20Err%20is%20Human%201999%20%20report%20brief.pdf

Institute for Safe Medication Practices: Examination of fatal error supports system-based approach to safety. March 16, 2010 (press release). (Referenced December 9, 2013.) www.ismp.org/pressroom/PR20100316.pdf

Institute for Safe Medication Practices: ISMP survey on drug shortage "gray market" shows widespread impact on hospitals. August 25, 2011 (press release). (Referenced December 10, 2013.) www.ismp.org/pressroom/PR20110825.pdf

Institute for Safe Medication Practices: ISMP survey shows prescription time guarantees may lead to errors. September 17, 2012 (press release). (Referenced December 10, 2013.) www.ismp.org/pressroom/PR20120917.pdf

Institute for Safe Medication Practices: ISMP Launches new vaccine error reporting program. December 11, 2012 (press release). (Referenced December 10, 2013.) www.ismp.org/pressroom/PR20121211.pdf

Institute for Safe Medication Practices: Survey shares pharmacist, technician perspectives on compounded sterile product management. January 24, 2013 (press release). (Referenced December 10, 2013.) www.ismp.org/pressroom/PR20130124.pdf

Institute for Safe Medication Practices: ISMP launches consensus-based medication safety best practices. December 6, 2013 (press release). (Referenced December 9, 2013.) www.ismp.org/pressroom/PR20131206.pdf

Institute for Safe Medication Practices: The National Medication Errors Reporting Program (ISMP MERP) (website). (Referenced December 10, 2013.) www.ismp.org/orderforms/reporterrortoISMP.asp

James JT: A new, evidence-based estimate of patient harms associated with hospital care, *J Patient Saf* 9:122, 2013. (doi: 10.1097/PTS.0b013e3182948a69). (Referenced April 10, 2014.) http://journals.lww.com/journalpatientsafety/Fulltext/2013/09000/A_New,_Evidence_based_Estimate_of_Patient_Harms.2.aspx

Kim GR, Chen AR, Arceci RJ et al: Error reduction in pediatric chemotherapy: computerized order entry and failure modes and effects analysis, *Arch Pediatr Adolesc Med* 2006;160:495, 2006 (doi:10.1001/archpedi.160.5.495) (Referenced December 10, 2013.)

Lifshin L, Nimmo C: Developing and maintaining up-to-date training for pharmacy technicians. *Am J Health Syst Pharm* 58:968, 2001. (Referenced November 25, 2013.) www.ashp.org/DocLibrary/Accreditation/RTP-TechDevelopTraining.aspx

Lowery M: Pharmacy mistake blamed for heparin overdoses at Texas hospital. *Drug Topics: Voice of the Pharmacist* (online). July 11, 2008. (Referenced November 25, 2013.) http://drugtopics.modernmedicine.com/drug-topics/news/clinical/hospitalhealth-system-pharmacy/pharmacy-mistake-blamed-heparin-overdoses-t

Mizner JJ: *Pharmacy technician certification examination*, ed 3, St Louis, 2014, Elsevier.

National Association of Boards of Pharmacy: United States Pharmacopeial Convention joins Anti-Counterfeiting Campaign. (online). December 4, 2013. (Referenced December 10, 2013.) www.nabp.net/news/united-states-pharmacopeial-convention-joins-anti-counterfeiting-campaign

National Coordinating Council for Medication Error Reporting and Prevention: Council recommendations: recommendations to reduce medication errors associated with verbal medication orders and prescriptions. Revised February 24, 2006. (Referenced April 9, 2014.) www.nccmerp.org/council/council2001-02-20.html

National Coordinating Council for Medication Error Reporting and Prevention: Moving into the second decade: developing recommendations and offering tools. (Referenced December 10, 2013.) www.nccmerp.org/pdf/fifteen_Year_report.pdf

National League for Nursing: Medication errors injure 1.5 million people and cost billions of dollars annually; report offers comprehensive strategies for reducing drug-related mistakes (press release). (Referenced December 10, 2013.) www.nln.org/newsreleases/iom_08_06.pdf

Oregon News: Adult prescription dispensed to four year old. *Oregon State Board of Pharmacy Newsletter*, February 2009. (Referenced December 10, 2013.) www.nabp.net/news/oregon-news-adult-prescription-dispensed-to-four-year-old

Pray WS, Van Dusen V: Medication errors: causes, prevention, liability, and the apology (CE). *Drug Topics: Voice of the Pharmacist* (online). February 15, 2011. (Referenced December 10, 2013.) via http://drugtopics.modernmedicine.com/drug-topics/news/modernmedicine/modern-medicine-feature-articles/medication-errors-causes-preventi-0

Preventing errors with pediatric patients. *The American Nurse*. (Referenced January 11, 2014.) www.theamericannurse.org/index.php/2012/10/05/preventing-errors-with-pediatric-patients/

Radwan C: Pharmacy technicians face states' scrutiny, regulation. *Drug Topics: Voice of the Pharmacist* (online). August 25, 2009. (Referenced December 10, 2013.) via http://drugtopics.modern medicine.com/drugtopics/Associations/Pharmacy-technicians -face-states-scrutiny-regulati/ArticleStandard/Article/detail/ 621364

Reckmann MH, Westbrook JI, Koh Y et al: Does computerized provider order entry reduce prescribing errors for hospital inpatients? A systematic review. *J Am Med Inform Assoc* 16:613, 2009. (doi10.1197/jMI.M3050). (Referenced November 15, 2013.) http://jamia.bmj.com/content/16/5/613.abstract

Rybolt B: CVS will pay $650,000 to resolve prescription medication errors in N.J. N.J.com (blog post). February 25, 2013. (Referenced December 9, 2013.) http://blog.nj.com/independent press_impact/print.html?entry=/2013/02/cvs_nj_division_of _consumer_af.html

Skerrett PJ: Multitasking: a medical and mental hazard. (blog post). Harvard Health Blog. January 7, 2012. (Referenced December 9, 2013.) www.health.harvard.edu/blog/multitasking -a-medical-and-mental-hazard-201201074063

The Merck manual home health handbook (online). Drug errors. (Referenced July 15, 2013.) www.merckmanuals.com/home/ drugs/overview_of_drugs/drug_errors.html?qt=medication%20 errors&alt=sh

Vivian JC: Criminalization of medication errors, *US Pharm* 34:66, 2009. (Referenced December 9, 2013.) www.uspharmacist.com/ content/d/pharmacy%20law/c/16572/

West D, Hastings J, Earley A: An economic justification of the use of dispensing technologies in independent community pharmacies. National Community Pharmacists Association (Referenced December 9, 2013.) www.ncpafoundation.org/ downloads/asset_upload_file169_7723.pdf

Websites Referenced

Florida Board of Pharmacy. Registered Pharmacy Technician Requirements. (Referenced May 15, 2014.) http://floridas pharmacy.gov/licensing/registered-pharmacy-technician/

FreeCE.Com. Pharmaceutical Education Consultants. Medication Error Prevention. A Guide for Pharmacists (Referenced May 15, 2014.) http://www.freece.com/freece/CECatalog_Details. aspx?ID=c3800910-420b-4d15-9b55-2e2a065bd29d

Institute for the Ages. Demographic Transition Facts. (Referenced June 10, 2014.) www.institutefortheages.org/facts-on-aging/

Institute for Healthcare Improvement. Reconcile Medications at All Transition Points. (Referenced May 15, 2014.) www.ihi.org/ knowledge/Pages/Changes/ReconcileMedicationsatAll TransitionPoints.aspx

Institute for Healthcare Improvement. Reconcile Medications in Outpatient Settings. (Referenced May 15, 2014.) www.ihi.org/ knowledge/Pages/Changes/ReconcileMedicationsinOutpatient Settings.aspx

Institute for Healthcare Improvement. How to Guide: Prevent Adverse Drug Events (Medication Reconciliation. (Referenced May 15, 2014.) www.ihi.org/knowledge/Pages/Tools/Howto GuidePreventAdverseDrugEvents.aspx

2014-15 Targeted Medication Safety Best Practices for Hospitals. (Referenced July 2, 2014.) http://www.ismp.org/tools/best practices/default.aspx

SECTION 2
Pharmacology and Medications

SECTION OUTLINE

Therapeutic Agents for the Nervous System

Joshua J. Neumiller

OBJECTIVES

Upon completing this chapter, you should be able to do the following:

1. Describe the major components of the nervous system, including components of the central nervous system and peripheral nervous system.
2. List the primary symptoms of conditions associated with dysfunction of the central nervous system and peripheral nervous system.
3. Discuss other conditions associated with the nervous system and their clinical features.
4. Recognize drugs used to treat the conditions associated with the nervous system.
5. Write the generic and trade names for the drugs discussed in this chapter.
6. List appropriate auxiliary labels when filling prescriptions for drugs discussed in this chapter.

TERMS AND DEFINITIONS

Alzheimer's disease (AD) A progressive form of dementia that affects memory, thinking, and behavior

Attention deficit/hyperactivity disorder (ADHD) A physiological brain disorder that affects the ability to engage in quiet, passive activities or to focus one's attention; attributable to an imbalance of neurotransmitters in the brain

Autonomic nervous system A branch of the nervous system that carries out "automatic" bodily functions; it is composed of the sympathetic and parasympathetic systems

Blood-brain barrier (BBB) A barrier that exists in the brain as a result of special permeability characteristics of the capillaries that supply brain cells; these capillaries prevent certain solutes or chemicals from being transferred from the blood to the brain

Bradykinesia Slowed movement

Brainstem A section of the brain consisting of the medulla oblongata, pons, and midbrain, which connect the forebrain and cerebrum to the spinal cord

Central nervous system (CNS) Consists of the brain and spinal cord; it acts to coordinate sensory and motor control of body functions

Cerebellum A structure located posterior to the pons and medulla oblongata; it is responsible for posture, balance, and voluntary muscle movement

Cerebrospinal fluid (CSF) Clear watery fluid that is continually produced and absorbed that flows in the ventricles of the brain and around the surface of the brain and spinal cord

Epilepsy A brain disorder marked by repeated seizures over time

Extrapyramidal symptoms (EPS) Often result from taking antipsychotic medications and include parkinsonism, dystonia, and tremors

Hemorrhagic stroke A stroke caused by the rupture of a blood vessel in the brain

Homeostasis The tendency of the body to maintain stability, such as with body temperature

Insomnia Difficulty falling or staying asleep

Ischemic stroke A stroke caused by blockage of a blood vessel in the brain

Multiple sclerosis (MS) An autoimmune disorder that affects nerves in the CNS; it leads to impaired motor function

Myasthenia gravis A neuromuscular disorder leading to weakness of the skeletal muscles

Neuron The basic building block and cell of the nervous system

Parasympathetic nervous system (PSNS) A division of the autonomic nervous system that functions during restful situations

Parkinson's disease (PD) A movement disorder with the classic symptoms of tremor, rigidity, bradykinesia, and postural instability

Peripheral nervous system (PNS) The division of the nervous system outside the brain and spinal cord

Polyneuropathy A neurological disorder that occurs when many nerves throughout the body malfunction; it can be associated with painful neuropathy

Psychosis A mental illness characterized by loss of contact with reality; it may be a true mental illness, may be due to an underlying medical condition (e.g., dementia, drug withdrawal syndromes), or may be induced by substances such as medications, recreational drugs, or poisons

Schizophrenia A disorder characterized by inappropriate emotions and unrealistic thinking

Somatic nervous system The motor neurons of the peripheral nervous system that control voluntary actions of the skeletal muscles and provide sensory input (touch, hearing, sight)

Sympathetic nervous system (SNS) A division of the autonomic nervous system that functions during stressful situations; the "fight or flight" part of the autonomic nervous system

Tardive dyskinesia (TD) A type of dyskinesia (unwanted, involuntary rhythmic movements) attributed as a potential side effect of taking dopamine antagonists such as phenothiazines or other medications (e.g., metoclopramide); the symptoms may continue even after discontinuation of the offending drug

Select Common Drugs Prescribed for Neurological Conditions

Trade Name	Generic Name	Pronunciation
Myasthenia Gravis		
Mestinon	pyridostigmine	(pie-rid-o-**stig**-meen)
Imuran	azathioprine	(ay-za-**thye**-oh-preen)
Peripheral Neuropathy		
Cymbalta	duloxetine	(du-**lox**-uh-teen)
Effexor	venlafaxine	(**ven**-la-fax-een)
Neurontin	gabapentin	(**ga**-ba-**pen**-tin)
Zostrix	capsaicin	(cap-**say**-sin)
Epilepsy		
Tegretol	carbamazepine	(kar-ba-**maz**-e-peen)
Depakote	divalproex sodium	(di-val-**pro**-ex so-de-um)
Lamictal	lamotrigine	(la-**mow**-tri-jeen)
Keppra	levetiracetam	(**lee**-ve-ti-**ra**-se-tam)
Trileptal	oxcarbazepine	(**ox**-kar-**baz**-e-peen)
Dilantin	phenytoin	(**fen**-i-toyn)
Gabitril	tiagabine	(tye-**ag**-a-been)
Topamax	topiramate	(toe-**pir**-uh-mate)
Alzheimer's Disease		
Aricept	donepezil	(do-**nay**-pa-zil)
Razadyne	galantamine	(gal-**an**-ta-meen)
Exelon	rivastigmine	(ri-va-**stig**-meen)
Namenda	memantine	(meh-**man**-teen)
Parkinson's Disease		
Sinemet	levodopa/carbidopa	(**lee**-vo-**doe**-pa/**car**-bih-**doe**-pa)
Mirapex	pramipexole	(pram-i-**pex**-ole)
Requip	ropinirole	(row-**pin**-i-**role**)
Neupro	rotigotine	(row-**tig**-oh-teen)
Symmetrel	amantadine	(ah-**man**-ta-deen)
Comtan	entacapone	(en-**tak**-a-pone)
Zelapar	selegiline	(se-**le**-ja-leen)
Azilect	rasagiline	(ras-**aj**-il-een)
Multiple Sclerosis		
Avonex, Rebif	interferon beta-1a	(in-tur-**fear**-on **bay**-ta won ay)
Betaseron	interferon beta-1b	(in-tur-**fear**-on **bay**-ta won bee)
Copaxone	glatiramer	(gla-**tir**-a-mer)
Ampyra	dalfampridine	(dal-**fam**-pri-**deen**)
Gilenya	fingolimod	(fin-**gol**-i-mod)

Continued

Select Common Drugs Prescribed for Neurological Conditions—cont'd

Trade Name	Generic Name	Pronunciation
Tysabri	natalizumab	(na-ta-**liz**-yoo-mab)
Novantrone	mitoxantrone	(mye-toe-**zan**-trone)
Migraine Headache		
Imitrex	sumatriptan	(**soo**-mah-**trip**-tan)
Relpax	eletriptan	(el-e-**trip**-tan)
Frova	frovatriptan	(**al**-mo-**trip**-tan)
Axert	almotriptan	(**nar**-a-**trip**-tan)
Maxalt	rizatriptan	(**rye**-za-**trip**-tan)
Zomig	zolmitriptan	(**zol**-mi-**trip**-tan)
Depression		
Prozac	fluoxetine	(floo-**ox**-e-teen)
Paxil	paroxetine	(pa-**rox**-e-teen)
Celexa	citalopram	(si-**tal**-oh-pram)
Lexapro	escitalopram	(**es**-sye-**tal**-oh-pram)
Zoloft	sertraline	(**sir**-tra-leen)
Cymbalta	duloxetine	(du-**lox**-uh-teen)
Effexor	venlafaxine	(**ven**-la-fax-een)
Pristiq	desvenlafaxine	(des-**ven**-la-**fax**-een)
Elavil	amitriptyline	(am-uh-**trip**-tah-leen)
Tofranil	imipramine	(im-**ip**-ra-meen)
Pamelor	nortriptyline	(nor-**trip**-ti-leen)
Wellbutrin	bupropion	(bew-**pro**-pe-on)
Anxiety Disorders		
Xanax	alprazolam	(al-pra-**zoe**-lam)
Valium	diazepam	(dye-**az**-e-pam)
Ativan	lorazepam	(lor-**a**-ze-pam)
Serax	oxazepam	(ox-**a**-ze-pam)
BuSpar	buspirone	(byoo-**spye**-rone)
Schizophrenia		
Haldol	haloperidol	(**hal**-oh-**pear**-uh-dol)
Zyprexa	olanzapine	(oh-lan-**zah**-peen)
Risperdal	risperidone	(ris-**per**-ih-done)
Abilify	aripiprazole	(**ar**-i-**pip**-ra-zole)
Seroquel	quetiapine	(kwe-**tye**-a-peen)
Geodon	ziprasidone	(zi-**pray**-si-done)
Fanapt	iloperidone	(**eye**-loe-**per**-i-done)
Latuda	lurasidone	(loo-**ras**-i-done)
Invega	paliperidone	(pal-ee-**per**-i-done)
Bipolar Disorder		
Eskalith	lithium	(**lith**-e-um)
Lamictal	lamotrigine	(la-**moe**-tri-jeen)
Zyprexa	olanzapine	(oh-lan-**zah**-peen)
Seroquel	quetiapine	(kwe-**tye**-a-peen)
Risperdal	risperidone	(ris-**per**-uh-done)
Geodon	ziprasidone	(zi-**pray**-si-done)
Depakote	valproic acid	(val-**pro**-ik-**a**-sid)
Insomnia		
Restoril	temazepam	(tem-**az**-e-pam)
Halcion	triazolam	(try-**az**-oh-lam)
Lunesta	eszopiclone	(es-zoe-**pik**-lone)
Sonata	zaleplon	(**zal**-e-plon)
Ambien	zolpidem	(zole-**pi**-dem)

Select Common Drugs Prescribed for Neurological Conditions—cont'd

Trade Name	Generic Name	Pronunciation
Rozerem	ramelteon	(ra-**mel**-tee-on)
Benadryl	diphenhydramine	(**dye**-fen-**hye**-dra-meen)
Unisom	doxylamine	(dox-**il**-uh-meen)

Attention Deficit/Hyperactivity Disorder (ADHD)

Ritalin	methylphenidate	(meth-il-**fen**-i-date)
Dexedrine Spansule	dextroamphetamine	(dex-troe-am-**fet**-uh-meen)
Focalin	dexmethylphenidate	(dex-meth-il-**fen**-i-date)
Adderall	amphetamine/dextroamphetamine	(am-**fet**-a-meen/**dex**-troe-am-**fet**-uh-meen)
Vyvanse	lisdexamfetamine	(lis-**dex**-am-**fet**-uh-meen)
Strattera	atomoxetine	(**a**-toe-**mox**-e-teen)

The nervous system is a complex bodily system responsible for controlling and coordinating numerous functions in the body, including both conscious and unconscious activities. Nerves enable the body to perform internal functions involuntarily, such as regulation of the heartbeat, the digestive system breaking down a meal, or the brain interpreting visual signals from the eyes. The complex functions of the nervous system are better understood when the divisions of the nervous system are described in terms of their specific functions. We begin with common medical terminology associated with the nervous system and an overview of the main branches of the nervous system, describing some of the basic functions of each branch. An understanding of the nervous system is important to understand how medications are used to treat conditions associated with the nervous system. Select medical conditions that affect the nervous system are discussed, along with common medications used clinically to treat those conditions.

The Nervous System

The nervous system coordinates the activities of the body and enables us to interact with our environment. The nervous system, through the actions of nerves, allows us to detect and respond to stimuli, which are changes that occur either within the body or in the outside environment. The nervous system is critical in maintaining **homeostasis** in the body. A nice analogy for understanding the nervous system is to think of it as a complex, mainframe computer system with its network of nerves connected to the body, much as the Internet is connected to millions of homes. The mainframe (central nervous system) is connected to computers (target sites) that interpret the signals; likewise, the computer extensions can send messages to the mainframe computer,

where they can be interpreted such that the body can respond (Figure 15-1).

The **central nervous system (CNS)** is composed of the brain, the brainstem, and the spinal cord. The **peripheral nervous system (PNS)** is located outside the CNS and consists of the afferent (sensory) and efferent (motor) branches. The afferent (sensory) division transmits impulses from the body's organs and tissues to the CNS, where they are interpreted. The efferent (motor) division then relays the interpreted impulses to the appropriate organ and triggers an effect. The efferent division is further divided into the **somatic nervous system** and the **autonomic nervous system**. The somatic system relays motor impulses to skeletal muscles throughout the body, and the autonomic system transmits motor impulses to smooth muscle (e.g., the muscle surrounding the blood vessels), cardiac muscle (i.e., the heart), and glandular tissue. The autonomic nervous system consists of two main branches: the sympathetic nervous system (SNS) and the parasympathetic nervous system (PSNS), which are described later in the chapter.

Remember, although the nervous system has many divisions, all the components described in this chapter are considered one organ system (Figure 15-2). We begin with a discussion of the smallest functional part of the nervous system, the neuron.

 Tech Note!

The nervous system is composed of the CNS and the PNS. The CNS consists of the brain, brainstem, and spinal cord. The PNS carries messages from the body to the CNS, where they are interpreted. Then impulses are relayed from the brain and spinal cord outward to the rest of the body, where they trigger an effect. The PNS is divided into the somatic and autonomic divisions.

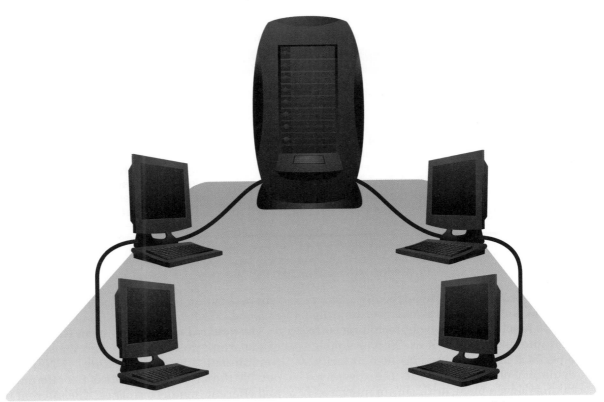

FIGURE 15-1 The nervous system is analogous to a mainframe computer (central nervous system) that communicates with other computers farther away (peripheral nervous system).

Neurons

The smallest unit of the nervous system is the **neuron**. Billions of neurons run throughout our bodies and carry messages back and forth in the nervous system. Neurons are composed of four main sections: the cell body, the dendrites, the axon, and the nerve terminal (see Figure 15-3). As neurons branch out, forming a network of relay stations, they allow nerve impulses to travel from one neuron to another via small gaps called *synapses.* The dendrites are extensions that receive electrical impulses from the previous neuron's nerve terminal. The cell body processes the electrical message before it enters the axon. Many axons are covered by a special form of insulation called a *myelin sheath;* it consists of phospholipids and proteins and serves to accelerate impulse conduction (Figure 15-3).

Nerve Transmission

If we follow the conduction of a chemical message from one neuron to another, we would notice that three basic changes occur in the cell membrane: polarization, depolarization, and repolarization. When the cell is in a resting state, there is an overall negative charge inside the neuron that consists of potassium ions (positive) and chloride ions (negative). The

outside of the neuron is more positive, with sodium as the positive charge. At this point, the cell is polarized and waiting to be excited. When a neurotransmitter activates the cell membrane, an influx of sodium ions occurs, changing the negative charge inside the cell to a positive charge. This is called *depolarization.* The cell restores the resting state by allowing the inside positive charges (potassium ions) to escape. As the transition back to the resting state occurs, the cell actively transports the sodium back to the outside and allows the potassium to reenter the cell. The cell repolarizes, bringing it full circle and back to the resting stage (Figure 15-4).

So, what is a neurotransmitter? Simply stated, neurotransmitters (NTs) are chemicals that are located in and released by neurons. They provide impulses that are emitted and sent from one nerve cell to another. NTs can either excite or inhibit other nerve cells or tissues in the body, and they are used by the nervous system to communicate a message. NTs work by binding to receptors for which they specifically activate (much like a lock and key) to trigger a response (Figure 15-5). Although many different types of NTs have been discovered, only a few of the primary ones are discussed here and in the following chapters. The impairment of NT function in the brain and in the periphery can cause various

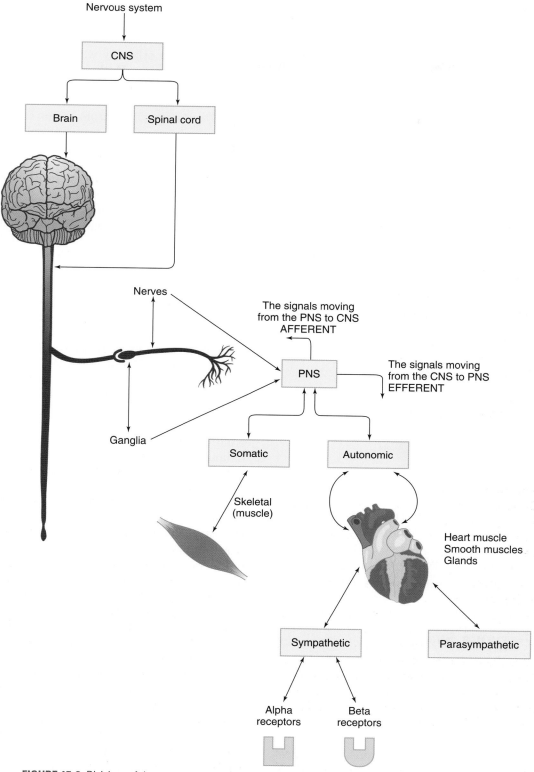

FIGURE 15-2 Divisions of the nervous system include the somatic and autonomic branches. The somatic division sends and receives impulses to and from the muscles, whereas the autonomic system regulates both the sympathetic and parasympathetic systems. *CNS,* Central nervous system; *PNS,* peripheral nervous system.

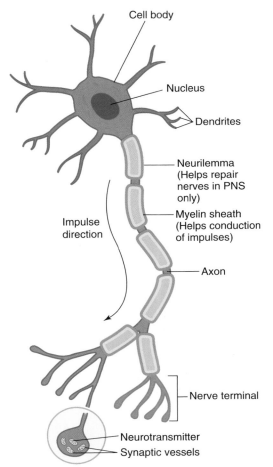

FIGURE 15-3 Neuron. Impulses travel down the axon into the nerve terminal, where they are released into the synaptic space between each neuron. Impulses then are transmitted to the following neuron via the dendrites, which extend out of the cell body. The spaces between segments of the myelin sheath are known as the *nodes of Ranvier.*

physical and mental disorders, which are discussed in this chapter.

Central Nervous System

The CNS is composed of the spinal cord, the brainstem, and the brain. The following sections provide an overview of the primary functions of the CNS.

Brain

The brain is composed of several sections. The largest area of the brain is the cerebral cortex, which is composed of gray matter that lies over white matter. Gray matter consists of neuron cell bodies and dendrites and is where most of the neuronal activity takes place. The gray matter is where language, memory, and cognitive functions occur. The white matter consists of bundles of nerve fibers. The white matter functions to communicate between other areas of the cerebral cortex and brain. The cerebral cortex is divided into the left and right hemispheres (*hemi* meaning half). The two halves can communicate with each other by way of the corpus callosum (bundles of axons). Each of the two hemispheres is divided further into four different lobes, each having specific functions:

- *Frontal lobe:* Controls motor function, parts of speech, emotions, problem solving, reasoning, and planning
- *Parietal lobe:* Important in orientation, recognition, sensation, and understanding language
- *Occipital lobe:* Important in control of perception and interpretation related to vision
- *Temporal lobe:* Important in receiving and integrating auditory stimuli and regulating emotion, personality, and behavior

The **brainstem** connects the brain to the spinal cord and consists of three main areas: the midbrain, pons, and medulla oblongata. These three areas are linked to many of the nerves in the brain (Figure 15-6). Above the brainstem is the thalamus. The thalamus is a type of relay station that is involved in the transmission of messages between the brain and the spinal cord. The thalamus sends messages to the appropriate area in the cerebral cortex. At the back of the brain, near the brainstem, is the **cerebellum**; this highly folded part of the brain is responsible for precise movements, such as maintaining balance and posture and coordinating movement.

When discussing medications for the treatment of neurologic disorders, it is important to discuss the blood-brain barrier. The **blood-brain barrier (BBB)** serves a protective function as it works to prevent certain molecules and substances from entering and possibly damaging the brain. In this way, the brain is independently protected from the rest of the body. A typical property of the BBB is the ability to protect the brain from bacteria that may be in the bloodstream. However, if an infection does occur in the brain, it is difficult to treat because defensive antibodies are too large to pass the BBB. Unfortunately, certain viruses can easily pass the BBB because they are extremely small and often attach themselves to circulating immune cells that do cross into the brain. In terms of medications, certain properties make medicines more or less likely to cross the BBB. In general, small molecules that are lipophilic, or "fat loving," are more likely to be able to pass through the BBB.

Spinal Cord

The spinal cord (Figure 15-7), located inside the vertebral column, serves as a pathway from the brain to the peripheral nervous system. The spinal nerves are protected by the vertebrae. Within the vertebrae

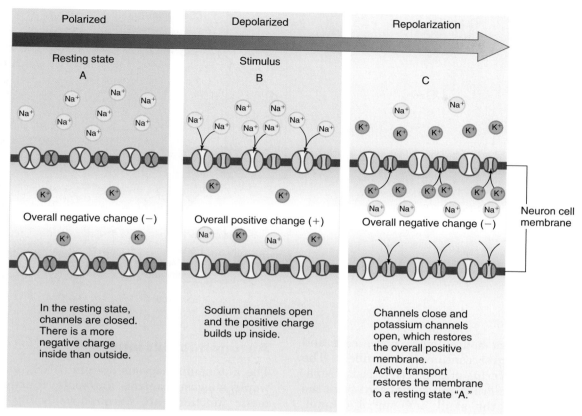

FIGURE 15-4 Neuronal impulse transfer cycle.

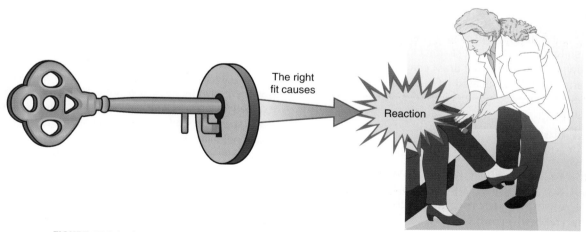

FIGURE 15-5 Lock-and-key mechanism. As the knee is tapped, impulses are sent to and from the brain. The neurotransmitters affect specific receptors that are interpreted. The reaction sent via neurotransmitters is to jerk the knee.

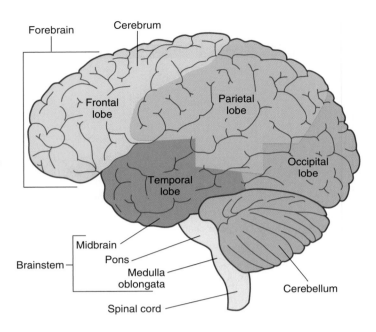

FIGURE 15-6 Lobes of the brain, cerebellum, and brainstem, which are all part of the central nervous system.

an inner gray matter houses many nerve cells and an outer white matter contains nerve fibers. The meninges, a thin covering of connective tissue, separate and protect the brain and spinal cord from the bony structures of the skull and spinal column, respectively. The brain and spinal cord also are cushioned by a watery liquid called the **cerebrospinal fluid (CSF)**.

 Tech Note!

The nerves of the brain crisscross so that the left side of the brain controls the right side of the body. Therefore, people suffering from a stroke (blocked or diminished blood flow) on one side of the brain can lose the ability to move parts of the body located on the opposite side.

Cranial Nerves

Twelve pairs of cranial nerves originate from the brain (Figure 15-8). These nerves have specific functions and are designated by Roman numerals. The numbers represent the order in which the fibers are located in the brain from front to back. Most of these nerves have sensory and motor fibers, with three sets having sensory fibers only. Table 15-1 lists the primary functions of each set of cranial nerves, I to XII, respectively.

Peripheral Nervous System

The PNS is divided into the autonomic and somatic systems, each having specific functions. These systems and their functions are described in the following sections.

Autonomic System

The autonomic nervous system (ANS), as its name would suggest, controls automatic functions. Automatic functions are unconscious bodily functions, such as heartbeat and breathing. The autonomic nervous system is subdivided further into two main branches, the sympathetic and parasympathetic nervous systems (see Figure 15-2). These systems regulate functions of the organs, tissues, and blood vessels (Figure 15-9).

 Tech Note!

The autonomic system is an involuntary branch of the PNS. The autonomic system is divided into sympathetic and parasympathetic divisions. The sympathetic system releases the neurotransmitter norepinephrine when we are stressed, and the parasympathetic system releases acetylcholine when we are at rest.

Sympathetic Nervous System

The function of the **sympathetic nervous system (SNS)** is to respond to stressful situations; it is associated with the "fight or flight" response. During the fight-or-flight stress response, the SNS shuts down the nonessential systems of the body. This redirects energy to other areas, such as the muscular system. The SNS also sends impulses to various organs and tissues for other emotional situations, such as when a person experiences anxiety. When you have an interview for a new job and your palms get sweaty, your heart rate increases, and your breathing becomes quick and shallow, you are experiencing a sympathetic reaction. Again, as part of the

the effects of activation of these receptors with a sympathomimetic agent.

Parasympathetic Nervous System

The **parasympathetic nervous system (PSNS)** can be thought of as the opposite of or counterbalance to the SNS. One of the main functions of the PSNS is activation of the digestive system. This function includes secreting acidic juices, increasing peristalsis, and inducing insulin release from the pancreas. The PSNS functions while we rest and is inhibited only when the sympathetic system overrides it during periods of intense stress, as discussed previously.

The main neurotransmitter of the PSNS is acetylcholine. Acetylcholine is an important NT in both the CNS and PNS. Two types of cholinergic agents (agents that activate the PSNS) are those that mimic acetylcholine and those that stop the destruction of acetylcholine by the enzyme acetylcholinesterase. Because these cholinergic drugs mimic the PSNS, they are referred to as *parasympathomimetics*, whereas drugs that inhibit the cholinergic reaction by blocking the receptor are called *anticholinergics*. Parasympathetic receptors, which respond to acetylcholine, are located on smooth and cardiac muscle cells and in other areas of the body (see Figure 15-9).

Somatic System

The somatic system is a network of nerves that relay messages to the CNS from the outside world and return messages to the body. The spinal and cranial nerves are part of the somatic system. This system regulates the motor nerves that control voluntary actions of the skeletal muscles and impulses from sensory receptors. Receptor sites are sensitive to a stimulus and include smell, taste, touch, and hearing.

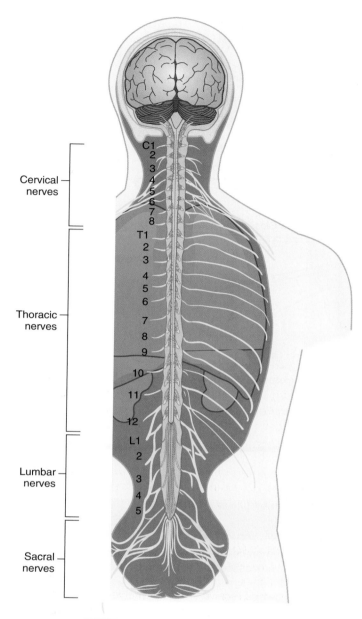

Cervical nerves

C1
2
3
4
5
6
7
8

Thoracic nerves

T1
2
3
4
5
6
7
8
9
10
11
12

Lumbar nerves

L1
2
3
4
5

Sacral nerves

FIGURE 15-7 Segments of the spinal cord.

Conditions of the Nervous System and Their Treatments

Dysfunction of the nervous system produces a multitude of conditions. Because so many conditions, disorders, and diseases can affect the brain and nervous system, only a sample of the major disorders and the medications used to treat them are discussed in detail.

Diseases and Conditions of the Peripheral Nervous System

Myasthenia Gravis

Myasthenia gravis is a rare autoimmune disorder that affects the transmission of electrical impulses from the CNS to muscles throughout the body. This

autonomic nervous system, the SNS response is an instinctive, or autonomic, reaction.

The main NTs of the SNS are norepinephrine and epinephrine. Four main types of receptors respond to these NTs. Alpha-1 receptors are located in peripheral blood vessels, the heart, and the eyes. Alpha-2 receptors are located primarily on smooth muscle. Beta-1 receptors are located primarily in heart muscle, and beta-2 receptors are located in the respiratory system, blood vessels, and elsewhere in the body. Drugs that mimic natural SNS neurotransmitters are referred to as *sympathomimetics* or *adrenergics,* and drugs used to block their actions are called *sympatholytics* or are named after the specific receptor they inhibit (e.g., beta-blockers). Table 15-2 lists

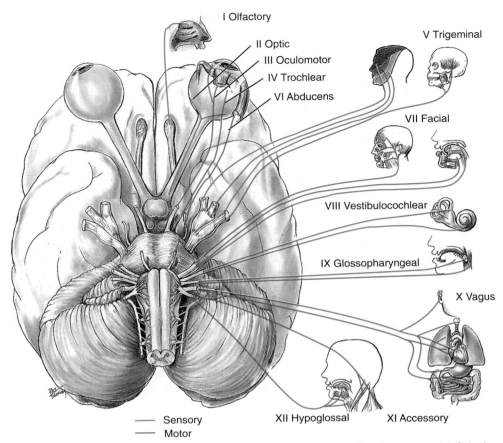

I Olfactory
II Optic
III Oculomotor
IV Trochlear
VI Abducens
V Trigeminal
VII Facial
VIII Vestibulocochlear
IX Glossopharyngeal
X Vagus
XII Hypoglossal
XI Accessory

— Sensory
— Motor

FIGURE 15-8 Cranial nerves. (From Applegate E: *The anatomy and physiology learning system,* ed 4, St Louis, 2010, Saunders.)

TABLE 15-1

Primary Functions of the Cranial Nerves

Cranial Nerve Number	Cranial Nerve Name	Function
I	Olfactory	Associated with smell. Mucous membranes in the nose transmit information to a region in the cerebral cortex that processes and then sends a response to the sensory information.
II	Optic	Associated with vision. The optic nerves receive an image that is captured by the retina. These messages travel via the optic nerve through the thalamus to the visual cortex, where they are processed.
III	Oculomotor	Oculomotor muscles are involved in movement of specific regions of the eye and eyelid.
IV	Trochlear	The trochlear nerves control another area of the eye involved in eye movement.
V	Trigeminal	Located in the brainstem; provides sensation to the face, scalp, nasal mucous membranes, mouth, and eyes. It is also responsible for sensation in the skin and muscles of the jaw.
VI	Abducens	Another cranial nerve involved in eye movement.
VII	Facial	Involved in sensation of taste in the front of the tongue. Linked to face and head muscles; results in facial expressions.
VIII	Vestibulocochlear	Linked to inner ear (hearing) and responsible for sense of balance.
IX	Glossopharyngeal	Linked to sinus, back of tongue, soft palate, parotid gland, and reflexive control of the heart. Also plays a role in swallowing.
X	Vagus	Extends from the brainstem through the neck and then through the chest and abdominal cavity. Involved in functions such as swallowing, breathing, speaking, heartbeat, and digestion. Linked to other nerves, receiving messages from the ear, pharynx, esophagus, chest, and abdominal area.
XI	Spinal accessory	Composed of two divisions. The cranial branch controls muscles of the pharynx, larynx, and palate, contributing to swallowing and movement of the digestive tract. The spinal branch is involved in muscle movement of the upper shoulders, head, and neck.
XII	Hypoglossal	The hypoglossal nerve controls the muscles of the tongue.

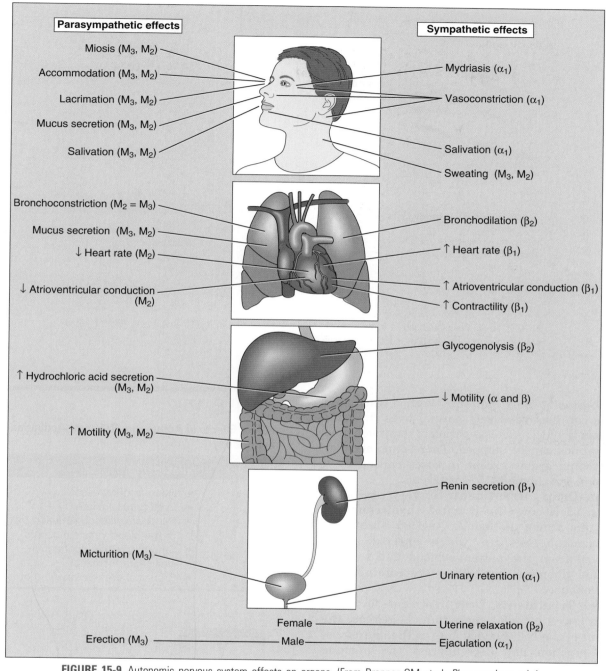

Parasympathetic effects

Miosis (M$_3$, M$_2$)

Accommodation (M$_3$, M$_2$)

Lacrimation (M$_3$, M$_2$)

Mucus secretion (M$_3$, M$_2$)

Salivation (M$_3$, M$_2$)

Bronchoconstriction (M$_2$ = M$_3$)

Mucus secretion (M$_3$, M$_2$)

↓ Heart rate (M$_2$)

↓ Atrioventricular conduction (M$_2$)

↑ Hydrochloric acid secretion (M$_3$, M$_2$)

↑ Motility (M$_3$, M$_2$)

Micturition (M$_3$)

Erection (M$_3$)

Sympathetic effects

Mydriasis (α$_1$)

Vasoconstriction (α$_1$)

Salivation (α$_1$)

Sweating (M$_3$, M$_2$)

Bronchodilation (β$_2$)

↑ Heart rate (β$_1$)

↑ Atrioventricular conduction (β$_1$)

↑ Contractility (β$_1$)

Glycogenolysis (β$_2$)

↓ Motility (α and β)

Renin secretion (β$_1$)

Urinary retention (α$_1$)

Female — Uterine relaxation (β$_2$)

Male — Ejaculation (α$_1$)

FIGURE 15-9 Autonomic nervous system effects on organs. (From Brenner GM et al: *Pharmacology*, ed 4, Philadelphia, 2014, Saunders.)

results in musculoskeletal weakness affecting areas such as the muscles of the throat, eye, and eyelid, in addition to muscles that voluntarily control facial movement. Although the muscles in the face, eyes, and mouth are most commonly affected, the disease can affect other areas. Vocal and visual difficulties may occur, and drooping of the eyelids is a common symptom. Muscles are easily fatigued and take a much longer time to recover from activity. This is a chronic disease that if not treated worsens over time. Myasthenia gravis is caused by the production of anti–acetylcholine receptor (nicotinic receptor) anti-bodies that diminish signals from the nerves to the muscles, leading to the characteristic muscle fatigue seen in this condition (Figure 15-10). Accordingly, diagnostic tests can confirm the disease, including a blood test that detects acetylcholine receptor antibodies.

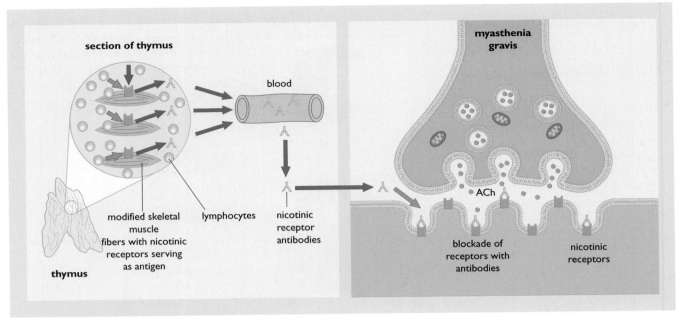

FIGURE 15-10 Postulated source of antigen and antibody production in myasthenia gravis. (From Page CP et al: *Integrated pharmacology,* ed 3, Philadelphia, 2006, Mosby.)

Prognosis. Most patients with myasthenia gravis can lead relatively normal lives. In some patients the disease has a period of remission, and medications can be stopped. There is no cure for myasthenia gravis except in cases caused by a tumor in the thymus (15% of cases).

Non–Drug Treatment. Surgery is performed to remove the thymus (thymectomy) if a thymic tumor is found. Another treatment is plasmapheresis, in which antibodies are removed from the patient's blood and healthy immune globulins (antibodies) are administered intravenously.

Drug Treatments. Drug treatments for myasthenia gravis include agents that (1) increase the amount of the NT acetylcholine at the neuromuscular junction and (2) suppress the immune system. Anticholinesterase medications (e.g., pyridostigmine) are frequently used to treat myasthenia gravis. These drugs work by inhibiting the destruction of acetylcholine by the enzyme acetylcholinesterase. They improve neuronal transmission and increase muscle strength. Side effects of these medications may occur because of overstimulation of the parasympathetic nervous system, resulting in nausea, vomiting, diarrhea, and severe abdominal pain. Immunosuppressant drugs (e.g., azathioprine, cyclosporine, or prednisone) may be administered to slow the progression of the disease by reducing the formation of anti–acetylcholine receptor antibodies.

TABLE 15-2

Select Effects of Adrenergic Receptor Activation in the Body

Receptor	Effects
alpha-1	• Heart rate increases • Eyes (pupils) dilate • Peripheral vasoconstriction (narrowing of the blood vessels) occurs
alpha-2	• Smooth muscle contraction
beta-1	• Heart rate increases
beta-2	• Bronchial dilation (opening of airway)

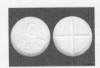

GENERIC NAME: pyridostigmine
TRADE NAME: Mestinon
INDICATION: Myasthenia gravis
ROUTE OF ADMINISTRATION: Oral; injection
COMMON ADULT DOSAGE: *Oral:* 60-1500 mg per day in divided doses
MECHANISM OF ACTION: Potentiates the actions of acetylcholine by inhibition of acetylcholinesterase
SIDE EFFECTS: Dizziness, headache, diarrhea, flatulence
AUXILIARY LABEL:
• Take with food or milk.

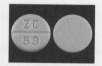

GENERIC NAME: azathioprine
TRADE NAME: Imuran
INDICATION: Autoimmune disease
ROUTE OF ADMINISTRATION: Oral
COMMON ADULT DOSAGE: 2-3 mg/kg/day
MECHANISM OF ACTION: Inhibits the production of
  anti–acetylcholine receptor antibodies
SIDE EFFECTS: Nausea, vomiting, increased risk of
  infection

Polyneuropathy

Polyneuropathy is typically characterized by distal loss of sensation, burning, or weakness, depending on the nerves involved. Polyneuropathy has a number of causes, including diabetes mellitus, alcohol abuse, and human immunodeficiency virus (HIV) infection, among others. Polyneuropathy also can be a side effect of certain medications. One of the most common forms of polyneuropathy is diabetic neuropathy. Diabetic neuropathy is thought to be caused by a variety of metabolic, vascular, and hormonal factors that lead to nerve damage. Prevention of diabetic neuropathy is the cornerstone of management, and the management of blood sugar is important to the prevention of this condition. Symptoms of diabetic polyneuropathy (which often involves the feet) can include an array of symptoms, from numbness to tingling to pain in the feet.

Prognosis. Polyneuropathies, in general, are conditions that slowly progress over time. As noted under Drug Treatments, many polyneuropathies (e.g., painful diabetic polyneuropathy) are difficult to treat. In other cases, however, the condition can be self-limited, and symptoms spontaneously improve in some cases.

Non–Drug Treatment. In addition to drug therapy, transcutaneous electrical nerve stimulation (TENS) has demonstrated benefits in some studies of patients with painful diabetic polyneuropathy. Foot care, in the form of daily foot inspections, is also critical to prevent ulceration, infection, and amputation.

Drug Treatments. Painful diabetic polyneuropathy is characteristically difficult to treat. People often try multiple therapies before they find a medicine or combination of medicines that

works well for them. Drugs used for the treatment of painful diabetic polyneuropathy include antidepressant agents (e.g., duloxetine, venlafaxine, and amitriptyline), anticonvulsants (e.g., gabapentin and pregabalin), narcotic pain medications (e.g., oxycodone and tramadol), anesthetic medications (e.g., lidocaine), and over-the-counter medicines (e.g., capsaicin creams).

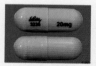

GENERIC NAME: duloxetine
TRADE NAME: Cymbalta
INDICATION: Diabetic neuropathy
ROUTE OF ADMINISTRATION: Oral
COMMON ADULT DOSAGE: 60 mg daily
MECHANISM OF ACTION: Inhibits the reuptake of both
  serotonin and norepinephrine, thus increasing the
  availability of these neurotransmitters
SIDE EFFECTS: Dizziness, increased blood pressure,
  headache
AUXILIARY LABEL:
• Administer without regard to meals.

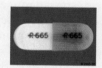

GENERIC NAME: gabapentin
TRADE NAME: Neurontin
INDICATION: Neuropathic pain
ROUTE OF ADMINISTRATION: Oral
COMMON ADULT DOSAGE: 900-1800 mg/day in divided
  doses
MECHANISM OF ACTION: Increases the gamma-
  aminobutyric acid (GABA) response (GABA is the
  primary inhibitory NT in the CNS)
SIDE EFFECTS: Fatigue, peripheral edema
AUXILIARY LABEL:
• Administer without regard to meals.

GENERIC NAME: capsaicin cream
TRADE NAME: Zostrix
INDICATION: Diabetic polyneuropathy

ROUTE OF ADMINISTRATION: Topical
COMMON ADULT DOSAGE: Apply to the affected area two to four times daily
MECHANISM OF ACTION: Depletion of substance P in peripheral sensory neurons; substance P is the primary chemical mediator of pain impulses from the periphery to the CNS
SIDE EFFECTS: Skin irritation (burning, stinging, and itching)
AUXILIARY LABEL:
- Avoid contact with eyes and mucous membranes.

Diseases and Conditions of the Central Nervous System

Epilepsy

Epilepsy is a seizure disorder marked by hyperexcitability in some of the nerve cells in the brain. The two main types of seizures are partial seizures and generalized seizures. Partial seizures affect only one hemisphere of the brain and may result in relatively mild symptoms. Generalized seizures affect both hemispheres and have different levels of intensity, ranging from petit mal seizures (the least violent) to grand mal seizures, which are longer and more intense. Children with epilepsy often have petit mal seizures, causing them to stare into the distance for a time. In grand mal seizures, also known as *tonic-clonic seizures,* the person loses consciousness and falls to the ground; a period of widespread muscle spasms (tonic phase) is followed by a period of muscle relaxation (clonic phase). Injuries can occur, depending on where and when the seizure takes place. The person having the seizure does not remember the episode. Table 15-3 outlines various seizure types.

Prognosis. Although there is no known cure for epilepsy, most people live relatively normal lives with drug treatment or surgical intervention. Social stigmas are associated with this condition that can cause embarrassment and frustration. Women must consult with their physicians about the risks of taking seizure medications while pregnant.

Non–Drug Treatment. If medication does not control seizures, surgery may be necessary to remove lesions in the brain; however, surgery is not always an effective treatment approach.

Drug Treatments. Monotherapy (one drug) or polytherapy (more than one drug) may be prescribed. Anticonvulsants (Table 15-4) are normally prescribed to reduce the number of seizures. Anticonvulsants prevent abnormal impulses in the CNS by inhibiting one or more of the ions involved in nerve conduction, such as sodium, calcium, or potassium. Drug interactions are common with the anticonvulsants, and it is important that pharmacy technicians and pharmacists be on the lookout for drug interaction warnings when processing anticonvulsant prescriptions. Benzodiazepines (discussed with the treatment of anxiety) are also used for the treatment of epilepsy.

GENERIC NAME: carbamazepine
TRADE NAME: Tegretol, Tegretol-XR
INDICATION: Generalized tonic-clonic, partial seizures
ROUTE OF ADMINISTRATION: Oral
COMMON ADULT DOSAGE: 200-1200 mg/day in divided doses
MECHANISM OF ACTION: Blocks sodium channels, inhibiting repetitive firing of neurons
SIDE EFFECTS: Dizziness, drowsiness, dry mouth, headache
AUXILIARY LABELS:
- May cause dizziness or drowsiness.
- Take with food.
- Do not stop taking abruptly.

GENERIC NAME: phenytoin
TRADE NAME: Dilantin, Phenytek
INDICATION: Partial seizures, tonic-clonic seizures, status epilepticus
ROUTE OF ADMINISTRATION: Oral; injection
COMMON ADULT DOSAGE: 4-7 mg/kg/day
MECHANISM OF ACTION: Decreases the seizure threshold through effects on sodium channels
SIDE EFFECTS: Dizziness, insomnia, nausea, vomiting, headache
AUXILIARY LABEL:
- Do not stop taking abruptly.

GENERIC NAME: ethosuximide
TRADE NAME: Zarontin

TABLE 15-3

Types of Seizures

Type	Description
Partial Seizures	
Simple partial motor type	Involves stiffening or jerking in one extremity followed by a tingling sensation in the same area. Consciousness is not normally lost, although the seizure may progress to a generalized seizure.
Simple partial sensory type	Involves perceptual distortion, including hallucinations.
Complex partial type	Effects vary and may include purposeless behavior. The patient experiences an aura immediately before the seizure begins that may include a pungent smell, nausea, a dreamy sensation, an unusual taste, or a visual disturbance. Behavior changes may include glassy stare, picking at one's clothing, aimless wandering, lip-smacking or lip-chewing motions, and unintelligible speech. Symptoms may last seconds to 20 minutes. Mental confusion may continue after seizure.
Generalized Seizures	
Absence (petit mal)	Brief change in level of consciousness, indicated by blinking or rolling of the eyes, a blank stare, and slight mouth movements. Patient retains posture. Seizures normally last no longer than 10 seconds, although they may repeat often throughout the day. Most often affects children.
Myoclonic (bilateral massive epileptic myoclonus)	Brief, involuntary muscular jerks of the body or extremities.
Tonic-clonic (grand mal)	Typically starts with a loud cry attributable to air rushing from the lungs through the vocal cords; the patient falls to the ground and loses consciousness, and the body stiffens and then alternates between spasms and relaxation phases.
Akinetic seizure	General loss of postural tone and temporary loss of consciousness; also known as *drop attack;* often occurs in children.
Status epilepticus	Continuous seizure that can occur in all types of seizures and may be accompanied by a loss of consciousness and respiratory distress; a life-threatening event. May occur as a result of abrupt withdrawal of anticonvulsant medications, head trauma, encephalopathy, or septicemia caused by meningitis.

TABLE 15-4

Select Anticonvulsants for the Treatment of Epilepsy

Medication Class	Generic Name	Brand Name	Common Adult Oral Dose
Anticonvulsants	carbamazepine	Tegretol, Tegretol XR	400-1200 mg per day
	divalproex sodium	Depakote, Depakote ER	10-60 mg/kg per day
	ethosuximide	Zarontin	500-1500 mg per day
	lacosamide	Vimpat	100-400 mg per day
	lamotrigine	Lamictal	50-400 mg per day
	levetiracetam	Keppra	1000-3000 mg per day
	oxcarbazepine	Trileptal	600-2400 mg per day
	phenytoin	Dilantin	4-7 mg/kg per day
	tiagabine	Gabitril	32-56 mg per day
	topiramate	Topamax	50-1600 mg per day
	vigabatrin	Sabril	1000-1500 mg per day
	zonisamide	Zonegran	100-600 mg per day

INDICATION: Absence seizures
ROUTE OF ADMINISTRATION: Oral
COMMON ADULT DOSAGE: 250 mg twice daily initially, titrated up to 1.5 g given in two divided doses
MECHANISM OF ACTION: Treats seizures through effects on calcium channels
SIDE EFFECTS: Drowsiness, nausea, vomiting, headache
AUXILIARY LABELS:
- May cause dizziness or drowsiness.
- Do not stop taking abruptly.

GENERIC NAME: diazepam (C-IV)
TRADE NAME: Valium, Diastat Rectal Gel
INDICATION: Status epilepticus, intermittent treatment of generalized tonic-clonic seizures
ROUTE OF ADMINISTRATION: Oral; rectal gel; injection
COMMON ADULT DOSAGE: *Oral:* 2-10 mg two to four times daily
MECHANISM OF ACTION: Benzodiazepine (binds to benzodiazepine receptor and activates GABA inhibitory response)
SIDE EFFECTS: Drowsiness
AUXILIARY LABELS:
- May cause dizziness or drowsiness.
- For rectal use only (Diastat Rectal Gel).
- Do not stop taking abruptly.
- Do not drink alcohol.
- Caution: Federal law prohibits the transfer of this drug to any person other than the patient for whom it was prescribed.

Alzheimer's Disease

Alzheimer's disease (AD) is a progressive disease associated with memory loss, confusion, impaired judgment, personality changes, disorientation, and loss of language skills. AD is most common in the elderly, although it can occasionally occur in younger adults. Although multiple types of dementia (progressive conditions of deteriorating cognitive function) have been recognized, AD is the most common and accounts for 50% to 70% of cases. People with AD have been shown to have decreased acetylcholine production in the brain, which is why acetylcholinesterase inhibitors are frequently used to treat AD.

Currently, three major categories of AD have been described: early stage, mid-stage, and late stage. Not all patients experience the onset and progression of AD in the same way, but a classification of disease progression is sometimes helpful for the family and physician monitor the severity of the disease. Additionally, seven specific stages are often used to classify the progression of AD (Table 15-5).

Prognosis. Although medication may slow the progression of AD in some cases, no treatments are available to stop the progression of the disease. AD affects every individual differently as it progresses. The deterioration of normal functions, such as swallowing, the inability to move, and the total absence of communicative or cognitive skills, are seen in late-stage AD.

Non–Drug Treatment. In addition to the use of drugs to help slow the progression of AD, skilled care is often needed for individuals in the later stages. Education is important for the patient, family, and friends to help them understand the progression and effects of AD and have realistic expectations for treatment.

Drug Treatment. Two classifications of drugs have been approved for use by the U.S. Food and Drug Administration (FDA) to treat AD: acetylcholinesterase inhibitors (which prevent the breakdown of acetylcholine) and memantine (Table 15-6). Drug treatment may help delay progression of the disease, but it typically does not result in improvements in memory or other symptoms of AD.

Parkinson's Disease

Parkinson's disease (PD) is a progressive disorder of the basal ganglia and is associated with the loss or deficiency of the NT dopamine. The basal ganglia are a group of cells in the medulla of the cerebrum. The function of the basal ganglia is to regulate skeletal muscle activity and body movement. The overall degeneration of dopamine-producing neurons instigates the symptoms of Parkinson's disease (Figure 15-11). Because PD is a progressive disease, the severity of symptoms becomes more pronounced over time. The hallmark symptoms of PD can be remembered by the acronym TRAP, which stands for *t*remor, *r*igidity, *a*kinesia (or **bradykinesia**), and *p*ostural instability. Over time, physical movement slows in people with PD to the point that they can become wheelchair bound. Other problems, such as swallowing and speech difficulties, constipation, and even cognitive impairment, are associated with PD. Although the cause of PD is unknown, its development has been linked to genetics and environmental influences.

TABLE 15-5

Stages Associated with Alzheimer's Disease (AD)*

Stage	Symptom	Description
1	No impairment or normal functioning	Normal function; person does not show signs or symptoms of disease.
2	Very mild decline	Earliest signs of AD. Person is aware of memory loss; forgets familiar words and the location of common household items. No signs of AD seen upon physician's examination and within family unit or friends.
3	Mild cognitive decline	Signs appear as problems of memory loss continue. May not be able to remember names of people; reads less because of a decrease in memory retention; loses more items, including those that are valuable; and exhibits a decline in planning or organizational skills. Presence of disease becomes measurable in a clinical/medical interview.
4	Moderate cognitive decline	Mild or early-stage AD; deficiencies become evident as condition progresses. Decreased knowledge of recent occasions or current events in the world; cannot perform tasks related to more complex cognitive functions, such as managing finances, planning dinner functions, or performing mathematical calculations (e.g., counting backwards by 7). Person suffers reduced memory of personal history and may become withdrawn from individuals and group situations.
5	Moderately severe cognitive decline	Moderate or mild-stage AD; may include major gaps in memory and in daily activities. Person may not remember home address or phone number, may not remember day of week or month of year, and has trouble performing basic math manipulations (counting backwards by 2s). Still, person knows own name and names of immediate family members; does not require assistance with functions such as eating or using the toilet.
6	Severe cognitive decline	Moderately severe or mid-stage AD. Characterized by significant personality changes (e.g., becomes suspicious of caretakers, has hallucinations), exhibits wandering behavior, occasionally forgets names of family members, cannot dress self or go to the toilet (increasing episodes of incontinence). May experience a disruption in sleep-wake cycle and may begin repetitive behaviors such as hand-wringing or shredding tissues.
7	Very severe cognitive decline	Severe or late-stage AD. Last stage of AD; person loses the ability to speak, control movements, or respond to environment. Eventually may lose ability to feed self, use the toilet, walk without assistance, or sit without support. May not be able to smile or hold head up, and as reflexes continue to decline, muscles become rigid and swallowing is impaired.

*Although this is a guide to the stages of AD, not all individuals show these signs in this order, and the rate at which AD progresses varies from person to person.

TABLE 15-6

Select Medications Approved for the Treatment of Alzheimer's Disease

Medication Class	Generic Name	Brand Name	Common Side Effects	Common Dose Range
Acetylcholinesterase Inhibitors	donepezil galantamine	Aricept Razadyne	• Gastrointestinal side effects • Weight loss • Slowed heart rate	• 5-23 mg daily • *Immediate release:* 4-12 mg twice daily • *Extended release:* 8-24 mg once daily
	rivastigmine	Exelon		• *Oral:* 3-6 mg by mouth twice daily • *Patch:* 4.6-9.5 mg/24 hours
N-Methyl-D-Aspartate (NMDA) Receptor Antagonist	memantine	Namenda	• Dizziness • Headache • Fatigue	• *Immediate release:* 10 mg twice daily • *Extended release:* 28 mg once daily

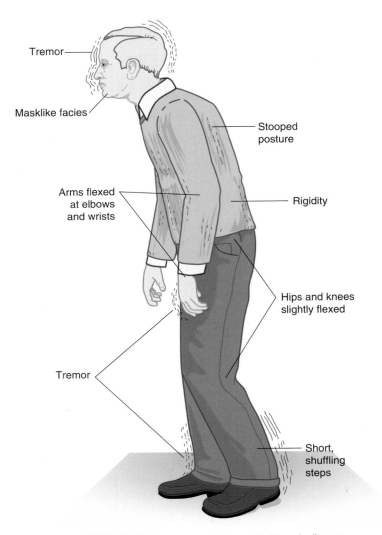

Tremor

Masklike facies

Stooped posture

Arms flexed at elbows and wrists

Rigidity

Hips and knees slightly flexed

Tremor

Short, shuffling steps

FIGURE 15-11 Symptoms and signs of Parkinson's disease.

Prognosis. The course of PD can vary from person to person. Typically this is a slow, progressive disorder that affects the person over several years. Many people can live somewhat normally with the help of medications, exercise, and maintenance of overall good health. As the disease progresses, however, management of the disease with medications becomes increasingly difficult in most cases.

Non–Drug Treatment. Non–drug treatments include lifestyle interventions, various types of therapy, and surgery. As mentioned previously, PD is a disease that leads to slowing of movement. Accordingly, staying active is incredibly important for people with PD to maintain their functionality. Working with physical therapy, occupational therapy, and speech therapy also can help maintain functionality with activities of daily living, movement, and speech. For individuals with advanced disease who are unable to control their symptoms well with medical therapy, a surgical procedure known as deep brain stimulation (DMS) can be performed. In this surgery, electrodes are inserted into certain areas in the brain that can help some people better control their motor (movement) symptoms.

Drug Treatment. Several medications are currently used for the treatment of the motor symptoms of PD (Table 15-7). Levodopa/carbidopa is the "gold standard" treatment for PD, although a variety of different medication regimens can be used. Because PD can be difficult to differentiate clinically from other movement disorders, administration of PD medications (e.g., levodopa/carbidopa) is often used to assist in diagnosing the disease.

Tech Note!

People with PD are very in tune with their medication needs. Many physicians allow people with PD to dose their medications according to their symptoms on any given day. Because of this, people with PD are often much less regimented with their medication instructions than are people receiving treatment for other medical conditions.

TABLE 15-7

Select Medications Approved for the Treatment of Parkinson's Disease (PD)

Generic Name	Brand Name	Common Side Effects	Common Dose Range
Levodopa/Carbidopa			
Levodopa is converted to dopamine in the central nervous system (CNS), which helps manage the motor symptoms of PD; carbidopa blocks the peripheral conversion of levodopa to dopamine so that it can reach the CNS.			
levodopa/carbidopa	Sinemet, Sinemet CR	• Nausea • Confusion • Dizziness • Hallucinations • Dyskinesia	• 25-100 mg 3 times daily titrated to effect; dose and frequency can vary significantly based on individual needs
Dopamine Agonists			
Dopamine agonists mimic the actions of dopamine in the CNS to help treat the motor symptoms of PD.			
pramipexole	Mirapex, Mirapex XL	• Nausea • Vomiting • Peripheral Edema • Hallucinations • Compulsive behavior	• *Immediate release:* 0.375-4.5 mg given 3 times daily • *XL:* 0.375-4.5 mg once daily
ropinirole	Requip, Requip XL		• *Immediate release:* 0.75-24 mg day given 3 times daily • *XL:* 2-24 mg once daily
rotigotine	Neupro		• *Patch:* 2-8 mg/day
Amantadine			
Amantadine may increase dopamine availability in the CNS; it also may help due to its anticholinergic effects.			
amantadine	Symmetrel	• Nausea • Vomiting • Peripheral edema	• 100-400 mg daily given 1-2 times daily
Catechol-O-Methyltransferase (COMT) Inhibitors			
Prevents the peripheral conversion of levodopa by the enzyme COMT.			
entacapone	Comtan	• Red discoloration of body fluids • Diarrhea • Abdominal pain • Dry mouth	• 200 mg with each dose of levodopa/carbidopa
tolcapone	Tasmar		• 100-200 mg given 3 times daily
Monoamine Oxidase-B Inhibitors (MAO$_B$-I)			
Inhibition of MAO-B decreases the metabolism of dopamine in the CNS.			
selegiline	Eldepryl, Zelapar	• Nausea • Dizziness • Headache • Insomnia	• *Eldepryl:* 5 mg twice daily or 10 mg in the morning • *Zelapar:* 1.25-2.5 mg daily in the morning
rasagiline	Azilect		• 0.5-1 mg daily
Anticholinergics			
Anticholinergic activity reduces the excessive cholinergic activity present in PD.			
benztropine	Cogentin	• Constipation • Dry mouth • Blurred vision • Urinary retention • Confusion	• 1-6 mg per day divided twice daily
trihexyphenidyl	Artane		• 1-15 mg daily given in divided doses

GENERIC NAME: levodopa/carbidopa
TRADE NAME: Sinemet, Sinemet CR
INDICATION: Parkinson's disease
ROUTE OF ADMINISTRATION: Oral
COMMON ADULT DOSAGE: Doses very individualized, based on patient's needs
MECHANISM OF ACTION: Levodopa is converted to dopamine in the CNS, which helps manage the motor symptoms of PD. Carbidopa prevents the peripheral conversion of levodopa to dopamine so more levodopa can penetrate the CNS
SIDE EFFECTS: Nausea, dizziness, hallucinations, dyskinesia (excessive, uncontrolled movements)
AUXILIARY LABEL:
• May cause dizziness or drowsiness.

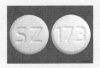

GENERIC NAME: pramipexole
TRADE NAME: Mirapex, Mirapex XL
INDICATION: Parkinson's disease, restless leg syndrome
ROUTE OF ADMINISTRATION: Oral
COMMON ADULT DOSAGE: 1.5-4.5 mg per day in divided doses
MECHANISM OF ACTION: Dopamine agonist (mimics the actions of dopamine)
SIDE EFFECTS: Nausea, peripheral edema, hallucinations, compulsive behavior
AUXILIARY LABEL:
• May cause dizziness or drowsiness.

GENERIC NAME: rotigotine
TRADE NAME: Neupro
INDICATION: Parkinson's disease (can be used with other antiparkinsonian agents), restless leg syndrome
ROUTE OF ADMINISTRATION: Transdermal patch
COMMON ADULT DOSAGE: 4- to 8-mg patch daily (available in 1-, 2-, 3-, 4-, 6-, and 8-mg patches)

MECHANISM OF ACTION: Dopamine agonist (mimics the actions of dopamine)
SIDE EFFECTS: Nausea, peripheral edema, hallucinations, compulsive behavior, application site irritation
AUXILIARY LABEL:
• May cause dizziness or drowsiness.

Multiple Sclerosis

Multiple sclerosis (MS) is a chronic neurological condition that affects the integrity of the myelin sheath on neurons in the CNS. Myelin covers the axon portion of neurons and helps facilitate proper nerve transmission throughout the nervous system. MS is an autoimmune disorder in which cells of the immune system break down the myelin sheath (Figure 15-12). After they are damaged by the immune system, the myelin sheaths are replaced by plaques of sclerotic (hard) tissue. When this occurs, the electrical impulses cannot pass from one neuron to another effectively, leading to impaired movements and other neurological deficits. As with many conditions discussed in this chapter, the course of MS can be quite variable from one individual to the next; therefore, a series of MS "types" (Table 15-8) often is used to describe the clinical course. Symptoms can range from mild to severe and may include muscle weakness, abnormal sensations such as numbness or tingling over any part of the body, vision changes, and loss of coordination.

Prognosis. The prognosis depends largely on the disease pattern and severity of MS. Those who have frequent attacks initially or who are older than age 40 before symptoms occur tend to have a poor prognosis.

Non–Drug Treatment. Physical and occupational therapy can assist with recovering and maintaining functionality in the long term and after attacks. Maximizing strength and balance is critical to avoiding falls and other potential problems.

Drug Treatment. The first treatment is disease-modifying immunotherapy (e.g., the use of interferons) to slow and minimize progression of the disease. Symptomatic short-term treatment with steroids (antiinflammatory agents) to manage flare-ups is also used. Dalfampridine is an agent that can be used to improve walking in people with MS. Medications of significant importance are those used to treat fatigue, spasticity, tremors, pain, depression, and other common conditions seen in people with MS.

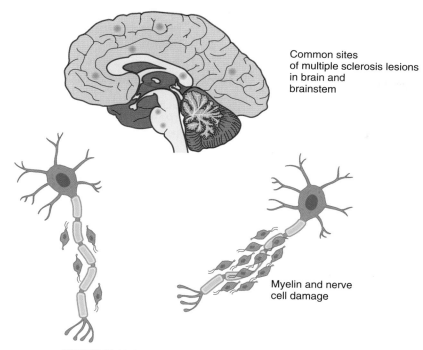

Common sites of multiple sclerosis lesions in brain and brainstem

Myelin and nerve cell damage

FIGURE 15-12 Multiple sclerosis lesions in the brain and brainstem.

TABLE 15-8

Disease Patterns or "Types" of Multiple Sclerosis (MS)

Pattern	Description
Relapsing-remitting MS	Individuals with this type of MS experience attacks (i.e., flare-ups or relapses) of worsening neurological function. These can be followed by complete recovery periods (remission). This is the most common type of MS, affecting approximately 85% of MS patients. Most patients eventually enter a secondary progressive phase.
Primary progressive MS	Individuals diagnosed with this type of MS have slowly worsening neurological functions from the onset of the disease. There are no distinct relapses or remissions. Approximately 10% of people suffer from this type of MS.
Secondary progressive MS	In this type of MS the disease worsens more steadily, with or without occasional flare-ups, recovery periods, or plateaus. Many people develop this type of MS after an initial period of relapsing-remitting MS.
Progressive relapsing MS	With this type of MS, people experience a steadily worsening disease from the onset of the condition and episodes of deteriorating neurological functions with each attack. A recovery period may or may not occur, and there are no remission periods.

GENERIC NAME: interferon beta-1a
TRADE NAME: Avonex
INDICATION: Multiple sclerosis
ROUTE OF ADMINISTRATION: Intramuscular (IM) injection

COMMON ADULT DOSAGE: 30 mcg every week
MECHANISM OF ACTION: Inhibits the production of proinflammatory mediators responsible for triggering autoimmune reactions in MS
SIDE EFFECTS: Dizziness, headache, stomach pain, runny/stuffy nose, depression
AUXILIARY LABELS:
- For intramuscular use only.
- May cause dizziness.
- Refrigerate.

GENERIC NAME: interferon beta-1a
TRADE NAME: Rebif
INDICATION: Multiple sclerosis
ROUTE OF ADMINISTRATION: Subcutaneous (SUBCUT) injection
COMMON ADULT DOSAGE: 22 or 44 mcg three times weekly
MECHANISM OF ACTION: Inhibits the production of proinflammatory mediators responsible for triggering autoimmune reactions in MS
SIDE EFFECTS: Headache, weakness or muscle pain, insomnia, injection site reactions, depression
AUXILIARY LABELS:
• For subcutaneous use only.
• Refrigerate.

 Tech Note!
Interferon agents should be used cautiously in people with depression.

GENERIC NAME: interferon beta-1b
TRADE NAME: Betaseron
INDICATION: Multiple sclerosis
ROUTE OF ADMINISTRATION: SUBCUT injection
COMMON ADULT DOSAGE: 0.25 mg every other day
MECHANISM OF ACTION: Inhibits the production of proinflammatory mediators responsible for triggering autoimmune reactions in MS
SIDE EFFECTS: Headache, weakness or muscle pain, insomnia, injection site reactions, depression
AUXILIARY LABELS:
• For subcutaneous use only.
• Refrigerate.

GENERIC NAME: glatiramer
TRADE NAME: Copaxone
INDICATION: Multiple sclerosis
ROUTE OF ADMINISTRATION: SUBCUT injection
COMMON ADULT DOSAGE: 20 mg daily
MECHANISM OF ACTION: Modifies immune processes responsible for MS; the exact mechanism is unknown
SIDE EFFECTS: Injection site edema, rash, infection
AUXILIARY LABELS:
• For subcutaneous use only.
• Refrigerate.

GENERIC NAME: dalfampridine
TRADE NAME: Ampyra
INDICATION: For improved walking in people with MS
ROUTE OF ADMINISTRATION: Oral
COMMON ADULT DOSAGE: 10 mg twice daily
MECHANISM OF ACTION: Potassium channel blocker; mechanism of its benefit in MS is unknown
SIDE EFFECTS: Insomnia, constipation, dizziness, headache, seizures
AUXILIARY LABEL:
• Do not divide, crush, chew, or dissolve tablets.

Migraine Headache

Migraine headaches are episodic, severe headaches that are frequently associated with nausea and/or light and sound sensitivity. The triggers for migraines can vary from one person to the next but can range from hormonal changes (e.g., before menstruation, during pregnancy, and with contraceptive use) to foods, stress, bright lights, and other changes in the environment. In some cases, no identifiable cause is found. Drugs may also influence the frequency and severity of migraines. Serotonin is thought to be involved in the development of migraine, and interestingly, serotonin agonists (drugs that activate serotonin receptors) are frequently used in the treatment of migraine. Migraine headaches are relatively common and are estimated to affect approximately 12% of the population.

Prognosis. No cure exists for migraine headaches. A variety of medications can be taken once a migraine occurs (some of which are listed in the following drug monographs), and a number of treatments can be tried to prevent migraines (prophylactic therapy). Although finding the right drug or combination of drugs to control migraines adequately may be difficult, once the correct medication has been determined, migraines can be managed effectively and will not interfere with the patient's lifestyle.

Non–Drug Treatment. Non–drug treatment includes using preventive measures (i.e., avoidance of triggers) and following an exercise regimen. Headache diaries can be very helpful in identifying triggers.

Drug Treatments. For mild to moderate migraines the first line of treatment typically involves nonsteroidal antiinflammatory drugs (NSAIDs) or combination analgesics. For people who do not respond to NSAIDs, migraine-specific agents, such as triptans, are indicated. Some triptans (e.g., sumatriptan) are available in non-oral formulations for people who experience nausea and vomiting and cannot use an oral medication. People who experience frequent migraines can use prophylactic medications, including blood pressure medications (i.e., beta-blockers, calcium channel blockers), antidepressants (e.g., tricyclic antidepressants [TCAs], selective serotonin reuptake inhibitors [SSRIs]), some anticonvulsants (e.g., topiramate), and others. These may be prescribed as monotherapy or polytherapy, depending on the individual. Narcotic pain medications are also used in some instances.

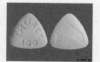

GENERIC NAME: sumatriptan
TRADE NAME: Imitrex
INDICATION: Migraine
ROUTE OF ADMINISTRATION: Oral; nasal spray; SUBCUT injection
COMMON ADULT DOSAGE: *Oral:* 25-100 mg upon onset of migraine, dose may be repeated if necessary (not to exceed 200 mg); *nasal spray:* 1 spray into nostril, may repeat in 2 hours (alternate nostrils) × 1 (max

40 mg/24 hr); *SUBCUT injection:* 6 mg, dose may be repeated if necessary (max 12 mg/24 hr)
MECHANISM OF ACTION: Binds serotonin receptors, leading to inhibited vasodilation and inflammation
SIDE EFFECTS: Dizziness, nausea, tiredness
AUXILIARY LABELS:
- May cause dizziness or drowsiness.
- Take with water.

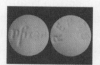

GENERIC NAME: eletriptan
TRADE NAME: Relpax
INDICATION: Migraine
ROUTE OF ADMINISTRATION: Oral
COMMON ADULT DOSAGE: 20-40 mg initial dose, may repeat dose in 2 hours if needed (max 80 mg/24 hr)
MECHANISM OF ACTION: Binds serotonin receptors, leading to inhibited vasodilation and inflammation
SIDE EFFECTS: Dizziness, nausea, tiredness
AUXILIARY LABELS:
- May cause dizziness or drowsiness.
- Take with water.

Stroke

A stroke is the disruption of blood flow to the brain due to blockage of an artery or to hemorrhage (i.e., a **hemorrhagic stroke**). Although stroke has several causes, most strokes are **ischemic strokes**. This is a decrease of blood flow to the brain when blood vessels are blocked by a clot or become too narrow. The brain is then deprived of oxygen, and brain cells can die. Although the disruption is specific to the vascular system, it directly affects the nervous system (NS) and the functions associated with the NS (see Chapter 18 for a detailed discussion of medications used to prevent strokes and heart attacks). The severity of damage to the brain depends on the size of the blockage and how much brain tissue is harmed. The effects can range from weakness of a limb to paralysis of one side of the body to loss of the ability to speak. Several symptoms may occur when a person has a stroke. The most common effects include a severe headache, dizziness, visual difficulties, loss of balance or difficulty moving one side of the body, and weakness in the muscles of the facial area that can cause difficulty in speaking.

Prognosis. The prognosis depends on the severity of the damage to the brain. One of the most important factors affecting the outcome is the time that elapses before treatment begins. If a stroke is suspected, it is important to call 911 and to begin treatment as soon as possible. Quick treatment may reduce long-term symptoms. Depending on how quickly the stroke is treated and the severity of the blockage, some patients never fully recover. Most people require a strong support system; often family members become caregivers for the stroke patient.

Non–Drug Treatment. Patients often require extensive physical and/or speech therapy to regain functionality. This may take place in a rehabilitation hospital, an outpatient center, or the home. Support groups frequently can help the survivor cope with the emotional aspect of this condition.

Drug Treatment. Patients who have had an ischemic stroke and who present to the emergency department quickly after the onset of symptoms may be treated with antithrombotic medications ("clot busters") to limit the potential damage to the brain. Hemorrhagic strokes may require neurosurgery. Most of the medical treatment for ischemic strokes is aimed at prevention of future strokes. Treatment includes a range of medications that prevent blood from forming blockages, in addition to drugs that control cholesterol levels. Chapter 18 presents a detailed description of preventive agents for stroke and heart attack.

Other Conditions Associated with the Nervous System

Depression

The World Health Organization lists major depression among the most burdensome diseases in the world. In the United States, the lifetime prevalence of major depression is approximately 16%, and this incidence increases in those with chronic medical conditions such as diabetes and heart disease. There are many types of depression, ranging in severity from minor depression to major depression with thoughts of suicide. Other specific types of depression include postpartum depression (after pregnancy) and seasonal affective disorder (SAD) (depression during the winter months). Major depression can be very difficult to treat and can interfere with a person's ability to function normally; activities such as sleeping, eating, working, studying, and forms of enjoyment are disrupted. Many times this type of depression is associated with a serious illness or anxiety disorder, as noted previously.

A variety of antidepressant medications are used in the treatment of depression; these medications increase levels of NTs in the brain. Under normal circumstances, these NTs stimulate the brain as they are released and are then reabsorbed by the brain cells, where they are broken down by an enzyme called *monoamine oxidase* (MAO). Because NTs are believed to be deficient in people with depression, antidepressant medications work to increase the amount of NTs available in the brain.

Prognosis. Depression can be treated effectively in most cases using psychotherapy and/or antidepressant medications. The prognosis of any given case largely depends on the severity of depression in that individual and his or her support systems. Both short-term and long-term treatment options are available.

Non–Drug Treatment. Psychotherapy can help for short- or long-term depression. Support groups and other social-based therapies can be very helpful. Other forms of treatment include behavioral and cognitive therapy. Electroconvulsive therapy is an option for severe cases of ongoing depression that are not relieved by medications or traditional therapy sessions. For seasonal depression, light treatment may help alleviate symptoms.

Drug Treatments. Agents commonly used to treat depression include SSRIs, serotonin/norepinephrine reuptake inhibitors (SNRIs), TCAs, and monoamine oxidase inhibitors (MAOIs). These agents help increase the levels of serotonin and norepinephrine in the brain. These classes of antidepressants have variable effects in terms of efficacy, side effects, and the types of conditions they are used to treat. A serious side effect common to all antidepressants is the increased risk of suicidal thinking and behavior in children, adolescents, and young adults with major depressive disorder. MAOIs also have a very large number of side effects and cannot be taken with other antidepressants or with many other medications and foods. Table 15-9 presents a description of select antidepressants.

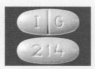

GENERIC NAME: sertraline
TRADE NAME: Zoloft

TABLE 15-9

Select Medications Approved for the Treatment of Depression

Generic Name	Brand Name	Common Side Effects	Common Dose Range
Selective Serotonin Reuptake Inhibitors (SSRIs)			
SSRIs increase the amount of serotonin available in the central nervous system (CNS).			
citalopram	Celexa	• Dizziness	• 10-40 mg daily
escitalopram	Lexapro	• Headache	• 10-20 mg daily
fluoxetine	Prozac, Prozac Weekly	• GI side effects	• 10-80 mg daily
		• Weight gain	• 90 mg weekly
paroxetine	Paxil, Paxil CR	• Sleep disturbances	• *Immediate release:* 10-50 mg daily
		• Increased risk of suicidal thinking and behavior in children, adolescents, and young adults with major depressive disorder	• *CR:* 12.5-62.5 mg daily
sertraline	Zoloft		• 25-200 mg daily
Serotonin Norepinephrine Reuptake Inhibitors (SNRIs)			
SNRIs increase the amount of serotonin and norepinephrine available in the CNS.			
desvenlafaxine	Pristiq	• Same as SSRIs	• 50-400 mg daily
duloxetine	Cymbalta		• 40-60 mg daily
venlafaxine	Effexor, Effexor XR		• *Immediate release:* 75-225 mg daily in divided doses
			• *XR:* 37.5-225 mg once daily
Tricyclic Antidepressants (TCAs)			
TCAs primarily increase the availability of norepinephrine and serotonin in the CNS.			
amitriptyline	Elavil	• Sedation	• 10-200 mg daily in single or divided doses
doxepin	Sinequan	• Drowsiness	• 25-300 mg daily in single or divided doses
nortriptyline	Aventyl	• Weight gain	• 10-150 mg daily in single or divided doses
		• Suicidal ideation	
		• Anticholinergic side effects	
Monoamine Oxidase Inhibitors (MAOIs)			
Inhibition of the MAO enzyme leads to increased availability of neurotransmitters such as norepinephrine and dopamine.			
phenelzine	Nardil	• Hypertensive crisis	• 45-90 mg daily in divided doses
		• Orthostatic hypotension	
		• Drowsiness	
		• Constipation	
		• Confusion	
Bupropion			
Bupropion increases the availability of dopamine in the CNS.			
bupropion	Wellbutrin, Wellbutrin SR, Wellbutrin XL, Aplenzin	• Insomnia	• *Immediate release:* 200-300 mg daily in divided doses
		• Dizziness	• *SR:* 150-400 mg daily in divided doses
		• Headache	• *XL:* 150-450 mg daily
		• Increased seizure risk	
Trazodone			
Trazodone increases the availability of serotonin in the CNS.			
trazodone	Desyrel	• Drowsiness	• 150-400 mg daily in divided doses
		• Dizziness	
		• Confusion	
		• Orthostatic hypotension	
Vilazodone			
Vilazodone increases the availability of serotonin in the CNS and is a 5-hydroxytryptamine receptor partial agonist.			
vilazodone	Viibryd	• Drowsiness	• 10-40 mg daily
		• Dizziness	
		• Insomnia	
		• Fatigue	
		• Abnormal dreams	

INDICATION: Depression, OCD, panic disorder, PTSD, social anxiety disorder
ROUTE OF ADMINISTRATION: Oral tablet; oral solution
COMMON ADULT DOSAGE: 25-200 mg once daily
MECHANISM OF ACTION: SSRI (increases the amount of serotonin available in the CNS)
SIDE EFFECTS: Insomnia, dizziness, drowsiness, sexual dysfunction, headache, constipation
AUXILIARY LABEL:
- Do not drink alcohol.

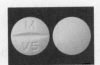

GENERIC NAME: venlafaxine
TRADE NAME: Effexor, Effexor XR
INDICATION: Depression, anxiety disorder
ROUTE OF ADMINISTRATION: Oral
COMMON ADULT DOSAGE: 75-225 mg/day
MECHANISM OF ACTION: SNRI (increases the amount of serotonin and norepinephrine available in the CNS)
SIDE EFFECTS: Dry mouth, increased blood pressure, dizziness, drowsiness
AUXILIARY LABELS:
- May cause dizziness and drowsiness.
- Do not drink alcohol.

GENERIC NAME: amitriptyline
TRADE NAME: Elavil
INDICATION: Depression
ROUTE OF ADMINISTRATION: Oral
COMMON ADULT DOSAGE: 25-300 mg daily
MECHANISM OF ACTION: TCA (increases the amount of serotonin and norepinephrine available in the CNS)
SIDE EFFECTS: Drowsiness, dry mouth, blurred vision, dizziness
AUXILIARY LABELS:
- May cause dizziness and drowsiness.
- Take with food.
- Do not drink alcohol.

GENERIC NAME: bupropion
TRADE NAME: Wellbutrin, Wellbutrin SR, Wellbutrin XL
INDICATION: Depression, seasonal affective disorder, nicotine withdrawal
ROUTE OF ADMINISTRATION: Oral
COMMON ADULT DOSAGE: *Wellbutrin:* 100-150 mg three times daily; *Wellbutrin SR:* 150-200 mg once or twice daily; *Wellbutrin XL:* 150-450 mg/day once daily
MECHANISM OF ACTION: Miscellaneous antidepressant, increases the amount of dopamine available in the CNS
SIDE EFFECTS: Dizziness, drowsiness, hallucinations, seizures
AUXILIARY LABEL:
- May cause dizziness and drowsiness.
SPECIAL NOTE: Another form of bupropion, Zyban, is used for smoking cessation; patients should not take Wellbutrin and Zyban together.

Anxiety Disorders

Anxiety is characterized by unease and fear typically associated with an event or a situation that may have an unknown outcome. Anxiety is a normal physiologic reaction. It becomes problematic when it becomes so severe that it interferes with daily personal and social interactions. Anxiety can be so severe in some individuals that it elicits panic attacks or compulsive behaviors. Anxiety can be expressed as a feeling of fear or dread, with symptoms ranging from a rapid heart rate to trembling. Anxiety disorders can be divided into several different types; the diagnosis of each type is specific to the patient's symptoms. These range from panic disorders, such as post-traumatic stress disorder (PTSD) and **phobias**, to personality disorders, such as obsessive-compulsive disorder (OCD). Some types of anxiety disorders include the following:

- *Generalized anxiety disorder (GAD):* This is a frequent condition in which a person experiences constant anxiety and worries continuously about common problems in life (e.g., money or relationships) over a period of 6 months or longer.
- *Social anxiety disorder:* Also referred to as *social phobia,* this is a condition in which the person experiences constant anxiety and extreme fear regarding being around others. The person with social anxiety disorder attempts to avoid situations in which he or she is exposed

to groups of people or needs to speak or interact with people. The avoidance stems from overwhelming fears of being humiliated, being judged, and feeling uncomfortable; the condition disrupts the person's daily life and normal daily activities.

- *Panic disorder:* An anxiety disorder in which the person experiences recurrent panic attacks. The attacks can be triggered by a situational event from the person's past. During a panic attack, the person experiences severe apprehension, fear, and terror, in addition to physical complaints such as dizziness, heart palpitations, or shakiness. Severe panic disorders can lead to phobias and PTSD.
- *PTSD:* This condition follows any incident that is either traumatic or terrifying to the person who experienced the event. Sights, sounds, and even smells can prompt flashbacks, nightmares, and constant memories. Soldiers returning from war are a common group suffering from PTSD. Other people who may suffer from PTSD include rape victims, those exposed to violence, and those diagnosed with a life-threatening medical illness. The symptoms of PTSD can occur at any time after the precipitating event.
- *Phobias:* Phobias are marked by an irrational, persistent fear of situations, people, or things. The person suffering from a phobia experiences several symptoms, including a rapid heart rate, shortness of breath, and trembling. Treatment ranges from psychotherapy to antianxiety medications.

Prognosis. With proper diagnosis and treatment, including medication and ongoing therapy, people with anxiety disorders can live relatively normal lives.

Non–Drug Treatments. Most people require psychotherapy and behavioral therapy, which can help the individual learn to resist the urges, compulsions, or other triggers that cause the abnormal response.

Drug Treatments. Primary medications used include antianxiety agents (e.g., benzodiazepines) and SSRIs.

GENERIC NAME: alprazolam (schedule IV [C-IV])
TRADE NAME: Xanax, Xanax XR

INDICATION: Anxiety disorders
ROUTE OF ADMINISTRATION: Oral
COMMON ADULT DOSAGE: 0.25-0.5 mg three times daily up to a maximum of 4 mg/day in divided doses
MECHANISM OF ACTION: Binds benzodiazepine receptors leading to CNS depression
SIDE EFFECTS: Drowsiness, dizziness, dry mouth
AUXILIARY LABELS:
- May cause dizziness and drowsiness.
- Avoid alcohol.
- Caution: Federal law prohibits the transfer of this drug to any person other than the patient for whom it was prescribed.

 Tech Note!

All benzodiazepine medications are schedule IV medications.

GENERIC NAME: buspirone
TRADE NAME: BuSpar
INDICATION: Anxiety disorders
ROUTE OF ADMINISTRATION: Oral
COMMON ADULT DOSAGE: 7.5-30 mg twice daily
MECHANISM OF ACTION: Not well understood, but suppresses serotonergic activity while enhancing noradrenergic and dopaminergic activity. The net effect is improvement in anxiety symptoms
SIDE EFFECTS: Drowsiness, dizziness, nausea
AUXILIARY LABEL:
- May cause dizziness and drowsiness.

Bipolar Disorder

Bipolar disorder is characterized by excessive mood swings that range from manic (high) to depressive (low) states. Specific symptoms of mania include agitation, hyperactivity, inflated self-esteem, risky or reckless behavior, and decreased sleep requirements. The depression phase can include fatigue, loss of self-esteem, suicidal thoughts, social withdrawal from family and friends, and eating and sleeping disturbances. The goal of treatment is to stabilize the mood and minimize these wide-ranging fluctuations from mania and depression.

Prognosis. With proper medications the symptoms of bipolar disorder can be controlled, although many people stop taking their medications once they feel better (manic stage). A strong support system is needed for continuing treatment.

Non–Drug Treatment. Psychotherapy can be used to help with the depressive phase. For those whose depressive state cannot be controlled by medications, electroconvulsive therapy may be an alternative form of treatment.

Drug Treatment. Treatment primarily involves the use of mood-stabilizing drugs such as lithium and anticonvulsants (e.g., carbamazepine, divalproex, lamotrigine). Although the complete mechanism for lithium is not understood fully, it is believed to alter behavior by enhancing the uptake of serotonin and norepinephrine by nerve cells. This sets lithium apart from all the other psychiatric drugs, because it does not cause any major CNS changes such as sedation, feelings of euphoria, or depression.

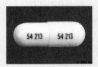

GENERIC NAME: lithium
TRADE NAME: Eskalith
INDICATION: Bipolar disorder
ROUTE OF ADMINISTRATION: Oral
COMMON ADULT DOSAGE: 600 mg three times daily; doses vary based on laboratory results of serum lithium levels
MECHANISM OF ACTION: Mechanism is unknown, but efficacy is believed to be due to effects on NTs such as serotonin
SIDE EFFECTS: Dizziness, drowsiness, tremor, nausea, vomiting, diarrhea
AUXILIARY LABELS:
- May cause dizziness and drowsiness.
- Take with food or milk.

SPECIAL NOTE: All patients taking lithium must have their blood levels monitored regularly for toxicity. It may take several weeks to see the desired effect of this agent.

Schizophrenia

Schizophrenia is a psychiatric disorder involving chronic or episodic **psychosis**. Schizophrenia is commonly associated with impaired social and occupational functioning and is among the most socially and economically disabling medical conditions, according to the World Health Organization. People with schizophrenia commonly exhibit both positive symptoms and negative symptoms. Positive symptoms can include hallucinations, delusions, and disorganized speech, whereas negative symptoms can include depressed mood and impairments in attention, memory, and high-level functioning. A diagnosis of schizophrenia is made based on the presence of the symptoms mentioned, in addition to diminished social and/or occupational dysfunction for at least 6 months.

Although the exact of cause of schizophrenia is unknown, the disorder is believed to have a strong genetic component. That being said, several environmental risk factors also have been associated with the development of schizophrenia, such as living in an urban area, immigration, experiencing obstetrical complications, and being born in the late winter to early spring, which is thought to reflect exposure to influenza virus during neural development. Additionally, people with schizophrenia have higher rates of other psychiatric disorders, such as depression, anxiety disorders, and substance abuse, compared with individuals without schizophrenia.

Prognosis. The prognoses for people with schizophrenia can be quite diverse. Although some studies have shown the prognosis to be quite poor, other studies have reported that certain subsets of people with schizophrenia can achieve fairly good outcomes in terms of symptoms, employment, and functioning. The goal of treatment is to minimize symptoms and maximize functionality and independence.

Non–Drug Treatments. Both professional counseling and a strong support system are keys to the success of treatment; however, drug therapy is necessary to adequately manage positive and negative symptoms of the disease.

Drug Treatments. Drug treatments focus on eliminating the symptoms of the disease, improving quality of life, and allowing the patient to live a productive life. Treatments are determined based on the phases of schizophrenia: acute, stabilizing, maintenance, or recovery phase. Often various medications and/or strengths of agents must be used before the most effective combination for the patient is found; this is because everyone responds differently to medications. Antipsychotic agents are used to treat schizophrenia and are often categorized as first generation (sometimes called "typical" antipsychotics) and second generation ("atypical" antipsychotics). A particularly devastating adverse reaction that can occur while taking antipsychotic medications is tardive dyskinesia (TD). The symptoms include involuntary movement of the facial muscles, tongue, jaw, and head. If these symptoms appear, the medication must be stopped immediately because these effects can be irreversible. Extrapyramidal symptoms (EPS) can also occur, which are side effects that mimic Parkinson's disease. This happens because antipsychotic medications block the effects of dopamine, essentially causing a drug-induced parkinsonism. Antipsychotic medications are likewise associated with weight gain and an increased incidence of type 2 diabetes. Long-acting antipsychotics (decanoates) can be given once monthly (usually by a nurse or physician) for schizophrenia. These depot agents, which tend to have a slower onset of action (24 to 72 hours after injection) and longer duration of action (average of 3 to 4 weeks), can be useful in the chronic management of schizophrenia symptoms. Examples of antipsychotic medications are provided in the following drug monographs.

As noted previously, people with schizophrenia are at higher risk for other psychiatric disorders. Accordingly people with schizophrenia are also commonly treated with other medications, such as the following:

- *Antianxiety medications:* Agents such as clonazepam (Klonopin) and diazepam (Valium) may be used to reduce anxiety and nervousness.
- *Anticonvulsant medications:* Agents such as carbamazepine (Tegretol) and valproate (Depakote) can help stabilize and reduce the symptoms during a relapse.
- *Antidepressants:* Various SSRIs (e.g., sertraline [Zoloft] or citalopram [Celexa]) or TCAs (e.g., nortriptyline [Pamelor]) can be used to help treat the depressive symptoms often experienced by people with schizophrenia.

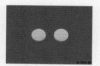

GENERIC NAME: haloperidol
TRADE NAME: Haldol
INDICATION: Schizophrenia, acute psychosis
ROUTE OF ADMINISTRATION: Oral; solution for injection; suspension for injection (long-acting)
COMMON ADULT DOSAGE: Dose can vary depending on individual and dosage form; maximum oral dose is

100 mg per day; maximum 450 mg per month of haloperidol decanoate (long-acting suspension); maximum dose of solution for injection dependent on clinical response and tolerability
MECHANISM OF ACTION: First-generation antipsychotic (blocks dopamine receptors)
SIDE EFFECTS: Extrapyramidal symptoms, drowsiness, confusion, tardive dyskinesia
AUXILIARY LABEL:
- May cause dizziness and drowsiness.

GENERIC NAME: clozapine
TRADE NAME: Clozaril, Fazaclo
INDICATION: Schizophrenia
ROUTE OF ADMINISTRATION: Oral
COMMON ADULT DOSAGE: 12.5 mg once or twice daily, with increased increments of 25-50 mg once daily; max 300-450 mg per day in divided doses
MECHANISM OF ACTION: Second-generation antipsychotic (blocks dopamine receptors)
SIDE EFFECTS: Hematologic effects, drowsiness, dizziness, headache, extrapyramidal symptoms
AUXILIARY LABELS:
- May cause dizziness and drowsiness.
- Take with or without food.
- Do not drink alcohol.

 Tech Note!

Clozapine is associated with a risk of hematologic effects, including agranulocytosis. Because of this, clozapine is available only through a monitoring and distribution system to ensure that patients are receiving the appropriate blood monitoring for this medication.

GENERIC NAME: olanzapine
TRADE NAME: Zyprexa, Zyprexa Zydis, Zyprexa Relprevv
INDICATION: Schizophrenia, agitation
ROUTE OF ADMINISTRATION: Oral; IM injection

COMMON ADULT DOSAGE: *Oral:* 5-20 mg daily; *IM injection:* 150-300 mg every 2 weeks or 405 mg every 4 weeks

MECHANISM OF ACTION: Second-generation antipsychotic (blocks dopamine receptors)

SIDE EFFECTS: Drowsiness, weight gain, headache, dizziness, extrapyramidal symptoms

AUXILIARY LABELS:
- May cause dizziness and drowsiness.
- Do not swallow; let dissolve in mouth (orally disintegrating tablet [ODT] form).
- Do not drink alcohol.

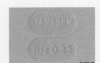

GENERIC NAME: risperidone

TRADE NAME: Risperdal, Risperdal M-Tab, Risperdal Consta

INDICATION: Schizophrenia

ROUTE OF ADMINISTRATION: Oral; IM injection

COMMON ADULT DOSAGE: *Oral:* 1 mg twice daily up to 8 mg once daily to twice daily; *IM injection:* 12.5-50 mg every 2 weeks

MECHANISM OF ACTION: Second-generation antipsychotic (blocks dopamine receptors)

SIDE EFFECTS: Drowsiness, weight gain, headache, dizziness, extrapyramidal symptoms

AUXILIARY LABELS:
- May cause dizziness or drowsiness.
- Do not swallow; let dissolve in mouth (ODT form).
- Do not drink alcohol.

GENERIC NAME: aripiprazole

TRADE NAME: Abilify, Abilify Discmelt

INDICATION: Schizophrenia, agitation, depression, bipolar disorder

ROUTE OF ADMINISTRATION: Oral

COMMON ADULT DOSAGE: 10-15 mg once daily

MECHANISM OF ACTION: Second-generation antipsychotic (blocks dopamine receptors)

SIDE EFFECTS: Drowsiness, weight gain, headache, dizziness, extrapyramidal symptoms

AUXILIARY LABELS:
- May cause dizziness or drowsiness.
- Do not swallow; let dissolve in mouth (ODT form).
- Do not drink alcohol.

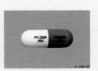

GENERIC NAME: ziprasidone

TRADE NAME: Geodon

INDICATION: Schizophrenia, agitation, bipolar disorder

ROUTE OF ADMINISTRATION: Oral; IM injection

COMMON ADULT DOSAGE: *Oral:* 20-80 mg twice daily; *IM injection:* 10-20 mg (max 40 mg per day)

MECHANISM OF ACTION: Second-generation antipsychotic (blocks dopamine receptors)

SIDE EFFECTS: Drowsiness, weight gain, headache, dizziness, extrapyramidal symptoms

AUXILIARY LABELS:
- May cause dizziness or drowsiness.
- Do not drink alcohol.

Insomnia

People with **insomnia** have impaired daytime functioning due to a difficulty initiating sleep or maintaining sleep, or they experience poor-quality sleep. A person is considered to have insomnia when all three of the following factors are present:
- The person complains of difficulty initiating sleep, difficulty maintaining sleep, or waking up too early.
- The sleep difficulty occurs even though the person has an adequate opportunity to sleep.
- The impairment in sleep causes difficulties in daytime functioning.

Insomnia is one of the most common medical complaints; an estimated 30% to 50% of the population has insomnia. Sleeping difficulties may need to be treated, depending on how often they occur and the impact the sleep loss has on daily functioning. Insomnia can affect all age groups, but the prevalence increases with age and is more common in women than men. Causes for insomnia range from stressful situations, sleep interruptions, and pain. Insomnia can also be related to medication use, which is an important consideration for pharmacists when counseling patients about over-the-counter agents to treat insomnia. Various illnesses also can affect sleep patterns and sleep quality, such as sleep apnea, acid reflux disease, Parkinson's disease, and Alzheimer's disease. In people with insomnia, it is important to identify and correct the cause of the insomnia, if possible.

Prognosis. Depending on the cause of the insomnia, most people can be treated effectively by modification of risk factors, adopting nonpharmacological practices to help with sleep, or the use of medications.

Non–Drug Treatment. Good sleeping hygiene is a focus of behavioral therapy to treat insomnia. Behavioral therapy includes regular exercise, maintaining a consistent sleep schedule, avoiding alcohol and caffeine intake after certain times of the day, and keeping the bedroom quiet and at the right temperature. Relaxation therapy techniques, such as dimming lights, listening to soft music, and meditating before retiring, can also be helpful.

Drug Treatment. Many OTC drugs are available for people suffering from mild cases of insomnia. The main ingredients in OTC products for insomnia are antihistamines, such as diphenhydramine and doxylamine. Because the main side effect of antihistamines is sedation, products containing diphenhydramine, for example, can be very effective for people who have difficulty falling asleep. It is important to remember that OTC treatments for insomnia are intended to treat short-term insomnia. For people experiencing insomnia that continues over a longer period, a prescription medication may be needed. OTC products containing diphenhydramine (e.g., Tylenol PM) are generally not recommended in the elderly because they can cause confusion and increase the risk of falls.

Several types of prescription medications can be used to treat insomnia, including benzodiazepines, nonbenzodiazepines, and certain antidepressants. Although these medications can be effective, they are best used in combination with non–drug treatments (as described previously). The elderly must be especially careful when combining OTC sleeping agents with their other prescription medications. Examples of medications used to treat insomnia are provided in Table 15-10.

 Tech Note!
Although nonbenzodiazepine prescription medications were first marketed in the United States as not having the same side effects as benzodiazepines, they can produce many of the same side effects.

GENERIC NAME: temazepam (C-IV)
TRADE NAME: Restoril
INDICATION: Insomnia
ROUTE OF ADMINISTRATION: Oral
COMMON ADULT DOSAGE: 15-30 mg at bedtime
MECHANISM OF ACTION: Bind benzodiazepine receptors leading to CNS depression
SIDE EFFECTS: Drowsiness, dizziness, dry mouth, amnesia
AUXILIARY LABELS:
- May cause dizziness and drowsiness.
- Do not drink alcohol.
- Caution: Federal law prohibits the transfer of this drug to any person other than the patient for whom it was prescribed.

GENERIC NAME: eszopiclone (C-IV)
TRADE NAME: Lunesta
INDICATION: Insomnia
ROUTE OF ADMINISTRATION: Oral
COMMON ADULT DOSAGE: 1-3 mg at bedtime
MECHANISM OF ACTION: Modulates the GABA system of the CNS leading to sedation
SIDE EFFECTS: Drowsiness, dizziness, headache, amnesia
AUXILIARY LABELS:
- May cause dizziness and drowsiness.
- Do not drink alcohol.
- Caution: Federal law prohibits the transfer of this drug to any person other than the patient for whom it was prescribed.

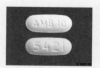

GENERIC NAME: zolpidem (C-IV)
TRADE NAME: Ambien, Ambien CR, Zolpimist, Edular, Intermezzo

TABLE 15-10

Select Medications Used for the Treatment of Insomnia

Medication Class	Generic Name	Brand Name	Common Side Effects	Common Dose Range
Benzodiazepines	flurazepam temazepam triazolam	Dalmane Restoril Halcion	• Drowsiness • Dizziness • Confusion • Fatigue • Amnesia	• 15-30 mg at bedtime • 7.5-30 mg at bedtime • 0.125-0.5 mg at bedtime
Nonbenzodiazepine Hypnotics	eszopiclone zaleplon zolpidem	Lunesta Sonata Ambien Ambien CR Zolpimist Edluar Intermezzo	• Drowsiness • Dizziness • Confusion • Fatigue • Amnesia	• 1-3 mg at bedtime • 5-20 mg at bedtime • 5-10 mg at bedtime • 6.25-12.5 mg at bedtime • 1-2 sprays (5-10 mg) orally (PO) at bedtime • 5-10 mg sublingually (SL) at bedtime • 1.75-3.5 mg SL once per night for middle-of-the-night awakening
Melatonin Receptor Agonists	ramelteon melatonin*	Rozerem Melatonin	• Drowsiness • Dizziness • Fatigue • Rebound insomnia • Drowsiness • Dizziness • Abdominal pain • Nightmares	• 8 mg within 30 min of bedtime • 0.3-6 mg at bedtime
Antihistamines	diphenhydramine* doxylamine*	Benadryl Unisom	• Dizziness • Drowsiness • Dry mouth • Confusion	• 12.5-50 mg at bedtime • 25 mg at bedtime

*Available over-the-counter.

INDICATION: Insomnia
ROUTE OF ADMINISTRATION: Various oral dosage forms
COMMON ADULT DOSAGE: *Immediate release:* 10 mg at bedtime; *CR:* 12.5 mg at bedtime
MECHANISM OF ACTION: Modulates the GABA system of the CNS leading to sedation
SIDE EFFECTS: Drowsiness, dizziness, confusion, fatigue, amnesia
AUXILIARY LABELS:
• May cause dizziness and drowsiness.
• Do not drink alcohol.
• Caution: Federal law prohibits the transfer of this drug to any person other than the patient for whom it was prescribed.

Attention Deficit/Hyperactivity Disorder

Attention deficit/hyperactivity disorder (ADHD) is a physiological brain disorder in which the person has difficulty focusing his or her attention or engaging in quiet, passive-type behavior, or both. Boys are three times as likely as girls to be diagnosed with ADHD, which affects 3% to 5% of school-age children. The symptoms and signs include impulsive, explosive, or irritable behavior. Although intelligence is not affected, work performance in school is sporadic because of the lack of the ability to focus on a task. An older child or adult describes symptoms in terms of being easily distracted by irrelevant thoughts, sounds, or sights. Daydreaming is also a common symptom and can affect the person's ability to meet deadlines, keep track of school or work materials, and finish assignments.

Prognosis. With proper treatment and understanding of ADHD, the outlook for a normal productive life is very good.

Non–Drug Treatment. Education is extremely important in understanding ADHD. This normally involves the participation of several people: parents, teachers, and therapists, in addition to the patient and physician. Treatment varies, depending on the child's symptoms and ability to

TABLE 15-11

Select Agents Approved for the Treatment of Attention Deficit/Hyperactivity Disorder (ADHD)

Trade Name	Generic Name	Dosage Forms	Notes
Ritalin, Ritalin LA, Ritalin SR	methylphenidate (C-II)	• Tablets • LA: capsules • SR: tablets	• *LA:* Capsule form may be opened and sprinkled on food, such as applesauce.
Concerta		• ER: tablets	• *SR:* Tablets; do not crush, chew, or divide.
Daytrana		• Transdermal patch	• Do not crush, chew, or divide tablets. • Apply topically once daily in the morning; remove after 9 hr.
Methylin		• Chewable tablets	
Metadate CD, Metadate ER		• Oral solution • CD: extended-release capsules • ER: extended-release tablets	• *CD:* Capsule form may be opened and sprinkled onto food, such as applesauce. • *ER:* Tablet; do not crush, chew, or divide.
Dexedrine Spansule, ProCentra Solution	dextroamphetamine (C-II)	• Tablets • Oral solution • Spansules (capsules)	• Do not crush, chew, or divide tablets or spansules.
Focalin, Focalin XR	dexmethylphenidate (C-II)	• Tablets • XR: capsules	• *XR:* Capsule form may be opened and sprinkled onto food, such as applesauce. • *Tablets:* Do not crush, chew, or divide.
Adderall, Adderall XR	amphetamine/ dextroamphetamine (C-II)	• Tablets • XR: capsules	• *XR:* Capsule form may be opened and sprinkled onto food, such as applesauce. • *Tablets:* Do not crush, chew, or divide.
Vyvanse	lisdexamfetamine (C-II)	• Capsules	• Capsules may be opened and entire contents dissolved in a glass of water. Do not divide dose.
Strattera	atomoxetine	• Capsules	• May be taken with or without food. May be discontinued without tapering dose. Capsules should not be opened.

function at home and in school. Behavior modification, coaching, and supportive psychotherapy can help the patient cope with the disorder. To develop a treatment plan, parents are urged to understand the types of professionals available to treat the condition.

Drug Treatment. In certain cases the use of medications may be beneficial (Table 15-11). Stimulants and atomoxetine are the most commonly used drugs currently. Common CNS stimulants used include Ritalin (methylphenidate) and amphetamines such as Dexedrine (dextroamphetamine). For those who are prescribed these agents, it is important to note that they are schedule II (C-II) drugs, and patients can develop physical dependence (a continued need to take the medication).

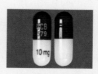

GENERIC NAME: methylphenidate (C-II)
SELECT TRADE NAMES: Ritalin, Concerta, Daytrana, Methylin

INDICATION: ADHD

ROUTE OF ADMINISTRATION: Oral; transdermal patch

COMMON DOSAGE: Doses vary, depending on dosage form and patient's age

MECHANISM OF ACTION: Mechanism in ADHD not clearly understood. It is believed to be due to modulation of serotonin effects in the brain via changes in dopamine transport

SIDE EFFECTS: Dizziness, drowsiness, headache, loss of appetite, nausea, nervousness, trouble sleeping

AUXILIARY LABELS:
- May cause dizziness and drowsiness.
- Do not drink alcohol.
- Do not take MAOIs while using this medication.
- Do not stop medication abruptly.
- Caution: Federal law prohibits the transfer of this drug to any person other than the patient for whom it was prescribed.

DO YOU REMEMBER THESE KEY POINTS?

- Names of the major components and divisions of the nervous system and their functions
- The primary symptoms of the various neurological conditions associated with the nervous system discussed
- Medications used to treat the various nervous system conditions discussed
- The generic and trade names for the drugs discussed in this chapter
- The appropriate auxiliary labels that should be used when filling prescriptions for drugs discussed in this chapter

REVIEW QUESTIONS

Multiple Choice Questions

1. Neurons are made of the following components *except:*
   A. Dendrites
   B. Cell body
   C. Nerve terminals
   D. Amino acids

2. Which of the following is a rare autoimmune disorder that affects the transmission of electrical impulses from the CNS to muscles throughout the body?
   A. Myasthenia gravis
   B. Alzheimer's disease
   C. Parkinson's disease
   D. Multiple sclerosis

3. The autonomic nervous system can be broken down into the _____ and _____.
   A. parasympathetic nervous system; sympathetic nervous system
   B. parasympathetic nervous system; somatic nervous system
   C. peripheral nervous system; somatic nervous system
   D. central nervous system; sympathetic nervous system

4. The part of the brain that controls memory, reason, and language skills is the:
   A. Medulla oblongata
   B. Cerebellum
   C. Cerebral cortex
   D. Brainstem

5. _____ affect the sympathetic system, whereas _____ affect the parasympathetic system.
   A. Cholinergics, anticholinergics
   B. Cholinergics, adrenergics
   C. Adrenergics, antiadrenergics
   D. Adrenergics, cholinergics

6. Which of the following medications is a dopamine agonist?
   A. Rasagiline
   B. Benztropine
   C. Rotigotine
   D. Amantadine

7. Which of the following medications for Alzheimer's disease is available as a patch?
   A. Donepezil
   B. Memantine
   C. Galantamine
   D. Rivastigmine

8. The illness that is marked by extremes in elevated and depressed moods is defined as:
    A. Schizophrenia
    B. Bipolar disorder
    C. Depression
    D. All of the above

9. An important auxiliary label to include on a benzodiazepine bottle would be:
    A. Take in the morning
    B. Take on an empty stomach
    C. May cause dizziness and drowsiness
    D. Take as directed

10. Which of the following medication classes should be used cautiously in people with depression?
    A. Dopamine agonists
    B. Interferons
    C. SSRIs
    D. Antipsychotics

11. SSRIs inhibit the reuptake of which of the following neurotransmitters?
    A. Norepinephrine
    B. Epinephrine
    C. Serotonin
    D. Dopamine

12. Which of the following is *not* a classic symptom of Parkinson's disease?
    A. Tremor
    B. Rigidity
    C. Postural instability
    D. Diarrhea

13. Which of the following is *not* used to treat insomnia?
    A. Trazodone
    B. Zolpidem
    C. Dexmethylphenidate
    D. Diphenhydramine

14. Sumatriptan (Imitrex) is available in which of the following dosage forms for the treatment of migraine?
    A. Tablet
    B. Injection
    C. Nasal spray
    D. All of the above

15. Which of the following conditions is *not* considered an anxiety disorder?
    A. PTSD
    B. Phobia
    C. OCD
    D. Schizophrenia

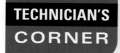

TECHNICIAN'S CORNER

Using a drug reference resource, look up a medication from each of the SSRI, SNRI, TCA, and MAOI antidepressant medication classes and familiarize yourself with the types of medical conditions they are used to treat in addition to depression.

Bibliography

Applegate E: *The anatomy and physiology learning system*, ed 4, St Louis, 2010, Saunders.

Clinical Pharmacology Online: (Referenced August 19, 2014.) www.clinicalpharmacology.com.

Damjanov I: *Pathology for the health professions*, ed 4, St Louis, 2011, Saunders.

Fishback JL: *Pathology*, ed 3, Philadelphia, 2005, Mosby.

Huether SE: *Understanding pathophysiology*, ed 5, St Louis, 2012, Mosby.

Scanlon V, Sanders T: *Essentials of anatomy and physiology*, ed 5, Philadelphia, 2007, FA Davis.

Solomon EP: *Introduction to human anatomy and physiology*, ed 3, St Louis, 2009, Saunders.

Thibodeau G, Patton K: *Structure and function of the body*, ed 13, St Louis, 2007, Mosby.

Thibodeau GA, Patton KT: *Anatomy and physiology*, ed 8, St Louis, 2012, Mosby.

Therapeutic Agents for the Endocrine System

Joshua J. Neumiller

OBJECTIVES

Upon completing this chapter, you should be able to do the following:

1. Name the major endocrine glands of the body.
2. Describe the locations and functions of the endocrine glands discussed.
3. List the primary symptoms of conditions associated with dysfunction of the principal endocrine glands discussed.
4. Recognize drugs used to treat the endocrine conditions discussed.
5. Write the generic and trade names for the drugs discussed in this chapter.
6. List appropriate auxiliary labels when filling prescriptions for drug discussed in this chapter.

TERMS AND DEFINITIONS

Acromegaly A condition caused by excessive growth hormone production during adulthood

Addison's disease A condition resulting in a decrease in levels of adrenocortical hormones (e.g., mineralocorticoids and glucocorticoids), which causes symptoms such as muscle weakness and weight loss

Adrenal cortex A portion of the adrenal gland that secretes steroids, including mineralocorticoids, glucocorticoids, and sex steroids

Adrenal medulla A portion of the adrenal gland that synthesizes and secretes the catecholamines norepinephrine and epinephrine

Aldosterone The principal mineralocorticoid in the body that maintains sodium and potassium homeostasis by stimulating the kidneys to conserve sodium and excrete potassium

Calcitonin A thyroid hormone that helps to regulate blood concentrations of calcium and phosphate and promotes the formation of bone

Catecholamines Hormones produced in the brainstem, nervous system, and adrenal glands that help the body respond to stress and prepare the body for the "fight or flight" response; they are important in regulating heart rate, blood pressure, and nervous system functions

Comorbidity A concomitant, but not necessarily related, medical condition existing simultaneously with another condition

Cretinism A condition in which the development of the brain and body is inhibited by a congenital lack of thyroid hormone secretion

Endocrine glands Glands in the body that produce hormones that enter the bloodstream to reach their target site or act at target sites near the site of hormone release

Endocrinologist A physician who specializes in the treatment of conditions involving the endocrine system

Exocrine glands Glands in the body that produce hormones that are sent to the target organ or tissue via a tube or duct

Exophthalmos Prominence (protrusion) of the eyeball out of the orbit; bilateral presentation is commonly caused by increased thyroid hormone

Gastroparesis Delayed gastric emptying

Gigantism A condition associated with excessive production of growth hormone during childhood or adolescence that results in excessive height and growth of body tissues

Glucometer A device used to test blood sugar levels in people with diabetes mellitus

Goiter A condition in which the thyroid gland is enlarged because of a lack of iodine; it can be either a simple goiter or a toxic goiter (i.e., resulting from a tumor)

Graves disease A condition caused by hypersecretion of thyroid hormones; symptoms include diffuse goiter, exophthalmos, and skin changes

Homeostasis The equilibrium pertaining to the balance of the body with respect to fluid levels, pH level, osmotic pressures, and concentrations of various substances

Hormones Chemical substances produced and secreted by an endocrine duct into the bloodstream that result in a physiological response at a specific target tissue

Hyperglycemia Elevated concentration of glucose in the blood

Hypertension Elevated blood pressure

Hyperthyroidism Excessive secretion of thyroid hormone

Hypocalcemia Low concentration of calcium in the blood

Hypoglycemia Excessively low concentration of glucose in the blood

Hypokalemia Low concentration of potassium in the blood

Hypopituitary dwarfism Short stature due to a deficiency in growth hormone during childhood

Insulin resistance Resistance of the tissues of the body (skeletal muscle and fat) to the effects of insulin; insulin resistance is associated with the development of type 2 diabetes mellitus

Myxedema A condition associated with a decrease in overall thyroid function in adults; also known as *hypothyroidism*

Oogenesis Production or development of an egg

Orthostatic hypotension Low blood pressure that occurs upon standing up

Ovulation Release of an egg from the ovary

Pancreas An endocrine gland that produces both insulin and glucagon

Parenteral A term indicating administration of a substance by a route other than by mouth

Peripheral neuropathy Damage to nerves of the peripheral nervous system

Thyroxine (T$_4$) A thyroid hormone derived from tyrosine (amino acid) that influences the metabolic rate

Triiodothyronine (T$_3$) A thyroid hormone that helps regulate growth and development and controls metabolism and body temperature; it is mainly produced through the metabolism of thyroxine

Type 1 diabetes mellitus (T1DM) A form of diabetes mellitus associated with an absolute deficiency of insulin production by the pancreas; people with T1DM require insulin therapy

Type 2 diabetes mellitus (T2DM) A form of diabetes mellitus associated with insulin resistance and a relative deficiency of insulin; people with T2DM can be treated with oral therapies, non-insulin injectable medications, and insulin

Vasopressin Another term used for antidiuretic hormone (ADH)

Common Drugs Prescribed for Endocrine Conditions

Trade Name	Generic Name	Pronunciation
Treatment of Syndrome of Inappropriate Antidiuretic Hormone Secretion (SIADH)		
Declomycin	demeclocycline	(**dem**-e-kloe-**sye**-kleen)
Treatment of Diabetes Insipidus		
Pitressin	vasopressin	(**vay**-soe-**pres**-in)
DDAVP	desmopressin acetate	(**dez**-mo-**pres**-in **as**-e-tate)
Treatment of Acromegaly and Gigantism		
Sandostatin	octreotide	(ok-**tree**-oh-tide)
Treatment of Hyperthyroidism		
PTU	propylthiouracil	(pro-pull-thigh-oh-**yoor**-ah-sill)
Tapazole	methimazole	(meth-**em**-ah-zoll)
Treatment of Hypothyroidism		
Armour Thyroid	desiccated thyroid	(**des**-eh-kate-ed **thigh**-roid)
Synthroid, Levoxyl	levothyroxine	(lee-vo-**thigh**-rox-een)
Cytomel	liothyronine	(lie-oh-**thigh**-row-neen)
Thyrolar	liotrix	(lee-ow-**tricks**)
Treatment of Hyperparathyroidism		
Rocaltrol	calcitriol	(**kal**-si-**trye**-ole)
Hectorol	doxercalciferol	(dock-sir-kal-**sih**-fer-all)
Zemplar	paricalcitol	(par-ee-**cal**-sih-tahl)
Sensipar	cinacalcet	(sin-ah-**cal**-set)
Treatment of Cushing's Syndrome		
Lysodren	mitotane	(**mye**-toe-tane)
Metopirone	metyrapone	(me-**teer**-a-pone)
Treatment of Addison's Disease		
Florinef	fludrocortisone acetate	(floo-**droe**-kor-ti-sone **as**-see-tate)
Cortef	hydrocortisone	(hye-droe-**kor**-ti-sone)

Continued

Common Drugs Prescribed for Endocrine Conditions—cont'd

Trade Name	Generic Name	Pronunciation
Medrol	methylprednisolone	(**meth**-il-pred-**nis**-oh-lone)
Solu-Medrol	methylprednisolone sodium succinate	(**meth**-il-pred-**nis**-oh-lone **so**-de-um **suck**-sin-ate)
Orapred	prednisolone	(pred-**nis**-oh-lone)
Deltasone	prednisone	(**pred**-ni-sown)

Insulin for Treatment of Diabetes Mellitus
Rapid Acting

Humalog	insulin lispro	(**in**-su-lin **lis**-pro)
NovoLog	insulin aspart	(**in**-su-lin **as**-part)
Apidra	insulin glulisine	(**in**-su-lin **gloo**-lis-een)

Short Acting

Humulin R, Novolin R	regular insulin	(**reg**-yoo-lar **in**-su-lin)

Intermediate Acting

Humulin N, Novolin N	isophane insulin (NPH)	(**eye**-soe-fane)

Long Acting

Levemir	insulin detemir	(**de**-te-mir)
Lantus	insulin glargine	(**glar**-jeen)

Oral Antidiabetic Drugs for Treatment of Type 2 Diabetes Mellitus (T2DM)
Biguanide

Glucophage	metformin	(met-**four**-men)

Alpha-Glucosidase Inhibitors

Precose	acarbose	(**ay**-car-bose)
Glyset	miglitol	(**mig**-li-tol)

Meglitinides

Prandin	repaglinide	(re-**pag**-lih-nide)
Starlix	nateglinide	(na-**teg**-lih-nide)

Sulfonylureas

Amaryl	glimepiride	(gly-**mep**-ir-ide)
Glucotrol	glipizide	(**glip**-eh-zyed)
Micronase, DiaBeta	glyburide	(**glye**-burr-eyed)

Thiazolidinedione

Actos	pioglitazone	(pye-oh-**glit**-ah-zone)

DPP-4 Inhibitors

Januvia	sitagliptin	(**sye**-ta-**glip**-tin)
Onglyza	saxagliptin	(**sax**-a-**glip**-tin)
Tradjenta	linagliptin	(**lin**-a-**glip**-tin)
Nesina	alogliptin	(**al**-oh-**glip**-tin)

Incretin Mimetics

Byetta	exenatide	(ex-**en**-a-tide)
Victoza	liraglutide	(**lir**-a-**gloo**-tide)
Bydureon	exenatide suspension	(ex-**en**-a-tide)

SGLT-2 Inhibitors

Invokana	canagliflozin	(kan-uh-**glif**-loh-zin)
Farxiga	dapagliflozin	(dap-a-**glif**-loh-zin)

The endocrine system is responsible for the production and secretion of **hormones** from various glands in the body. The Greek word *orme* means "to excite." This is exactly what hormones do; they activate specific target cells and organs to elicit a response. Many different types of hormones are produced in different glands. **Endocrinologists** are physicians who specialize in the study of glands and hormones. In this chapter we discuss the location and function of the major glands and hormones of the body. Major conditions affecting the endocrine system are discussed, along with the types of medications used to treat them. All medication dosages listed are based on adult dosage unless otherwise stated.

Anatomy of the Endocrine System

Figure 16-1 illustrates the principal endocrine glands in the body. As shown in the figure, three glands are located in the head: the pituitary gland, hypothalamus, and pineal gland. The pituitary gland produces hormones that affect other glands and specific organs of the body and regulates the thyroid gland, adrenal cortex, and the gonads (ovaries and testes). The hypothalamus, located above the pituitary gland, secretes hormones that regulate the secretion of

other hormones by the pituitary gland. The pineal gland, located behind and below the hypothalamus, is involved in controlling circadian rhythms, sleep-wake patterns and other body functions, primarily through the production of the hormone melatonin.

Located at the base of the neck, the thyroid gland produces three hormones that affect metabolism: **thyroxine (T_4)**, **triiodothyronine (T_3)**, and **calcitonin**. The parathyroid glands, positioned slightly behind and above the thyroid gland, secrete a hormone called *parathyroid hormone (PTH)*, which helps maintain adequate calcium levels. Located lower in the chest is the thymus, which secretes hormones that play an important role in the immune system of the body. The two adrenal glands are located in the abdominal area, one gland positioned above each kidney. The adrenal glands secrete specific hormones (epinephrine and norepinephrine) linked to the stress responses of the body.

The largest gland is the **pancreas**. The pancreas is responsible for the production and secretion of hormones from groupings of cells known as "islets of Langerhans." The islets of Langerhans contain alpha-cells that produce glucagon and beta-cells that produce insulin. Sex hormones are produced in the gonads. In women, the ovaries secrete hormones such as estrogen and progesterone, and in men, the main hormone secreted from the testes is testosterone. A detailed discussion of sex hormones is presented in Chapter 22.

Description of Hormones and Glands

Hormones are responsible for many different human functions, including emotions. The actions of hormones are classified by the distance they travel. Autocrine hormones act on the same cell from which they are secreted; for example, interleukin-2 stimulates T cells (part of the immune system). Endocrine hormones, in contrast, influence cells that are located farther away. The endocrine hormones are the focus of this chapter.

Glands have two mechanisms of action, endocrine or exocrine. Hormones produced by **endocrine glands** either enter the bloodstream to reach their target site or act at target sites near the site of hormone release. Hormones produced by **exocrine glands** are sent to the target organ or tissue via a tube or duct. An example of a tube or duct that secretes outwardly to the surface of the skin is the duct of the sweat glands. Because of this difference, endocrine glands do not have ducts.

Structure and Function of Hormones

Hormones of the endocrine system are classified as proteins, steroids, and amines (Figure 16-2).

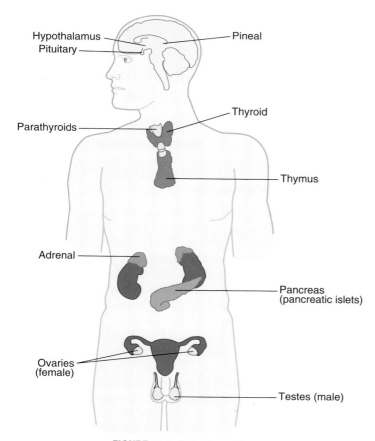

Hypothalamus
Pituitary
Pineal
Parathyroids
Thyroid
Thymus
Adrenal
Pancreas (pancreatic islets)
Ovaries (female)
Testes (male)

FIGURE 16-1 Endocrine anatomy.

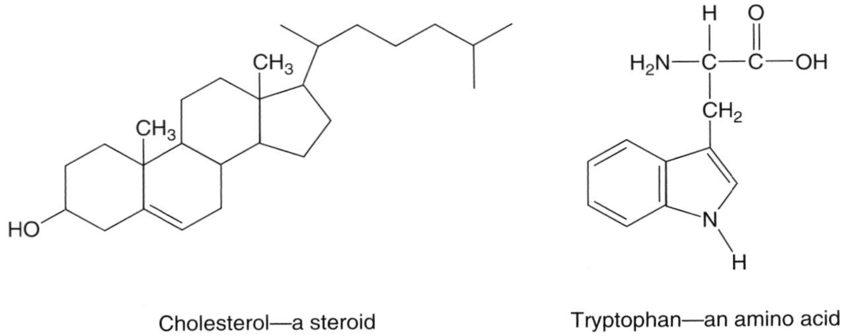

Cholesterol—a steroid

Tryptophan—an amino acid

FIGURE 16-2 Structures of a steroid and an amino acid.

Proteins include insulin, growth hormone (GH), and calcitonin. Steroids include cortisol and aldosterone from the adrenal cortex, estrogen and progesterone from the ovaries, and testosterone from the testes. The hormones thyroxine, epinephrine, and norepinephrine are examples of amines.

Hormone levels are balanced and maintained in a normal range through a feedback system with a mechanism similar to that of your home thermostat. However, hormones in general can be considered specialized keys that unlock specific doors. When the key enters the lock, a reaction takes place. As the hormone travels through the body, it does not react with any keyhole other than the ones it was made to fit. **Homeostasis** is disrupted if glands secrete too many or too few hormones; rather, a delicate balance must be maintained to produce the correct response. Accordingly, many hormones are regulated by sensitive "feedback loops" that control the amount of hormone produced by any given gland (see the following section, Mechanism of Action). Table 16-1 provides a list of endocrine glands, the hormones they produce, and the general functions of each hormone. If a gland produces too much or too little of a hormone, various conditions of the endocrine system may result. Hormones perform many functions throughout the body, including the following:

- Maintain homeostasis (i.e., maintain normal physiological limits by increasing and decreasing blood glucose levels for energy use)
- Prepare the body for an emergency situation (i.e., instigate the fight-or-flight reaction)
- Participate in the development of the reproductive system (i.e., cause sexual maturity and reproductive functions, such as menstruation and pregnancy)

Mechanism of Action

Receptor sites for hormones are located inside and outside of cells. Protein hormones fit into receptor sites outside cells, whereas steroid hormones enter into and attach to receptor sites inside the cell. Both

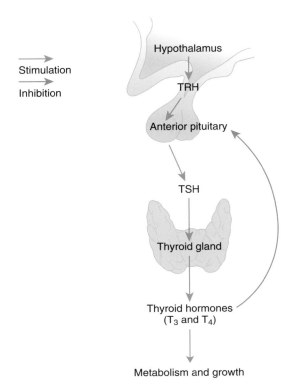

FIGURE 16-3 Regulation of thyroid hormone secretion by negative feedback. (From Solomon EP: *Introduction to human anatomy and physiology,* ed 3, St Louis, 2009, Saunders.)

mechanisms cause a reaction. The following three signaling pathways influence the endocrine system and the production of hormones:

- Negative feedback is the primary regulatory mechanism for maintaining homeostasis. In negative feedback, a stimulus results in actions that reduce the stimulus. Figure 16-3 provides an example of a negative feedback loop. In this example, an increase in the concentration of thyroid hormones (T_3 and T_4) above normal levels signals the anterior pituitary gland to reduce the production of thyroid-stimulating hormone (TSH). In essence, thyroid hormones are able to limit their own production by this negative feedback mechanism.

TABLE 16-1

Select Endocrine Glands, Hormones, and Their Functions

Hormone	Target Tissue	Function
Pituitary Gland		
Adrenocorticotropic hormone (ACTH)	Adrenal cortex	Stimulates secretion of adrenocortical hormones
Antidiuretic hormone (ADH)	Kidneys	Stimulates resorption of water (conserves water)
Follicle-stimulating hormone (FSH)	Gonads	Stimulates gonad growth and function
Growth hormone (GH)	Many tissue targets	Regulates growth of muscles, bones, and tissues
Luteinizing hormone (LH)	Gonads	Stimulates gonad growth and function
Oxytocin	Uterus and mammary glands	Stimulates uterine contractions during birth and milk ejection into the mammary ducts
Thyroid-stimulating hormone (TSH)	Thyroid gland	Promotes secretion of hormones from the thyroid gland
Pineal Gland		
Melatonin	Hypothalamus	Influences sleep-wake cycles
Thyroid Gland		
Calcitonin	Bone	Regulates calcium levels by inhibiting calcium release from bone
Thyroid hormones (T_4 and T_3)	Many tissue targets	Affects metabolism
Parathyroid Glands		
Parathyroid hormone (PTH)	Bone, kidneys, and digestive tract	Increases calcium levels by stimulating calcium release from bone, stimulating calcium resorption by the kidneys, and increasing calcium absorption from the intestines
Adrenal Glands		
Aldosterone	Kidneys	Regulates salt/water balance
Cortisol	Many tissue targets	Regulates metabolism of proteins, fats, and carbohydrates
Epinephrine	Skeletal muscle, heart, blood vessels, liver	Stimulates sympathetic nervous system
Norepinephrine	Skeletal muscle, heart, blood vessels, liver	Stimulates sympathetic nervous system
Pancreas		
Glucagon	Liver, adipose (fat) tissue	Increases levels of glucose in the blood
Insulin	Many tissue targets	Facilitates glucose uptake into the tissues, stimulates glycogen production, and stimulates fat storage
Ovaries		
Estrogens	Many tissue targets	Regulates menstrual cycle; develops and maintains female sex characteristics
Progesterone	Uterus, breast	Stimulates development of the uterine lining
Testes		
Testosterone	Many tissue targets	Influences sex-related characteristics in males and promotes sperm production

- Positive feedback may also occur; however, in positive feedback, a stimulus results in actions that further increase the stimulus. For example, during labor, specific hormones are released that promote continued release of more hormones until a result is achieved; contractions result in the birth of a baby.

- The third response system is via the nervous system. Stressful situations can alter the production and secretion of specific hormones that, when released, prepare the body for the situation. For example, if a person is in an emergency, the body requires more energy; therefore, hormones such as epinephrine may be released, giving the body an extra boost of energy.

Functions of the Endocrine Glands

Hypothalamus

Located in the brain below the thalamus, the hypothalamus is a small organ that links the nervous system to the endocrine system. The hypothalamus stimulates the pituitary gland by neuronal impulses and directly or indirectly regulates most endocrine activity. The hypothalamus plays a key role in the regulation of several functions, such as water balance, metabolism of fat and carbohydrates, body temperature, appetite, and emotions. In addition, this organ produces releasing or inhibiting hormones that regulate the anterior pituitary gland. Hormones from the hypothalamus are also sent to the pituitary gland, where they are both stored and secreted.

Pituitary Gland

The pituitary gland is analogous to the control tower of the endocrine system. As noted previously, the pituitary gland is situated close to the hypothalamus, which regulates the release of many hormones from the pituitary gland. As shown in Figure 16-4,

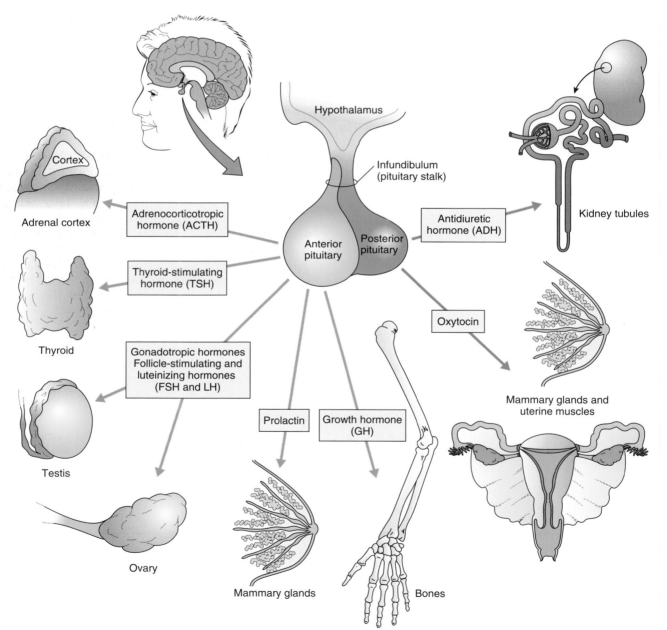

FIGURE 16-4 The pituitary gland is suspended from the hypothalamus by a stalk of neural tissue. (From Solomon EP: *Introduction to human anatomy and physiology,* ed 3, St Louis, 2009, Saunders.)

the gland is composed of two portions, the anterior and posterior lobes. Although small, the anterior lobe synthesizes hormones that stimulate many different organs. Table 16-1 summarizes the various hormones secreted from the pituitary gland, their target tissues, and their functions. Two hormones, oxytocin and antidiuretic hormone (ADH), are stored in the posterior portion of the pituitary gland. Oxytocin stimulates uterine contractions and cervical dilation during birth and lactation, and ADH (also known as **vasopressin**) affects the kidneys, cardiovascular system, and central nervous system. This entire pituitary system is regulated via negative feedback control from the nervous system (specifically the hypothalamus) and from the levels of other hormones.

Pineal Gland

The pineal gland is responsible for the production and secretion of melatonin. Melatonin is a hormone that facilitates the onset of sleep and influences biological rhythms and the onset of sexual maturity. The gland is affected by the retinal response to light, with exposure to light suppressing melatonin secretion.

 Tech Note!
Melatonin is available as an over-the-counter product to help with insomnia.

Thyroid Gland

The thyroid gland is located at the base of the neck (Figure 16-5). As mentioned previously, this gland is responsible for producing and secreting three hormones: T_4, T_3, and calcitonin. Iodine is necessary in the thyroid gland to synthesize T_4 and T_3; each hormone is named to indicate the number of iodine atoms in its structure. T_4 and T_3 are important in regulating the rate of metabolism of proteins, fats (lipids), and sugars (carbohydrates) throughout the body; therefore, they play an important role in the growth and homeostasis of the body. Calcitonin plays an active role in the regulation of calcium levels. Calcium is the major mineral found in bones. Calcium is also important for the proper functioning of muscle contractions, nerve impulses, and blood clotting. A constant level is maintained by three different hormones: calcitonin, vitamin D, and PTH. The function of calcitonin, specifically, is to inhibit the removal of calcium from bone.

Parathyroid Glands

Located behind the thyroid gland are the parathyroid glands (see Figure 16-5). The parathyroid organ is composed of two sets of secreting glands. These glands are the primary regulators of calcium levels in the blood through the release of PTH. PTH increases calcium levels by stimulating the release of calcium from the bones and by stimulating calcium reabsorption by the kidneys. PTH also activates vitamin D to increase the amount of calcium that is absorbed from the intestine. The parathyroid glands are regulated by the concentration of calcium in the blood and bodily fluids (Figure 16-6). When calcium levels are higher than normal in the blood, the parathyroid glands are inhibited and slow their release of PTH. When calcium levels in the blood fall,

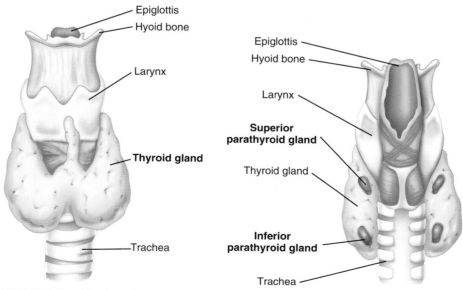

FIGURE 16-5 Thyroid and parathyroid glands. (From Thibodeau GA, Patton KT: *Anatomy and physiology,* ed 8, St Louis, 2012, Mosby.)

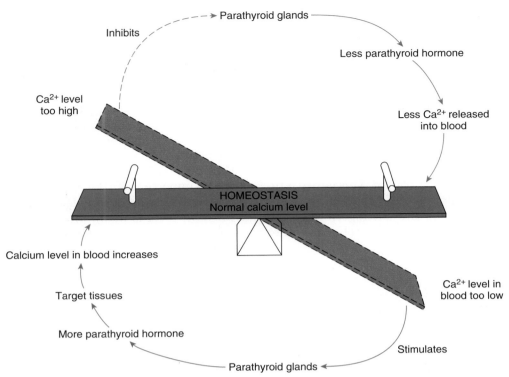

FIGURE 16-6 Calcium regulation by negative feedback. (From Solomon EP: *Introduction to human anatomy and physiology,* ed 3, St Louis, 2009, Saunders.)

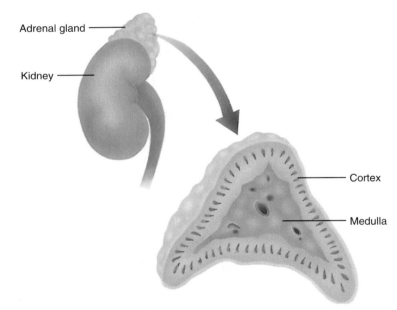

FIGURE 16-7 The paired adrenal glands are small, yellow masses of tissues that lie in contact with the upper ends of the kidneys. Each gland consists of a central medulla and an outer cortex. (From Solomon EP: *Introduction to human anatomy and physiology,* ed 3, St Louis, 2009, Saunders.)

however, more PTH is released. In this way, PTH is regulated by a negative feedback mechanism.

Adrenal Glands

The adrenal glands are located directly on top of each of the two kidneys (Figure 16-7). Each adrenal gland consists of a central portion, known as the **adrenal medulla**, and an outer region, called the **adrenal cortex**. The adrenal glands are important in helping the body cope with stress (Figure 16-8). The adrenal medulla synthesizes and secretes the **catecholamines** norepinephrine and epinephrine. These hormones are stored in the adrenal medulla until

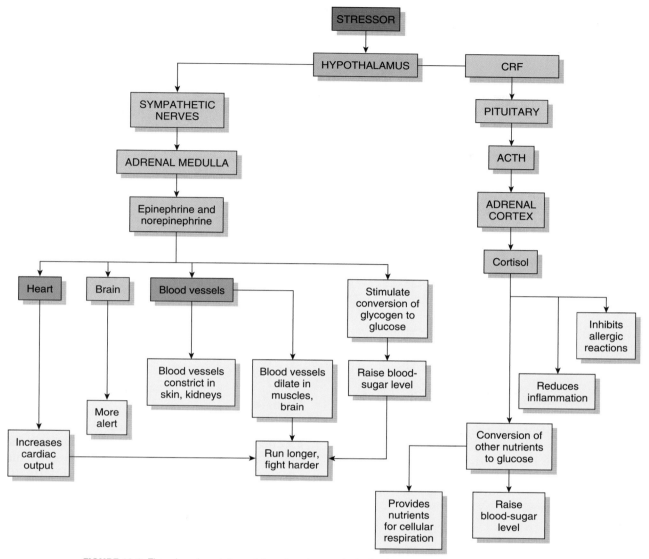

FIGURE 16-8 The adrenal medulla and the adrenal cortex both play important roles in helping the body cope with stress. (From Solomon EP: *Introduction to human anatomy and physiology,* ed 3, St Louis, 2009, Saunders.)

activated by the sympathetic nervous system (see Chapter 15 for a description of the nervous system). As mentioned previously, one of the functions of the endocrine system is to stimulate the fight-or-flight reaction. For instance, when the body encounters a stressful situation, it prepares itself for fight or flight, depending on the situation. When the sympathetic nervous system is activated, the heart rate increases and the blood vessels dilate to allow more blood to reach the skeletal muscles and to increase blood flow to the brain. Stored glucose is released into the bloodstream to fuel the body's increased metabolic rate. Epinephrine accounts for approximately 70% to 80% of the released catecholamines and norepinephrine 20% to 30%.

 Tech Note!

Norepinephrine is the same substance that is secreted as a neurotransmitter by neurons in the central nervous system.

The cortex of the adrenal glands produces three types of hormones: glucocorticoids, mineralocorticoids, and sex hormones (i.e., androgens or estrogens). Glucocorticoids, such as cortisol, affect the metabolism of lipids, carbohydrates, and proteins. They increase glucose levels, reduce inflammation, and increase the capacity to cope with stressful

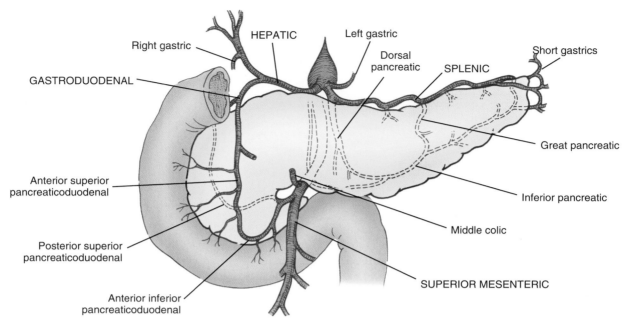

FIGURE 16-9 Pancreas. (From Rothrock JC: *Alexander's care of the patient in surgery,* ed 15, St Louis, 2015, Mosby.)

situations. Mineralocorticoids are crucial for regulating the salt and water balance in the body. The principal mineralocorticoid in the body is aldosterone, which maintains sodium and potassium homeostasis by stimulating the kidneys to conserve sodium and excrete potassium. The adrenal cortex also secretes small amounts of both androgens and estrogens in both men and women.

Pancreas

The pancreas is the largest organ of the endocrine system (Figure 16-9). It carries out both endocrine and exocrine functions in the body. The exocrine function of the pancreas is the secretion of digestive enzymes into the small intestine. The endocrine function of the pancreas is to maintain energy homeostasis throughout the body by regulating glucose (sugar) levels in the blood. The gland primarily accomplishes this by secreting both glucagon and insulin from cells in the islets of Langerhans. Glucagon is secreted in response to low blood glucose levels. This hormone triggers the liver to release stored glucose. When the blood glucose concentration is high, in contrast, insulin is released into the bloodstream. This hormone targets tissues such as the liver, muscle, and adipose tissues to take up glucose from the bloodstream, where it can be used as energy or stored for later use as glycogen. Because glucagon and insulin have opposite actions on blood glucose levels, they work together to maintain glucose homeostasis (Figure 16-10).

Ovaries

The two ovaries in women are responsible for the production (**oogenesis**) and secretion of one or, rarely, two eggs or more (**ovulation**) each month. Located on either side of the uterus (Figure 16-11), the ovaries sit above the uterus and are close to the fallopian tubes, which connect the two organs. Although ovulation begins at puberty, it is not possible to become pregnant until the menstrual cycle begins. The ability to have children ends as the levels of the responsible hormones (e.g., estrogen) decline until the ovarian cycle stops. The ovaries secrete the hormones estrogen and progesterone; the ovaries are the primary source of estrogen in women. The function of estrogen is the development of the breasts and genitals and the regulation of the menstrual cycle, which prepares the female for pregnancy. The anterior pituitary gland releases follicle-stimulating hormone (FSH), which triggers estrogen levels to increase, which in turn causes the secretion of luteinizing hormone (LH), another pituitary hormone. The combination of these two hormones triggers the cascade of events leading to ovulation.

Testes

The testes are responsible for the production and secretion of sperm (spermatogenesis). The testes are located in the scrotum (Figure 16-12). Sperm production begins before the age of puberty and decreases with age, although most men produce

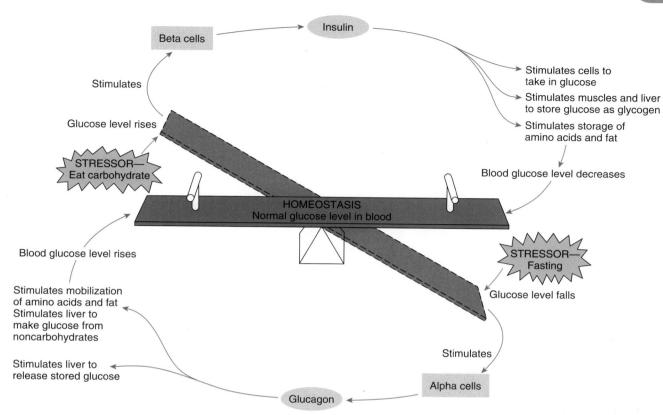

FIGURE 16-10 Regulation of blood glucose (sugar) level by insulin and glucagon. (From Solomon EP: *Introduction to human anatomy and physiology*, ed 3, St Louis, 2009, Saunders.)

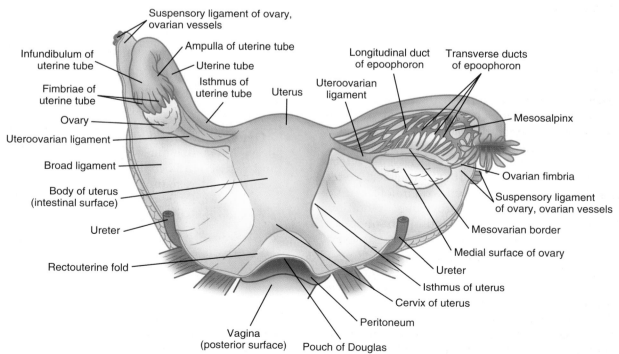

FIGURE 16-11 Ovaries. (From Rothrock JC: *Alexander's care of the patient in surgery*, ed 13, St Louis, 2007, Mosby.)

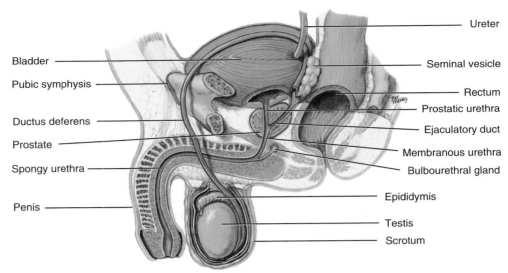

FIGURE 16-12 Testes. (From Applegate E: *The anatomy and physiology learning system,* ed 4, St Louis, 2010, Saunders.)

sperm throughout their lifetime. FSH is released as puberty begins, causing the stored, immature sperm cells to divide and mature. The production of testosterone in the testes is responsible for the growth of adjacent organs, such as the prostate gland, seminal vesicles, and vas deferens. Testosterone is also responsible for secondary sex characteristics, such as changes in voice pitch as a boy enters puberty and increased muscle development. A detailed discussion of sex hormones and reproductive health is presented in Chapter 22.

Conditions of the Endocrine System and Their Treatments

Many different types of conditions and illnesses can be associated with dysfunctions of the endocrine system. Many of these conditions are due to too much or too little production of a hormone by a gland of the endocrine system. Because hormones are critical to functions of other tissues and organs, diseases of the endocrine system can have a variety of effects throughout the body. Table 16-2 lists select conditions and/or illnesses associated with a defect in the endocrine system. As noted previously, conditions related to reproduction are covered in Chapter 22.

Conditions of the Pituitary Gland and Hypothalamus and Their Treatments

Syndrome of Inappropriate Antidiuretic Hormone Secretion

Syndrome of inappropriate antidiuretic hormone secretion (SIADH) is a disease of the posterior pituitary gland characterized by inappropriately high levels of secretion of ADH (vasopressin). ADH

is produced in the hypothalamus and stored in the posterior pituitary gland, and when needed, it is released into the bloodstream. SIADH is most commonly associated with tumors that secrete ADH, but it can also be due to brain injury or infections. SIADH is associated with increases in total body water due to increased water reabsorption by the kidneys, which also leads to hyponatremia (low sodium levels).

Prognosis. Symptoms typically resolve after treatment and correction of excess fluid and hyponatremia.

Non–Drug Treatment. Because SIADH can be caused by infections and other underlying conditions, it is important to address the primary reason contributing to its development. With resolution of hyponatremia, symptoms of hyponatremia can resolve after approximately 3 days of treatment.

Drug Treatment. Emergency treatment of severe hyponatremia with hypertonic saline and fluid restriction is critical. Demeclocycline can be used to treat resistant or chronic SIADH. Demeclocycline works by causing tubules in the kidney to develop resistance to the effects of ADH.

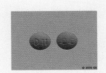

GENERIC NAME: demeclocycline
TRADE NAME: Declomycin

TABLE 16-2

Summary of Select Conditions Associated with the Endocrine System

Disease/Condition	Cause	Clinical Conditions/Characteristics
Conditions Associated with the Pituitary Gland		
Syndrome of inappropriate antidiuretic hormone secretion (SIADH)	↑ Antidiuretic hormone (ADH)	• ↑ Total body water
Diabetes insipidus	↓ ADH	• Hyponatremia • Thirst • Dehydration • Polyuria (frequent urination)
Hypopituitarism	Absence or deficiency of some or all pituitary hormones	• Panhypopituitarism • Hypopituitary dwarfism
Hypersecretion of growth hormone (GH)	↑ GH	• Gigantism • Acromegaly
Conditions Associated with the Thyroid Gland		
Hyperthyroidism	↑ Thyroid hormone (TH)	• Graves disease • Goiter
Hypothyroidism	↓ TH	• Cretinism • Myxedema
Conditions Associated with the Parathyroid Glands		
Hyperparathyroidism	↑ Parathyroid hormone (PTH)	• Hypercalcemia
Hypoparathyroidism	↓ PTH	• Hypocalcemia
Conditions Associated with the Adrenal Glands		
Cushing's disease; Cushing's syndrome	↓ Adrenocorticotrophic hormone (ACTH)	• Weight gain • Flushing of the face • Thinning of the hair • Acne
Hyperaldosteronism	↑ Aldosterone	• Hypertension • Hypokalemia
Addison's disease (primary adrenal insufficiency)	↓ Corticosteroids ↓ Mineralocorticoids ↑ ACTH	• Fatigue • Weight loss • Nausea • Syncope
Conditions Associated with the Pancreas		
Type 1 diabetes mellitus (T1DM)	Absolute insulin deficiency	• Hyperglycemia
Type 2 diabetes mellitus (T2DM)	Insulin resistance + relative insulin deficiency	• Hyperglycemia
Gestational diabetes	Insulin resistance during pregnancy	• Hyperglycemia

INDICATION: Off-label treatment of SIADH
ROUTE OF ADMINISTRATION: Oral
COMMON ADULT DOSAGE: 600-1200 mg daily given in three or four divided doses
MECHANISM OF ACTION: Causes the renal tubules to develop resistance to ADH
SIDE EFFECTS: Gastrointestinal (GI) upset
AUXILIARY LABEL:
• Take on an empty stomach with plenty of fluids.

Diabetes Insipidus

Diabetes insipidus is a rare disorder caused by a deficiency of ADH (vasopressin). Causes of this condition include brain tumors or infection of the meninges (meningitis) or brain (encephalitis), and hemorrhage in or around the pituitary gland. Kidneys that do not respond normally to the hormone cause the same type of condition and symptoms; this condition is known as *nephrogenic diabetes insipidus*. Symptoms of diabetes insipidus include excessive thirst, frequent urination (polyuria), and dehydration. It is important to note that diabetes insipidus is not the same as diabetes mellitus (discussed later).

Prognosis. Overall, the prognosis for diabetes insipidus is good, depending on the type and severity of the condition. Once it has been controlled with treatment, there are no limitations on activity or diet, including the intake of water.

Non–Drug Treatment. Treatment includes keeping a record of daily weight and prevention of dehydration. It is also suggested that the person wear a medical identification bracelet indicating his or her condition and prescribed medications.

Drug Treatment. Vasopressin and desmopressin acetate (synthetic forms of ADH) are typically prescribed to treat diabetes insipidus. Agents that can stimulate production of ADH (e.g., chlorpropamide, carbamazepine, and clofibrate) may also be used.

Hypopituitarism

Hypopituitarism (includes panhypopituitarism and dwarfism) involves a range of dysfunctions from absence of selective pituitary hormones to complete failure of hormonal functions. Accordingly, the signs and symptoms of hypopituitarism are variable and depend on which hormones are affected. Panhypopituitarism is characterized by partial or total failure in the secretion of all anterior pituitary hormones (corticotropin, TSH, LH, FSH, GH, and prolactin), in addition to the posterior pituitary hormone ADH. Partial hypopituitarism and complete hypopituitarism occur in both adults and children. A deficiency of GH in children may result in hypoglycemia and short stature, resulting in **hypopituitary dwarfism**. Corticotropin deficiency affects normal protein, carbohydrate, and lipid metabolism, resulting in **hypoglycemia**, fatigue, progressive emaciation (weight loss), and death.

Treatments include:

- Partial or total hypophysectomy (surgery)
- Radiation treatments
- Treatment with chemical agents

Signs and symptoms develop slowly over time and vary depending on the severity of the condition. In adults, impotence, infertility, decreased libido, diabetes insipidus, hypothyroidism, and adrenocortical insufficiency may occur. An interruption in growth or the onset of puberty may occur in children. Dwarfism is not apparent at birth but appears during the first 3 to 6 months of age.

Prognosis. The prognosis for hypopituitarism in children is good if the condition is treated early. With early diagnosis and treatment, the symptoms may be controlled or stopped.

Non–Drug Treatment. Surgery may be necessary in the event of a tumor, although medication may still be needed throughout the patient's lifetime.

Drug Treatment. Treatment of pituitary hypofunction is directed at the underlying cause and replacement of needed hormones; also, the age of the child determines the hormones involved in replacement therapy. In the event of a deficiency of adrenocorticotropic hormone (ACTH), hydrocortisone or prednisone may be administered. In TSH deficiency, L-thyroxine may be prescribed. However, doses of these agents depend on the age of the patient. For gonadotropin deficiency, steroid replacement therapy begins at puberty. GH replacement therapy may be prescribed in childhood through puberty.

Hypersecretion of Growth Hormone

Gigantism and acromegaly are two rare, progressive conditions that involve an increase in levels of GH. Hyperfunction of the pituitary gland can be caused by various tumor growths. If this condition is present in children, it is referred to as **gigantism**. The bones elongate, resulting in heights that have reached almost 9 feet. If this condition arises after normal bone growth has halted, it is called **acromegaly**, and symptoms involve increased size of the head, tongue, nose, hands, feet, and toes (Figure 16-13).

Prognosis. Patients with gigantism are susceptible to cardiovascular and respiratory complications. Persons with acromegaly are susceptible to diabetes mellitus and have increased risk for colon cancer.

Non–Drug Treatment. Treatment may involve removal of the tumor or growth causing excessive GH secretion, although any bone growth preceding removal cannot be reversed. Radiation therapy may also be used.

Drug Treatment. The goal of treatment with medications may include shrinking the pituitary mass, restoring secretory patterns and serum levels to their normal state, and retaining normal pituitary secretion of other hormones to prevent recurrence of the condition. Currently, octreotide, a somatostatin analogue, is the pharmacological treatment most often used for GH excess in children and adults. Other agents (e.g., lanreotide, pegvisomant, bromocriptine, and cabergoline) may also be used to treat gigantism and acromegaly.

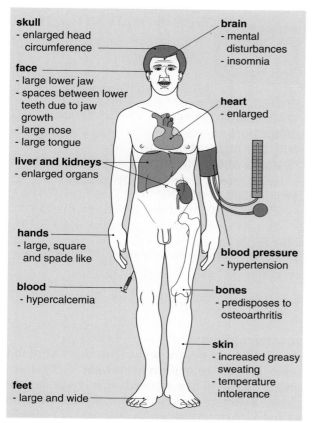

FIGURE 16-13 Features of acromegaly. (From Fishback JL: *Pathology,* ed 3, Philadelphia, 2005, Mosby.)

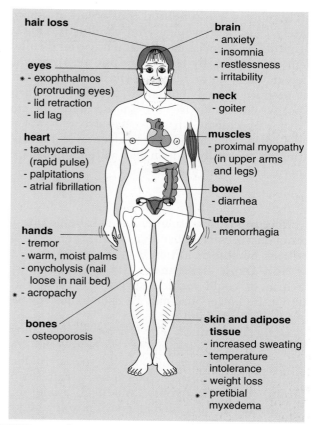

FIGURE 16-14 Summary diagram illustrating features of thyrotoxicosis. (From Fishback JL: *Pathology,* ed 3, Philadelphia, 2005, Mosby.)

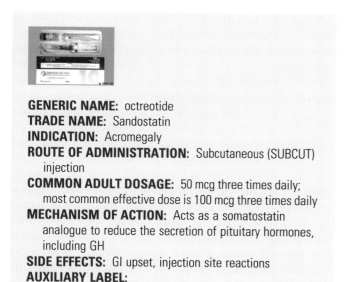

GENERIC NAME: octreotide
TRADE NAME: Sandostatin
INDICATION: Acromegaly
ROUTE OF ADMINISTRATION: Subcutaneous (SUBCUT) injection
COMMON ADULT DOSAGE: 50 mcg three times daily; most common effective dose is 100 mcg three times daily
MECHANISM OF ACTION: Acts as a somatostatin analogue to reduce the secretion of pituitary hormones, including GH
SIDE EFFECTS: GI upset, injection site reactions
AUXILIARY LABEL:
• Administer subcutaneously.

Conditions of the Thyroid Gland and Their Treatment

Hyperthyroidism

Thyrotoxicosis is a condition that results from increased thyroid hormones. **Hyperthyroidism** is a specific form of thyrotoxicosis caused by the oversecretion of hormones from the thyroid gland. Common diseases that cause hyperthyroidism include Graves disease and toxic multinodular goiter. **Graves disease** is the most common cause of hyperthyroidism and is an autoimmune disorder. The body manufactures antibodies to TSH receptors, leading to an increase in the production of T_4 and triiodothyronine T_3. The most common symptoms of Graves disease are diffuse thyroid enlargement (goiter), inflammation and enlargement of the tissues in the orbit of the eye (causing the eyes to bulge, a condition known as **exophthalmos**), and thickening of the skin over the lower legs (Figure 16-14). Graves disease is more common in women and occurs in less than 1% of the population in the United States.

A **goiter** gives the appearance of an enlarged neck and usually is caused by a nonmalignant tumor or nodules in or on the thyroid gland that are associated with excess production of thyroid hormone (see Figure 16-14). Goiters are painless and range in size from barely discernible to the size of a grapefruit. If the goiter is small, it is not normally treated because many goiters resolve on their own. If the goiter continues to grow, medications can be used; surgery generally is reserved for cases in which medication is ineffective.

Thyroiditis is a condition that occurs in approximately 1 out of 20 women after childbirth. This type of thyroid problem causes little, if any, gland enlargement and is usually temporary and resolves within a few months. Later, however, the thyroid gland may not produce enough hormones, resulting in chronic hypothyroidism. Viruses are another potential cause of hyperthyroidism, with the excessive amounts of T_3 and T_4 disappearing after the infection has resolved. Although hyperthyroidism has various causes, the general symptoms are the same.

Prognosis. Treatments are available for all common types of hyperthyroidism; therefore, the outlook for this condition is good.

Non–Drug Treatment. If a tumor exists, treatment could include surgery to remove the tumor. Radiation also may be used to destroy part of the thyroid gland.

Drug Treatment. For Graves disease, initial therapy with a beta-blocker can be used to ameliorate some of the symptoms of hyperthyroidism, such as palpitations, increased heart rate (tachycardia), tremors, anxiety, and heat intolerance. Antithyroid agents, such as methimazole and propylthiouracil (PTU), are also used to interfere with the thyroid gland's ability to make hormones. The most common treatment in the United States is the use of radioactive iodine, which destroys cells in the thyroid gland. It is important to remember that the use of radioactive iodine to destroy the thyroid gland often results in hypothyroidism that requires thyroid supplementation.

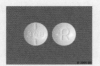

GENERIC NAME: propylthiouracil (PTU)
TRADE NAME: None
INDICATION: Hyperthyroidism
ROUTE OF ADMINISTRATION: Oral
COMMON ADULT DOSAGE: *Initial:* 300-400 mg daily in divided doses (initial dosage); *maintenance:* 100-150 mg daily
MECHANISM OF ACTION: Directly interferes with the first step in thyroid hormone synthesis, leading to a decrease in thyroid hormone production
SIDE EFFECTS: Nausea, headache, urticarial rash
AUXILIARY LABEL:
• Take as directed.

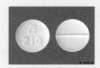

GENERIC NAME: methimazole
TRADE NAME: Tapazole
INDICATION: Hyperthyroidism
ROUTE OF ADMINISTRATION: Oral
COMMON ADULT DOSAGE: *Initial:* 15-60 mg daily in divided doses; *maintenance:* 5-30 mg daily
MECHANISM OF ACTION: Directly interferes with the first step in thyroid hormone synthesis, leading to a decrease in thyroid hormone production
SIDE EFFECTS: Fever, rash, itching
AUXILIARY LABEL:
• Take as directed.

Hypothyroidism

Hypothyroidism occurs when the thyroid gland is unable to secrete sufficient levels of T_3 and T_4. Primary causes of hypothyroidism include congenital defects, defective production of thyroid hormones, and loss of thyroid tissue after surgical or radioactive treatment for hyperthyroidism. Hypothyroidism due to a congenital deficiency is sometimes referred to as *thyroid dysgenesis.* The absence of the thyroid gland affects the growth of the child's body and the development of the nervous system. If the condition is not discovered early, the child's growth will be stunted (dwarfism), and the child will develop mental retardation (**cretinism**). Once hypothyroidism is diagnosed, thyroid medication must be administered for the lifetime of the patient, although any retardation that has already occurred is irreversible.

A lack of iodine in the diet can cause a deficiency in the production of thyroid hormones because iodine is necessary for the synthesis of T_3 and T_4. Hypothyroidism caused by iodine deficiency is not common in developed nations because of the addition of iodine to salt; therefore, patients with hypothyroidism rarely need iodine supplementation. Inflammation of the thyroid gland, known as *thyroiditis,* is an autoimmune condition. Hashimoto's thyroiditis is specifically discussed in Chapter 23.

Hypothyroidism is a common medical problem, and women older than age 35 are most commonly affected. Symptoms include increased sensitivity to cold, brittle fingernails, constipation, unexplained weight gain, among others (Figure 16-15). Hypothyroidism results in an overall decrease in energy and mental alertness. It can also be associated with the condition **myxedema**. Symptoms include skin that appears puffy and has a waxy appearance; the patient

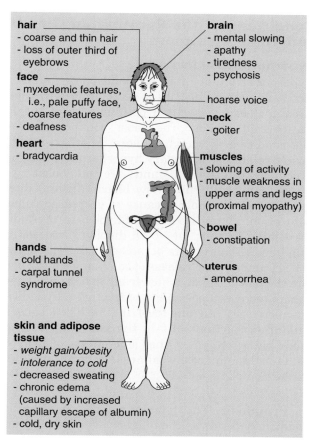

hair
- coarse and thin hair
- loss of outer third of eyebrows

face
- myxedemic features, i.e., pale puffy face, coarse features
- deafness

heart
- bradycardia

hands
- cold hands
- carpal tunnel syndrome

skin and adipose tissue
- *weight gain/obesity*
- *intolerance to cold*
- decreased sweating
- chronic edema (caused by increased capillary escape of albumin)
- cold, dry skin

brain
- mental slowing
- apathy
- tiredness
- psychosis

- hoarse voice

neck
- goiter

muscles
- slowing of activity
- muscle weakness in upper arms and legs (proximal myopathy)

bowel
- constipation

uterus
- amenorrhea

FIGURE 16-15 Summary diagram illustrating features of hypothyroidism in the adult. (From Fishback JL: *Pathology,* ed 3, Philadelphia, 2005, Mosby.)

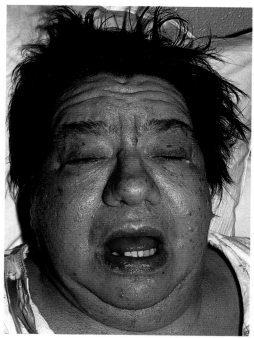

FIGURE 16-16 Myxedema. (From Huether SE: *Understanding pathophysiology,* ed 5, St Louis, 2012, Mosby.)

GENERIC NAME: desiccated thyroid (combined T_4-T_3 product)
TRADE NAME: Armour Thyroid, Westhroid
INDICATION: Hypothyroidism, goiter
ROUTE OF ADMINISTRATION: Oral
COMMON ADULT DOSAGE: 60-120 mg once daily
MECHANISM OF ACTION: Supplements missing thyroid hormone to normal (euthyroid) levels
SIDE EFFECTS: No major side effects if correct dosage is taken
AUXILIARY LABELS:
- Take as directed.
- Take with water on an empty stomach.

GENERIC NAME: levothyroxine sodium (T_4)
TRADE NAME: Synthroid, Levothroid, Levoxyl, Tirosint, Unithroid
INDICATION: Hypothyroidism

may also have dramatic changes in mental status if the condition is severe, such as myxedema coma (Figure 16-16).

Prognosis. If hypothyroidism is not treated, the symptoms may progress, although the condition is not normally life-threatening. When treated appropriately with medication, most patients do quite well.

Non–Drug Treatment. The main treatment for hypothyroidism caused by tumors is surgical removal of the tumor. In the case of thyroiditis, surgery may also be necessary to remove all or part of the thyroid gland.

Drug Treatment. Most patients with hypothyroidism do not have tumors and are managed with hormone replacement therapy. Thyroid hormone replacement agents need to be taken for life (one dose a day) due to the chronic nature of the condition. Levothyroxine is most commonly preferred by many medical physicians because of its ease of dosing (i.e., it uses one thyroid hormone, T_4).

ROUTE OF ADMINISTRATION: Oral
COMMON ADULT DOSAGE: 25-200 mcg once daily
MECHANISM OF ACTION: Supplements missing thyroid hormone to normal (euthyroid) levels
SIDE EFFECTS: No major effects if correct dosage is taken
AUXILIARY LABELS:
- Take as directed.
- Take with water on an empty stomach.

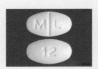

GENERIC NAME: liothyronine sodium (T₃)
TRADE NAME: Cytomel, Triostat
INDICATION: Hypothyroidism
ROUTE OF ADMINISTRATION: Oral
COMMON ADULT DOSAGE: 25-100 mcg once daily
MECHANISM OF ACTION: Supplements missing thyroid hormone to normal (euthyroid) levels
SIDE EFFECTS: No major effects if correct dosage is taken
AUXILIARY LABELS:
- Take as directed.
- Take with water on an empty stomach.

 Tech Note!

Liothyronine (T₃) is sometimes used off-label to augment antidepressant therapy in patients who have not had an adequate response to antidepressant therapy.

GENERIC NAME: liotrix (combined T₄-T₃ product)
TRADE NAME: Thyrolar
INDICATION: Hypothyroidism
ROUTE OF ADMINISTRATION: Oral
COMMON ADULT DOSAGE: 25-100 mcg (based on T₄ content) taken once daily
MECHANISM OF ACTION: Supplements missing thyroid hormone to normal (euthyroid) levels
SIDE EFFECTS: No major effects if correct dosage is taken
AUXILIARY LABELS:
- Take as directed.
- Take with water on an empty stomach.

Conditions of the Parathyroid Glands and Their Treatment

Hyperparathyroidism

Hyperparathyroidism is a condition in which an increased amount of PTH is secreted into the bloodstream; it can arise from one or more of the four parathyroid glands. The most common cause of this condition is benign tumors. Another condition closely related is secondary hyperparathyroidism, in which the parathyroid glands are compensating for chronic **hypocalcemia** (low blood calcium) due to renal failure or another cause of decreased calcium absorption. These two forms of hyperparathyroidism are similar in that they both display increased calcium levels. This occurs because the increased levels of PTH promote the release of calcium from the bones into the bloodstream, which leads to bone weakening and an increased possibility of fractures. In addition, the increased calcium level in the blood causes a buildup of calcium salts in the kidneys, which can cause kidney stones. Other side effects of hypercalcemia include muscle weakness, lethargy, and heart conduction changes.

Prognosis. The prognosis for hyperparathyroidism depends on the diagnosis of the condition. In some cases, after removal of all or part of the affected gland, functioning may return to normal. Other patients may need to monitor their calcium intake for life. For those with renal failure, continuous dialysis may be necessary until a kidney transplant is received.

Non–Drug Treatment. Treatment depends on the underlying cause. If the hyperparathyroidism is due to a tumor, surgical removal of the tumor may be necessary. In addition, removal of several of the parathyroid glands may be necessary. If the hyperparathyroidism is caused by improper kidney function, transplantation or dialysis may be necessary to limit the disease process. Other treatments may include reducing calcium levels by increasing fluid intake and/or limiting dietary intake of calcium.

Drug Treatment. A variety of medications have been used in patients with hyperparathyroidism, although not all of them necessarily carry an indication for this purpose. Medications used for the treatment of osteoporosis have been used for hyperparathyroidism, such as the bisphosphonates, raloxifene, and estrogen/progestin therapy (a detailed discussion of these agents is presented in Chapter 17). Other medications, such as the calcimimetics and vitamin D analogues, suppress PTH or counteract the effects of hyperparathyroidism at the level of the PTH receptor.

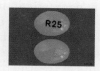

GENERIC NAME: calcitriol
TRADE NAME: Calcijex, Rocaltrol
INDICATION: Hyperparathyroidism, hypocalcemia
ROUTE OF ADMINISTRATION: Oral; intravenous
COMMON ADULT DOSAGE: *Oral:* 0.25-0.5 mcg daily; *IV:* 1-2 mcg three times weekly
MECHANISM OF ACTION: Calcitriol is another name for the active form of vitamin D, which is important in maintaining calcium balance and regulating PTH levels
SIDE EFFECTS: Hypercalcemia
AUXILIARY LABEL:
• Protect from light.

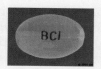

GENERIC NAME: doxercalciferol
TRADE NAME: Hectorol
INDICATIONS: Hyperparathyroidism
ROUTE OF ADMINISTRATION: Oral; intravenous
COMMON ADULT DOSAGE: *Oral:* 1-3.5 mcg daily
MECHANISM OF ACTION: Doxercalciferol is metabolized in the liver to active vitamin D, which is important in maintaining calcium balance and regulating PTH levels
SIDE EFFECTS: Hypercalcemia
AUXILIARY LABEL:
• Take with or without food.

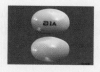

GENERIC NAME: paricalcitol
TRADE NAME: Zemplar
INDICATION: Hyperparathyroidism
ROUTE OF ADMINISTRATION: Oral; intravenous
COMMON ADULT DOSAGE: *Oral:* 1-2 mcg daily *or* 2-4 mcg three times per week
MECHANISM OF ACTION: Inhibits PTH secretion
SIDE EFFECTS: Hypercalcemia
AUXILIARY LABEL:
• Take with or without food.

GENERIC NAME: cinacalcet
TRADE NAME: Sensipar
INDICATION: Hyperparathyroidism, hypercalcemia
ROUTE OF ADMINISTRATION: Oral
COMMON ADULT DOSAGE: *Oral:* 60-360 mg daily in divided doses
MECHANISM OF ACTION: Mimics calcium at calcium-sensing receptors on the parathyroid gland, leading to a reduction in PTH secretion
SIDE EFFECTS: GI symptoms
AUXILIARY LABEL:
• Take with food.

Hypoparathyroidism

Malfunctioning of the parathyroid glands can cause hypoparathyroidism. Hypoparathyroidism is most commonly due to damage to the parathyroid glands during thyroid surgery. The result is hypocalcemia, which, in turn, reduces vitamin D levels in the body. Symptoms include muscle spasms, irregular heart contractions, and alteration of normal nerve conduction.

Prognosis. The prognosis for hypoparathyroidism is good with chronic replacement therapy.

Non–Drug Treatment. The only treatment for hypoparathyroidism is administration of the supplemental medications calcium and vitamin D.

Drug Treatment. Treatment is directed at correcting the hypocalcemia. Acute treatment can involve **parenteral** administration of calcium, with long-term treatment involving the use of calcium and vitamin D supplements. Chapter 17 presents a detailed discussion of calcium and vitamin D supplements.

Conditions of the Adrenal Glands and Their Treatment

As discussed previously, each adrenal gland consists of two portions, a cortex and a medulla. We first discuss disorders of the adrenal cortex, which range from overproduction to underproduction of steroids. The three types of steroids produced are mineralocorticoids, glucocorticoids, and sex steroids. A decrease in secretion of these steroids can affect the levels of sodium, potassium, and chloride in the body; can alter carbohydrate metabolism; or can cause sexual problems (discussed in Chapter 22).

Cushing's Disease

Cushing's disease is caused by excessive secretion of adrenocorticotropic hormone (ACTH) from the anterior pituitary gland. Cushing's disease is more common in adults and is two to three times more common in women than in men. Cushing's syndrome is an uncommon disorder that occurs whenever there is too much cortisol in the system, regardless of the cause. Cushing's syndrome is the most common complication of Cushing's disease. As cortisol is released from the adrenal glands, symptoms develop that can include weight gain, flushing of the face, thinning of the hair, and acne (Figure 16-17). Other symptoms include overall weakness, fatigue, and slow-healing injuries.

In approximately 70% of cases of Cushing's syndrome, the cause is overproduction of corticotropin. Three etiologies are associated with excess corticotropin production: hypersecretion of corticotropin from the pituitary glands; the presence of a corticotropin-releasing tumor in another organ; or overmedication with corticosteroids (e.g., transplant recipients, people with rheumatoid arthritis, and individuals with severe asthma who must take corticosteroids as part of their treatment).

Prognosis. After removal of a nonmalignant tumor, patients with Cushing's disease have a good prognosis. For patients taking corticosteroids for inflammatory conditions, the disadvantages must be weighed against the benefits of treatment with the corticosteroids.

Non–Drug Treatment. Adrenal gland tumors that cause Cushing's syndrome also require surgery. After excision of the tumor, medication may be necessary. Patients with Cushing's disease require either surgical excision of the tumor or radiation therapy.

Drug Treatment. If the condition continues after surgery, patients with Cushing's syndrome may require drug therapy (e.g., mitotane or metyrapone) that reduces cortisol levels.

Hyperaldosteronism

Hyperaldosteronism is characterized by excessive **aldosterone** secretion by the adrenal glands. Aldosterone promotes the excretion of potassium and the retention of sodium and water. Hyperaldosteronism can be primary or secondary in nature. Primary hyperaldosteronism is due to an abnormality of the adrenal cortex, whereas secondary hyperaldosteronism is caused by a stimulus outside the adrenal glands. **Hypertension** (high blood pressure) and hypokalemia (low blood potassium) are the hallmarks of primary hyperaldosteronism.

Prognosis. The prognosis for hyperaldosteronism is good after identification and treatment of the underlying cause and management of the hypertension and hypokalemia.

Non–Drug Treatment. If an aldosterone-secreting tumor is present, surgical removal of the tumor is required.

Drug Treatment. Drug therapy for the management of hypertension and use of potassium supplements to rectify any existing hypokalemia are required.

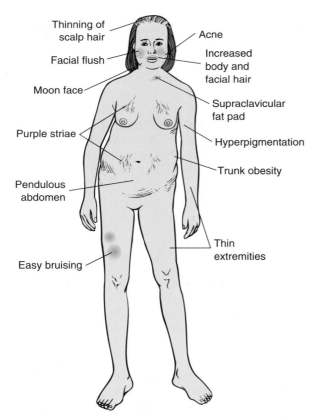

Thinning of scalp hair
Acne
Facial flush
Increased body and facial hair
Moon face
Supraclavicular fat pad
Purple striae
Hyperpigmentation
Pendulous abdomen
Trunk obesity
Easy bruising
Thin extremities

FIGURE 16-17 Symptoms of Cushing's disease. (From Huether SE: *Understanding pathophysiology*, ed 5, St Louis, 2012, Mosby.)

Addison's Disease

Addison's disease, which is associated with inadequate corticosteroid and mineralocorticoid synthesis and elevated serum ACTH, is a rare hormonal disorder caused by a deficiency of cortisol. In approximately 70% of those with Addison's disease, autoimmune disease causes dysfunction of the adrenal cortex. Symptoms begin gradually and include fatigue, weight loss, nausea, and syncope (fainting).

Prognosis. Depending on the cause of Addison's disease, it is possible to correct the cortisol levels, although the replacement therapy must be taken for the patient's lifetime. If left untreated, Addison's disease can be life-threatening.

Non–Drug Treatment. Surgery may be indicated for tumor removal. In addition, the patient may need to balance both potassium and sodium intake in the daily diet. Monitoring daily weight and recording daily intake and output of fluids also may be necessary.

Drug Treatment. Treatment consists of replacement therapy with oral glucocorticoids and mineralocorticoids.

Tech Note!

Long-term corticosteroid treatment can lead to hyperglycemia and the development of type 2 diabetes mellitus.

Mineralocorticoid

GENERIC NAME: fludrocortisone acetate
INDICATION: Addison's disease
ROUTE OF ADMINISTRATION: Oral
COMMON ADULT DOSAGE: 0.1 mg three times weekly to 0.2 mg daily
MECHANISM OF ACTION: Mimics the actions of aldosterone
SIDE EFFECTS: GI upset, edema, hypertension
AUXILIARY LABEL:
• Take with food to minimize GI upset.

Glucocorticoids

GENERIC NAME: hydrocortisone
TRADE NAME: Cortef
INDICATION: Addison's disease, inflammation
ROUTE OF ADMINISTRATION: Oral
COMMON ADULT DOSAGE: 20-240 mg daily given in divided doses

MECHANISM OF ACTION: Antiinflammatory, antipruritic, and vasoconstrictive effects
SIDE EFFECTS: GI upset, hyperglycemia, increased risk of fracture
AUXILIARY LABEL:
• Take with food.
SPECIAL NOTE: Additional dosage forms include the following injectables: hydrocortisone acetate, hydrocortisone sodium succinate (e.g., A-Hydrocort, Solu-Cortef). Dosages vary, depending on the condition treated and the individual's response.

GENERIC NAME: methylprednisolone
TRADE NAME: Medrol
INDICATION: Inflammation, Addison's disease
ROUTE OF ADMINISTRATION: Oral
COMMON ADULT DOSAGE: 4-48 mg daily in divided doses
MECHANISM OF ACTION: Antiinflammatory, antipruritic, and vasoconstrictive effects
SIDE EFFECTS: GI upset, hyperglycemia, increased risk of fracture
AUXILIARY LABEL:
• Take with food.
SPECIAL NOTE: Methylprednisolone dose packs are available in 21-tablet sets and are commonly dispensed to slowly taper the patient off the medication or to a maintenance level of continued medication.

GENERIC NAME: methylprednisolone sodium succinate
TRADE NAME: Solu-Medrol
INDICATION: Addison's disease, inflammation
ROUTE OF ADMINISTRATION: Intramuscular; intravenous
COMMON ADULT DOSAGE: *IM* or *IV:* 10-40 mg
MECHANISM OF ACTION: Antiinflammatory, antipruritic, and vasoconstrictive effects
SIDE EFFECTS: GI upset, hyperglycemia, osteoporosis, cataracts, Cushing's syndrome

GENERIC NAME: prednisolone
TRADE NAME: Orapred
INDICATION: Addison's disease, Inflammation
ROUTE OF ADMINISTRATION: Oral
COMMON ADULT DOSAGE: 5-60 mg once daily
MECHANISM OF ACTION: Antiinflammatory, antipruritic, and vasoconstrictive effects
SIDE EFFECTS: GI upset, hyperglycemia, osteoporosis, cataracts, Cushing's syndrome
AUXILIARY LABEL:
- Take with food.

SPECIAL NOTE: Syrup must be measured in calibrated dose cup, oral syringe, or measuring spoon.

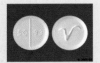

GENERIC NAME: prednisone
INDICATION: Addison's disease, Inflammation
ROUTE OF ADMINISTRATION: Oral
COMMON ADULT DOSAGE: morning: 5 mg; evening: 2.5 mg
MECHANISM OF ACTION: Antiinflammatory, antipruritic, and vasoconstrictive effects
SIDE EFFECTS: GI upset, hyperglycemia, osteoporosis, cataracts, Cushing's syndrome
AUXILIARY LABEL:
- Take with food.

Conditions Affecting the Adrenal Medulla

Most of the conditions that affect the adrenal medulla result from tumor growth. The main types of tumor that affect the adrenal medulla are pheochromocytomas. Pheochromocytomas continually secrete catecholamines, which can result in hypertension. With surgical removal, the hypertension is relieved and the patient's prognosis is generally good. Medical therapy is typically used to stabilize the blood pressure before, during, and after surgery.

Endocrine Conditions of the Pancreas and Their Treatments

The pancreas is responsible for the production and release of insulin and glucagon. Insulin is important in the transportation of glucose into cells, where it is then either used for energy or stored as glycogen. Insulin also stimulates protein synthesis and releases fatty acids from adipose (fat) tissue. Conditions associated with **hyperglycemia**, or an increase in blood glucose, are known as *diabetes mellitus*.

Diabetes Mellitus

One of the best-known conditions of the endocrine system is diabetes mellitus (DM). DM is a chronic disease associated with hyperglycemia. The two most common types are **type 1 diabetes mellitus (T1DM)** and **type 2 diabetes mellitus (T2DM)**. It is estimated that 26 million people in the United States are living with DM, 7 million of who are not aware that they have the disease.

Type 1 Diabetes Mellitus. T1DM is caused by the destruction of or a defect in the beta-cells of the pancreas. This results in an inability of the pancreas to synthesize and secrete insulin, leading to an absolute insulin deficiency in people with T1DM. Because people with T1DM are unable to produce insulin, the use of exogenous insulin is required for treatment. The classic symptoms of hyperglycemia that can lead to a diagnosis of T1DM include polyuria (frequent urination), polydipsia (excessive thirst), and polyphagia (excessive appetite). The loss of glucose via urination can cause dehydration, weight loss, fatigue, and extreme hunger.

Type 2 Diabetes Mellitus. Most people with DM have T2DM. As mentioned, T1DM is due to an absolute deficiency of insulin; T2DM, however, is due to **insulin resistance**, or a decreased ability of the tissues to respond to the effects of insulin. Insulin resistance increases with obesity; therefore, most T2DM patients are obese. Adults are most commonly affected by T2DM; however, the increasing prevalence of obesity in children has resulted in an increased diagnosis of T2DM in children. Because of the insulin resistance associated with T2DM, the beta-cells of the pancreas are forced to work harder to produce insulin to compensate for the insulin resistance and keep the blood sugars from becoming elevated. Over time, the beta-cells begin to fail, and people with T2DM start to produce less insulin, thus requiring many people with T2DM to take insulin injections to manage their blood sugar.

T2DM is a metabolic disease associated with a number of other **comorbidities**. The following conditions are commonly associated with T2DM:
- Obesity
- Lack of physical activity
- Hypertension (high blood pressure)
- History of gestational DM
- Older than age 45 years
- Strong family history of T2DM
- Hyperlipidemia (elevated cholesterol levels)

Gestational Diabetes Mellitus. Gestational diabetes mellitus (GDM) occurs in women during pregnancy, with blood glucose levels usually returning to normal after childbirth. GDM is associated only with pregnancy; weight gain and an increase in the concentrations of estrogen and placental hormones, which antagonize insulin, are its two precipitating factors. The effects may last only through the pregnancy period, although the condition must be treated through diet and possibly the use of medications. Poor management of GDM can lead to complications with the pregnancy and health problems for the child after birth. Some patients with gestational diabetes will have risk factors to develop T2DM later in life. For more information on gestational diabetes, visit the website *www.diabetes.org/gestational-diabetes.jsp*.

Prognosis. With proper treatment and management of DM, a person can lead a normal life. Thorough education regarding lifestyle, medications, and monitoring are essential to optimizing treatment outcomes.

People with DM are at risk for a variety of complications if their condition is not well controlled, which can affect both the quality and longevity of life. Some complications associated with DM include:
- Macrovascular disease (cardiac disease, including risk for heart attack and stroke)
- Erectile dysfunction (impotence)
- **Gastroparesis**
- Increased infections of the skin (feet), urinary tract (UTIs), and vagina (vaginitis)
- Nephropathy (kidney disease)
- **Orthostatic hypotension**
- **Peripheral neuropathy**
- Retinopathy (eye disease)

Non–Drug Treatment. An important first-line treatment for patients with DM are lifestyle changes that include increased physical activity and a healthful diet, which can help maintain blood glucose levels and lead to weight loss (which may help reduce insulin resistance in people with T2DM). Many people with DM can benefit from periodic visits with a dietitian. Daily foot checks are also important to monitor for any mechanical damage to the feet that can lead to infection or ulceration.

Drug Treatments. A variety of medications are available to treat DM. For T1DM, insulin given by subcutaneous injections or infusion is required. Synthetic insulin products produced in laboratories are the primary (and essential) treatment option for patients with T1DM, and many T2DM patients require insulin therapy, particularly as their disease progresses and their beta-cells lose the ability to produce insulin. The main categories of insulin used therapeutically are rapid- and short-acting, intermediate-acting, long-acting, and mixed-acting insulin. These categories are related to how fast and how long the insulin products work in the body. Table 16-3 provides an overview of currently available single insulin products, and Table 16-4 lists currently available premixed insulin products. Insulin products differ in their onset of action (how fast they work) and duration of action (how long they work). Great care should be taken when dispensing insulin products to patients to ensure accurate prescription filling, sufficient counseling, and adequate patient understanding. Many of the products have similar names and are available in similar doses but have very different onsets and durations of action.

People with T2DM are often treated with oral agents and noninsulin injectable medications to manage their blood glucose levels. The drugs listed in Table 16-5 are examples of noninsulin agents that can be used to manage T2DM. Of note, the injectable medication pramlintide can be used in people with either T1DM or T2DM. Because so many new agents are being marketed, it is important for technicians always to stay abreast of the various agents being used.

Combination Agents. Because many people with T2DM require multiple medications to achieve their treatment goals, a variety of combination products are available to reduce the number of pills patients need to take on a daily basis. Table 16-6 provides a list of combination oral products currently on the market for the treatment of T2DM.

Blood Glucose Meters. People with DM are often asked to monitor their blood glucose levels with a **glucometer** by taking a drop of blood using a small needle called a lancet. Although the finger is the most common location used for blood sampling, some meters allow blood to be taken from the forearm, thigh, or fleshy part of the hand (this is known as "alternate site testing"). The blood is placed on a test strip that is inserted into the glucometer. Glucometers display a digital number on the screen that indicates the current blood glucose level. A wide range of blood glucose meters is available, including meters with large font size for people with poor eyesight, and even glucometers that talk to the user.

Regardless of the type of meter chosen, it is important to keep the meter clean and the test strips in proper condition.

TABLE 16-3

Currently Available Single Insulin Products for the Treatment of Diabetes Mellitus

Generic Name	Trade Name	Availability	Onset of Action	Duration of Action
Rapid-Acting Insulin Products				
Insulin lispro	• Humalog • Humalog KwikPen	• 3-mL and 10-mL vials • 5 (3-mL) cartridges • 5 (3-mL) prefilled pens	5-15 min	4-6 hr
Insulin aspart	• NovoLog • NovoLog FlexPen	• 10-mL vial • 5 (3-mL) cartridges • 5 (3-mL) prefilled pens		
Insulin glulisine	• Apidra • Apidra SoloStar	• 10-mL vial • 5 (3-mL) cartridges • 5 (3-mL) prefilled pens		
Short-Acting Insulin Products				
Regular human insulin	• Humulin R • Humulin R Pen • Novolin R	• 3-mL and 10-mL vials • 5 (3-mL) prefilled pens • 10-mL vial	0.5-1 hr	6-10 hr
Intermediate-Acting Insulin Products				
NPH insulin (Humulin N)	• Humulin N • Novolin N	• 3-mL and 10-mL vials • 5 (3-mL) prefilled pens • 10-mL vial	1-2 hr	10-16 hr
Long-Acting Insulin Products				
Insulin detemir	• Levemir • Levemir FlexPen	• 10-mL vial • 5 (3-mL) prefilled pens	3-4 hr	14-24 hr
Insulin glargine	• Lantus • Lantus SoloStar	• 10-mL vial • 5 (3-mL) cartridges • 5 (3-mL) prefilled pens	2-4 hr	~24 hr

TABLE 16-4

Currently Available Premixed Insulin Products*

Generic Name	Trade Name
Insulin lispro protamine + insulin lispro	• Humalog Mix 50/50 • Humalog Mix 50/50 KwikPen • Humalog Mix 75/25 • Humalog Mix 75/25 KwikPen
Insulin aspart protamine + insulin aspart	• NovoLog Mix 70/30 • NovoLog Mix 70/30 FlexPen
NPH insulin + regular human insulin	• Humulin 70/30 • Humulin 70/30 Pen • Novolin 70/30

*The fractions listed in premixed insulins (e.g., 70/30) indicate the ratio of long-acting insulin to rapid- or short-acting insulin.

TABLE 16-5

Noninsulin Medications for the Treatment of Diabetes Mellitus

Medication Class	Generic Name	Trade Name	Common Side Effects	Common Dose Range	Labeling/Storage/Miscellaneous Information
Insulin Sensitizers					
Biguanide	metformin	Glucophage Riomet	• Gastrointestinal (GI) upset	• 500-2550 mg 1-3 times daily (max 2550 mg/day)	• Take by mouth with food • First-line treatment for T2DM
	metformin XR	Glucophage XR	• Nausea • Diarrhea	• 500-2000 mg once daily with evening meal	
	metformin XR	Fortamet	• Flatulence • Alterations in taste	• 500-2500 mg once daily with evening meal (max 2500 mg/day)	
	metformin XR	Glumetza		• 1000-2000 mg once daily with evening meal (max 2000 mg/day)	
Thiazolinedione	pioglitazone	Actos	• Weight gain • Fluid retention	• 15-45 mg daily once daily (max 45 mg/day)	• Take by mouth with or without food
Insulin Secretagogues					
Sulfonylureas	glimepiride	Amaryl	• Weight gain	• 1-8 mg once daily (max 8 mg/day)	• Take by mouth with meals
	glipizide	Glucotrol	• Hypoglycemia	• 5-40 mg once or twice daily (max 40 mg/day)	
	glipizide XL	Glucotrol XL	• GI upset	• 5-20 mg once daily (max 20 mg/day)	
	glyburide	Diabeta, Micronase		• 2.5-20 mg once or twice daily with first meal of the day (max 20 mg/day)	
	micronized glyburide	Glynase		• 1.5-12 mg once daily with first meal of the day (max 12 mg/day)	
Meglitinides	nateglinide	Starlix	• Weight gain • Hypoglycemia	• 60-120 mg orally three times daily before meals (max 360 mg/day)	• Take by mouth within 30 min of start of meal
	repaglinide	Prandin		• 0.5-4 mg orally three to four times daily before meals (max 16 mg/day)	

Continued

TABLE 16-5

Noninsulin Medications for the Treatment of Diabetes Mellitus—cont'd

Medication Class	Generic Name	Trade Name	Common Side Effects	Common Dose Range	Labeling/Storage/Miscellaneous Information
Other Oral Medications					
Alpha-Glucosidase Inhibitors	acarbose	Precose	• GI upset • Flatulence • Weight loss	• 25-100 mg orally three times daily with meals (max 150 mg/day if body weight ≤60 kg; max 300 mg/day if body weight >60 kg)	• Take by mouth with food
	miglitol	Glyset		• 25-100 mg orally three times daily with meals (max 300 mg/day)	
Dipeptidyl Peptidase-4 (DPP-4) Inhibitor	sitagliptin saxagliptin linagliptin alogliptin	Januvia[a] Onglyza Tradjenta Nesina	• Sinusitis • GI upset • Headache	• 25-100 mg orally once daily (max 100 mg/day) • 2.5-5 mg once daily (max 5 mg/day) • 5 mg daily • 6.25-25 mg orally once daily (max 25 mg/day)	
Sodium-Glucose Co-transporter 2 (SGLT2) Inhibitors	canagliflozin dapagliflozin empagliflozin	Invokana Farxiga Jardiance	• Genital fungal infections • Increased urination • Orthostasis	• 100-300 mg orally once daily by mouth (max 300 mg/day) • 5-10 mg orally once daily (max 10 mg/day) • 10-25 mg orally once-daily (max 25 mg/day)	• *Canagliflozin:* Not recommended if eGFR <45 mL/min/1.73 m² • *Dapagliflozin:* Not recommended if eGFR <60 mL/min/1.73 m² • *Empagliflozin:* Not recommended if eGFR ≤45 mL/min/1.73m²
Non-Insulin Injectable Medications					
Incretin Mimetics	exenatide liraglutide exenatide suspension albiglutide	Byetta Victoza Bydureon Tanzeum	• Weight loss • GI upset • Nausea/vomiting • Hypoglycemia	• 5-10 mcg SUBCUT twice a day • 0.6-1.8 mg SUBCUT daily • 2 mg SUBCUT once weekly • 20-50 mg SUBCUT once weekly	• Give doses within 1 hr of meals • Give in combination with other oral agents • Administer once daily without regard to meals • Administer once weekly • Administer once weekly
Synthetic Amylin Analog	pramlintide	Symlin	• Hypoglycemia • GI upset	• 15-120 mcg SUBCUT immediately before large meals (max 120 mcg/dose)	• Only for use in patients with DM using mealtime insulin • Can be used in both T2DM and T1DM

DM, Diabetes mellitus; *eGFR*, estimated glomerular filtration rate; *qid*, four times daily; *SUBCUT*, subcutaneously; *T1DM*, type 1 diabetes mellitus; *T2DM*, type 2 diabetes mellitus; *tid*, three times daily.

TABLE 16-6

Combination Oral Agents for the Treatment of Type 2 Diabetes Mellitus

Trade Name	Generic Name
Metaglip	glipizide-metformin
Glucovance	glyburide-metformin
Jentadueto	linagliptin-metformin
Kombiglyze XR	saxagliptin-metformin
Janumet	sitagliptin-metformin
Kazano	alogliptin-metformin
Oseni	alogliptin-pioglitazone
Duetact	pioglitazone-glimepiride
ActoPlus Met, ActoPlus Met XR	pioglitazone-metformin
PrandiMet	repaglinide-metformin

DO YOU REMEMBER THESE KEY POINTS?

- Names of the major endocrine glands of the body
- The locations and functions of the endocrine glands discussed
- The primary symptoms of the various endocrine conditions discussed
- Medications used to treat the various endocrine conditions discussed
- The generic and trade names for the drugs discussed in this chapter
- The appropriate auxiliary labels that should be used when filling prescriptions for drugs discussed in this chapter

REVIEW QUESTIONS

Multiple Choice Questions

1. Three glands located in the head are the:
   A. Pineal, pituitary, and pancreas
   B. Hypothalamus, pituitary, and pineal
   C. Pituitary, exocrine, and endocrine
   D. None of the above
2. The islets of Langerhans are found in which gland?
   A. Pineal
   B. Thalamus
   C. Pancreas
   D. Adrenal
3. The condition that affects children suffering from hypothyroidism is known as:
   A. Aphasia
   B. Cretinism
   C. Myxedema
   D. None of the above
4. Glimepiride is used to treat:
   A. Type 2 diabetes
   B. Type 1 diabetes
   C. Both type 1 and type 2 diabetes
   D. None of the above

5. Which combination drug does *not* have metformin as a main ingredient?
   A. ActoPlus Met
   B. Duetact
   C. Glucovance
   D. Metaglip
6. Vasopressin is another term for which of the following hormones?
   A. Antidiuretic hormone
   B. Calcitonin
   C. Follicle-stimulating hormone
   D. Growth hormone
7. Sandostatin (octreotide) is used to treat which of the following conditions?
   A. Acromegaly
   B. Type 2 diabetes mellitus
   C. Cretinism
   D. Hyperparathyroidism
8. Graves disease is the most common cause of:
   A. Hypothyroidism
   B. Hypopituitarism
   C. Hypergonadism
   D. Hyperthyroidism

9. Levothyroxine is the drug of choice to treat which of the following conditions?
   - **A.** Hyperthyroidism
   - **B.** Diabetes mellitus
   - **C.** Hypoparathyroidism
   - **D.** Hypothyroidism

10. Cushing's disease is caused by excessive secretion of:
    - **A.** Antidiuretic hormone
    - **B.** Adrenocorticotropic hormone
    - **C.** Follicle-stimulating hormone
    - **D.** Growth hormone

11. Hyperaldosteronism is associated with which of the following?
    - **A.** Hypertension
    - **B.** Hyperkalemia
    - **C.** Both A and B
    - **D.** None of the above

12. Insulin can be used to treat which of the following?
    - **A.** Type 1 diabetes mellitus
    - **B.** Type 2 diabetes mellitus
    - **C.** Gestational diabetes
    - **D.** All of the above

13. Which of the following is primarily considered a mineralocorticoid?
    - **A.** Methylprednisolone
    - **B.** Hydrocortisone
    - **C.** Prednisone
    - **D.** Fludrocortisone acetate

14. Which of the following is considered the first-line agent for the treatment of type 2 diabetes mellitus?
    - **A.** Metformin
    - **B.** Glipizide
    - **C.** Pioglitazone
    - **D.** Insulin

15. Which of the following hormones is *not* secreted by the pituitary gland?
    - **A.** Antidiuretic hormone
    - **B.** Insulin
    - **C.** Follicle-stimulating hormone
    - **D.** Growth hormone

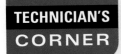
TECHNICIAN'S CORNER

Using a drug reference book or online drug resource, determine which agents in Table 16-5 are associated with causing hypoglycemia (low blood sugar).

Bibliography

Applegate E: *The anatomy and physiology learning system*, ed 4, St Louis, 2010, Saunders.

Clinical Pharmacology Online. (Referenced August 19, 2014.) www.clinicalpharmacology.com.

Damjanov I: *Pathology for the health professions*, ed 4, St Louis, 2011, Saunders.

Fishback JL: *Pathology*, ed 3, Philadelphia, 2005, Mosby.

Huether SE: *Understanding pathophysiology*, ed 5, St Louis, 2012, Mosby.

Scanlon V, Sanders T: *Essentials of anatomy and physiology*, ed 5, Philadelphia, 2007, FA Davis.

Solomon EP: *Introduction to human anatomy and physiology*, ed 3, St Louis, 2009, Saunders.

Thibodeau G, Patton K: *Structure and function of the body*, ed 13, St Louis, 2007, Mosby.

Thibodeau GA, Patton KT: *Anatomy and physiology*, ed 8, St Louis, 2012, Mosby.

Therapeutic Agents for the Musculoskeletal System

Joshua J. Neumiller

OBJECTIVES

Upon completing this chapter, you should be able to do the following:

1. Describe the major components of the musculoskeletal system.
2. List the primary symptoms of conditions associated with the musculoskeletal system.
3. Recognize drugs used to treat the conditions associated with the musculoskeletal system.
4. Write the generic and trade names for the drugs discussed in this chapter.
5. List appropriate auxiliary labels when filling prescriptions for drugs discussed in this chapter.

TERMS AND DEFINITIONS

Analgesic A drug that acts to relieve pain

Antipyretic A drug used to prevent or reduce fever

Arthroplasty Surgical reconstruction or replacement of a joint

Bone fracture A break or rupture of a bone

Bone marrow A fatty network of connective tissue that fills the cavities of bones

Cancellous bone A meshwork of spongy bone typically found at the core of vertebral bones in the spine and the ends of long bones; also called *spongy bone*

Compact bone Rigid bone, which constitutes most of the skeleton; also known as *cortical bone*

Cyclooxygenase (COX) Either of two related enzymes that control the production of prostaglandins

Euphoria A feeling or state of intense excitement and happiness

Fascicles A bundle of structures, such as muscle fibers

Gout A painful form of arthritis characterized by defective metabolism of uric acid

Ligament A fibrous connective tissue that connects to bones

Miosis Constriction of the pupil of the eye

Motor nerve A nerve carrying impulses from the brain or spinal cord to a muscle or gland

Muscle fiber Muscle cell

Neuromuscular junction The junction between a nerve fiber and the muscle it supplies

Opioid analgesic An analgesic medication that activates opioid receptors

Osteoarthritis (OA) Degeneration of joint cartilage and the underlying bone

Osteoporosis A medical condition in which the bones become brittle and fragile from loss of bone density and poor microarchitecture

Prostaglandin A mediator responsible for the features of inflammation, such as swelling, pain, stiffness, redness, and warmth

Resorption The process or action by which something is reabsorbed, such as bone resorption in the development of osteoporosis

Reye's syndrome A life-threatening metabolic disorder in young children of uncertain cause but sometimes precipitated by aspirin use

Skeletal muscle Muscle that is connected to the skeleton to form part of the mechanical system that moves the limbs and other parts of the body

Skeletal system The hard structure (bones and cartilages) that provides a frame for the body

Spongy bone Meshwork of spongy bone typically found at the core of vertebral bones in the spine and the ends of long bones, also known as *cancellous bone*

Subchondral bone Bone located below the cartilage, particularly within a joint

Synovium A thin membrane in synovial (freely moving) joints that lines the joint capsule and secretes synovial fluid

Tendon A flexible but inelastic cord of strong fibrous collagen tissue that attaches a muscle to a bone

Uric acid The water-insoluble end product of purine metabolism; deposition of uric acid as crystals in the joints and kidneys causes gout

Common Drugs for the Musculoskeletal System

Trade Name	Generic Name	Pronunciation
Salicylates		
Bayer	aspirin	(**ass**-pur-in)
Nonsteroidal Antiinflammatory Drugs (NSAIDs)		
Aleve, Naprosyn	naproxen sodium	(nah-**prox**-sin **sow**-dee-um)
Indocin	indomethacin	(in-doe-**meth**-ah-sin)
Lodine	etodolac	(ee-toe-**doe**-lak)
Mobic	meloxicam	(me-**lox**-i-cam)
Advil	ibuprofen	(**eye**-bue-**proe**-fen)
Toradol	ketorolac	(**key**-toh-**role**-ak)
Voltaren	diclofenac	(dye-**kloe**-fen-ak)
Cyclooxygenase-2 Inhibitors (COX-2 Inhibitors)		
Celebrex	celecoxib	(**sel**-e-**kox**-ib)
Opioid Analgesics		
Percocet (C-II)	oxycodone/acetaminophen	(**ox**-e-koe-done/a-**seet**-ah-**min**-oh-fen)
Lortab (C-II)	hydrocodone/acetaminophen	(hye-droe-**koe**-done/a-**seet**-ah-**min**-oh-fen)
Tylenol w/Codeine (C-III)	acetaminophen/codeine	(a-**seet**-ah-**min**-oh-phen/**koe**-deen)
Dilaudid (C-II)	hydromorphone	(**hye**-droe-**mor**-fone)
Duragesic (C-II)	fentanyl	(**fen**-ta-nil)
Demerol (C-II)	meperidine	(me-**per**-ih-deen)
Miscellaneous Analgesics		
Ultram (C-IV)	tramadol	(**tram**-a-dol)
Nucynta (C-II)	tapentadol	(ta-**pen**-ta-dol)
Osteoporosis Medications		
Fosamax	alendronate	(a-**len**-dro-nate)
Actonel	risedronate	(rih-**sed**-ro-nayt)
Boniva	ibandronate	(eye-**ban**-dro-nate)
Evista	raloxifene	(ra-**lox**-i-feen)
Prolia	denosumab	(den-**oh**-sue-mab)
Gout Medications		
Colcrys	colchicine	(**kol**-chi-seen)
Zyloprim	allopurinol	(al-loh-**pure**-i-nole)
Uloric	febuxostat	(feb-**ux**-loh-stat)
Benuryl	probenecid	(proe-**ben**-a-sid)
Skeletal Muscle Relaxants		
Flexeril	cyclobenzaprine	(sye-kloe-**ben**-za-preen)
Robaxin	methocarbamol	(meth-oh-**kar**-ba-mal)
Soma (C-IV)	carisoprodol	(kar-eh-soe-**proe**-dole)
Lioresal	baclofen	(**bak**-loe-fen)
Neuromuscular Blockers		
Nimbex	cisatracurium	(sis-**at**-ra-**kure**-ee-um)
Norcuron	vecuronium	(**vek**-ue-**roe**-nee-um)
Tracium	atracurium	(at-rah-**cure**-ih-um)
Pavulon	pancuronium	(pan-kure-**oh**-nee-um)

Anatomy and Physiology of the Skeletal System

The **skeletal system** has several important physiologic functions in the body. Primarily, it provides structural support for the body and protection for many of the organs in the body. For example, the skull contains and protects the brain, and the ribs provide protection for the heart and lungs. Bones also facilitate movement. Muscles are attached to bones by **tendons**, which allow us to use our bones as levers to move and exert muscular forces. Bones are held together at joints by **ligaments**, which allow bones to articulate at areas such as the knee and elbow (Figure 17-1).

Long bones, such as the femur in the leg, also contain **bone marrow** (Figure 17-2). Bone marrow is crucial because it is where the blood cells of the hematologic system are produced (see Chapter 26). Bones also serve as storage banks for minerals such as calcium and phosphorus because these minerals are very important to a variety of bodily functions. When calcium levels are high in the blood, calcium is stored in the bones by cells called osteoblasts. Conversely, when calcium levels are low, calcium is removed from the bones by cells called osteoclasts.

This is an important concept that is discussed later in the section on osteoporosis.

The two main types of bone are compact bone and spongy bone. **Compact bone**, also known as *cortical bone,* is very dense and located near the surface of the bones, where there is the greatest need for strength. **Spongy bone**, on the other hand, is typically located on the inner part of bones and is composed of a network of thin strands of bone known as *trabeculae.* The spongy bone (sometimes referred to as **cancellous bone**) is where the bone marrow can be found (Figure 17-3).

Anatomy and Physiology of Skeletal Muscle

The body has three types of muscle: skeletal muscle, smooth muscle, and cardiac muscle. This chapter focuses on skeletal muscle. As mentioned previously, **skeletal muscles** are attached to bones and help facilitate movement, such as walking, talking, and chewing food.

It is important to understand how skeletal muscle works to best understand the medicines that work by affecting skeletal muscle contraction. Each skeletal muscle is composed of hundreds to thousands of

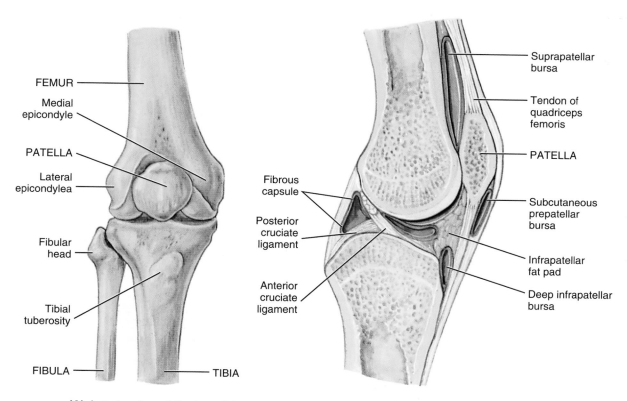

(A) Anterior view of the knee joint.   **(B)** Sagittal section of the knee joint.

FIGURE 17-1 The knee joint is a complex synovial joint. (From Solomon EP: *Introduction to human anatomy and physiology,* ed 3, St Louis, 2009, Saunders.)

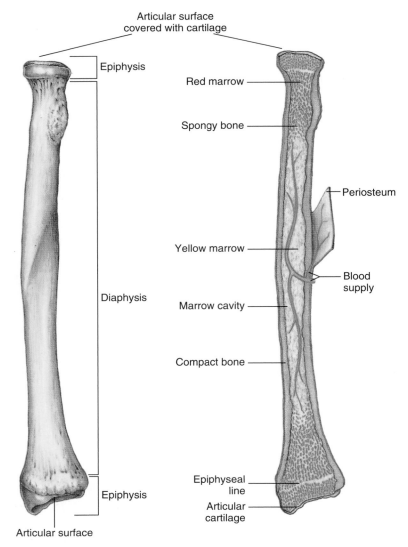

Articular surface
covered with cartilage

Epiphysis

Red marrow

Spongy bone

Periosteum

Diaphysis

Yellow marrow

Blood
supply

Marrow cavity

Compact bone

Epiphysis

Epiphyseal
line

Articular
cartilage

Articular surface

(A) The structure of a typical long bone.　　**(B)** Internal structure of a long bone.

FIGURE 17-2 Anatomy of a bone. (From Solomon EP: *Introduction to human anatomy and physiology,* ed 3, St Louis, 2009, Saunders.)

muscle cells called **muscle fibers**. These fibers are in turn grouped into bundles called **fascicles**. A group of fascicles makes up a muscle (Figure 17-4). Each muscle fiber is composed of threadlike structures called *myofibrils,* which are made up of tiny structures known as myofilaments. These actin and myosin myofilaments are how muscles are able to contract. Actin and myosin filaments in the muscle ratchet along one another, causing the filament to shorten (Figure 17-5). This shortening of the filaments corresponds to muscle contraction.

So what signals actin and myosin filaments in the skeletal muscle to contract? **Motor nerves** are nerves that carry signals from the central nervous system (CNS) to skeletal muscles, telling them to

contract. A given motor nerve can signal anywhere from one to several hundred muscle fibers. The point where a motor neuron meets and signals the skeletal muscle is known as the **neuromuscular junction** (Figure 17-6).

Common Conditions Affecting the Musculoskeletal System

A variety of musculoskeletal conditions can affect the bones, skeletal muscles, or both; this chapter focuses on common musculoskeletal conditions frequently encountered in the ambulatory care setting. Select other musculoskeletal disorders, such as rheumatoid arthritis (see Chapter 23), are covered separately.

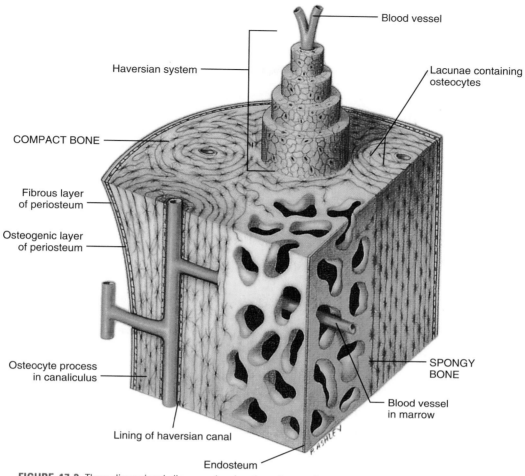

FIGURE 17-3 Three-dimensional diagram showing the microscopic structure of bone. (From Solomon EP: *Introduction to human anatomy and physiology,* ed 3, St Louis, 2009, Saunders.)

Osteoarthritis

Osteoarthritis (OA) is a disease associated with aging that affects articular cartilage, which is the cartilage that lines the joints (Figure 17-7). Osteoarthritis is the most common form of joint disease. Risk factors for osteoarthritis include increasing age, obesity, repetitive joint overuse, and joint trauma. Genetic and environmental factors may also play a role. Advanced age is one of the strongest risk factors associated with OA. In the elderly, it is a major cause of disability and health care expenditures. X-ray changes of osteoarthritis of the knee or hip are evident in most people over 60 years of age. The changes in cartilage strength and structure lead to cracking and erosion of cartilage and hypertrophy of **subchondral bone**. Loss of normal cushioning from cartilage upsets the interaction between **synovium**, cartilage, and bone.

Osteoarthritis differs from rheumatoid arthritis in several important respects. Unlike rheumatoid arthritis, there is generally no systemic illness associated with osteoarthritis. Joint involvement is asymmetric, with morning stiffness typically lasting less than 30 minutes upon rising. Osteoarthritis primarily affects weight-bearing joints. The joints that are usually involved include those of the hand, foot, knee, hip, and spine. Classic symptoms of osteoarthritis include pain on joint use and limitations of motion. Short-duration joint stiffness in the morning is also common.

Prognosis. Although there is no known cure for OA, there are many treatments and ways to slow the progression of this disease. Although the prognosis is highly dependent on the severity of the osteoarthritis, nonpharmacological and pharmacological treatment can help significantly in maintaining quality of life and functionality.

Non–Drug Treatment. Treatment of patients with osteoarthritis should focus on controlling pain and other symptoms to minimize disability and maintain quality of life. In addition to education of the patient and family, nonpharmacological interventions should include physical and

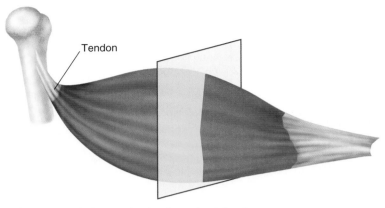

(A) The muscle is attached to bone by a tendon.

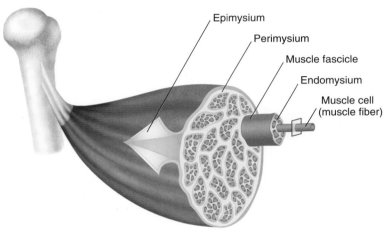

(B) The muscle is surrounded by a connective tissue covering—the epimysium. The muscle consists of fascicles—bundles of muscle fibers. Each fascicle is wrapped in connective tissue—the perimysium. Individual muscle fibers are surrounded by endomysium.

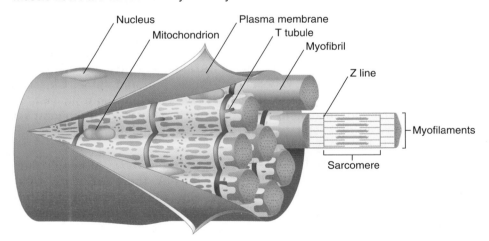

(C) Part of a muscle fiber showing the myofibrils. Myofibrils are threadlike structures composed of actin and myosin filaments. One myofibril is magnified and shown in detail to illustrate the filaments. The regular pattern of overlapping filaments gives skeletal and cardiac muscle their striated appearance. The Z lines mark the ends of the sarcomeres.

FIGURE 17-4 Muscle structure. (From Solomon EP: *Introduction to human anatomy and physiology,* ed 3, St Louis, 2009, Saunders.)

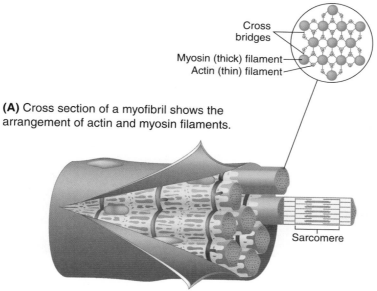

(A) Cross section of a myofibril shows the arrangement of actin and myosin filaments.

(B) Part of a muscle fiber showing the location of the filaments.

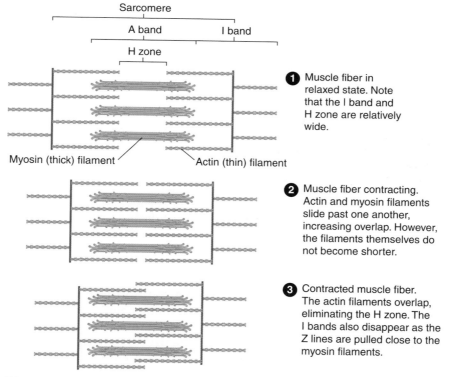

1. Muscle fiber in relaxed state. Note that the I band and H zone are relatively wide.

2. Muscle fiber contracting. Actin and myosin filaments slide past one another, increasing overlap. However, the filaments themselves do not become shorter.

3. Contracted muscle fiber. The actin filaments overlap, eliminating the H zone. The I bands also disappear as the Z lines are pulled close to the myosin filaments.

(C) A muscle contracts (shortens) when actin and myosin filaments slide past one another. The amount of overlap between actin and myosin filaments increases.

FIGURE 17-5 Muscle contraction. (From Solomon EP: *Introduction to human anatomy and physiology,* ed 3, St Louis, 2009, Saunders.)

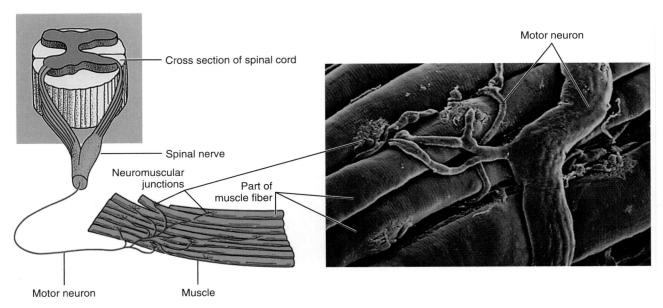

(A) Each nerve fiber controls many muscle fibers.

(B) Scanning electron micrograph of neuromuscular junctions (100x). Note how the motor neuron branches to innervate several muscle fibers.

FIGURE 17-6 Nerve fibers from a motor nerve transmit impulses to muscle fibers. (From Solomon EP: *Introduction to human anatomy and physiology,* ed 3, St Louis, 2009, Saunders.)

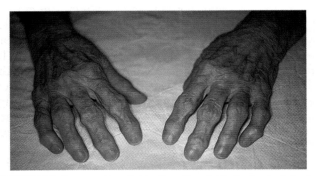

FIGURE 17-7 Severe osteoarthritis. (From Swartz M: *Textbook of physical diagnosis: history and examination,* ed 7, St Louis, 2014, Saunders.)

occupational therapy, regular exercise, and weight loss, if needed. Obesity is considered the biggest modifiable risk factor. Surgical options for the treatment of osteoarthritis include knee irrigation, arthroscopic lavage, osteotomy, and total joint **arthroplasty.**

Drug Treatment. Pharmacological treatment of osteoarthritis typically relies on the use of analgesics and nonsteroidal antiinflammatory drugs (NSAIDs) initially to minimize pain signals originating from the joints (Figure 17-8). Acetaminophen is often the first agent recommended for osteoarthritis pain. Oral and topical NSAIDs also are used. For severe pain, narcotic analgesics may be prescribed. Another option is steroid injections into the aching joint, although this treatment is for short-term use only because it can damage the joint.

Although acetaminophen, NSAIDs, and opioid analgesics can be used for a variety of pain conditions, they are discussed in detail here largely in the context of the treatment of OA. The student should be aware that these analgesic agents can be used at a variety of doses for mild, moderate, and severe pain. The prescribing information contains dosing recommendations for other pain disorders and conditions.

Acetaminophen

Acetaminophen, often abbreviated APAP in the United States, is both an **analgesic** and an **antipyretic.** An important difference between acetaminophen and aspirin is that acetaminophen does not have peripheral antiinflammatory properties or inhibitory effects on platelet function. As mentioned previously, acetaminophen is widely considered the analgesic of choice for osteoarthritis, largely because when compared with NSAIDs, acetaminophen has fewer hematologic, gastrointestinal (ulcer), and renal effects. That being said, acetaminophen use is not without risks. Misuse of acetaminophen is considered the single most common cause of acute liver failure in the United States. Many of these cases are unintentional, however, because many products contain acetaminophen, making it easy to take more

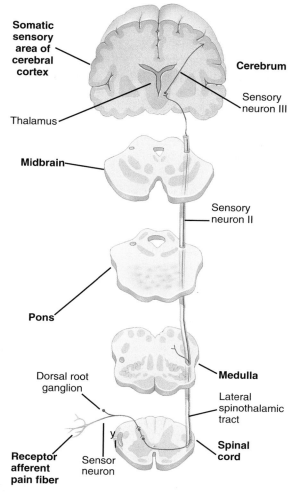

FIGURE 17-8 Pain route. (From Potter PA, Perry AG: *Fundamentals of nursing*, ed 8, St Louis, 2012, Mosby.)

than the general daily limit of 3000 mg. Table 17-1 provides information on acetaminophen and other nonopioid analgesic medications.

 Tech Note!

A multitude of prescription and over-the-counter (OTC) products contain acetaminophen. Consumers should be reminded of this when purchasing a prescription or OTC product.

GENERIC NAME: acetaminophen
TRADE NAME: Tylenol (over the counter [OTC])
INDICATION: Musculoskeletal pain, osteoarthritis, headache, fever
ROUTE OF ADMINISTRATION: Oral; rectal; intravenous
COMMON ADULT DOSAGE: 500-1000 mg as needed (max 3000 mg daily) for most formulations and routes

---

MECHANISM OF ACTION: Inhibits cyclooxygenase-1 (COX-1) and COX-2 in the CNS
SIDE EFFECTS: Nausea, vomiting, constipation, liver damage

 Tech Note!

Acetaminophen (Tylenol) is not an antiinflammatory agent. Although it does affect cyclooxygenase enzymes in an inhibitory way by relieving pain and fever, it works in the CNS and does not alleviate inflammation in the periphery.

Aspirin

In England in the early 1800s, it was reported that the bark of the willow tree was effective as a pain, fever, and inflammation reducer. Many cultures had known this for centuries, but it was not until the early 1800s that the medical community began to isolate the active ingredients. Henri Leroux, a French chemist, determined that a bitter glycoside was responsible for the medicinal properties of the bark. This chemical was referred to as *salicin*. Salicin can be broken down into two compounds, glucose (sugar) and salicylic alcohol. Salicylic alcohol ultimately can be broken down into acetylsalicylic acid (ASA). The first company to market this miracle agent was the Bayer Company in 1899; the company called its new wonder drug *aspirin*. Since then, many new drugs have been introduced into the marketplace that work similarly; however, aspirin is still a popular drug because it is effective and inexpensive.

Although aspirin has proven to be an effective agent for treating fever, pain, and inflammation, it generally should not be given to children, especially those with flulike symptoms. This is because aspirin use in this population has been associated with the development of Reye's syndrome. **Reye's syndrome**, which may occur following chickenpox or an upper respiratory tract viral infection, is a childhood disease that causes vomiting, lethargy, and encephalopathy, which can lead to coma and death.

The maximum dose for aspirin in adults is 4 g per day. A common side effect is upset stomach. Aspirin is an effective inhibitor of platelet aggregation. Accordingly, one of the most common uses of aspirin is the prevention of strokes or heart attacks. Many people with a risk for heart attacks and strokes (e.g., people with diabetes) take a daily aspirin. Because aspirin inhibits platelets, this therapy has risks. Aspirin can increase the risk of bleeding, and this should be considered before it is used. Aspirin should particularly be used cautiously in combination with anticoagulants, such as warfarin (see Chapter 18).

TABLE 17-1

Select Nonopioid Analgesic Medications

Generic Name	Trade Name	Common Side Effects	Common Dose Range	Comments
Acetaminophen (APAP)				
acetaminophen	Tylenol	• Nausea • Vomiting • Headache • Liver toxicity	• *IR:* 500 mg PO 1-2 tablets every 6 hr • *ER:* 650 mg PO 2 tablets every 8 hr	Maximum daily dose of 3000 mg daily
Nonsteroidal Antiinflammatory Drugs (NSAIDs)				
aspirin	Bayer, Ecotrin	• Nausea • Dyspepsia • Gastrointestinal ulcer • Reye's syndrome	• 325-650 mg PO every 4 hr or 81 mg PO once daily (max 4 g/day)	Antiplatelet effect usually lasts about 14 days
ibuprofen naproxen	Advil, Motrin Naprosyn, EC Naprosyn (delayed release)	• Rash • Heartburn • Nausea • Dizziness • Fluid retention	• 400-800 mg PO every 6-8 hr • *IR:* 250-500 mg PO twice daily • *DR:* 375-500 mg PO twice daily	
naproxen sodium oxaprozin	Aleve Daypro	• Gastrointestinal ulcer • Hypertension • Acute renal failure • Liver toxicity	• 220-440 mg PO twice daily (max 660 mg/day) • 600-1200 mg PO daily	Long duration allows for once daily dosing.
diclofenac	Cataflam, Voltaren, Voltaren XR	• Similar to NSAIDs listed above	• *IR:* 50 mg PO two or three times daily • *DR:* 75 mg PO twice daily • *XR:* 100 mg PO once or twice daily	
etodolac	Lodine, Lodine XL		• *IR:* 400-500 mg PO twice daily • *XL:* 400-1000 mg PO once daily	
indomethacin	Indocin, Indocin SR		• *IR:* 25-50 mg PO 2-3 times daily • *SR:* 75 mg PO once or twice daily	Rectal suppositories available
nabumetone	Relafen		• 1000 mg PO in 1-2 doses daily	Long duration allows for once daily dosing
meloxicam	Mobic		• 7.5 mg PO once daily (max 15 mg/day)	
COX-2 Selective Inhibitor				
celecoxib	Celebrex	• Nausea • Diarrhea • Headache • Hypertension • Acute renal failure • Thrombotic events	• 200 mg PO daily in 1-2 divided doses	Less risk of gastrointestinal ulcer

DR, Delayed release; *ER,* extended release; *IR,* immediate release; *PO,* orally; *SR,* sustained release; *XR,* extended release.

GENERIC NAME: aspirin
TRADE NAME: Bayer (OTC)
INDICATION: Headache, fever, mild pain, thromboembolism prophylaxis
ROUTE OF ADMINISTRATION: Oral
COMMON ADULT DOSAGE: 81-325 mg as needed (max 4 g per day)

MECHANISM OF ACTION: Inhibits COX-1 and COX-2 enzymes; inhibits platelet aggregation via inhibition of thromboxane-A2 (TXA2)
SIDE EFFECTS: Nausea, indigestion, increased bleeding risk
AUXILIARY LABEL:
• Take with food or milk.

Tech Note!

Aspirin is also known by its chemical name, acetylsalicylic acid (ASA). This chemical inhibits prostaglandins, thus reducing inflammation and helping to decrease pain and fever. Many physicians prescribe 81 to 325 mg per day for antiplatelet effects, which reduces blood clotting.

Nonsteroidal Antiinflammatory Drugs

Aspirin is a salicylate drug and was the prototype agent for the newer NSAIDs. Although NSAIDs have a chemical structure different from aspirin, a close similarity exists between their structures. All of these agents have analgesic, antipyretic, and anti-inflammatory properties that make them popular in the retail marketplace. Naturally occurring and exogenous steroids are able to help reduce inflammation by binding to steroid receptors. In contrast, NSAIDs suppress inflammation by inhibiting the enzyme cyclooxygenase, which is responsible for **prostaglandin** synthesis. **Cyclooxygenase (COX)** is an enzyme involved in the pathway that synthesizes prostaglandins and other compounds. COX is a substance found in all tissues, where it helps regulate many processes. Cyclooxygenase has two forms, cyclooxygenase-1 (COX-1) and cyclooxygenase-2 (COX-2). COX-1 is present in most tissues and assists with many normal body functions, including protecting gastric mucosa and promoting platelet aggregation. COX-2 is found mainly at sites of tissue injury, where it helps sensitize receptors to pain and mediates inflammation. COX-2 also is located in the brain, where it affects fever and pain perception. Therefore, COX-1 can be considered an enzyme involved in maintaining normal metabolic processes, whereas COX-2 is associated with processes in which pain and discomfort are present.

By inhibiting prostaglandin synthesis, NSAIDs not only suppress inflammation, but also help treat pain. NSAIDs can be used for mild to moderate pain and inflammation.

NSAIDs also have an antipyretic effect by acting on the hypothalamus (the body thermostat). More than one dozen NSAIDs are available in prescription form, with a handful of others available over the counter (see Chapter 27). Wide variations have been documented among different NSAIDs, even if they are related and in the same chemical family (see Table 17-1).

NSAIDs are used to treat many different types of conditions and chronic illnesses, such as the following:

- Muscle pain
- Rheumatoid arthritis (RA)
- Joint pain (e.g., OA)
- Dysmenorrhea

Millions of people use OTC and prescription NSAIDs to treat various inflammatory conditions. However, overuse of these agents can cause major problems. NSAIDs can worsen stomach problems, such as gastroesophageal reflux disease (GERD). They also can cause gastrointestinal (GI) ulcers and bleeding. All NSAIDs should be taken with food to prevent stomach irritation.

GENERIC NAME: ibuprofen
TRADE NAME: Motrin, Advil (OTC)
INDICATION: Analgesia, fever, inflammatory conditions
ROUTE OF ADMINISTRATION: Oral; intravenous
COMMON ADULT DOSAGE: 200-800 mg every 6-8 hours (max 3200 mg/day) for oral and IV products
MECHANISM OF ACTION: Inhibits COX-1 and COX-2 enzymes
SIDE EFFECTS: GI ulceration, increased risk of bleeding, increased blood pressure, renal impairment
AUXILIARY LABELS:
- May cause dizziness or drowsiness.
- Take with food or milk.

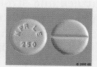

GENERIC NAME: naproxen
TRADE NAME: Aleve (OTC), Naprosyn (Rx)
INDICATION: Analgesia, fever, inflammatory conditions
ROUTE OF ADMINISTRATION: Oral
COMMON ADULT DOSAGE: 250-500 mg twice daily (max 1500 mg/day)
MECHANISM OF ACTION: Inhibits COX-1 and COX-2 enzymes
SIDE EFFECTS: GI ulceration, increased risk of bleeding, increased blood pressure, renal impairment
AUXILIARY LABELS:
- May cause dizziness or drowsiness.
- Take with food or milk.

GENERIC NAME: meloxicam
TRADE NAME: Mobic
INDICATION: Osteoarthritis, rheumatoid arthritis
ROUTE OF ADMINISTRATION: Oral
COMMON ADULT DOSAGE: 7.5-15 mg once daily

MECHANISM OF ACTION: Inhibits COX-1 and COX-2 enzymes
SIDE EFFECTS: GI ulceration, increased risk of bleeding, increased blood pressure, renal impairment
AUXILIARY LABELS:
- Shake the suspension well before use.
- Take with or without food.

Cyclooxygenase-2 Inhibitors

As mentioned previously, cyclooxygenase has two forms, COX-1 and COX-2. First-generation NSAIDs inhibit COX-1 and COX-2 enzymes, which results in a decrease in inflammation, pain, and fever. Unfortunately, inhibiting COX-1 enzymes has serious side effects, such as gastric ulceration, bleeding, and renal damage. The theory behind COX-2–selective inhibitors is that they could treat pain and inflammation without the risk of nonselective agents that also inhibit COX-1. Unfortunately, selective COX-2 inhibition has not been shown to be greatly advantageous in reducing NSAID-related side effects. Agents such as rofecoxib (Vioxx) and valdecoxib (Bextra) (both of which were COX-2 inhibitors) were withdrawn from the market because of safety concerns, including the potential for an increased risk of cardiovascular events, such as heart attack and stroke. COX-2 inhibitors are now usually reserved for patients intolerant of traditional NSAID agents. Celecoxib (Celebrex) is currently the only COX-2 inhibitor approved for use in the United States.

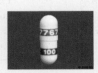

GENERIC NAME: celecoxib
TRADE NAME: Celebrex
INDICATION: Osteoarthritis (OA), rheumatoid arthritis (RA)
ROUTE OF ADMINISTRATION: Oral
COMMON ADULT DOSAGE: *OA:* 200 mg daily or 100 mg twice daily; *RA:* 100-200 mg twice daily
MECHANISM OF ACTION: Selective inhibition of COX-2
SIDE EFFECTS: Nausea, abdominal pain, cardiovascular events
AUXILIARY LABEL:
- Take with food or milk.

Topical Over-the-Counter Pain Relievers

Topical products can also be helpful in the management of osteoarthritis and muscle strains. Products containing menthol and methyl salicylate (e.g., Bengay, IcyHot), trolamine salicylate (Aspercreme), and camphor plus menthol (Tiger Balm) are widely used. It is important that people use these products only on intact skin.

Opioid Analgesics

Opioid analgesics play an important role in pain management through their mechanism of action on opioid receptors in the brain. The three main types of opioid receptors in the brain are mu, kappa, and delta opioid receptors. Analgesia with opioids is mediated through changes in the perception of pain at the level of the spinal cord and CNS (Figure 17-9). Many of the opioids used clinically are mu-receptor agonists; morphine is considered the prototypical opioid pain medication. Activation of mu-receptors produces analgesia, **miosis** (pupillary constriction), respiratory depression, **euphoria**, decreased gastrointestinal motility, and physical dependence. Opioid

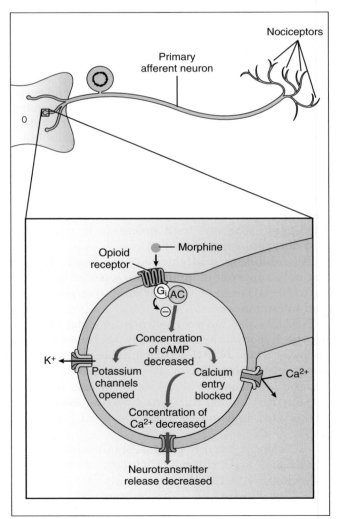

FIGURE 17-9 Mechanism of opioid action in the spinal cord. (From Brenner GM et al: *Pharmacology,* ed 4, Philadelphia, 2014, Saunders.)

medications are controlled substances, and the schedule depends on the agent and formulation. Because opioid medications cause sedation and respiratory depression, overdose with these medications is potentially life-threatening. Opioid antagonists, such as naloxone and naltrexone, can be used to reverse the effects of opioid agonists by competing for opioid receptor sites. Table 17-2 provides an overview of select opioid agonists and antagonists.

AUXILIARY LABELS:
- May cause dizziness or drowsiness.
- Avoid alcohol.
- Caution: Federal law prohibits the transfer of this drug to any person other than the patient for whom it was prescribed.

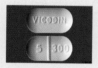

GENERIC NAME: hydrocodone/APAP
TRADE NAME: Vicodin, Lortab, Norco (C-II)
INDICATION: Moderate to severe pain
ROUTE OF ADMINISTRATION: Oral
COMMON ADULT DOSAGE: 1-2 tablets every 4-6 hours as needed for pain
MECHANISM OF ACTION: Hydrocodone activates opioid receptors; APAP inhibits COX-1 and COX-2
SIDE EFFECTS: Constipation, drowsiness, dependence
AUXILIARY LABELS:
- May cause dizziness or drowsiness.
- Avoid alcohol.
- Caution: Federal law prohibits the transfer of this drug to any person other than the patient for whom it was prescribed.
SPECIAL NOTE: Maximum dose of APAP is 4 g/day.

 Tech Note!

For opioid medications available in combination with acetaminophen, the maximum amount of medication that can be taken per day is limited by the amount of acetaminophen (maximum 3000 mg daily). Some individuals (e.g., those with liver disease) may be advised to take a smaller daily amount of acetaminophen (e.g., 2000 to 3000 mg daily).

GENERIC NAME: oxycodone
TRADE NAME: Roxicodone (C-II)
INDICATION: Moderate to severe pain
ROUTE OF ADMINISTRATION: Oral
COMMON ADULT DOSAGE: 5-15 mg every 4-6 hours as needed initially, then titrated to effect
MECHANISM OF ACTION: Activation of opioid receptors
SIDE EFFECTS: Constipation, drowsiness, dependence

GENERIC NAME: fentanyl
TRADE NAME: Duragesic, Fentora, Onsolis, Actiq, Lazanda, ABSTRAL, SUBSYS (C-II)
ROUTE OF ADMINISTRATION: Oral; transdermal; intranasal; intravenous; sublingual
INDICATION: Moderate to severe pain, general anesthesia
COMMON ADULT DOSAGE: Dose is highly variable based on dosage form and baseline opioid use
MECHANISM OF ACTION: Activation of opioid receptors
SIDE EFFECTS: Constipation, drowsiness, dependence
AUXILIARY LABELS:
- May cause dizziness or drowsiness.
- Avoid alcohol.
- Caution: Federal law prohibits the transfer of this drug to any person other than the patient for whom it was prescribed.

Osteoporosis

Osteoporosis is defined as a systemic skeletal disease characterized by low bone mass and microarchitectural deterioration of bone tissue. These changes in the bone lead to bone fragility and susceptibility to **bone fracture**. Osteoporosis occurs most commonly in postmenopausal women, although male osteoporosis has gained attention as a growing public health concern.

Bone is constantly being broken down (a process known as **resorption**) and rebuilt. Osteoclasts are a type of bone cell that invades the surface of the bone and erodes it. In doing so, osteoclasts create a cavity on the surface of the bone. Osteoblasts, or bone-forming cells, then fill in the cavity with new bone, which contains collagen and minerals such as calcium and phosphorus. Osteoclast and osteoblast activity is physiologically coupled so that bone that is resorbed is replaced. Osteoporosis occurs when bone resorption outpaces the laying down of new bone. Figure 17-10 depicts this remodeling process and illustrates the mechanism of action by which many of the drugs used to treat osteoporosis work.

Recall that the human skeleton is composed of cortical bone, which is relatively dense and compact, and cancellous bone, which consists of a lattice

TABLE 17-2

Select Opioid Analgesics and Opioid Receptor Antagonists

Medication Class	Generic Name	Trade Name	Common Side Effects	Common Starting Dose Range
Opioid Analgesics	codeine + acetaminophen (C-III)	NA	• Drowsiness • Constipation • Nausea • Vomiting • Itchiness (pruritus) • Respiratory depression	• 30-60 mg PO every 4-6 hr
	hydrocodone + acetaminophen (C-II)	Lortab, Norco, Vicodin		• 5-10 mg PO every 6 hr
	oxycodone (C-II)	Roxicodone, OxyContin (ER), Percocet		• *IR:* 5-15 mg PO every 4-6 hr • *ER:* 10 mg PO twice daily

	morphine (C-II)	MS-Contin, Kadian SR		• *IR:* 2-10 mg IV every 2-4 hr *or*
				  • 2-10 mg IM every 3-4 hr *or*
				  • 10-30 mg PO every 4 hr
				• *ER:* 15-30 mg PO 1-2 times daily

	hydromorphone (C-II)	Dilaudid		• *IR:* 0.3-1 mg IV every 2-4 hr *or*
				  • 0.3-1 mg IM/SUBCUT every 3-4 hr *or*
				  • 2-4 mg PO every 3-4 hr
				• *ER:* 8 mg PO every 24 hr

	oxymorphone (C-II)	Opana, Numorphan		• 0.5-1.5 mg IV/IM/SUBCT every 4-6 hr *or* • 5-10 mg PO every 4-6 hr
	fentanyl (C-II)	Duragesic		• 10-50 mcg IV/SUBCUT every 1-2 hr *or* • *Patch:* 12-25 mcg/72hr
	meperidine (C-II)	Demerol		• 50-150 mg PO/IV/SUBCUT every 3-4 hr prn
	methadone (C-II)	Dolophine		• 1.25-5 mg IV/SUBCUT/IM every 4-8 hr *or* • 2.5-10 mg PO every 4-8 hr
Partial Opioid Agonist	buprenorphine (C-III)	Buprenex, Subutex	• Sedation • Hypotension • Respiratory depression • Headache • Sweating	• 0.3 mg IM/IV every 6-8 hr as needed *or* • *Patch:* 5 mcg/hr applied once every 7 days
Mixed Opioid Agonists	nalbuphine	Nubain	• Sedation • Dizziness • Headache • Nausea • Dry mouth • Palpitations • Pain • Tremors • Withdrawal symptoms	• 10 mg/70 kg IV/IM every 3-6 hr (max 20 mg/dose and 160 mg/day)
Opioid Antagonists (Reversal Agents)	naloxone	Narcan		• 2 mg IM/IV every 2-3 min until reversal (after 10 mg with no reversal, search for other causes)
	naltrexone	Vivitrol	• Syncope • Headache • Insomnia • Dizziness • Nausea • Injection site reaction	• 25 mg PO daily, then 50 mg PO daily once a day thereafter *or* • 380 mg IM once every 4 wk

ER, Extended release; *IM,* intramuscular; *IV,* intravenous; *PO,* oral; *SUBCUT,* subcutaneous.

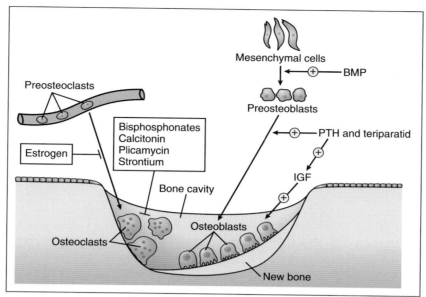

FIGURE 17-10 Effects of drugs and hormones on bone remodeling. (From Brenner GM et al: *Pharmacology,* ed 4, Philadelphia, 2014, Saunders.)

network that is commonly called "spongy" bone and also known as trabecular bone. Cancellous bone is found in vertebrae, ribs, the pelvis, and the ends of long bones and is very metabolically active. Roughly 25% of all trabecular bone turns over annually. In essence, every 5 to 10 years, a completely new skeleton is formed. When the rate of bone resorption exceeds the rate of new bone formation, bone mineral density begins to decrease and bone (particularly spongy bone) becomes weakened and prone to fracture. Although fractures can occur anywhere, fractures of the hip and long bones (e.g., the femur) are associated with the most morbidity and mortality. Vertebral fractures, however, are the most common and can lead to kyphosis (Figure 17-11), or a bent over, stooped posture.

Prognosis. The prognosis of osteoporosis can be good when the condition is treated with dietary changes, exercise, and medication. According to the National Osteoporosis Foundation, approximately 10 million people have osteoporosis, and 34 million are estimated to have low bone mass, which can lead to osteoporosis. The cost to the health care system in 2005 was approximately $19 billion and is expected to rise to $25.3 billion by the year 2025.

Non–Drug Treatments. Primary prevention of osteoporosis must start early in life, through a healthy lifestyle involving physical activity, a healthy diet, and refraining from smoking. Exercise helps to increase bone density, as does an

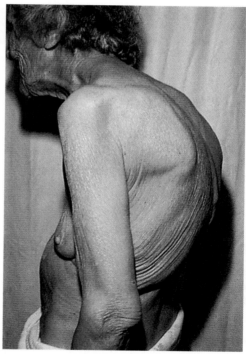

FIGURE 17-11 Kyphosis. (From McCance KL: *Pathophysiology: the biologic basis for disease in adults and children,* ed 6, St Louis, 2010, Mosby.)

adequate intake of calcium and vitamin D. Calcium requirements can be met by drinking milk, eating cheese, or taking calcium supplements.

Drug Treatments. Treatment of osteoporosis focuses on reducing the risk of fracture, decreasing bone loss, preserving normal bone remodeling, and maintaining quality of life. Some agents, such as the bisphosphonates and raloxifene, are indicated for both prevention and treatment. Others, such as calcitonin, are used only for treatment of osteoporosis. An adequate intake of vitamin D and calcium are critical cotherapies. Table 17-3 provides a summary of select agents approved for the treatment of osteoporosis.

INDICATION: Osteoporosis, osteoporosis prophylaxis, Paget's disease
ROUTE OF ADMINISTRATION: Oral
COMMON ADULT DOSAGE: 5-10 mg daily or 35-70 mg weekly
MECHANISM OF ACTION: Inhibits osteoclast activity to slow bone resorption
SIDE EFFECTS: Abdominal pain, muscle pain, osteonecrosis of the jaw (ONJ)
AUXILIARY LABEL:
• Take as directed.

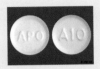

GENERIC NAME: alendronate
TRADE NAME: Fosamax

TABLE 17-3

Select Medications for the Treatment of Osteoporosis

Medication Class	Generic Name	Trade Name	Common Side Effects	Common Dose Range
Bisphosphonates	alendronate	Fosamax	• Abdominal pain • Muscle pain	• 5-10 mg PO daily or • 35-70 mg PO weekly
	ibandronate	Boniva	• Rash • Flulike symptoms	• 150 mg PO monthly or • 3 mg IV bolus every 3 months
	risedronate	Actonel	• Osteonecrosis of the jaw (ONJ) • Atypical femur fractures • Atrial fibrillation	• 5 mg PO daily or • 35 mg PO weekly or • 150 mg PO monthly
	zoledronic Acid	Reclast	• Injection site reactions • Bone pain • Nausea/vomiting • Fatigue	• 5 mg IV every 1-2 yr
Calcitonin Hormone Analogue	calcitonin salmon	Fortical, Miacalcin	• Nosebleeds • Rhinitis • Flushing	• 200 units (1 spray) in one nostril daily, switching nostrils daily or • 100 units IM/SUBCUT every other day
Selective Estrogen Receptor Modulator (SERM)	raloxifene	Evista	• Hot flashes • Leg cramps • Joint pain • Increased triglycerides • Increased risk of clots	• 60 mg PO daily
Parathyroid Hormone Analogue	teriparatide	Forteo	• Hypercalcemia • Hypercalciuria • Hypotension • Nausea • Dizziness	• 20 mcg SUBCUT daily for up to 2 yr
Monoclonal Antibody	denosumab	Prolia	• Headache • Diarrhea • Vomiting • Dizziness	• 60 mg SUBCUT once every 6 mo
Supplementation	vitamin D and calcium	Citracal, Caltrate	• Stomach upset • Constipation • Kidney stones	• 1000-1200 mg of calcium and 400-800 international units of vitamin D by mouth

IM, Intramuscular; *IV,* intravenous; *PO,* oral; *SUBCUT,* subcutaneous.

GENERIC NAME: raloxifene
TRADE NAME: Evista
INDICATION: Osteoporosis treatment, osteoporosis prophylaxis
ROUTE OF ADMINISTRATION: Oral
COMMON ADULT DOSAGE: 60 mg daily
MECHANISM OF ACTION: Selective estrogen receptor modulator (SERM): activates estrogen receptors in some tissues and antagonizes estrogen receptors in other tissues
SIDE EFFECTS:
- Hot flashes, leg cramps, increased risk of thrombosis

Gout

Gout is a form of arthritis that occurs when **uric acid** builds up in the blood, leading to the development of uric acid crystals in the joint, which in turn leads to inflammation and pain (Figure 17-12). Ninety percent of patients with gout have trouble excreting uric acid, and 10% are overproducers. Acute gout flares are intensely painful inflammatory arthritic attacks that typically involve a single joint but can affect multiple joints.

The overall prevalence of gout is about 6 in 1000 in men and 1 in 1000 in women, but prevalence increases with age. Other than hyperuricemia, common risk factors for gout are obesity, hypertension, and renal insufficiency. Drugs that impair the renal excretion of uric acid that have been linked to gout include alcohol, diuretics, and levodopa, among others. Whenever a patient presents with new-onset or exacerbated gout, the pharmacist should review the drug regimen for medications that may be contributory.

Prognosis. The prognosis for gout can be good if contributing factors can be identified and resolved to prevent recurrent gout attacks.

Medications can both help prevent and treat acute gouty arthritis (Table 17-4).

Non–Drug Treatment. A variety of nonpharmacological interventions can reduce the risk of gout attacks. Weight loss, abstaining from alcohol, and adopting a diet low in pruines (e.g., avoiding meats such as beef, lamb, and pork) can be particularly beneficial.

Drug Treatment. Initial treatment goals for patients with gout focus on alleviating the inflammation and pain associated with acute attacks. Therapies include colchicine, NSAIDs, and corticosteroids. Maintaining low uric acid levels by using uricosuric drugs or xanthine oxidase inhibitors may prevent recurrent attacks.

Other Select Medication Classes That Affect the Musculoskeletal System

Skeletal Muscle Relaxants

Skeletomuscular pain can arise from a number of causes. Although everyone experiences some pain at one time or another, severe injury or chronic pain may require additional care. Treatments generally include drug therapies (e.g., analgesics, muscle relaxers) and physical therapy. For severe injuries. surgery may be an option if medications and physical therapy prove ineffective for treating the condition and maintaining quality of life and functionality. Skeletal muscle relaxants are often used for injuries of the musculoskeletal system and work by reducing muscle tone (Table 17-5).

GENERIC NAME: carisoprodol
TRADE NAME: Soma (C-IV)
INDICATION: Musculoskeletal pain
ROUTE OF ADMINISTRATION: Oral
COMMON ADULT DOSAGE: 250-350 mg three to four times daily
MECHANISM OF ACTION: Blocks neuronal signaling, leading to muscle relaxation
SIDE EFFECTS: Dizziness, drowsiness, vertigo, headache
AUXILIARY LABELS:
- May cause dizziness or drowsiness.
- Avoid alcohol.
- Caution: Federal law prohibits the transfer of this drug to any person other than the patient for whom it was prescribed.

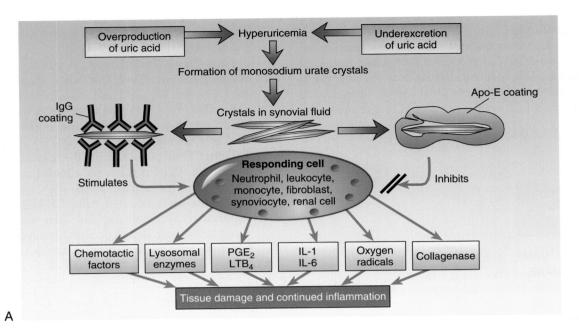

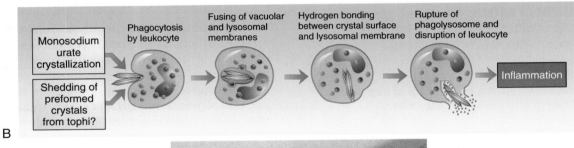

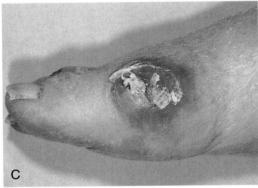

FIGURE 17-12 Pathogenesis of acute gouty arthritis. (From McCance KL: *Pathophysiology: the biologic basis for disease in adults and children,* ed 6, St Louis, 2010, Mosby.)

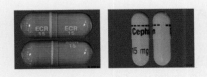

GENERIC NAME: cyclobenzaprine
TRADE NAME: Flexeril, Amrix
INDICATION: Muscle spasm
ROUTE OF ADMINISTRATION: Oral

COMMON ADULT DOSAGE: *Immediate release:* 5-10 mg three times daily; *extended release:* 15-30 mg once daily
MECHANISM OF ACTION: Reduces muscle spasm by a direct effect on the CNS
SIDE EFFECTS: Dizziness, drowsiness, blurred vision, dry mouth, constipation
AUXILIARY LABELS:
- May cause dizziness or drowsiness.
- Avoid alcohol.

TABLE 17-4

Select Agents for the Treatment of Gout

Medication Class	Generic Name	Trade Name	Common Side Effects	Common Dose Range
NSAIDs	ibuprofen	Advil, Motrin	• Nausea • Dizziness • Fluid retention • Gastrointestinal ulcer • Hypertension • Acute renal failure	• 400-800 mg PO twice daily
	naproxen	Naprosyn		• 500 mg PO twice daily
	indomethacin	Indocin		• 50 mg PO 3 times daily *or* • 75 mg PO twice daily
Antigout Agent	colchicine	Colcrys	• Nausea • Vomiting • Diarrhea	• 1.2 mg (2 tabs) PO, then 0.6 mg (1 tab) PO 1 hr later *or* • 0.5-0.6 mg PO twice daily for chronic use to prevent an attack
Corticosteroids	prednisone	Deltasone	• Fluid retention • High blood pressure • Increased blood sugar	• 30-50 mg PO daily for 1-2 days, then taper off over 7-10 days
	triamcinolone	Kenalog		• 20-40 mg INJ (intraarticular)
	methylprednisolone	Depo-Medrol		• 4-80 mg INJ (intraarticular)
Xanthine Oxidase Inhibitor	allopurinol	Zyloprim	• Nausea • Diarrhea • Rash	• 100-300 mg PO daily
	febuxostat	Uloric		• 40-80 mg PO daily
Uricosuric Agent	probenecid	Benuryl	• Stomach upset • Rash • Dizziness • Flushing	• 250 mg PO twice daily for 1 wk, then 500 mg PO twice daily (max 2 g/day)

INJ, Injection; *IV,* intravenous; *PO,* oral; *tabs,* tablets.

TABLE 17-5

Select Skeletal Muscle Relaxants

Medication Class	Generic Name	Trade Name	Common Side Effects	Common Dose Range
Skeletal Muscle Relaxant	cyclobenzaprine	Flexeril	• Drowsiness • Dry mouth • Dizziness • Fatigue	• *IR:* 5 mg PO 3 times daily • *ER:* 15 mg PO once daily
	methocarbamol	Robaxin		• 1.5 g PO 4 times daily for 2-3 days, then reduce to 4-4.5 g/day divided into 3-6 doses *or* • 1 g IV/IM every 8 hr
	carisoprodol (C-IV)	Soma		• 250-350 mg 3 times daily and at bedtime
	baclofen	Lioresal		• 5 mg PO 3 times daily (max 80 mg/day)
	metaxalone	Skelaxin		• 800 mg PO 3-4 times daily

ER, Extended release; *IM,* intramuscular; *IR,* immediate release; *IV,* intravenous; *PO,* oral.

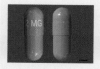

GENERIC NAME: tizanidine
TRADE NAME: Zanaflex
INDICATION: Spasticity associated with conditions such as multiple sclerosis and spinal cord injury

ROUTE OF ADMINISTRATION: Oral
COMMON ADULT DOSAGE: 4-8 mg every 6-8 hours as needed
MECHANISM OF ACTION: Activates central alpha-2 receptors to reduce spasmodic activity
SIDE EFFECTS: Dizziness, drowsiness, dry mouth
AUXILIARY LABELS:
• May cause dizziness or drowsiness.
• Avoid alcohol.

TABLE 17-6

Select Neuromuscular Blocking Agents

Type	Generic Name	Brand Name	Duration	Common Dose Range
Depolarizing	succinylcholine	Anectine	2-3 min	• *Initial:* 1-1.5 mg/kg intravenously (IV) • *Maintenance:* variable
Nondepolarizing	cisatracurium	Nimbex	20-35 min	• *Initial:* 0.15-0.2 mg/kg IV • *Maintenance:* variable
	vecuronium	Norcuron	60-90 min	• *Initial:* 0.08-0.1 mg/kg IV • *Maintenance:* variable
	rocuronium	Zemuron	30-60 min	• *Initial:* 0.6-1.2 mg/kg IV • *Maintenance:* variable
	atracurium	Tracrium	30-60 min	• *Initial:* 0.4-0.5 mg/kg IV • *Maintenance:* variable
	pancuronium	Pavulon	2-3 hr	• *Initial:* 0.06-0.1 mg/kg IV • *Maintenance:* variable

 Tech Note!

Studies have shown that the pharmacokinetics of tizanidine capsules and tablets vary enough to cause differences in efficacy and side effects if the patient changes dosage forms. Patients should be warned about potential differences in clinical effect if they are switching from one dosage form to another.

Neuromuscular Blockers

Neuromuscular blocking agents are used with anesthetics when a patient is undergoing surgery. Neuromuscular blockers relax skeletal muscles to induce paralysis. They are used to help place the patient on a ventilator and to suppress the patient's spontaneous breathing once a ventilator is in place. These agents can be divided into two major categories, depolarizing and nondepolarizing neuromuscular blockers. Depolarizing agents, such as succinylcholine, mimic the effects of the neurotransmitter acetylcholine. By mimicking acetylcholine, succinylcholine competes with acetylcholine for the cholinergic receptors to cause prolonged depolarization. The depolarization is prolonged because succinylcholine is not rapidly degraded by acetylcholinesterase. This prolonged depolarization results in skeletal muscle paralysis.

Nondepolarizing agents also compete with acetylcholine but do not have any agonist activity at receptors. Instead, nondepolarizing agents block receptor activation by acetylcholine and thus prevent transmission of impulses leading to muscle relaxation. The type of neuromuscular blocker used depends on the duration of anesthesia required (Table 17-6). The action of the blocking agent can be prolonged with additional, smaller dosages. Pharmacy technicians may be responsible for filling floor stock orders for these medications for the operating room.

 Tech Alert!

Remember the following sound-alike, look-alike drugs:
- alendronate, risedronate, ibandronate
- Trandate versus Tridrate

DO YOU REMEMBER THESE KEY POINTS?

- Names of the major components of the musculoskeletal system and their functions
- The primary symptoms of the various musculoskeletal conditions discussed
- Medications used to treat the various musculoskeletal conditions discussed
- The generic and trade names for the drugs discussed in this chapter
- The appropriate auxiliary labels that should be used when filling prescriptions for drugs discussed in this chapter

REVIEW QUESTIONS

Multiple Choice Questions

1. Muscles are attached to bones by:
   A. Tendons
   B. Muscle fibers
   C. Ligaments
   D. Fascia

2. Acetaminophen (Tylenol) has all of the following pharmacologic actions *except:*
   A. Antiinflammatory
   B. Antipyretic
   C. Analgesic
   D. Acetaminophen has all of the above actions.

3. Celecoxib (Celebrex) is a selective inhibitor of:
   A. COX-1
   B. COX-2
   C. Mu opioid receptors
   D. Kappa opioid receptors

4. _____ are cells that resorb bone.
   A. Osteophytes
   B. Osteoblasts
   C. Osteoclasts
   D. Osteosarcomas

5. Which of the following is a selective estrogen receptor modulator (SERM) used to treat osteoporosis?
   A. Alendronate
   B. Raloxifene
   C. Denosumab
   D. Calcitonin salmon

6. Which of the following can be administered once weekly?
   A. Alendronate
   B. Raloxifene
   C. Denosumab
   D. Calcitonin salmon

7. Which of the following can be administered intranasally?
   A. Alendronate
   B. Raloxifene
   C. Denosumab
   D. Calcitonin salmon

8. Which of the following side effects is *not* characteristic of opioid analgesics?
   A. Miosis
   B. Euphoria
   C. Diarrhea
   D. Respiratory depression

9. Which of the following is a neuromuscular blocker?
   A. Fentanyl
   B. Ibuprofen
   C. Pancuronium
   D. Carisoprodol

10. The maximum recommended daily dose of acetaminophen for people who are otherwise healthy (do not have liver disease) is:
    A. 1000 mg
    B. 2000 mg
    C. 3000 mg
    D. 8000 mg

11. Which of the following is a parathyroid hormone analogue for the treatment of severe osteoporosis?
    A. Alendronate
    B. Teriparatide
    C. Denosumab
    D. None of the above

12. Fentanyl can be administered by which of the following routes?
    A. Oral
    B. Transdermal
    C. Intravenous
    D. All of the above

13. Which of the following drugs for the treatment of gout is a "uricosuric" agent?
    A. Probenecid
    B. Allopurinol
    C. Febuxostat
    D. Colchicine

14. Which of the following is associated with precipitating Reye's syndrome in children?
    A. Acetaminophen
    B. Ibuprofen
    C. Aspirin
    D. Naproxen

15. Osteoarthritis is considered:
    A. An immune system disease
    B. A degenerative joint disease
    C. An acute allergic reaction
    D. All of the above

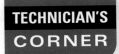

Mary Price presents to the pharmacy and reports having recently had an ultrasound screening exam on her heel to check her bone mineral density (BMD). She says that the exam result was abnormal, and she was instructed to speak with her physician about it. Ms. Price is curious about what medications she can take to prevent osteoporosis.

Using a comprehensive drug reference, look up which medications and/or supplements are used for osteoporosis prophylaxis and familiarize yourself with potential side effects associated with these medications.

Bibliography

Clinical Pharmacology Online. (Referenced August 19, 2014.) www.clinicalpharmacology-ip.com.

Damjanov I: *Pathology for the health professions*, ed 4, St Louis, 2011, Saunders.

Fishback JL: *Pathology*, ed 3, Philadelphia, 2005, Mosby.

McCance KL: *Pathophysiology: the biologic basis for disease in adults and children*, ed 6, St. Louis, 2010, Mosby.

Patton KT et al: *Mosby's handbook of anatomy and physiology*, St Louis, 2000, Mosby.

Price SA et al: *Pathophysiology: clinical concepts of disease processes*, ed 6, St Louis, 2003, Mosby.

Solomon EP: *Introduction to human anatomy and physiology*, ed 3, St Louis, 2009, Saunders.

Thompson JM et al: *Mosby's clinical nursing*, ed 5, St Louis, 2001, Mosby.

UpToDate Online. (Referenced August 19, 2014.) www.uptodate.com.

Therapeutic Agents for the Cardiovascular System

Joshua J. Neumiller

OBJECTIVES

Upon completing this chapter, you should be able to do the following:

1. Describe the major components of the cardiovascular system.
2. List the primary symptoms of conditions associated with dysfunction of the cardiovascular system.
3. Recognize drugs used to treat the conditions associated with the cardiovascular system discussed in this chapter.

4. Write the generic and trade names for the drugs discussed in this chapter.
5. List appropriate auxiliary labels when filling prescriptions for drugs discussed in this chapter.

TERMS AND DEFINITIONS

Aldosterone A steroid hormone secreted by the adrenal cortex that regulates the salt and water balance in the body

Aneurysm A balloonlike bulge or dilation of an artery due to weakening of the arterial wall

Angina Chest pain due to an inadequate supply of oxygen to the heart muscle

Angiotensin II A peptide hormone that causes vasoconstriction and a subsequent increase in blood pressure

Anticoagulant An agent used to prevent the formation of blood clots

Antihyperlipidemics A diverse group of pharmaceuticals used in the treatment of hyperlipidemia

Aorta The great arterial trunk that carries blood from the heart to be distributed to tissues of the body

Arrhythmia An abnormal or irregular heart rhythm

Arteriosclerosis A condition characterized by thickening, loss of elasticity (hardening), and calcification of the arterial walls

Artery A vessel that carries oxygenated blood from the heart to the tissues of the body

Atherosclerosis A process of progressive thickening and hardening of the walls of medium-sized and large arteries as a result of fat deposits on their inner lining

Atrium The entry chamber on both sides of the heart

Blood pressure The pressure of the blood within the arteries

Capillary An extremely small vessel that connects the ends of the smallest arteries (arterioles) to the smallest veins (venules), where

exchange of nutrients, waste products, oxygen (O_2), and carbon dioxide (CO_2) occurs

Cardiac muscle A type of muscle tissue found only in the heart

Cardiac output (CO) The amount of blood the heart pumps through the circulatory system in a minute

Coagulation Solidification or change from a fluid state to a solid state, as in the formation of a blood clot

Coronary artery Either of two arteries that arise from the aorta (one from the left side and one from the right side) and supply the tissues of the heart itself

Diastole The period when the heart is in a state of relaxation and dilation

Embolus A clump of material, often a blood clot, that travels from one part of the body to another and obstructs a blood vessel; an embolus can consist of any material, including bacteria or air

Endocardium The thin membrane that lines the interior of the heart; the inner layer of the heart wall

Enzyme A protein that accelerates a reaction by reducing the amount of energy required to initiate the reaction

Epicardium The outer layer of the heart wall; the inner layer of the pericardium

Essential hypertension The most common form of hypertension; it occurs in the absence of any evident cause

Fibrates A class of antihyperlipidemic drugs primarily effective at lowering triglycerides

Heart failure (HF) Inability of the heart to keep up with the demands on it and, specifically, failure of the heart to pump blood with normal efficiency

High-density lipoprotein (HDL) A lipoprotein of blood plasma that is composed of a high proportion of protein with little triglyceride and cholesterol; it is associated with a decreased probability of developing atherosclerosis

Hyperlipidemia Also known as *hypercholesterolemia*—a condition marked by an increase in cholesterol in the bloodstream that can lead to atherosclerosis, or hardening of the arteries

Hypertension High blood pressure

Hypotension Low blood pressure

Low-density lipoprotein (LDL) A molecule that is a combination of lipid (fat) and protein; it is associated with an increased probability of developing atherosclerosis

Lumen A channel within a tube (e.g., a blood vessel)

Myocardial infarction (MI) The death of myocardial tissue due to sudden deprivation of oxygenated blood flow, often as a result of a blood clot plugging a coronary artery; also known as a *heart attack*

Myocardium The middle muscular layer of the heart wall; it consists of cardiac muscle tissue

Nicotinic acid A member of the vitamin B complex; also known as *niacin*

Nitrates A class of drugs used to treat heart conditions, such as angina

Orthostatic hypotension A temporary lowering of blood pressure, usually related to standing up suddenly

Pericardium A fluid-filled membrane that surrounds the heart; also called the *pericardial sac*

Peripheral resistance Vascular resistance to the flow of blood in peripheral arterial vessels

Pulmonary artery One of the two vessels formed as terminal branches of the pulmonary trunk; they convey unaerated blood to the lungs

Renin A protein released by the kidney in response to low sodium levels or blood volume

Secondary hypertension Hypertension that results from an underlying identifiable cause

Statin An informal term for HMG-CoA reductase inhibitors, which are used for the treatment of hyperlipidemia, primarily to lower LDL cholesterol

Stent A tube designed to be inserted into a vessel or passageway to keep it open

Stroke The sudden death of some brain cells due to lack of oxygen when blood flow to the brain is impaired by blockage (ischemic stroke) or rupture (hemorrhagic stroke) of an artery to the brain

Syndrome A set of conditions that occur together

Systole The period when the heart is contracting; specifically, when the left ventricle of the heart contracts

Tachycardia A rapid heart rate, usually defined as greater than 100 beats per minute

Thrombin An enzyme formed in coagulating blood from prothrombin; thrombin reacts with fibrinogen and converts it to fibrin, which is essential in the formation of blood clots; thrombin levels are tested by performing a prothrombin time or partial thromboplastin time blood test

Thrombolytic A medication used to break up a thrombus or blood clot

Thrombosis The formation or presence of a blood clot in a blood vessel

Transient ischemic attack (TIA) A neurological event in which the signs and symptoms of a stroke appear but resolve within a short time

Triglyceride The major form of fat stored by the body; it consists of three molecules of fatty acid combined with a molecule of the alcohol glycerol

Vasoconstriction Narrowing of the blood vessels that results from contraction of the muscular walls of the vessels

Vasodilation Widening of blood vessels that results from relaxation of the muscular walls of the vessels

Vein A vessel that carries deoxygenated blood to or toward the heart

Vena cava One of the two large veins that carry deoxygenated blood from the upper (superior vena cava) and lower (inferior vena cava) parts of the body to the right atrium of the heart

Ventricle One of the two lower chambers of the heart

Select Common Drugs Prescribed for Cardiovascular Conditions

Trade Name	Generic Name	Pronunciation
Alpha-Blockers		
Cardura	doxazosin	(dok-**sah**-zoh-sin)
Hytrin	terazosin	(tur-**ah**-zoh-sin)
Minipress	prazosin	(**pra**-zoh-sin)
Antiarrhythmics		
Betapace, Betapace AF	sotalol	(soe-**ta**-lol)
Cordarone, Pacerone	amiodarone	(**a**-mi-**oh**-da-rone)
Norpace	disopyramide	(dye-so-**peer**-a-mide)
Pronestyl, Procanbid	procainamide	(pro-**cane**-ah-mide)
Quinidex	quinidine	(**kwin**-ah-deen)
Rythmol	propafenone	(proe-pa-**feen**-none)
Tikosyn	dofetilide	(doe-**fet**-ah-lide)

Select Common Drugs Prescribed for Cardiovascular Conditions—cont'd

Trade Name	Generic Name	Pronunciation
ACE Inhibitors		
Accupril	quinapril	(**kwin**-ah-pril)
Altace	ramipril	(rah-**mi**-pril)
Capoten	captopril	(**cap**-tow-pril)
Lotensin	benazepril	(ben-**ayz**-ah-pril)
Monopril	fosinopril	(foe-**sin**-oh-pril)
Prinivil, Zestril	lisinopril	(lih-**sin**-oh-pril)
Vasotec	enalapril	(eh-**nal**-ah-pril)
Angiotensin Receptor Blockers (ARBs)		
Atacand	candesartan	(kan-de-**sar**-tan)
Avapro	irbesartan	(erb-ba-**sar**-tan)
Cozaar	losartan	(low-**sar**-tan)
Diovan	valsartan	(val-**sar**-tan)
Micardis	telmisartan	(tel-meh-**sar**-tan)
Teveten	eprosartan	(eh-pro-**sar**-tan)
Beta-Blockers (BBs)		
Brevibloc	esmolol	(**es**-mo-lol)
Inderal	propranolol	(pro-**pran**-oh-lol)
Lopressor	metoprolol	(meh-toe-**pro**-lol)
Tenormin	atenolol	(uh-**ten**-oh-lol)
Trandate	labetalol	(lah-**bet**-ah-lol)
Visken	pindolol	(**pin**-doe-lol)
Calcium Channel Blockers (CCBs)		
Calan, Isoptin	verapamil	(ver-**ap**-ah-mill)
Cardene	nicardipine	(nye-**kar**-di-peen)
Cardizem	diltiazem	(dill-**tie**-ah-zem)
Norvasc	amlodipine	(am-**low**-di-peen)
Plendil	felodipine	(fe-**low**-di-peen)
Procardia	nifedipine	(nye-**feh**-di-peen)
Anticoagulants		
Coumadin	warfarin	(**war**-far-in)
Heparin	heparin	(heh-**par**-in)
Direct Thrombin Inhibitor		
Pradaxa	dabigatran	(**da**-bi-**gat**-ran)
Low-Molecular-Weight Heparins (LMWHs)		
Fragmin	dalteparin	(**dal**-te-**par**-in)
Lovenox	enoxaparin	(ee-nox-**ap**-a-rin)
Antiplatelet Agents		
Aggrenox	aspirin/dipyridamole	(**as**-pir-rin/dye-peer-**id**-a-mole)
Ecotrin	aspirin	(**as**-pir-rin)
Plavix	clopidogrel	(kloh-**pid**-oh-grel)
Nitrates		
Imdur, Monoket	isosorbide mononitrate	(**eye**-soe-**sor**-bide **mon**-oh-**nye**-trate)
Isordil	isosorbide dinitrate	(**eye**-soe-**sor**-bide dye-**nye**-trate)
Nitrostat, Tridil	nitroglycerin	(**nye**-troe-**glis**-sir-rin)
Antihyperlipidemic Agents		
Lovaza	omega-3-acid ethyl esters	(oh-**may**-ga 3 **as**-id **eth**-il **es**-ters)
Niacor	niacin	(**nye**-a-sin)

Continued

Select Common Drugs Prescribed for Cardiovascular Conditions—cont'd

Trade Name	Generic Name	Pronunciation
Zetia	ezetimibe	(eh-**zet**-eh-mibe)
Lopid	gemfibrozil	(gem-**fib**-row-**zil**)
Antara, Lipofen, Tricor	fenofibrate	(**fen**-no-**fye**-brate)
TriLipix, Fibricor	fenofibric acid	(**fen**-oh-fye-**brik** as-id)
Zocor	simvastatin	(sym-vah-**stat**-in)
Lipitor	atorvastatin	(a-**tor**-vah-stat-in)
Mevacor	lovastatin	(low-**vah**-stat-in)
Pravachol	pravastatin	(**pra**-vah-stat-in)
Crestor	rosuvastatin	(row-**soo**-vah-stat-in)
Lescol	fluvastatin	(**floo**-vah-stat-in)
Colestid	colestipol	(koe-**les**-ti-pole)
Questran	cholestyramine	(koe-**les**-teer-a-meen)
WelChol	colesevelam	(**koe**-le-**sev**-e-lam)
Diuretics		
Aldactone	spironolactone	(spear-**on**-oh-**lak**-tone)
Ezride, Microzide	hydrochlorothiazide	(hye-dro-klor-o-**thy**-zide)
Bumex	bumetanide	(byew-**met**-ah-nide)
Demadex	torsemide	(**tore**-se-mide)
Diamox	acetazolamide	(ah-see-ta-**zole**-a-mide)
Diuril	chlorothiazide	(klor-oh-**thye**-a-zide)
Dyrenium	triamterene	(try-**am**-tur-reen)
Lasix	furosemide	(feur-**oh**-sah-myde)
Zaroxolyn	metolazone	(meh-**tole**-uh-zone)
Thrombolytics		
Activase	alteplase (t-PA)	(**al**-teh-**place**)
Retavase	reteplase	(reh-**teh**-place)
TNKase	tenecteplase	(ten-**ek**-teh-place)

The cardiovascular system is a network of many complex interactions. These interactions involve the blood, lungs, kidneys, arteries, and veins of the body and the heart muscle itself. We begin with an overview of the anatomy of the heart, followed by the most common conditions that affect the heart. The last section of the chapter discusses the treatments available for heart conditions, with particular emphasis on the medications used. Pharmacy technicians fill many prescriptions for heart medications over their careers, and it is important to learn basic information about the classifications to assist the pharmacist.

Anatomy of the Heart and Vasculature System

The heart is located in the chest cavity between the lungs. The heart is a large muscle that initiates systemic arterial pulse waves, causing blood to circulate throughout the body and supply it with nutrition and oxygen (Figure 18-1). The muscle that composes the heart is called **cardiac muscle**. Extending from the heart are large blood vessels called **arteries**. These

arteries flow into smaller vessels called *arterioles* and ultimately into very small blood vessels called **capillaries**. From the capillaries, oxygen and nutrients are exchanged throughout the tissues of the body.

A normal heart beats 60 to 100 times per minute and is about the size of a person's fist. The heart is surrounded by connective tissue called the **pericardium**, which in turn is anchored by ligaments to the chest wall and diaphragm. The heart wall is composed of three main layers:

1. **Endocardium** (inner layer): The endocardium has a smooth, accordion pleat–like surface, which allows the heart wall to collapse when it contracts.
2. **Myocardium** (middle muscular layer): The myocardium is the heart muscle that contracts to facilitate a heartbeat.
3. **Epicardium** (outer layer): The epicardium is the outer layer of the heart wall. The coronary arteries that supply the heart with oxygenated blood and the coronary veins that return deoxygenated blood to the heart are located in the epicardium.

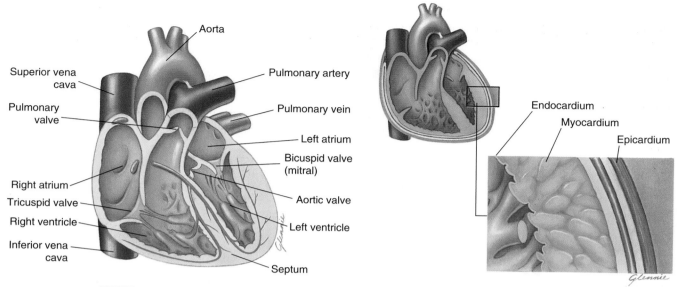

FIGURE 18-1 Anatomy of the heart. (From Gerdin J: *Health careers today*, ed 5, St Louis, 2012, Mosby.)

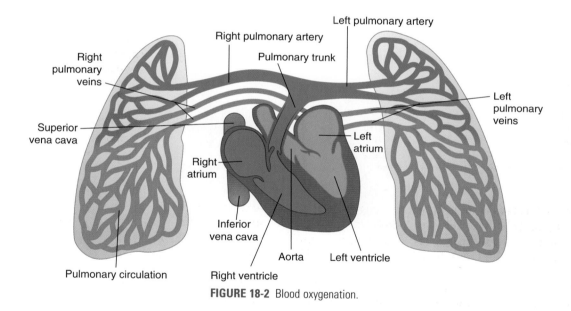

FIGURE 18-2 Blood oxygenation.

Oxygenation

The heart has two sides, each of which is composed of two chambers (Figure 18-2). The first two chambers are the right **atrium** and the right **ventricle**. Blood circulates through the body, exchanging oxygen, nutrients, and other substances in tissues and organs. The blood returns to the heart via two large **veins** called the superior **vena cava** and the inferior vena cava. The superior vena cava transports blood from the upper portion of the body, and the inferior vena cava carries blood from the lower portion of the body back to the heart. From the vena cava, blood is emptied into the right atrium and then travels into the right ventricle. During a heartbeat, the right ventricle contracts, expelling blood into the

pulmonary arteries; the pulmonary arteries carry blood to the lungs, where blood is fully oxygenated by the air we breathe (see Chapter 19). Interestingly, the pulmonary arteries carry deoxygenated blood, whereas most other arteries in the body carry oxygenated blood. The left atrium of the heart receives the fully oxygenated blood from the lungs via the pulmonary veins. Once again, and unique to the respiratory system, pulmonary veins carry oxygenated blood, whereas veins in other parts of the body carry deoxygenated blood. Blood then passes into the left ventricle. The left ventricle contracts, expelling the blood through the **aorta** and outward through the vasculature to the tissues of the body (Figure 18-3). Although the heart is an efficient organ, it still

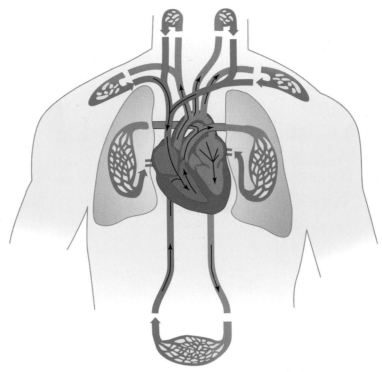

FIGURE 18-3 Circulation of blood through the body.

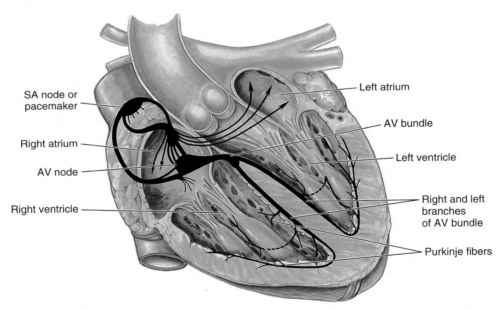

FIGURE 18-4 Conduction system of the heart. (From Solomon EP: *Introduction to human anatomy and physiology,* ed 3, St Louis, 2009, Saunders.)

must be oxygenated, just as other organs are. The main arteries that supply blood to the heart are called the **coronary arteries**.

Cardiac Conduction System

The cardiac conduction system provides the electrical charge that makes the heart pump. This system regulates the rate by which the heart beats and facilitates heart rhythm. This cardiac conduction system is operated by two nodes, the sinoatrial (SA) node and the atrioventricular (AV) node (Figure 18-4). The SA node, in the upper right atrium wall, is where the impulse begins. The signal then proceeds down to the AV node, in the septum between the right atrium and the right ventricle. From the AV node the impulse is conducted to the ventricles to initiate a ventricular beat.

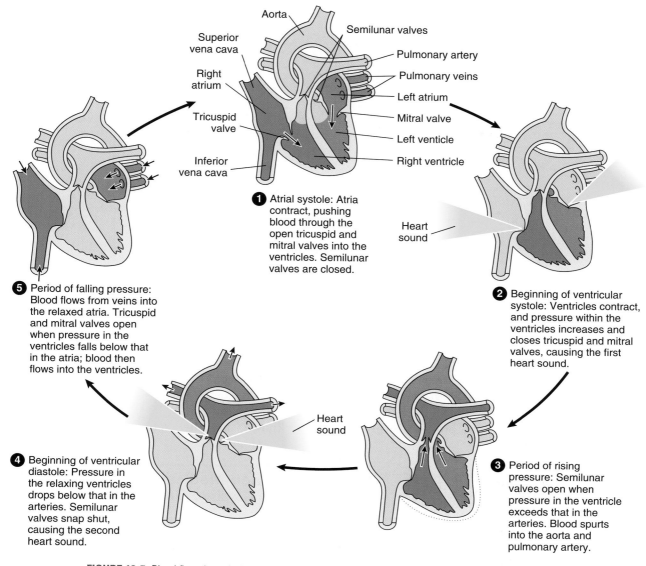

FIGURE 18-5 Blood flow through the heart during the cardiac cycle. (From Solomon EP: *Introduction to human anatomy and physiology,* ed 3, Philadelphia, 2009, Saunders.)

The Cardiac Cycle

The series of events that occur for one complete heartbeat is called the *cardiac cycle.* This cycle is composed of two sequences (Figure 18-5):

1. **Systole:** The myocardium squeezes blood from the heart chamber into the pulmonary artery or aorta.
2. **Diastole:** Blood is allowed to refill the chambers (relaxation). During diastole, the atria contract to pack 20% more blood into the ventricles. Most of the body's blood supply is cycled every minute through the heart.

Regulation of the Heart and Vasculature

The parasympathetic and sympathetic branches of the autonomic nervous system have opposite effects on the heart rate (see Chapter 15). The parasympathetic nervous system acts to slow the heart, whereas the sympathetic nervous system acts to increase the heart rate. In response to exercise or emotional stress, the adrenal glands release norepinephrine and epinephrine, which increase the heart rate.

Blood pressure is the force exerted by the blood against the inner walls of the blood vessels. The flow of blood depends on the heart rate and force of contractions. When the heart works harder to increase **cardiac output (CO)**, blood flow increases, causing a rise in blood pressure and vice versa. Blood flow is also affected by the volume of blood in the circulatory system. For example, blood pressure can fall if a person becomes dehydrated. On the other hand, an increase in blood volume can lead to an increase in blood pressure. A blood pressure

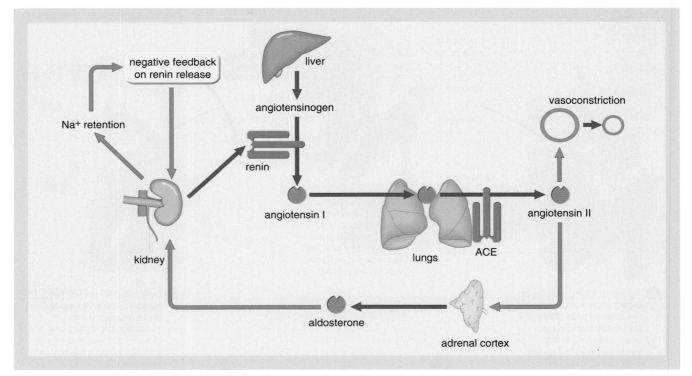

FIGURE 18-6 Renin-angiotensin-aldosterone system. *ACE,* Angiotensin-converting enzyme. (From Page C et al: *Integrated pharmacology,* ed 3, St Louis, 2006, Mosby.)

reading is expressed as systolic pressure over diastolic pressure.

 Tech Note!
Remember that fluid volume in the body can change based on salt intake. This is why people with edema are often placed on salt-restricted diets.

Peripheral resistance is resistance to blood flow caused by the viscosity of the blood and by the amount of force required to pump blood through the vessels. When the peripheral resistance increases, blood pressure increases. As the diameter of blood vessels decreases (**vasoconstriction**), peripheral resistance increases. **Vasodilation**, on the other hand, is an increase in blood vessel diameter that results in a decrease in peripheral resistance.

Hormones are also important in regulating blood pressure. In response to low blood pressure, the kidneys release **renin**. This **enzyme** acts on a plasma protein (angiotensinogen), initiating a series of reactions that produces **angiotensin II**, a hormone that causes vasoconstriction. Angiotensin II also acts indirectly to maintain blood pressure by signaling the adrenal glands to increase their output of **aldosterone**. This hormone increases the retention of sodium by the kidneys, resulting in greater fluid retention and increased blood volume. This system

is known as the renin-angiotensin-aldosterone system (Figure 18-6).

Common Medication Classes Used to Treat Cardiac Conditions

Because many different agents are used to treat heart conditions (e.g., coronary artery disease) and their causes (e.g., hypertension and high cholesterol levels), it is important to understand not only the types of medications, but also their mechanisms of action and possible side effects. Before discussing individual conditions of the cardiovascular system, let's first discuss some common drug classes used to treat cardiac conditions and how they work. Many of these drugs are used to treat multiple cardiovascular conditions. An easy way to remember the types of medications used to treat the heart conditions discussed in this chapter is the mnemonic "ABCD" (*a*ngiotensin-converting enzyme [ACE] inhibitors, *b*eta-blockers, *c*alcium channel blockers, and *d*iuretics). These are the common classifications of agents used to treat heart conditions, although not necessarily in the order in which they are prescribed. Although more classifications of agents are available (which are discussed throughout the chapter), ABCD is a simplified way to remember the four classes mentioned. Table 18-1 provides an overview of these and other classes of medications commonly used to treat cardiovascular disease.

TABLE 18-1

Select Drug Classes Used in the Treatment of Cardiovascular Conditions

Drug Classification	General Use	Generic Name	Trade Name	General Effect
Angiotensin-converting enzyme (ACE) inhibitors	Hypertension	benazepril lisinopril captopril ramipril fosinopril moexipril	Lotensin Prinivil Capoten Altace Monopril Univasc	Prevent blood vessel constriction
Beta-blockers	Hypertension	nadolol metoprolol pindolol bisoprolol acebutolol	Corgard Lopressor Visken Zebeta Sectral	Reduce workload of the heart
Calcium channel blockers	Hypertension	verapamil diltiazem nifedipine	Calan, Isoptin Cardizem Adalat, Procardia	Increase blood flow and decrease vessel constriction in the heart
Bile acid sequestrants	Hypercholesterolemia	cholestyramine colestipol	Prevalite, Questran Colestid	Lower cholesterol
Statins	Hypercholesterolemia	atorvastatin lovastatin pravastatin simvastatin	Lipitor Mevacor Pravachol Zocor	
Diuretics	Hypertension, edema	hydrochlorothiazide chlorothiazide furosemide bumetanide spironolactone triamterene metolazone	Ezride, Microzide Diuril Lasix Bumex Aldactone Dyrenium Zaroxolyn	Reduce fluid volume
Nitrates	Angina	nitroglycerin isosorbide dinitrate	Nitrostat, Nitro-Dur Dilatrate-SR, Isordil	Relax blood vessels, allowing more blood to reach the heart
Antiplatelet agents	Thrombosis Thrombosis	aspirin clopidogrel	Ecotrin Plavix	Prevent blood clot formation

Angiotensin-Converting Enzyme Inhibitors

ACE inhibitors are a group of agents that help reduce blood pressure by dilating arteries. Recall from Figure 18-6 that angiotensin I is converted to angiotensin II by the angiotensin-converting enzyme. ACE inhibitors effectively inhibit the production of angiotensin II and thus the vasoconstriction it causes. The net effect of ACE inhibitors is peripheral vasodilation and lowering of blood pressure.

 Tech Note!

A potential side effect of ACE inhibitors is the characteristic "ACE inhibitor cough." This tends to be a dry, hacking cough that does not resolve over time. People who develop this cough sometimes need to be switched to an alternative class of medications (frequently angiotensin II receptor blockers).

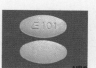

GENERIC NAME: lisinopril
TRADE NAME: Prinivil, Zestril
INDICATION: Acute myocardial infarction, heart failure, hypertension
ROUTE OF ADMINISTRATION: Oral
COMMON ADULT DOSAGE: 10-40 mg once daily
MECHANISM OF ACTION: ACE inhibitor (prevents the conversion of angiotensin I to angiotensin II, thus leading to vasodilation)
SIDE EFFECTS: Dizziness, headache, dry cough
AUXILIARY LABEL:
- May cause dizziness/drowsiness.

GENERIC NAME: benazepril
TRADE NAME: Lotensin
INDICATION: Hypertension
ROUTE OF ADMINISTRATION: Oral
COMMON ADULT DOSAGE: 5-40 mg taken in 1 or 2 doses
MECHANISM OF ACTION: ACE inhibitor (prevents the conversion of angiotensin I to angiotensin II, thus leading to vasodilation)
SIDE EFFECTS: Dizziness, headache, dry cough
AUXILIARY LABEL:
- May cause dizziness/drowsiness.

Angiotensin II Receptor Antagonists

Angiotensin II receptor antagonists, also known as *angiotensin II receptor blockers (ARBs)*, work by inhibiting the effects of angiotensin II on angiotensin II receptors. The net effects are very similar to those of ACE inhibitors, including a reduction in blood pressure due to a net vasodilation.

 Tech Note!
One of the main clinical differences between ACE inhibitors and ARBs is that ARBs very rarely cause a dry cough as a side effect, while patients taking ACE inhibitors frequently experience a dry cough.

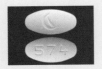

GENERIC NAME: losartan
TRADE NAME: Cozaar
INDICATION: Hypertension, stroke prophylaxis, proteinuria, diabetic nephropathy
ROUTE OF ADMINISTRATION: Oral
COMMON ADULT DOSAGE: 25-100 mg once daily or divided twice daily
MECHANISM OF ACTION: Antagonizes angiotensin II receptors, blocking the vasoconstrictive effects of angiotensin II
SIDE EFFECTS: Dizziness, nausea, muscle pain

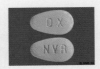

GENERIC NAME: valsartan
TRADE NAME: Diovan
INDICATION: Hypertension, heart failure
ROUTE OF ADMINISTRATION: Oral
COMMON ADULT DOSAGE: 80-320 mg once daily
MECHANISM OF ACTION: Antagonizes angiotensin II receptors, blocking the vasoconstrictive effects of angiotensin II
SIDE EFFECTS: Dizziness, nausea, muscle pain

 Tech Note!
Generic drug names can often provide a clue to the drug class to which they belong. ARBs often end in "-artan," whereas ACE inhibitors end in "-pril." Beta-blockers typically end in "-lol."

Beta-Blockers

Beta-blockers are effective because they block both norepinephrine and epinephrine from binding to beta-adrenergic receptors. Blocking these receptors reduces the heart rate, which can help lower blood pressure and regulate the heartbeat in people with **tachycardia**. Beta-blockers act at two sites, the beta-1 and beta-2 receptor sites. Beta-1 receptors are located in the heart, and beta-2 receptors are located in the lungs and arteries. The actions of beta-blocker medications can be specific or nonspecific. Nonspecific agents affect both beta-1 and beta-2 receptors, whereas specific beta-blockers affect only beta-1 receptors in the heart and have little action in the lungs.

A nonspecific agent, which affects both beta-1 and beta-2 receptors, would not be recommended for a patient who has been diagnosed with asthma or another type of respiratory problem because blocking beta-2 receptors in the lungs and bronchi leads to constriction of the airways (see Chapter 19). For this reason, beta-1–selective beta-blockers are often preferred for treating cardiovascular conditions.

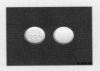

GENERIC NAME: atenolol
TRADE NAME: Tenormin

INDICATION: Hypertension, angina, myocardial infarction
ROUTE OF ADMINISTRATION: Oral
COMMON ADULT DOSAGE: *Oral:* 25-100 mg once daily
MECHANISM OF ACTION: Cardioselective beta-1 receptor blocker
SIDE EFFECTS: Dizziness, drowsiness, fatigue
AUXILIARY LABEL:
* May cause dizziness/drowsiness.

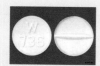

GENERIC NAME: metoprolol
TRADE NAME: Lopressor, Toprol XL
INDICATION: Hypertension, angina, myocardial infarction, heart failure
ROUTE OF ADMINISTRATION: Oral; intravenous
COMMON ADULT DOSAGE: *Immediate release (IR):* 12.5-50 mg twice daily; *XL:* 50-200 mg per day
MECHANISM OF ACTION: Cardioselective beta-1 receptor blocker
SIDE EFFECTS: Dizziness, drowsiness, fatigue
AUXILIARY LABEL:
* May cause dizziness/drowsiness.

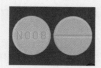

GENERIC NAME: propranolol
TRADE NAME: Inderal, Inderal LA
INDICATION: Hypertension, angina, atrial fibrillation, tremor, migraine prophylaxis
ROUTE OF ADMINISTRATION: Oral; intravenous
COMMON ADULT DOSAGE: *IR for hypertension:* 40-80 mg three times daily; *LA:* 80-160 mg once daily
MECHANISM OF ACTION: Nonselective beta-receptor blocker
SIDE EFFECTS: Dizziness, drowsiness, fatigue
AUXILIARY LABEL:
* May cause dizziness/drowsiness.

 Tech Note!

Propranolol is a beta-blocker that readily crosses the blood-brain barrier (BBB). Because of this, propranolol is used for a variety of central nervous system (CNS) conditions, including migraine prophylaxis and treatment of some tremors.

Calcium Channel Blockers

Calcium channel blockers (CCBs) act by reducing the calcium intake of the heart muscle and the blood vessels. This leads to a relaxation of smooth muscle in the vasculature, which in turn leads to vasodilation and a decrease in blood pressure. The two main categories of CCBs are dihydropyridines and nondihydropyridines. Dihydropyridine CCBs (e.g., nifedipine and amlodipine) have a greater effect on the peripheral vasculature and are used primarily to treat high blood pressure. Diltiazem and verapamil, the two currently available nondihydropyridine CCBs, affect the heart in addition to the vasculature; for this reason, these CCBs are also used to treat arrhythmias.

GENERIC NAME: diltiazem
TRADE NAME: Cardizem CD, Cardizem LA, Cardizem SR, Dilacor XR, Tiazac Select
INDICATION: Angina, hypertension, atrial fibrillation
ROUTE OF ADMINISTRATION: Oral; intravenous
COMMON ADULT DOSAGE: Dose is highly variable, depending on dosage form and condition treated
MECHANISM OF ACTION: Blocks calcium channels, leading to relaxation of muscle and vasodilation
SIDE EFFECTS: Dizziness, headache, gingival hyperplasia, arrhythmias
AUXILIARY LABEL:
* May cause dizziness.

GENERIC NAME: amlodipine
TRADE NAME: Norvasc
INDICATION: Hypertension, angina
ROUTE OF ADMINISTRATION: Oral
COMMON ADULT DOSAGE: 5-10 mg once daily
MECHANISM OF ACTION: Blocks calcium channels, leading to relaxation of muscle and vasodilation
SIDE EFFECTS: Dizziness, drowsiness, peripheral edema
AUXILIARY LABEL:
* May cause dizziness/drowsiness.

Conditions Affecting the Cardiovascular System

Diseases and conditions affecting the health of the cardiovascular system include hypertension, heart failure, hypercholesterolemia, arrhythmias, and congenital heart disease, among others. Cardiovascular disease is rampant in the United States and other countries. An exhaustive review of cardiovascular diseases is beyond the scope of this chapter; however, the following sections provide an overview of conditions commonly encountered in both the ambulatory and inpatient settings.

Common Conditions

Hypertension

Hypertension, or high blood pressure, is a prevalent problem in the United States, affecting millions of Americans. This disease also is known as the "silent killer" because usually there are no obvious signs of its presence. When a cause for hypertension cannot be established, the person is considered to have **essential hypertension**. Of those with hypertension, approximately 19 out of 20 have essential hypertension, and 1 out of 20 has an identifiable cause, such as medications, certain kidney diseases (e.g., renal artery stenosis), and diseases of the adrenal glands (e.g., Cushing's syndrome), to name a few. Hypertension with a known cause is called **secondary hypertension**. Some people with severe hypertension may have symptoms such as nosebleeds and/or headaches; however, most people do not have any symptoms. This is the reason it is important to monitor blood pressure, which is measured with a blood pressure cuff that measures blood pressure in millimeters of mercury (mmHg). Whatever the cause of hypertension, the result is that the heart must work much harder to pump blood through the vascular system to provide oxygen and nutrients to the body. Four stages of blood pressure have been described (Box 18-1).

 Tech Note!

Patients with hypertension should be informed by their physicians and pharmacists that many OTC agents can affect their blood pressure. These include nonsteroidal antiinflammatory drugs (NSAIDs), antihistamines, decongestants, and ingredients in many different cold and allergy remedies.

Prognosis. With proper diet (and medications, if necessary), hypertension can be effectively controlled.

BOX 18-1

Classification of Blood Pressure

Classification	Systolic Pressure (mmHg)	Diastolic Pressure (mmHg)
Normal	90-119	60-79
Prehypertension	120-139	80-89
Stage 1 hypertension	140-159	90-99
Stage 2 hypertension	≥160	≥100

Non–Drug Treatment. Individuals should have their blood pressure measured regularly throughout their lifetime to identify hypertension early so that nonpharmacological strategies can be used to manage the condition. Research suggests that even a mild case of hypertension can lead to problems later in life because of the extra work placed on the heart.

Many risk factors for hypertension cannot be changed, such as a family history of the disease. However, the following lifestyle changes can help manage hypertension:

- Maintaining a healthy weight
- Engaging in regular physical activity
- Avoiding high-sodium foods, such as potato chips, pickles, canned soups, and processed meat (e.g., bacon, cold cuts), in addition to table salt
- Increasing the daily intake of fruits and vegetables
- Limiting alcohol intake (no more than two drinks per day for men and one per day for women)
- Reducing stress through daily relaxation techniques
- Stopping or avoiding smoking

Drug Treatment. If the desired blood pressure cannot be achieved through lifestyle modifications, medications may be prescribed. The first-line therapy for most people with hypertension is thiazide diuretics; however, under certain circumstances other medications may be selected first. Although diuretics are commonly the first-line drug, other agents frequently are used as monotherapy or combination therapy, such as ACE inhibitors, beta-blockers, and calcium channel blockers, as previously described. In addition to reviewing the information previously presented on these classes of medications, see Table 18-2 for information on select agents used in the treatment of hypertension.

TABLE 18-2

Select Medications Used for the Treatment of Hypertension

Medication Class	Generic Name	Trade Name	Common Side Effects	Common Dose Range
Angiotensin-Converting Enzyme (ACE) Inhibitors	benazepril	Lotensin	• Cough • Hyperkalemia • Angioedema • Hypotension	• 20-80 mg orally (PO) divided into 1-2 doses daily
	lisinopril	Prinivil, Zestril		• 5-40 mg PO once daily
	captopril	Capoten		• 25 mg PO 2-3 times daily
	ramipril	Altace		• 2.5-5 mg PO once daily (max 20 mg)
	enalapril	Vasotec		• 2.5-40 mg PO in 1-2 divided doses daily
Beta-Blockers	nadolol	Corgard	• Bradycardia • Fatigue • Atrioventricular (AV) block • Dizziness • Hypotension	• 40-120 mg PO once daily
	metoprolol	Lopressor Toprol-XL		• 100-450 mg/day PO in 2-3 divided doses daily
	atenolol	Tenormin		• 50-100 mg PO once daily
	propranolol	Inderal		• 25-50 mg PO once daily (max 100 mg)
	labetalol	Trandate		• 40-160 mg PO in 2-3 divided doses daily
				• 100-400 mg PO twice daily *or*
	carvedilol	Coreg		• 20 mg intravenous (IV) push over 2 min
				• 3.125-6.25 mg PO twice daily *or*
				• *Extended release:* 20-40 mg PO once daily (max 80 mg)
Angiotensin Receptor Blockers (ARBs)	losartan	Cozaar	• Hyperkalemia • Orthostatic hypotension	• 25-100 mg PO in 1-2 divided doses
	valsartan	Diovan		• 80-320 mg PO once daily
	olmesartan	Benicar		• 20-40 mg PO once daily
	candesartan	Atacand		• 8-32 mg PO 1-2 times daily
Direct Renin Inhibitor	aliskiren	Tekturna	• Rash • Hyperkalemia • Diarrhea	• Initially 150 mg PO once daily, may increase to a max of 300 mg PO once day
Calcium Channel Blockers: Dihydropyridines	nifedipine	Adalat, Procardia	• Dizziness • Headache • Constipation • Peripheral edema • Gingival overgrowth	• 30-60 mg PO once daily extended release (max 120-180 mg/day)
	amlodipine	Norvasc		• 5-10 mg PO once daily
	nicardipine	Cardene		• 20-40 mg PO 3 times daily
Calcium Channel Blockers: Nondihydropyridines	diltiazem	Cardizem	• Bradycardia • Edema • AV block • Dizziness • Headache • Pain	• 180-420 mg PO once daily (max 540 mg/day)
	verapamil	Calan		• *Immediate release:* 80-320 mg/day PO in 2 divided doses daily • *Extended release:* 120-360 mg/day PO in 1-2 divided doses daily
Loop Diuretics	furosemide	Lasix	• Hypokalemia • Hypotension • Headache • Weakness	• 20-80 mg PO 1-2 times daily
	bumetanide	Bumex		• 0.5-1 mg PO 1-2 times daily (max 10 mg/day)
Thiazide Diuretics	hydrochlorothiazide (HCTZ)	Microzide	• Hypokalemia • Hyponatremia • Hyperglycemia • Hypotension • Photosensitivity	• 12.5-50 mg PO in 1-2 doses daily (max 200 mg daily)
	chlorothiazide	Diuril		• 12.5-50 mg PO once daily (max 100-200 mg daily)
	metolazone	Zaroxolyn		• 2.5-10 mg PO once daily (max 20 mg daily)

Continued

TABLE 18-2

Select Medications Used for the Treatment of Hypertension—cont'd

Medication Class	Generic Name	Trade Name	Common Side Effects	Common Dose Range
Potassium-Sparing Diuretics	spironolactone	Aldactone	• Hyperkalemia • Gynecomastia • Decreased libido	• 25-200 mg/day PO in 1-2 divided doses
	triamterene	Dyrenium	• Hyperkalemia • Hypotension • Muscle cramps	• 100-300 mg PO 1-2 times daily (max 300 mg daily)
Alpha-1 Receptor Blockers	doxazosin	Cardura	• Orthostasis • Reflex tachycardia • Headache	• 1 mg PO once daily, then titrate upward to a goal of 4-8 mg PO once daily
		Cardura XL (extended release)	• Dizziness	• 4 mg PO once daily with breakfast, then titrate upward to 8 mg PO once daily
	terazosin	Hytrin		• 1 mg PO at bedtime, then titrate upward prn; most patients need 10 mg (max 20 mg/day)
	prazosin	Minipress		• 1 mg PO 2-3 times daily
Alpha-2 Adrenergic Agonists	methyldopa	Aldomet	• Rebound hypertension if withdrawn too fast • Sedation • Dry mouth • Hepatitis	• 250-1000 mg/day PO in 2 divided doses (max 3 g/day)
	clonidine	Catapres		• *Immediate release:* 0.1-0.8 mg/day PO in 2 divided doses daily • *Extended release:* 0.17-0.52 mg PO once daily • Patch form is available

Hypotension

Hypotension, by definition, is low blood pressure. One of the more common problems that people experience is orthostatic hypotension. This occurs because a large amount of blood remains in the lower extremities (ankles and feet). When a person stands quickly, the blood returning to the heart is decreased considerably, and the body responds by increasing the heartbeat, compensating for the lack of blood flow. This results in a feeling of lightheadedness. Symptoms of hypotension include syncope (fainting) and/or dizziness. For people who have chronic hypotension, physicians may recommend nondrug therapies and/or may prescribe medication to help increase blood pressure.

Prognosis. With proper medical treatment and lifestyle changes, hypotension can be effectively controlled in most cases.

Non–Drug Treatment. Adjustments in medications may alleviate hypotension resulting from medication use. Increasing salt intake can additionally help raise blood pressure; however, this can be done only if an increase in salt does not affect any comorbid medical conditions. Drinking more water helps increase fluid volume in the bloodstream and relieves dehydration. For people with orthostatic hypotension, moving or standing up slowly can help minimize symptoms. Compression stockings can also be used to help prevent the pooling of blood in the legs.

Drug Treatment. The two most common drugs used to treat postural hypotension are fludrocortisone (which increases blood volume) and midodrine (which raises blood pressure).

 Tech Note!

Many people who experience hypotension have a disease associated with the development of hypotension, such as Parkinson's disease. Also, many patients who experience hypotension are actually experiencing a drug side effect.

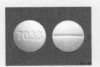

GENERIC NAME: fludrocortisone
TRADE NAME: Florinef
INDICATION: Orthostatic hypotension, Addison's disease, adrenocortical insufficiency

ROUTE OF ADMINISTRATION: Oral
COMMON ADULT DOSAGE: 0.1-0.2 mg once daily
MECHANISM OF ACTION: Mimics the actions of aldosterone, leading to sodium and water retention that increases blood pressure
SIDE EFFECTS: Weakness, muscle cramps, osteoporosis, fragile skin
AUXILIARY LABEL:
• Take with food or milk.

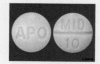

GENERIC NAME: midodrine
TRADE NAME: ProAmatine
INDICATION: Orthostatic hypotension
ROUTE OF ADMINISTRATION: Oral
COMMON ADULT DOSAGE: 10 mg three times per day
MECHANISM OF ACTION: Activates alpha-1 receptors in the vasculature, leading to vasoconstriction and an increase in blood pressure
SIDE EFFECTS: Headache, urinary retention, chills

Hyperlipidemia

Hyperlipidemia (also known as *hypercholesterolemia*) is an increase in cholesterol in the bloodstream that can lead to **atherosclerosis**, or hardening of the arteries. Atherosclerosis increases the incidence of angina, heart attack, and stroke. When discussing fats (lipids) in the body, it is important to recognize that cholesterol is only one type of lipid and that it performs many vital functions, including the synthesis of steroid hormones and cell membranes. When people eat foods that are high in fat and cholesterol, they often are ingesting too much, which leads to a buildup of these fats in the body. In addition to diet, hyperlipidemia also can result from certain inherited conditions. The most widespread genetically associated disorder is familial hypercholesterolemia. Blood tests are used to measure serum levels of different forms of cholesterol, such as **low-density lipoproteins (LDLs)** and **high-density lipoproteins (HDLs)**. The function of LDL is to carry cholesterol to the tissues, where it becomes lodged in blood vessel walls and contributes to atherosclerosis. HDL, or "good cholesterol," removes cholesterol from the arteries and transports it to the liver. **Triglycerides** (TGs) are another form of cholesterol that has been linked to the development of atherosclerosis. Figure 18-7 illustrates the development of an atherosclerotic plaque, which is a complex interplay between the

vasculature, cholesterol, and cells of the immune system.

Prognosis. In severe cases, bypass surgery or cardiac stenting may be indicated for individuals experiencing symptoms of ischemia from atherosclerosis.

Non–Drug Treatment. By eating a healthy diet and engaging in regular physical activity, many people can lower their cholesterol levels. Diet and lifestyle changes (exercise, weight control, and cessation of smoking) are a critical initial approach for patients without other major risk factors for heart disease. People with significant risk factors for heart disease and stroke (or those with familial hyperlipidemia) may incorporate drug treatments immediately, along with diet and lifestyle changes, to reduce their risk of serious cardiovascular events.

Drug Treatment. Antihyperlipidemic agents are some of the most widely used medications in the United States. Antihyperlipidemic agents include HMG-CoA reductase inhibitors (also known as "statins"), bile acid sequestrants, fibrates, niacin, and ezetimibe (Table 18-3).

The **statins** specifically inhibit an enzyme responsible for one of the first steps in the overall conversion of fats into cholesterol. They raise HDL levels and reduce LDL and TG levels; therefore, these drugs are the most widely used agents for the treatment of hyperlipidemia.

GENERIC NAME: lovastatin
TRADE NAME: Mevacor, Altoprev
INDICATION: Hypercholesterolemia, myocardial infarction prophylaxis
ROUTE OF ADMINISTRATION: Oral
COMMON ADULT DOSAGE: *Immediate release:* 10-80 mg once daily at bedtime; *Altoprev:* 10-60 mg once daily at bedtime
MECHANISM OF ACTION: Inhibits the enzyme HMG-CoA reductase, which is responsible for one of the first steps in the overall conversion of fats into cholesterol
SIDE EFFECTS: Muscle pain, liver toxicity, nausea, constipation
AUXILIARY LABELS:
• Take with meals.
• Take in the evening.

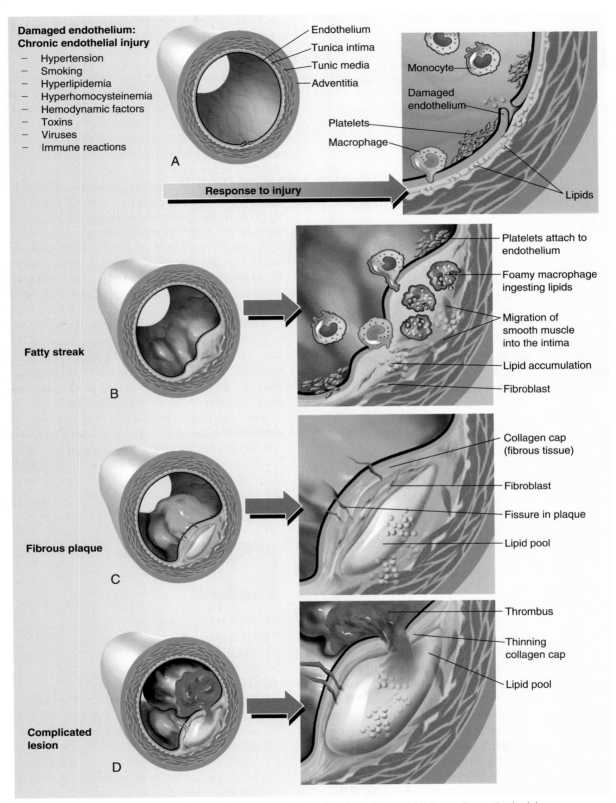

Damaged endothelium: Chronic endothelial injury
- Hypertension
- Smoking
- Hyperlipidemia
- Hyperhomocysteinemia
- Hemodynamic factors
- Toxins
- Viruses
- Immune reactions

Endothelium
Tunica intima
Tunic media
Adventitia

A

Monocyte
Damaged endothelium
Platelets
Macrophage
Lipids

Response to injury

Fatty streak

B

Platelets attach to endothelium
Foamy macrophage ingesting lipids
Migration of smooth muscle into the intima
Lipid accumulation
Fibroblast

Fibrous plaque

C

Collagen cap (fibrous tissue)
Fibroblast
Fissure in plaque
Lipid pool

Complicated lesion

D

Thrombus
Thinning collagen cap
Lipid pool

FIGURE 18-7 Progression of atherosclerosis. (From Huether S, McCance K: *Understanding pathophysiology,* ed 5, St Louis, 2012, Mosby.)

TABLE 18-3

Select Medications Used for the Treatment of Hyperlipidemia

Medication Class	Generic Name	Trade Name	Common Side Effects	Common Dose Range
Nicotinic Acid	niacin*	Niacor, Niaspan ER	• Flushing • Itching • Dyspepsia • Hyperglycemia • Hyperuricemia	• *Immediate release:* 4.5 g/day PO in 3 divided doses • *ER:* 1-2 g PO once daily
Bile Acid Sequestrants	cholestyramine	Questran	• Upset stomach • Bloating	• 8-16 g/day PO divided into 2 doses (max 24 g/day)
	colestipol	Colestid	• Constipation • Headache	• *Granules:* 5-30 g/day PO in 1-2 divided doses • *Tablets:* 2-16 g/day PO in 1-2 divided doses
	colesevelam	WelChol		• 3.75 g PO once daily or • 1.875 g PO twice daily
HMG-CoA Reductase Inhibitors (Statins)	atorvastatin lovastatin pravastatin simvastatin rosuvastatin fluvastatin	Lipitor Mevacor Pravachol Zocor Crestor Lescol	• Headache • Upset stomach • Liver toxicity • Muscle pain	• 10-80 mg PO once daily • 20-80 mg PO once daily • 10-80 mg PO once daily • 5-40 mg PO once daily • 5-40 mg PO once daily • 20-80 mg PO once daily
Fibrates	gemfibrozil fenofibrate	Lopid Tricor	• Myopathy • Upset stomach • Abdominal pain • Diarrhea	• 600 mg PO twice daily • 48-145 mg PO once daily
Cholesterol Absorption Inhibitors	ezetimibe	Zetia	• Headache • Angioedema • Fatigue • Diarrhea • Upper respiratory infection	• 10 mg PO once daily
Omega-3 Fatty Acids	fish oil	Lovaza	• Nausea • Vomiting • Weight gain • Prolonged bleeding	• 4 g PO divided into 1-2 doses daily

*Taking 325 mg of aspirin before niacin helps reduce flushing and itching.

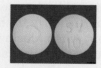

GENERIC NAME: simvastatin
TRADE NAME: Zocor
INDICATION: Hypercholesterolemia, myocardial infarction prophylaxis, stroke prophylaxis
ROUTE OF ADMINISTRATION: Oral
COMMON ADULT DOSAGE: 5-40 mg once daily in the evening
MECHANISM OF ACTION: Inhibits the enzyme HMG-CoA reductase, which is responsible for one of the first steps in the overall conversion of fats into cholesterol

SIDE EFFECTS: Muscle pain, liver toxicity, nausea, constipation
AUXILIARY LABELS:
• Take with meals.
• Take in the evening.

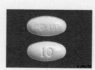

GENERIC NAME: atorvastatin
TRADE NAME: Lipitor

INDICATION: Hypercholesterolemia, myocardial infarction prophylaxis, stroke prophylaxis
ROUTE OF ADMINISTRATION: Oral
COMMON ADULT DOSAGE: 10-80 mg once daily in the evening
MECHANISM OF ACTION: Inhibits the enzyme HMG-CoA reductase, which is responsible for one of the first steps in the overall conversion of fats into cholesterol
SIDE EFFECTS: Muscle pain, liver toxicity, nausea, constipation
AUXILIARY LABELS:
- Take with meals.
- Take in the evening.

Bile acid sequestrants, such as cholestyramine, increase the loss of cholesterol through the gastrointestinal (GI) tract. They do this by binding to bile acids in the GI tract and preventing their reabsorption. Because bile acids are made from cholesterol, the loss of bile acids through the feces has a net effect of lowering cholesterol levels in the body.

GENERIC NAME: cholestyramine
TRADE NAME: Questran, Questran Light, Prevalite
INDICATION: Hypercholesterolemia
ROUTE OF ADMINISTRATION: Oral (powder)
COMMON ADULT DOSAGE: Initially, 4 g once or twice daily before meals (maximum 24 g per day in divided doses)
MECHANISM OF ACTION: Binds to bile acids in the GI tract, preventing their reabsorption and thus lowering cholesterol levels
SIDE EFFECTS: Constipation, flatulence
AUXILIARY LABELS:
- Take before meals.
- Take with plenty of fluids.
SPECIAL NOTE: The powder form should be mixed into 60 to 180 mL of liquid. Other medications should be taken 4 to 6 hours apart from cholestyramine to avoid interference with absorption.

Fibrates, such as gemfibrozil and fenofibrate, are less effective at lowering LDL cholesterol but can increase HDL levels and lower TGs. Because of this,

Tech Note!

The bile acid sequestrant colesevelam (Welchol) is approved for the treatment of hyperlipidemia and type 2 diabetes mellitus. The mechanism of action of colesevelam in helping to lower blood glucose levels is not entirely clear.

they are frequently used in combination with statins in people with persistently low HDL and high TG levels. The exact mechanism by which fibrates affect cholesterol is not known.

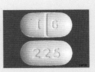

GENERIC NAME: gemfibrozil
TRADE NAME: Lopid
INDICATION: Hyperlipidemia, hypertriglyceridemia
ROUTE OF ADMINISTRATION: Oral
COMMON ADULT DOSAGE: 600 mg twice daily administered 30 minutes before morning and evening meals
MECHANISM OF ACTION: Exact mechanism is not known
SIDE EFFECTS: Dyspepsia, abdominal pain, diarrhea, liver toxicity
AUXILIARY LABEL:
- Take with food.

Nicotinic acid (niacin), which is a B-complex vitamin, reduces LDL and TG levels and increases HDL levels. Although the exact mechanism by which niacin treats hyperlipidemia is unknown, the effect is believed to be due to niacin's role as a vitamin. Another effect of niacin is dilation of the blood vessels that supply cutaneous blood flow, particularly to the face, neck, and chest. Because of this, when niacin is used at therapeutic doses, it can cause the characteristic "niacin flush." This flush can result in headaches, pain, and pruritus in some people.

GENERIC NAME: nicotinic acid
TRADE NAME: Niacor, Niaspan
INDICATION: Hyperlipidemia, hypertriglyceridemia
ROUTE OF ADMINISTRATION: Oral
COMMON ADULT DOSAGE: *Niacor:* 1-2 g three times daily with meals; *Niaspan:* 500 mg at bedtime initially, then 1-2 g per day at bedtime

MECHANISM OF ACTION: Exact mechanism is not known
SIDE EFFECTS: Photosensitivity, niacin flush
AUXILIARY LABEL:
- May cause photosensitivity.

 Tech Note!

"Nonflushing" forms of niacin are available for people who experience a niacin flush. Aspirin (unless otherwise contraindicated) can also be taken before niacin to help minimize flushing symptoms.

Ezetimibe (Zetia) is an oral medication approved for use as monotherapy or in combination with statins or fenofibrate for the treatment of hyperlipidemia. Ezetimibe works by inhibiting the absorption of cholesterol from the GI tract.

GENERIC NAME: ezetimibe
TRADE NAME: Zetia
INDICATION: Hyperlipidemia
ROUTE OF ADMINISTRATION: Oral
COMMON ADULT DOSAGE: 10 mg once daily
MECHANISM OF ACTION: Inhibits the absorption of cholesterol from the GI tract
SIDE EFFECTS: Abdominal pain, fatigue, dizziness, headache
SPECIAL NOTE: Ezetimibe can be given at the same time as statins but should be given at least 2 hours before or 4 hours after a bile acid sequestrant.

Coronary Artery Disease

Coronary artery disease (CAD) is a condition in which the arteries of the heart do not receive proper oxygenation, often due to narrowing of the arteries as a result of atherosclerosis. Symptoms can include hypertension, angina pectoris, hyperlipidemia, and myocardial infarction (Figure 18-8).

Atherosclerosis is a **syndrome** (more than one condition) that affects arterial blood vessels. Inflammation occurs as a result of the lifelong buildup of small plaques, mainly composed of lipids, and the clumping of platelets (see Figure 18-7). Over time, small injuries can occur in the vessel wall. When damage occurs to the arterial wall, the body responds by sending macrophages and T lymphocytes to fight the plaques; however, instead of eliminating plaques, these lymphocytes increase the blockage. This cycle continues, potentially causing total blockage of a vessel that can result in a heart attack or stroke. **Arteriosclerosis** is a condition that results from thickening, loss of elasticity (hardening), and calcification of the arterial walls. Hypertension, hyperlipidemia, diabetes mellitus, and normal aging all contribute to the progression of arteriosclerosis. Patients with atherosclerosis often also have arteriosclerosis.

CAD is one of the leading causes of death in both men and women. This may be due partially to the fact that after their first heart attack, many people do not make the necessary changes in lifestyle or adhere to their medication regimen to avoid further complications. With both proper medication and lifestyle changes, many people can live with CAD and reduce their risk factors for heart attack and stroke. Because CAD blocks blood flow to areas of the heart muscle, a primary symptom of the disease is **angina** due to a lack of oxygen to the myocardium.

Angina Pectoris. Angina pectoris results from a decrease in blood flow to the heart, which causes

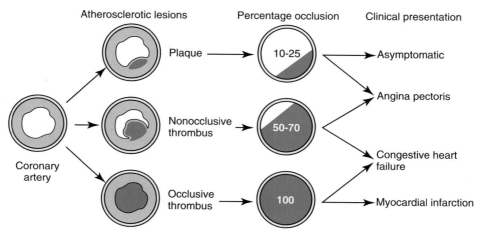

FIGURE 18-8 Narrowing of the coronary artery may cause different clinical symptoms, depending on the extent of occlusion and the speed at which it develops. (From Damjanov I: *Pathology for the health professions,* ed 4, Philadelphia, 2011, Saunders.)

chest pain or a sense of pressure. The pain can vary from minor to severe. Decreased blood flow can be caused by factors such as hardening of the arteries (atherosclerosis), hypertension, and cigarette smoking. Environmental and genetic influences also can play a role in acquiring angina (chest pain). The three types of angina are:

- Stable angina
- Variant angina
- Unstable angina

In classic stable (chronic) angina, the person can experience short ischemic episodes. Patients often describe a pressure in their chest, which they may describe as "an elephant sitting on my chest." This pain can occur in the chest, neck, arms, teeth, and jaw. This form of angina is precipitated by exertion and generally occurs after a set level of physical activity. Many times this type of angina attack occurs after exercise, excessive activity, or emotional stress; therefore, the episodes are usually predictable.

Variant angina (also called *Prinzmetal's* or *vasospastic angina*) may not be related to atherosclerosis; instead, the patient experiences spasms of the coronary artery that can occur spontaneously. These spasms effectively narrow the **lumen** (or cavity) of the artery, thus reducing blood flow to the heart.

Variant angina does not necessarily occur after physical exercise or stress and is less predictable than stable angina.

Unstable angina, which may worsen in a person with a known history of angina attacks, can occur at rest. For people with preexisting angina, unstable angina may develop when their symptoms become more severe in pattern compared with the patient's usual symptoms. Unstable angina may be due to the rupture of an atherosclerotic plaque. Because unstable angina may be a sign of an impending heart attack, it requires immediate medical attention.

Prognosis. The prognosis for angina depends on the type of angina and the severity of the condition. A history of heart conditions, such as arrhythmias or heart attacks, also influences the outcome and treatment approach.

Non–Drug Treatment. Modifying behaviors to lessen angina attacks include smoking cessation, stress reduction, weight loss, lowering blood pressure and cholesterol levels, and controlling any underlying conditions (e.g., hypertension). Surgical procedures may be used to relieve occlusion in some patients. Angioplasty (Figure 18-9) or

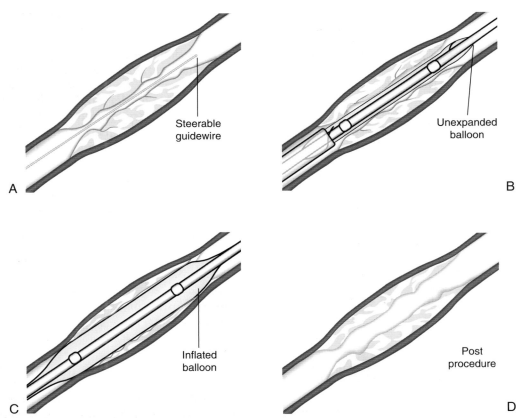

FIGURE 18-9 Coronary angioplasty procedure. (From Sole ML et al: *Introduction to critical care nursing,* ed 6, Philadelphia, 2013, Saunders.)

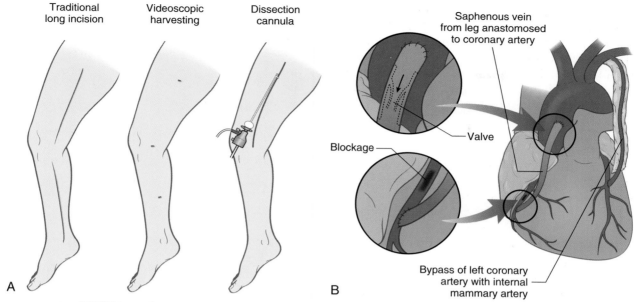

FIGURE 18-10 Coronary artery bypass graft surgery. (From Sole ML et al: *Introduction to critical care nursing,* ed 6, Philadelphia, 2013, Saunders.)

TABLE 18-4

Select Common Nitrate Agents

Trade Name	Generic Name	Normal Usage
Tridil	nitroglycerin (NTG) solution for injection	Emergency management of acute angina
NTG in D₅W	nitroglycerin + dextrose solution for injection	Emergency management of acute angina
Nitrostat	nitroglycerin (sublingual tablet)	Treatment of acute angina
NitroMist	nitroglycerin (sublingual spray)	Treatment of acute angina
Nitro-Time	nitroglycerin (extended-release capsule)	Routine medication for stable angina
Nitro-Dur, Minitran	nitroglycerin (transdermal patch)	Routine medication for stable angina
Imdur	isosorbide mononitrate	Routine medication for stable angina
	isosorbide dinitrate (sublingual tablet	Treatment of acute angina
Dilatrate SR, Isochron	isosorbide dinitrate (extended-release capsule)	Routine medication for stable angina

coronary artery bypass graft (CABG) (Figure 18-10) are two such surgical procedures that can be used. Angioplasty is the insertion and inflation of a small balloon into the affected area, which removes and/or stabilizes the plaque. In the CABG procedure, a piece of healthy blood vessel is taken from another part of the body and grafted to bypass the affected vessel in the heart. Stent placement is another intervention often used to widen arteries to improve coronary blood flow. A **stent** is a small, cylindrical device that is inserted into the affected artery, providing a framework to hold the artery open. The stent is placed by inserting a catheter through a vein and guiding the stent to the affected site. Stents can be uncoated or coated with a slow-release medication that keeps the artery from clotting and ultimately closing.

Drug Treatment. Nitrates, calcium channel blockers, and beta-blockers are commonly used to treat and prevent angina symptoms. For people with symptoms of angina, the most commonly prescribed antianginal agent is nitroglycerin. Millions of individuals carry nitroglycerin sublingual tablets in their pockets or purses in the event of an acute angina attack. Nitroglycerin has many dosage forms, including capsules, topical patches, ointments and creams, and sublingual sprays. The sublingual tablets and injectable forms are used for emergencies.

Nitrates (Table 18-4) are vasodilators; that is, they dilate the arteries to permit an increase of blood flow to the heart muscle. They also reduce the workload of the heart. Isosorbide dinitrate, isosorbide mononitrate, and nitroglycerin are the

Doctor David Gall
1000 Archway
St. Louis, MO
ph: 816-555-5555

Patient name: _R. Jones-Lewis_

Address: _106 Nutree Way_   Date: _1-30-XX_

R: NTG 0.4mg sl #100

Take 1 sl q 5 min x3

if no relief call 911

D. Gall
Dr. Signature

Refills: _6_   DEA # _____

FIGURE 18-11 Nitroglycerin sublingual tablet prescription.

common nitrate agents used for the treatment of angina. Both isosorbide dinitrate and nitroglycerin are available as sublingual tablets, which are effective because of their rapid absorption. Figure 18-11 shows a common sublingual nitroglycerin prescription order for the treatment of an acute angina attack.

Nitroglycerin sublingual tablets must be kept in a dry area and in the original light-protected glass container to prevent the active agent from deteriorating. Another form for acute relief is translingual nitroglycerin spray. The patient sprays metered doses under the tongue, with a maximum of three sprays in a 15-minute period. Sublingual dosages are kept at the patient's bedside in an institution, or constantly with the ambulatory individual, for emergency relief of angina attacks. In the hospital, nitroglycerin is often given by intravenous (IV) infusion for a variety of circumstances, including the treatment of unstable angina.

Longer acting nitrate dosage forms are available for chronic treatment of angina to prevent attacks. Transdermal dosage forms (nitroglycerin) or oral dosage forms (e.g., nitroglycerin, isosorbide dinitrate, and isosorbide mononitrate) are available. The nitroglycerin transdermal patches normally are applied once daily in the morning and are removed at bedtime to reduce the possibility of tolerance to the medication. Ointment tubes are available in 60-g, 30-g, and 1-g unit dose sizes. The ointment is squeezed onto the paper in increments of ½ inch to 2 inches (similar to toothpaste placed on a toothbrush), then placed on the chest.

Other agents commonly used for the chronic treatment of angina include beta-blockers and calcium channel blockers, which reduce heart ischemia by mechanisms different from those of nitrate agents.

 Tech Note!

When filling a prescription for nitroglycerin sublingual tablets (e.g., Nitrostat), never take the tablets out of the amber glass container in which they are packaged, so that the nitroglycerin is protected from degradation by light. Instead, place the glass container in a larger plastic vial on which the label is attached. Nitroglycerin should also be packaged with a non-childproof cap so that people can readily open the vial if experiencing chest pain or a heart attack.

Thrombotic Events

The formation of a clot in a vessel, blocking blood flow, is known as **thrombosis**. Coagulation (blood clotting) is a normal body function aimed at stopping hemorrhage and starting the healing process. Unfortunately, our bodies also can form unwanted blood clots. This clotting can occur because of an overactive clotting mechanism (genetic), can result from narrowing of the arteries (as in people with atherosclerosis), or may be due to prolonged inactivity. An **embolus** (plural, emboli) is a blood clot that has broken away from the thrombus (main clot) and has traveled through the body to another area, where it can become lodged and create a blockage. Thrombi and emboli can precipitate myocardial infarction, stroke, or deep vein thrombosis (DVT).

Prognosis. If the thrombus/embolus is treated quickly, the prognosis can be good. In certain cases warfarin or low-dose heparin may need to be taken for a prolonged period.

Non–Drug Treatment. Wearing support stockings and standing and walking on a regular basis to facilitate circulation in the lower extremities are potential nonpharmacological means to minimize the risk of developing a clot.

Drug Treatment. Depending on the severity of the clot, either an anticoagulant (to prevent clotting) or a thrombolytic (to break up or dissolve the clot) can be used. Thrombolytics are given parenterally under the supervision of a physician. These must be used soon after a clot occurs, before the affected organ or tissue is damaged (such as the brain in the case of a stroke). Table 18-5 provides an overview of anticoagulants, antiplatelet agents, and thrombolytics.

Clots are formed by fibrin, a protein that holds blood cells together to make a blood clot. Heparin inhibits thrombosis by accelerating the activity of antithrombin III to inactivate **thrombin**. This impedes the **coagulation** mechanism. Patients admitted to the hospital with a myocardial infarction or stroke may be administered an IV heparin drip to prevent blood coagulation. Heparin is effective and is intended for short-term use in a hospital setting.

GENERIC NAME: heparin
TRADE NAME: Hep-Lock

TABLE 18-5

Select Anticoagulant and Antiplatelet Agents

Medication Class	Generic Name	Trade Name	Common Adult Dose
Vitamin K Antagonist (VKA)	warfarin	Coumadin	PO; dose titrated to goal INR
Anticoagulant-Heparin	heparin	Hep-Lock	5000 units IV every 8-12 hr
Low-Molecular Weight Heparins (LMWHs)	dalteparin	Fragmin	2500-5000 units SUBCUT every 24 hr
	enoxaparin	Lovenox	30 mg SUBCUT every 12 hr
Antiplatelet Agents	aspirin/dipyridamole	Aggrenox	1 tablet (25/200 mg) PO twice daily
	aspirin	Ecotrin	81-325 mg PO once daily
	clopidogrel	Plavix	75 mg PO once daily
	cilostazol	Pletal	100 mg PO twice daily
	ticlopidine	Ticlid	250 mg PO twice daily
	ticagrelor	Brilinta	90 mg PO twice daily
	prasugrel	Effient	*Loading dose:* 60 mg PO, then 10 mg once daily
Factor Xa Inhibitors	fondaparinux	Arixtra	2.5 mg SUBCUT once daily
	rivaroxaban	Xarelto	20 mg PO once daily
	apixaban	Eliquis	2.5 mg PO twice daily for set number of days (2-4 wk average)
Direct Thrombin Inhibitors	bivalirudin	Angiomax	*Bolus:* 0.1 mg/kg IV, then 0.25 mg/kg/hr
	lepirudin	Refludan	*Bolus:* 0.4 mg/kg IV, then 0.15 mg/kg/hr (max bolus 44 mg; max infusion 16.5 mg/hr)
	argatroban		2 mcg/kg/min IV adjusted until steady-state aPTT achieved
	dabigatran	Pradaxa	150 g PO twice daily
Glycoprotein IIb/IIIa Inhibitors	abciximab	ReoPro	*Bolus:* 0.25 mg/kg IV
	eptifibatide	Integrilin	180 mcg/kg IV over 1-2 min
	tirofiban	Aggrastat	*Initial:* 0.4 mcg/kg/min for 30 min, then 0.1 mcg/kg/min
Thrombolytics	alteplase (t-PA)	Activase	0.9 mg/kg IV infusion over 1 hr (varying protocols/indications)
	reteplase	Retavase	10 units IV over 2 min with a second dose 30 min later
	tenecteplase	TNKase	*Bolus:* 30-50 mg IV (weight based) over 5 seconds

aPTT, Activated partial thromboplastin time; *INR,* international normalized ratio; *IV,* intravenously; *PO,* orally; *SUBCUT,* subcutaneously.

INDICATION: Treatment and prevention of clot formation
ROUTE OF ADMINISTRATION: Injection (intravenous, subcutaneous)
COMMON ADULT DOSAGE: Dosing is highly variable depending on patient factors and indication
MECHANISM OF ACTION: Inhibits thrombosis by accelerating the activity of antithrombin III to inactivate thrombin
SIDE EFFECTS: Hemorrhage, injection site reactions

Another type of **anticoagulant** is warfarin. Unlike heparin, orally administered warfarin is indicated for long-term use and is usually taken once daily. Warfarin interferes with the synthesis of vitamin K–dependent coagulation factors (II, VII, IX, and X) in the liver. Prothrombin time and international normalized ratio (INR) tests must be done to monitor how long it takes the blood to form clots while the patient is taking this medication. It is vital that a patient not be overdosed on warfarin, or the patient can experience potentially life-threatening bleeding. Warfarin is notorious for interacting with other prescription medications, OTC products, herbals, and even food. People receiving warfarin are often monitored on a regular basis.

Some patients are treated in the hospital and/or discharged home with a low-molecular-weight heparin (LMWH), such as enoxaparin, which is administered as a subcutaneous injection (see Table 18-5). The dosage depends on the indication for use and also on the patient's weight. LMWHs are frequently used as "bridge therapy" after orthopedic surgeries while people are started on warfarin. Bridge therapy means that the LMWH is used to prevent clot formation until the warfarin achieves a therapeutic level.

Tech Note!

Foods such as broccoli contain a large amount of vitamin K, which may counteract the effectiveness of warfarin. Other foods high in vitamin K include liver, brussels sprouts, spinach, Swiss chard, coriander, collards, and cabbage. Patients should try to keep the amount of vitamin K in their diets at a stable level. For example, people who normally do not eat broccoli and who begin to take warfarin should avoid starting to consume large amounts of broccoli (or other vegetables with vitamin K) because this will counteract the effectiveness of warfarin. Consistency is the key.

GENERIC NAME: warfarin
TRADE NAME: Coumadin, Jantoven
INDICATION: Prevention of clot formation
ROUTE OF ADMINISTRATION: Oral
COMMON ADULT DOSAGE: Dose varies depending on treatment goals and response—a common starting dose is 2-5 mg daily
MECHANISM OF ACTION: Interferes with the synthesis of vitamin K–dependent coagulation factors to prevent clot formation
SIDE EFFECTS: Hemorrhage
AUXILIARY LABEL:
- Avoid alcohol.

Although warfarin is widely used for long-term prevention of clots for people undergoing various forms of surgery or for people with atrial fibrillation, another medication, dabigatran (Pradaxa), was recently introduced to the market. This medication, a direct thrombin inhibitor, works by inhibiting thrombin to prevent thrombin-induced platelet aggregation and the development of a clot. Dabigatran has the potential advantage over warfarin of not requiring routine monitoring (see Table 18-5 for more information about dabigatran and other direct thrombin inhibitors).

GENERIC NAME: dabigatran
TRADE NAME: Pradaxa
INDICATION: Stroke prophylaxis, embolism prophylaxis in people with atrial fibrillation
ROUTE OF ADMINISTRATION: Oral
COMMON ADULT DOSAGE: 75-150 mg twice daily
MECHANISM OF ACTION: Inhibits thrombin to prevent thrombin-induced platelet aggregation and the development of a clot
SIDE EFFECTS: Hemorrhage
AUXILIARY LABEL:
- Do not repackage or store capsules in any other container.

Myocardial Infarction. If coronary blood flow to an area of the heart becomes entirely blocked because of a thrombus or embolism, that area of heart muscle cannot receive the necessary oxygen. This results in the death of that part of the heart muscle, a condition known as **myocardial infarction (MI)**, commonly referred to as a heart attack. The onset of an MI is experienced differently from person to person and may not be treated quickly if the patient is unaware that his or her symptoms indicate a heart attack. Depending on the severity of the blockage, the patient may have an MI from which he or she can recover over time or a massive MI that weakens the heart permanently or may even result in death.

Prognosis. Many people survive an MI because of prompt medical treatment. Several classes of drugs can be used to manage various conditions, and lifestyle changes can reduce the chances of recurrence of an MI. Some patients are at high risk for heart arrhythmia, heart failure, or other complications after an MI.

Non–Drug Treatment. The many medications available for post-MI patients have been discussed previously in this chapter. Cardiac rehabilitation, dietary changes, and reduction of risk factors (e.g., cessation of smoking) are all important actions to implement after a heart attack. However, if the patient's MI was severe or if the condition of the coronary arteries is such that the blockages present place the patient at high risk, an intervention such as bypass surgery may be necessary (as discussed previously).

Drug Treatment. After an MI, drug treatment goals are to reduce mortality (risk of death) of the patient and to prevent reinfarction. After an MI, the heart undergoes structural changes, and another major goal of drug therapy is to maximize and preserve the remaining function of the left ventricle and to avoid heart arrhythmia and heart failure. Many medications are used, including beta-blockers, ACE inhibitors, statins, aspirin, and other antiplatelet medications (e.g., clopidogrel [Plavix]). The treatments chosen depend on the individual patient's history, type of infarction, and the types of procedures that may have been performed. Table 18-6 provides an overview of potential treatments that can be used during an acute MI and for maintenance therapy after an MI.

Transient Ischemic Attacks and Strokes. **Transient ischemic attacks (TIAs)** are caused by a short period of reduced oxygenation to the brain that can be due to atherosclerotic cerebrovascular disease. TIAs are similar to strokes, except that the duration of a TIA is much shorter and typically no permanent loss of function occurs. Transient attacks may last only a few minutes or may occur many times over the span of a day. If atherosclerotic plaque forms a clot, a thrombus can form that eventually may obstruct the vessel, causing a stroke. TIAs sometimes are referred to as mini-strokes and are considered a precursor to a stroke.

The two types of strokes are ischemic (clot) strokes and hemorrhagic (bleeding) strokes. Hemorrhagic strokes occur when weakened vessels, or **aneurysms**, in the brain rupture. When a vessel ruptures, blood flows into areas of the brain, causing damage; additional injury is caused by the lack of oxygenated blood flow to areas of the brain where it is needed. Most of the symptoms of TIAs and strokes may appear rapidly; they include vision or hearing problems, weakness on one or both sides of the body, dizziness, slurred speech, and sudden, severe headache.

Prognosis. As mentioned, a TIA may be a precursor to a stroke. If a patient presents with TIA symptoms, certain diagnostic tests can be performed to determine the likelihood of more TIAs or even an impending stroke. Common diagnostic tests include computed tomography (CT) and magnetic resonance imaging (MRI) scans.

Non–Drug Treatment. As for other cardiovascular diseases discussed previously, reducing the factors that contribute to the underlying causes is one of the changes that must be made. This includes smoking cessation, reducing fat and alcohol consumption, weight loss if necessary, engaging in physical activity, and eating a balanced diet. Nonfatal strokes are one of the most common causes of disability, resulting in possible brain damage and the necessity for physical and occupational therapy.

Drug Treatment. TIAs are treated by improving arterial blood flow to the brain so that a stroke can be avoided. In the case of a TIA, patients may be treated with antiplatelet medication (e.g., aspirin) to reduce the risk of clot formation or with anticoagulants (e.g., warfarin). Usually the last resort is carotid artery surgery to remove arterial plaques.

The main agents used to treat an acute ischemic stroke in progress are thrombolytics, such as tissue plasminogen activator (t-PA, Activase), if indicated. Therapy must be given within 3 hours of the onset of the symptoms of the event, after the patient has been evaluated to rule out intracranial bleeding (see Table 18-5).

TABLE 18-6

Select Agents Used in the Treatment of Acute Coronary Syndrome/Myocardial Infarction

Medication Class	Generic Name	Trade Name	Common Dose Range
Vasodilator/Antianginal	nitroglycerin	Nitrostat	• 400 mcg sublingual (SL) or spray every 5 min (max 3 doses) • *Patch:* 0.4-0.8 mg/hr (12-14 hr patch on, then 10-12 hr patch off)
	isosorbide mononitrate	Imdur	• *Immediate release (IR):* 5-20 mg orally (PO) twice daily • *Extended release (ER):* 30-60 mg PO once daily in the morning (max 240 mg/dose)
	isosorbide dinitrate	Isordil	• *IR:* 5-20 mg PO 2-3 times daily • *ER:* 40 mg 1-2 times daily
Opioid	morphine	MS Contin	• 2-8 mg intravenously (IV) every 5-15 min after nitroglycerin
Gas	oxygen	NA	• 2-4 L/min via nasal cannula for first 6 hr
Vasodilator/Antianginal	nitroglycerin	Nitrostat	• 400 mcg SL or spray every 5 min (max 3 doses)
Beta-Blocker	metoprolol	Lopressor	• 50-100 mg PO twice daily or 5 mg IV slow push over 5 min (max 15 mg)
Anticoagulant-Heparin Glycoprotein IIb/IIIa Inhibitors	heparin abciximab eptifibatide tirofiban	Hep-Lock ReoPro Integrilin Aggrastat	• 5000 units IV every 8-12 hr • *Bolus:* 0.25 mg/kg IV • 180 mcg/kg IV over 1-2 min • *Initial:* 0.4 mcg/kg/min for 30 min, then 0.1 mcg/kg/min
Thrombolytic	alteplase (t-PA)	Activase	• 0.9 mg/kg IV infusion over 1 hr (varying protocols/indications)
Antiplatelet (in Combination with Aspirin)	clopidogrel ticagrelor prasugrel	Plavix Brilinta Effient	• 75 mg PO once daily • 90 mg PO twice daily • *Loading dose:* 60 mg PO, then 10 mg once daily

Arrhythmia

As previously discussed, the heart beats in a regular rhythm. This is accomplished via special fibers that run throughout the heart. The pacemaker is located in the SA node. Many factors influence the efficient operation of the pacemaker, including chemical balance. If an imbalance results from chemicals (e.g., electrolytes) or oxygen deprivation, irregular heartbeats, or **arrhythmias**, can occur. Medications can also cause arrhythmias. Depending on the severity of the arrhythmia, acute care may or may not be required. Some patients may require chronic use of medications to help maintain the heart's normal rhythm.

Non–Drug Treatment. Identifying the root cause of an arrhythmia is an important aspect of care. If the arrhythmia is caused by medications or some other cause that can be addressed, addressing the causative factor should be a primary approach to treatment. In severe cases in which medications cannot correct the rhythm, a pacemaker implant may be necessary.

Drug Treatment. The medications used in treating arrhythmias are called antiarrhythmic agents. Quinidine sulfate, procainamide, amiodarone, sotalol, and verapamil are some common agents that may be prescribed. Table 18-7 provides select examples of antiarrhythmic medications.

Prognosis. The outcome of an arrhythmia depends on its location and severity. Arrhythmias originating in the atrium may ultimately be controlled with medications or other treatment. Ventricular tachycardia or fibrillation is generally more serious.

 Tech Note!

Serious medication errors can occur because of the similar names of quinidine and quinine. Quinine is an antimalarial agent; quinidine is an antiarrhythmic. These two medications are often close to one another on a pharmacy shelf and have been mistaken for one another.

TABLE 18-7

Select Agents Used in the Treatment of Arrhythmias

Generic Name	Trade Name	Common Side Effects	Common Dose Range*
sotalol	Betapace, Betapace AF	• Depression • Dizziness • Stomach upset	• 80-160 mg orally (PO) twice daily
amiodarone	Cordarone, Pacerone	• Photosensitivity • Hypotension	• 5-7 mg/kg intravenously (IV) over 30-60 min, then 1.2-1.8 g/day continuous infusion *or* • 600-800 mg/day PO in divided doses until 10 g total, then 200-400 mg daily
digoxin	Lanoxin	• Dizziness • Headache • Heart block • Nausea • Visual disturbances	• 0.125-0.5 mg PO once daily • 0.1-0.4 mg IV or intramuscularly (IM) once daily
disopyramide	Norpace	• Dry mouth • Constipation	• *Immediate release (IR):* 100 mg PO every 6 hr • *Extended release (ER):* 200 mg PO every 12 hr
procainamide	Pronestyl, Procanbid	• Hypotension • Taste changes	• 50 mg/kg/day IM divided into doses every 3-6 hr *or* • 50 mg/min IV repeated prn every 5 min until a total of 1 g
quinidine	Quinidex	• Diarrhea • Lightheadedness • Hypotension	• *IR:* 200-400 mg PO every 6 hr • *ER:* 300 mg PO every 8-12 hr
propafenone	Rythmol	• Dizziness • Stomach upset • Bronchospasm	• *IR:* 150 mg PO every 8 hr (max 300 mg/8 hr) • *ER:* 225 mg PO twice daily (max 450 mg/dose)
dofetilide	Tikosyn	• Hypotension • Bradycardia • Dizziness	• 500 mcg PO twice daily
flecainide	Tambocor	• Dizziness • Headache • Blurred vision	• 100-200 mg PO twice daily
dronedarone	Multaq	• Bradycardia • Stomach upset • Rash	• 400 mg PO twice daily
lidocaine	Xylocaine	• Seizures • Psychosis	• *Bolus:* 1-1.5 mg/kg IV/intraosseously (IO) • *Infusion:* 1-4 mg/min IV

*Dosing can vary depending on type and severity of arrhythmia.

Heart Failure

Heart failure (HF) is a progressive disease in which the heart cannot pump enough blood to meet the oxygen and nutrient demands of the body. Several treatments are available to help patients with HF, but there is no cure. Edema is a characteristic component of HF because the kidneys compensate for the lack of blood flow by retaining more fluid in the body. This fluid increases the heart's workload, further weakening it. Eventually the heart can no longer pump adequately. A variety of cardiovascular conditions that have already been discussed can contribute to the development of HF, including hypertension, MI, and CAD. Other conditions that may cause HF include valvular heart disease, congenital heart defects, cardiomyopathy, and endocarditis. Symptoms of HF include fatigue, shortness of breath (SOB) during activities of daily living or when lying down, peripheral edema, and pulmonary edema.

Prognosis. HF can be treated in several ways, although certain conditions associated with the onset of HF often cannot be reversed. Through the use of medications and lifestyle changes, the life span of a person with HF can be greatly improved.

Non–Drug Treatment. A number of changes can influence the severity of HF. Such nonpharmacological treatments include reduction of salt intake, cessation of smoking, loss of weight, rest and modification of daily activities, and reduction of stress. If valvular or congenital heart disease is the source of a patient's heart failure, surgery may correct the defects and improve heart function.

Drug Treatment. The goal of all drug treatments is to improve the ease and efficiency of heart function. One of the most common treatments used in HF is digoxin. Additional agents include ACE inhibitors, ARBs, beta-blockers, and diuretics (Table 18-8). Digoxin, which is a cardiac glycoside, increases the force of the heartbeat. Diuretics are almost always used to help lower blood pressure and manage the edema associated with HF.

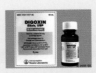

GENERIC NAME: digoxin
TRADE NAME: Lanoxin
INDICATIONS: Heart failure, atrial fibrillation
ROUTE OF ADMINISTRATION: Oral; injection
COMMON ADULT DOSAGE: 0.125-0.25 mg once daily
MECHANISM OF ACTION: Inhibits Na-K-ATPase pump, leading to an increase in intracellular calcium in cardiac muscle, which in turn leads to more forceful heart contractions

TABLE 18-8

Select Agents Used in the Treatment of Heart Failure

Medication Class	Generic Name	Trade Name	Common Side Effects	Common Dose Range
Acute Heart Failure **Loop Diuretic**	furosemide	Lasix	• Hypokalemia • Hypotension • Headache • Weakness	• 40-180 mg intravenously (IV) (max 360 mg)
Vasodilator	nitroglycerin	Nitrostat	• Hypotension • Headache • Flushing • Peripheral edema	• 5-10 mcg/min IV infusion, titrate upward to effect
	nitroprusside	Nitropress	• Hypotension • Flushing	• 5-300 mcg/min IV (max 400 mcg/min)
Natriuretic Peptide, B-Type	nesiritide	Natrecor	• Hypotension • Headache • Nausea	• *Bolus:* 2 mcg/kg IV, then 0.01 mcg/kg/min continuous infusion
Adrenergic Agonist	dobutamine	Dobutrex	• Increased heart rate • Increased blood pressure • Chest pain • Fever • Headache	• 2.5-20 mcg/kg/min IV infusion (max 40 mcg/kg/min)
Phosphodiesterase Enzyme Inhibitor	milrinone	Primacor	• Ventricular arrhythmia • Hypotension • Headache • Chest pain	• 0.375 mcg/kg/min IV infusion
Chronic Heart Failure **ACE Inhibitors**	benazepril	Lotensin	• Cough • Hyperkalemia • Angioedema • Hypotension	• 20-80 mg orally (PO) divided into 1-2 doses daily
	lisinopril	Prinivil, Zestril		• 5-40 mg PO once daily
	captopril	Capoten		• 25 mg PO 2-3 times daily
	ramipril	Altace		• 2.5-5 mg PO once daily (max 20 mg)
	enalapril	Vasotec		• 2.5-40 mg PO in 1-2 divided doses daily

TABLE 18-8

Select Agents Used in the Treatment of Heart Failure—cont'd

Medication Class	Generic Name	Trade Name	Common Side Effects	Common Dose Range
Beta-Blockers	metoprolol	Toprol XL	• Bradycardia • Fatigue • Dizziness • Hypotension • Nausea	• 12.5-25 mg PO once daily (target 200 mg/day)
	carvedilol	Coreg		• 3.125-6.25 mg PO twice daily *or* • *ER:* 20-40 mg PO once daily (max 80 mg)
Loop Diuretic	furosemide	Lasix	• Hypokalemia • Hypotension • Headache • Weakness • Cross-sensitivity to sulfa	• 20-80 mg PO 1-2 times daily (titrate to achieve dry weight goal)
Thiazide Diuretics	hydrochlorothiazide (HCTZ)	Microzide	• Hypokalemia • Hyponatremia • Hyperglycemia • Hypotension • Photosensitivity	• 12.5-50 mg PO in 1-2 doses daily (max 200 mg daily)
	metolazone	Zaroxolyn		• 2.5-10 mg PO once daily (max 20 mg daily)
Cardiac Glycoside	digoxin	Lanoxin	• Dizziness • Mental disturbances • Headache • Nausea • Visual disturbances	• 0.125-0.5 mg PO once daily
Aldosterone Inhibitors	spironolactone	Aldactone	• Hyperkalemia • Hyponatremia • Gynecomastia • Decreased libido	• 12.5-25 mg/day PO once daily
	eplerenone	Inspra		• 25-50 mg PO 1-2 times daily (max 100 mg daily)
Vasodilators	hydralazine	Apresoline	• Chest pain • Flushing • Anxiety • Rash	• 10-25 mg PO 3 times daily (target 75 mg/dose)
	isosorbide dinitrate	Isordil	• Headache • Lightheadedness • Hypotension	• 40 mg PO 4 times daily

SIDE EFFECTS: Nausea, vomiting, diarrhea, dizziness, visual changes (if toxic levels reached)

AUXILIARY LABELS:
• Take as prescribed.
• Do not stop taking medication without consulting physician.

A variety of diuretic agents can be used to help reduce edema in people with HF. With thiazides and loop diuretics, an important consideration is the large amount of potassium lost in the urine. For this reason, the use of both classes of drugs may require potassium supplementation, although this is more commonly seen with loop diuretics. Potassium-sparing diuretics, on the other hand, lead to the retention of potassium. These agents include diuretics such as triamterene and spironolactone. Chapter 21 presents a detailed discussion of diuretics.

 Tech Note!

The antidote for an overdose of digoxin or symptomatic toxicity is digoxin immune Fab (e.g., Digibind). This agent binds to the digoxin molecule, and the drug is excreted from the body. This treatment must be done in the emergency department, and the antidote is available in injectable form only.

 Tech Alert!

Remember the following sound-alike, look-alike drugs:
Cardene versus Cardizem
Cardene SR versus Cardizem SR
nicardipine versus nifedipine versus nimodipine
Lotensin versus Lioresal

DO YOU REMEMBER THESE KEY POINTS?

- Names of the major components of the cardiovascular system and their functions
- The primary symptoms of the various cardiovascular conditions discussed
- Medications used to treat the various cardiovascular conditions discussed

- The generic and trade names for the drugs discussed in this chapter
- The appropriate auxiliary labels that should be used when filling prescriptions for drugs discussed in this chapter

REVIEW QUESTIONS

Multiple Choice Questions

1. The artery responsible for supplying the heart muscle with oxygen is called the:
   A. Pulmonary artery
   B. Aorta
   C. Coronary artery
   D. Myocardial passageway

2. A cardiac condition in which fluids can build up within tissues is known as:
   A. Myocardial infarction
   B. Angina pectoris
   C. Heart failure
   D. Hypertension

3. Factor(s) that may affect the development of atherosclerosis is (are):
   A. Lifestyle
   B. Family history
   C. Smoking
   D. All of the above

4. In "ACE inhibitors," ACE stands for:
   A. Activating coronary electrical
   B. Altering and converting enzyme
   C. Angiotensin-converting enzyme
   D. Angina-converting enzyme

5. Beta-blockers are effective for cardiac conditions because they work by:
   A. Blocking receptor sites in the heart
   B. Blocking receptor sites in the heart and kidneys
   C. Activating receptor sites in the heart and lungs
   D. Activating receptor sites in the heart and kidneys

6. Which instruction is *not* necessary patient information for taking oral nitroglycerin medications?
   A. Take with food
   B. Keep medication in the original container
   C. Take as needed for chest pain; maximum 3 times in 15 minutes; if no relief after the first dose, then call 911
   D. Keep medication out of direct sunlight

7. t-PA is classified as a:
   A. Vasoconstrictor
   B. Vasodilator
   C. Prophylaxis thrombolytic
   D. Thrombolytic

8. The four chambers of the heart are:
   A. Right and left: upper and lower atrium
   B. Right and left: atrium and superior and inferior venae cavae
   C. Right and left: atrium and ventricle
   D. None of the above

9. Which of the following is used to dissolve blood clots?
   A. Heparin
   B. Aspirin
   C. t-PA
   D. Warfarin

10. Which of the following diuretics is associated with hyperkalemia (elevated potassium levels)?
    A. Furosemide
    B. Bumetanide
    C. Hydrochlorothiazide
    D. Spironolactone

11. Fondaparinux (Arixtra) is a(n):
    A. Vitamin K antagonist
    B. Factor Xa inhibitor
    C. LMWH
    D. Direct thrombin inhibitor

12. Nitrostat is a brand name for:
    A. Diltiazem
    B. Verapamil
    C. Atenolol
    D. Nitroglycerin

13. Which of the following is *not* a calcium channel blocker?
    A. Verapamil
    B. Metolazone
    C. Nifedipine
    D. Diltiazem

14. Which of the following is a bile acid sequestrant?
    A. Niacin
    B. Colesevelam
    C. Simvastatin
    D. Fenofibrate

15. Which of the following would be used to treat deep vein thrombosis (DVT)?
    A. Anticoagulants
    B. Thrombolytics
    C. Calcium channel blockers
    D. Both A and B

TECHNICIAN'S CORNER

Mrs. Lewis arrives at the pharmacy with several prescriptions. Using a comprehensive drug reference, such as *Drug Facts and Comparisons*, look up the medications listed and determine which conditions may be affecting Mrs. Lewis. In addition, classify each of the medications and transcribe the prescription into lay terms as though you were preparing a prescription label.

Zocor 5 mg qd, #30
Digoxin 0.125 mg qd, #30
Furosemide 40 mg bid, #60
K-Dur 20 mEq bid, #60
Albuterol INH 1 to 2 puffs prn SOB, #17g
NTG 0.4 mg sl tab prn cp, 1 q 5/min, max 3 tabs over 15/min; call 911 if chest pain unrelieved after first dose, 4/#25s
Atenolol 25 mg qd, #30

Bibliography

Clinical Pharmacology Online. (Referenced August 19, 2014.) www.clinicalpharmacology-ip.com.

Damjanov I: *Pathology for the health professions*, ed 4, St Louis, 2011, Saunders.

Fishback JL: *Pathology*, ed 3, Philadelphia, 2005, Mosby.

Huether S, McCance K: *Understanding pathophysiology*, ed 5, St Louis, 2012, Mosby.

McCance KL: *Pathophysiology: the biologic basis for disease in adults and children*, ed 6, St Louis, 2010, Mosby.

Page C et al: *Integrated pharmacology*, ed 3, 2006, Mosby.

Patton KT et al: *Mosby's handbook of anatomy and physiology*, St Louis, 2000, Mosby.

Price SA et al: *Pathophysiology: clinical concepts of disease processes*, ed 6, St Louis, 2003, Mosby.

Sole ML et al: *Introduction to critical care nursing*, ed 6, St Louis, 2013, Saunders.

Solomon EP: *Introduction to human anatomy and physiology*, ed 3, St Louis, 2009, Saunders.

UpToDate Online. (Referenced August 19, 2014.) www.uptodate.com.

Therapeutic Agents for the Respiratory System

Joshua J. Neumiller

OBJECTIVES

Upon completing this chapter, you should be able to do the following:

1. Describe the major components of the respiratory system.
2. List the primary symptoms of conditions associated with dysfunction of the respiratory system.
3. Recognize prescription and over-the-counter (OTC) drugs used to treat conditions of the lower and upper respiratory system.
4. Write the generic and trade names for the drugs discussed in this chapter.
5. List appropriate auxiliary labels when filling prescriptions for drugs discussed in this chapter.

TERMS AND DEFINITIONS

Allergen A substance that causes an allergic reaction

Alveoli Tiny air sacs in the lungs where the exchange of oxygen and carbon dioxide takes place

Anticholinergic An agent that inhibits the physiological action of acetylcholine

Antihistamine A drug or other compound that inhibits the effects of histamine; used especially in the treatment of allergies

Antitussive A drug that can decrease the coughing reflex of the central nervous system

Aspiration The drawing of a foreign substance into the respiratory tract during inhalation

Bronchi Any of the major air passages of the lungs that diverge from the windpipe

Bronchioles Any of the small branches into which a bronchus divides in the respiratory tract

Cilia Short, microscopic, hairlike structures

Decongestant A drug that shrinks the swollen membranes in the nasal cavity, making it easier to breathe

Diaphragm A dome-shaped, muscular partition separating the thorax from the abdomen that plays a major role in breathing

Dyspnea Difficult or labored breathing

Expectorant A drug that helps remove mucous secretions from the respiratory system; it loosens and thins sputum and bronchial secretions for ease of expectoration

Expiration The act of breathing out; exhalation

Influenza A respiratory tract infection caused by an influenza virus

Inspiration The act of breathing in; inhalation

Prophylactic Treatment given before an event or exposure to prevent the occurrence of a condition or symptom

Sputum Fluid (mucus) that is expectorated from the lungs and bronchial tissues

Select Common Drugs Used for Conditions of the Respiratory System

Trade Name	Generic Name	Pronunciation
Antihistamines		
Allegra	fexofenadine	(**fex**-oh-**fen**-a-deen)
Zyrtec	cetirizine	(se-**tir**-a-zeen)
Anticholinergics—Oral Inhalers		
Atrovent HFA	ipratropium bromide	(**ip**-rah-**troe**-pee-um/**bro**-mide)
Spiriva	tiotropium	(tye-oh-**troe**-pee-um)
Mucolytic		
Mucomyst	acetylcysteine	(a-**seet**-ill-**sis**-teen)
Bronchodilators		
Proventil HFA, Ventolin HFA	albuterol	(al-bu-**ter**-ol)
Foradil Aerolizer	formoterol	(for-**moe**-ter-ol)
Serevent Diskus	salmeterol	(sal-**meh**-ter-ol)
Xopenex HFA	levalbuterol	(leh-val-**byoo**-ter-ol)
Inhaled Corticosteroids		
Azmacort	triamcinolone	(try-am-**sin**-oh-lone)
AeroBid	flunisolide	(flew-**nis**-oh-lide)
Beclovent	beclomethasone	(beck-low-**meth**-ah-sone)
Flovent Diskus/Flovent HFA	fluticasone	(floo-**tic**-ah-sone)
Pulmicort Flexhaler	budesonide	(byoo-**des**-oh-nide)
Mast Cell Stabilizer		
Intal	cromolyn	(**krom**-oh-lin)
Nasal Corticosteroids		
Nasonex	mometasone	(moe-**met**-a-sone)
Rhinocort	budesonide	(byoo-**dess**-oh-nide)
Flonase	fluticasone	(floo-**tic**-ah-sone)
Immunomodulator		
Xolair	omalizumab	(**oh**-ma-**liz**-yoo-mab)
Leukotriene Inhibitors		
Singulair	montelukast	(mon-tea-**loo**-cast)
Accolate	zafirlukast	(zay-fur-**loo**-cast)
Xanthine		
Theo-Dur	theophylline	(thee-**off**-ah-lin)
Antitubercular Agents		
	isoniazid	(eye-**soe**-nye-a-**zid**)
Myambutol	ethambutol	(e-tham-**byoo**-tole)
	pyrazinamide	(peer-ah-**zin**-a-mide)
Rifadin	rifampin	(rif-am-**pin**)
	streptomycin	(strep-**toe**-mye-sin)

The lungs and airways play an important role in the body. The respiratory system is composed of many structures, each having specific functions (Figure 19-1). For example, the lungs facilitate the absorption of oxygen from the air we breathe during inhalation and also the removal of carbon dioxide from the body during exhalation. The fine hairs of the nose and the mucosal lining of the bronchi act as filters to trap dust, microorganisms, and foreign particles. These unwanted particles are engulfed in mucus, propelled by cilia to the throat, and swallowed. In addition, the nose helps to heat and humidify cold, dry air so that it is more compatible with our body temperature. This chapter

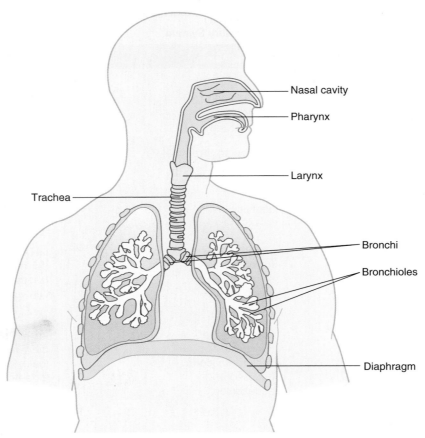

FIGURE 19-1 Diagram of the respiratory system.

discusses the structure and functions of the respiratory system, the events involved in the act of respiration, and the conditions that affect the respiratory system and their treatment.

Structure and Function of the Respiratory System

The respiratory system resembles a large, multi-branched tree that has been inverted. The large trunk is analogous to the trachea, and the two main branches of the tree represent the **bronchi** (Figure 19-1). The smaller branches are the **bronchioles**, and the leaves are the alveolar sacs, where gas exchange takes place (Figure 19-2). When discussing the respiratory system, it is useful to discuss its structure and function in two parts, the upper and lower respiratory tract. Let's first focus on the upper respiratory tract. The primary functions of the upper respiratory tract are to filter, warm, and moisten air before it enters the lower respiratory tract.

Upper Respiratory System

The upper respiratory system is composed of the nose and nasal cavities, the pharynx (i.e., the throat), and

the larynx (i.e., the voice box) (Figure 19-3). A mucosal lining covers the inside of the respiratory tract, forming a protective barrier that serves as an air purification mechanism by trapping inhaled irritants such as dust and pollens. The nasal septum separates the interior of the nose into two distinct cavities that are lined by a mucous membrane with microscopic, hairlike structures called **cilia**. The function of the mucous membrane is to warm and moisten inhaled air. The nose also functions as the sensory organ for the sense of smell and acts as a drainage system for tears from the eye. The pharynx is shared by the respiratory and digestive systems; food passes into the esophagus, and air flows through the trachea, also known as the *windpipe*. The tonsils, composed of lymphatic tissue (see Chapter 23), are located in the pharynx.

The larynx is also called the voice box because it contains the vocal cords responsible for speech. Compared with men, women have a much smaller larynx, and it does not protrude from the neck. This cartilage (usually visible only in men) is referred to as the "Adam's apple." The epiglottis, a thin, leaf-shaped structure made of elastic cartilage (see Figure 19-3), is located at the entrance of the larynx. Its function is to obstruct the trachea automatically, similar to a trapdoor, when swallowing takes place to keep food,

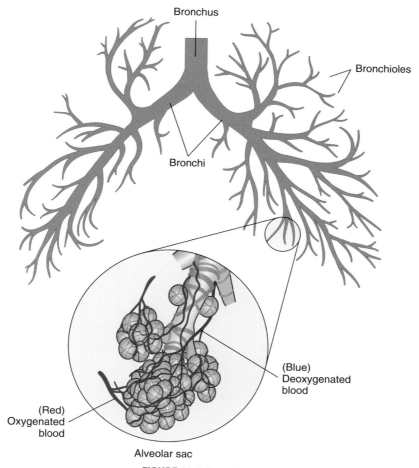

FIGURE 19-2 Bronchial tree.

liquid, and saliva from entering the airway. If food enters the trachea rather than the esophagus, choking can occur.

 Tech Note!

In people who have swallowing difficulties (e.g., individuals with Parkinson's disease), food, liquids, and medications can make their way into the trachea instead of the esophagus. This is known as **aspiration**, which can lead to serious health problems, such as aspiration pneumonia.

Lower Respiratory System

The lower respiratory system is composed of the trachea, bronchial tree, and lungs. The trachea (windpipe) is lined with a mucous membrane that traps airborne particles; the cilia then propel the particles upward, where they are swallowed. The trachea branches into two structures. called the *right bronchus* and the *left bronchus*, leading to the right and left lungs, respectively. The trachea is reinforced with rings of cartilage so that it does not collapse when the neck is bent (see Figure 19-3).

Each of the two bronchi that branch out from the trachea in turn split into smaller bronchi and bronchioles. The function of the bronchioles is to distribute air throughout the lungs and into the **alveoli**. Respiration occurs in the alveoli, and oxygen and carbon dioxide pass between the tiny capillaries surrounding the alveoli and the air in them. Oxygen diffuses from the alveoli into the bloodstream for use by the body, and carbon dioxide passes from the blood into the alveoli for exhalation.

The lungs fill the chest cavity, except for the space occupied by the heart and large vessels, and their main function is breathing and facilitation of gas exchange. The lungs are divided into lobes, three in the right lung and two in the left lung (Figure 19-4). The lungs are separated from each other by the mediastinum, the region of the thoracic cavity in which the heart is located. The left lung has an indentation on its surface, called the *cardiac notch*, to accommodate the apex of the heart. At the base of the chest cavity is a major respiratory muscle called the **diaphragm**, which is critical in facilitating both inspiration and expiration. This large, dome-shaped muscle separates the chest cavity from the abdominal cavity. It contracts and flattens during

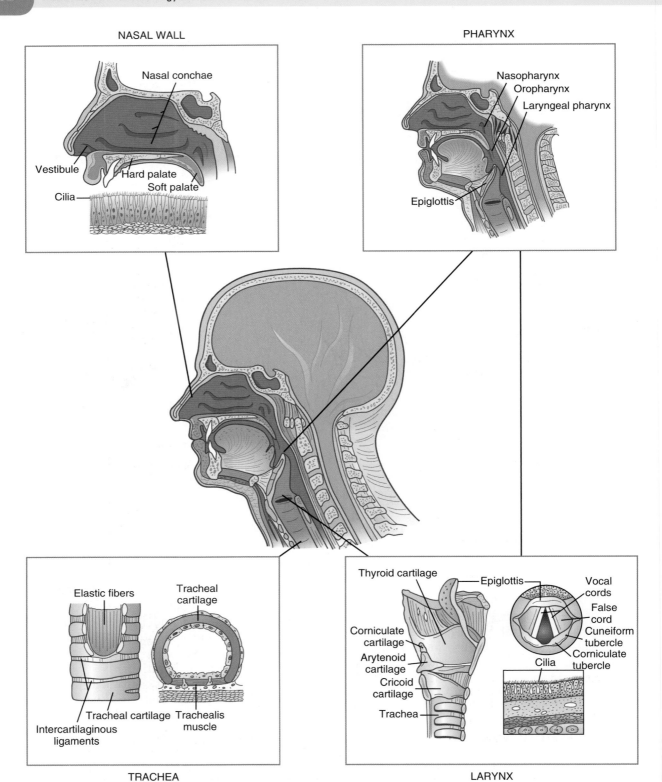

FIGURE 19-3 Structures of the upper airway. (From McCance KL: *Pathophysiology: the biologic basis for disease in adults and children,* ed 6, St Louis, 2010, Mosby.)

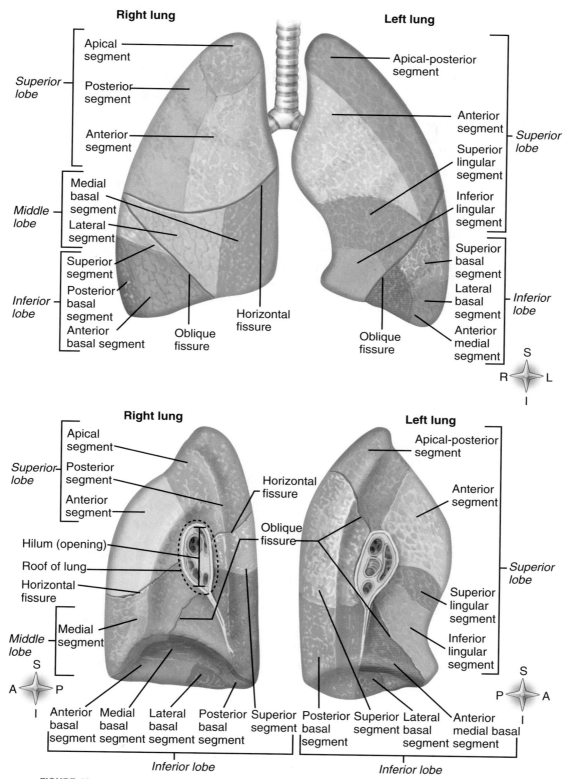

FIGURE 19-4 Lobes and segments of the lungs. (From Patton KT et al: *Mosby's handbook of anatomy and physiology,* St Louis, 2000, Mosby.)

inspiration, and it relaxes during exhalation. A variety of other muscles, in addition to the diaphragm, are important in the breathing process, as discussed in the next section.

Respiration

The act of respiration can be divided into two distinct phases, **inspiration**, the movement of air into the lungs; and **expiration**, the movement of air out of the lungs. Changes in the size and shape of the chest cavity (or thorax) during respiration cause a change in air pressure that forces air to move into and out of the lungs (Figure 19-5). As a person actively inhales (inspiration), the muscles of the diaphragm and intercostal muscles contract, resulting in an increase in the size of the thoracic cavity. Because of this increased volume of the chest cavity, the pressure inside the lungs is lower than the atmospheric pressure, resulting in air flowing into the lungs. Expiration, on the other hand, occurs as the chest relaxes and the thorax returns to its resting size and shape. The reduction in the size of the thoracic cavity causes the pressure in the thorax to increase, which allows air to be expelled from the lungs. Breathing is an involuntary mechanism, meaning that you do not have to think about it; the body automatically exhales and inhales when needed. The respiratory control center, located in the medulla in the brainstem, automatically controls the rate and depth of breathing, depending on the oxygen needs of the body.

Tech Note!
The average respiratory rate for adults is 12 to 18 breaths per minute, whereas a 6- to 12-year-old child's rate is higher at 18-30 breaths per minute. The infant rate from birth to one year can range from 30 to 60 breaths per minute.

Breathing rates vary, depending on the size of the person. The breathing rates of small children, for example, can be twice as fast as those of adults. The normal amount of air expelled from the lungs in a typical exhalation is approximately 500 mL, or 0.5 L, for an average adult, although the total lung capacity is more than 5 L of air. The elasticity of the lungs allows the capacity to vary widely, depending on the need for oxygen. Table 19-1 lists common medical terms used to describe different types of breathing dysfunction.

Tech Note!
Some medications can alter respiratory rates. For example, opioids (e.g., morphine) can suppress the respiratory rate.

TABLE 19-1

Medical Terms Used to Describe Various Types of Breathing Dysfunction

Condition	Description
Apnea	Respiration stops
Bradypnea	Abnormally slow respiratory rate
Cyanosis	Discoloration of the skin (blue-gray) due to lack of oxygenation
Dyspnea	Labored or difficult respiration
Hyperventilation	Deep and rapid respiration
Hypopnea	Shallow breathing and/or abnormally low respiratory rate
Orthopnea	Labored or difficult respiration while lying down
Tachypnea	Rapid respiratory rate

Gas Exchange

The air we breathe is composed of approximately 21% oxygen, 79% nitrogen, and less than 0.5% carbon dioxide. As we breathe, the lungs exchange inspired oxygen for carbon dioxide (waste), which in turn is expired. In the alveolus, each oxygen molecule is able to move across the thin membrane into red blood cells that are passing closely by in blood vessels on the other side of the membrane. These red blood cells drop off carbon dioxide molecules before picking up oxygen molecules. The carbon dioxide molecules then move out of the lung capillary blood supply into the alveolar sacs and out of the body via expired air. The newly oxygenated red blood cells are pumped to the tissues and organs of the body by the heart (Figure 19-6).

The regulation of respiration permits the body to adjust to varying demands for oxygen supply and carbon dioxide removal, as previously discussed. This is done efficiently with help from the respiratory center in the medulla oblongata. The exchange of oxygen and carbon dioxide also helps keep the pH of the blood balanced. The body uses some carbon dioxide to make bicarbonate, which maintains the blood pH close to 7.4, a level needed to sustain life. Because of this important role of carbon dioxide, conditions that result in abnormal respiration can result in acid-base disorders that sometimes require treatment.

Disorders and Conditions of the Respiratory System

Conditions of the Upper Respiratory System

Many conditions affect the respiratory system. Some may be genetic, and others may be attributable to

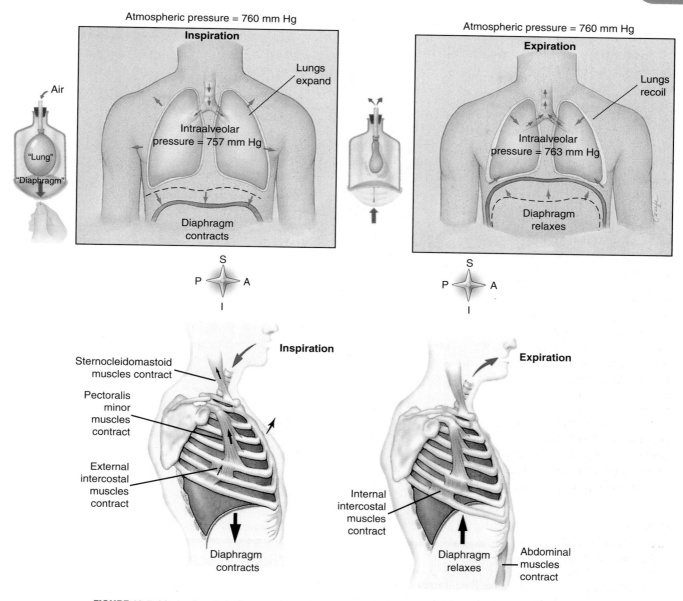

FIGURE 19-5 Mechanics of ventilation. (From Patton KT et al: *Mosby's handbook of anatomy and physiology,* St Louis, 2000, Mosby.)

contagious infections, habits (e.g., smoking), and other environmental factors. The symptoms of a respiratory illness are noticeable because of the abnormal breathing and coughing symptoms that typically accompany such conditions. Although upper respiratory illnesses are diverse, similar types of medications are used to treat most of these conditions, which are often infectious. These include antitussives, analgesics, and antipyretics, among others. For more severe conditions, which may involve bacterial infection or allergy, antibiotics and corticosteroids may be prescribed. Table 19-2 lists common conditions of the upper respiratory system, symptoms, and medications used for their treatment. The following sections describe the causes, symptoms and treatment of typical upper respiratory tract

disorders. Many agents can be purchased over the counter for symptomatic management (see Chapter 27 for additional information).

Common Cold

The common cold is a self-limiting illness that encompasses a group of diseases caused by a variety of viruses. The common cold is the most frequent acute illness in the United States and other industrialized countries. Common symptoms of this mild upper respiratory infection include nasal congestion and rhinorrhea (runny nose), sneezing, sore throat, cough, fever, headache, and fatigue. Efforts to reduce the transmission of the common cold usually focus on preventive measures to help limit the spread of viruses, such as good hygiene (e.g., hand washing

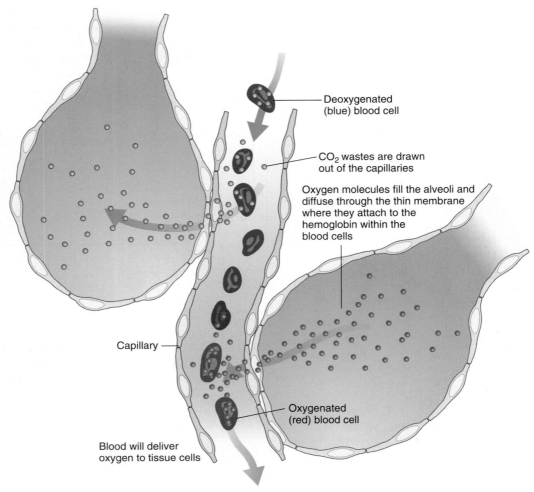

FIGURE 19-6 Exchange of oxygen and carbon dioxide.

TABLE 19-2

Common Conditions of the Upper Respiratory System

Conditions	Common Symptoms	Medications for Symptomatic Management
Common cold (viral)	Stuffy nose, sore throat, sneezing, headache, muscle aches	Decongestants, antihistamines, analgesics
Influenza (viral)*	Fever, chills, headache, muscle aches, fatigue, cough	Analgesics, antipyretics
Strep throat (bacterial)	Fever, headache, sore throat	Antibiotics, analgesics, antipyretics
Bronchitis (bacterial or viral)*	Cough, shortness of breath, fatigue, chest pain	Bronchodilators, analgesics
Allergic rhinitis	Stuffy nose, congestion	Antihistamines, nasal corticosteroids
Sinusitis	Stuffy nose, headache, congestion	Antihistamines, nasal corticosteroids

*Can affect both the upper and lower respiratory tract.

and/or use of hand sanitizers) and proper sneezing techniques.

Prognosis. The average incidence of the common cold ranges from five to seven episodes per year in preschool children to two or three episodes per year in adults. With rest and time, a cold runs its course. In some individuals, colds can exacerbate chronic conditions such as asthma, emphysema, and bronchitis.

Non–Drug Treatment. Drinking plenty of water and getting enough rest are important components of non–drug treatment of the common cold. To help relieve congestion that worsens at night, a vaporizer may be used. Gargling with warm saline can help provide relief from a sore throat.

Drug Treatment. Common symptomatic treatments include decongestants, antihistamines, antitussives, and expectorants. These are available in a variety of dosage forms, such as liquids, lozenges, nasal sprays, and oral tablets and capsules. Examples of common agents used to manage the symptoms of the common cold are outlined in the following text. A more detailed discussion of OTC products for the treatment of the common cold can be found in Chapter 27. In general, product selection should be aimed at the specific symptoms that are troublesome to the individual.

Antihistamines are agents that can be used to help alleviate rhinorrhea and sneezing. However, their use is limited due to side effects, such as sedation and drying of the mucous membranes (eyes, nose, and mouth).

GENERIC NAME: diphenhydramine (OTC)
TRADE NAME: Benadryl
INDICATION: Cough, allergic rhinitis, rhinorrhea, insomnia
ROUTE OF ADMINISTRATION: Oral; topical; injectable
COMMON ADULT DOSAGE: *Oral dose for common cold:* 12.5-50 mg every 4-6 hours (not to exceed 300 mg every 24 hours)
MECHANISM OF ACTION: Blocks the effects of histamine at histamine-1 (H_1) receptors
SIDE EFFECTS: Drowsiness, dry mouth, dizziness, confusion

Antitussives are medications that can be used to suppress a cough. Because the common cold can be associated with cough in some cases, antitussives are sometimes used for symptomatic management. However, the American College of Chest Physicians does not recommend the use of cough suppressants for cough associated with upper respiratory infections. Antitussives are available by prescription and OTC.

GENERIC NAME: dextromethorphan (OTC)
TRADE NAME: Delsym
INDICATION: Cough
ROUTE OF ADMINISTRATION: Oral
COMMON ADULT DOSAGE: 10-20 mg every 4 hours or 30 mg every 6-8 hours
MECHANISM OF ACTION: Believed to suppress the cough center in the medulla of the brain
SIDE EFFECTS: Drowsiness, dizziness, fatigue

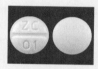

GENERIC NAME: promethazine/codeine
TRADE NAME: Phenergan with Codeine (C-V)
INDICATION: Cough, common cold
ROUTE OF ADMINISTRATION: Oral
COMMON ADULT DOSAGE: 5 mL every 4-6 hours, not to exceed 30 mL in 24 hours, or 10 mg/6.25 mg per 5 mL syrup
MECHANISM OF ACTION: Codeine suppresses the cough center in the medulla, and promethazine primarily antagonizes H_1 receptors
SIDE EFFECTS: Constipation, drowsiness, respiratory depression
AUXILIARY LABELS:
- May cause drowsiness.
- May cause dizziness.
- Caution: Federal law prohibits the transfer of this drug to any person other than the patient for whom it was prescribed.

Expectorants, such as guaifenesin, break up thick mucous secretions of the lungs or bronchi so that they can be easily expelled from the respiratory tract by coughing. Patients should be counseled to increase fluid intake after taking expectorants to assist with thinning of mucosal secretions.

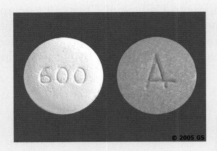

GENERIC NAME: guaifenesin (OTC)
TRADE NAME: Mucinex
INDICATION: Cough, congestion
ROUTE OF ADMINISTRATION: Oral
COMMON ADULT DOSAGE: 200-400 mg (10-20 mL) every 4 hours (max 2400 mg/day)
MECHANISM OF ACTION: Increases the ability to clear phlegm and bronchial secretions by reducing their viscosity
SIDE EFFECTS: Diarrhea, drowsiness, dizziness, headache

Decongestants affect the adrenergic receptors of the vascular smooth muscle, leading to constriction of blood vessels and a decrease in mucus production. Many decongestants are available as OTC products. These products generally should be avoided by people with hypertension.

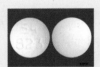

GENERIC NAME: pseudoephedrine
TRADE NAME: Sudafed
INDICATION: Nasal congestion, common cold, allergic rhinitis
ROUTE OF ADMINISTRATION: Oral; intranasal
COMMON ADULT DOSAGE: 30-60 mg every 4-6 hours
MECHANISM OF ACTION: Adrenergic agonist that activates alpha- and beta-adrenergic receptors, leading to vasoconstriction to reduce nasal congestion
SIDE EFFECTS: Increased blood pressure, insomnia, restlessness
SPECIAL NOTE: Pseudoephedrine is now a regulated drug. Because of the misuse of a key component used in making the street drug methamphetamine, quantities sold are now limited across the United States

GENERIC NAME: phenylephrine (OTC)
TRADE NAME: Sudafed PE (oral); Neo-Synephrine (nasal)
INDICATION: Nasal congestion
ROUTE OF ADMINISTRATION: Oral; intranasal
COMMON ADULT DOSAGE: *Oral:* 10 mg every 4-6 hours; *intranasal:* 1 to 2 sprays every 4 hours
MECHANISM OF ACTION: Adrenergic agonist that activates alpha- and beta-adrenergic receptors, leading to vasoconstriction to reduce nasal congestion
SIDE EFFECTS: Dizziness, insomnia, increased blood pressure, rebound congestion

 Tech Note!

Many decongestants can actually contribute to worsening of nasal congestion as a result of a phenomenon known as *rebound congestion*. This is particularly common with some OTC nasal inhaler medications, such as oxymetazoline (Afrin) and phenylephrine (Neo-Synephrine). Because of the risk of rebound congestion, decongestants should not be overused and patients should follow the instructions for duration of use.

Cromolyn sodium is a synthetic compound that was originally produced in the search for an improved bronchodilator. Although it was not found to have bronchodilating properties, cromolyn does inhibit antigen-induced bronchospasm. Because of this, cromolyn is used as a **prophylactic** agent for the treatment of asthma and as a nasal preparation to treat seasonal allergic rhinitis and nasal congestion. Some evidence suggests that cromolyn may improve symptoms of the common cold.

GENERIC NAME: cromolyn sodium
TRADE NAME: Nasalcrom (nasal) available OTC, Opticrom (ophthalmic), Gastrocrom (oral)
INDICATION: Asthma prophylaxis, seasonal allergic rhinitis, nasal congestion
ROUTE OF ADMINISTRATION: Intranasal; inhaled; ophthalmic; oral
COMMON ADULT DOSAGE: *Intranasal:* 1 spray into each nostril three to four times daily

MECHANISM OF ACTION: Inhibits degranulation of mast cells of the immune system, preventing the release of histamine and inhibiting inflammation

SIDE EFFECTS: Sneezing, nasal irritation

AUXILIARY LABEL:
- [Nasal formulations]: Shake well.

Allergies

An allergy is an abnormal response of the immune system to an unrecognized, typically harmless substance. This response does not occur in all people and varies widely. In certain people the allergic response can be severe to life-threatening. Types of **allergens** vary widely and include pollens, animal dander, foods, medications, chemicals, or environmental pollutants. Allergies are one of the most common types of respiratory problems, experienced by approximately 50 million people in the United States alone. Symptoms and reactions include rash, hives, itching, and nasal congestion. Severe reactions can cause stomach pain, vomiting, wheezing, shortness of breath (SOB), hypotension (low blood pressure), swelling of the throat, and anaphylactic shock if left untreated.

Prognosis. If treated properly, most allergic reactions can be controlled and managed symptomatically. If the allergen is identified, allergy shots can be used to lessen symptoms.

Non–Drug Treatment. Avoiding specific allergens is the best way to prevent an allergic reaction. If a reaction occurs, the type and severity of the allergic response determines whether treatment can be handled with or without medications. For allergic reactions caused by allergens in the home, removing the allergen is a good first step. Using a humidifier and/or air purifier may lessen the concentrations of an airborne allergen. Foods and medications that need to be avoided should be documented in the individual's medical record and pharmacy profile, and in certain cases wristbands should be worn that list life-threatening allergies. Exposure to outdoor allergens can be lessened by wearing a face mask or by staying indoors on days in which environmental pollutants or pollen levels are high.

Drug Treatments. Many of the medications used for allergies mimic those used to treat the common cold. Allergy medications include oral, intranasal, ophthalmic, and topical antihistamines and/or decongestants (Table 19-3). Many

TABLE 19-3

Select Prescription Medications for the Treatment of Allergies

Medication Class	Generic Name	Trade Name	Common Side Effects	Common Dose Range
Inhaled Corticosteroids	beclomethasone	Beconase AQ, Qnasl	• Cough • Headache • Nasal burning • Nasal dryness	• 1-2 sprays in each nostril twice daily
	budesonide	Rhinocort Aqua		• 1 spray in each nostril once daily
	flunisolide	Nasarel		• 2 sprays in each nostril twice daily
	fluticasone	Veramyst		• 2 sprays in each nostril once daily *or* • 1 spray in each nostril twice daily
	mometasone	Nasonex		• 2 sprays in each nostril once daily
	triamcinolone	Nasacort AQ		• 2 sprays in each nostril once daily
Antihistamines	desloratadine	Clarinex, Clarinex RediTabs	• Cough • Dizziness	• 5 mg once daily
	fexofenadine	Allegra, Allegra ODT		• 60 mg twice daily; 180 mg once daily
	levocetirizine	Xyzal		• 2.5-5 mg once daily
	olopadine	Patanase		• 2 sprays in each nostril twice daily
	triprolidine	Zymine, Zymine XR		• 2.5 mg every 4-6 hr
Leukotriene Receptor Antagonist	montelukast	Singulair	• Fatigue • Dyspepsia • Dizziness • Headache	• 10 mg once daily

allergy medications can be obtained without a prescription as OTC drugs. Most OTC antihistamines cause drowsiness as a side effect; however, OTC medications now are available that either have a mild sedative effect or cause no sedation at all (see Chapter 27). Other agents require a prescription, such as oral corticosteroids, intranasal or respiratory corticosteroids, leukotriene inhibitors, and epinephrine. In life-threatening cases, injectable epinephrine may be used to open the airways.

GENERIC NAME: fexofenadine
TRADE NAME: Allegra
INDICATION: Allergic rhinitis, urticaria
ROUTE OF ADMINISTRATION: Oral
COMMON ADULT DOSAGE: 60 mg twice daily or 180 mg once daily
MECHANISM OF ACTION: Selective H_1 receptor blocker
SIDE EFFECTS: Headache, vomiting, dizziness, fatigue
AUXILIARY LABEL:
- Take with water.

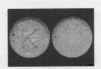

GENERIC NAME: desloratadine
TRADE NAME: Clarinex
INDICATION: Allergic rhinitis, urticaria, pruritus
ROUTE OF ADMINISTRATION: Oral
COMMON ADULT DOSAGE: 5 mg once daily
MECHANISM OF ACTION: Selective H_1 receptor blocker
SIDE EFFECTS: Headache, dry mouth, fatigue, dizziness
AUXILIARY LABEL:
- Do not crush or chew tablet.

Rhinitis

Rhinitis is irritation and inflammation of the mucous membranes lining the nasal passage. It is caused by several different factors, including colds, influenza, allergens (as described previously), air pollution, or strong odors (e.g., perfume, chemicals, or even certain medications). Rhinitis is either acute (e.g., colds or flu) or chronic (e.g., continuous or seasonal exposure to allergens). Common symptoms include runny and itchy nose, sneezing, congestion, and postnasal drip. Postnasal drip is due to the accumulation of mucus

in the back of the nose and throat. Drinking plenty of fluids can thin the mucus associated with postnasal drip and aid in its expectoration. Additional symptoms may include coughing, runny or watery eyes, and headache.

Prognosis. Rhinitis caused by colds or the flu is normally short-lived, subsiding over several days, whereas chronic rhinitis is a continuing condition that may require chronic treatment or intermittent treatment during allergy season.

Non–Drug Treatments. Cold or flu viruses causing rhinitis can be treated with OTC saline irrigation products. When used as an irrigating solution, saline can help relieve postnasal drip symptoms. For rhinitis resulting from exposure to allergens, symptoms can be lessened through several actions, including use of air purifiers or humidifiers in the home, using cotton bedding, keeping windows closed during pollen season, and avoiding live plants in the home, depending on the type of allergy. Animals that cause allergies should be bathed often to minimize shedding of dander.

Drug Treatments. In addition to the treatments discussed previously for rhinitis (e.g., decongestants and antihistamines), steroid nasal sprays, such as beclomethasone, flunisolide, budesonide, mometasone, and fluticasone, can be used to reduce inflammation in the sinuses.

GENERIC NAME: triamcinolone
TRADE NAME: Nasacort AQ (available OTC)
INDICATION: Allergic rhinitis
ROUTE OF ADMINISTRATION: Intranasal
COMMON ADULT DOSAGE: 2 sprays into each nostril once daily
MECHANISM OF ACTION: Corticosteroid (produces antiinflammatory and vasoconstrictive effects that help treat rhinitis symptoms)
SIDE EFFECTS: Dry mouth, nasal dryness, cough, nasal irritation
AUXILIARY LABEL:
- Shake well before use.

GENERIC NAME: fluticasone
TRADE NAME: Flonase
INDICATION: Allergic rhinitis
ROUTE OF ADMINISTRATION: Intranasal

COMMON ADULT DOSAGE: 1 or 2 sprays into each nostril once daily.

MECHANISM OF ACTION: Corticosteroid (produces antiinflammatory and vasoconstrictive effects that help treat rhinitis symptoms)

SIDE EFFECTS: Headache, nosebleed, cough, nasal irritation

AUXILIARY LABEL:
- Shake well before use.

Influenza

A more severe type of viral respiratory illness is known as the flu, or **influenza** (Figure 19-7). Influenza infects the respiratory system, including the nose, throat, bronchial tubes, and lungs. Influenza is responsible for millions of dollars of lost wages and health care costs annually, and it can be a potentially fatal infection in the very young, the elderly, and people who are immunocompromised.

Prognosis. With proper treatment, most people recover from influenza; however, the very old and young and those with a weakened immune system can experience a slow recovery or even death. Obtaining a flu vaccine annually is the best way to avoid or lessen the risk of contracting influenza.

Non–Drug Treatment. Normally the best remedy is bed rest and drinking plenty of fluids.

Drug Treatment. For severe influenza, antivirals may be prescribed at the early onset of symptoms (usually within 48 hours) to help shorten the course or lessen the severity of the illness. They can also be used as prophylaxis upon exposure to somebody with the virus (Table 19-4). Some strains of influenza are resistant to antiviral medications, however. Vaccines are commonly given during the peak flu season. Chapter 23 presents a detailed discussion of vaccines.

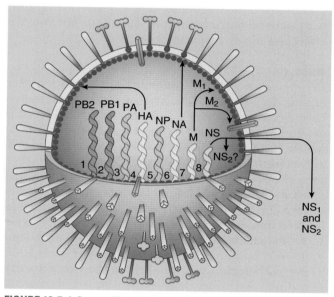

FIGURE 19-7 Influenza. (From Goldman M: *Procedures in cosmetic dermatology series: photodynamic therapy,* ed 2, St Louis, 2008, Saunders.)

TABLE 19-4

Select Agents for the Treatment and/or Prophylaxis of Influenza

Medication Class	Generic Name	Trade Name	Indications	Common Dose Range
Adamantane Antivirals	amantadine	Symmetrel	• Influenza A virus infection • Influenza prophylaxis • Parkinson's disease	• *Influenza A virus infection:* 200 mg/day in 1-2 doses • *Influenza prophylaxis:* 200 mg/day in 1-2 doses; begin as soon as possible after exposure and continue for at least 10 days
	rimantadine	Flumadine	• Influenza A virus infection • Influenza prophylaxis	• *Influenza A virus infection:* 100 mg twice daily • *Influenza prophylaxis:* 100 mg twice daily
Neuraminidase Inhibitors	oseltamivir	Tamiflu	• Influenza A virus infection • Influenza B virus infection • Influenza prophylaxis	• *Influenza A or B virus infection:* 75 mg twice daily for 5 days • *Influenza prophylaxis:* 75 mg daily for 10 days to 6 wk
	zanamivir	Relenza	• Influenza A virus infection • Influenza B virus infection • Influenza prophylaxis	• *Influenza A or B virus infection:* 10 mg (2 oral inhalations) twice daily for 5 days • *Influenza prophylaxis:* 10 mg (2 oral inhalations) once daily for 28 days

Tech Note!

Antibiotics are not appropriate for treating viral infections such as colds and influenza. Antibiotic means "against life," and viruses are not living because they require a host cell to reproduce. Prescribing antibiotics for viral infections contributes to the development of resistant strains of bacteria.

Conditions of the Lower Respiratory System

Conditions and disorders of the lower respiratory tract generally originate from the lungs but can also affect the upper respiratory system.

Asthma

Asthma is a chronic inflammatory condition that affects the airways. It is one of several obstructive lung diseases that share some clinical characteristics of chronic obstructive pulmonary disease (COPD), which is described later (Figure 19-8). The classic signs of asthma include intermittent **dyspnea** (shortness of breath), cough, and wheezing. In people with asthma, the muscles around the bronchioles contract, narrowing the air passages so that air cannot be inhaled properly. In addition to this increase of resistance to airflow, the condition is worsened by edema and secretion of mucus into the airway (Figure 19-9). These pathological changes lead to the characteristic crackling and wheezing sounds heard during an asthma attack. Because asthma is an inflammatory disease, certain triggers can cause inflammation of the airways, leading to the production of mucus and bronchiole constriction previously mentioned. The most common triggers of asthma attacks are encounters with allergens, such as animals or environmental irritants, exercise, and stress.

Prognosis. The prognosis for this disease is highly dependent on the severity of the individual's asthma. Prophylactic and rescue agents can be used effectively to manage the condition.

Non–Drug Treatments. Management of asthma begins with patient education aimed at avoiding allergens and irritants that trigger asthmatic attacks. Calming techniques can help patients relax during an asthma attack.

Drug Treatments. Two general categories of medications are used in the management of asthma: those used for prophylaxis (or maintenance) and those used when an attack occurs (abortive therapies) (Table 19-5). Metered dose inhalers are often prescribed, and it is important for patients to learn how to use them properly so that they obtain the correct dosage of medication (Figure 19-10).

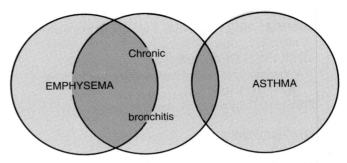

FIGURE 19-8 Interrelationship between the disease entities making up COPD. (From Price SA et al: *Pathophysiology: clinical concepts of disease processes,* ed 6, St Louis, 2003, Mosby.)

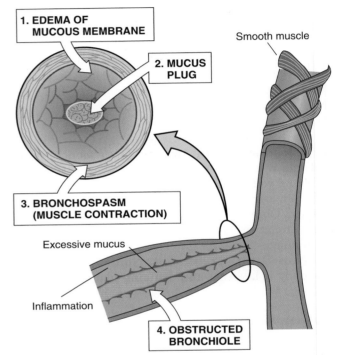

FIGURE 19-9 Asthma obstruction. (From Moscou K, Snipe K: *Pharmacology for pharmacy technicians,* ed 2, St Louis, 2013, Mosby.)

Tech Note!

Spacers (a generic term) may be used with certain inhalers. Spacers are manufactured tubes that attach to the inhaler and have a one-way valve to allow the patient to inhale, not exhale, into the device; this allows more of the drug to reach the lungs. Spacers can be helpful for patients who have difficulty timing the actuation of their inhalers with inhalation. Some medications are also formulated as dry powder inhalers, which do not require patients to time their inhalation.

Corticosteroids. Corticosteroids act as antiinflammatory medications and thus lessen the constriction of the bronchial tubes. Most can be given twice daily

TABLE 19-5

Select Common Agents Used in the Treatment of Asthma and/or Chronic Obstructive Pulmonary Disease

Generic Name	Trade Name	Indications	Common Side Effects
Inhaled Steroids			
Exert antiinflammatory actions to reduce inflammation in the airways			
beclomethasone	Qvar	Asthma	• Dry mouth
budesonide	Pulmicort Flexhaler, Pulmicort Respules	Asthma	• Cough
			• Thrush
fluticasone	Flovent Diskus, Flovent HFA	Asthma	
Short-Acting Beta-Agonists			
Activate beta-2 receptors in the lung, leading to relaxation of the bronchial smooth muscle, in turn leading to bronchodilation and an increase in bronchial airflow			
albuterol beta-2 selective	ProAir HFA, Ventolin HFA, Accuneb, VoSpire ER	Asthma Acute bronchospasm	• Headache • Nervousness
levalbuterol beta-2 selective	Xopenex, Xopenex HFA	Asthma Acute bronchospasm	• Dizziness • Insomnia • Tremor • Cough
Long-Acting Beta-Agonists			
Activate beta-2 receptors in the lung, leading to relaxation of the bronchial smooth muscle, in turn leading to bronchodilation and an increase in bronchial airflow			
arformoterol beta-2 selective	Brovana	Chronic obstructive pulmonary disease (COPD)	• Headache • Cough
formoterol beta-2 selective	Foradil Aerolizer, Perforomist	Asthma COPD	• Upper respiratory tract infection
salmeterol beta-2 selective	Serevent Diskus	Asthma COPD	
Inhaled Anticholinergics			
Block the effects of acetylcholine, leading to bronchial smooth muscle relaxation			
ipratropium	Atrovent HFA	COPD Bronchospasm prophylaxis	• Nausea • Vomiting
tiotropium	Spiriva	COPD Bronchospasm prophylaxis	• Dizziness • Drowsiness
Methylxanthines			
Relax the smooth muscle of the bronchial airways and pulmonary blood vessels			
theophylline	Elixophyllin, Theochron, Theo-24, Uniphyl	Asthma COPD Asthma prophylaxis	• Nausea • Vomiting • Insomnia • Dizziness • Seizures
Leukotriene Receptor Antagonists			
Inhibit the effects of leukotrienes to reduce bronchial smooth muscle contraction, airway edema, and mucus formation			
montelukast	Singulair	Asthma Bronchospasm prophylaxis	• Headache • Heartburn
zafirlukast	Accolate	Asthma Bronchospasm prophylaxis	• Nausea • Fatigue
Phosphodiesterase-4 (PDE4) Inhibitor			
Inhibits the enzyme PDE4, an effect that is thought to reduce inflammation			
roflumilast	Daliresp	COPD	• Insomnia • Anxiety • Diarrhea • Nausea

Continued

TABLE 19-5

Select Common Agents Used in the Treatment of Asthma and/or Chronic Obstructive Pulmonary Disease—cont'd

Generic Name	Trade Name	Indications	Common Side Effects
Anti-IGE Antibody *Blocks the inflammatory effects of IgE* omalizumab	Xolair	Asthma	• Injection site reactions • Rash • Hypersensitivity reactions
Mast Cell Stabilizer *Inhibits degranulation of mast cells of the immune system, preventing the release of histamine and inhibiting inflammation* cromolyn sodium	Intal	Asthma Bronchospasm prophylaxis	• Throat irritation • Cough • Headache
Mucolytic Agent *Reduces the viscosity of mucus secreted in the lungs and aids in the removal of these secretions through coughing and/ or drainage* acetylcysteine	Mucomyst	COPD	• Airway irritation • Drowsiness • Fever

Combination Products	
Generic Name (Brand Name)	**Indications**
albuterol/ipratropium (Combivent Respimat, Duoneb)	COPD
budesonide/formoterol (Symbicort)	Asthma COPD
formoterol/mometasone (Dulera)	Asthma
fluticasone/salmeterol (Advair Diskus, Advair HFA)	Asthma COPD

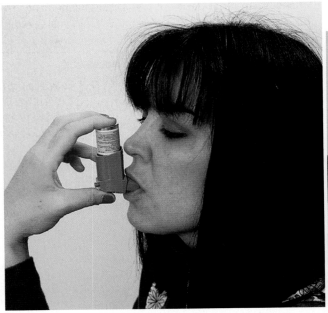 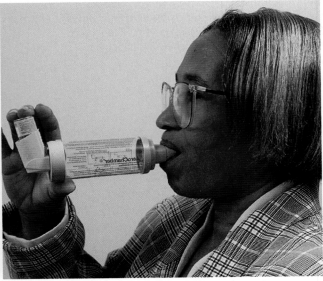

FIGURE 19-10 A, Proper use of an inhaler. **B,** Inhaler with spacer (e.g., AeroChamber). (From Elkin MK, Perry AG, Potter PA: *Nursing interventions and clinical skills,* ed 4, St Louis, 2007, Elsevier.)

and in some patients may be effective in once daily doses. Inhaled corticosteroids are a mainstay of the chronic management of asthma. Oral corticosteroids are also used for acute asthma exacerbations but are reserved for short courses of treatment due to the side effects associated with taking these medications orally.

GENERIC NAME: triamcinolone acetonide
TRADE NAME: Azmacort
INDICATION: Asthma prophylaxis (maintenance therapy)
ROUTE OF ADMINISTRATION: Inhalation
COMMON ADULT DOSAGE: 2 puffs (150 mcg) three or four times daily
MECHANISM OF ACTION: Antiinflammatory actions to reduce inflammation in the airways
SIDE EFFECTS: Bronchospasm, cough
AUXILIARY LABELS:
- Shake well.
- Take as directed.

GENERIC NAME: salmeterol xinafoate powder
TRADE NAME: Serevent Diskus
INDICATION: Asthma maintenance
ROUTE OF ADMINISTRATION: Inhalation
COMMON ADULT DOSAGE: 50 mcg (1 inhalation) twice daily
MECHANISM OF ACTION: Activation of beta-2 receptors in the lung leads to relaxation of the bronchial smooth muscle, which in turn leads to bronchodilation and an increase in bronchial airflow
SIDE EFFECTS: Headache, cough, upper respiratory tract infection
AUXILIARY LABEL:
- Use as directed.

GENERIC NAME: fluticasone propionate
TRADE NAME: Flovent HFA, Flovent Diskus
INDICATION: Asthma prophylaxis (maintenance therapy)
ROUTE OF ADMINISTRATION: Inhalation
COMMON ADULT DOSAGE: *Flovent HFA:* 88 mcg (2 sprays) twice daily; *Flovent Diskus:* 100 mcg twice daily
MECHANISM OF ACTION: Antiinflammatory actions to reduce inflammation in the airways
SIDE EFFECTS: Bronchospasm, cough
AUXILIARY LABELS:
- [Flovent HFA]: Shake well.
- Take as directed.

 Tech Note!

A variety of inhaler devices are available on the market. Metered dose inhalers (MDIs) are delivery devices that propel medication into the lungs through the use of a propellant. Although chlorofluorocarbons (CFCs) had been used traditionally as a propellant MDIs now use hydrofluoroalkane (HFA) because it is better for the environment. Because MDIs propel the drug when actuated, patients need to "time" their breath with activation of the inhaler. Albuterol inhalers are a common example of MDIs. Dry powder inhalers (DPIs) do not require coordinated timing for patients to use the product correctly. DPIs often use blisters that are punctured and subsequently inhaled by the patient. Tiotropium (Spiriva HandiHaler) is an example of a DPI.

Leukotriene Receptor Antagonists (Leukotriene Inhibitors). Leukotriene inhibitors are used in asthma to reduce the inflammatory actions of leukotrienes that induce bronchial smooth muscle contraction, airway edema, and mucus formation.

Long-Acting Beta-Agonists. Many people with asthma are treated with maintenance medications, such as inhaled corticosteroids and long-acting beta-agonists, which are frequently used in combination. The airways contain beta-receptors, and when these receptors are activated, the smooth muscle surrounding the airways relaxes, opening the airways. Nonselective beta-agonists and the high doses of beta-2–selective agonists used for asthma treatment have the side effect of tachycardia due to beta-1 receptor stimulation.

GENERIC NAME: montelukast
TRADE NAME: Singulair, Singulair Chewable Tablet
INDICATION: Asthma, allergic rhinitis, bronchospasm prophylaxis

ROUTE OF ADMINISTRATION: Oral
COMMON ADULT DOSAGE: 10 mg once daily in the evening
MECHANISM OF ACTION: Inhibits the effects of leukotrienes to reduce bronchial smooth muscle contraction, airway edema, and mucus formation
SIDE EFFECTS: Headache, heartburn, nausea, fatigue
AUXILIARY LABEL:
- [Chewable tablets]: Chew tablet well prior to swallowing.

Short-Acting Beta-Agonists. As described previously, the activation of beta-2 receptors in the lungs relaxes the bronchial smooth muscle, leading to bronchodilation and a resultant increase in bronchial airflow. In addition to long-acting beta-agonists, short-acting agents are routinely used by people with asthma as "rescue" inhalers. These agents, most notably albuterol, can be used on a scheduled basis or as needed to help with worsening of asthma symptoms. Short-acting beta-agonists are most commonly used as metered inhalers and as solutions for use in nebulizers.

GENERIC NAME: albuterol
TRADE NAME: Proventil HFA, Ventolin HFA, AccuNeb
INDICATION: Asthma, acute bronchospasm, bronchospasm prophylaxis
ROUTE OF ADMINISTRATION: Inhalation; oral
COMMON ADULT DOSAGE: *MDI:* 2 puffs every 4-6 hours or as needed; *nebulizer:* 0.63-1.25 mg three or four times daily as needed
MECHANISM OF ACTION: Activates beta-2 receptors in the lung, leading to relaxation of the bronchial smooth muscle, which in turn leads to bronchodilation and an increase in bronchial airflow
SIDE EFFECTS: Headache, nervousness, dizziness, insomnia, tremor, cough, tachycardia
AUXILIARY LABELS:
- [Inhalers]: Shake well before using.
- May cause dizziness.

Anticholinergics. Ipratropium is widely used in the management of asthma. This medication is an **anticholinergic** drug that blocks the effects of acetylcholine, which leads to bronchial smooth muscle relaxation. Ipratropium is often used in combination with albuterol.

GENERIC NAME: ipratropium
TRADE NAME: Atrovent HFA, Atrovent Nasal Spray, Atrovent Nasal Forte
INDICATION: Bronchospasm prophylaxis, COPD, rhinorrhea
ROUTE OF ADMINISTRATION: Inhalation; intranasal
COMMON ADULT DOSAGE: *MDI:* 2 sprays (17 mcg/spray) three or four times daily; *nebulizer:* 500 mcg three or four times daily
MECHANISM OF ACTION: Blocks the effects of acetylcholine, which leads to bronchial smooth muscle relaxation
SIDE EFFECTS: Nausea, vomiting, dizziness, drowsiness
AUXILIARY LABELS:
- [Atrovent Nasal Spray]: Shake well before using.
- May cause dizziness.

Chronic Obstructive Pulmonary Disease

COPD is a term used to describe a group of pulmonary diseases of long duration that are characterized by increased resistance to airflow. Depending on its characteristics and presentation, asthma can sometimes fall into the broad category of COPD. The three general types of COPD are chronic bronchitis, emphysema, and asthma (if airflow is not completely reversible). Any long-term lung condition or exposure to lung irritants that damages the lungs can contribute to the development of COPD. Emphysema causes the destruction of the alveolar walls, eventually leading to a loss of elasticity of the lungs. This can be caused by smoking, by exposure to environmental hazards (e.g., asbestos and fiberglass) or, in rare cases, by a genetic predisposition. Because normal exhalation requires elastic recoil of the lungs, the affected lungs allow air to be inhaled, but the individual cannot exhale all the air. Figure 19-11 provides a graphical representation of the pathology and changes within the lung with the various forms of COPD.

Prognosis. COPD is a chronic condition associated with physical impairment, debility, and decreased quality of life. It can lead to death. With proper management, however, people with COPD can continue to lead productive lives.

Non–Drug Treatment. Smoking cessation is an important aspect of non–drug therapy. In extreme cases, a lung transplant may be needed to remove parts of the affected lung.

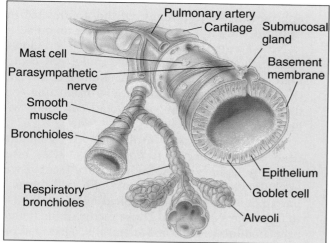

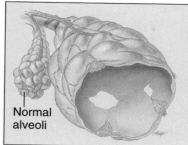

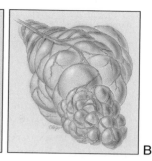

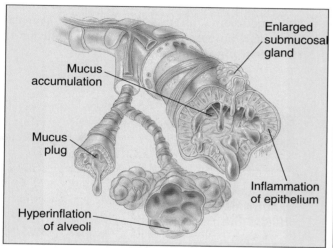

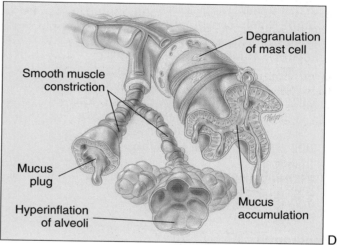

FIGURE 19-11 Airway obstruction. **A,** The normal lung. **B,** Emphysema. **C,** Chronic bronchitis. **D,** Bronchial asthma. (From Huether S, McCance K: *Understanding pathophysiology,* ed 5, St. Louis, 2012, Mosby.)

Drug Treatment. Given the interrelationship between asthma and COPD, many of the medications discussed previously for the treatment of asthma are also used in COPD. Additional examples of combination products used in the management of COPD are listed below and in Table 19-5.

MECHANISM OF ACTION: Combination product containing an inhaled corticosteroid and long-acting beta-agonist

SIDE EFFECTS: Throat irritation, fungal infection, headache, nausea, dizziness

AUXILIARY LABEL:
- [Advair HFA]: Shake well before use.

GENERIC NAME: fluticasone/salmeterol
TRADE NAME: Advair HFA, Advair Diskus (powder)
INDICATION: COPD, asthma
ROUTE OF ADMINISTRATION: Inhalation
COMMON ADULT DOSAGE: *MDI:* 2 inhalations twice daily; *Diskus:* 1 inhalation twice daily

GENERIC NAME: formoterol/budesonide
TRADE NAME: Symbicort
INDICATION: COPD, asthma
ROUTE OF ADMINISTRATION: Inhalation

COMMON ADULT DOSAGE: 2 inhalations twice daily

MECHANISM OF ACTION: Combination product containing an inhaled corticosteroid and long-acting beta-agonist

SIDE EFFECTS: Throat irritation, fungal infection, headache, nausea, dizziness

AUXILIARY LABEL:
- Shake well before using.

GENERIC NAME: ipratropium/albuterol

TRADE NAME: Combivent Respimat, DuoNeb

INDICATION: COPD, bronchospasm

ROUTE OF ADMINISTRATION: Inhalation

COMMON ADULT DOSAGE: *MDI:* 1 inhalation four times daily; *nebulizer:* 3 mL four times daily

MECHANISM OF ACTION: Combination product containing an anticholinergic and short-acting beta-agonist

SIDE EFFECTS: Tachycardia, dry mouth, dizziness, insomnia

AUXILIARY LABEL:
- Shake well before using.

Pneumonia

Pneumonia is an infection that causes acute inflammation in the airways of the lung, blocking them with thick mucus. One lobe (or many lobes) of one lung may be affected, or both lungs may be affected. The source of this infection can be bacterial, viral, fungal, protozoal, or, in rare cases, parasitic. A form of pneumonia known as *aspiration pneumonia* can be caused by aspirating food, fluids, or other foreign substances into the lungs. Once organisms such as bacteria or viruses enter the lung, they multiply. As the body tries to fight the infection, fluid and pus fill the lungs, making breathing difficult. The most common bacterial organism causing community-acquired pneumonia is *Streptococcus pneumoniae*, which is associated with a rapid onset of pneumonia. Older adults are at high risk, especially after an injury that requires them to remain in bed. People who are immunocompromised also are at higher risk of developing pneumonia.

Prognosis. Most people recover from pneumonia with rest, hydration, and medications, if appropriate for treatment. Of those admitted to a hospital, only a fraction die from pneumonia.

Non–Drug Treatment. As noted previously, rest and proper hydration are important components of non–drug therapy. Avoidance of irritants that may otherwise compromise breathing (e.g., dust, cigarette smoke, allergens) can help with breathing.

Drug Treatment. Antibiotics are frequently used to treat bacterial pneumonia. Less often, fungal infections occur, and they are treated with antifungals and other agents. For all types of pneumonia, respiratory medications may be used to treat the symptoms. These medications include bronchodilators and corticosteroids, described previously for the treatment of asthma and COPD. The medications used for the treatment of bacterial pneumonia often depend on the causative organism; numerous antibiotics are used for the treatment of pneumonia.

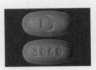

GENERIC NAME: azithromycin

TRADE NAME: Zithromax

INDICATION: Pneumonia, community-acquired pneumonia, miscellaneous bacterial infections

ROUTE OF ADMINISTRATION: Oral; intravenous (IV)

COMMON ADULT DOSAGE: *Oral:* 500 mg on day 1, followed by 250 mg once daily on days 2 through 5; *IV:* 500 mg for 2 days, then 500 mg orally daily to complete a 7- to 10-day course

MECHANISM OF ACTION: Macrolide antibiotic (inhibits bacterial protein synthesis)

SIDE EFFECTS: Diarrhea, nausea, vomiting, abdominal pain, anorexia

AUXILIARY LABEL:
- Take until gone.

GENERIC NAME: levofloxacin

TRADE NAME: Levaquin

INDICATION: Pneumonia, community-acquired pneumonia, miscellaneous bacterial infections

ROUTE OF ADMINISTRATION: Oral; intravenous

COMMON ADULT DOSAGE: 750 mg daily for 5 days or 500 mg daily for 7-14 days

MECHANISM OF ACTION: Fluoroquinolone antibiotic (inhibits bacterial DNA synthesis)

SIDE EFFECTS: Diarrhea, nausea, vomiting, abdominal pain, dyspepsia, tendinitis

AUXILIARY LABELS:

- Take at least 2 hours before or after any antacid or multivitamin.
- Take until gone.

Tech Note!

Fluoroquinolone antibiotics, such as Levaquin, have a boxed warning associating them with an increased risk of tendonitis and tendon rupture.

Tuberculosis

Tuberculosis (TB) is a leading cause of morbidity and mortality worldwide and at one time was the leading cause of death in the United States. The management of TB can be difficult because the causative organism, *Mycobacterium tuberculosis,* is resistant to many drugs. Although this bacterium typically infects the lungs to cause TB, it can also infect other organs, such as the kidneys, brain, and spine. Overall, the main goals of TB treatment include eradicating the bacteria that cause the infection with antibiotic medications, preventing the development of drug resistance, and preventing relapse of the disease. Because TB is highly contagious, health care workers and other at-risk individuals are frequently tested for the illness with a tuberculin skin test (also known as a PPD skin test). Figure 19-12 shows an example of a positive PPD skin test result. A PPD skin test essentially shows whether a person has developed an immune response to *M. tuberculosis.* People test positive if they have an active TB infection, if they were exposed to TB in the past, or if they received the bacille Calmette-Guérin (BCG) vaccine against TB (which is not given in the United States).

Prognosis. Tuberculosis can be cured if the prescribed medications are taken as directed. If left untreated, a TB infection can result in morbidity and death.

Non–Drug Treatment. No non–drug treatments can be used to cure TB. Good hygiene should be used to prevent transmission of TB because it is extremely contagious.

Drug Treatment. Most of the primary antituberculin agents are bactericidal (Table 19-6). This means that they kill *M. tuberculosis.* These agents are often used in combination for a course of treatment lasting many months. **Sputum** tests are often required to confirm whether treatment can be stopped. Although the medications used to treat tuberculosis are effective, many patients do not continue to take the medication as prescribed due to the long duration of treatment required to clear the infection completely. For this reason, patients must be educated by their physicians and pharmacists about the importance of finishing their medication regimen to eradicate the infection.

GENERIC NAME: isoniazid (INH)
INDICATION: TB infection, TB prophylaxis
ROUTE OF ADMINISTRATION: Oral; injectable
COMMON ADULT DOSAGE: 5 mg/kg (up to 300 mg) once daily for up to 6 months
MECHANISM OF ACTION: Inhibits mycobacterial cell wall synthesis
SIDE EFFECTS: Diarrhea, abdominal pain, nausea, vomiting, hepatitis
AUXILIARY LABELS:

- Take on an empty stomach.
- Take as directed.

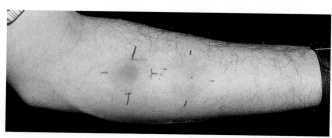

FIGURE 19-12 Positive result on a tuberculosis test. (From Zitelli BJ, Davis HW: *Atlas of pediatric physical diagnosis,* ed 6, Philadelphia, 2007, Saunders.)

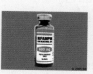

GENERIC NAME: rifampin
TRADE NAME: Rifadin
INDICATION: TB infection, meningococcal infection prophylaxis
ROUTE OF ADMINISTRATION: Oral; injectable
COMMON ADULT DOSAGE: 600 mg once daily

TABLE 19-6

Select Medications Used in the Treatment of Tuberculosis

Generic Name	Trade Name	Common Adult Oral Dosages*
ethambutol	Myambutol	• 15-25 mg/kg orally (PO) daily • 50 mg/kg PO twice weekly • 25-30 mg/kg PO 3 times weekly
ethionamide isoniazid (INH) pyrazinamide (PZA)	Trecator	• 15-20 mg/kg PO once daily or in divided doses • 5 mg/kg (intramuscularly) IM or PO daily for up to 6 months • 15-30 mg/kg PO daily • 50-70 mg/kg PO twice weekly
rifabutin	Mycobutin	• 5 mg/kg PO once daily for 2 months initially in combination, followed by 5 mg/kg 2 times per week in combination with isoniazid for an additional 4 months
rifampin rifapentine streptomycin	Rifadin Priftin	• 600 mg PO or IV once daily • 600 mg PO twice weekly for 2 months • 1 g or 15 mg/kg IM daily for 2-3 months, then 1 g IM 2-3 times weekly for up to 1 year

*Agents are typically used in combination regimens due to drug resistance.

MECHANISM OF ACTION: Inhibits bacterial and mycobacterial RNA synthesis
SIDE EFFECTS: Nausea, vomiting, cramps, diarrhea, orange to reddish discoloration of urine and other bodily fluids
AUXILIARY LABELS:
• Take at least 1 hour prior to or 2 hours after a meal.
• Take as directed.

Lung Cancer

Lung cancer is the most common cancer worldwide. Lung cancer became the most common cause of cancer deaths in men in the 1950s and the leading cause of cancer death in women in the mid-1980s. Due to a decrease in smoking rates, death rates from lung cancer have decreased in recent years. As the name suggests, lung cancer refers to malignancies of the airways. About 95% of all lung cancers are classified as either small cell lung cancer (SCLC) or non–small cell lung cancer (NSCLC). This classification is important in terms of treatment and prognosis.

Prognosis. As with any form of cancer, the stage of disease, presence of metastases, and other patient-specific factors determine the prognosis for lung cancer.

Non–Drug Treatment. Aside from smoking cessation, lung cancers can be treated with radiation and surgical resection for surgical candidates.

Drug Treatment. Chemotherapy is a primary treatment modality for a variety of types and stages of lung cancer. Chemotherapy additionally plays a role as adjuvant therapy after surgical resection. A variety of chemotherapeutic agents can be used to treat lung carcinomas.

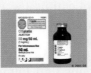

GENERIC NAME: cisplatin
TRADE NAME: Platinol
INDICATION: NSCLC, bladder cancer, mesothelioma, ovarian cancer, testicular cancer
ROUTE OF ADMINISTRATION: Injectable
COMMON ADULT DOSAGE: Dosage varies based on cancer stage, patient's weight, and combination therapies used
MECHANISM OF ACTION: Inhibits DNA synthesis
SIDE EFFECTS: Allergic reactions, mouth sores, infection, diarrhea

GENERIC NAME: vinorelbine
TRADE NAME: Navelbine
INDICATION: NSCLC
ROUTE OF ADMINISTRATION: Injectable

COMMON ADULT DOSAGE: Dosage varies based on cancer stage, patient's weight, and combination therapies used
MECHANISM OF ACTION: Inhibits cell division by interfering with microtubule formation
SIDE EFFECTS: Myelosuppression, neuropathy, fatigue

 Tech Alert!
Remember the following sound-alike, look-alike drugs:
diphenhydramine versus dicyclomine or dimenhydrinate
epinephrine versus ephedrine
Alupent versus Atrovent
albuterol versus atenolol

DO YOU REMEMBER THESE KEY POINTS?

- Names of the major components of the respiratory system and their functions
- The primary symptoms of the various upper and lower respiratory tract conditions discussed
- Medications used to treat the various respiratory conditions discussed
- The generic and trade names for the drugs discussed in this chapter
- The appropriate auxiliary labels that should be used when filling prescriptions for drugs discussed in this chapter

REVIEW QUESTIONS

Multiple Choice Questions

1. The process of gas exchange in the lungs takes place specifically in the:
   A. Brainstem
   B. Brain
   C. Medulla
   D. Alveoli

2. The large, dome-shaped muscle that separates the chest cavity from the abdominal cavity is the:
   A. Larynx
   B. Diaphragm
   C. Bronchus
   D. Trachea

3. The main function(s) of the cilia in the upper respiratory tract is (are):
   A. To smell
   B. To catch foreign material
   C. To warm and moisten air molecules
   D. Both A and C

4. The function of gas exchange includes all of the following *except*:
   A. Balancing the pH of the body
   B. Oxygenation of the bloodstream
   C. Discarding unused carbon dioxide
   D. Exchanging nitrogen for carbon dioxide

5. Oseltamivir (Tamiflu) is approved to treat:
   A. Influenza
   B. COPD
   C. Asthma
   D. Lung cancer

6. COPD is a term used to describe a group of pulmonary diseases of long duration that are characterized by increased resistance to airflow, which includes all of the following *except*:
   A. Emphysema
   B. Postnasal drip
   C. Chronic bronchitis
   D. Asthma

7. Albuterol is classified as a(n):
   A. Inhaled corticosteroid
   B. Long-acting beta-agonist
   C. Short-acting beta-agonist
   D. Inhaled anticholinergic

8. Tuberculosis (TB) is caused by which of the following microorganisms?
   A. *Mycobacterium tuberculosis*
   B. *Staphylococcus aureus*
   C. *Streptococcus pneumoniae*
   D. *Haemophilus influenzae*

9. Dextromethorphan is classified as a(n):
   A. Antitussive
   B. Antihistamine
   C. Corticosteroid
   D. Mucolytic

10. The act of respiration can be divided into two distinct phases: _____, the movement of air into the lungs, and _____, the movement of air out of the lungs.
    A. inspiration; expiration
    B. expiration; inspiration
    C. inspiration; absorption
    D. expiration; absorption

11. Which class of medications used in the treatment of asthma is associated with the development of thrush as a side effect?
    A. Short-acting beta-agonists
    B. Long-acting beta-agonists
    C. Inhaled corticosteroids
    D. Inhaled anticholinergics

12. What is the brand name for fexofenadine?
    A. Nasarel
    B. Clarinex
    C. Allegra
    D. Singulair

13. Which of the following medications for the treatment of asthma is given as an injection and is associated with injection site reactions as a common side effect?
    A. Zafirlukast (Accolate)
    B. Omalizumab (Xolair)
    C. Cromolyn sodium (Nasalcrom)
    D. Tiotropium (Spiriva)

14. Which of the following is an inhaled anticholinergic for the treatment of COPD?
    A. Ipratropium (Atrovent HFA)
    B. Salmeterol (Serevent Diskus)
    C. Tiotropium (Spiriva)
    D. Both A and C

15. Agents that break up thick mucous secretions of the lungs or bronchi so that they can be expelled from the system through coughing are called:
    A. Mucolytics
    B. Antitussives
    C. Expectorants
    D. Both A and C

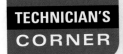

TECHNICIAN'S CORNER

Many conditions of the respiratory tract discussed in this chapter are treated symptomatically with OTC products such as diphenhydramine, guaifenesin, and pseudoephedrine. Using a drug reference, identify key contraindications to these products and patients who should avoid using them.

Bibliography

Clinical Pharmacology Online. (Referenced August 19, 2014.) www.clinicalpharmacology-ip.com.

Damjanov I: *Pathology for the health professions*, ed 4, St Louis, 2011, Saunders.

Fishback JL: *Pathology*, ed 3, Philadelphia, 2005, Mosby.

Goldman M: *Procedures in cosmetic dermatology series: photodynamic therapy*, ed 2, St Louis, 2008, Saunders

McCance KL: *Pathophysiology: the biologic basis for disease in adults and children*, ed 6, St Louis, 2010, Mosby.

Moscou K, Snipe K: *Pharmacology for pharmacy technicians*, ed 2, St Louis, 2013, Mosby.

Patton KT et al: *Mosby's handbook of anatomy and physiology*, St. Louis, 2000, Mosby.

Solomon EP: *Introduction to human anatomy and physiology*, ed 3, St. Louis, 2009, Saunders.

UpToDate Online. (Referenced August 19, 2014.) www.uptodate.com.

Therapeutic Agents for the Gastrointestinal System

Joshua J. Neumiller

OBJECTIVES

Upon completing this chapter, you should be able to do the following:

1. Describe the major components of the gastrointestinal system.
2. List the primary symptoms of conditions associated with dysfunction of the gastrointestinal system.
3. Recognize prescription and over-the-counter (OTC) drugs discussed for the treatment of conditions associated with the gastrointestinal system.

4. Write the generic and trade names for the drugs discussed in this chapter.
5. List appropriate auxiliary labels when filling prescriptions for drugs discussed in this chapter.

TERMS AND DEFINITIONS

Absorption In the gastrointestinal system, the processes that cause the movement of nutrients, fluids, and medications from the gastrointestinal tract into the bloodstream

Amino acids Molecules that are the building blocks of proteins

Antiemetics A drug effective in the treatment of nausea and vomiting

Carbohydrates Chemical compounds that contain carbon, hydrogen, and oxygen; examples include sugars, glycogen, starches, and cellulose

Chyme The soupy mixture (semifluid consistency) that results after food has mixed with stomach acids and digestive enzymes as it passes into the duodenum (first part of the small intestine)

Digestion The mechanical, chemical, and enzymatic action of breaking food into molecules that can be used in metabolism

Emesis A medical term for vomiting

Excretion Elimination of waste products and other remnants of metabolism, primarily through stools and urine

Fistulae Permanent abnormal passageways between two organs in the body or between an organ and the exterior of the body

Ingestion The act of taking in food, liquid, or other substances (e.g., medications)

Peristalsis The contraction and relaxation of the tubular muscles of the esophagus, stomach, and intestines that move substances from the mouth to the anus

Surface area The amount of an object's surface that is in contact with its surroundings

Common Drugs for the Gastrointestinal System

Trade Name	Generic Name	Pronunciation
Gastroesophageal Reflux Disease (GERD)		
Axid	nizatidine	(nye-**zah**-tih-deen)
Pepcid	famotidine	(fa-**mo**-tih-deen)
Tagamet	cimetidine	(sy-**meh**-tih-deen)
Zantac	ranitidine	(ra-**nih**-tih-deen)
AcipHex	rabeprazole	(rah-**beh**-prah-zole)
Dexilant	dexlansoprazole	(dex-**lan**-soe-prah-zole)
Nexium	esomeprazole	(es-o-**meh**-prah-zole)
Prevacid	lansoprazole	(lan-**sew**-prah-zole)
Prilosec	omeprazole	(oh-**meh**-prah-zole)
Protonix	pantoprazole	(pan-**toe**-prah-zole)
Zegerid	omeprazole/sodium bicarbonate	(oh-**meh**-prah-zole/**so**-dee-um by-**kar**-bow-nate)
Constipation		
Citrucel	methylcellulose	(meth-ill-**cell**-you-lows)
Constulose	lactulose	(**lak**-tyoo-lose)
Colace	docusate sodium	(**dok**-yoo-sate sow-dee-um)
Dulcolax	bisacodyl	(by-saw-**co**-dill)
FiberCon	calcium polycarbophil	(**kal**-ce-uhm **pol**-ee-**kar**-bow-phyl)
Fleet	mineral oil	(min-**uh**-ral oy-il)
Glycerin, Babylax, Colace Glycerin	glycerin anhydrous	(**glis**-ir-in)
Metamucil	psyllium	(**sill**-ee-um)
MiraLax	polyethylene glycol 3350	(**pol**-ee-**eth**-il-een **glye**-kol)
Phillips' Milk of Magnesia	magnesium hydroxide	(mag-**nee**-see-um/hye-**drock**-side)
Senokot, Ex-Lax	senna	(**sen**-ah)
Amitiza	lubiprostone	(loo-**bee**-pros-tone)
Diarrhea		
Imodium AD	loperamide	(low-**pear**-ah-myde)
Lomotil	diphenoxylate/atropine	(die-fen-**ox**-i-late/at-row-peen)
Pepto-Bismol	bismuth subsalicylate	(**biz**-muth sub-suh-**li**-suh-late)
Severe Diarrhea Predominant–Irritable Bowel Syndrome		
Lotronex	alosetron	(a-**low**-se-tron)
Nausea/Vomiting		
Antivert	meclizine	(**meck**-la-zeen)
Dramamine	dimenhydrinate	(die-men-**hi**-dra-nate)
Transderm Scop	scopolamine	(sko-**pole**-la-meen)
Compazine	prochlorperazine	(pro-klor-**pear**-ah-zeen)
Phenergan	promethazine	(pro-**meth**-a-zeen)
Tigan	trimethobenzamide	(try-meth-oh-**ben**-za-mide)
Aloxi	palonosetron	(**pal**-oh-**noe**-seh-tron)
Anzemet	dolasetron	(doe-**la**-seh-tron)
Kytril	granisetron	(gra-**ni**-seh-tron)
Zofran	ondansetron	(on-**dan**-seh-tron)
Reglan	metoclopramide	(mea-toe-**clow**-prah-myde)
Flatulence		
Mylicon	simethicone	(sye-**meth**-i-cone)

The digestive tract extends from the mouth to the anus. It processes ingested substances, such as food and fluids, so they can be absorbed and used by the body. Foods are broken down from large substances into smaller substances that can be absorbed readily into the bloodstream and used for energy production, in protein synthesis, and as enzymes for essential metabolic reactions. As food is broken down, nutrients are absorbed and nonessential food elements are excreted through the feces or urine. This chapter reviews the anatomy and physiology of the gastrointestinal tract and discuss medications used to treat select conditions that affect this system.

Form and Function of the Gastrointestinal System

The gastrointestinal (GI) system carries out four main functions in the body: digestion, absorption, metabolism, and **excretion**. Various organs in the GI system perform these functions 24 hours a day. The GI system is controlled by the parasympathetic nervous system (see Chapter 15). When we are at rest, the parasympathetic nervous system, which is responsible for the "rest and digest" functions of the body, is at work in the GI system. Each organ in the GI tract completes specific tasks. In addition to discussing the anatomy and function of the stomach and intestinal tract, this chapter discusses additional organs that are important in the GI system, such as the tongue, salivary glands, liver, pancreas, and gallbladder. These auxiliary (also called *ancillary* or *accessory*) organs play important roles in the GI system to that assist with **digestion**.

Anatomy and Physiology of the Gastrointestinal System

When they think about the GI system, most people consider the stomach the primary organ. However, by the time food has arrived at the stomach, the process of digestion has already begun. Let us begin by looking at the overall system of the GI tract (Figure 20-1). The organs discussed in this chapter, in sequence, are the mouth, salivary glands, pharynx, and esophagus (**ingestion** and digestion); followed by the stomach and small intestine (digestion and nutrient absorption); the large intestine (reabsorption of water and electrolytes and storage of feces); and finally the rectum and anus (elimination). Auxiliary organs and their functions in the GI system are also discussed.

Ingestion

The mouth begins the process of digestion by physically breaking down food into smaller pieces through the act of chewing. In addition to the action of the teeth chewing food into smaller pieces, salivary glands begin to secrete enzymes that initiate the chemical breakdown of food. The mouth has three pairs of salivary glands that are responsible for the beginning of food digestion: sublingual, submandibular, and parotid glands. The sublingual and submandibular glands are located below the tongue and jaw, respectively. Each parotid gland is located immediately in front of the ear (Figure 20-2).

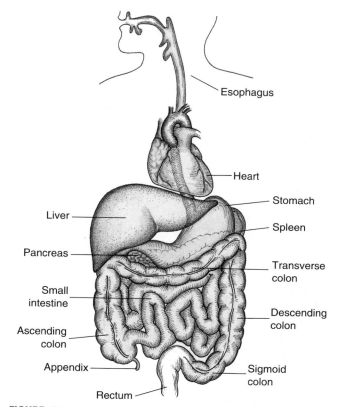

FIGURE 20-1 Anatomy of the gastrointestinal system (including the mouth, pharynx, esophagus, stomach, and intestines). (From Potter PA, Perry AG: *Fundamentals of nursing,* ed 8, St Louis, 2013, Mosby.)

Another function of saliva besides the enzymatic breakdown of food is to moisten the esophagus to assist with swallowing. With help from the tongue, the food is swallowed and makes its way into the pharynx (i.e., the throat) and then the esophagus. **Peristalsis** is involuntary muscle contraction and relaxation, which begins in the esophagus to propel food downward into the stomach. As the food arrives in the stomach, it enters an acidic environment in which further chemical breakdown of food and nutrients occurs. Figure 20-3 shows the pH (a measure of acidity) of the stomach related to other liquids and products.

 Tech Note!

The level of acidity in the stomach is important in the absorption of many drugs and minerals. A variety of drug interactions can occur between acid-lowering medications (e.g., proton pump inhibitors) and medications that require an acidic environment in the stomach for proper absorption.

When activated by food, gastric juices are secreted in the stomach. The gastric juices are composed of hydrochloric acid and a variety of enzymes. The

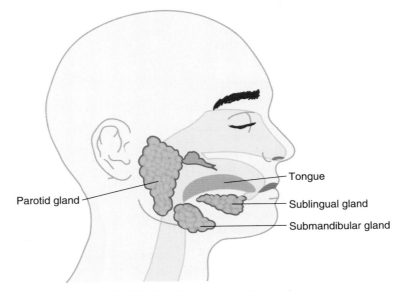

FIGURE 20-2 Major glands of the mouth.

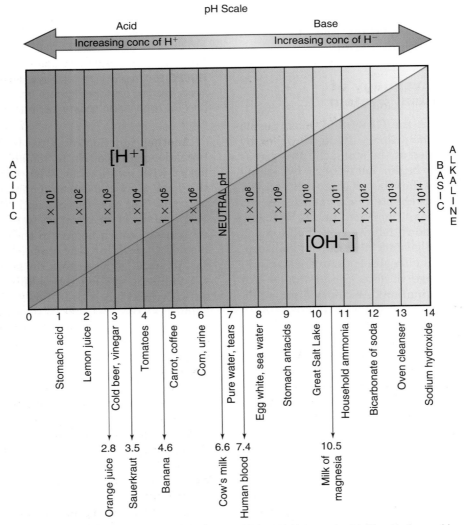

FIGURE 20-3 The pH scale ranges from 1 (the most acidic) to 14 (the most basic). The pH of normal human blood is 7.4, approximately the midpoint of the range.

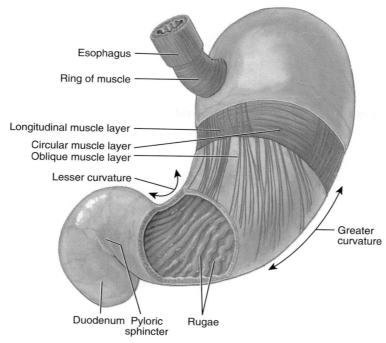

FIGURE 20-4 Structure of the stomach. (From Solomon EP: *Introduction to human anatomy and physiology,* ed 3, St Louis, 2009, Saunders.)

enzymatic function of the stomach is important because it allows the intestines to absorb the nutrients and chemicals and use them for metabolic processes in the body. The acidic environment of the stomach can also destroy many medications; therefore, several medications need a special coating for protection. Some medications (e.g., parenteral medications, such as insulin) need to be administered in a totally different form to bypass the stomach and its acidic environment. To help balance this extremely acidic pH, the inner mucosal lining of the stomach is alkaline for protection. An additional protective mucosal lining prevents the acid from eating through the stomach wall.

The stomach itself is composed of several different types of muscle that aid in the digestion process by churning and mixing the stomach contents (Figure 20-4). When the churning function of the stomach, in conjunction with the enzymes and acid of the stomach, has converted the solid substances ingested into small pieces, the acidic, semifluid mixture that remains is referred to as **chyme**. Chyme exits the stomach and passes through the pyloric sphincter, a muscle that serves as an opening into the small intestine, for further digestion and absorption of nutrients (Figure 20-4).

Absorption

Absorption of nutrients takes place primarily in the small intestine. The vitamins and minerals move through the lining of the gut. Molecules of glucose,

amino acids, and fatty acids are absorbed and begin to circulate through the bloodstream for delivery to the cells of the body.

The small intestine, which is about 6 m long, is responsible for the final steps in the digestion of food. The materials that are not digested or absorbed from the small intestine pass into the large intestine. The structure of the small intestine is congruent with its function; that is, to absorb nutrients from the foods we eat. To do this, it must be able to make contact with as much of the broken-down food as possible and for as long as possible. The small intestine is able to accomplish this because it is extremely long and composed of many folds, which increase its absorptive **surface area** (Figure 20-5).

The small intestine can be divided further into three sections: the duodenum, jejunum, and ileum. Each has a specific function and contribution to the breakdown and absorption of food. The duodenum, located at the beginning of the small intestine, is about 25 cm long. It also is connected to the liver and pancreas, from which it receives secretions that mix with the chyme from the stomach. In addition to the liver and pancreas, the gallbladder aids in the digestion of food. The gallbladder releases bile to help in the dispersion of fats. The next section of the small intestine is the jejunum, which is much longer (about 2.5 m). The ileum, the most distal section, is about 3.5 m long.

Most of the absorption of food and oral drugs takes place in these three sections of the small intestine. Intestinal secretions have a more alkaline pH than

Segment of jejunum

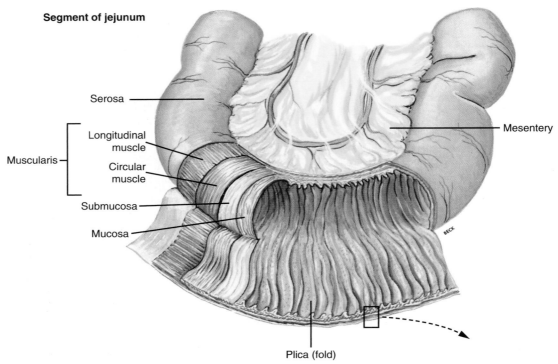

FIGURE 20-5 Wall of the small intestine. (From Patton KT et al: *Mosby's handbook of anatomy and physiology,* St Louis, 2000, Mosby.)

the stomach, which allows for good absorption of nutrients. Various enzymes continue to break down specific foods, such as sugar, protein, and fat. Nutrients and drugs absorb into the bloodstream from the small intestine through several processes, including diffusion and active transport. Various transport processes available in the walls of the small intestine help carry important nutrients and drugs to the bloodstream. Each villus (a fingerlike projection; see Figure 20-5) on the surface of the small intestine has a network of capillaries and fine lymphatic vessels. The epithelial cells of these villi transport nutrients and drugs from the lumen into the capillaries. Any substances that are not absorbed or remain undigested pass into the large intestine.

Excretion

The large intestine follows the small intestine. Although the large intestine is much larger in diameter, it is not as long as the small intestine (it is only about 1.5 m). Although some absorption continues in the large intestine, it is largely limited to water and electrolytes. The substances moving through this portion of the intestine are transformed into solid fecal matter as water and electrolytes are resorbed.

The main organs involved in excretion are the rectum and anus. The rectum is the shortest section

of the intestinal tract and connects to the anal canal. The time required for normal passage of fecal material can range from 3 to 5 days. In the anal canal, the internal anal sphincter is under involuntary control and is responsible for the urge to defecate. The external anal sphincter is under voluntary control, giving the person control of the bowels.

Auxiliary Organ Functions

The chemical contribution of the auxiliary organs (pancreas, liver, and gallbladder) to digestion is only one of their many functions. All three organs have ducts that lead to the duodenum. In the duodenum, the enzymes from the pancreas meet the contents from the stomach and actively metabolize various foods. Foods such as proteins, **carbohydrates**, and fats must be converted from complex molecules to simple molecules. Proteins are large molecules that are broken down into smaller peptides and amino acids. Carbohydrates arrive in the stomach as large sugar molecules and are converted into disaccharides; in the duodenum, they are further broken down into monosaccharides and are absorbed and used for energy. Fats begin their process of digestion in the duodenum, where they encounter bile, which is produced by the liver and stored in the gallbladder. These long carbon chains of fat are more difficult to metabolize. They are first made water soluble by a

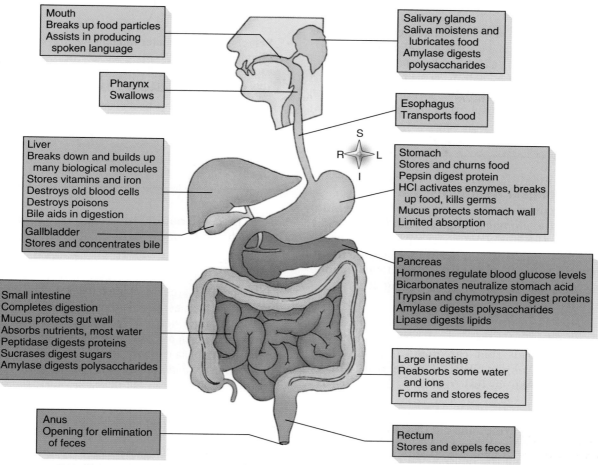

FIGURE 20-6 Summary of digestive function. (From Patton KT, et al: *Mosby's handbook of anatomy and physiology,* St Louis, 2000, Mosby.)

process called *emulsification* and then are broken down further by enzymes called *lipases.*

Figure 20-6 provides a summary of the anatomy and function of the GI tract as they have been discussed in this section.

Conditions Affecting the Gastrointestinal System

Numerous conditions can affect the GI system. These conditions affect different areas of the GI tract and may include any of the structures from the mouth to the anus. Conditions that affect digestion include commonly occurring and recurring conditions, such as heartburn, upset stomach, and gastroesophageal reflux disease (GERD). In the upper and lower bowels, constipation or diarrhea may occur in both acute and chronic forms. More severe illnesses, such as inflammatory bowel diseases (Crohn's disease and ulcerative colitis) and ulcers, can be exacerbated by consistent stress. Other GI condi-

tions can be caused by bacterial infections and tumors. This chapter focuses on relatively common conditions associated with the GI tract that affect patients the pharmacy technician is likely to encounter. Examples of drugs used to treat each specific condition also are discussed.

Conditions Primarily Associated with the Stomach

The high acid content of stomach fluids causes a number of commonly experienced GI conditions. These conditions are known more commonly as upset stomach, indigestion, or heartburn. Antacids are normally used for occasional dyspepsia (upset stomach) or heartburn. They reduce the acidity of the stomach. Most remedies for relief of these occasional symptoms may be purchased over the counter (see Chapter 27). Other conditions of the stomach include GERD and peptic ulcers. Stomach disorders may require prescribed medications if OTC agents do not adequately relieve the symptoms.

Gastroesophageal Reflux Disease

GERD can occur when the upper sphincter (opening) at the top of the stomach relaxes. This allows acidic contents from the stomach to back up into the esophagus, possibly resulting in a burning sensation in the chest or throat. Risk factors for GERD can include obesity, smoking, and pregnancy, among others.

Prognosis. With the use of medications and avoidance of foods that can make the condition worse, the outlook for GERD is quite good. Many people can make a full recovery from GERD symptoms.

Non–Drug Treatments. Avoiding foods that may bring about symptoms of GERD is an important aspect of treatment. Another non–drug approach is raising the head of the bed if the person's GERD symptoms are prominent while he or she is lying down. If medication and diet are not effective, surgery is an option; however, surgery is rarely needed because of the effectiveness of medical management.

Drug Treatments. In addition to antacids, histamine-2 (H_2) antagonists are used to treat GERD and ulcers. Agents such as cimetidine and ranitidine block H_2 receptors in the lining of the stomach. Proton pump inhibitors (PPIs) are a third type of agent used for the treatment of GERD. PPIs inhibit gastric acid production in the stomach lining by blocking the final enzymatic reaction before acid secretion. All three classes of these medications are available over the counter, but some H_2 antagonists and PPIs require a prescription.

Antacids. Antacids include aluminum carbonate, sodium bicarbonate, calcium carbonate, magnesium hydroxide, and aluminum hydroxide. These ingredients each chemically neutralize acid to increase the pH level in the stomach (make it less acidic). Table 20-1 lists examples of single-ingredient antacids, and Table 20-2 provides a list of key antacid products

TABLE 20-1

Select Over-the-Counter Antacid Agents (Single Ingredient)

Active Ingredient	Dosage Form	Strength
aluminum hydroxide	Oral suspension	320 mg/5 mL
magnesium hydroxide (Phillips' Milk of Magnesia)	Oral suspension	400 mg/5 mL
	Chewable tablets	311 mg
	Soft chew	500 mg

used in combination to treat GERD and related stomach conditions.

Histamine-2 Antagonists. H_2-antagonists bind to H_2-receptor sites, reducing acid secretion. They are well-tolerated agents: rare side effects of histamine antagonists include drowsiness, headache, and rash. Prescription formulations typically are stronger than OTC formulations. Although most of the prescription agents have normal dosages approved by the U.S. Food and Drug Administration (FDA) for specific medical conditions, many physicians allow patients to take an H_2-antagonist on an as-needed basis for occasional indigestion.

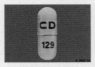

GENERIC NAME: ranitidine
TRADE NAME: Zantac
INDICATION: GERD, erosive esophagitis, gastric ulcer, duodenal ulcer treatment and prophylaxis (OTC for heartburn and indigestion)
ROUTE OF ADMINISTRATION: Oral; intravenous
COMMON ADULT DOSAGE: *Oral Rx dose for GERD:* 150 mg twice daily; *IV dose for most conditions:* Up to 200 mg/day

TABLE 20-2

Select Over-the-Counter Combination Antacids

Active Ingredients	Trade Name	Dosage Form OTC	Strength of Active Ingredients
aluminum hydroxide (AlOH) and magnesium trisilicate	Gaviscon	Chewable tablets	AlOH 80 mg, magnesium trisilicate 20 mg
aluminum hydroxide and magnesium hydroxide (MgOH)	Mag-Al; Mylanta Ultimate Strength Suspension	Suspension	AlOH 225 mg + MgOH 200 mg/5 mL
aluminum hydroxide, magnesium hydroxide, and simethicone	Almacone	Chewable tablets	AlOH 200 mg, MgOH 200 mg, simethicone 20 mg
	Maalox Regular Strength Antacid; Mylanta	Suspension	AlOH 200 mg, MgOH 200 mg, simethicone 20 mg/5 mL
	Mintox Maximum Strength	Suspension	AlOH 400 mg, MgOH 400 mg, simethicone 40 mg/5 mL
sodium bicarbonate, acetaminophen (APAP), and citric acid	Bromo Seltzer	Effervescent granules	Sodium bicarbonate 3.5 g, APAP 650 mg, citric acid 2.67 g
sodium bicarbonate, aspirin, and citric acid	Alka-Seltzer	Effervescent tablets	Sodium bicarbonate 1700 mg, aspirin 325 mg, citric acid 1000 mg
sodium bicarbonate, citric acid, and potassium bicarbonate	Alka-Seltzer Gold	Effervescent tablets	Sodium bicarbonate 1050 mg, citric acid 1000 mg, potassium bicarbonate 344 mg

MECHANISM OF ACTION: Competitively inhibits the binding of histamine to H_2-receptors on gastric parietal cells to reduce gastric acid secretion.

SIDE EFFECTS: Constipation, nausea, abdominal pain

AUXILIARY LABEL (RX):
- May administer without regard to meals.

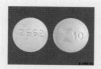

GENERIC NAME: famotidine

TRADE NAME: Pepcid, Pepcid AC

INDICATION: GERD, erosive esophagitis, gastric ulcer, duodenal ulcer treatment and prophylaxis (OTC for heartburn and indigestion)

ROUTE OF ADMINISTRATION: Oral; intravenous

COMMON ADULT DOSAGE: *Oral Rx dose for GERD:* 20 mg twice daily; *IV dose:* variable depending on indication and setting

MECHANISM OF ACTION: Competitively inhibits the binding of histamine to H_2-receptors on gastric parietal cells to reduce gastric acid secretion

SIDE EFFECTS: Headache, dizziness, constipation

AUXILIARY LABEL (RX):
- May cause dizziness and drowsiness.
- [Suspension]: Shake well.

Proton Pump Inhibitors. PPIs are used primarily in the treatment of GERD and peptic ulcers. Most of these agents are available as a delayed-release form and can be taken once daily. The mechanism of action for all PPIs is blocking gastric acid secretion in the stomach. Currently, the only PPI products available over the counter are Prilosec OTC, Prevacid 24HR, Zegerid OTC, and Nexium 24HR.

Table 20-3 provides a summary of select H_2-antagonists and PPIs for the treatment of GERD.

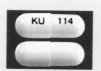

GENERIC NAME: omeprazole

TRADE NAME: Prilosec

INDICATION: Gastric ulcer, duodenal ulcer, GERD, erosive esophagitis; OTC for frequent heartburn occurring 2 or more days per week for up to 2 weeks

ROUTE OF ADMINISTRATION: Oral

COMMON ADULT DOSAGE: Dosage varies, depending on the severity of the condition; a common dose is 20 mg once daily; *OTC dosage:* 20 mg daily for up to 14 days

MECHANISM OF ACTION: Prevents gastric acid secretion from parietal cells of the stomach

TABLE 20-3

Select Histamine-2 Antagonists and Proton Pump Inhibitors for the Treatment of Gastroesophageal Reflux Disease

Medication Class	Generic Name	Trade Name	Common Side Effects	Common Dose Range
Histamine-2 Antagonists	cimetidine famotidine nizatidine ranitidine	Tagamet Pepcid Axid Zantac	• Constipation • Nausea • Abdominal pain	• 800 mg twice daily • 20 mg twice daily for up to 6 wk • 150 mg twice daily for up to 12 wk • 150 mg twice daily
Proton Pump Inhibitors (PPIs)	dexlansoprazole esomeprazole lansoprazole omeprazole omeprazole + sodium bicarbonate pantoprazole rabeprazole	Dexilant Nexium Prevacid Prilosec Zegerid Protonix Aciphex	• Diarrhea • Nausea • Headache • Abdominal pain • Increased risk of fractures	• 30 mg once daily for up to 4 wk • 20 mg once daily for up to 4 wk • 15-30 mg once daily for up to 8 wk • 20 mg once daily for up to 4 wk • 20 mg once daily for up to 4 wk • 40 mg once daily for up to 8 wk • 20 mg once daily for up to 4 wk

SIDE EFFECTS: Diarrhea, nausea, headache, stomach pain, increased risk of fractures

AUXILIARY LABELS (RX):
• Take before meals.
• Do not crush or chew.

GENERIC NAME: lansoprazole
TRADE NAME: Prevacid, Prevacid 24HR
INDICATION: GERD, duodenal ulcer, gastric ulcer, prophylaxis for nonsteroidal antiinflammatory drug (NSAID)–induced ulcer, erosive esophagitis
ROUTE OF ADMINISTRATION: Oral; intravenous
COMMON ADULT DOSAGE: Dosage varies, depending on the severity of the condition; common dose is 15-30 mg once daily
MECHANISM OF ACTION: Prevents gastric acid secretion from parietal cells of the stomach
SIDE EFFECTS: Diarrhea, nausea, headache, stomach pain, increased risk of fractures
AUXILIARY LABELS:
• Take before meals.
• Do not crush or chew.

GENERIC NAME: pantoprazole
TRADE NAME: Protonix
INDICATION: GERD, erosive esophagitis
ROUTE OF ADMINISTRATION: Oral; intravenous
COMMON ADULT DOSAGE: Dosage varies, depending on the severity of the condition; a common dose is 40 mg once daily
MECHANISM OF ACTION: Prevents gastric acid secretion from parietal cells of the stomach
SIDE EFFECTS: Diarrhea, nausea, headache, stomach pain, increased risk of fractures
AUXILIARY LABEL:
• Do not crush or chew.

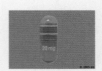

GENERIC NAME: esomeprazole
TRADE NAME: Nexium, Nexium 24HR

INDICATION: GERD, duodenal ulcer, erosive esophagitis, and prophylaxis for NSAID-induced ulcer

ROUTE OF ADMINISTRATION: Oral; intravenous

COMMON ADULT DOSAGE: Dosage varies, depending on the severity of the condition; a common dose is 20 mg once daily

MECHANISM OF ACTION: Prevents gastric acid secretion from parietal cells of the stomach

SIDE EFFECTS: Diarrhea, nausea, headache, stomach pain, increased risk of fractures

AUXILIARY LABELS:

- Take 1 hour before meals on an empty stomach.
- Do not crush or chew.

Tech Note!

Patients often need assistance in determining how to treat upset stomach and/or heartburn. Pharmacists should be consulted because they can differentiate between common problems and possible conditions that may be the underlying cause of the patient's symptoms. A pharmacist either can suggest the proper treatment or can refer the patient to his or her physician for an evaluation. In addition, because many OTC stomach agents can interact with prescription medications, it is important that most patients avoid self-treatment, which could cause more harm than good.

Peptic Ulcer Disease

Peptic ulcer disease (PUD) is a chronic condition that causes sores (ulcers) in the lining of the stomach and/or duodenum (Figure 20-7). Occasionally ulcers may also appear in the esophagus. The main symptom of PUD is abdominal pain that is often relieved by ingesting food or taking antacids. Drugs (e.g.,

NSAIDs) and bacterial infection *(Helicobacter pylori)* are the leading causes of PUD because they damage the lining of the stomach, duodenum, or esophagus and cause ulcerations. The bacterium *H. pylori*, a contributor in most cases of peptic ulcer, may be acquired through infected water or food and by person-to-person contact. *H. pylori* is commonly treated with a combination of two antibiotics and a PPI.

Prognosis. With proper treatment of PUD using antibiotics and acid-reducing medications, the incidence of relapse can be quite low. If ulcers are associated with NSAID use, it is important that the person avoid future NSAID use to prevent relapse.

Non–Drug Treatment. One of the most important ways to reduce the possibility of contracting *H. pylori* is to wash your hands. This reduces the spread of the bacteria. Avoid long-term use of NSAIDs when possible; NSAIDs can cause ulcers by interfering with the protective prostaglandins in the stomach. If NSAID therapy is needed, some agents may be taken to prevent ulcers (e.g., PPIs). Cigarette smoking not only contributes to ulcer formation, but also increases the risk of ulcer complications, such as ulcer bleeding and perforation; therefore, smoking cessation can be helpful. Many conditions can coexist, and care providers may recommend ingestion of a bland diet, avoidance of aggravating foods, and/or use of stress reduction techniques.

Drug Treatments. PUD caused by *H. pylori* typically indicates use of antibiotics as a course of treatment. The bacterium can embed itself into the mucosal lining of the stomach, duodenum, and

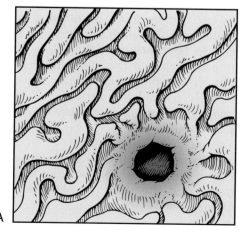

A   ENDOSCOPIC VIEW

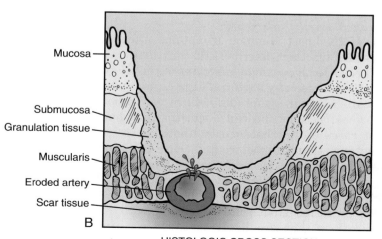

B   HISTOLOGIC CROSS SECTION

Mucosa
Submucosa
Granulation tissue
Muscularis
Eroded artery
Scar tissue

FIGURE 20-7 Peptic ulcer. (From Damjanov I: *Pathology for the health professions,* ed 4, St. Louis, 2011, Saunders.)

TABLE 20-4

First-Line Recommendations for the Treatment of *Helicobacter pylori* Infection

Patient Characteristic	Regimen (Adult Oral Dosage)*
Patients who: 1. Are not allergic to penicillin 2. Have not previously received a macrolide antibiotic	10- to 14-day course of: • Standard-dose protein pump inhibitor (PPI) twice daily • Clarithromycin 500 mg twice daily • Amoxicillin 1000 mg twice daily
Patients who: 1. Are allergic to penicillin 2. Have not previously received a macrolide or metronidazole or are unable to tolerate bismuth quadruple therapy	10-14 day course of: • Standard-dose PPI twice daily • Clarithromycin 500 mg twice daily • Metronidazole 500 mg twice daily
Patients who: 1. Are allergic to penicillin or have failed one course (above) of *H. pylori* treatment	10-14 day course of: • Bismuth subsalicylate 525 mg four times daily • Metronidazole 250 mg four times daily • Tetracycline 500 mg four times daily • Standard-dose PPI twice daily OR 10-14 day course of: • Bismuth subsalicylate 420 mg four times daily • Metronidazole 375 mg four times daily • Tetracycline 375 mg four times daily • Standard-dose PPI twice daily

*Dosing recommendations from the American College of Gastroenterology.
From Chey WD, Wong BCY: American college of gastroenterology guideline on the management of *Helicobacter pylori* infection, *Am J Gastroenterol* 102:1808-1825, 2007.

rectum. Table 20-4 provides a summary of currently approved regimens for the treatment of *H. pylori*–associated ulcers. Treatments may consist of two, three, or four agents to be given simultaneously. PPIs are often added to promote ulcer healing. A variety of antacids can be used for relief of abdominal pain.

Conditions Primarily Associated with the Intestines

Two of the most common symptoms affecting the intestinal tract are diarrhea and constipation. These can be caused by various infections of the GI system. Infections caused by bacteria, viruses, and parasites typically result in symptoms of diarrhea. Tumors and other obstructions can cause constipation; however, most cases of diarrhea or constipation are isolated symptoms that can be treated with OTC medications. In addition, medications are among the most common causes of diarrhea or constipation; therefore, to alleviate potential problems, many physicians prescribe stool softeners along with routine medications that are likely to cause constipation. Chronic inflammatory bowel conditions, such as ulcerative colitis and Crohn's disease, can also produce symptoms such as diarrhea but are more

long-term in nature and associated with long-term complications.

Patients who require a bowel resection, such as for the removal of a tumor, may be required to wear an ileostomy or colostomy bag. Ostomy bags are attached to the abdomen with adhesive strips; wearing an ostomy bag allows the patient to empty the intestinal contents into the bag through the stoma (ostomy opening). The site of the ostomy varies, depending on the location of the resection. Because the intestinal tract is responsible for most nutrient absorption, if the ostomy site is close to the stomach, fewer nutrients can be absorbed through the intestine and must be provided to the patient. Other than having to empty the ostomy bag a few times during the day and changing the tubing occasionally, a person can live a relatively normal life with an ostomy. Some specialty pharmacies provide ostomy care supplies. The types of ostomies are:

- *Colostomy:* Surgical creation of an opening (stoma) in the abdominal wall to allow feces to pass from the bowel through the opening rather than through the anus. A colostomy may be temporary or permanent (e.g., cancer of the colon or rectum).
- *Ileostomy:* A surgical opening made in the ileum onto the abdominal wall to allow for the passage of feces. Performed in cases of cancer of the

colon, severe or recurrent Crohn's disease, or ulcerative colitis.

Another common condition is excess gas in the intestines, which can cause pain and distention of the stomach or intestines; this can be both uncomfortable and embarrassing. The source of gas is the intestinal bacteria that normally coat the intestines. As the bacteria digest the foods we eat (sugars, starch, cellulose), they produce hydrogen and/or methane as a by-product. OTC agents are available to treat this condition.

Inflammatory Bowel Disease

Inflammatory bowel disease comprises two major disorders, Crohn's disease and ulcerative colitis. Although both conditions fall under the umbrella of IBD, they have distinct clinical characteristics that differentiate them (Figure 20-8). Crohn's disease and ulcerative colitis are discussed individually. Table 20-5 provides information on select agents used for the treatment of these conditions.

Crohn's Disease. Crohn's disease is a chronic inflammatory disease of the intestines that can cause ulcerations in the small and large intestinal lining; however, it can affect the digestive tract anywhere from the mouth to the anus. As mentioned previously, Crohn's disease is closely related to ulcerative colitis, and together they constitute inflammatory bowel disease. Although the exact cause of Crohn's disease is unknown, both autoimmune and genetic factors are thought to play a role in its development. Symptoms include cramping, tenderness, flatulence, nausea, fever, and diarrhea. In contrast to ulcerative colitis, Crohn's disease can result in inflammation and ulceration throughout the thickness of the bowel (transmural) that can result in the formation of microperforations and **fistulae** in the bowel (Figure 20-9).

Prognosis. The prognosis for Crohn's disease depends on the severity of the condition. With proper lifestyle changes and medication to control the disorder, the outcome can be good.

Non–Drug Treatment. Effective treatment often requires lifestyle changes, such as physical rest and a restricted diet. Trigger foods must be identified and avoided. In debilitated patients, parenteral nutrition may be necessary to maintain nutritional status while resting the bowels. Vitamin B_{12} injections, along with various supplements and the elimination of dairy products, may be prescribed. Surgery (colectomy with ileostomy) may be necessary to correct bowel perforation, massive hemorrhage, fistulae, or acute intestinal obstruction.

Drug Treatment. To control inflammation, agents such as 5-aminosalicylates (5-ASA), sulfasalazine (Azulfidine), and mesalamine (Asacol) are normally prescribed first. Corticosteroids (prednisone) and immunomodulators, such as azathioprine (Imuran) and tacrolimus (Prograf), may be prescribed if 5-ASA drugs are not effective or if the condition is severe. Biological agents, such as infliximab (Remicade) and adalimumab (Humira),

Comparison of the basic features of Crohn's disease and ulcerative colitis		
	Crohn's disease	**Ulcerative colitis**
Prevalence in U.S.	~30–50 per 100,000 in U.S.	~80 per 100,000
Site	Any part of GI system but typically terminal ileum	Colon and rectum only
Macroscopic: • disease continuity • bowel wall • ulcers	Discontinuous Thickened with strictures and adhesions Deep fissures form basis of fistulae	Continuous Not thickened Flat based; do not extend to submucosa
Microscopic: • pattern of inflammation • crypt pattern	Transmural Focal Granulomas (in 60% of cases) Little distortion	Mucosal and submucosal Diffuse No granulomas Distorted in long-standing disease; crypt abscesses
Anal lesions	Present in 75%; anal fistulae; ulceration or chronic fissure	Present in < 25%
Frequency of fistula	10–20% of cases	Uncommon
Risk of developing cancer	Slightly increased	Significantly increased

FIGURE 20-8 Comparison of the basic features of Crohn's disease and ulcerative colitis. (From Fishback JL: *Pathology,* ed 3, Philadelphia, 2005, Mosby.)

TABLE 20-5

Select Agents for the Treatment of Inflammatory Bowel Disease

Medication Class	Generic Name	Trade Name	Common Side Effects	Comments
5-Aminosalicylates	mesalamine (5-ASA) sulfasalazine	Apriso, Pentasa, Asacol, Rowasa, Canasa Azulfidine	• Dizziness • Abdominal pain • Rectal irritation with rectal formulations	• Approved by the U.S. Food and Drug Administration (FDA) for ulcerative colitis • Used off-label for Crohn's disease
	balsalazide	Colazal		• FDA-approved for ulcerative colitis
Tumor Necrosis Factor (TNF)-Alpha Inhibitors	adalimumab certolizumab pegol infliximab	Humira Cimzia Remicade	• Nausea • Infusion/Injection site reactions • Increased risk of infection • Diarrhea	• FDA-approved for Crohn's disease • FDA-approved for Crohn's disease and ulcerative colitis
Alpha-4 Integrin Antagonist	natalizumab	Tysabri	• Allergic reactions • Increased risk of infection • Rash	• FDA-approved for Crohn's disease

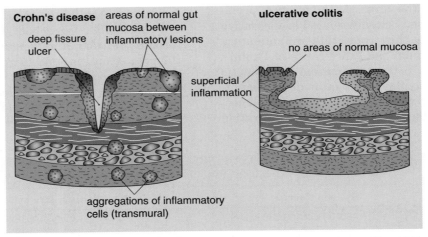

FIGURE 20-9 Depth and distribution of lesions in the bowel wall in Crohn's disease. (From Fishback JL: *Pathology,* ed 3, Philadelphia, 2005, Mosby.)

may also be prescribed. If infection occurs because of the overgrowth of bacteria in the small intestine, antibiotics may be prescribed. Antidiarrheals are used to control diarrhea, and fluid/electrolyte replacement is necessary to counteract any resulting dehydration.

Ulcerative Colitis. Ulcerative colitis causes inflammation and sores in the lining of the large intestine or colon. Ulcerative colitis affects only the colon and rectum, whereas Crohn's disease can affect the

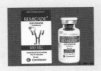

GENERIC NAME: infliximab
TRADE NAME: Remicade
INDICATION: Crohn's disease, ulcerative colitis, rheumatoid arthritis
ROUTE OF ADMINISTRATION: Intravenous (IV) infusion

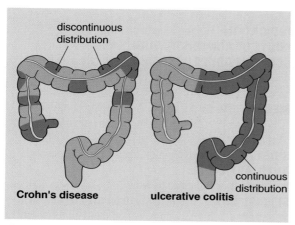

FIGURE 20-10 Comparisons of distribution of lesions along the bowel in Crohn's disease and ulcerative colitis. (From Fishback JL: *Pathology,* ed 3, Philadelphia, 2005, Mosby.)

COMMON ADULT DOSAGE: 5 mg/kg infused IV and then 2 and 6 weeks later; followed by maintenance regimen of 5 mg/kg every 8 weeks thereafter

MECHANISM OF ACTION: Inhibits the proinflammatory cytokine tumor necrosis factor (TNF)–alpha to reduce the inflammatory response

SIDE EFFECTS: Nausea, infusion site reactions, increased risk of infection, diarrhea

AUXILIARY LABELS:
- For infusion only.
- Keep vials refrigerated before use.

SPECIAL NOTE: Infliximab is usually administered by a physician or nurse in a medical setting. Each prescription for Remicade is accompanied by an extra patient information sheet, called a *Medication Guide.*

entire GI system (Figure 20-10). Symptoms of ulcerative colitis include stomach pain, cramps, bloody diarrhea, or bleeding from the rectum. Some people may experience fever, loss of appetite, and weight loss. Because the symptoms associated with ulcerative colitis are often seen in other, related conditions, it is important to rule out an infectious cause.

Prognosis. The course of ulcerative colitis typically involves intermittent exacerbations alternating with periods of symptomatic remission.

Non–Drug Treatment. Treatment can include many lifestyle changes, such as adjusting dietary intake to avoid triggers, using stress reduction techniques, and having a strong support system. In severe cases, surgery may be necessary.

Drug Treatment. Depending on the severity of the symptoms, various agents can be prescribed. For mild symptoms, antidiarrheals, corticosteroids, or 5-ASA may be used for a short time. For moderate to severe symptoms, both corticosteroids and aminosalicylates may be prescribed. Many of the medications used for ulcerative colitis are the same as those used for Crohn's disease (see Table 20-5).

GENERIC NAME: mesalamine (5-ASA)

TRADE NAME: Asacol

INDICATION: Mild to moderate ulcerative colitis, Crohn's disease

ROUTE OF ADMINISTRATION: Oral; rectal

COMMON ADULT DOSAGE: *Ulcerative colitis—oral tablet (Asacol):* 800 mg three times a day for 6 weeks; *rectal suppository (Asacol):* 500 mg suppository administered two times daily; *rectal enema (mesalamine):* 4 g (rectal instillation) once a day for 3 to 6 weeks or until remission is achieved

MECHANISM OF ACTION: Inhibition of the cyclooxygenase (COX) enzyme to reduce inflammation in the bowel

SIDE EFFECTS: Abdominal pain, nausea, vomiting, rectal irritation with rectal formulations

AUXILIARY LABELS:
- [Oral ER products]: Administer whole; do not open, crush or chew.
- [Suspension enema]: Shake well before using. For rectal use only.
- [Suppository]: For rectal use only.

Irritable Bowel Syndrome

IBS is a functional GI condition characterized by chronic abdominal pain and altered bowel habits. IBS is the most commonly diagnosed GI condition and affects men, women, young patients, and the elderly. IBS is believed to account for 25% to 50% of all referrals to gastroenterology offices. Abdominal pain associated with IBS can range from mild to debilitating, and altered bowel habits can range from episodic diarrhea, constipation, and alternating diarrhea and constipation.

Prognosis. Although there is no cure for IBS, the prognosis is good with supportive treatment and avoidance of known triggers.

Non–Drug Treatment. Avoiding specific irritants and triggers is one of the leading non–drug treatments; irritants can include foods or stress factors. A high-fiber diet can help control constipation. Foods that may cause symptoms of IBS include gas-producing foods, sugarless chewing gum and candy, coffee, and alcohol. It is also believed that food allergies may play a role in the development of IBS, and food allergies are sometimes evaluated in severe cases of IBS. Stress management techniques, along with regular exercise, can help in many cases.

Drug Treatment. Often antispasmodics (dicyclomine) are prescribed to manage IBS; however, if this agent is used over a long period the patient may become dependent. Other agents used to treat various symptoms of IBS include antidiarrheals (e.g., Lomotil, Imodium), which slow intestinal movements; bile acid sequestrants (e.g., cholestyramine), which prevent bile acids from stimulating the colon and thereby relieve diarrhea; and alosetron (Lotronex) for patients with diarrhea-type IBS who have not responded to other treatments. Antidepressants or antianxiety agents may also be prescribed to treat symptoms of depression or anxiety that often accompany this condition. Patients with constipation-type IBS may respond to lubiprostone (Amitiza).

GENERIC NAME: dicyclomine
TRADE NAME: Bentyl
INDICATION: IBS
ROUTE OF ADMINISTRATION: Oral
COMMON ADULT DOSAGE: 20 mg four times daily
MECHANISM OF ACTION: Believed to reduce muscular tone in the GI tract to decrease muscle spasms
SIDE EFFECTS: Drowsiness, dizziness, blurred vision, constipation
AUXILIARY LABELS:
• May be administered without regard to meals.
• Avoid alcohol.

GENERIC NAME: alosetron
TRADE NAME: Lotronex

INDICATION: Diarrhea-prominent IBS
ROUTE OF ADMINISTRATION: Oral
COMMON ADULT DOSAGE: 0.5 mg twice daily for 4 weeks; may be increased to 1 mg twice daily if well tolerated
MECHANISM OF ACTION: Antagonizes serotonin receptors (5-HT3), which diminishes pain and decreases diarrhea
SIDE EFFECTS: Constipation, drowsiness, headache
AUXILIARY LABEL:
• Take with a full glass of water.
SPECIAL NOTE: This agent is to be used in women suffering from IBS who have had diarrhea for at least 6 months. It has not been shown to be effective in men with IBS.
SPECIAL NOTE: Infrequent but serious adverse effects have occurred with the use of Lotronex, including ischemic colitis and severe constipation that may result in hospitalization and, in rare cases, blood transfusion, surgery, and death.
SPECIAL NOTE: The patient must read and sign a patient-physician agreement form before receiving a prescription.

GENERIC NAME: lubiprostone
TRADE NAME: Amitiza
INDICATION: IBS with constipation in women, idiopathic constipation
ROUTE OF ADMINISTRATION: Oral
COMMON ADULT DOSAGE: 8-24 mcg twice daily with food and water
MECHANISM OF ACTION: Increases intestinal fluid secretion by activating chloride channels in the GI tract, leading to softer stools and increased motility of the GI tract
SIDE EFFECTS: Nausea, vomiting, headache, diarrhea
AUXILIARY LABEL:
• Take with food and water.

 Tech Note!
The main differences between irritable bowel syndrome and inflammatory bowel disease are that IBS is not considered a disease and does not involve inflammation. IBS is a functional disorder with no known structural cause, so it can be diagnosed only by its symptoms.

Diarrhea

An abnormal increase in the frequency, fluidity, or volume of bowel movements is considered diarrhea. Abdominal cramping, gas, and general discomfort may accompany diarrhea. Diarrhea is often broken down into two main types, acute and chronic. Acute is short term (often caused by viral and bacterial infections), whereas chronic symptoms continue for longer periods; chronic diarrhea generally is considered to be diarrhea lasting for at least 1 month. Diarrhea can stem from a multitude of causes, including disorders of the colon (colitis), GI tumors, metabolic disorders, and infectious causes. In severe cases of infectious diarrhea, the number of stools may reach 20 or more per day. Although treatment depends on the cause, the symptoms of diarrhea can be treated with antidiarrheal agents.

As diarrhea continues, vital fluids and electrolytes are lost through the intestines. Death can occur if fluids and electrolytes are not replaced (diarrhea is a significant cause of death worldwide). People who are most susceptible to this danger are older adults and young children. Diarrhea is a symptom in many conditions; therefore, if symptoms are not controlled with OTC agents within a few days, diagnosis may be necessary for proper treatment. However, evaluation by a physician should be sought for children younger than 3 years, patients who also have a fever, and anyone experiencing diarrhea for longer than 2 days.

Prognosis. In many cases diarrhea is short-lived and resolves without treatment. In other cases, treatment with medication is required. The prognosis largely depends on the underlying cause of the diarrhea.

Non–Drug Treatments. Resting and drinking clear fluids (e.g., oral rehydrating solutions, such as Pedialyte) until the diarrhea subsides are commonly suggested to prevent dehydration and electrolyte loss.

Drug Treatments. Several agents, OTC and prescription, are used to manage diarrhea. OTC drugs include medications such as Kaopectate, FiberCon, and Pepto-Bismol. Several prescription drugs are also available for the treatment of diarrhea (Table 20-6). Agents such as diphenoxylate/atropine (Lomotil) are generally reserved for short-term use because they can become less effective with continued use.

GENERIC NAME: diphenoxylate/atropine (C-V)
TRADE NAME: Lomotil
INDICATION: Diarrhea
ROUTE OF ADMINISTRATION: Oral
COMMON ADULT DOSAGE: 5 mg four times daily, then 2.5 mg two or three times per day as needed (max 20 mg/day)
MECHANISM OF ACTION: Slows intestinal motility to treat diarrhea
SIDE EFFECTS: Dry mouth, dizziness, drowsiness, constipation
AUXILIARY LABELS:
- May cause dizziness and drowsiness.
- Caution: Federal law prohibits the transfer of this drug to any person other than the patient for whom it was prescribed.

TABLE 20-6

Select Agents for the Treatment of Diarrhea

Generic Name	Trade Name	Common Side Effects	Common Dose Range
atropine/ diphenoxylate (C-V)	Lomotil	• Dry mouth • Dizziness • Drowsiness • Constipation	• 5 mg four times daily, then 2.5 mg 2-3 times per day prn (max 20 mg/day)
bismuth subsalicylate	Pepto Bismol (OTC)	• Dark stools • Tongue discoloration	• 2 tablets or 30 mL (liquid) prn, not to exceed 8 doses in 24 hr
loperamide	Imodium (OTC)	• Dizziness • Drowsiness • Dry mouth	• 4 mg initially for loose stool (max 8 mg/day for 2 days for an acute episode)
psyllium	Metamucil (OTC)	• Abdominal pain • Flatulence • Nausea	• 2.4 g in 240 mL of fluid twice daily

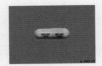

GENERIC NAME: loperamide
TRADE NAME: Imodium, Imodium AD (OTC)
INDICATION: Diarrhea
ROUTE OF ADMINISTRATION: Oral
COMMON ADULT DOSAGE: 4 mg initially after loose
stool (max 8 mg/day for 2 days for an acute episode)
MECHANISM OF ACTION: Slows GI motility
SIDE EFFECTS: Dizziness, drowsiness, dry mouth

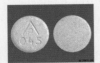

GENERIC NAME: bismuth subsalicylate
TRADE NAME: Pepto-Bismol (OTC)
INDICATION: Diarrhea, dyspepsia, heartburn
ROUTE OF ADMINISTRATION: Oral
COMMON ADULT DOSAGE: 2 tablets or 30 mL (liquid)
as needed, not to exceed 8 doses in 24 hours
MECHANISM OF ACTION: Antidiarrheal effect is
believed to be due to inhibition of prostaglandin
synthesis
SIDE EFFECTS: Stools may appear grayish black; tongue
discoloration
AUXILIARY LABEL: NOTE: Remember this is a salicylate
and should be used cautiously in those with salicylate
allergy.

Constipation

Constipation is a condition in which the feces are hard and dry and bowel movements are infrequent or irregular. Many people have a bowel movement once a day to several times daily, whereas others may normally have fewer bowel movements. The ease of the bowel movement is more important than the frequency when defining constipation in an individual. Most people can treat temporary constipation themselves through dietary changes or OTC agents; however, if other symptoms are present (weight loss, abdominal pain, or rectal bleeding), a more serious condition may be the cause. Certain medications can cause constipation, such as narcotic pain medications (e.g., codeine, oxycodone), antidepressants (e.g., amitriptyline, imipramine), anticonvulsants (e.g., phenytoin, carbamazepine), calcium channel blockers (e.g., diltiazem, nifedipine, verapamil), and aluminum-containing antacids.

Prognosis. Constipation can be managed in most cases by either dietary modifications or medications. Increased physical activity also may be helpful. When constipation is a symptom of a more serious disease, such as a tumor, surgery or chemotherapy may be necessary to treat the underlying condition.

Non–Drug Treatments. Non–drug treatments suggested to avoid constipation include the ingestion of adequate dietary fibers (such as those found in fruits and vegetables) in the daily diet. Roughage also aids in good digestion and elimination. In addition to a well-balanced meal plan, drinking plenty of water helps prevent constipation.

Drug Treatments. A variety of medications are used for the treatment of constipation (Table 20-7). Stool softeners pull water and fatty compounds into the intestine to aid in elimination. Hyperosmotic agents work by osmosis, increasing pressure in the bowels by absorbing water, similar to bulk-forming agents. Stimulant laxatives work by increasing peristalsis in the intestines (specifically the colon), which forces the contents to be expelled. People who constantly take stimulant laxatives eventually may become dependent on them; therefore, it is recommended that stimulant laxatives be used on a short-term basis when used OTC. Enemas can also be used to treat constipation.

> **Tech Note!**
> Bowel evacuants are also used to empty the intestines before a procedure or surgery. The solutions contain polyethylene glycol and replacement electrolytes because the intestines are not able to absorb the necessary ions from the expelled fecal material. Typically, the patient must drink approximately 2 to 4 L (2000 to 4000 mL) of solution within a relatively short time. Staying at home is recommended after administration of bowel evacuants because of the rapid onset of action and the need for frequent elimination.

Bulk-Forming Laxatives. Bulk-forming agents (e.g., psyllium) function by absorbing water from the body to increase the moisture and overall bulk of the stools, allowing for easier elimination. A positive aspect of these agents is that they can be taken over long periods and can be used for both constipation and diarrhea. Because of this, these agents are often referred to as "bowel stabilizing" agents. Examples of bulk-forming agents include polycarbophil (FiberCon) and methylcellulose (Citrucel).

TABLE 20-7

Select Agents for the Treatment of Constipation

Medication Class	Generic Name	Trade Name	Common Side Effects	Common Adult Dose
Bulk-Forming Laxatives	methylcellulose	Citrucel (OTC)	• Abdominal pain • Flatulence • Nausea	• 2 g in 8 oz water given 1-3 times daily
	psyllium	Metamucil (OTC)		• 2.4 g in 240 mL water given 1-3 times daily
Stool Softener (Emollient Laxative)	docusate	Colace (OTC)	• Gastrointestinal (GI) cramping • Abdominal pain	• 240 mg daily
Osmotic Laxatives	polyethylene glycol	MiraLax (OTC)	• Abdominal pain • Cramping • Flatulence • Nausea	• 17 g of powder in 120-240 mL fluid once daily
Stimulant Laxatives	bisacodyl senna	Bisac-Evac (OTC) Senokot (OTC)	• GI irritation • Nausea • Abdominal cramping • Tolerance/dependence	• 10-15 mg daily • 1-2 tablets twice daily
Miscellaneous	lubiprostone	Amitiza	• Nausea • Vomiting • Headache • Diarrhea	• 8-24 mcg twice daily with food and water
Combination Products	docusate/senna	Senna Plus (OTC)	• See individual ingredients above	• 2-4 tablets daily until bowel movements are normalized

GENERIC NAME: psyllium (OTC)
TRADE NAME: Metamucil
INDICATION: Constipation
ROUTE OF ADMINISTRATION: Oral
COMMON ADULT DOSAGE: 1 tablespoon daily in 8 ounces of water or juice
MECHANISM OF ACTION: Absorbs liquid into the GI tract, leading to increased bulk of the stool, which facilitates peristalsis and bowel motility
SIDE EFFECTS: Bloating, gas, abdominal cramping
SPECIAL NOTE: Should be taken with at least 8 ounces of fluid to prevent choking.

GENERIC NAME: docusate (OTC)
TRADE NAME: Colace
INDICATION: Constipation
ROUTE OF ADMINISTRATION: Oral; rectal (enema)
COMMON ADULT DOSAGE: *Oral:* 50-240 mg once daily
MECHANISM OF ACTION: Stool softener, lowers the surface tension of the feces, allowing water and lipids to penetrate the stool
SIDE EFFECTS: GI cramping, abdominal pain

Emollient Laxatives (Stool Softeners). Docusate improves the ability of water in the colon to penetrate and mix with stool. The increased water content softens the stool. Often stool softeners are used as a preventive measure rather than to treat constipation. These agents work gently and are very effective.

Stimulant Laxatives. Stimulant laxatives cause the muscles of the small intestine and colon to propel their contents rapidly. They also increase the content of water in the stool, either by reducing the absorption of water in the colon or by causing additional secretion of water in the small intestines. Examples of stimulants include senna compounds and castor oil.

GENERIC NAME: bisacodyl (OTC)
TRADE NAME: Dulcolax
INDICATION: Constipation
ROUTE OF ADMINISTRATION: Oral; rectal (suppository or enema)
COMMON ADULT DOSAGE: 10 mg orally or rectally once daily as needed
MECHANISM OF ACTION: Increases intestinal motility by irritating the GI mucosa
SIDE EFFECTS: Abdominal pain, dizziness, nausea, perianal irritation (rectal use)

GENERIC NAME: senna (OTC)
TRADE NAME: Senokot
INDICATION: Constipation (also used for constipation from opioid agents)
ROUTE OF ADMINISTRATION: Oral
COMMON ADULT DOSAGE: Dosage depends on preparation
MECHANISM OF ACTION: Increases intestinal motility by irritating the GI mucosa
SIDE EFFECTS: GI irritation, nausea, abdominal cramping

Osmotic Laxatives. These agents are compounds that remain in GI tract and retain water that is already in the colon. The result is softening of the stool. Examples include polyethylene glycol (MiraLax) and lactulose (Constulose).

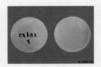

GENERIC NAME: polyethylene glycol (OTC)
TRADE NAME: MiraLax
INDICATION: Constipation
ROUTE OF ADMINISTRATION: Oral

COMMON ADULT DOSAGE: 17 g powder in 120-240 mL fluid once daily
MECHANISM OF ACTION: Osmotic agent that binds water and causes it to be retained in the stool
SIDE EFFECTS: Abdominal pain, cramping, flatulence, nausea

Flatulence

Flatulence is normally caused by the by-products (nitrogen, carbon dioxide, methane) of the microbial breakdown of certain foods. Sugars (lactose, sorbitol, fructose) and starches (rice, wheat, certain vegetables) may pose a problem because they may be difficult to digest. People who are lactose intolerant lack the enzyme lactase. This enzyme is located in the lining of the intestines, and without it the person cannot metabolize the carbohydrate lactose; this results in poor digestion of milk products.

Another cause of flatulence may be poor absorption of foods in the small intestine, which allows more undigested food to reach the bacteria in the colon. Sometimes the bacteria are present in the small intestine, where the food has not had a chance to be digested, and bacteria begin producing gas. Symptoms are discomfort (bloating) and pain in the abdominal cavity.

Prognosis. With proper treatment, flatulence can be greatly reduced. However, the patient should be educated that flatulence is a normal digestive process that everyone experiences, although levels of gas production may vary.

Non–Drug Treatment. For individuals with lactose intolerance, using soy products is an option. Alternatively, people who are lactose intolerant can ingest replacement enzymes (lactase supplements) similar to those found in the lining of the intestines. Eliminating trigger foods that cause gas can lessen symptoms. For pancreatic insufficiency, specific enzyme replacements can be taken with meals. Beano, an OTC product, contains an enzyme (alpha-d-galactosidase) that helps to break down sugars in vegetables so they can be absorbed, thus eliminating gas in the intestines.

Drug Treatment. OTC medications used for the treatment of gas typically contain simethicone as the primary ingredient. This medication is available in tablets, chewable tablets, and liquid for children.

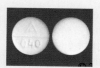

GENERIC NAME: simethicone
TRADE NAME: Gas-X, Phazyme (OTC)
INDICATION: For the relief of gas and abdominal distention caused by gas
ROUTE OF ADMINISTRATION: Oral
COMMON ADULT DOSAGE: 40-125 mg up to four times daily after meals and at bedtime as needed
MECHANISM OF ACTION: Reduces the surface tension of gas bubbles, preventing gas pockets
SIDE EFFECTS: None reported

Miscellaneous Conditions of the Gastrointestinal System

Nausea and Vomiting

Emesis is another term for vomiting. This violent reaction of the body is controlled by the medulla oblongata in the brain. Known as the chemoreceptor trigger zone (CTZ), or nausea zone, this small area of the brainstem can be activated by smell, pain, medication, motion sickness (originating in the inner ear), and even emotions. When the CTZ is activated, chemical signals are sent via the nervous system to the vomit center, which then relays the message to the stomach, where muscles of the diaphragm, stomach, esophagus, and salivary glands work together to cause the vomiting reflex.

Although most people have experienced nausea and vomiting, it is usually an isolated event. Other causes of emesis include food or drug poisoning, overconsumption of alcohol, or a postsurgical reaction to anesthesia. People who are subjected to certain chemotherapeutic agents as a part of cancer treatment must deal with extreme nausea and vomiting. The chemotherapy agents activate the CTZ, causing emesis as a common side effect.

Prognosis. If vomiting goes untreated, severe dehydration and a decrease in electrolyte levels (potassium, sodium), in addition to alkalosis, may occur, requiring a longer recovery period. Treating the underlying cause or condition normally alleviates emesis.

Non–Drug Treatments. Depending on the reason for vomiting, certain non–drug treatments can be effective. To prevent transfer of infectious causes of vomiting, avoid undercooked foods and wash hands before eating. If nausea occurs, eating a soda cracker or toast can sometimes help. One of the most important considerations is that dehydration can occur with continued vomiting; replacing the lost liquids and electrolytes is a vital aspect of treatment.

Drug Treatments. Drugs used to treat vomiting are referred to as **antiemetics**. Most antiemetics require a prescription. Agents that do not affect the CTZ can be purchased over the counter and usually are used for motion sickness. Depending on the underlying cause or causes of the emesis, it may be treated with or without medications. Medications include anticholinergics, antidopaminergics, H_1-antihistamines, cannabinoids (dronabinol), corticosteroids (dexamethasone, methylprednisolone), and benzodiazepines (lorazepam). Agents such as corticosteroids, serotonin antagonists, and benzodiazepines are often used before emetic chemotherapies to prevent emesis.

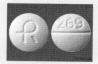

GENERIC NAME: metoclopramide
TRADE NAME: Reglan
INDICATION: Nausea and vomiting, gastroparesis
ROUTE OF ADMINISTRATION: Oral; intravenous
COMMON ADULT DOSAGE: *Nonchemotherapeutic dose:* 5-10 mg before meals and at bedtime as needed; *chemotherapeutic dosage:* 10 mg in 50 mL of normal saline over 30 minutes; given once before chemotherapy treatment, may repeat every 2 hours for two doses or every 3 hours for three doses
MECHANISM OF ACTION: Antagonism of dopamine receptors in the CTZ
SIDE EFFECTS: Diarrhea, drowsiness, fatigue, parkinsonism
AUXILIARY LABEL:
• May cause dizziness and drowsiness.

 Tech Note!
Because metoclopramide blocks dopamine receptors in the brain, it should not be used in patients with Parkinson's disease. Metoclopramide actually has a boxed warning for the possibility of tardive dyskinesia due to its effects on dopamine receptors.

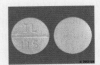

GENERIC NAME: prochlorperazine
TRADE NAME: Compazine, Compro
INDICATION: Nausea and vomiting, schizophrenia
ROUTE OF ADMINISTRATION: Oral; intravenous (IV) or intramuscular (IM); rectal
COMMON ADULT DOSAGE: *Oral:* 5 mg three to four times daily as needed; *IV or IM:* 5 to 10 mg every 3 or 4 hours (max 40 mg per day); *rectal:* 25 mg every 12 hours
MECHANISM OF ACTION: Blocks dopamine receptors in the mesolimbic system
SIDE EFFECTS: Dizziness, drowsiness, dry mouth, extrapyramidal side effects
AUXILIARY LABEL:
• May cause dizziness and drowsiness.

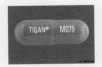

GENERIC NAME: trimethobenzamide
TRADE NAME: Tigan
INDICATION: Nausea and vomiting
ROUTE OF ADMINISTRATION: Oral; intramuscular (IM)
COMMON ADULT DOSAGE: *Oral:* 300 mg three to four times daily; *IM:* 200 mg three to four times daily
MECHANISM OF ACTION: Believed to act on the CTZ; however, the exact mechanism is unknown
SIDE EFFECTS: Dizziness, drowsiness, diarrhea, headache, blurred vision
AUXILIARY LABEL:
• May cause dizziness and drowsiness.

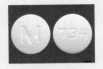

GENERIC NAME: ondansetron
TRADE NAME: Zofran, Zofran ODT
INDICATION: Nausea and vomiting (including chemotherapy induced)
ROUTE OF ADMINISTRATION: Oral; intravenous
COMMON ADULT DOSAGE: *Oral:* 8 mg 30 minutes before chemotherapy treatment, then 8 mg 8 hours after dose, followed by 8 mg every 12 hours for several days;

IV: 0.15 mg/kg infused over 15 minutes beginning 30 minutes before the initiation of chemotherapy
MECHANISM OF ACTION: Blockade of serotonin 5-HT3 receptors in the chemoreceptor trigger zone
SIDE EFFECTS: Fever, headache, constipation, diarrhea
AUXILIARY LABEL:
• Take as directed.

GENERIC NAME: meclizine
TRADE NAME: Antivert, Bonine (OTC)
INDICATION: Nausea and vomiting, motion sickness, vertigo
ROUTE OF ADMINISTRATION: Oral
COMMON ADULT DOSAGE: 12.5-50 mg 1 hour before exposure to stimulus
MECHANISM OF ACTION: H_1-receptor antagonist; anticholinergic
SIDE EFFECTS: Dizziness, drowsiness, dry mouth
SPECIAL NOTE: Meclizine is also available in 25- and 50-mg tablets but requires a prescription.

Colorectal Cancer

Colorectal cancer (CRC) is a relatively common form of cancer with a high mortality rate. Although the mortality rate has been decreasing by about 3% per year since 1990, CRC is still the second most common cause of cancer-related death in the United States. Initial symptoms of CRC can include abdominal pain, a change in bowel habits, blood in the stool, weakness, anemia, and weight loss.

Prognosis. As noted, CRC is the second most common cause of cancer-related death in the United States. The pathologic stage of the cancer at diagnosis is the best indicator of the long-term prognosis for both colon and rectal cancer; therefore, early detection is optimal for a favorable prognosis.

Non–Drug Treatments. Surgery is considered the only curative modality for localized CRC and is often used for treatment of cancers localized to the colon/rectal wall and/or regional lymph nodes, although some cases are considered nonoperable.

Drug Treatments. A variety of chemotherapeutic agents are used in CRC.

GENERIC NAME: bevacizumab
TRADE NAME: Avastin
INDICATION: Colorectal cancer, non-small cell lung cancer, renal cell cancer
ROUTE OF ADMINISTRATION: Intravenous
COMMON ADULT DOSAGE: 5-10 mg/kg every 14 days in combination with 5-fluorouracil–based chemotherapy
MECHANISM OF ACTION: Binds vascular endothelial growth factor (VEGF) to decrease the formation of new blood vessels to the tumor
SIDE EFFECTS: Allergic reactions, mouth sores, infection, chest pain

GENERIC NAME: oxaliplatin
TRADE NAME: Eloxatin
INDICATION: Colorectal cancer
ROUTE OF ADMINISTRATION: Intravenous
COMMON ADULT DOSAGE: Dosage varies based on cancer stage, patient weight, and combination therapies used
MECHANISM OF ACTION: Inhibits DNA synthesis
SIDE EFFECTS: Allergic reactions, mouth sores, infection, diarrhea

GENERIC NAME: irinotecan
TRADE NAME: Camptosar
INDICATION: Colorectal cancer
ROUTE OF ADMINISTRATION: Intravenous
COMMON ADULT DOSAGE: Dosage varies by weight and other combination chemotherapeutic agents used
MECHANISM OF ACTION: Inhibits DNA synthesis
SIDE EFFECTS: Allergic reactions, mouth sores, infection, diarrhea

 Tech Alert!

Remember these sound-alike, look-alike drugs:
simethicone versus cimetidine
hydroxyzine versus hydralazine
Prevacid versus Pravachol or Prinivil
metoclopramide versus metolazone
ranitidine versus amantadine
Zantac versus Zofran

DO YOU REMEMBER THESE KEY POINTS?

- Names of the major organs of the gastrointestinal system and their functions
- The primary symptoms of the various GI conditions discussed
- Medications used to treat the various GI conditions discussed
- The generic and trade names for the drugs discussed in this chapter
- The appropriate auxiliary labels that should be used when filling prescriptions for drugs discussed in this chapter

REVIEW QUESTIONS

Multiple Choice Questions

1. The primary functions of the gastrointestinal system include all of the following *except*:
   A. Digestion
   B. Absorption
   C. Secretion
   D. All of the above are GI functions
2. The small intestines are composed of the following segments *except*:
   A. Duodenum
   B. Jejunum
   C. Colon
   D. Ilium
3. Bile is made by the _____ and stored by the _____.
   A. gallbladder; liver
   B. liver; gallbladder
   C. gallbladder; pancreas
   D. liver; pancreas
4. Which of the following is a proton pump inhibitor (PPI)?
   A. Ranitidine
   B. Omeprazole
   C. Sucralfate
   D. Aluminum hydroxide

5. Bentyl (dicyclomine) is frequently used for which condition?
   A. Constipation
   B. Ulcerative colitis
   C. Irritable bowel syndrome (IBS)
   D. None of the above

6. A person diagnosed with gastroesophageal reflux disease may receive which of the following medications?
   A. Calcium carbonate
   B. Ranitidine
   C. Omeprazole
   D. All of the above

7. Of the following medications used for the treatment of diarrhea, which is a C-V controlled substance?
   A. Imodium (loperamide)
   B. Bismuth subsalicylate
   C. Lomotil (atropine + diphenoxylate)
   D. None of the above

8. Which of the following is available for purchase as an OTC product?
   A. Protonix
   B. AcipHex
   C. Prevacid 24HR
   D. Asacol

9. Inflammatory bowel disease is composed of the following:
   A. Diarrhea and constipation
   B. Ulcerative colitis and irritable bowel syndrome
   C. Irritable bowel syndrome and diarrhea
   D. Ulcerative colitis and Crohn's disease

10. *Helicobacter pylori* is commonly associated with which of the following GI conditions?
    A. Peptic ulcer disease (PUD)
    B. Crohn's disease
    C. Ulcerative colitis
    D. GERD

11. The chemoreceptor trigger zone (CTZ) is an important target for medications used in the treatment of:
    A. Nausea and vomiting
    B. Inflammatory bowel disease
    C. PUD
    D. IBS

12. Which of the following is used for the treatment of flatulence?
    A. Bismuth subsalicylate
    B. Simethicone
    C. Loperamide
    D. Famotidine

13. Colorectal cancer is currently the _____ most common cause of cancer-related death in the United States.
    A. Second
    B. Third
    C. Fourth
    D. Fifth

14. Which of the following is used for the treatment of constipation and is a "stool softener"?
    A. Senna
    B. Docusate
    C. MiraLax (polyethylene glycol)
    D. Psyllium

15. Which of the following would *not* be used to prevent emesis?
    A. Pepto-Bismol
    B. Meclizine
    C. Docusate sodium
    D. Both A and C

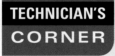

TECHNICIAN'S CORNER

1. A patient arrives at your pharmacy to fill a prescription. The prescription reads: codeine 30 mg; take one to two tablets every 4 to 6 hours as needed for pain. The quantity indicates #100.
   What over-the-counter medication or medications were probably prescribed by the physician or will be suggested by the pharmacist at the time of consultation? Why?

2. A patient who tested positive for *Helicobacter pylori* arrives at the pharmacy and gives you a prescription for the following agents:
   Clarithromycin
   Omeprazole
   Metronidazole
   What would be the recommended strengths and the dosing of these medications? Also, give the length of time the medications should be taken. How is a stop date determined for these medications?

Bibliography

Clinical Pharmacology Online. (Referenced August 19, 2014.) www.clinicalpharmacology-ip.com.

Damjanov I: *Pathology for the health professions*, ed 4, St Louis, 2011, Saunders.

Fishback JL: *Pathology*, ed 3, Philadelphia, 2005, Mosby.

Patton KT et al: *Mosby's handbook of anatomy and physiology*, St Louis, 2000, Mosby.

Potter PA, Perry AG: *Fundamentals of nursing*, ed 8, St Louis, 2013, Mosby.

Solomon EP: *Introduction to human anatomy and physiology*, ed 3, St Louis, 2009, Saunders.

UpToDate Online. (Referenced August 19, 2014.) www.uptodate.com.

Therapeutic Agents for the Renal System

Joshua J. Neumiller

OBJECTIVES

Upon completing this chapter, you should be able to do the following:

1. Describe the major components of the renal and urological systems.
2. List the primary symptoms of conditions associated with dysfunction of both the renal and urological systems.
3. Recognize prescription and over-the-counter drugs used to treat the conditions associated with the renal and urological systems as discussed in this chapter.

4. Write the generic and trade names for the drugs discussed in this chapter.
5. List appropriate auxiliary labels when filling prescriptions for drugs discussed for the treatment of conditions associated with the renal and urological systems.

TERMS AND DEFINITIONS

Acidosis Increase in the blood's acidity, resulting from the accumulation of acid or loss of bicarbonate; the pH of blood is lowered

Alkalosis Increase in the blood's alkalinity, resulting from the accumulation of alkali or reduction of acid content; the pH of blood is elevated

Anion A negatively charged ion

Cation A positively charged ion

Chronic kidney disease (CKD) A condition that reduces the kidneys' ability to function properly

Collecting duct A series of tubules in the kidneys that connect the nephrons to the ureter

Dialysate The fluid into which material passes by way of the membrane in dialysis

Dialysis The passage of a solute through a semipermeable membrane to remove toxic materials and to maintain fluid, electrolyte, and pH levels of the body when the kidneys are malfunctioning

Diuretic An agent that increases urine output and excretion of water from the body

Edema A condition characterized by the collection of excess of watery fluid in the cavities or tissues of the body

Erythropoietin A hormone secreted by the kidneys that increases the rate of production of red blood cells

Interstitial space Small, narrow spaces between tissues

Ions Atoms or molecules with a net electrical charge (positive or negative)

Lithotripsy Treatment with ultrasound shock waves to break a kidney stone into small particles

Micturition Urination

Nephron The filtering unit of the kidneys

Nosocomial infection An infection that originates in the hospital or institutional setting

Osmosis The diffusion of water from low solute concentrations to higher solute concentrations across a semipermeable membrane

Peritonitis Inflammation of the peritoneum, typically caused by bacterial infection

Plasma The colorless fluid portion of blood

Renal artery One of the pair of arteries that branch from the abdominal aorta; each kidney has one renal artery

Renal vein The vein in which filtered blood from the kidneys is sent back into the body's circulatory system; each kidney has one renal vein

Renin An enzyme secreted by and stored in the kidneys that promotes the production of the protein angiotensin

Stress incontinence Involuntary emission of urine when pressure in the abdomen suddenly increases

Tubular reabsorption The conservation of protein, glucose, bicarbonate, and water from the glomerular filtrate by the tubules

Tubular secretion A function of the nephron in which ions, toxins, and water are secreted into the collecting duct to be excreted

Ureteroscopy Examination of the upper urinary tract, usually performed with an endoscope passed through the urethra

Urethritis Inflammation of the urethra

Urge incontinence Incontinence of urine due to involuntary bladder contractions that result in an urgent need to urinate

Urinary acidification The conversion of urine to a more acidic content

Urolithiasis Solid mineral deposits that form stones in the urinary tract

Common Drugs Used to Treat the Renal and Urinary Systems

Trade Name	Generic Name	Pronunciation
Loop Diuretics		
Bumex	bumetanide	(byew-**meh**-tah-nide)
Demadex	torsemide	(**tore**-sea-myde)
Edecrin	ethacrynic acid	(eth-a-**krin**-ik **as**-id)
Lasix	furosemide	(fyoor-**oh**-sah-myde)
Osmotic Diuretic		
Osmitrol	mannitol	(**man**-ah-tol)
Potassium-Sparing Diuretics		
Aldactone	spironolactone	(spir-own-oh-**lak**-tone)
Dyrenium	triamterene	(try-**am**-tur-een)
Midamor	amiloride	(ah-mill-or-ide)
Thiazide and Thiazide-Like Diuretics		
Microzide	hydrochlorothiazide	(hye-droe-klor-oh-**thy**-a-zide)
Thalitone	chlorthalidone	(klor-**thal**-ah-doan)
Zaroxolyn	metolazone	(me-**toe**-lah-zone)
Chronic Kidney Disease Agents		
Common Phosphorus Binding Agents		
PhosLo	calcium acetate	(**kal**-see-uhm **ass**-eh-tate)
Renagel, Renvela	sevelamer	(se-**vel**-a-mer)
Hematopoietic Agents (for Anemia in Chronic Renal Failure)		
Epogen, Procrit	epoetin alfa	(eh-**poh**-ee-tin **al**-fah)
Aranesp	darbepoetin alfa	(dar-be-**poh**-e-tin **al**-fa)
Iron Supplement		
Feosol	ferrous sulfate	(fair-**us** sul-**fate**)
Vitamin D Analog		
Rocaltrol	calcitriol	(**kal**-si-**trye**-ol)
Antibiotics to Treat Urinary Tract Infections (UTIs)		
Cipro	ciprofloxacin	(sip-roe-**flox**-a-sin)
Keflex	cephalexin	(cef-a-**lex**-in)
Macrobid	nitrofurantoin	(**nye**-troe-fue-**ran**-toin)
Bactrim	sulfamethoxazole/trimethoprim	(sul-fa-meth-**ox**-a-zole/trye-**meth**-oh-prim)
Agents for the Treatment of Overactive Bladder (OAB)		
Ditropan, Oxytrol, Gelnique	oxybutynin	(**ox**-i-**bue**-ti-nin)
Toviaz	fesoterodine	(**fes**-oh-**ter**-oh-deen)
Detrol	tolterodine	(tol-**ter**-oh-deen)
Vesicare	solifenacin succinate	(sol-ee-**fen**-a-sin **suhk**-suh-neyt)
Enablex	darifenacin	(dar-e-**fen**-a-sin)
Sanctura	trospium chloride	(trose-**pee**-um **klor**-ide)

The kidneys are the major organs of both the renal and urinary systems. The kidneys are responsible for maintenance of the chemical composition of electrolytes, fluids, and tissues in the body, including acid-base balance, preservation of normal blood pressure, and production of hormones such as the active form of vitamin D, renin, and erythropoietin. This chapter discusses the location and function of the various components of the renal and urological systems and provides an overview of the treatment of common conditions that can affect these systems.

Anatomy and Physiology of the Renal and Urological Systems

The kidneys are located inside the upper abdominal cavity, with one kidney positioned on each side of the vertebral column (Figure 21-1). The right kidney is located a little lower than the left kidney because the liver is positioned directly above it. The kidneys are shaped much like a kidney bean, with a small indentation called the *hilus*. Blood enters the kidneys at the hilus from the **renal artery** (Figure 21-2). Blood is then filtered in the kidney as it passes through a series of structures. Important **ions**, such as sodium and chloride, are reabsorbed into the body and circulatory system. The **renal vein** and ureter leave the kidney at the hilus. The renal vein returns the blood to the body after it has undergone the filtration process in the kidney. The ureters carry wastes removed from the blood to the bladder, where the waste is stored for excretion as urine (Figure 21-1).

The bladder is similar to a holding tank that can expand, depending on the volume of urine it contains. When the bladder becomes full, we feel the

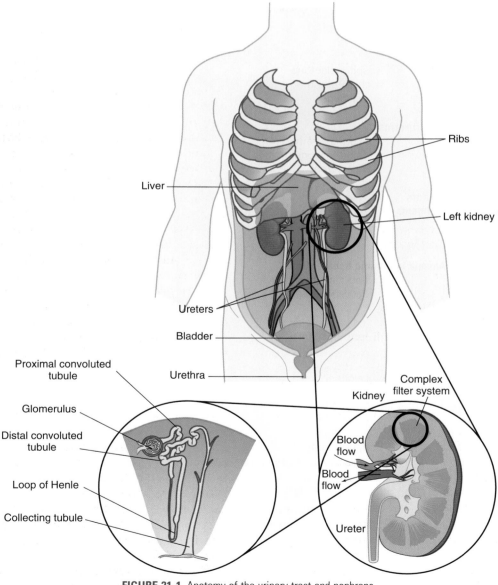

FIGURE 21-1 Anatomy of the urinary tract and nephrons.

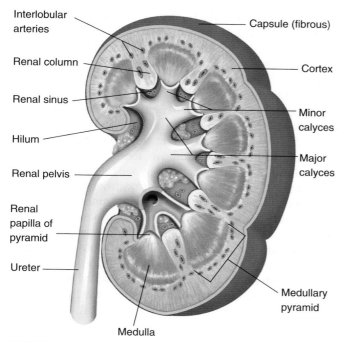

FIGURE 21-2 Kidney structure. (From McCance KL: *Pathophysiology: the biologic basis for disease in adults and children,* ed 6, St Louis, 2010, Mosby.)

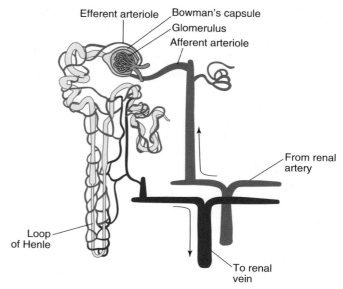

FIGURE 21-3 Nephron anatomy.

urge to urinate. The urine is eliminated through the urethra, a short tube leading from the bladder to the outside of the body.

Function of the Kidneys

The kidneys play a crucial role in the body and regulate a variety of bodily processes. Waste products are constantly being developed by the body as by-products of normal metabolism by active tissues (e.g., muscles) and from the digestion of the food we eat. Ultimately the blood is filtered as it passes through the kidneys, which remove these wastes, and the cleansed blood (and other vital components, such as proteins) is returned to the body. Waste products filtered out of the blood by the kidneys enter the urinary system and are ultimately excreted through the urine.

Excretion is one of the four major important metabolic functions of the body. These four functions are:

- *Absorption:* The intake of liquids, solids, and gases into the body
- *Distribution:* The way in which chemicals, nutrients, and drugs are separated and sent throughout the body to their target organs and tissues
- *Metabolism:* The chemical changes and reactions that occur in the body system; metabolism includes anabolism (building up processes) and catabolism (breaking down processes)
- *Excretion:* The elimination of chemicals and substances from the body system

Normal urinary output for an adult is 1 to 2 L per day. Urine contains urea, which is produced by the liver. Urea is a form of nitrogen that, upon standing for a time in the presence of oxygen, changes to ammonia, which causes the characteristic smell of urine. As mentioned, another important function of the kidneys is balancing the fluid and electrolyte content of the body. The kidneys balance ions in the blood and eliminate excess ions through excretion in the urine. The fluid that is filtered out of the blood by the kidneys, referred to as *filtrate,* is composed of water, ions (e.g., sodium, potassium, chloride), glucose (sugar), and small proteins. If electrolyte concentrations fall out of balance, which can occur if the kidneys are not filtering appropriately, conditions such as metabolic acidosis or **alkalosis** can develop. **Acidosis** occurs when too many free hydrogen ions (H^+) are present in the fluids of the body, and alkalosis occurs when there is either retention of bicarbonate (HCO_3^-) or excessive loss of hydrogen ions. Although the kidneys are only about the size of a fist, they manage to filter about 45 gallons of blood daily.

Nephron Function

The functional unit of the kidney is the **nephron.** Nephrons are primarily responsible for the regulation of fluids, solutes, and wastes in the body. Each kidney contains millions of microscopic nephrons (Figure 21-3). Each nephron is shaped like an inverted pyramid, and its tubules have many twists and turns. The nephrons actively filter the blood 24 hours a day. The following is a systematic look at the filtering process as the flow of blood enters the kidney (Figure 21-3).

1. The renal artery enters the kidney and divides into progressively smaller vessels until it becomes

the afferent arterioles. Blood then passes from the afferent arterioles into a cluster of capillaries called the *glomerulus*. Each glomerulus is surrounded by a double-layered epithelial cup that resembles a baseball glove; this structure is called *Bowman's capsule*.

2. Blood cells, platelets, and large proteins cannot pass through the capillaries of the glomerulus into Bowman's capsule. Only plasma can pass through the glomerulus. **Plasma** is the liquid component of blood, which is mostly water. However, some of the components of plasma (e.g., albumin and antibodies) are too large to leave the capillaries. Other components of plasma include toxins, which may accumulate in the blood. These are frequently very small and can leave the capillaries easily and enter Bowman's capsule.

3. The filtrate from Bowman's capsule travels down the descending tubule (also called the *proximal convoluted tubule*). It then completes a U-turn through the *loop of Henle*, and returns up the ascending tubule (called the *distal convoluted tubule*).

4. As the filtrate passes through the nephron tubules, various nutrients, water, and important chemical ions (e.g., sodium, chloride, and potassium) are pulled out of the filtrate (i.e., reabsorbed) and returned to the plasma to be used by the body. At the same time, other ions in the tubules (e.g., those in excess) are excreted.

5. The filtrate, now called urine, travels from the nephrons to the **collecting ducts**.

6. The collecting ducts empty directly into the ureter.

7. The ureter extends from the hilus of each kidney directly to the bladder.

8. The bladder empties the urine into the urethra for elimination.

 Tech Note!

Sodium is an important electrolyte that helps conduct nerve impulses and balance fluid in the body; sodium content is regulated through reabsorption in the kidneys.

Tubular Reabsorption

An important function of the nephrons is carrying out **tubular reabsorption**. As mentioned before, the filtrate produced in the nephron contains water, ions, glucose, and other molecules that are small enough to pass through the glomerulus. Some molecules in the filtrate eventually are excreted in urine; however, others, such as glucose (sugar), water, sodium, chloride, and amino acids, are still needed by the body. This is where tubular reabsorption comes in. The nephrons can reabsorb these small molecules so that they can reenter the plasma for use by the body. This process takes place at various

points along the proximal convoluted tubule, distal convoluted tubule, and loop of Henle (Figure 21-4). This concept is very important to understanding how diuretic medications (used in the treatment of edema and hypertension) work.

Tubular reabsorption is a critical process that enables the kidneys to carry out another important function; regulation of the acid-base balance of the body. Two mechanisms affect the balance of ions. The first is ion exchange. Sodium ions are pulled out of the tubules and are exchanged for hydrogen ions. As sodium accumulates on the outside of the proximal convoluted tubules, it creates an osmotic gradient, and water molecules are drawn toward the higher concentration of sodium in an effort to equilibrate the sodium concentration. The movement of water molecules is called **osmosis** (Figure 21-5). The overall effect is a decrease in excreted water. Ion exchange also can take place in the distal convoluted tubule. As sodium ions exit the distal convoluted tubule, they are exchanged for potassium ions. The loop of Henle has a different transport mechanism, called *active transport* (see Figure 21-4). Instead of an exchange of ions, there is a one-way uptake of sodium and chloride from the loop of Henle. These ions return to the circulatory system. Overall, most of the sodium that enters the renal system is reabsorbed.

Tubular Secretion

Tubular secretion is another major function of the nephrons. This function takes place throughout the nephron. Various ions, toxins, and water are secreted into the collecting duct. First, molecules such as toxins, water-soluble molecules, and excess or unnecessary chemicals (including some medications) are excreted. The second function of secretion is to allow the kidneys to regulate the pH of the blood through **urinary acidification**. This is why urine has a pH of 4 to 5, whereas the pH of blood is maintained at approximately 7.4.

As hydrogen ions are taken into the nephron, they combine with other molecules to produce bicarbonate. This is released into the bloodstream, where it regulates the overall pH of the body, helping to maintain homeostasis. Bicarbonate is a buffer. A buffer has the ability to bind hydrogen (which creates a basic environment) or release hydrogen (which creates an acidic environment), balancing the pH of the blood. To put it another way, an acid can release hydrogen ions, whereas a base can remove hydrogen ions by binding to them. The extra hydrogen ions are taken into the tubules and eventually excreted.

The kidneys are also responsible for the production of **renin**, an enzyme that plays a role in maintaining water balance in the body. When the body is under stress (causing a loss of fluids), the kidneys

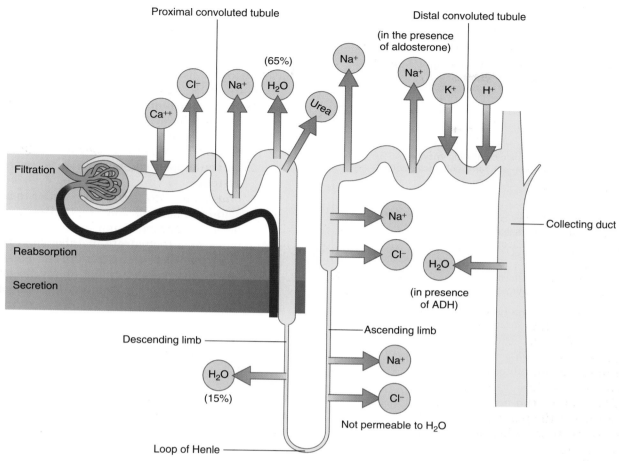

FIGURE 21-4 Tubular reabsorption and secretion.

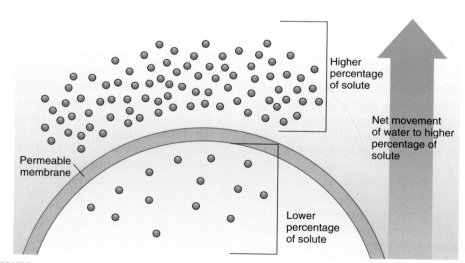

FIGURE 21-5 Osmotic gradient: the smaller water molecules gravitate toward the highly concentrated sodium ions.

secrete renin. The renin is released into the bloodstream, where it transforms angiotensinogen into angiotensin I, which circulates throughout the system. Angiotensin I is transformed in the liver to angiotension II. The formation of angiotensin II

activates the adrenal cortex, which begins to excrete aldosterone (a hormone); the aldosterone circulates back to the kidneys, where it activates the kidneys to increase the reabsorption of fluids (Figure 21-6). This overall effect increases the volume of fluids

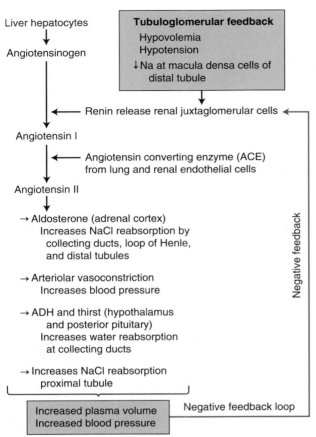

FIGURE 21-6 Renin-angiotensin-aldosterone system. (From McCance KL: *Pathophysiology: the biologic basis for disease in adults and children,* ed 6, St Louis, 2010, Mosby.)

throughout the body, which increases blood pressure to protect against dehydration.

Importance of Electrolytes

An important function of the kidneys is to maintain homeostasis by balancing the levels of electrolytes in the body. To understand the importance of the kidneys' regulation of electrolytes, it is important to understand some of the functions of these ions in the body:

- **Cations**
  - *Calcium (Ca^{2+}):* Bone and teeth formation, cell membrane integrity, cardiac conduction, nerve impulse conduction, muscle contraction, hormone secretion
  - *Potassium (K$^+$):* Necessary for glycogen (sugar) deposits in the liver (to maintain blood sugar levels) and skeletal muscles (for energy); aids in nerve impulse and cardiac conduction; helps in contraction in skeletal and smooth muscles
  - *Magnesium (Mg^{2+}):* Aids in cardiac and skeletal muscle excitability, enzyme activities, and neurochemical activities

- *Sodium (Na$^+$):* Maintains water balance, nerve impulse transmission, and regulation of acid-base balance; participates in cellular chemical reactions
- **Anions**
  - *Chloride (Cl$^-$):* The main anion in the transport of sodium, hydrogen, and potassium; essential to acid-base balance
  - *Bicarbonate (HCO$_3^-$):* The most important chemical that acts as a buffer; it is essential for the proper acid-base balance for the body system
  - *Phosphate (PO$_4^{3-}$):* Aids as a buffer to balance acid-base regulation in cells; promotes normal neuromuscular action and participates in carbohydrate metabolism; essential for formation and strength of bones and teeth; also necessary for many biochemical pathways (e.g., production of energy, cell division)

Conditions Affecting the Renal and Urological Systems

It seems as though it would be impossible for individuals to survive without the constant functioning of both kidneys; however, many people live with just one kidney. The kidneys are so efficient that as little as 20% of a kidney needs to function for a person to survive. In spite of the kidneys' resiliency and efficiency, it is still very important for people to closely monitor their diet, medications, and activities to maintain kidney health. It is reassuring to know, however, that many people can live normal lives with only one kidney or partial kidney function. In some cases, however, dialysis or even kidney transplantation may be necessary.

Although not discussed in this chapter in detail, other conditions that can affect the renal and urinary systems in general include blockages or infections of the kidney, ureter, bladder, or urethra. If residual urine does not leave the bladder, infection can easily result. Drinking plenty of water is one of the most effective ways of taking care of the urinary system because it helps to flush the body of toxins and other unwanted chemicals.

Common Conditions Associated with the Renal and Urological Systems

As noted previously, a variety of conditions can affect the renal and urological systems, ranging from blockages to infections to chronic conditions. This section describes some of the more common disorders associated with the renal and urological systems and discusses medications commonly used to treat these conditions.

TABLE 21-1

Stages of Chronic Kidney Disease

Stage	Severity	GFR Range (mL/min)	Symptoms
1	Kidney damage with normal or increased GFR	≥90	Usually absent, mild hypertension
2	Kidney damage with a mild decrease in GFR	60-89	Mild hypertension
3	Moderate decrease in GFR	30-59	Mild hypertension
4	Severe decrease in GFR	15-29	Moderate hypertension, hyperphosphatemia, anemia
5	End-stage renal disease (ESRD)	<15	Severe hypertension, hyperphosphatemia, anemia

Resource: National Kidney Foundation. KDOQI clinical practice guidelines for chronic kidney disease: evaluation, classification, and stratification. (Referenced September 6, 2014.) https://www.kidney.org/professionals/kdoqi/guidelines_ckd/p4_class_g1.htm.
GFR, Glomerular filtration rate.

Chronic Kidney Disease

Chronic kidney disease (CKD) is the progressive loss of renal function. Diabetes mellitus and uncontrolled hypertension are the most common causes of CKD in adults in the United States. Other potential causes of CKD include kidney diseases such as glomerulonephritis, pyelonephritis, and vascular disorders. Kidney function, in general, decreases with age; older individuals have CKD more often than younger adults. As a kidney ages, it is less able to compensate for fluid imbalances in the body. Depending on the level of disease, CKD is stratified into five stages, based on the glomerular filtration rate (GFR), which is a measure of how well the kidneys are filtering (Table 21-1). The progression of CKD is thought to be associated with a series of common changes in the kidneys, including glomerular hypertension and hyperfiltration, glomerulosclerosis, and inflammation of the tubules.

As renal failure progresses, every part of the body can be affected due to the buildup of waste products and an imbalance of fluids. Early symptoms include fatigue, headache, shortness of breath (SOB), sudden weight changes, and edema. Symptoms can progress to include a variety of other systemic symptoms (Table 21-2). Anemia is a common symptom of more advanced CKD because the kidneys produce the hormone **erythropoietin**. When kidney function declines, less erythropoietin is produced, leading to a decrease in red blood cell production and the development of anemia.

Prognosis. The gradual decline of kidney function in people with CKD is often asymptomatic initially but can progress to cause volume overload, metabolic acidosis, hypertension,

TABLE 21-2

Select Systemic Effects of Chronic Kidney Disease

System	Effect
Cardiovascular	Hypertension, heart failure
Respiratory	Pulmonary edema, dyspnea
Gastrointestinal	Nausea, vomiting, gastrointestinal bleeding
Endocrine	Hyperparathyroidism, osteomalacia
Immunologic	Suppressed immunological responses, increased infection risk
Nervous	Fatigue, peripheral neuropathy

anemia, and bone disease. These outcomes can lead to morbidity in this patient population, but studies show that not all people with early CKD experience a progression of loss of kidney function; therefore, the prognosis can be highly variable. When the disease does progress, however, people with CKD have a substantially increased risk of cardiovascular disease and risk of death. In fact, the risk of death in people with CKD is higher than the risk of progression to dialysis.

Non–Drug Treatment. Dietary management is very important in the treatment of CKD. The intake of foods high in phosphates (e.g., colas) and dairy products (e.g., milk, cheese) is often limited in these patients. For those with significant edema and/or hypertension, moderation of sodium intake is important. Protein restriction may also be warranted, with studies showing that this may help reduce damage to the kidneys.

Dialysis is a procedure in which waste products are removed from the blood of patients with end-stage renal disease (ESRD). Dialysis is used to compensate for a lack of filtration by the kidneys to remove waste products from the blood and balance electrolytes and fluid volume. Two major methods are used today, hemodialysis and peritoneal dialysis. Although each of these types of dialysis has drawbacks, they are life-sustaining treatments. Negative aspects of dialysis include the additional medications that patients must take to further balance pH and fluids, the inconvenience of having to be stationary for a length of time during a dialysis session, and the fact that even sophisticated machinery cannot perform as efficiently as the body's own kidneys.

Hemodialysis requires the patient to visit a clinic or hospital for treatment. A vein shunt (needle puncture with a reinforced opening) is used to connect the patient's bloodstream to the dialysis machine. The dialysis machine uses a mechanical filtration system to clean a small but steady stream of blood from the patient's body. Although the length of treatment varies, traditional hemodialysis normally takes 3 hours or longer two or three times weekly.

Peritoneal dialysis is an alternative to hemodialysis. The patient's bloodstream is connected to a bag of osmotic solution. A catheter plug is implanted into the abdominal cavity for administration and removal of a solution known as **dialysate**. The osmotic solution (dialysate) flows into the peritoneal cavity. The peritoneal membrane is a thin lining that encases the organs of the abdomen, including the stomach, liver, spleen, and kidneys. The osmotic solution works in the same fashion as the sodium gradient works in the kidneys. As the solution is allowed to fill the cavity, wastes are pulled into the solution, where they can be drained from the cavity into an empty bag attached to the outside of the abdominal wall. This treatment usually is done several times daily to keep toxin levels to a minimum. Treatment can be done at home; however, peritoneal dialysis can also be performed in clinics if the patient cannot afford a home health nurse for assistance (Figure 21-7). It is important that aseptic technique be used when performing this type of dialysis to prevent **peritonitis**, an infection in the abdominal cavity.

Nocturnal hemodialysis is another form of dialysis that allows the patient to receive treatment while sleeping. Dialysis treatment is done using the help of a portable peritoneal or hemodialysis machine, 8 to 12 hours per night. Patients do not have to wait between treatments, which is when they begin to feel the effects of toxic buildup; in addition, patients do not have to spend several hours immobilized at a dialysis clinic. If dialysis is done in a home setting, the patient must be able to troubleshoot problems with the machinery if

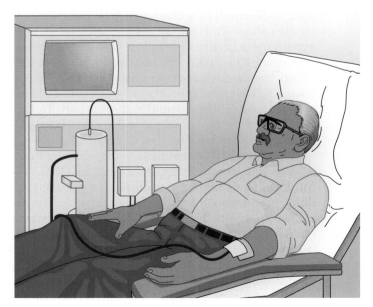

Hemodialysis

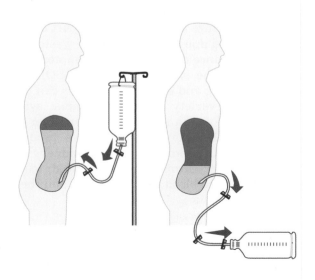

Continuous ambulatory peritoneal dialysis

FIGURE 21-7 Two types of dialysis.

there is a malfunction. Finally, the patient usually must have a home health nurse to help with the treatment.

Drug Treatment. People receiving dialysis have to be careful of their fluid and salt intake. With any of these treatments, a loss of ions and nutrients must be replaced with supplements each time dialysis is performed. One of the most common side effects of ESRD is anemia, as previously described. For this condition, iron and erythropoietin are often used. Iron supplements can increase the oxygen-carrying capacity of the hemoglobin in red blood cells. Hemoglobin is a protein in the red blood cells that carries oxygen with the help of iron. Other medications may include vitamin supplements, antihypertensives, and phosphorus-lowering medications such as calcium carbonate, calcium acetate, and sevelamer. Vitamin D supplements are often used because the kidneys are important in the synthesis of the active form of vitamin D, which places people with CKD at risk of having weak bones.

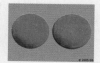

GENERIC NAME: ferrous sulfate (OTC)
TRADE NAME: None
INDICATION: Iron deficiency anemia
ROUTE OF ADMINISTRATION: Oral
COMMON ADULT DOSAGE: 325 mg one to three times per day
MECHANISM OF ACTION: Increases iron concentrations in the blood to help increase the production of red blood cells
SIDE EFFECTS: Constipation, black stools

GENERIC NAME: epoetin alfa
TRADE NAME: Epogen, Procrit
INDICATION: Anemia
ROUTE OF ADMINISTRATION: Subcutaneous (SUBCUT); intravenous (IV)
COMMON ADULT DOSAGE: 50-100 units/kg IV or SUBCUT three times weekly initially, dose adjusted based on response and hemoglobin levels

MECHANISM OF ACTION: Stimulates the production of red blood cells, mimics the action of endogenous erythropoietin
SIDE EFFECTS: Hypertension, headache, injection site reactions, rash
AUXILIARY LABELS:
- Refrigerate.
- Do not shake.
- Protect from light.

GENERIC NAME: darbepoetin alfa
TRADE NAME: Aranesp
INDICATION: Anemia
ROUTE OF ADMINISTRATION: Subcutaneous; intravenous
COMMON ADULT DOSAGE: 0.45 mcg/kg IV or SUBCUT once weekly or 0.75 mcg/kg every 2 weeks initially, with dose adjustments based on response and hemoglobin levels in adults receiving hemodialysis
MECHANISM OF ACTION: Stimulates the production of red blood cells, mimics the action of endogenous erythropoietin
SIDE EFFECTS: Hypertension, headache, injection site reactions, rash
AUXILIARY LABELS:
- Refrigerate.
- Do not shake.
- Protect from light.

GENERIC NAME: calcium carbonate (OTC)
TRADE NAME: Tums
INDICATION: Hyperphosphatemia
ROUTE OF ADMINISTRATION: Oral
COMMON ADULT DOSAGE: 500-2000 mg three times daily with meals; adjusted based on calcium and phosphate levels
MECHANISM OF ACTION: Binds to dietary phosphate in the gastrointestinal (GI) tract to inhibit its absorption, reducing phosphate levels
SIDE EFFECTS: Constipation

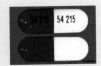

GENERIC NAME: calcium acetate (Rx)
TRADE NAME: PhosLo
INDICATION: Hyperphosphatemia
ROUTE OF ADMINISTRATION: Oral
COMMON ADULT DOSAGE: 1334 mg (2 tablets or gel caps) three times daily with meals; adjusted based on calcium and phosphate levels
MECHANISM OF ACTION: Binds to dietary phosphate in the GI tract to inhibit its absorption, reducing phosphate levels
SIDE EFFECTS: Constipation
AUXILIARY LABELS:
- Protect from moisture.
- Take with meals.

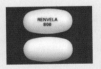

GENERIC NAME: sevelamer (Rx only)
TRADE NAME: Renagel, Renvela
INDICATION: Hyperphosphatemia
ROUTE OF ADMINISTRATION: Oral
COMMON ADULT DOSAGE: 800-1600 mg three times daily with meals; dose based on phosphate levels
MECHANISM OF ACTION: Binds to dietary phosphate in the GI tract to inhibit its absorption, reducing phosphate levels
SIDE EFFECTS: Headache, heartburn, diarrhea
AUXILIARY LABELS:
- Protect from moisture.
- Take with meals.

GENERIC NAME: calcitriol
TRADE NAME: Rocaltrol
INDICATION: Renal osteodystrophy
ROUTE OF ADMINISTRATION: Oral
COMMON ADULT DOSAGE: 0.25-1 mcg/day for most patients; based on serum calcium levels and other parameters

MECHANISM OF ACTION: Active form of vitamin D; does not require activation by the kidneys
SIDE EFFECTS: Hypercalcemia (elevated calcium levels)
AUXILIARY LABEL:
- Do not crush or chew.

Kidney Stones

Kidney stones are small aggregations of material (usually calcium, magnesium, or uric acid salts) that form in the kidney and/or urinary tract. Hundreds of thousands of Americans experience a condition known as **urolithiasis** (kidney stones) every year. Although stones are most common in people between the ages of 20 and 55, they can affect anyone. One of the first signs of a kidney stone is pain during urination. Kidney stones often pass naturally through the urine without treatment. For stones that cannot be easily passed, medical treatment is often necessary. In severe cases, kidney stones can actually cause a blockage in the urinary tract, which is a serious medical situation. Symptoms that may occur with a blockage can include fever, vomiting, blood in the urine, and extreme flank, back, and/or abdominal pain. Different types of stones can form at different locations in the urinary tract (Figure 21-8).

Prognosis. Patients have several options for kidney stone removal and prevention. Through dietary changes and medication, people can limit the possible development of future stones.

Non–Drug Treatment. If the stone is small enough, no treatment may be needed other than pain management and fluid intake while the stone passes through the urinary tract. For larger stones, a variety of procedures can be used, based on the composition of the stone. **Lithotripsy** is the use of shock waves to break up kidney stones. **Ureteroscopy** can also be used. In this procedure, a ureteroscope, which is a lighted instrument that can be inserted through the urethra, is used to retrieve the stone or stones with the help of an attached camera and endoscopic instruments. More invasive surgical procedures may be used to retrieve stones, depending on their size and location. Drinking plenty of water is important in treatment and prevention because this helps to flush out any small stones and may help prevent the formation of future stones.

Drug Treatments. Analgesics can be used for relieving pain; common over-the-counter (OTC) drugs that can be used include a variety of nonsteroidal antiinflammatory drugs (NSAIDs) and acetaminophen. Calcium channel blockers (CCBs)

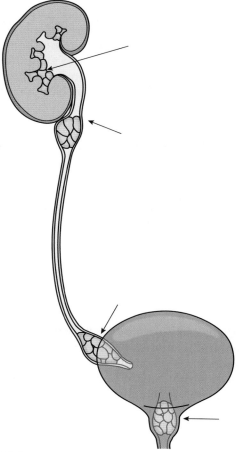

FIGURE 21-8 Common locations of kidney stones. (From Monahan F et al: *Phipps' medical-surgical nursing: health and illness perspectives,* ed 8, St Louis, 2007, Mosby.)

(e.g., nifedipine) and alpha-blockers (e.g., tamsulosin) can be used to accelerate the passage of stones. The mechanism of action of CCBs is unclear; however, it is known that they act on the ureter. Agents used to prevent calcium stones include thiazide diuretics and potassium citrate. Agents to prevent formation of uric acid stones are allopurinol and potassium citrate.

GENERIC NAME: allopurinol
TRADE NAME: Zyloprim
INDICATION: Kidney stones, gout
ROUTE OF ADMINISTRATION: Oral
COMMON ADULT DOSAGE: 200-300 mg once daily or in divided doses

MECHANISM OF ACTION: Inhibits the enzyme xanthine oxidase, which blocks the production of uric acid
SIDE EFFECTS: Nausea, vomiting, dyspepsia, rash
AUXILIARY LABELS:
• May cause dizziness/drowsiness.
• Take with a full glass of water.

GENERIC NAME: potassium citrate
TRADE NAME: Urocit-K
INDICATION: Kidney stones, renal tubular acidosis
ROUTE OF ADMINISTRATION: Oral
COMMON ADULT DOSAGE: 10-20 mEq three times daily with meals (max 100 mEq/day)
MECHANISM OF ACTION: Increases urine pH and citrate concentrations in the urine to produce urine that is less likely to lead to crystallization of stones
SIDE EFFECTS: Nausea, vomiting, diarrhea, gas
AUXILIARY LABEL:
• Take with food.

Edema

Edema is a buildup of fluid in tissues of the body. Edema can occur in the extremities (peripheral edema), the lungs (pulmonary edema), and other areas of the body. Fluids are normally stored in the blood and **interstitial spaces** (spaces around cells). As a result of various conditions, fluids can accumulate in other tissues, leading to edema (Box 21-1). The two general types of peripheral edema are pitting edema and nonpitting edema. Pitting is observed when an indentation on the surface of the skin can be made by applying pressure (Figure 21-9); this is often associated with high-salt diets and/or heart failure (HF). (Chapter 18 presents a more detailed discussion of edema associated with HF.) Nonpitting edema does not leave a skin indentation and can prove more difficult to treat due to the underlying cause.

Prognosis. In some cases edema may be a temporary condition that corrects itself within a couple of days. Causes of temporary edema can include high altitude, exercise, or medication. For individuals who have chronic forms of edema, medications and dietary modifications can be used to help control this condition. People with HF

BOX 21-1

Select Causes of Edema

Chronic venous insufficiency: Attributable to poor blood flow caused by a weakness in the veins; often seen in older and obese people

Cirrhosis: Chronic hepatic disease characterized by destruction and fibrotic regeneration of hepatic cells.

Heart failure: Decreased ability to function properly because of overload. Can occur after myocardial infarction or be due to CHF, cardiomyopathy, or coronary artery disease (CAD)

High salt intake: Can cause fluids to be retained in cells if kidneys cannot eliminate excess sodium and fluids

Kidney disease: Inability of the kidneys to function properly in regulation of fluids. Due to hypertension, diabetes, or any condition affecting any part of the renal system

Thrombophlebitis: Inflammation of the veins due to clot formation. Can be caused by trauma, inactivity, or varicose veins

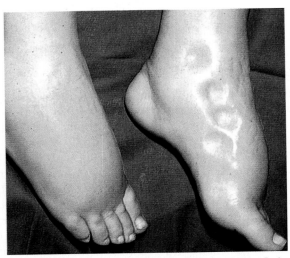

FIGURE 21-9 Pitting edema. (From Bloom A, Ireland J, Watkins P: *A colour atlas of diabetes,* ed 2, St Louis, 1992, Mosby.)

typically take chronic medications to manage their edema.

Non–Drug Treatment. As mentioned previously, sodium restriction can be helpful in managing edema. Elevating the legs above chest additionally can help move the fluid toward the heart and reduce peripheral edema for some patients. Support stockings can be worn to help deter the buildup of excess fluids in the legs.

Drug Treatment. Whether edema is treated with medications depends on its underlying cause.

For example, medication-induced edema is not likely to respond to diuretic treatment. For this reason, it is important to determine the cause of the edema, not just manage the symptoms. For most causes of edema, the main drugs prescribed are diuretics. Classes of **diuretics** include the thiazides, thiazide-like agents, loop diuretics, potassium-sparing diuretics, carbonic anhydrase inhibitors, and osmotic diuretics. Each classification is discussed, along with its drug action and an example of each medication. The normal dosage given is an adult maintenance dose for the treatment of edema (Table 21-3). Certain diuretics (e.g., loop diuretics, thiazides, and potassium-sparing agents) are also commonly used for the treatment of chronic hypertension because they lower blood pressure by reducing blood volume, cardiac output, and systemic vascular resistance.

Thiazides and Thiazide-like Agents. Thiazides (e.g., hydrochlorothiazide) and thiazide-like diuretics (e.g., metolazone) act by inducing an equal increase in the urinary excretion of the ions sodium and chloride. These agents accomplish this by inhibiting the normal process of reabsorption of sodium and chloride in the distal convoluted tubule. They also lower the urinary excretion of calcium and increase the loss of potassium. Because of the loss of potassium, a potassium supplement may be taken concurrently with this type of medication if it is prescribed chronically, unless other drugs that preserve potassium are used at the same time. Thiazides can also be used for hypertension and to prevent the formation of kidney stones, as previously mentioned.

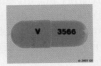

GENERIC NAME: hydrochlorothiazide (HCTZ)
TRADE NAME: Microzide
INDICATION: Edema, hypertension
ROUTE OF ADMINISTRATION: Oral
COMMON ADULT DOSAGE: 12.5-50 mg daily or intermittently
MECHANISM OF ACTION: Increases the excretion of sodium, chloride, and water by inhibiting sodium ion transport across the renal tubules
SIDE EFFECTS: Hypotension, photosensitivity, increased blood sugar, increased uric acid
AUXILIARY LABEL:
• May cause photosensitivity.

TABLE 21-3

Select Diuretic Medications

Generic Name	Trade Name	Common Side Effects	Common Dose Range
Loop Diuretics			
Inhibit sodium and chloride reabsorption in the loop of Henle and on the proximal and distal tubules			
furosemide	Lasix	• Hypotension • Headache • Weakness	• 10-80 mg orally or intravenously (PO/IV) 1-2 times daily (max 600 mg/day)
bumetanide	Bumex		• 0.5-1 mg PO/IV 1-2 times daily (max 10 mg/day)
torsemide	Demadex		• 5-20 mg PO/IV once daily (max 200 mg)
ethacrynic acid	Edecrin		• 50-200 mg/day PO in 1-2 divided doses (max 400 mg daily)
Thiazide-Type Diuretics			
Block reabsorption of sodium and chloride ions, increasing the amount of sodium crossing the distal tubule and thus increasing water excretion through the kidneys			
hydrochlorothiazide (HCTZ)	Microzide	• Low blood pressure • Photosensitivity	• 12.5-50 mg PO in 1-2 doses daily (max 200 mg daily)
chlorthalidone	Thalitone		• 12.5-50 mg PO once daily (max 100-200 mg daily)
metolazone	Zaroxolyn		• 2.5-10 mg PO once daily (max 20 mg daily)
Potassium-Sparing Diuretics			
Inhibit sodium reabsorption at distal convoluted tubule, cortical collecting tubule, and collecting duct and reduce potassium excretion			
triamterene	Dyrenium	• Low blood pressure • Muscle cramps • Headache	• 50-100 mg PO 1-2 times daily (max 300 mg daily)
amiloride	Midamor		• 5-10 mg PO 1-2 times daily (max 20 mg daily)
Aldosterone Antagonists/Potassium-Sparing Diuretics			
Compete against aldosterone for receptors in the distal renal tubules, which increases sodium and water excretion while retaining potassium			
spironolactone	Aldactone	• Gynecomastia • Decreased libido • Nausea • Vomiting • Diarrhea • Hypotension	• 25-200 mg/day PO in 1-2 divided doses
eplerenone	Inspra		• 50 mg PO 1-2 times daily (max 100 mg daily)
Carbonic Anhydrase Inhibitors			
Inhibit the reabsorption of bicarbonate in the proximal convoluted tubule and increase the excretion of water, sodium, and potassium			
acetazolamide	Diamox	• Hypokalemia • Hyponatremia • Metabolic acidosis • Hyperglycemia • Flushing • Hypotension	• 250-500 mg PO 1-2 times daily (max 1000 mg daily)

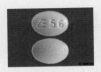

GENERIC NAME: metolazone
TRADE NAME: Zaroxolyn
INDICATION: Edema, hypertension
ROUTE OF ADMINISTRATION: Oral
COMMON ADULT DOSAGE: 2.5-20 mg daily
MECHANISM OF ACTION: Increases the excretion of chloride, sodium, and water by inhibiting sodium transport across the renal tubule
SIDE EFFECTS: Hypotension, photosensitivity, increased blood sugar, increased uric acid
AUXILIARY LABEL:
- May cause photosensitivity.

Loop Diuretics. Loop diuretics inhibit reabsorption of sodium and chloride in the proximal convoluted tubule, distal convoluted tubule, and loop of Henle. Because of the strong action of these agents, a great deal of potassium is lost with urination. Potassium supplements are often needed to maintain potassium levels and are typically prescribed at the same time as a loop diuretic. Loop diuretics normally are prescribed to be taken early in the day to avoid excessive nocturia.

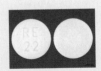

GENERIC NAME: furosemide
TRADE NAME: Lasix
INDICATION: Edema, hypertension, pulmonary edema
ROUTE OF ADMINISTRATION: Oral; intravenous
COMMON ADULT DOSAGE: 10-80 mg orally once daily; dose can vary by indication and practice setting.
MECHANISM OF ACTION: Inhibits sodium and chloride resorption in the ascending limb of the loop of Henle
SIDE EFFECTS: Dehydration, low potassium levels, hypotension
AUXILIARY LABELS:
- May cause dizziness.
- May cause photosensitivity.

Potassium-Sparing Agents. Because potassium-sparing agents function primarily in the distal convoluted tubule and inhibit sodium reabsorption, which reduces potassium loss, they do not cause large amounts of potassium to be excreted in the urine. With these types of agents, it is recommended that patients avoid consuming large quantities of potassium-rich foods; in addition, as is also true for loop diuretics, monitoring of potassium levels is an important aspect of treatment.

GENERIC NAME: spironolactone
TRADE NAME: Aldactone
INDICATION: Edema, hypertension, heart failure
ROUTE OF ADMINISTRATION: Oral
COMMON ADULT DOSAGE: 25-200 mg per day
MECHANISM OF ACTION: Inhibits the effects of aldosterone on the distal renal tubules
SIDE EFFECTS: Drowsiness, gynecomastia, high potassium levels (hyperkalemia)
AUXILIARY LABEL:
- May cause dizziness and drowsiness.

GENERIC NAME: triamterene
TRADE NAME: Dyrenium
INDICATION: Edema, ascites, hypokalemia
ROUTE OF ADMINISTRATION: Oral
COMMON ADULT DOSAGE: 50-100 mg twice daily
MECHANISM OF ACTION: Inhibits sodium-potassium ion exchange in the distal renal tubule, causing diuresis
SIDE EFFECTS: Nausea, headache, fatigue, hyperkalemia
AUXILIARY LABEL:
- Take with food.

Osmotic Diuretics. Osmotic diuretics inhibit tubular reabsorption of water by increasing the osmolarity of the glomerular filtrate. They are used for prophylaxis of acute renal failure when the GFR is reduced. The only osmotic agent used for the treatment of edema is mannitol (Osmitrol), which forces urine production in people with acute kidney failure. The increased urine production helps to prevent progression to CKD and also contributes to elimination of toxic substances from the body. The dosage is based on the patient's weight, and the medication is given intravenously.

 Tech Alert!

Mannitol is available only as an injectable solution. Mannitol must be stored at a temperature of 15° to 30°C (59° to 86°F); it has a tendency to crystallize at lower temperatures because of its high sugar content (e.g., the solution is supersaturated at room temperature). If mannitol crystallizes, it can be placed for short periods in 70°C water and periodically shaken vigorously. The vials cannot be warmed in a microwave because they may explode.

Urinary Tract Infection

A urinary tract infection (UTI) is an infection (either bacterial or fungal) of any part of the urinary tract (kidneys, bladder, ureters, and/or urethra). The most common cause of a UTI is the bacterium *Escherichia coli (E. coli)* acquired from the colon. If the infection is focused in the urethra, it is called **urethritis**. *Cystitis* indicates infection/inflammation of the bladder, and *pyelonephritis* is infection/inflammation of the kidney. Sexually transmitted diseases (STDs) are another cause of UTIs. People with various preexisting conditions may be more likely to have infections. Immunocompromised people are at risk because of a weakened immune system, and people with uncontrolled diabetes are at increased risk due to the elevated glucose levels in the urine. Symptoms vary with each type of infection but can include a painful, burning sensation when urinating, fever, lack of urine output, cloudy or bloody urine, nausea, and vomiting. Confusion is another possible symptom associated with UTIs.

Prognosis. The prognosis for UTIs is good if proper treatment is administered. For people experiencing frequent UTIs, prophylactic therapy may be necessary.

Non–Drug Treatment. Several precautions can be taken to minimize the risk of UTI. These include wiping from front to back after urination or defecation, making sure the genital area is cleaned both before and after sexual intercourse, and urinating after intercourse.

Drug Treatment. Antimicrobial agents are the main course of treatment for most UTIs. Select antibiotics for bacterial infections, in addition to other agents used for the symptomatic management of UTIs, are presented in Table 21-4. For symptomatic fungal urinary tract infections,

fluconazole (Diflucan) or other antifungal agents may be prescribed. Even though most symptoms resolve after the initiation of antibiotic therapy, it is important that the entire course of medication be finished to reduce the risk of recurrence or development of antibiotic resistance.

 Tech Note!

An infection that is acquired by the patient while in the hospital or an institutional setting is a **nosocomial infection.** Many nosocomial urinary tract infections are caused by catheterization or cystoscopic examinations. Regardless of the cause, it is important to determine the specific organism so that the proper medication can be prescribed. A new term used to describe this type of infection that may replace "nosocomial infection" in the near future is "health care–associated infection" (HAI).

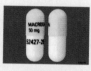

GENERIC NAME: nitrofurantoin
TRADE NAME: Macrobid, Macrodantin
INDICATION: UTI, cystitis
ROUTE OF ADMINISTRATION: Oral
COMMON ADULT DOSAGE: *Macrobid:* 100 mg twice daily for 7 days; *Macrodantin:* 50-100 mg four times daily for 7 days or for at least 3 days after resolution of infection
MECHANISM OF ACTION: Inhibits bacterial carbohydrate metabolism and cell wall formation
SIDE EFFECTS: Nausea, diarrhea, abdominal pain, drowsiness
AUXILIARY LABEL:
• Take until gone.

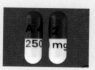

GENERIC NAME: cephalexin
TRADE NAME: Keflex
INDICATION: UTI, pneumonia, otitis media, other infections
ROUTE OF ADMINISTRATION: Oral
COMMON ADULT DOSAGE: 500 mg twice daily for 7 to 14 days

TABLE 21-4

Select Agents Used in the Treatment of Urinary Tract Infections*

Medication Class	Generic Name	Trade Name	Common Dose Range
Sulfonamide	sulfamethoxazole/ trimethoprim	Bactrim DS	• *DS:* 1 tablet (800 mg sulfamethoxazole/160 mg trimethoprim) orally (PO) 2 times daily for 3 days
Nitrofuran Antibacterial	nitrofurantoin	Macrobid	• 100 mg PO 2 times daily for 5 days
Fluoroquinolone	ciprofloxacin	Cipro	• 250 mg PO 2 times daily for 3 days
Fluoroquinolone	levofloxacin	Levaquin	• 250 mg PO 2 times daily for 3 days
Penicillin	amoxicillin/clavulanate	Augmentin	• 875 mg/125 mg PO 2 times daily for 10 days
Cephalosporin	cephalexin	Keflex	• 500 mg PO 2 times daily for 7 days
Penicillin and Aminoglycoside	ampicillin + gentamicin	Omnipen + Garamycin	• 1-2 g ampicillin intravenously (IV) every 6 hr with 1.5 mg/kg gentamicin IV every 8 hr
Urinary Analgesic	phenazopyridine	Pyridium	• 200 mg PO 3 times daily after meals as needed (prn) for 2 days
Urinary Antispasmodic	flavoxate	Urispas	• 100-200 mg PO 3-4 times daily; reduce dose as symptoms improve

*The treatment of urinary tract infections (UTIs) is tailored to specific organisms when applicable, and the duration and strength of therapy depends on the severity and location of the infection, in addition to the patient's age and history of UTIs.

MECHANISM OF ACTION: Inhibits bacterial cell wall synthesis
SIDE EFFECTS: Nausea, vomiting, diarrhea, dizziness
AUXILIARY LABELS:
- May cause dizziness.
- Take until gone.

 Tech Note!

The medication phenazopyridine is a urinary analgesic frequently used to treat pain associated with UTIs. It is available OTC and by prescription under a number of different brand names. One side effect is its tendency to turn urine orange or reddish in color, which should be noted with an auxiliary label on the prescription formulation.

Urinary Incontinence

A common condition that affects millions of Americans is incontinence, which is the loss of control of urination and/or defecation. This chapter discusses the issue of urinary incontinence, often referred to as *overactive bladder (OAB)*. Older adults, especially females, are more prone to this condition; women who have multiple pregnancies tend to develop this condition later in life because of the stretching of pelvic muscles during childbirth.

Micturition is the medical term used to describe urination. Although the bladder can store almost 1 L of fluid, receptors are triggered when the bladder is approximately half full to tell us that it is time to empty the bladder. Even after urinating, a small amount of urine (approximately 100 mL) always remains in the bladder. When a person coughs or sneezes, enough force may be placed on the bladder to release a small amount of urine. This is called **stress incontinence**. Weight gain also can intensify this type of condition. **Urge incontinence** is involuntary urination resulting from a sudden, uncontrollable impulse to urinate. Urge incontinence has several causes, such as decreased bladder capacity, infection, or irritation. In addition, increased fluid intake, including alcohol or caffeine ingestion, can increase the risk.

Prognosis. Often incontinence can be overcome if the patient seeks help from his or her physician. If incontinence cannot be corrected by nonpharmacological means or with the use of medication, certain medical procedures, including surgery, can be used.

Non–Drug Treatment. The most common non–drug therapy for most types of incontinence is pelvic muscle (Kegel) exercises. This is an exercise that involves strengthening of the pelvic floor muscles. The exercise requires that the patient tighten the muscles around the pelvis in the same fashion as he or she would to hold urine. The exercise regimen typically prescribed is three sets of 8 to 12 slow-velocity contractions sustained for 6 to 8 seconds each. These exercises are performed three or four times per week and continued for 15 to 20 weeks.

Drug Treatment. Anticholinergic medications are frequently used for the management of urge incontinence (Table 21-5).

TABLE 21-5

Select Antimuscarinic Medications* Used in the Treatment of Urinary Incontinence

Generic Name	Trade Name	Common Side Effects	Common Dose Range
oxybutynin	Ditropan Ditropan XL (extended release) Gelnique (gel formulation) Oxytrol (transdermal patch)	• Dry mouth (highest incidence with overactive bladder [OAB] medications) • Constipation • Confusion	• 5 mg orally (PO) 2-4 times daily • 5-30 mg PO once daily • 3% or 10%; apply correct gel content once daily to thigh, abdomen, or shoulder • *Patch:* 3.9 mg/day applied 2 times a week.
tolterodine	Detrol Detrol LA (extended release)	• Dry mouth • Constipation • Confusion	• 2 mg PO 2 times daily • 4 mg PO once daily
trospium	Sanctura Sanctura XR	• Dry mouth • Constipation • Confusion	• 20 mg PO 2 times daily, 1 hr before meals • 60 mg PO once daily, 1 hr before a meal
darifenacin	Enablex	• Constipation • Dry mouth • Confusion	• 7.5-15 mg PO once daily
solifenacin	Vesicare	• Dry mouth • Constipation • Confusion	• 5-10 mg PO once daily
fesoterodine	Toviaz	• Increased heart rate • Dry mouth • Constipation • Confusion	• 4-8 mg PO once daily

*Antimuscarinics inhibit the action of acetylcholine on smooth muscle, creating an antispasmodic effect.

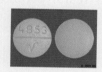

GENERIC NAME: oxybutynin
TRADE NAME: Ditropan, Ditropan XL, Oxytrol (Patch), Gelnique (topical gel), Oxytrol for Women (OTC Patch)
INDICATION: OAB
ROUTE OF ADMINISTRATION: Oral; transdermal
COMMON ADULT DOSAGE: *Tablet:* 5 mg two to three times daily; *extended-release tablets:* 5-30 mg once daily; *patch:* apply patch every 3-4 days; *Gel:* apply 1 packet topically once daily
MECHANISM OF ACTION: Relaxes bladder smooth muscle
SIDE EFFECTS: Dizziness, drowsiness, confusion, blurred vision, dry mouth, constipation
AUXILIARY LABELS:
• May cause dizziness/drowsiness.
• [Ditropan XL]: Do not crush, break, or chew.
• [Transdermal patch or gel]: For topical use only.

GENERIC NAME: tolterodine
TRADE NAME: Detrol, Detrol LA
INDICATION: OAB, urinary urgency
ROUTE OF ADMINISTRATION: Oral
COMMON ADULT DOSAGE: *Detrol:* 1-2 mg twice daily; *Detrol LA:* 2-4 mg once daily
MECHANISM OF ACTION: Relaxes bladder smooth muscle
SIDE EFFECTS: Dizziness, drowsiness, confusion, blurred vision, dry mouth, constipation
AUXILIARY LABELS:
• May cause dizziness.
• [Detrol LA]: Do not crush, break, or chew.

 Tech Alert!
Remember the following sound-alike, look-alike drugs:
chlorthalidone versus chlorothiazide
Bumex versus Buprenex
furosemide versus torsemide
metolazone versus metoclopramide
Ditropan versus diazepam

DO YOU REMEMBER THESE KEY POINTS?

- The anatomy of the renal and urological systems, and the names of their anatomical components
- The primary symptoms of the various conditions associated with the renal and urological systems
- Medications used to treat the various renal and urological conditions discussed

- The generic and trade names for the drugs discussed in this chapter
- The appropriate auxiliary labels that should be used when filling prescriptions for drugs discussed in this chapter

REVIEW QUESTIONS

Multiple Choice Questions

1. Blood enters the kidneys through the:
   A. Renal fascia
   B. Renal artery
   C. Renal vein
   D. Hilus

2. All of the following are components of the nephron *except:*
   A. The glomerulus
   B. The urethra
   C. Bowman's capsule
   D. The loop of Henle

3. When taking loop diuretics, it is often necessary to take which of the following supplements?
   A. Potassium
   B. Calcium
   C. Multivitamins
   D. All of the above

4. Which of the following is *not* a loop diuretic?
   A. Furosemide
   B. Chlorthalidone
   C. Bumetanide
   D. Torsemide

5. Buffers have the ability to prevent:
   A. Large changes in pH
   B. Edema
   C. Renal failure
   D. Blood loss

6. Plasma is a component of:
   A. Buffers
   B. Water
   C. Blood
   D. Dialysis

7. Chronic kidney disease (CKD) has ____ stages.
   A. 3
   B. 4
   C. 5
   D. 6

8. Which of the following is *not* indicated for the treatment of urinary incontinence?
   A. Oxybutynin
   B. Allopurinol
   C. Tolterodine
   D. Trospium chloride

9. Mannitol (Osmitrol) falls into which of the following categories?
   A. Loop diuretic
   B. Osmotic diuretic
   C. Thiazide diuretic
   D. Potassium-sparing diuretic

10. Which of the following classifications include diuretics?
    A. Blood formers
    B. Thiazides
    C. Carbonic anhydrase inhibitors
    D. Both B and C

11. Loop diuretics and thiazides:
    A. Have a slow mechanism of action
    B. Cause a loss of potassium
    C. Cause a loss of sodium
    D. Must be taken with a potassium-sparing agent

12. Which of the following is used to treat hyperphosphatemia in CKD?
    A. Sevelamer
    B. Calcitriol
    C. Epoetin alfa
    D. Hydrochlorothiazide

13. Which of the following is a serious infection that is a risk of peritoneal dialysis if aseptic technique is not used?
    A. Otitis media
    B. UTI
    C. Peritonitis
    D. Cystitis

14. Which of the procedures can be used to treat certain kidney stones?
    A. Lithotripsy
    B. Ureteroscopy
    C. Surgery
    D. All of the above

15. Which of the following is *not* a potassium-sparing agent?
    A. Spironolactone
    B. Furosemide
    C. Amiloride
    D. Both B and C

TECHNICIAN'S CORNER

Using a drug information resource, look up the various clinical indications, in addition to edema, that are treated with the diuretics discussed in this chapter.

Bibliography

Bloom A, Ireland J, Watkins P: *A colour atlas of diabetes*, ed 2, St Louis, 1992, Mosby.

Clinical Pharmacology Online. (Referenced September 6, 2014.) www.clinicalpharmacology-ip.com.

Damjanov I: *Pathology for the health professions*, ed 4, St Louis, 2011, Saunders.

Fishback JL: *Pathology*, ed 3, Philadelphia, 2005, Mosby.

McCance KL: *Pathophysiology: the biologic basis for disease in adults and children*, ed 6, St Louis, 2010, Mosby.

Monahan F et al: *Phipps' medical-surgical nursing: health and illness perspectives*, ed 8, St Louis, 2007, Mosby.

National Kidney Foundation. Chronic Kidney Disease 2006: A guide to select NKF KDOQI guidelines and recommendations, 2006. (Referenced September 6, 2014.) http://www.kidney.org/professionals/kls/pdf/Pharmacist_CPG.pdf

Patton KT et al: *Mosby's handbook of anatomy and physiology*, St Louis, 2000, Mosby.

Solomon EP: *Introduction to human anatomy and physiology*, ed 3, St Louis, 2009, Saunders.

UpToDate Online. (Referenced September 6, 2014.) www.uptodate.com.

Therapeutic Agents for the Reproductive System

Joshua J. Neumiller

OBJECTIVES

Upon completing this chapter, you should be able to do the following:

1. Describe the anatomy and physiology of the reproductive system.
2. List the primary signs and symptoms of common conditions associated with the reproductive system.
3. Recognize prescription and over-the-counter drugs used to treat common conditions of the reproductive system discussed in this chapter.
4. Write the generic and trade names for the drugs discussed in this chapter.
5. List appropriate auxiliary labels when filling prescriptions for drugs discussed in this chapter.

TERMS AND DEFINITIONS

Abortifacient Any treatment that causes abortion of a fetus

Androgen Male hormone

Benign A condition, tumor, or growth that is not cancerous and therefore will not metastasize (spread)

Benign prostatic hyperplasia (BPH) Enlargement of the prostate

Depot An area of the body where a substance can accumulate or be stored for later distribution

Endometrium The mucous membrane lining the inner wall or layer of the uterus

Erectile dysfunction (ED) Inability of a man to maintain an erection sufficient for satisfying sexual activity

Estrogen Any of a group of anabolic sex hormones that promote the development and maintenance of female sexual characteristics

Fallopian tube A narrow tube that connects the ovary to the uterus

Fertilization The process by which a sperm unites with an ovum

Gametes Sex cells, or ova and sperm

Mammary gland The milk-producing gland of women

Menopause Cessation of menstruation; a natural phenomenon in which a woman passes from a reproductive state to a nonreproductive state

Menses The time of menstruation

Negative feedback A self-regulating mechanism in which the output of a system has input or control on the process; in this case, the stimulus results in reactions that reduce the effects of the stimulus

Nocturia Urination at night

Oocyte (ovum) The female reproductive germ cell, more commonly known as an egg

Ovaries The female reproductive organs in which ova, or eggs, are produced

Palliative Something that brings relief but does not cure

Pelvic inflammatory disease (PID) Inflammation of the female genital tract, accompanied by fever and lower abdominal pain

Progesterone An anabolic sex hormone that stimulates the uterus to prepare for pregnancy

Prostate A gland surrounding the neck of the bladder in males that produces a fluid component of semen

Sperm (plural, spermatozoa) The male reproductive germ cell

Spermatogenesis The development of sperm in the testes

Spermicide An agent that kills sperm

Teratogen Any agent that causes abnormal embryonic or fetal development

Testes The male reproductive organs that produce sperm

Testosterone An anabolic sex hormone produced in the testes that stimulates the development of male sexual characteristics

Uterus The organ in the lower abdomen of a woman where gestation of a fetus occurs

Select Common Drugs for the Treatment of Conditions Affecting the Male and Female Reproductive Systems

Trade Name	Generic Name	Pronunciation
Androgens		
Androderm	testosterone	(tes-**toss**-ter-own)
Testred, Android	methyltestosterone	(meth-ill-tes-**toss**-ter-own)
Alpha-Adrenergic Blockers		
Flomax	tamsulosin	(tam-**sue**-lo-sin)
Uroxatral	alfuzosin	(al-**fue**-zoe-sin)
5-Alpha Reductase Inhibitors		
Avodart	dutasteride	(doo-**tas**-ter-ide)
Proscar	finasteride	(fin-**ass**-ter-ide)
Estrogens		
Estrace, Estraderm	estradiol	(ess-tra-**dye**-ol)
Ogen, Ortho-Est	estropipate	(ess-troe-**pye**-pate)
Premarin	conjugated estrogens	(kon-juh-**gat**-ed **ess**-troe-gens)
Prempro, Premphase	conjugated estrogens/ medroxyprogesterone	(kon-juh-**gat**-ed **ess**-troe-gens/me-drox-see-proe -**jess**-ter-own)
Progestins		
Prometrium	progesterone	(pro-**jess**-ter-own)
Micronor	norethindrone	(nor-**eth**-in-drone)
Ovrette	norgestrel	(nor-**jess**-trel)
Provera	medroxyprogesterone	(me-drox-see-proe-**jess**-ter-owne)
Oral Contraceptives		
Monophasic Combinations		
Alesse, Levlen	ethinyl estradiol/levonorgestrel	(**eth**-in-ill ess-tra-**dye**-ol/**lev**-o-nor-**jess**-trel)
Demulen	ethinyl estradiol/ethynodiol diacetate	(**eth**-in-ill ess-tra-**dye**-ol/eh-the-no-**dye**-ol di-**as**-ah-tate)
Desogen, Ortho-Cept	ethinyl estradiol/desogestrel	(**eth**-in-ill ess-tra-**dye**-ol/des-o-**ges**-trel)
Lo/Ovral, Ovral	ethinyl estradiol/norgestrel	(**eth**-in-ill ess-tra-**dye**-ol/nor-**jess**-trel)
Ortho-Cyclen	ethinyl estradiol/norgestimate	(**eth**-in-ill ess-tra-**dye**-ol/nor-**jess**-ti-mate)
Ortho Evra Patch	ethinyl estradiol/norgestimate	(**eth**-in-ill ess-tra-**dye**-ol/nor-**jess**-ti-mate)
Ortho-Novum 1/35	ethinyl estradiol/norethindrone	(**eth**-in-ill ess-tra-**dye**-ol/nor-**eth**-in-drone)
Ortho-Novum 1/50	mestranol/norethindrone	(**mess**-tra-nol/nor-**eth**-in-drone)
Yasmin 28, Yaz	drospirenone/ethinyl estradiol	(dro-**spy**-re-nown/**eth**-in-ill **ess**-tra-dye-ol)
Biphasic Combination		
Ortho-Novum 10/11	ethinyl estradiol/norethindrone	(**eth**-in-ill ess-tra-**dye**-ol/nor-**eth**-in-drone)
Triphasic Combinations		
Ortho Tri-Cyclen/ TriNessa/Tri-Sprintec	ethinyl estradiol/norgestimate	(**eth**-in-ill ess-tra-**dye**-ol/nor-**jess**-ti-mate)
Ortho-Novum 7/7/7	ethinyl estradiol/norethindrone	(**eth**-in-ill ess-tra-**dye**-ol/nor-**eth**-in-drone)
Triphasil	ethinyl estradiol/levonorgestrel	(**eth**-in-ill ess-tra-**dye**-ol/**lev**-o-nor-**jess**-trel)
Long-Acting Contraceptives		
Depo-Provera	medroxyprogesterone	(me-drock-see-pro-**jess**-ter-own)
Infertility Medications		
Clomid	clomiphene	(**kloe**-mi-feen)
Crinone, Prochieve, Endometrin	progesterone	(pro-**jess**-ter-own)
Follistim AQ	follitropin beta (r-FSH)	(fol-**li**-troe-**pin** bet-ah)
Luveris	lutropin alfa (r-LH)	(lou-**tro**-peen **aal**-fa)
Ovidrel	choriogonadotropin alfa (r-HCG)	(kor-**ee**-oh-goe-nad-oh-**troe**-pin **al**-fa)

Continued

Select Common Drugs for the Treatment of Conditions Affecting the Male and Female Reproductive Systems—cont'd

Trade Name	Generic Name	Pronunciation
Emergency Contraceptive		
Plan B, Plan B One-Step, Next Choice	levonorgestrel	(**lev**-o-nor-**jess**-trel)
Drugs for Endometriosis		
Lupron	leuprolide	(loo-**pro**-lide)
Synarel	nafarelin	(**naf**-a-rell-in)
Zoladex	goserelin	(**goe**-ser-a-lin)
Drugs for Erectile Dysfunction		
Cialis	tadalafil	(tah-**dal**-ah-fill)
Levitra, Staxyn	vardenafil	(var-**den**-ah-fill)
Viagra	sildenafil	(sil-**den**-ah-fil)
Drugs Used for Reproductive System Infections/Sexually Transmitted Diseases		
Flagyl	metronidazole	(met-row-**nih**-dah-zole)
Valtrex	valacyclovir	(val-a-**sye**-kloe-veer)
Zovirax	acyclovir	(a-**sye**-kloe-veer)
Examples of Drugs for Vaginal Fungal Infections		
Diflucan	fluconazole	(floo-**kon**-ah-zole)
Vagistat-1	tioconazole	(**tye**-oh-**kon**-ah-zole)

The male and female reproductive systems operate interdependently with other systems, such as the endocrine system (which provides the hormones responsible for the maturation, development, and regulation of the reproductive system) and the urinary system. In men and women, the functions of reproduction are divided between the primary, secondary, and accessory organs. The primary reproductive organs are the gonads (ovaries or testes), which are necessary to produce the **gametes** (sex cells, namely the *ova* and **sperm**). The gonads are also responsible for the secretion of the hormones that provide gender characteristics of the male or female. The secondary reproductive organs include the structures necessary for transport and sustenance of eggs and sperm, and the organs necessary for the growth of the developing fetus in the female. Accessory organs include ducts, glands, and external genitalia. Hormones largely control the functions of the reproductive system. **Estrogen** and **testosterone** are present in both men and women, although their effects are somewhat different because of the different concentrations present in each gender (Table 22-1). This chapter reviews the anatomy and physiology of the female and male reproductive systems, select common reproductive conditions in both genders, and treatments for the conditions discussed.

Female Reproductive System

The two **ovaries** in women are responsible for the production (oogenesis) and secretion of one or, in rare cases, two eggs or more (ovulation) each month. Located on either side of the **uterus**, the ovaries sit above the uterus and are attached to the fallopian tubes, which connect the ovary to the uterus (Figure 22-1). Although ovulation begins at puberty, it is not possible to become pregnant until the menstrual cycle begins. The ability to have children ends as the levels of the responsible hormones (e.g., estrogen) decline, until the ovarian cycle stops. The ovaries, which secrete the hormones estrogen and progesterone, are the primary source of estrogen in women. The function of estrogen is the development of breasts and genitals and the regulation of the menstrual cycle, which prepares the female for pregnancy. The anterior pituitary gland releases follicle-stimulating hormone (FSH), which triggers estrogen levels to increase; this in turn causes the secretion of luteinizing hormone (LH), another pituitary hormone. The combination of these two hormones triggers the cascade of events that causes ovulation (Figure 22-2).

After puberty the female ovary matures one or more eggs each month. At birth the female ovary contains all the eggs available for the woman's lifetime. Thus women do not produce viable eggs

TABLE 22-1

Select Hormones Affecting the Reproductive System and Their Functions

Hormone	Gender	Functions
Androgens	Male	• Steroid hormone that stimulates and controls development and maintenance of male characteristics
	Female	• Precursor to estrogens in women
Testosterone	Male	• Stimulates growth and maturation of male reproductive organs
		• Triggers development of secondary sex characteristics (pubic and facial hair, enhanced hair growth on chest and other areas)
		• Stimulates sperm production
		• Responsible for sex drive
		• Voice changes
		• Skin changes (thicker skin, acne)
		• Bone and skeletal muscle growth (affects size and mass)
		• Affects production of gonadotropin-releasing hormone in the hypothalamus
	Female	• Responsible for sex drive
Gonadotropin-releasing hormone (GnRH)	Male	• Stimulates luteinizing hormone, which then stimulates gonadal secretion of testosterone, estrogen, and progesterone; sex steroids inhibit secretion of GnRH (negative feedback system)
	Female	• Same as in male
Luteinizing hormone (LH)	Male	• Stimulates secretion of sex steroids from gonads
		• Stimulates synthesis and secretion of testosterone; this is converted into estrogen
	Female	• Secretion of steroid hormones progesterone and estradiol
Progesterone	Female	• Necessary for maintenance of pregnancy and luteinization of ovarian follicles
	Male	• Not applicable
Follicle-stimulating hormone (FSH)	Female	• Stimulates ovarian follicles, producing many mature gametes (eggs)
	Male	• Maturation of sperm production

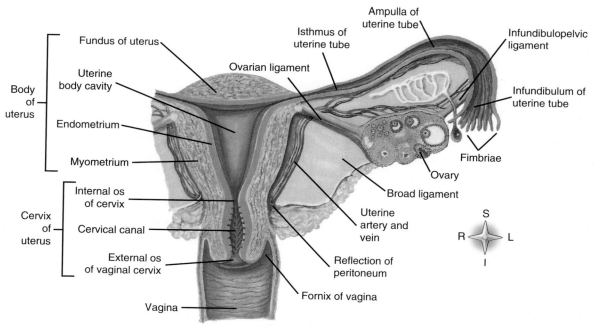

FIGURE 22-1 Female pelvic organs. (From Patton KT et al: *Mosby's handbook of anatomy and physiology,* St Louis, 2000, Mosby.)

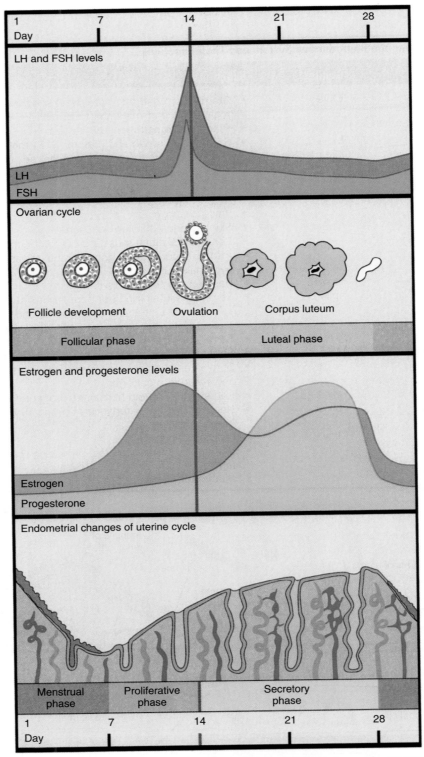

FIGURE 22-2 The normal menstrual cycle consists of a proliferative (follicular) phase and a secretory (luteal) phase. (From Damjanov I: *Pathology for the health professions,* ed 4, St Louis, 2011, Saunders.)

throughout their lifetime. When an egg is mature, it is gathered by the ovarian fimbriae at the opening to the **fallopian tubes**. The fimbriae are in constant motion to sweep the egg into the fallopian tube. At ovulation their activity increases, and currents generated in the peritoneal fluid are created to propel the egg into the fallopian tube. During the next 7 days, the **oocyte (ovum)** is moved down the fallopian tube, where it may become fertilized by sperm. Because an ovum is viable only for 24 to 38 hours,

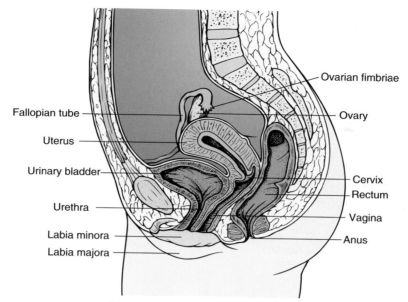

FIGURE 22-3 Female reproductive system.

fertilization usually occurs in the fallopian tube. The fallopian tubes exit into the uterus, which either houses the fertilized ovum or sloughs the ovum and **endometrium** during **menses** if fertilization has not occurred. This cycle begins at puberty and continues until menopause (Figure 22-3).

Gonadotropin-releasing hormone (GnRH) secreted from the hypothalamus acts on the anterior pituitary gland to secrete FSH and LH, the hormones necessary for ovulation (see Table 22-1). These hormones are controlled by **negative feedback** and are secreted in cycles (Figure 22-4), unlike the continuous secretion of sex hormones in males (discussed later). The levels of hormones peak when a woman is in her 20s and gradually decline throughout the remainder of her life.

The **mammary glands** (or breasts) are accessory organs of the female reproductive system. Breast tissue is also regulated by hormonal secretions. At puberty the increase in estrogen stimulates the development of glandular tissue, causing an accumulation of adipose tissue, and progesterone stimulates the development of the duct system used during milk production and secretion (Figure 22-5).

Conditions Affecting the Female Reproductive System

The principal medications that affect the female reproductive system are hormones. Some agents stimulate secretions, whereas others inhibit or counteract the actions of other hormones. Medication therapy for conditions of the reproductive tract can be complicated. Even male hormones are used to treat endometrial or breast cancer, endometriosis,

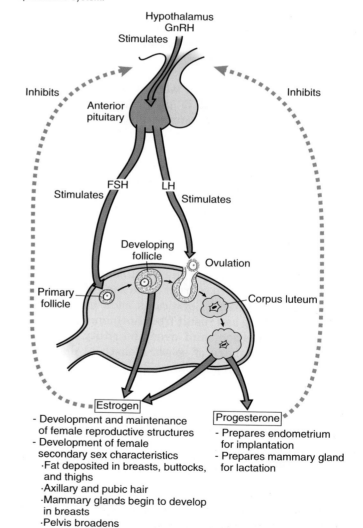

FIGURE 22-4 Function of the ovaries in response to hormone stimulation. *FSH,* Follicle-stimulating hormone; *GnRH,* gonadotropin-releasing hormone; *LH,* luteinizing hormone.

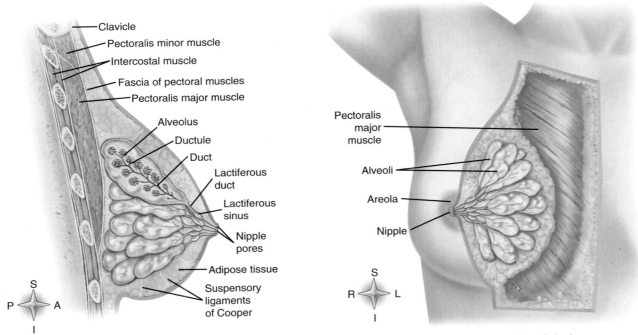

FIGURE 22-5 Female breast. (From Patton KT et al: *Mosby's handbook of anatomy and physiology,* St Louis, 2000, Mosby.)

and fibrocystic disease in women. When discussing hormonal therapies, it is important to remember that the hypothalamus cannot distinguish between hormones naturally produced by the body and those administered as medications; therefore, the body reacts to synthetic and naturally occurring hormones in the same manner. (This chapter discusses male and female sex hormones; Chapter 16 presents a review of other hormones of the endocrine system.) Table 22-2 provides a summary of hormonal therapies used to treat select female reproductive conditions.

Estrogens are one of the most common forms of medical therapy used to treat conditions of the female reproductive system. Conditions such as abnormal uterine bleeding can result from hormone imbalance, abnormal ovulation, and even infertility. Box 22-1 presents a summary of select menstrual disorders. In women, estrogens are used for a multitude of purposes and may be used to treat hypogonadism, to increase the possibility of contraception, and to relieve symptoms of menopause (natural or surgical). Estrogens support the development and maintenance of the reproductive organs and the secondary sex characteristics, and they have profound influences on the menstrual cycle.

The primary oral estrogen products in use clinically are conjugated estrogens and estradiol. Estrogens are also available in several forms; some forms are unique, such as implants, vaginal inserts, and transdermal systems. The most common forms are oral and injectable preparations (water based or oil

---

BOX 22-1

Menstrual Disorders

Amenorrhea: Absence of menstrual periods
Dysmenorrhea: Abdominal pain attributable to menstrual cramping
Hypomenorrhea: Low menstrual flow over a short menstrual period
Menorrhagia: Heavy menstrual flow over a long menstrual period
Oligomenorrhea: Light and infrequent menstrual periods
Polymenorrhea: Frequent menstruation
Premature menopause: Loss of ovarian function before age 40
Premenstrual syndrome: A group of symptoms that occur before the onset of menstruation (e.g., bloating, edema, headache, mood swings, and breast discomfort)

---

based). The oil-based injectable estrogen medications, called **depot** medications, are prepared to prolong the medication's action. Transdermal preparations are applied to the skin to provide continuous release of the medication. Drug-laden vaginal rings are pressed into the vaginal canal for the continuous release of medications into the local tissues. Other locally administered estrogens include vaginal inserts and creams that provide absorption of hormones at the site of application. The choice of

TABLE 22-2

Select Hormonal Therapies for the Treatment of Certain Female Reproductive Conditions

Medication Class	Generic Name	Brand Name	Common Side Effects	Common Dose Range
Endometriosis **Gonadotropin-Releasing Hormone**	leuprolide	Lupron	• Hot flashes • Night sweats • Amenorrhea • Vaginal atrophy • Vaginitis • Headaches • Bone density decrease	• 3.75 mg intramuscularly (IM) once a month (max 6 months) • 1 200-mcg/spray into one nostril in the morning and into the other nostril in the evening; started between days 2 to 4 of the cycle and used for no longer than 6 months • 3.6 mg subcutaneously (SUBCUT) monthly • 200-800 mg/day orally (PO) in 2 divided doses
	nafarelin	Synarel		
	goserelin	Zoladex		
Androgen	danazol	Danocrine	• Edema • Flushing • Hypertension • Acne • Hair loss/growth • Pain • Eosinophilia	
Infertility **Gonadotropin-Ovulation Stimulator**	menotropins	Menopur	• Headache • Abdominal pain • Injection site reaction • Nausea	• 75-150 units IM/SUBCUT daily for first 5 days (max 450 units and/or 12 days)
	urofollitropin (FSH)	Bravelle	• Headache • Hypertension • Acne • Breast tenderness • Hot flashes	• 150-450 units IM/SUBCUT for the first 5 days (max 12 days)
	choriogonadotropin alfa (r-HCG)	Ovidrel	• Ovarian cyst • Abdominal pain • Pain • Nausea	• 250 mcg SUBCUT given once after the last dose of an FSH agent
	lutropin alfa (r-LH)	Luveris	• Headache • Fatigue • Breast pain • Nausea • Constipation • Ovarian enlargement	• 75 units SUBCUT daily (max 14 days)
Selective Estrogen Receptor Modulator (SERM)–Ovulation Stimulator	clomiphene	Clomid	• Headache • Hot flashes • Bloating/discomfort • Visual changes	• 50 mg PO once daily for 5 days (begin on or about day 5 in the cycle; can be repeated 30 days later if needed)
Progestin	progesterone	Crinone	• Somnolence • Headache • Nervousness • Depression • Breast enlargement • Constipation • Nausea • Genital discomfort	• 90 mg intravaginal gel applied 1-2 times daily

Continued

TABLE 22-2

Select Hormonal Therapies for the Treatment of Certain Female Reproductive Conditions—cont'd

Medication Class	Generic Name	Brand Name	Common Side Effects	Common Dose Range
Dopamine Agonist	bromocriptine	Parlodel	• Dizziness • Nausea • Constipation • Rhinitis • Fatigue	• 2.5-15 mg PO once daily
Hormone Replacement Therapy				
Estrogen Derivative	estradiol	Estrace, Gynodiol	• Nausea • Vomiting • Swollen breasts	• 0.5-2 mg PO once daily (3 wk on, then 1 wk off, cycle)
		Estraderm	• Edema • Decreased sex drive	• *Patch:* 0.05-1 mg, replaced twice weekly
		Estring	• Bleeding • Clots • Depression	• 7.5 mcg released from inserted ring daily; replace every 90 days
	esterified estrogen	Menest		• 1.25 mg PO daily (3 wk on, then 1 wk off, cycle)
	conjugated estrogens	Premarin		• 0.3 mg PO daily (or cyclically)
	estropipate	Ogen		• 0.75-6 mg PO daily (often cyclically)
Estrogen and Progestin Combination	conjugated estrogens and medroxyprogesterone	Prempro	• Headache • Nausea • Swollen breasts • Changes in weight/appetite • Decreased sex drive • Stomach pain	• 0.3/1.5-0.625/5 mg PO once daily
	estradiol and levonorgestrel	Climara Pro	• Depression • Breast pain • Vaginal bleeding • Site reaction • Upper respiratory infection	• *Patch:* 0.045/0.015 mg; replace/apply 1 patch weekly

FSH, Follicle-stimulating hormone; *r-HCG,* recombinant human chorionic gonadotropin; *r-LH,* recombinant luteinizing hormone.

preparation to be used depends on the reason for use, the benefits versus the risks of treatment, the cost, the reliability of the patient to use it correctly, and convenience. Adverse effects of estrogens in females may include photosensitivity, nausea, vomiting, and bloating. Dysmenorrhea, breast tenderness and enlargement, and increased susceptibility to thrombotic disease are also risks of estrogen treatment.

As mentioned previously, male hormones can be used for treating certain female breast tumors that grow faster in the presence of estrogen. **Androgens** suppress the effects of estrogen, thus preventing rapid growth of these tumors. For women with endometriosis, androgens can cause suppression of the endometrium and thus prevent the excessive uterine bleeding associated with the disease. Women receiving androgen therapy for prolonged periods can experience amenorrhea or menstrual irregularities. Hot flashes, headaches, sleep disorders, increased libido, vaginitis, and masculinization are also found. Changes in the voice (lowering of the voice) are often permanent, whereas other symptoms, such as loss of breast mass, increased facial and body hair, and increased muscle mass, may reverse when the testosterone therapy is discontinued.

Progesterone, naturally occurring as progestin, is the female hormone secreted from day 14 through day 28 of the menstrual cycle. This hormone has many functions, including changing the secretions of the cervix and reducing uterine contractility. Other actions include stimulating the development of ducts and glands of the breasts in preparation for lactation. Synthetic progestins are used more frequently than natural forms because synthetic forms are more effective. Synthetic forms are either injected or administered orally, and the action of synthetic progestin is prolonged over that of progesterone. Progestins are used for treating amenorrhea and abnormal uterine bleeding from hormone imbalances, for contraception, in combination with estrogen hormone replacement therapy (HRT) to prevent endometrial overgrowth if the woman has an intact uterus, and as therapy for renal and endometrial cancer. When combined with oral estrogen, the dosage of progestin is measured in milligrams, whereas the estrogen component is measured in micrograms. Used to treat infertility, progesterone and progesterone-like products stimulate the development of ova and subsequent ovulation. The side effects associated with progestins include weight gain, stomach pain and cramping, swelling of the face and legs, headaches, mood swings, anxiety, weakness, rashes, acne, and insomnia. Menstrual changes and breast tenderness may occur.

GENERIC NAME: progesterone
TRADE NAME: Prometrium, Crinone, Endometrin
INDICATION: Amenorrhea, contraception, abnormal uterine bleeding, estrogen replacement therapy (ERT), infertility
ROUTE OF ADMINISTRATION: Injectable; vaginal; oral
COMMON ADULT DOSAGE: Varies by indication and dosage form
MECHANISM OF ACTION: Induces secretory activity in the endometrium in preparation for implantation of a fertilized egg and aids in maintenance of a pregnancy; suppresses midcycle surge of LH to prevent pregnancy
SIDE EFFECTS: Weight gain, cramping, headache, insomnia
AUXILIARY LABEL:
• Use as directed.

GENERIC NAME: medroxyprogesterone
TRADE NAME: Provera (oral), Depo-Provera (injection), Depo-SubQ Provera 104 (injection)
INDICATION: Amenorrhea, contraception, abnormal uterine bleeding, endometrial cancer, endometriosis, ERT, renal cell cancer

ROUTE OF ADMINISTRATION: Oral; injection (intramuscular [IM], subcutaneous [SUBCUT])
COMMON ADULT DOSAGE: *Oral:* 2-10 mg once daily for 5 to 10 days for amenorrhea and abnormal bleeding or cyclically with estrogen HRT; *Depo-Provera:* 150 mg deep IM every 3 months as a contraceptive or Depo-SubQ Provera 104 mg SUBCUT every 3 months
MECHANISM OF ACTION: Primary contraceptive effect involves inhibition of gonadotropin secretion to prevent follicular maturation and ovulation
SIDE EFFECTS: Breakthrough bleeding, breast tenderness, insomnia, bloating, nausea
AUXILIARY LABEL:
• Take as directed.

Common Conditions

The following sections provide specific information on women's health issues, such as female hypogonadism, pelvic inflammatory disease, infertility, contraception, and menopause.

Female Hypogonadism

Female hypogonadism is the lack of production of estrogen in the ovaries. In childhood the symptoms include a lack of menstruation and breast development and short height. If this condition occurs during puberty, symptoms include loss of menstruation, hot flashes, loss of body hair, and decreased libido. In adult women, hypogonadism can cause infertility and early menopause. Menopause is a natural transition that occurs between the ages of 50 and 60 years. The effects of menopause increase the risk of osteoporosis and heart disease after menopause is complete.

Turner's syndrome, a type of female hypogonadism, is caused by a genetic defect. Symptoms in infants include swollen hands and feet and a wide, webbed neck (Figure 22-6). In older females, symptoms may include drooping eyelids, absent or incomplete development at puberty (small breasts, scant pubic hair), absence of menstruation, short height, and vaginal dryness. Hormonal therapies can improve the body image of an individual with Turner's syndrome, but infertility cannot be reversed with treatment.

Prognosis. Hormonal therapies can improve body image and fertility in some forms of female hypogonadism, but infertility cannot be reversed in all forms of congenital hypogonadism.

Non–Drug Treatments. Although the proper functioning of the female reproductive system is not required to sustain the woman's life, many

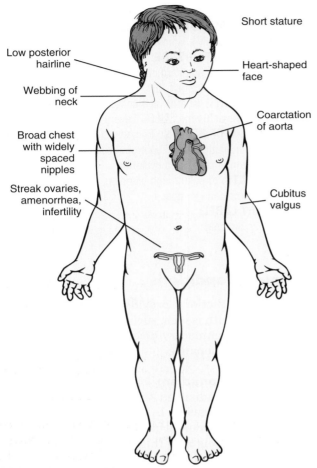

Short stature

Low posterior hairline

Heart-shaped face

Webbing of neck

Coarctation of aorta

Broad chest with widely spaced nipples

Streak ovaries, amenorrhea, infertility

Cubitus valgus

FIGURE 22-6 Typical features of Turner's syndrome. (From Damjanov I: *Pathology for the health professions,* ed 4, St Louis, 2011, Saunders.)

Infertility

An evaluation for the treatment of infertility is typically initiated after 1 year of regular unprotected intercourse in women under age 35 and after 6 months of unprotected intercourse in women over the age of 35. Anovulation is a cause of infertility that can be corrected by pharmacological treatment in many cases. Agents are given to promote maturation of the ovarian follicle and to stimulate ovulation. Endometriosis attributable to pelvic inflammatory disease can obstruct the fallopian tubes. Women with irregular menstrual cycles or no menstruation may also have problems with infertility.

Prognosis. The prognosis for infertility depends on the ages of the partners, the cause of the condition, the methods of treatment or assisted reproduction techniques used, and other factors.

Non–Drug Treatment. Surgery may correct fertility problems originating from structural abnormalities of the fallopian tubes, uterus, or ovaries. Another treatment that may help with infertility is assisted reproductive technology (ART), which uses in vitro fertilization, embryo transfer, and both egg and sperm transfer. The likelihood of success depends on several factors, including the woman's age. In the case of ART, hormonal medications are used to control and direct the ovulation and implantation cycles. Male infertility may be treated with medications or by using alternative techniques, such as sperm donation.

Drug Treatment. Hormone treatment is most commonly used to treat infertility. Agents such as clomiphene and progesterone can be used. Table 22-2 and the following drug monographs present examples of hormonal treatments used for female infertility.

women still desire the ability to conceive and bear offspring. The only non–drug treatment would be to prevent or deter possible causes of conditions that result in hypogonadism. In addition, maintaining ideal body weight, eating a healthy diet, refraining from smoking, and adhering to an exercise regimen may improve infertility.

Drug Treatments. Hormone replacement therapies can be used to diminish the symptoms of hypogonadism. Estrogen and progestin are used for hormone replacement and may help ovarian stimulation; low-dose testosterone may increase sex drive. Estrogen is available in tablet form, topical lotions or gels, or as transdermal patches. Testosterone is available in injectable form, gels, or topical patches (discussed in more detail later). In the case of Turner's syndrome, estrogen, progestin, and other hormone therapy are normally started around puberty to trigger breast and pubic hair growth and to ensure proper stature; no treatment restores fertility (see Table 22-2 for select hormone replacement therapies).

GENERIC NAME: clomiphene
TRADE NAME: Clomid, Serophene
INDICATION: Infertility
ROUTE OF ADMINISTRATION: Oral
COMMON ADULT DOSAGE: 50 mg tablet once daily for 5 days (initial cycle therapy)
MECHANISM OF ACTION: Stimulates FSH and LH secretion by increasing GnRH levels, leading to follicular development in the ovaries

SIDE EFFECTS: Hot flashes, dizziness, breast tenderness, fatigue, headache
AUXILIARY LABEL:
* Take as directed.

 Tech Note!
In rare cases, you may be presented with prescriptions for clomiphene (Clomid) and menotropins (Menopur) prescribed to a man. These agents are sometimes used off-label for the treatment of oligospermia (low sperm concentration in the semen), which is a cause of infertility in males.

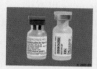

GENERIC NAME: menotropins
TRADE NAME: Menopur, Repronex
INDICATION: Hypogonadism, infertility
ROUTE OF ADMINISTRATION: Injectable (intramuscular [IM], subcutaneous [SUBCUT])
COMMON ADULT DOSAGE: 225 units (international units) of FSH/LH activity IM or SUBCUT once daily initially; adjust to response by no more than 150 units/day (max 450 units/day)
MECHANISM OF ACTION: Contains purified preparations of human FSH and LH, which act to stimulate follicle maturation and ovulation
SIDE EFFECTS: Headache, nausea, diarrhea, abdominal cramping
AUXILIARY LABEL:
* Take as directed.

Contraception

Oral Contraceptives. Oral contraceptives are used as a means of birth control by preventing fertilization of an ovum. Contraception may be accomplished through pharmacological methods, such as oral contraceptives, or with other medical devices, such as vaginal rings, patches, or intrauterine devices. Nonpharmacological methods, such as surgery, the rhythm method, and mechanical devices, also may be used. Of the different methods of birth control, the oral contraceptives have the highest incidence of side effects, ranging from nausea and vomiting to menstrual abnormalities to thrombotic complications. Concurrent cigarette smoking increases the risk of serious cardiovascular effects. Barrier methods have

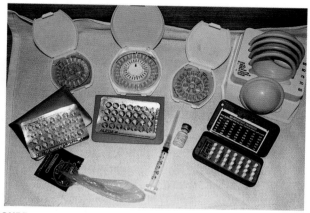
FIGURE 22-7 Common contraceptives, including barrier and medicinal methods: condoms, diaphragm, oral contraceptives, and parenteral contraceptives.

the fewest side effects but may not be as effective as hormone-based medications (Figure 22-7).

 Tech Note!
Oral contraceptives provide no protection against sexually transmitted diseases; this is an important point to make when providing patient education.

Combination oral contraceptives consist of estrogen and progestin to inhibit ovulation. The progestin-only contraceptives are called "mini-pills." The combination contraceptives are the most frequently prescribed contraceptives and are highly effective. The combination medications are available in monophasic, biphasic, triphasic, and estrophasic formulas. In the monophasic regimen, the daily doses of estrogen and progestin remain constant throughout the menstrual cycle. In the biphasic regimen, the estrogen dose remains constant but the progestin dose is increased in the second half of the cycle. Triphasic regimens divide the menstrual cycle into three phases, and the amount of progestin changes in each phase. The estrophasic cycle has a constant amount of progestin, and the estrogen component is increased gradually throughout the cycle. Phasic oral contraceptives are intended to mimic the female body's natural cycle while lessening side effects of the birth control pills.

The effectiveness of oral contraceptives depends on the woman taking the medication as prescribed. Usually, the medication is started on the fifth day of the menstrual cycle and should be taken at the same time of day for 21 days. If a single dose of a combination oral contraceptive is missed, the chance of ovulation is small. However, the risk of pregnancy increases with each dose missed. If one dose is missed, it should be taken as soon as it is remembered and the next pill should be taken on the regular schedule. This

TABLE 22-3

Select Contraceptive Products

Medication Class	Generic Name (Progestin)	Brand Name	Common Dose or Duration
Oral Combination (Estrogen and Progestin) Pills	desogestrel	Ortho-Cept, Kariva, Desogen, etc.	• Taken orally (PO) every day about the same time
	drosperinone	Yasmin, Yaz	
	ethynodiol diacetate	Zovia, Demulen, Kelnor	
	levonorgestrel	Alesse, Lessina, Portia	
	norethindrone	Ovcon, Brevicon, Necon	
	norethindrone acetate	Junel, Loestrin, Microgestin	
	norgestimate	Sprintec, Ortho Tri Cyclen	
	norgestrel	Cryselle, Ovral, Ogestrel	
Oral Progestin Only	norethindrone	Micronor, Nor-QD	• Taken PO every day about the same time
Injection (Progestin Only)	medroxyprogesterone acetate	Depo-SubQ	• Subcutaneous (SUBCUT) injection every 3 months
		Depo-Provera	• Intramuscular (IM) injection every 3 months
Intrauterine System (Progestin Only)	levonorgestrel	Mirena	• Effective for 5 years
Transdermal Combination (Estrogen and Progestin) Patch	norelgestromin	Ortho Evra	• Apply 1 patch for 3 wk, followed by 1 wk patch free; repeat cycle
Vaginal Ring (Estrogen and Progestin)	etonogestrel	NuvaRing	• Ring remains in vagina for 3 wk and then is removed for 1 wk; user repeats cycle
Implantable Device (Progestin Only)	etonogestrel	Implanon	• Effective for 3 years
Emergency Oral (Progestin Only)	levonorgestrel	Plan-B, Plan B One-Step	• 1 tablet as soon as possible within 72 hr of unprotected sexual intercourse, then a second tablet 12 hr later

may mean taking two pills in 1 day or in the same dose. If two doses are missed, two tablets should be taken on each of the next 2 days. If subsequent doses of birth control pills are missed, it is always a good idea to use a barrier method of contraception for the remainder of the cycle to avoid unplanned pregnancy.

Some of the side effects of oral contraceptives include nausea, vomiting, mood changes, appetite changes, changes in sex drive, and headaches. Women taking combination oral contraceptives may also experience breast tenderness; however, women taking progestin-only pills do not seem to experience as much breast tenderness or nausea. Some of the risks of combination oral contraceptives include thromboembolism (including myocardial infarction and stroke), and the risks are often increased in women who smoke. Table 22-3 provides a list of select oral and non–oral contraceptive products.

Other Contraceptive Products. Many contraceptive products are taken orally, but some are available in other dosage forms to allow for nonoral administration (see Table 22-3). An advantage of some nonoral products is that they can help individuals who may have trouble remembering to take a pill every day. Injectable products, for example, can be effective for 3 months. Some nonoral contraceptive dosage forms include the following:

- *Etonogestrel (NuvaRing):* Similar to the traditional oral contraceptive but administered by a ring inserted into the vagina that can be left in place for up to 3 weeks
- *Levonorgestrel (Mirena):* Intrauterine device (IUD) that contains only progestin; contraceptive action lasts up to 5 years
- *Norelgestromin (Ortho Evra):* Contraceptive patch that can be applied weekly for 3 weeks, followed by 1 week patch free

GENERIC NAME: ethinyl estradiol; norelgestromin
TRADE NAME: Ortho Evra
ROUTE OF ADMINISTRATION: Transdermal patch
COMMON ADULT DOSAGE: *Patch:* Applied weekly for 3 weeks; the fourth week is patch free
MECHANISM OF ACTION: Suppresses the hypothalamic-pituitary system, reducing the secretion of GnRH
SIDE EFFECTS: Nausea, breast tenderness, headache, dizziness, menstrual irregularity
AUXILIARY LABELS:
- Apply topically.
- Take as directed.

 Tech Note!

The current recommendation for contraceptive transdermal patches, such as Ortho Evra, is to apply the patch to the upper arm, back, abdomen, or buttock. The patch should be applied and worn for 1 week and then removed; a new patch should be applied on the same day of the week that the first patch was applied. The fourth week should be patch free.

GENERIC NAME: medroxyprogesterone
TRADE NAME: Depo-Provera (injection), Depo-SubQ Provera 104 (injection)
INDICATION: Amenorrhea, contraception, abnormal uterine bleeding, endometrial cancer, endometriosis, estrogen replacement therapy (ERT), renal cell cancer
ROUTE OF ADMINISTRATION: Injection
COMMON ADULT DOSAGE: *Depo-Provera:* 150 mg deep IM every 3 months as a contraceptive; *Depo-SubQ Provera:* 104 mg SUBCUT every 3 months
MECHANISM OF ACTION: Primary contraceptive effect involves inhibition of gonadotropin secretion to prevent follicular maturation and ovulation
SIDE EFFECTS: Breakthrough bleeding, breast tenderness, insomnia, bloating, nausea

GENERIC NAME: levonorgestrel intrauterine system
TRADE NAME: Mirena
INDICATION: Contraception, heavy menstrual bleeding (menorrhagia)

ROUTE OF ADMINISTRATION: Intrauterine
COMMON ADULT DOSAGE: Insert one system into the uterus; each system is effective for 5 years, at which time a new system is inserted
MECHANISM OF ACTION: Levonorgestrel in the IUD is thought to contribute to contraception by thickening cervical mucus, inhibiting sperm survival, and altering the endometrium
SIDE EFFECTS: Menstrual irregularities, abdominal pain

Other contraceptive products include **spermicides**. These contraceptives are available as foam, jelly, gel, cream, suppository, and vaginal film. The correct use of a spermicide is essential for contraceptive efficacy. The spermicide must be applied before, but no more than 1 hour in advance of, sexual intercourse. Spermicides may be purchased without a prescription and must be applied each time intercourse is anticipated.

Barrier devices are nonpharmacological methods of birth control, although a prescription is written for cervical caps and diaphragms to ensure proper fitting. These devices include male and female condoms, cervical caps, and diaphragms. The most commonly used barrier method is the male condom. Three materials are used in the manufacture of male condoms: latex, polyurethane, and lamb intestine. The female condom is a loose-fitting tubular polyurethane pouch with flexible rings at both ends, and the diaphragm is a soft rubber cap with a metal spring that fits over the cervix. Before a diaphragm is inserted, it should be filled with spermicide to block the cervix completely. The cervical cap, another contraceptive device, is a small cup-shaped barrier that fits directly over the cervical rim and is held in place by suction.

Another product that is available as an emergency form of contraception is commonly known as the "morning-after pill," which prevents conception and pregnancy after intercourse. Morning-after pills are contraceptives formulated of high-dose progestin only or both estrogen and progestin. The combined form of emergency contraception is about 75% effective, but one almost universal side effect is nausea and vomiting. Therefore, progestin-only emergency contraception, which is less likely to cause nausea, is more popularly used. A product known as Plan B One-Step contains a large dose of levonorgestrel and requires only a single dose within 72 hours of intercourse. Progestin-only emergency contraception is more effective than a combined estrogen and progestin regimen, primarily because it is better tolerated.

Emergency contraception products do have some risk associated with them and should not be used as a regular means of birth control.

RU-486, or mifepristone (Mifeprex), is more commonly known as the abortion pill. RU-486 acts as an antiprogestin. Because progesterone is necessary for establishment and maintenance of pregnancy, RU-486 acts as an antagonist to progesterone and prevents the maintenance of the pregnancy. For safety, this medication must be used within the first 7 weeks of pregnancy. Because of the **abortifacient** effects of the medication, RU-486 must be administered by a qualified health care professional in the prescriber's office.

Menopause

As previously described, estrogen and progesterone secretion responds to hormones released from the anterior pituitary gland. GnRH (from the hypothalamus) stimulates FSH and LH (from the anterior pituitary gland) to cause the ovaries to secrete estrogen and progesterone. Unlike testosterone in the male, these hormones follow cyclical patterns each month, beginning at puberty and continuing until menopause, when hormone secretion decreases. During perimenopause, the ovaries gradually reduce estrogen production.

Menopause is a natural loss of the production of hormones normally synthesized by the ovaries that occurs with age. Although this is not a "disease," the symptoms associated with menopause, such as hot flashes, can lead women to seek hormone replacement therapy (HRT).

cancer when combination medications are not used. If a patient does not have a uterus, estrogen alone is prescribed.

The use of HRT for menopausal symptoms is particularly controversial. Although effective in treating menopausal symptoms such as hot flashes, mood swings, and night sweats, HRT has been shown to increase a women's risk of developing breast cancer, stroke, blood clots, and heart disease. Understandably, findings caused confusion among women and health care professionals, with many women discontinuing HRT or deciding not to initiate HRT. Currently, many practitioners prescribe HRT to be used as a short-term therapy to help women with the most severe menopausal symptoms. HRT must be initiated with a thorough understanding of the benefits, risks, family health factors, personal health risks, and preferences of the individual.

Estrogen therapy has many side effects; therefore, the smallest dose should be given for the shortest time necessary. All estrogens have a Pregnancy Category X rating because they can act as **teratogens**. Teratogenic agents cause birth defects by causing abnormal development of the embryo or fetus during pregnancy. Table 22-2 and the following drug monographs present examples of HRT products.

Prognosis. Uncomfortable but not life-threatening, the symptoms of menopause can last for many years.

Non–Drug Treatments. Some lifestyle changes that can lessen the symptoms associated with menopause include weight reduction, consuming a healthy diet, smoking cessation, physical activity, and stress reduction techniques. Additionally, many herbal and other naturopathic treatments can be used for the management of menopause.

Drug Treatments. Estradiol is the major natural estrogen that is produced by the ovaries. Estradiol is used for hormone replacement therapy in the naturally postmenopausal woman or in women who have had their ovaries surgically removed. Estradiol is usually combined with a progestin in a woman with an intact uterus because of the increased risk of endometrial overgrowth and the potential risk for endometrial

GENERIC NAME: estradiol

TRADE NAME: Estrace (oral), Divigel, Estrasorb, EstroGel, Alora, Climara, (transdermal), Femring, Vagifem (vaginal), Depo-Estradiol (injectable)

INDICATION: Menopausal symptoms, female hypogonadism

ROUTE OF ADMINISTRATION: Oral; transdermal (patches, lotions, or gels); vaginal; injectable

COMMON ADULT DOSAGE: Varies widely by dosage form and route of delivery

MECHANISM OF ACTION: Supplements estrogen to treat menopausal symptoms associated with a decline in estrogen levels

SIDE EFFECTS: Nausea, vomiting, breast tenderness, dizziness, abnormal vaginal bleeding, thrombotic events

AUXILIARY LABEL:

- Use as directed.

GENERIC NAME: esterified estrogen
TRADE NAME: Menest
INDICATION: Menopausal symptoms, female hypogonadism, atrophic vaginitis, osteoporosis prophylaxis
ROUTE OF ADMINISTRATION: Oral
COMMON ADULT DOSAGE: 0.3-1.25 mg once daily
MECHANISM OF ACTION: Supplements estrogen to treat menopausal symptoms associated with a decline in estrogen levels
SIDE EFFECTS: Nausea, vomiting, breast tenderness, dizziness, abnormal vaginal bleeding, thrombotic events
AUXILIARY LABEL:
• Use as directed.

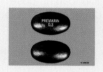

GENERIC NAME: conjugated estrogens
TRADE NAME: Premarin
INDICATION: Menopausal symptoms, osteoporosis prophylaxis, female hypogonadism, atrophic vaginitis
ROUTE OF ADMINISTRATION: Oral; vaginal; injectable
COMMON ADULT DOSAGE: Varies widely by dosage form and route of delivery
MECHANISM OF ACTION: Supplements estrogen to treat menopausal symptoms associated with a decline in estrogen levels
SIDE EFFECTS: Nausea, vomiting, breast tenderness, dizziness, abnormal vaginal bleeding, thrombotic events
AUXILIARY LABEL:
• Use as directed.

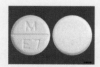

GENERIC NAME: estropipate
TRADE NAME: None
INDICATION: Menopausal symptoms, osteoporosis prophylaxis, female hypogonadism, atrophic vaginitis
ROUTE OF ADMINISTRATION: Oral
COMMON ADULT DOSAGE: 0.75-6 mg once daily

MECHANISM OF ACTION: Supplements estrogen to treat menopausal symptoms associated with a decline in estrogen levels
SIDE EFFECTS: Nausea, vomiting, breast tenderness, dizziness, abnormal vaginal bleeding, thrombotic events
AUXILIARY LABEL:
• Take as directed.

Pelvic Inflammatory Disease

Inflammation of the female reproductive organs is referred to as **pelvic inflammatory disease (PID)**. PID is a severe inflammation of the uterine lining, fallopian tubes, or ovaries that can cause chronic pain and permanent infertility. Tubal ectopic pregnancy (i.e., the egg attaches to and grows in the fallopian tube) occurs six to 10 times more often in women who have a history of PID. Ectopic pregnancy is a serious condition that is normally fatal to the fetus and may be life-threatening to the mother.

Often PID occurs due to a sexually transmitted disease (STD), although this is not exclusively the case. An untreated infection of the genital tract may result in PID. The length of time for the infection to occur ranges from days to months. Symptoms include abnormal or increased vaginal discharge, bleeding between periods, painful menstruation, painful urination/bowel movements, fever, painful intercourse, and pain in the upper right abdomen. PID can require hospitalization in severe cases, such as for women who do not respond to oral antibiotics.

The following are risk factors for PID:
• *History of PID:* Prior episodes of PID, especially those caused by gonorrhea and chlamydia, increase a woman's risk for future PID.
• *Age:* PID occurs most frequently among those 15 to 25 years of age.
• *Multiple sex partners:* Women who have multiple sex partners or whose partner has multiple sex partners have an increased risk of contracting PID.

Prognosis. With rapid diagnosis, treatment, and prevention methods, the outlook for PID is good. For women with a history of PID, the risk for a subsequent episode is increased; therefore, prevention is a key factor.

Non–Drug Treatments. The use of barrier contraceptives, in addition to screening young women and their sexual partners for sexually transmitted diseases (e.g., chlamydia), may be beneficial in PID prevention.

Drug Treatments. Specific antimicrobials are prescribed to target the causative microbe

TABLE 22-4

Select Treatment Regimens for Pelvic Inflammatory Disease (PID)

Oral Regimen A*

Ceftriaxone 250 mg intramuscularly (IM) single dose	plus	Doxycycline 100 mg orally (PO) twice daily for 14 days	with or without	Metronidazole 500 mg PO twice daily for 14 days

Oral Regimen B*

Cefoxitin 2 g IM single dose and probenecid 1 g PO single dose	plus	Doxycycline 100 mg PO twice daily for 14 days	with or without	Metronidazole 500 mg PO twice daily for 14 days

Oral Regimen C*

Ceftizoxime or cefotaxime 1 g IM as single dose	plus	Doxycycline 100 mg PO twice daily for 14 days	with or without	Metronidazole 500 mg PO twice daily for 14 days

Parenteral Regimen A*

Cefotetan 2 g intravenously (IV) every 12 hr	or	Cefoxitin 2 g intravenously (IV) every 6 hours	plus	Doxycycline 100 mg PO or IV every 12 hr

Parenteral Regimen B*

Clindamycin 900 mg IV every 8 hr			plus	Gentamicin loading dose IV/IM (2 mg/kg), followed by 1.5 mg/kg every 8 hr

Parenteral A or B to Be Followed with:

Doxycycline 100 mg PO three times daily for 14 days	or	Clindamycin 450 mg PO four times daily for 14 days		

Alternative Parenteral Regimens*

Ampicillin/sulbactam (Unasyn) 3 g IV every 6 hr			plus	Doxycycline 100 mg PO or IV every 12 hr for 14 days

*Regimens are optional so that the physician can determine the best course of treatment.

(bacteria, protozoa, or fungi). If the patient is treated at home, oral medications are typically prescribed. If hospitalization is necessary, therapy is usually initiated with intravenous antibiotics, antiprotozoals, or antifungals. Different combinations of medications have been recommended for the treatment of PID by the Centers for Disease Control and Prevention (CDC). As outlined in Table 22-4, a variety of regimens is recommended for consideration by the treating physician. depending on whether the condition is treated in the inpatient or ambulatory setting.

Male Reproductive System

The two **testes** in men (Figure 22-8) are responsible for the production and secretion of sperm (**spermatogenesis**). The **testes** are located in the scrotum. **Sperm** production begins before the age of puberty and declines with age, although most men produce sperm throughout their lifetime. FSH is released as puberty begins and causes the stored immature sperm cells to divide and mature. Each sperm contains one half of the genetic material that is contributed to a new life during reproduction. The production of **testosterone** (also from the testes) is responsible for the growth of adjacent organs: prostate gland, seminal vesicles, vas deferens, and others. Testosterone is also responsible for secondary sex characteristics, such as changes in voice pitch as a boy enters puberty and increased muscle development. This hormone also affects the differences in the physiques of men and women.

In the male, the reproductive system is closely tied to the urinary system (Figure 22-9). The urethra passes through the penis, is surrounded by the prostate gland, and is responsible for voiding urine from the body, in addition to serving as the exit route for sperm upon ejaculation. After sperm are formed, they mature and are stored in the

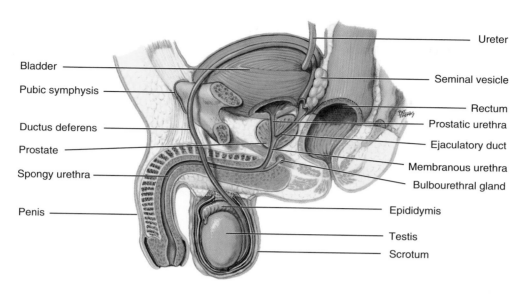

FIGURE 22-8 Testes. (From Applegate E: *The anatomy and physiology learning system,* ed 4, St Louis, 2011, Saunders.)

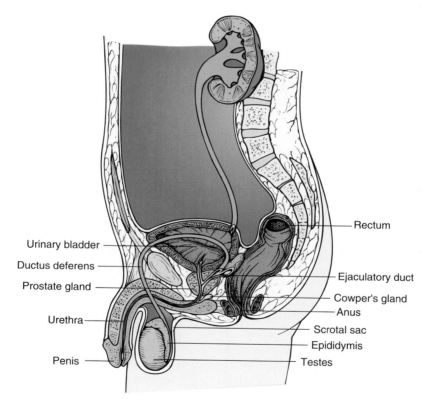

FIGURE 22-9 Male reproductive system.

epididymis (a series of tightly coiled tubes wrapped around the back of the testes) and then travel into the vas deferens (a muscular tube that extends from the epididymis to the ejaculatory duct), where peristaltic movements transport the sperm into the ejaculatory duct.

The **prostate** is about the size and shape of a walnut. It encircles part of the urethra, the tube that carries urine out of the bladder and through the penis. The secretions of the prostate gland both enhance the motility and viability of sperm and provide a slightly alkaline environment that endures

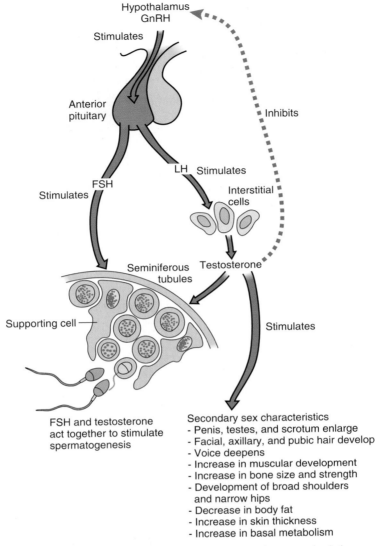

FIGURE 22-10 Function of the testes in response to hormone stimulation.

the acidic environment of the vagina. The sperm and fluids pass through the urethra in the penis for ejaculation during sexual intercourse.

Male sex hormones are stimulated by the release of GnRH from the hypothalamus. GnRH then travels to the anterior pituitary and causes it to secrete LH (also called *interstitial cell–stimulating hormone*) in the male, and FSH. Interstitial cell–stimulating hormone then promotes the growth of interstitial cells in the testes and stimulates the cells to secrete testosterone. Testosterone and FSH stimulate spermatogenesis (creation of sperm) in the testicles (Figure 22-10).

Male sex hormones collectively are called **androgens**, and testosterone is the most abundant androgen. At puberty, androgens stimulate the formation of secondary male characteristics, such as increased muscle mass, deepening of the voice, and growth of facial hair. Although females produce testosterone,

the androgens play a less significant role in the development of female sexual characteristics and reproductive processes.

Conditions Affecting the Male Reproductive System

A number of conditions can affect the male reproductive system. With the implementation of diagnostic procedures, many of these conditions can be identified and treated. A wide variety of available medications can cure or mitigate diseases and conditions of the male reproductive system.

Common Conditions

Male Hypogonadism
The condition in which the male body cannot produce enough testosterone is referred to as hypogonadism.

This condition can occur in the fetus, during puberty, or at any time during adulthood. Hypogonadism can be caused by underdevelopment of the genitals (during fetal development), impaired growth (at puberty), infection (bacterial or viral), or injury to the glands that produce testosterone (tumors or trauma). Symptoms resulting from the lack of testosterone include fatigue, decreased sex drive, and difficulty concentrating.

Prognosis. With testosterone replacement therapy, the symptoms of male hypogonadism can be treated effectively.

Non–Drug Treatment. Stress reduction can minimize anxiety and help improve the man's attitude about this condition.

Drug Treatment. Androgens are used to treat male hypogonadism or infertility resulting from a low sperm count. The increase in the sperm count is achieved through increased secretion of testosterone, FSH, and interstitial cell–stimulating hormone. Different types of medication delivery systems can be used to promote puberty and development of secondary sex characteristics in children with male hypogonadism. Dosage forms include intramuscular (IM), transdermal, and oral dosage forms.

Androgens provide a sense of well-being, mental stability, and energy to those with male hypogonadism. Testosterone also provides the body with a resistance to fatigue. Natural testosterone that is used for medicinal purposes was originally obtained from the testes of bulls; however, the drug is now chemically synthesized. Because of the misuse and abuse potential of androgen products, the Drug Enforcement Administration (DEA) has placed these products on the schedule III list of controlled medications. Table 22-5 provides a list of select androgens used for the treatment of male hypogonadism. The use of testosterone products for age-related decreases in testosterone has become increasingly popular in recent years.

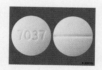

GENERIC NAME: methyltestosterone (C-III)
TRADE NAME: Testred, Android (capsules), Methitest (tablets)

TABLE 22-5

Select Androgen Supplements

Medication Class	Generic Name	Brand Name	Common Side Effects	Common Dose Range
Androgens	testosterone	Androderm	• Acne • Deep vein thrombosis • Edema • Hypertension • Hair loss/growth • Erections • Application/injection site reactions	• *Patch:* 5 mg placed on skin once daily (replaced for each new patch) • 1% applied once daily in the morning to shoulder/upper arms • 50-400 mg intramuscularly (IM) every 2-4 wk • 30 mg buccal tablet orally (PO) twice a day • 3-6 (75 mg) pellets implanted in subdermal fat every 3-6 months
		AndroGel		
		Depo-Testosterone Striant SR		
		Testopel		
	fluoxymesterone	Androxy	• Priapism • Edema • Acne • Hair growth • Prostate cancer	• 5-20 mg PO daily
Gonadotropin	human chorionic gonadotropin	Novarel	• Injection site reaction • Edema • Depression • Headache	• 500-1000 units IM 3 times/wk for 3 wk, followed by same dose twice a wk for 3 wk

INDICATION: *Men:* Androgen replacement therapy, male hypogonadism, delayed puberty, erectile dysfunction; *Women:* **Palliative** treatment of metastatic breast cancer

ROUTE OF ADMINISTRATION: Oral

COMMON ADULT DOSAGE: *Male hypogonadism:* 10-50 mg daily

MECHANISM OF ACTION: Supplements and replaces a lack of testosterone

SIDE EFFECTS: Acne, headache, nausea, weight gain, increased sex drive

AUXILIARY LABEL:
- Use as directed.
- Caution: Federal law prohibits the transfer of this drug to any person other than the patient for whom it was prescribed.

GENERIC NAME: testosterone (C-III)

TRADE NAME: Androderm

INDICATION: Androgen replacement therapy, male hypogonadism

ROUTE OF ADMINISTRATION: Transdermal (patch)

COMMON ADULT DOSAGE: 2.5 or 5 mg transdermal patch daily

MECHANISM OF ACTION: Supplements and replaces a lack of testosterone

SIDE EFFECTS: Topical irritation, acne, headache, nausea, weight gain, increased sex drive

AUXILIARY LABELS:
- Topical.
- Use as directed.
- Caution: Federal law prohibits the transfer of this drug to any person other than the patient for whom it was prescribed.

GENERIC NAME: testosterone (C-III)

TRADE NAME: AndroGel

INDICATION: Androgen replacement therapy, male hypogonadism

ROUTE OF ADMINISTRATION: Transdermal (gel)

COMMON ADULT DOSAGE: Initially 5 g of 1% gel applied once daily to skin of upper arms and/or abdomen (max 10 g of gel daily)

MECHANISM OF ACTION: Supplements and replaces a lack of testosterone

SIDE EFFECTS: Topical irritation, acne, headache, nausea, weight gain, increased sex drive

AUXILIARY LABELS:
- Topical.
- Use as directed.

- Caution: Federal law prohibits the transfer of this drug to any person other than the patient for whom it was prescribed.

Tech Note!

Secondary exposure of children to testosterone gel products has occurred. It is important that men using this product cover the application site and not hold small children such that transfer of the testosterone can occur.

Benign Prostatic Hypertrophy

Benign prostatic hypertrophy (BPH) is an enlargement of the prostate gland. The prostate gland is positioned between the bladder and urethra and encircles the urethra. When the prostate becomes enlarged, it makes urination difficult (Figure 22-11). This condition is termed "**benign**" because the enlargement of the prostate is not cancerous and therefore will not metastasize (spread). BPH occurs in approximately half of men by the age of 50. It is noncancerous and nonlethal, although it is disruptive to daily life. The goal of treatment for BPH is to relieve symptoms such as urinary hesitancy, a decrease in the stream of urine, postvoiding dribbling, frequency of urination, and **nocturia** and to prevent urinary tract infections.

Prognosis. Several treatments can be effective in lessening the symptoms of BPH. Treatments range from lifestyle changes to medication or surgery. Several procedures also may be available to reduce the enlarged prostate gland, thus relieving the symptoms of BPH.

Non–Drug Treatment. For mild symptoms of BPH, steps can be taken to attempt to diminish and/or determine the severity of the condition. These include avoiding smoking, alcohol, caffeine, and OTC antihistamines and decongestants, in addition to exercising regularly. Surgery is an option if the patient does not respond to medication. The physician physically removes excess tissue in the prostate gland. In another treatment, low-level radiofrequency waves are used to destroy the excess prostate tissue.

Drug Treatment. Two primary classes of drugs are used to treat BPH: 5-alpha reductase inhibitors and alpha-blockers (Table 22-6). 5-Alpha reductase inhibitors reduce the size of the prostate, although it can take up to 6 months to achieve maximum effectiveness. Alpha-blockers

thus reducing the growth of the prostate tissue. As mentioned previously, these agents can take several months to reach their full effect.

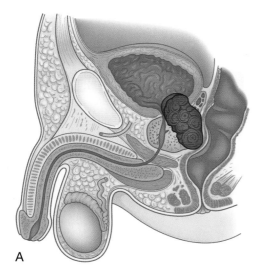

A

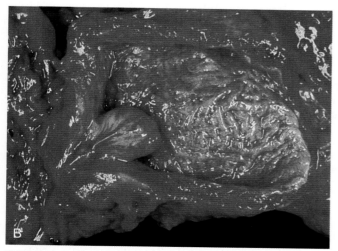

FIGURE 22-11 Benign prostatic hyperplasia (BPH). (From McCance KL: *Pathophysiology: the biologic basis for disease in adults and children,* ed 6, St Louis, 2010, Mosby.)

act quickly to lessen urinary symptoms of BPH, although they do not stop the overall process of prostate enlargement. Often the two medication classes are used concurrently to obtain the best results.

 Tech Note!
5-Alpha reductase inhibitors and alpha-blockers are commonly used together in men with BPH. A combination product on the market, dutasteride/tamsulosin (Jalyn) contains a drug from each of these classes.

5-Alpha Reductase Inhibitors. 5-Alpha reductase inhibitors block the conversion of testosterone to a more active androgen (5-alpha dihydrotestosterone [DHT]) that is known to increase the growth of cells,

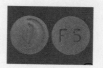

GENERIC NAME: finasteride
TRADE NAME: Proscar
INDICATION: BPH
ROUTE OF ADMINISTRATION: Oral
COMMON ADULT DOSAGE: 5 mg once daily
MECHANISM OF ACTION: Blocks the conversion of testosterone to a more active androgen (DHT) that is known to increase the growth of cells
SIDE EFFECTS: Erectile dysfunction, ejaculatory dysfunction, decrease in libido
AUXILIARY LABEL:
• Take as directed.

 Tech Note!
Finasteride is also available in a 1-mg dose under the brand name Propecia for the treatment of male pattern baldness.

GENERIC NAME: dutasteride
TRADE NAME: Avodart
INDICATION: BPH
ROUTE OF ADMINISTRATION: Oral
COMMON ADULT DOSAGE: 0.5 mg once daily
MECHANISM OF ACTION: Blocks the conversion of testosterone to a more active androgen (DHT) that is known to increase the growth of cells
SIDE EFFECTS: Erectile dysfunction, ejaculatory dysfunction, decrease in libido
AUXILIARY LABEL:
• Take as directed.

 Tech Note!
5-Alpha reductase inhibitors may cause birth defects; therefore, a woman who is pregnant or trying to become pregnant should avoid contact with crushed or broken tablets because the active drug can penetrate through the skin.

TABLE 22-6

Select Treatments for the Management of Benign Prostatic Hypertrophy (BPH)

Generic Name	Brand Name	Common Side Effects	Common Dose Range
5-Alpha Reductase Inhibitors Block the conversion of testosterone to dihydrotestosterone (DHT), which slows prostate growth and can shrink the prostate			
finasteride	Proscar	• Sexual dysfunction	• 5 mg orally (PO) once daily
dutasteride	Avodart	• Breast tenderness	• 0.5 mg PO once daily
		• Rash	
Alpha-1 Blockers Relax prostate smooth muscle, reducing bladder outlet resistance			
doxazosin	Cardura	• Orthostasis	• 1 mg PO once daily, then titrate upward to a goal of 4-8 mg PO once daily
		• Reflex tachycardia	
		• Headache	
	Cardura XL (extended release)	• Dizziness	• 4 mg PO once daily with breakfast, then titrate upward to 8 mg PO once daily
		• Abnormal ejaculation	
terazosin	Hytrin		• 1 mg PO at bedtime, then titrate upward prn; most patients need 10 mg (max 20 mg/day)
alfuzosin	Uroxatral	• Same side effect profile listed above, but with less orthostatic hypotension	• 10 mg PO once daily
tamsulosin	Flomax		• 0.4 mg PO once daily 30 min after the same meal each day
5-Alpha Reductase Inhibitors/Alpha-1 Blockers See mechanisms previously described for 5-alpha reductase inhibitors and alpha-1 blockers			
dutasteride and tamsulosin	Jalyn	• See side effects listed above	• 1 capsule (0.5 mg dutasteride/0.4 mg tamsulosin) PO once daily 30 minutes after the same meal each day
Phosphodiesterase Type 5 Inhibitors Increase cyclic guanosine monophosphate (cGMP) levels in the vascular smooth muscle cells, promoting relaxation and vasodilation			
tadalafil	Cialis	• Headache	• 5 mg PO once daily
		• Muscle aches	
		• Hypotension	

Alpha-Adrenergic Blockers. Alpha-blockers used in the treatment of BPH work selectively to inhibit alpha-1 receptor sites. Some of these agents (e.g., terazosin) are less selective for prostate tissue and are also used for the treatment of hypertension. Agents such as terazosin and doxazosin commonly cause orthostatic hypotension, so people should be careful when starting these agents to make sure they do not become lightheaded and fall. Other drugs (e.g., tamsulosin) have more targeted activity for the tissues of the prostate; however, these, too, pose a risk of causing orthostatic hypotension, dizziness, and falls. These agents treat the symptoms of BPH by relaxing smooth muscle tissue in the prostate and the bladder neck. This allows urine to flow out of the bladder more easily.

GENERIC NAME: terazosin
TRADE NAME: Hytrin
INDICATION: BPH, hypertension
ROUTE OF ADMINISTRATION: Oral
COMMON ADULT DOSAGE: 1 mg initially at bedtime; then increased to 2, 5, and then 10 mg once daily
MECHANISM OF ACTION: Relaxes smooth muscle tissue in the prostate and the bladder neck by blocking alpha receptors

TABLE 22-7

Select Causes of Erectile Dysfunction (ED)

Condition or Cause That Leads to ED	Effects
Prostatism	Enlargement of the prostate gland
Prostatitis	Inflammation of the prostate gland
Prostatocystitis	Inflammation of the prostate gland and bladder
Nerve damage	Injury to nervous system caused by trauma, surgery, or disease
Substance abuse	Alcohol leads to atrophy of testes, lowering testosterone levels; other drugs (e.g., heroin, cocaine, marijuana) contribute to ED
Low testosterone levels	Hypogonadism can lower sex drive and cause ED
Medications	Medications can have side effects that may cause sexual dysfunction, including ED, such as certain beta-blockers, calcium channel blockers, antidepressants, antihypertensive agents, antihistamines, H_2-antihistamines, and antiseizure medications
Depression/anxiety	Depression can cause or worsen ED due to stress, anxiety, low self-esteem, fears, guilty feelings
Cigarette smoking	Smoking can worsen atherosclerosis, which increases the possibility of ED

SIDE EFFECTS: Orthostatic hypotension, dizziness, drowsiness, blurred vision

AUXILIARY LABELS:
- May cause dizziness/drowsiness.
- Do not drive or perform any hazardous tasks until accustomed to side effects.

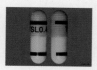

GENERIC NAME: tamsulosin
TRADE NAME: Flomax
INDICATION: BPH
ROUTE OF ADMINISTRATION: Oral
COMMON ADULT DOSAGE: 0.4-0.8 mg once daily; give ½ hour after the same meal each day
MECHANISM OF ACTION: Relaxes smooth muscle tissue in the prostate and the bladder neck by blocking alpha receptors
SIDE EFFECTS: Dizziness, blurred vision, diarrhea, headache
AUXILIARY LABELS:
- May cause dizziness/drowsiness.
- Do not drive or perform any hazardous tasks until you know how this drug affects you.

Erectile Dysfunction

Erectile dysfunction (ED) is the inability of the male to achieve or maintain an erection, commonly referred to as *impotence*. This is due to a lack of blood flowing to the penis rather than a lack of desire. This condition ranges from rarely occurring in a given individual to becoming a chronic problem. As a man ages, the probability of experiencing ED increases. As men age, they have an increased risk of developing not only prostate conditions but also other disease states that affect the ability to achieve an erection, such as diabetes, atherosclerosis, high blood pressure, and cardiovascular diseases. Additional causes of ED are listed in Table 22-7.

Prognosis. In many cases ED occurs only on rare occasions and does not pose a significant problem warranting treatment. Persistent ED can be a sign of a possible underlying problem. When a patient complains of ED, it is imperative that the physician identify and treat any underlying contributing conditions. With proper treatment and lifestyle changes, the frequency of episodes of ED may be reduced.

Non–Drug Treatments. Lifestyle changes such as reducing alcohol intake, smoking cessation, losing weight, and participating in an exercise program can be helpful, if appropriate. Nonpharmacological devices can also help treat ED. Vacuum devices (penis pumps) can be used to increase blood flow to the penis and initiate an erection. Psychotherapy in certain cases can also help the man overcome anxieties that may be contributing to psychogenic ED.

Drug Treatments. Sildenafil (Viagra), a phosphodiesterase inhibitor, was introduced in 1998 for the treatment of ED. This medication initially was researched for use as a cardiovascular agent

TABLE 22-8

Select Agents for the Treatment of Erectile Dysfunction

Medication Class	Generic Name	Brand Name	Common Side Effects	Common Dose Range
Phosphodiesterase-5 Inhibitors (PDE-5)	sildenafil	Viagra	• Flushing • Headache • Upset stomach • Hypotension • Priapism (lasting longer than 4 hr)	• 50 mg PO once daily 60 min before anticipated sexual activity
	vardenafil	Levitra Staxyn		• 10 mg 60 min before anticipated sexual activity
	tadalafil	Cialis		• 5-20 mg PO 30 min before anticipated sexual activity
Prostaglandin/ Vasodilator	alprostadil	Caverject	• Penile pain • Urethral burning • Headache • Scarring (injection) • Priapism	• 1.25-2.5 mcg intracavernous injection before sexual activity (dose is individualized and based on type/cause of erectile dysfunction)
		Muse		• 125-250 mcg intraurethral suppository administered prn for erection (max 2/day)

to lower blood pressure and treat angina pectoris. Today it is widely used to treat ED. Sildenafil (and other medications in this class) increases blood flow to the penis and causes penile rigidity. Possible side effects of phosphodiesterase inhibitors include headaches, flushing of the skin, gastrointestinal symptoms, nasal congestion, and diarrhea. Patients taking nitrates should not take sildenafil or related drugs concurrently because of the potential for dangerous decreases in blood pressure that can occur when these agents are combined. Table 22-8 lists select medications used to treat ED. You will note in the table that injectable and intraurethral products are also available to treat ED; however, these options are far less frequently used than oral ED medications.

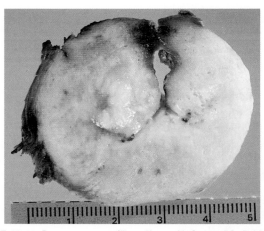

FIGURE 22-12 Prostate cancer. (From Kumar V, Cotran RS, Robbins SL: *Basic pathology,* ed 7, Philadelphia, 2003, Saunders.)

Prostate Cancer

Prostate cancer is a condition in which the cells in the prostate grow at an uncontrolled rate, forming tumors (Figure 22-12). This blocks the flow of urine through the prostate, and if left untreated, the cancer can metastasize through the body. Genetics seem to affect the onset of this condition; African American men are more likely to develop prostate cancer, as are men who have relatives with prostate cancer. Symptoms include nocturia, dysuria, blood in the urine or semen, painful ejaculation, and pain in the pelvis or lower back that does not subside. Prostate cancer has four stages, and staging of the cancer is necessary to determine the most effective treatment plan.

Prognosis. Although prostate cancer is a serious condition, advancements in treatment have improved outcomes for many individuals. Early diagnosis, increased public awareness, and new chemotherapy agents have increased the life span of men diagnosed with prostate cancer.

Non–Drug Treatment. Prostate cancer can be treated by performing surgery that removes the prostate (radical prostatectomy) or the testicles (orchidectomy). A partial removal of prostate tissue (transurethral resection of the prostate [TURP]) may be done to remove some of the cancer. Radiological treatment can be used to treat recurrent or advanced-stage prostate cancer.

TABLE 22-9

Select Hormonal Prostate Cancer Treatments

Type of Hormone Therapy	Generic Name	Trade Name	Effect in Men
Luteinizing hormone–releasing hormone (LHRH)	leuprolide	Lupron Depot	Blocks hormone production in testes
	goserelin	Zoladex	Blocks hormone production in testes
Antiandrogens	flutamide	Eulexin	Blocks effects of testosterone
	nilutamide	Nilandron	Blocks effects of testosterone

Drug Treatment. The treatment for prostate cancer is determined by the stage of the cancer. Hormone therapy is the most common medical treatment used for prostate cancer. The activity of hormones can be eradicated or reduced so that the cancerous cells stop reproducing. Antiandrogens and luteinizing hormone–releasing hormone (LHRH) agonists can cause a decrease in hormone activity and are the most common agents used. All of these treatments are usually started in stage 2 prostate cancer. Table 22-9 presents examples of hormonal medications used. For more advanced forms of prostate cancer, a variety of chemotherapeutic agents and regimens may be used.

Sexually Transmitted Diseases

Any disease that can be transmitted by sexual intercourse is considered to be a sexually transmitted disease. However, this does not mean that these diseases cannot be transmitted in other ways. For example, human immunodeficiency virus (HIV) can be spread either by intercourse or by the sharing of needles. Herpesvirus can be spread from a mother to a child through childbirth, and pubic lice and scabies can be transmitted from the sharing of towels or bedding and by close contact. Because STDs are embarrassing to patients, many do not seek treatment right away. Additionally, certain STDs (e.g., syphilis, herpes) can remain dormant (latent) for long periods, which results in more transference between partners until the symptoms become more obvious to the individual. Even then, many people are reluctant to provide the names of those who may be infected.

STDs can be caused by bacterial, viral, fungal, and protozoal organisms. If left untreated, some STDs can cause irreversible sterility, blindness, and even death. Several of these diseases, including chlamydia, gonorrhea, hepatitis, acquired immunodeficiency syndrome (AIDS), and syphilis, are on the list of Notifiable Infectious Diseases. If an individual is diagnosed as having one of the diseases on this list,

the medical practitioner is required by law to notify the local health department. This list of diseases is available from the CDC and is updated annually. Table 22-10 presents a list of the diseases that cause STDs, along with select drugs and dosage forms for the treatment of these diseases.

The symptoms of STDs vary according to disease and severity of infection. Chlamydia caused by the bacterium *Chlamydia trachomatis* can permanently damage a woman's reproductive organs; symptoms may be mild or even absent. Gonorrhea caused by the bacterium *Neisseria gonorrhoeae* also may have mild or no symptoms. Both chlamydia and gonorrhea can eventually cause pelvic inflammatory disease in women and epididymitis in men if left untreated; both are painful conditions that can lead to sterility. Early symptoms of HIV typically include fever, headache, fatigue, and rash; as the disease progresses, increased severity of these early symptoms may manifest, along with night sweats, chronic diarrhea, and chills. Genital herpes, which can lie dormant for months, years, or decades, causes small red bumps or blisters or a rash on the genitals. Hepatitis, which infects the liver, can cause fatigue, nausea, vomiting, darkening of the urine, or yellowing of the skin. Many of the symptoms of these diseases are not present in the early stages of the infection, making the transference of the infection more likely. Because infections are typically passed during sexual contact, protection and education are key components to preventing the spread of these diseases.

As mentioned, education is important in preventing the transmission of STDs. Some members of the general public may mistakenly believe that taking oral birth control or using contraceptive gels can protect against STDs, but this is not true. Some vaccines, such as Gardasil, can provide protection against certain human papillomavirus (HPV) infections but do not protect against all STDs. Research is currently under way to develop a vaccine against HIV; however, at this time there is no viable vaccine on the market. Because of the large amount of information and misinformation available to the public through a variety of media sources, patients may become confused about how to remain uninfected.

TABLE 22-10

Select Sexually Transmitted Diseases and Potential Treatments

Organism	Condition	Generic Name	Trade Name	Dose
Chlamydia trachomatis	Chlamydia	azithromycin	Zithromax	• 1 g orally (PO) once
		erythromycin	E-Mycin	• 500 mg PO 4 times daily for 7 days
		doxycycline	Vibramycin	• 100 mg PO twice daily for 7 days
		ofloxacin	Floxin	• 300 mg PO twice daily for 7 days
Neisseria gonorrhoeae	Gonorrhea	azithromycin	Zithromax	• 1 g PO once (if likely *Chlamydia* coinfection is not ruled out)
		cefixime	Suprax	• 400 mg PO once
		ceftriaxone	Rocephin	• 125 mg PO/intramuscularly (IM) once
Herpes simplex	Genital herpes	acyclovir	Zovirax	• 400 mg PO 3 times daily for 7-10 days
		famciclovir	Famvir	• 250 mg PO 3 times daily for 7-10 days
		valacyclovir	Valtrex	• 1 g PO twice daily for 10 days
Treponema pallidum	Syphilis	benzathine penicillin G	Bicillin L-A	• 50,000 units/kg IM (max 2.4 million units) once weekly for 3 wk
		azithromycin	Zithromax	• 2 g PO once
		tetracycline	Sumycin	• 500 mg PO 4 times daily for 14 days
Trichomonas vaginalis	Trichomoniasis vaginalis	metronidazole	Flagyl	• 2 gm PO once *or*
				• 500 mg PO once daily for 7 days
		tinidazole	Tinadamax	• 2 g PO once
Gardnerella vaginalis	Bacterial vaginitis	clindamycin	Cleocin, Cleocin Vaginal	• 300 mg PO twice daily for 7 days *or*
				• 2% cream applied daily for 7 days
		metronidazole	Flagyl, Metrogel Vaginal	• 500 mg PO twice daily for 7 days
Candida albicans	Vaginal candidiasis	butoconazole	Femstat, Femstat 3	• 1 applicator full (5 g) as a single dose
		clotrimazole	Gyne-Lotrimin	• 1 applicator full (2% [5 g]) as a single dose for 3 days
		fluconazole	Diflucan	• 150 mg PO as a single dose
		miconazole	Monistat	• 1200 mg vaginal suppository inserted for 1 day
		terconazole	Terazol 7, Terazol 3	• 0.8% cream 1 applicator full (5 g) daily at bedtime for 3 days
		tioconazole	Vagistat-1	• 1 applicator (about 4.6 g) intravaginally before bedtime as a single dose

The CDC, U.S. Public Health Department, and each state's public health department print brochures, produce videos, and maintain websites for up-to-date, reliable information. Tables 22-11 and 22-12 provide an overview of select agents used for the treatment of HIV and hepatitis, respectively.

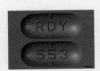

GENERIC NAME: valacyclovir
TRADE NAME: Valtrex
INDICATION: Herpes, varicella
ROUTE OF ADMINISTRATION: Oral

COMMON ADULT DOSAGE: *Herpes:* 500 mg twice daily for 3 days at the first sign or symptom of lesions; *Herpes zoster (Varicella):* 1 g three times daily for 7 days at the first sign of symptoms.
MECHANISM OF ACTION: Inhibits viral DNA synthesis
SIDE EFFECTS: Headache, nausea, abdominal pain, fatigue

 Tech Alert!
Remember these sound-alike, look-alike drugs:
  Cardura versus Coumadin and Cardene
  clomiphene versus clomipramine
  methyltestosterone versus methylprednisolone
  Provera versus Premarin
  Yasmin versus Yaz

TABLE 22-11

Select Agents for the Treatment of Human Immunodeficiency Virus (HIV) Infection and Acquired Immunodeficiency Syndrome (AIDS)*

Medication Class	Generic Name	Trade Name	Abbreviation	Common Dose Range
Nucleoside Reverse Transcriptase Inhibitors (NRTIs)	zidovudine	Retrovir	AZT	• 200 mg orally (PO) 3 times daily *or* • 300 mg PO twice daily
	didanosine	Videx	ddI	• Weight based: ≥60 kg: 400 mg PO daily; <60 kg: 250 mg PO daily
	lamivudine	Epivir	3TC	• 150 mg PO twice daily
	stavudine	Zerit	D4T	• Weight based: ≥60 kg: 40 mg PO twice daily; <60 kg: 30 mg PO twice daily
Nucleotide Reverse Transcriptase Inhibitor (NTRTI)	abacavir	Ziagen	ABC	• 300 mg PO twice daily
	emtricitabine	Emtriva	FTC	• 200 mg PO daily
	tenofovir	Viread	TFV	• 300 mg PO daily
Protease Inhibitors (PIs)	ritonavir	Norvir	RTV	• "Booster" for other PIs: 100-400 mg PO daily
	saquinavir	Invirase	SQV	• 1000 mg PO twice daily boosted with ritonavir 100 mg PO twice daily
	indinavir	Crixivan	IDV	• 800 mg PO every 8 hr
	nelfinavir	Viracept	NFV	• 750 mg PO three times daily *or* • 1250 mg PO twice daily
	amprenavir	Agenerase	APV	• 1200 mg PO twice daily
	lopinavir	Kaletra	LPV	• 400 mg PO twice daily boosted with RTV 100 mg PO twice daily
	atazanavir	Reyataz	ATV	• 400 mg PO daily *or* • 300 mg PO daily boosted with RTV 100 mg PO daily
	fosamprenavir	Lexiva	FPV	• 1400 mg PO twice daily *or* • 1400 mg PO daily boosted with RTV 200 mg PO daily
	tipranavir	Aptivus	TPV	• 500 mg PO twice daily boosted with RTV 200 mg PO twice daily
	darunavir	Prezista	DRV	• 600 mg PO twice daily boosted with RTV 100 mg PO twice daily
Non–Nucleoside Reverse Transcriptase Inhibitor (NNRTI)	nevirapine	Viramune	NVP	• 200 mg PO once daily for 14 days, then • 200 mg PO twice daily
	efavirenz	Sustiva	EFV	• 600 mg PO once daily at bedtime
	etravirine	Intelence	—	• 200 mg PO twice daily
Fusion Inhibitor	enfuvirtide	Fuzeon	T-20	• 90 mg subcutaneously (SUBCUT) twice daily
CCR5 Blocker	maraviroc	Selzentry	—	• 150-600 mg PO twice daily
Integrase Inhibitor	raltegravir	Isentress	—	• 400 mg PO twice daily

*Many of the medications are available in combination formulations, especially the NRTIs.

TABLE 22-12

Select Agents for the Treatment of Hepatitis B and C

Medication Class	Generic Name	Trade Name	Common Side Effects	Common Dose Range
Hepatitis B **Interferon**	interferon alfa-2b	Intron A	• Flulike symptoms • Depression • Headache • Injection site reactions	• 5 million units/day intramuscularly/ subcutaneously (IM/SUBCUT) *or* • 10 million units IM/SUBCUT 3 times/wk for 16 wk
	interferon alfa-2a pegylated	Pegasys		• 180 mcg SUBCUT once weekly for 48 wk
Nucleoside Reverse Transcriptase Inhibitors (NRTIs)	lamivudine	Epivir-HBV	• Fatigue • Headache • Nausea • Vomiting • Diarrhea	• 100 mg orally (PO) once daily
	telbivudine	Tyzeka	• Fatigue • Headache • Rash • Dizziness • Fever	• 600 mg PO once daily
	entecavir	Baraclude	• Headache • Nausea • Vomiting • Fatigue	• 0.5-1 mg PO once daily
Nucleotide Reverse Transcriptase Inhibitors (NTRTIs)	adefovir	Hepsera	• Headache • Abdominal pain • Diarrhea • Weakness • Hematuria	• 10 mg PO once daily
	tenofovir	Viread	• Insomnia • Depression • Pain • Nausea • Weakness	• 300 mg PO once daily
Hepatitis C **Interferon**	interferon alfa-2b	Intron A	• Flulike symptoms • Depression • Headache • Injection site reactions	• 5 million units/day IM/SUBCUT *or* • 10 million units IM/SUBCUT 3 times/wk for 16 wk
	interferon alfa-2a	Roferon-A		• 3 million units IM/SUBCUT 3 times/wk
	interferon alfa-2a pegylated	Pegasys		• 180 mcg SUBCUT once weekly for 48 wk
	interferon alfa-2b pegylated	PegIntron		• 1 mcg/kg SUBCUT weekly *or* • 1.5 mcg/kg SUBCUT weekly with Ribavirin
Antiviral	ribavirin	Rebetol	• Fatigue • Insomnia • Headache • Anemia • Hypotension	• 800-1200 mg/day PO in 2 divided doses
Protease Inhibitors	boceprevir	Victrelis	• Anemia • Taste changes • Fatigue	• 800 mg PO 3 times daily (added to PEG-INF + Ribavirin after 4 wk of dual therapy)
	telaprevir	Incivek	• Rash • Nausea • Insomnia	• 750 mg PO 3 times daily with food (added to PEG-INF + Ribavirin after 11 wk of dual therapy)

DO YOU REMEMBER THESE KEY POINTS?

- Names of the major anatomical components of the male and female reproductive systems and their functions
- The primary signs and symptoms of the various conditions discussed in this chapter
- Medications used to treat the various conditions discussed in this chapter

- The generic and trade names for the drugs discussed in this chapter
- The appropriate auxiliary labels that should be used when filling prescriptions for drugs discussed in this chapter

REVIEW QUESTIONS

Multiple Choice Questions

1. The primary female reproductive organs are:
   A. Uterus
   B. Ovaries
   C. Testes
   D. Both A and B
2. Male sex hormones are collectively called:
   A. Estrogens
   B. Androgens
   C. Progestins
   D. Testosterones
3. Testosterone is used to treat which condition?
   A. Hypogonadism in females
   B. Hypogonadism in males
   C. Breast and endometrial cancers in females
   D. Both B and C
4. Estrogens are used to treat which condition?
   A. Menopausal symptoms
   B. Hypogonadism in males
   C. Hypogonadism in females
   D. All of the above
5. Which medication class is used for the treatment of HIV/AIDS?
   A. Nucleoside reverse transcriptase inhibitors
   B. Protease inhibitors
   C. Non-nucleoside reverse transcriptase inhibitors
   D. All of the above
6. The brand name for tamsulosin is:
   A. Cardura
   B. Uroxatral
   C. Hytrin
   D. Flomax
7. How is clomiphene (Clomid) administered?
   A. Orally
   B. IM injection
   C. Intravaginally
   D. Transdermally
8. Medications used to treat benign prostatic hypertrophy include:
   A. 5-Alpha reductase inhibitors
   B. Estrogens
   C. Androgens
   D. Alpha-adrenergic blockers
   E. Both A and D

9. Which of the following is *not* a risk factor for pelvic inflammatory disease (PID)?
   A. Age
   B. Multiple sexual partners
   C. History of PID
   D. Hypertension
10. Pelvic inflammatory disease can be caused by:
    A. IUD usage
    B. STDs
    C. Bacterial infection
    D. All of the above
11. Gonorrhea may be treated with:
    A. Azithromycin
    B. Valacyclovir
    C. Acyclovir
    D. Both B and C
12. Interferons (e.g., Intron A, Pegasys) are used to treat which infectious disease?
    A. PID
    B. HIV
    C. Hepatitis
    D. Chlamydia
13. Which medication(s) is (are) associated with orthostatic hypotension?
    A. Doxazosin
    B. Finasteride
    C. Dutasteride
    D. All of the above
14. Which product is an intraurethral suppository for the treatment of erectile dysfunction?
    A. Caverject
    B. Muse
    C. Cialis
    D. Viagra
15. Medications and/or devices used to treat ED include:
    A. Sildenafil, vacuum devices, penile implants
    B. Cialis, Levitra, prostaglandin suppositories
    C. Atenolol, leuprolide, penile implants
    D. Both A and B

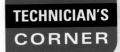

A 55-year-old male patient with diabetes mellitus, hypertension, and coronary artery disease presents a prescription to the pharmacy for sildenafil (Viagra). As the pharmacy technician, you review his medication history and find that he takes the following medications regularly:

Glucotrol-XL 5 mg daily
Metformin 500 mg tid
Tenormin 50 mg daily
Lipitor 20 mg q am
Isordil 10 mg bid

Using a drug reference resource, answer the following questions:

1. Is Viagra safe for dispensing with the previously listed medication history?
2. Which of the medications are in a correct dosage?
3. Which medications could be given with sildenafil?
4. Which are contraindicated with sildenafil, if any?
5. What should you as a pharmacy technician do if this prescription is presented for dispensing?

Bibliography

Applegate E: *The anatomy and physiology learning system*, ed 3, Philadelphia, 2006, Saunders.

Centers for Disease Control and Prevention (CDC): Sexually transmitted diseases (STDs). (Referenced September 6, 2014.) www.cdc.gov/std/treatment/2010/default.htm.

Clinical Pharmacology Online. (Referenced September 6, 2014.) www.clinicalpharmacology-ip.com.

Damjanov I: *Pathology for the health professions*, ed 4, St Louis, 2011, Saunders.

Fishback JL: *Pathology*, ed 3, Philadelphia, 2005, Mosby.

Huether S, McCance K: *Understanding pathophysiology*, ed 5, St Louis, 2012, Mosby.

McCance KL: *Pathophysiology: the biologic basis for disease in adults and children*, ed 6, St Louis, 2010, Mosby.

Page C et al: *Integrated pharmacology*, ed 3, 2006, Mosby.

Patton KT et al: *Mosby's handbook of anatomy and physiology*, St Louis, 2000, Mosby.

Price SA et al: *Pathophysiology: clinical concepts of disease processes*, ed 6, St Louis, 2003, Mosby.

Solomon EP: *Introduction to human anatomy and physiology*, ed 3, St Louis, 2009, Saunders.

Thibodeau GA, Patton KT: *Anatomy and physiology*, ed 8, St Louis, 2012, Mosby.

UpToDate Online. (Referenced September 6, 2014.) www.uptodate.com.

Therapeutic Agents for the Immune System

Joshua J. Neumiller

OBJECTIVES

Upon completing this chapter, you should be able to do the following:

1. Describe the organs and cells of the immune system and their roles.
2. List the primary signs and symptoms of common conditions associated with dysregulation of the immune system.
3. Differentiate between different types of immunizations.

4. Recognize prescription and over-the-counter drugs used to treat common conditions discussed in this chapter.
5. Write the generic and trade names for the drugs discussed in this chapter.
6. List appropriate auxiliary labels when filling prescriptions for drugs discussed in this chapter.

TERMS AND DEFINITIONS

Anaphylaxis An extreme, potentially life-threatening allergic reaction

Antibodies Complex molecules (immunoglobulins) made in response to the presence of an antigen (e.g., a protein of bacteria or other infecting organism) that neutralize the effect of the foreign substance

Antigen A substance that prompts the production of antibodies, resulting in an immune response

Antigen-presenting cell (APC) A cell of the immune system that presents antigens to lymphocytes to activate an immune response

Attenuated A term describing an altered or weakened live vaccine made from the disease organism against which the vaccine protects

Biological response modifier (BRM) An agent used to modify the body's immune response

Cytokine A protein that signals cells of the immune system

Hashimoto's thyroiditis An autoimmune disease leading to hypothyroidism

Hematopoiesis The formation of blood cells

Humoral immunity The immune response mediated by antibodies

Immunity A type of resistance to infection caused by an immune response from the body after exposure to antigens or administration of vaccines

Immunization The act of conferring immunity, such as with vaccination

Immunoglobulin An antibody

Inflammation A localized physical condition associated with red, swollen, hot, and often painful tissue

Innate immunity Natural immunity

Juvenile rheumatoid arthritis (JRA) Rheumatoid arthritis that affects children

Leukocyte A white blood cell (WBC)

Lymph node A structure that consists of many small, oval nodules that filter lymphatic fluid and fight infection; the site of lymphocyte, monocyte, and plasma cell production

Lymphocyte A mononuclear leukocyte found in the blood, lymph, and lymphoid tissues

Monocyte A phagocytic leukocyte

Phagocyte A cell of the immune system that engulfs cells, debris, and antigens

Plasma cell A cell of the immune system that secretes antibodies

Rheumatoid arthritis (RA) A progressive degenerative and crippling autoimmune disease of the joints

Spleen A lymphatic organ involved in the production and removal of blood cells and the storage of lymphocytes

Systemic A term meaning pertaining to the entire organism; "widespread" in contrast to "local"

Systemic lupus erythematosus (SLE) An autoimmune inflammatory disease of connective tissue with variable features, including fever, weakness, fatigue, and other systemic manifestations

Toxoid A type of vaccine in which a toxin has been rendered harmless but still invokes an antigenic response, improving immunity against the active toxin at some future date

Transplant rejection An immune response after tissue or organ transplantation

Vaccine A biological preparation that improves immunity to a particular disease by invoking an immune response and a "memory" of the response for future use

Vasodilation Widening of the vasculature, leading to increased blood flow

Virion A virus particle

Virus A microscopic, nonliving organism that replicates exclusively inside the host's cell using parts of the host cell, including DNA, ribosomes, and proteins

Select Vaccines That Affect the Immune System

Vaccine/Drug	Pronunciation
Immune Globulins	
Botulism immune globulin (BIG)	(**bot**-ue-lizm im-**myoon glob**-yoo-lin)
Cytomegalovirus immune globulin (CMV-IG)	(sye-toe-**meg**-a-lo-vye-rus im-**myoon glob**-yoo-lin)
Immune globulin G (IgG)	(im-**myoon glob**-yoo-lin)
Hepatitis B immune globulin (HBIG)	(hep-ah-**ty**-tiss **B** im-**myoon glob**-yoo-lin)
Rabies immune globulin (RIG)	(**ray**-beez im-**myoon glob**-yoo-lin)
Respiratory syncytial virus immune globulin (RSV-IG)	(**res**-pi-rah-tory sink-**tee**-ahl **vye**-rus im-**myoon glob**-yoo-lin)
Tetanus immune globulin (TIG)	(**tetn**-us im-**myoon** glob-yoo-lin)
Vaccinia immune globulin (VIG)	(vax-**in**-ee-a im-**myoon glob**-yoo-lin)
Varicella-zoster immune globulin (VZIG)	(var-ih-**sel**-ah-**zos**-ter im-**myoon glob**-yoo-lin)
Antitoxins	
Botulinum antitoxin	(**bot**-ue-li-um an-ti-**tok**-sin)
Diphtheria antitoxin	(**dip**-theer-ee-a an-ti-**tok**-sin)
Tetanus antitoxin	(**tet**-n-us an-ti-**tok**-sin)
Vaccines Against Viral Illness	
Influenza intranasal	(in-floo-**en**-za in-**tra**-naz-al)
Measles, mumps, rubella (MMR)	(**mee**-zels, **mumps**, roo-**bel**-a)
Poliovirus oral (OPV)	(**poe**-lee-oh)
Rotavirus oral	(**roe**-ta-vye-ris)
Smallpox (vaccinia)	(**small** pox)
Varicella (chickenpox)	(var-ih-**sel**-a)
Herpes zoster (varicella-zoster)	(her-**pees zos**-ter)
Avian influenza	(**a**-vee-an in-floo-**en**-za)
Hepatitis A	(hep-ah-**ty**-tiss **A**)
Hepatitis B	(hep-ah-**ty**-tiss **B**)
Human papillomavirus (HPV)	(hyoo-man **pap**-i-**lo**-ma-**vye**-rus)
Inactivated influenza virus injectable	(in-**ak**-ti-vay-ted in-**floo**-en-za **vye**-rus)
Japanese encephalitis virus	(**jap**-a-**neez** en-**cef**-a-**lye**-tis **vye**-rus)
Inactivated poliovirus (IPV)	(in-**ak**-ti-vay-ted **poe**-lee-oh-**vye**-rus)
Yellow fever	(yel-**oh** fee-**ver**)
Vaccines Against Bacterial Illness	
Anthrax vaccine	(**anth**-rax vax-**een**)
Haemophilus influenzae type b	(hee-**maw**-fil-us in-floo-**en**-za)
Lyme disease	(**lime** dis-**ese**)
Meningococcal	(me-**nin**-je-**kok**-al)
Plague	(**pla**-gwe)
Pneumococcal	(**noo**-moe-**kok**-al)
Typhoid	(**tye**-foid)

Select Immunosuppressive Agents for the Treatment of Autoimmune Disorders and Transplant Rejection

Trade Name*	Generic Name	Pronunciation
Azasan, Imuran	azathioprine	(ay-za-**thigh**-oh-preen)
CellCept, Myfortic	mycophenolate	(**mye**-koe-**fen**-oh-late)
Cytoxan	cyclophosphamide	(**sye**-kloe-**fos**-fa-mide)
Gengraf, Neoral, Sandimmune	cyclosporine	(**sye**-kloe-**spor**-en)
Prograf	tacrolimus	(ta-**kroe**-li-mus)
Rapamune	sirolimus	(sir-**oh**-li-mus)
Trexall	methotrexate	(meth-oh-**trex**-ate)
Orthoclone OKT3	muromonab-CD3	(**mue**-roe-**moe**-nab)
Simulect	basiliximab	(bass-ih-**lix**-ih-mab)
Zenapax	daclizumab	(dah-**klye**-zue-mab)

*Listing of trade names on the same row does not indicate that products are interchangeable in patient treatment regimens.

Human beings have always been plagued by bacterial and viral microbes that cause disease and death. In addition to these outside invaders, the body may need to defend against internal assailants, such as cancer cells or a misdirected attack from the immune system (i.e., autoimmune disease). Fortunately, with the development of vaccines and immune-modulating medications, morbidity and mortality resulting from infections and autoimmune disorders can now be better managed. This chapter describes the major functions of the immune system and discusses the rationale behind immunizations. It also covers the treatment of autoimmune disorders and transplant rejection.

Anatomy and Physiology of the Immune System

The body has a built-in defense mechanism that helps protect it from invading organisms. From birth, one of the most important functions of the body is to defend against invasion. The lymphatic system is important because it is involved in both immune cell production and proper functioning of the immune system (Figure 23-1). The lymphoid organs are sites of residence, proliferation, and differentiation of **lymphocytes** (e.g., T cells and B cells) and mononuclear **phagocytes** (e.g., macrophages). The many **lymph nodes** in the body contain a large number of lymphocytes, monocytes, and macrophages. Lymphatic veins, which collect interstitial fluid from the tissues and transport it back into the circulatory system as lymph, pass through lymph nodes in the body (Figure 23-2). As the lymph passes through the lymph nodes, the fluid is filtered of debris and microorganisms by immune cells in the node. In the case of an infection, lymphocytes in the lymph nodes are activated by the presence of microorganisms in the lymph to fight an infection. The bone marrow, thymus,

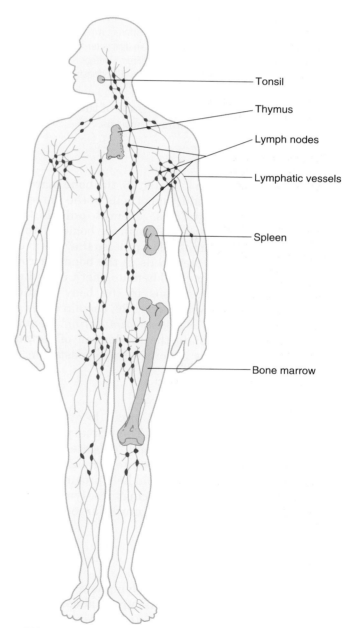

FIGURE 23-1 Overview of the major lymphatic organs of the body.

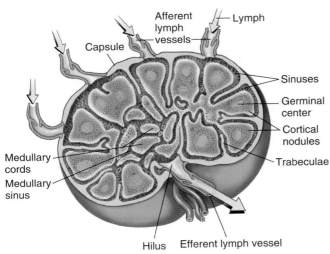

FIGURE 23-2 Cross section of a lymph node. Several afferent, valved lymphatics bring lymph to the node. A single efferent lymphatic leaves the node at the hilus. Note that the artery and vein also enter and leave at the hilus. Arrows show direction of lymph flow. (From Huether S, McCance K: *Understanding pathophysiology,* ed 5, St Louis, 2012, Mosby.)

tonsils, and spleen are larger organs of the lymphatic system, each having specific functions.

Bone Marrow

As discussed further in Chapter 26, the bone marrow is important in the production of cells in the immune and hematological systems. **Hematopoiesis,** or blood cell production, takes place in the bone marrow. Hematopoiesis is a complicated process that involves the differentiation of stem cells in the bone marrow into a variety of immune and hematopoietic cells that carry out different functions in the body (Figure 23-3). As is discussed in Chapter 26, certain types of medications, known as *colony-stimulating factors,* can be used to stimulate the production of certain types of cells that may be low in the bloodstream.

Thymus

The thymus is an important organ located in the upper chest (see Figure 23-1). The primary function of the thymus is to produce and "educate" lymphocytes, which ultimately circulate through lymph nodes and lymphatic tissues and help provide **immunity.** The thymus begins producing these lymphocytes before birth, and the organ is much larger in childhood than in adulthood.

Spleen

The **spleen** is the largest of the lymphoid organs and is located in the left side of the upper abdomen. The function of the spleen is to filter large amounts of blood cells as they reach the end of their life cycle.

The spleen is also important because it is the primary site for immune responses to blood-borne disease. The spleen is composed of two main areas: red pulp and white pulp (Figure 23-4). The red pulp contains macrophages and red blood cells that are being removed from circulation, and the white pulp contains lymphocytes (T cells and B cells). The spleen is estimated to contain approximately 25% of all of the lymphocytes in the body.

Cells and Mediators of the Immune System

The immune system is made up of a number of cells, each with its own specialized function (Figure 23-5). **Leukocytes,** or white blood cells (WBCs), and their functions are described briefly in the following list.

- *Neutrophils:* Neutrophils are the most abundant leukocyte in adults, accounting for approximately 55% of the total leukocyte count. Neutrophils are the first cells to the site of inflammation and act as phagocytes. Phagocytes are cells that ingest and destroy other cells (e.g., bacteria) and debris. Neutrophil cell counts are often used in laboratory testing to determine whether a person has an infection.
- *Eosinophils:* In healthy adults, eosinophils account for approximately 1% to 6% of WBCs. Eosinophils are important for fighting parasitic infections and allergic responses.
- *Macrophages:* Macrophages are powerful phagocytes that play a key role in immune and inflammatory responses. Immature macrophages, known as **monocytes,** are produced in the bone marrow and migrate to tissues where they mature and work to fight infections. Macrophages are also important because they ingest dead or defective cells in the body. Macrophages additionally act as **antigen-presenting cells (APCs)**; this means that when macrophages come in contact with an **antigen** (e.g., a bacterium) in the tissues, they migrate to the lymph nodes to signal T and B cells to gear up to fight the infection.
- *Mast cells:* Mast cells play a variety of roles in the immune system, including wound healing and defense against pathogens. However, mast cells are best known for their role in allergies and anaphylactic reactions (discussed later). Mast cells contain histamine, which they release during an allergic response.
- *Natural killer (NK) cells:* NK cells are a form of lymphocyte that specializes in killing tumor cells and some virus-infected cells as part of the innate immune response. NK cells are produced in the bone marrow and circulate in the bloodstream.
- *T cells:* T cells, or T lymphocytes, are important cells that contribute to the adaptive immune

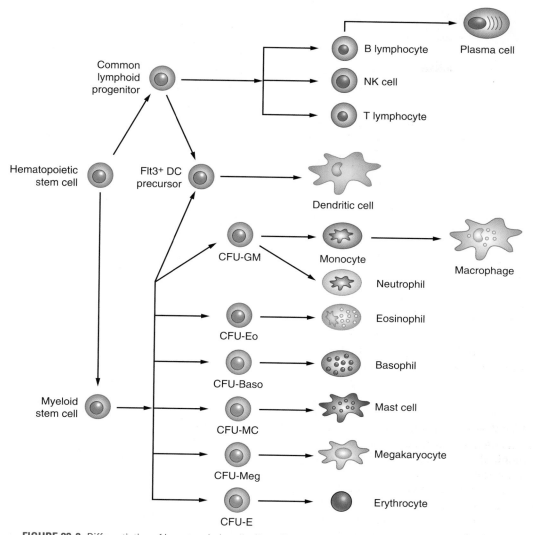

FIGURE 23-3 Differentiation of hematopoietic cells. (From Huether S, McCance K: *Understanding pathophysiology*, ed 5, St Louis, 2012, Elsevier.)

response. T cells are produced in the thymus and remain in the spleen and lymph nodes until they are activated by APCs to attack an invading pathogen.

- *B cells:* B cells, or B lymphocytes, are another important lymphocyte that acts as an antigen-presenting cell. B cells can also differentiate into **plasma cells** that produce **antibodies** against pathogen invaders to help clear an infection.

In addition to the select immune cells just described, cytokines are very important mediators that help drive immune responses. **Cytokines**, which are molecules secreted by a variety of cells (including immune cells), signal inflammation and the activation of immune responses. Cytokines such as tumor necrosis factor (TNF) and interleukin-1 (IL-1) help drive the inflammatory response (Figure 23-6). As is discussed later, medications that inhibit the effects of these cytokines can be used to treat conditions associated with chronic inflammation, such as in rheumatoid arthritis.

Types of Immunity

The immune response can be divided into two large categories, innate immunity and adaptive immunity (Figure 23-7). **Innate immunity** involves cells of the immune system that respond rapidly to an infection. Phagocytic cells (e.g., macrophages and neutrophils) migrate to the site of infection and begin to ingest bacteria or other antigens. These cells, in turn, release cytokines to facilitate the inflammatory response to infection. APCs at the inflammatory site process the antigen for presentation to lymphocytes in the lymph nodes, which helps to mount the adaptive immune response.

Lymphocytes are key cells in the adaptive immune response. Many lymphocytes remain in lymph nodes

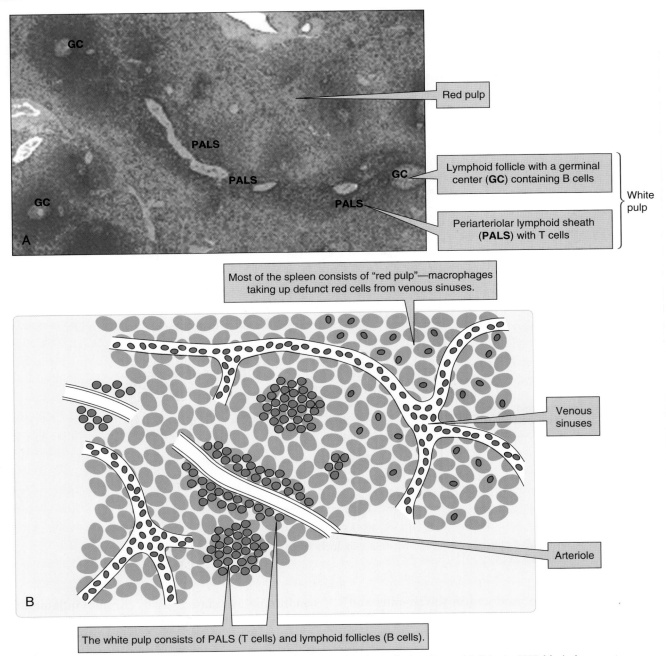

FIGURE 23-4 Spleen. (From Nairn R, Helbert M: *Immunology for medical students,* ed 2, St Louis, 2007, Mosby.)

and tissues, waiting to mount an immune response against invading pathogens. The two primary types of lymphocytes are T cells and B cells, which were described previously. B cells and their products, **immunoglobulins** (antibodies), contribute to **humoral immunity**, also known as *antibody-mediated immunity*. When activated, B cells become plasma cells that produce antibodies specific to an invading antigen. After an immune response, some of the B cells become memory cells that "remember" the invasion for a future date and can respond more

quickly to a repeated infection. T cells are also located in the lymph nodes and remain there until activated by an APC (Figure 23-8). When activated, T cells in the lymph node can then divide and expand to form an army of cells that can attack and eliminate the invading pathogen. This response can be a direct destruction of the attached cell and antigen, or the T cells can release a chemical signal that enlists the help of macrophages to destroy the invading antigen. As with B cells, memory T cells develop. Upon subsequent exposure to the same antigen, the memory

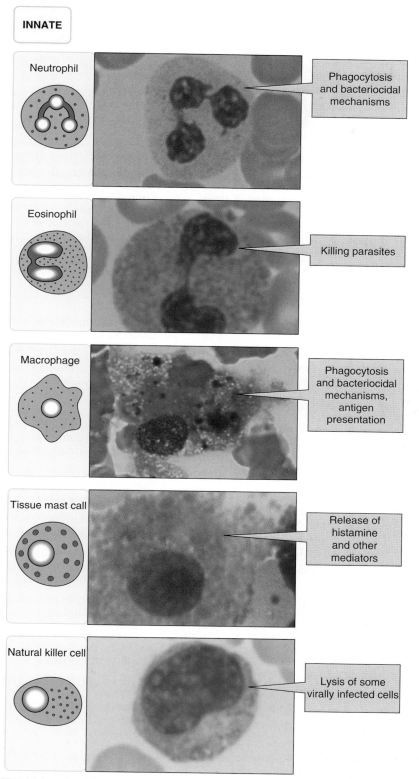

FIGURE 23-5 Major cells of the immune system. (From Nairn R, Helbert M: *Immunology for medical students,* ed 2, St Louis, 2007, Mosby.)

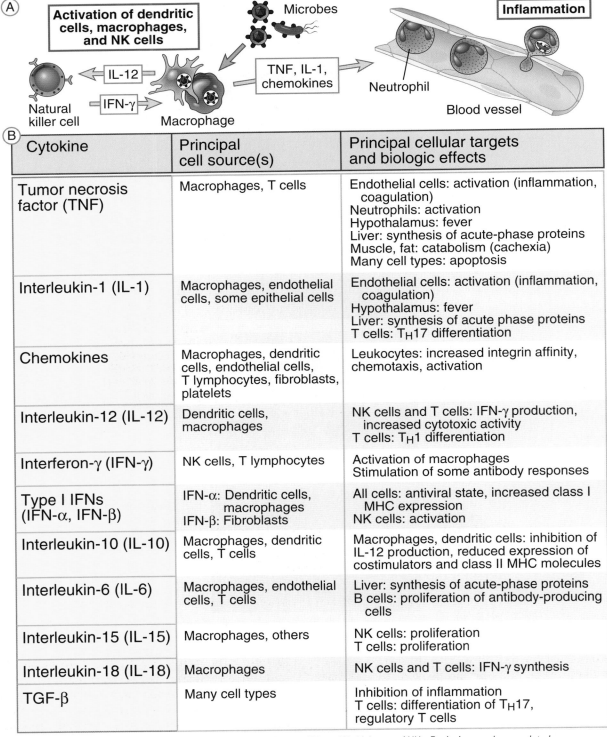

Cytokine	Principal cell source(s)	Principal cellular targets and biologic effects
Tumor necrosis factor (TNF)	Macrophages, T cells	Endothelial cells: activation (inflammation, coagulation) Neutrophils: activation Hypothalamus: fever Liver: synthesis of acute-phase proteins Muscle, fat: catabolism (cachexia) Many cell types: apoptosis
Interleukin-1 (IL-1)	Macrophages, endothelial cells, some epithelial cells	Endothelial cells: activation (inflammation, coagulation) Hypothalamus: fever Liver: synthesis of acute phase proteins T cells: T_H17 differentiation
Chemokines	Macrophages, dendritic cells, endothelial cells, T lymphocytes, fibroblasts, platelets	Leukocytes: increased integrin affinity, chemotaxis, activation
Interleukin-12 (IL-12)	Dendritic cells, macrophages	NK cells and T cells: IFN-γ production, increased cytotoxic activity T cells: T_H1 differentiation
Interferon-γ (IFN-γ)	NK cells, T lymphocytes	Activation of macrophages Stimulation of some antibody responses
Type I IFNs (IFN-α, IFN-β)	IFN-α: Dendritic cells, macrophages IFN-β: Fibroblasts	All cells: antiviral state, increased class I MHC expression NK cells: activation
Interleukin-10 (IL-10)	Macrophages, dendritic cells, T cells	Macrophages, dendritic cells: inhibition of IL-12 production, reduced expression of costimulators and class II MHC molecules
Interleukin-6 (IL-6)	Macrophages, endothelial cells, T cells	Liver: synthesis of acute-phase proteins B cells: proliferation of antibody-producing cells
Interleukin-15 (IL-15)	Macrophages, others	NK cells: proliferation T cells: proliferation
Interleukin-18 (IL-18)	Macrophages	NK cells and T cells: IFN-γ synthesis
TGF-β	Many cell types	Inhibition of inflammation T cells: differentiation of T_H17, regulatory T cells

FIGURE 23-6 Cytokines of innate immunity. (From Abbas AK, Lichtman AHH: *Basic immunology updated edition: functions and disorders of the immune system,* ed 4, Philadelphia, 2014, Saunders.)

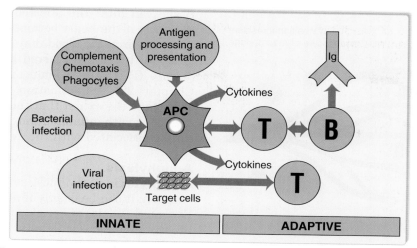

FIGURE 23-7 Innate and adaptive immunity. (From Nairn R, Helbert M: *Immunology for medical students,* ed 2, St Louis, 2007, Mosby.)

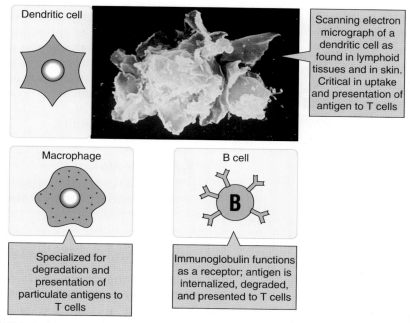

FIGURE 23-8 Antigen-presenting cells. (From Nairn R, Helbert M: *Immunology for medical students,* ed 2, St Louis, 2007, Mosby.)

cells produced from the first encounter are able to rapidly destroy the antigen and prevent the disease process.

The Inflammatory Response

Inflammation can be caused by infection, allergic reactions, or injury. Inflammation is a necessary response to bodily injury. Along with the obvious swelling effects of inflammation, other effects occur that are felt rather than seen. Thousands of years ago, the Romans described the symptoms of inflammation as redness, swelling, heat, pain, and eventual loss of function of the affected area. The body tries to repair the damage with the help of blood, cells, and natural chemicals. **Vasodilation** occurs during inflammation, allowing more blood to reach the affected area. As a result of the increased blood flow caused by vasodilation, the affected area becomes warmer, and edema (buildup of fluids) in the surrounding tissues may develop. A variety of immune cells previously described migrate to the inflamed area (Figure 23-9).

The cells of the body contain many different chemicals that play a role in inflammation. Each chemical has a specific job to perform. One such chemical found in many cells is an enzyme called *cyclooxygenase (COX).* This enzyme produces various hormones,

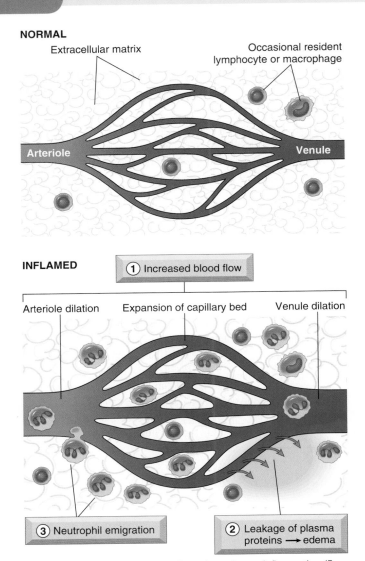

NORMAL

Extracellular matrix

Occasional resident lymphocyte or macrophage

Arteriole

Venule

INFLAMED

① Increased blood flow

Arteriole dilation

Expansion of capillary bed

Venule dilation

③ Neutrophil emigration

② Leakage of plasma proteins → edema

FIGURE 23-9 The major local manifestations of acute inflammation. (From Kumar V, Abbas AK: *Robbins and Cotran pathologic basis of disease,* ed 8, Philadelphia, 2010, Saunders.)

called *prostaglandins,* that are responsible for other chemical reactions that cause inflammation, pain, and increased temperature. Aspirin is one agent that inhibits COX pathways, thereby attenuating the production of prostaglandin. (See Chapter 17 to review other antiinflammatory medications.)

Inflammatory conditions can be either acute or chronic. Acute inflammation characteristically lasts a few days, and the body usually can recover without the aid of medications. Chronic inflammation can arise from an acute case of inflammation or from an injury. Chronic inflammation can occur locally, such as at a cut on the surface of the skin, or **systemically**, throughout the body. When inflammation becomes chronic, the site of injury may swell again, and a low-grade fever can result. Chronic inflammation can cause damage to the affected sites or internal organs. As the body heals, it may leave scar tissue. This scar

tissue can alter the affected area's physiology. For instance, if the heart becomes scarred, its ability to pump or circulate blood may be compromised. If the fallopian tubes are scarred by pelvic inflammatory disease (PID), the woman may become sterile (see Chapter 22). Inflammation also can damage the kidneys to the extent that the person requires dialysis. Along with inflammation, varying degrees of pain can be associated with the swelling that occurs.

Anaphylaxis

Anaphylaxis is the most severe case of an allergic reaction; it can be deadly if not treated immediately. For most people, allergies are inconvenient but not life-threatening; for others, a reaction can cause swelling of the airways within minutes. Most people have an allergic reaction to one agent or another in their lifetime, and it may occur more than once. Epinephrine is administered for the most severe reactions that cause swelling of the airways. Individuals who know they can suffer anaphylactic shock from a bee sting or other allergic reaction should always carry an epinephrine autoinjector (e.g., EpiPen or EpiPen Jr.) in case they are stung or have an allergic exposure. This device is available in packs of two injectors per kit in strengths of 0.15 mg for children and 0.3 mg for adults.

> **Tech Note!**
>
> For detailed information on the use of an EpiPen, visit this website: *www.epipen.com/how-to-use-epipen*.

Autoimmune Disorders

Although the immune system is very efficient in its ability to recognize and eliminate invaders, it sometimes can mistake normal body cells for foreign material and mount an immune response against healthy tissues; this is referred to as autoimmunity. There are a variety of autoimmune disorders. Type 1 diabetes mellitus (T1DM; see Chapter 16) is one example of an autoimmune disease. In T1DM, cells from the immune system attack and destroy the insulin-producing beta-cells of the pancreas. Therefore, people with T1DM require treatment with insulin to manage their blood glucose levels. Other autoimmune disorders include Crohn's disease (see Chapter 20), myasthenia gravis (see Chapter 15), and certain dermatological conditions (e.g., psoriasis). This chapter specifically discusses the treatment of systemic lupus erythematosus (SLE), rheumatoid arthritis (RA), Graves disease, and Hashimoto's thyroiditis (also known as *Hashimoto's disease*).

In the treatment of many autoimmune disorders, therapies aimed at suppressing the immune system are often used. Therapies known as **biological response modifiers (BRMs)** are targeted therapies that can "turn off" certain immune cells or neutralize cytokines in an effort to diminish the destructive inflammatory process. Table 23-1 provides a number of examples of BRMs and other immunomodulating agents used for the treatment of autoimmune disorders and cancers and for the prevention of organ transplant rejection.

Systemic Lupus Erythematosus

Systemic lupus erythematosus is a chronic inflammatory disease that can affect a variety of tissues and organs, including the joints, kidneys, skin, gastrointestinal tract, cardiovascular system, and nervous system. Nearly all people with SLE can experience a variety of symptoms that are somewhat nonspecific to the condition, such as fatigue, fever, and weight changes. Autoantibody production is a hallmark of SLE. Although the exact cause of the condition is unknown, a variety of conditions and events has been linked to SLE flares or first occurrence of symptoms. Such events include pregnancy, severe infections, exposure to ultraviolet light, and surgery.

Prognosis. The clinical course of SLE is highly variable and can be associated with periods of remission and chronic or acute relapses in symptoms. As mentioned previously, people with SLE can experience a variety of symptoms associated with inflammatory involvement of essentially any organ in the body. The prognosis for any given patient is highly dependent on the level and/or presence of severe organ dysfunction as a result of the inflammatory process associated with SLE. A variety of markers of disease activity has been described, such as antibody levels, the erythrocyte sedimentation rate (a measure of fibrosis), and other markers of inflammation that can help determine the severity of the condition and drive treatment decisions.

Non–Drug Treatment. A variety of nonpharmacological strategies can be used to treat SLE or minimize the occurrence of flares. Use of sunscreen to minimize exposure to ultraviolet light may be helpful, as may increased physical activity. Cigarette smoking has been associated with an increased risk of developing SLE, and smokers tend to have more active disease. Recommending smoking cessation for those who smoke may be beneficial. Because many of the therapies used to manage SLE are immunosuppressants, patients should be encouraged to update their immunizations before drug initiation. As is true with all autoimmune

disorders, rest, meditation, and avoidance of stress can be helpful non-drug interventions.

Drug Treatment. Because of the systemic nature of SLE, a variety of pharmacologic therapies is used to treat specific organ involvement. Agents such as nonsteroidal antiinflammatory drugs (NSAIDs), hydroxychloroquine, glucocorticoids, and immunosuppressive agents can be used. Immunosuppressive agents used in the management of SLE include cyclophosphamide, cyclosporine, tacrolimus, methotrexate, belimumab, and azathioprine, among others.

GENERIC NAME: belimumab
TRADE NAME: Benlysta
INDICATION: SLE
ROUTE OF ADMINISTRATION: Intravenous (IV)
COMMON ADULT DOSAGE: 10 mg/kg IV over 1 hour every 2 weeks for the first 3 doses, then every 4 weeks thereafter
MECHANISM OF ACTION: Inhibits B cells from becoming plasma cells and reduces B cell numbers
SIDE EFFECTS: Increased risk of infection, allergic reactions, infusion-related reactions

---

GENERIC NAME: azathioprine
TRADE NAME: Imuran
INDICATION: RA, prophylaxis of kidney transplant rejection, SLE
ROUTE OF ADMINISTRATION: Oral
COMMON ADULT DOSAGE: *SLE (off-label):* 2-3 mg/kg/ day in combination with prednisone
MECHANISM OF ACTION: Inhibits DNA and RNA synthesis, reducing the formation of immune cells and thus leading to immunosuppression
SIDE EFFECTS: Bone marrow suppression, nausea, vomiting, increased infection risk
AUXILIARY LABEL:
• Take as directed.

Rheumatoid Arthritis

Rheumatoid arthritis (RA) is an autoimmune form of arthritis that is painful and can lead to deformation of the bones and joints (Figure 23-10). More women than men are afflicted with RA. A form of RA,

Text continued on p. 594

TABLE 23-1

Select Biological Response Modifiers and Immunomodulators for Treatment of Autoimmune Disorders and Transplant Rejection Prophylaxis

Medication Class	Generic Name	Trade Name	Indications*	Common Side Effects	Common Dose Range†
Calcineurin Inhibitors	cyclosporine A	Gengraf, Sandimmune	Transplant rejections Rheumatoid arthritis Severe psoriasis	• Nephrotoxicity • Neurotoxicity • Gum hyperplasia	• 2.5-15 mg/kg/day orally (PO) divided twice daily
	tacrolimus	TAC, Prograf, FK506	Organ rejections Severe psoriasis Atopic dermatitis Systemic lupus erythematosus	• Nephrotoxicity • Neurotoxicity • Hypertension • Tremor • Headache	• 0.1-0.2 mg/kg/day PO divided twice daily
Antimetabolites	Mycophenolate	Cellcept	Solid organ transplant Myasthenia gravis Psoriasis	• Leukopenia • Thrombocytopenia • Nausea • Vomiting	• 250-1500 mg orally or intravenously (PO/IV) twice daily
	Azathioprine	Imuran	Renal transplant Rheumatoid arthritis Crohn's disease Ulcerative colitis Systemic lupus erythematosus	• Leukopenia • Thrombocytopenia • Nausea • Vomiting	• 50-150 mg PO daily
Rapamycin Inhibitors	sirolimus	Rapamune	Renal transplant	• Peripheral edema • Hypercholesterolemia • Anemia	• 6 mg PO on day 1 and then 2 mg PO once daily
	everolimus	Zortress	Pancreatic neuroendocrine tumors Renal transplant Renal cancers Breast cancer Subependymal giant cell astrocytoma (SEGA)	• Peripheral edema • Rash • Fever • Hypercholesterolemia • Anemia	• 10 mg PO once daily
Oral Disease-Modifying Antirheumatic Drugs (DMARDs)	methotrexate	Rheumatrex	Breast cancer Transplant Lymphoma Leukemia Osteosarcoma Psoriasis	• Alopecia • Photosensitivity • Nausea • Vomiting • Diarrhea • Leukopenia	• 7.5 mg PO once weekly (titrate up to 10-15 mg, max 20-30 mg/wk)
	sulfasalazine	Azulfidine	Rheumatoid arthritis Ulcerative colitis	• Rash • Abdominal pain • Nausea • Vomiting • Discolored urine	• *Initial:* 0.5-1 g PO 1-2 times daily for 1 wk (max 3 g/day); *Maintenance:* 2 g per day given in 2-3 divided doses

Category	Generic	Trade Name	Uses	Adverse Effects	Dosage
Glucocorticoids	prednisone	Deltasone	Rheumatoid arthritis Thyrotoxicosis Inflammatory pulmonary conditions	Hypertension Fluid retention Hypernatremia Osteoporosis Myopathy Cushing's syndrome Hyperglycemia	• 5-60 mg PO daily
	prednisolone dexamethasone	Orapred Decadron			• 5-7.5 mg PO daily initially • 0.75-9 mg in 2-4 divided doses (titrate as needed [prn])
Biological Response Modifiers: Tumor Necrosis Factor (TNF)-alpha Inhibitors	adalimumab	Humira	Crohn's disease Psoriasis Rheumatoid arthritis Ankylosing spondylitis	Injection site reactions Headache Sinusitis Hematological toxicities	• 40 mg subcutaneously (SUBCUT) every other week
	certolizumab	Cimzia	Crohn's disease Rheumatoid arthritis	Arthralgia Urinary tract infection (UTI) Infections Cancers	• 400 mg SUBCUT given at weeks 0, 2, and 4; then 200 mg SUBCUT every other week
	etanercept	Enbrel	Crohn's disease Psoriasis Rheumatoid arthritis	Injection site reactions Rhinitis Infections Cancers	• 50 mg SUBCUT weekly
	golimumab	Simponi	Psoriasis arthritis Rheumatoid arthritis Ankylosing spondylitis	Injection site reactions Infections Cancers	• 50 mg SUBCUT every month with methotrexate
	infliximab	Remicade	Crohn's disease Psoriasis Rheumatoid arthritis Ankylosing spondylitis Ulcerative colitis	Rash Abdominal pain Nausea Leukopenia	• 3 mg/kg IV at weeks 0, 2, and 6; then every 8 weeks
Biologic Response Modifiers: Interleukin Antagonists	anakinra	Kineret	Rheumatoid arthritis	Injection site reactions Nausea Diarrhea Neutropenia Infections	• 100 mg SUBCUT daily
	toclizumab	Actemra	Rheumatoid arthritis Systemic juvenile idiopathic arthritis	Hypertension Rash Diarrhea Elevated liver enzymes Neutropenia Cancers	• 4 mg/kg IV every 4 weeks (may increase to 8 mg/kg based on response; max 800 mg/infusion)
	basiliximab	Simulect	Solid organ transplant	Hypertension Edema Fever Abdominal pain UTI	• 20 mg IV on postoperative days 0 and 4

Continued

TABLE 23-1

Select Biological Response Modifiers and Immunomodulators for Treatment of Autoimmune Disorders and Transplant Rejection Prophylaxis—cont'd

Medication Class	Generic Name	Trade Name	Indications*	Common Side Effects	Common Dose Range†

Biologic Response Modifiers: Lymphocyte-Specific Agents	abatacept	Orencia	Juvenile idiopathic arthritis
			Rheumatoid arthritis
				• Nausea
				• Headache
				• UTI
					• Dosing is weight based
					• IV every 2 weeks, then every 4 weeks once at week 8
					  • <60 kg: 500 mg
					  • 60-100 kg: 750 mg
					  • >100 kg: 1000 mg

	belatacept	Nulojix	Kidney transplant rejection	• Edema • Diarrhea • Fever • Electrolyte imbalances • Infection	• 10 mg/kg IV on days 1 and 5 and end of weeks 4, 8, and 12
	rituximab	Rituxan	Non-Hodgkin's lymphoma Chronic lymphocytic leukemia Rheumatoid arthritis Wegener's granulomatosis Microscopic polyangiitis Transplant	• Infusion reaction • Neuropathy • Nausea • Rash • Fever • Fatigue • Tumor lysis syndrome	• 1000 mg IV infusion on days 1 and 15 with methotrexate
	belimumab	Benlysta	Systemic lupus erythematosus	• Nausea • Diarrhea • Infusion reactions	• 10 mg/kg IV every 2 weeks for 3 doses, then every 4 weeks
	glatiramer	Copaxone	Multiple sclerosis	• Pain/itching at injection site • Chest tightness • Flushing • Dyspnea	• 20 mg SUBCUT once daily

	Generic	Brand	Indications	Side Effects	Dosing
	natalizumab	Tysabri	Multiple sclerosis, Crohn's disease	• Flulike symptoms • Rash • Depression	• 300 mg IV infusion once every 4 weeks
	alemtuzumab	Campath	B-cell and T-cell cancers, Leukemias, Renal transplant	• Fever • Hypotension • Nausea • Rash • Vomiting	• 3 mg IV infusion on day 1, 10 mg IV infusion on day 3, then 30 mg/dose 3 times weekly for up to 12 weeks
Interferons	interferon beta-1b	Betaseron	Multiple sclerosis	• Injection site reaction • Injection site reaction • Flulike symptoms • Depression	• 0.25 mg SUBCUT every other day (titrate up to 1 mL every other day)
	interferon beta-1a	Avonex	Multiple sclerosis	• Flulike symptoms • Nausea • Leukopenia	• 30 mcg intramuscularly (IM) once weekly
		Rebif	Multiple sclerosis		• 22 or 44 mcg SUBCUT 3 times a week
Biological Response Modifier: Anthracenedione	mitoxantrone	Novantrone	Stem cell transplantation, Multiple sclerosis, Hodgkin's and non-Hodgkin's lymphoma, Prostate cancer, Acute nonlymphocytic leukemias	• Hepatotoxicity • Cardiotoxicity • Nausea • Vomiting • Diarrhea	• 12 mg/m^2 IV infusion every 3 months (max lifetime dose 140 mg/m^2)

*Indications listed include both FDA-approved and common off-label uses.
†Doses can vary depending on formulation and indication for use.

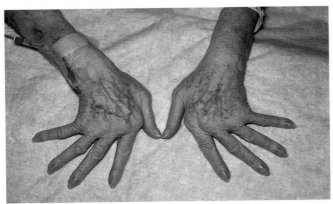

FIGURE 23-10 Severe rheumatoid arthritis. (From Swartz M: *Textbook of physical diagnosis: history and examination*, ed 6, Philadelphia, 2009, Saunders.)

known as **juvenile rheumatoid arthritis (JRA)**, affects children. In RA, inflammation in the joints leads to erosion and remodeling of the bones and cartilage, making movement extremely painful. As the disease progresses, deformity of the joints becomes irreversible. Therefore, treatment approaches to RA target both symptomatic management and prevention of joint destruction and disability. Treatment for RA includes physical therapy, medications (antiinflammatories and/or analgesics and disease-modifying antirheumatic drugs [DMARDs]), and diet.

Prognosis. Because RA has no known cure, the only recourse is to slow the progression of this disease, treat the pain associated with the condition, and minimize long-term disability.

Non–Drug Treatment. Treatments include increasing mobility and having the patient obtain psychological counseling if necessary. Physical and occupational therapy can help increase mobility and functionality to maintain independence. Physical activity can also help maintain flexibility and joint function.

Drug Treatment. Medications used to treat RA include NSAIDs, analgesics (nonnarcotic and narcotic), corticosteroids, and DMARDs. BRMs are a subcategory of DMARDs that are increasingly being used in early RA to minimize the progression of joint damage. BRMs modify the immune system through inhibition of cytokines and immune cells that contribute to inflammation and cell-mediated joint damage. Examples of DMARDs (including BRMs) are provided in the following monographs and in Table 23-1. For a general review of NSAIDs and other analgesics that are often used in RA, see Chapter 17.

GENERIC NAME: methotrexate
TRADE NAME: Rheumatrex
INDICATION: RA, JRA, various forms of cancer
ROUTE OF ADMINISTRATION: Oral; injectable
COMMON ADULT DOSAGE: *RA:* 7.5 mg PO once weekly or 2.5 mg PO every 12 hours for 3 doses once weekly
MECHANISM OF ACTION: Inhibits the enzyme dihydrofolate reductase, thus inhibiting cell proliferation and leading to immunosuppression
SIDE EFFECTS: Dizziness, fatigue, nausea, mouth ulcers, fever, increased risk of infection
AUXILIARY LABELS:
- Do not take if pregnant.
- Avoid alcohol.

 Tech Note!

It is important to remember that methotrexate is administered once weekly (or every 12 hours for 3 doses). A common pharmacy error is filling methotrexate to be taken daily. Always be sure to check the instructions for methotrexate when typing a prescription for this medication.

GENERIC NAME: etanercept
TRADE NAME: Enbrel
INDICATION: RA, JRA, psoriasis, psoriatic arthritis, ankylosing spondylitis
ROUTE OF ADMINISTRATION: Subcutaneous injection
COMMON ADULT DOSAGE: *RA:* 25 mg subcutaneously twice per week (3 to 4 days apart) *or* 50 mg weekly
MECHANISM OF ACTION: Inhibits the cytokine TNF, leading to decreased inflammation
SIDE EFFECTS: Nausea, vomiting, headache, diarrhea, injection site reactions, increased infection risk
AUXILIARY LABEL:
- Dispose of properly.

GENERIC NAME: adalimumab
TRADE NAME: Humira
INDICATION: RA, JRA, Crohn's disease, psoriasis, psoriatic arthritis, ulcerative colitis, ankylosing spondylitis
ROUTE OF ADMINISTRATION: Subcutaneous injection
COMMON ADULT DOSAGE: *RA:* 40 mg subcutaneously every other week
MECHANISM OF ACTION: Inhibits the cytokine TNF, leading to decreased inflammation
SIDE EFFECTS: Nausea, vomiting, headache, diarrhea, injection site reactions, increased infection risk
AUXILIARY LABEL:
• Dispose of properly.

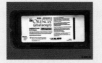

GENERIC NAME: abatacept
TRADE NAME: Orencia
INDICATION: RA, JRA
ROUTE OF ADMINISTRATION: Intravenous (IV) infusion; subcutaneous (SUBCUT) injection (powder for injection; solution for injection)
COMMON ADULT DOSAGE: *IV:* infusion based on body weight (<60 kg, give 500 mg; 60-100 kg, give 750 mg; >100 kg, give 1 g); given every 2 weeks for 3 doses, then every 4 weeks thereafter; *SUBCUT:* After a single IV dose, 125 mg SUBCUT within 1 day, followed by 125 mg SUBCUT weekly
MECHANISM OF ACTION: Inhibits T-cell activation, diminishing T-cell responses
SIDE EFFECTS: Headache, nausea, dizziness, injection site reactions, increased risk of infection
AUXILIARY LABEL:
• Dispose of properly.

Graves Disease

Graves disease is an autoimmune disorder that results in overstimulation of the thyroid gland, leading to a state of hyperthyroidism. In this condition, antibodies are produced by the immune system that bind to and activate thyroid-stimulating hormone (TSH) receptors in the thyroid gland, leading to an increased release of thyroid hormone.

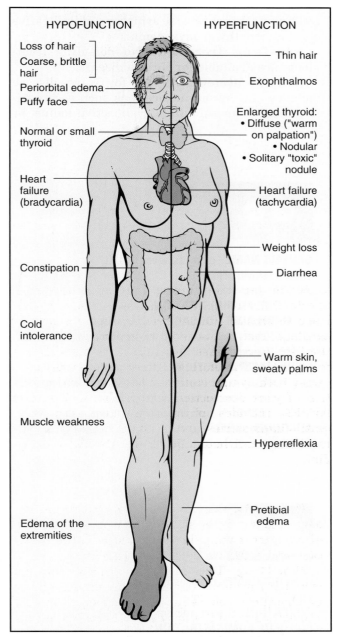

FIGURE 23-11 Clinical manifestations of hyperthyroidism and hypothyroidism. (From McCance KL: *Pathophysiology: the biologic basis for disease in adults and children,* ed 6, St Louis, 2010, Mosby.)

Graves disease is the underlying cause of 50% to 80% of cases of hyperthyroidism and is more commonly seen in women. A variety of clinical manifestations is associated with Graves disease (Figure 23-11).

Prognosis. The prognosis for Graves disease can be good if the condition is identified early and proper treatment is received. Although medication, radioactive iodine, and surgical interventions can effectively manage most symptoms, current treatments do not reverse symptoms of infiltrative ophthalmopathy or myxedema.

Non–Drug Treatment. No non–drug treatments are available for Graves disease.

Drug Treatment. Therapy for Graves disease includes antithyroid medications such as propylthiouracil or methimazole, radioactive iodine, or surgery.

GENERIC NAME: propylthiouracil (PTU)
TRADE NAME: None
INDICATION: Hyperthyroidism
ROUTE OF ADMINISTRATION: Oral
COMMON ADULT DOSAGE: *Initial dosage:* 300-400 mg daily in divided doses; *maintenance:* 100-150 mg daily
MECHANISM OF ACTION: Directly interferes with the first step in thyroid hormone synthesis, thus leading to a decrease in thyroid hormone production
SIDE EFFECTS: Nausea, headache, urticaria rash
AUXILIARY LABEL:
• Take as directed.

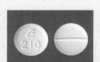

GENERIC NAME: methimazole
TRADE NAME: Tapazole
INDICATION: Hyperthyroidism
ROUTE OF ADMINISTRATION: Oral
COMMON ADULT DOSAGE: *Initial dosage:* 15-60 mg daily in divided doses; *Maintenance:* 5-30 mg daily
MECHANISM OF ACTION: Directly interferes with the first step in thyroid hormone synthesis, thus leading to a decrease in thyroid hormone production
SIDE EFFECTS: Fever, rash, itching
AUXILIARY LABEL:
• Take as directed.

Hashimoto's Thyroiditis

Hashimoto's thyroiditis, the most common cause of hypothyroidism in the United States, is characterized by autoimmune-mediated destruction of the thyroid gland. This autoimmune disease is believed to be due to a combination of genetic and environmental factors; infection, stress, pregnancy, iodine intake, and radiation exposure are known to be possible precipitating factors for Hashimoto's thyroiditis. (See Chapter 16 for a review of symptoms associated with hypothyroidism.)

Prognosis. The prognosis for Hashimoto's thyroiditis is good. Treatment involves thyroid supplementation to achieve a euthyroid state.

Non–Drug Treatment. No non–drug treatments are available for Hashimoto's thyroiditis.

Drug Treatment. Thyroid hormone replacement agents must be taken for life (one dose a day) because of the chronic nature of the condition. Levothyroxine is most commonly preferred by many physicians because of its ease of dosing (i.e., it contains one thyroid hormone, T_4). (See Chapter 16 for a detailed discussion of hypothyroidism treatment.)

Transplant Rejection

Another important use of immunosuppressive agents is in the management of organ transplant rejection. Because organ transplants involve the introduction of donated organs that are foreign to the recipient, a risk of transplantation is **transplant rejection.** In the process of transplant rejection, the host's immune system recognizes the transplanted organ as foreign and mounts an attack on it (Figure 23-12). In an effort to avoid transplant rejection, immunosuppressive drugs are used to suppress the immune system to keep the organ viable. Table 23-1 provides examples of agents used for transplant rejection prophylaxis. Nonpharmacological approaches to preventing infection are of utmost importance when immunosuppressive agents are used. Immunosuppressed individuals should be diligent in avoiding infection by avoiding people who are ill. In some instances the use of face masks and isolation precautions are warranted.

GENERIC NAME: sirolimus
TRADE NAME: Rapamune
INDICATION: Prophylaxis of kidney transplant rejection
ROUTE OF ADMINISTRATION: Oral
COMMON ADULT DOSAGE: *Initial:* 6 mg as soon as possible after transplantation; *Maintenance:* 2 mg once daily

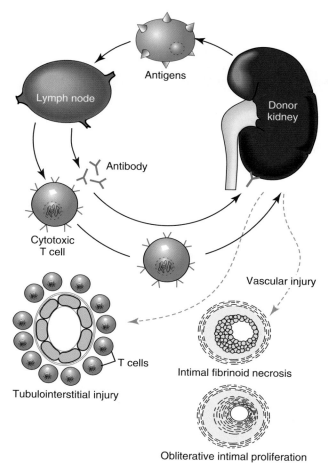

FIGURE 23-12 Transplant rejection is antibody mediated, cell mediated, or both. (From Damjanov I: *Pathology for the health professions*, ed 4, Philadelphia, 2011, Saunders.)

MECHANISM OF ACTION: Inhibition of T-cell activation and proliferation
SIDE EFFECTS: Hyperlipidemia, cough, pulmonary edema, increased risk of infection
AUXILIARY LABEL:
• Do not administer with grapefruit juice.

GENERIC NAME: belatacept
TRADE NAME: Nulojix
INDICATION: Prophylaxis of kidney transplant rejection
ROUTE OF ADMINISTRATION: Intravenous (IV)
COMMON ADULT DOSAGE: *Maintenance dose:* 5 mg/kg, rounded to the nearest 12.5-mg increment, IV over 30 minutes every 4 weeks
MECHANISM OF ACTION: Blocks the activation of T cells, inhibiting T-cell functions
SIDE EFFECTS: Increased risk of infection, diarrhea, nausea, vomiting, infusion reactions

---

Immunizations

Historically, thousands of children have died from diseases such as measles and mumps or have been physically scarred by the effects of polio. Although children still can contract these diseases today, they are seen less commonly, and death is rare because of the widespread use of **immunizations**. A variety of **vaccines** currently is available (Table 23-2).

> ## Tech Note!
> In rare cases, any vaccine may cause an allergic reaction; therefore, it is important to observe for any severe reactions after vaccination. With most vaccinations, a Vaccine Information Statement (VIS), published by the Centers for Disease Control and Prevention (CDC), is issued to the patient or legal caregiver of the patient receiving the vaccine. The VIS contains important information about the vaccine and its potential side effects. The law requires that the VIS be made available for certain vaccinations.

When children and adults are immunized, communities are better protected against diseases such as chickenpox, measles, and influenza. People with weakened immune systems, such as older adults, chemotherapy patients, transplant recipients, and individuals with acquired immunodeficiency syndrome (AIDS), are also at higher risk of developing and even dying from communicable diseases. Another high-risk group is individuals from countries where immunizations are not available. Because children are at high risk for catching and spreading many communicable diseases, a series of immunizations has been recommended to protect children and to promote community health (Table 23-3). In the United States, children cannot register for school unless they have proof of their immunizations or have obtained and filed appropriate medical or religious exemptions. A variety of immunizations is likewise recommended for adults (Table 23-4), such as annual influenza vaccines and herpes zoster vaccines to prevent shingles.

> ## Tech Note!
> Many hospitals require proof of childhood immunizations before hiring technicians or providing externships to technician students. Having your immunization records available helps you avoid blood tests that check for proof of previous immunizations.

The administration of vaccines results in the development of active acquired immunity. Vaccines can be either live or inactive. Live vaccines must be attenuated (weakened) so that they do not cause

TABLE 23-2

Vaccines Available in the United States (2012)

Vaccine	Trade Name	Type	Route	Comments
Adenovirus	Adenovirus	Live viral	Oral	Approved for military populations age 17 through 50 yr
Anthrax	BioThrax	Inactivated bacterial	IM	
DTaP	Daptacel, Infanrix	Inactivated bacterial	IM	Tetanus and diphtheria toxoids and acellular pertussis vaccine
DT	Generic	Inactivated bacterial toxoids	IM	Pediatric formulation (through age 6)
DTaP–IPV	Kinrix	Inactivated bacterial and viral	IM	Licensed for fifth (DTaP) and fourth (IPV) booster at 4-6 yr
DTaP–Hep B–IPV	Pediarix	Inactivated bacterial and viral	IM	Licensed for doses at 2, 4, and 6 mo (through age 6 yr); not licensed for boosters
DTaP–IPV/Hib	Pentacel	Inactivated bacterial and viral	IM	Licensed for four doses at 2, 4, 6, and 15-18 mo
Haemophilus influenzae type b (Hib)	PedvaxHIB	Inactivated bacterial	IM	
	ActHIB	Inactivated bacterial	IM	
	Hiberix	Inactivated bacterial	IM	Booster only
Haemophilus influenzae type b–hepatitis B	Comvax	Inactivated bacterial and viral	IM	Should not be used for Hep B birth dose
Hepatitis A (Hep A)	Havrix	Inactivated viral	IM	Pediatric and adult formulations available
Hepatitis A	Vaqta	Inactivated viral	IM	Pediatric and adult formulations available
Hepatitis B (Hep B)	Engerix-B	Inactivated viral	IM	Pediatric and adult formulations available; pediatric formulation not licensed for adults
	Recombivax HB	Inactivated viral	IM	Pediatric, adult, and dialysis formulations available; 2 pediatric doses = 1 adult dose
Hepatitis A–hepatitis B	Twinrix	Inactivated viral	IM	Pediatric dose of Hep A + adult dose of Hep B; minimum age 18 yr; 3-dose routine series
Herpes zoster (shingles)	Zostavax	Live attenuated viral	SUBCUT	Licensed for ≥50 yr
Human papillomavirus (HPV)	Gardasil	Inactivated viral	IM	Licensed for males and females 9 through 26 yr
	Cervarix	Inactivated viral	IM	Licensed for females 10 through 26 yr
Influenza (trivalent, types A and B)	Fluarix	Inactivated viral	IM	Minimum age 3 yr
	Fluvirin	Inactivated viral	IM	Minimum age 4 yr
	Fluzone	Inactivated viral	IM	Age range, 6 mo–3 yr, depending on amount in prefilled syringe
	Fluzone High-Dose	Inactivated viral	IM	Licensed for ≥65 yr
	Fluzone Intradermal	Inactivated viral	Intradermal	Age range 18 through 64 yr
	FluLaval	Inactivated viral	IM	Minimum age 18 yr
	Afluria	Inactivated viral	IM	Minimum age 6 mo
	Agriflu	Inactivated viral	IM	Minimum age 18 yr
	FluMist	Live attenuated viral	Intranasal	Age range 2 through 49 yr
Japanese encephalitis	Ixiaro	Inactivated viral	IM	Licensed for ≥17 yr; 2-dose series
Measles-mumps-rubella	M-M-R II	Live attenuated viral	SUBCUT	Minimum age 12 mo

TABLE 23-2

Vaccines Available in the United States (2012)—cont'd

Vaccine	Trade Name	Type	Route	Comments
Measles-mumps-rubella-varicella	ProQuad	Live attenuated viral	SUBCUT	Age range 1 through 12 yr
Meningococcal	Menomune	Inactivated bacterial	SUBCUT	Minimum age 2 yr
	Menactra	Inactivated bacterial	IM	Age range 9 mo through 55 yr
Pneumococcal	Menveo	Inactivated bacterial	IM	Age range 2 through 55 yr
	Pneumovax 23	Inactivated bacterial	SUBCUT or IM	Minimum age 2 yr
	Prevnar 13	Inactivated bacterial	IM	Age ranges 6 mo through 5 yr and ≥50 yr
Polio	Ipol	Inactivated viral	SUBCUT or IM	Trivalent, types 1, 2, 3
Rabies	Imovax Rabies, RabAvert	Inactivated viral	IM	
Rotavirus	Rota Teq, Rotarix	Live viral	Oral	*Rota Teq:* First dose between 6 wk and 14 wk 6 days; complete 3-dose series by 8 mo *Rotarix:* Same as for Rota Teq but in a 2-dose series
Tetanus (reduced) Diphtheria	Decavac, Tenivac	Inactivated bacterial toxoids	IM	Adult formulation (≥7 yr)
Tetanus (reduced) Diphtheria (reduced) Pertussis	Boostrix, Adacel	Inactivated bacterial	IM	Tetanus and diphtheria toxoids and pertussis vaccine; minimum age 10 yr *Adacel:* Acellular (age range 11-64 yr)
Tetanus toxoid	(Generic)	Inactivated bacterial toxoid	IM	May be used for adults or children
Typhoid	Typhim Vi	Inactivated bacterial	IM	
	Vivotif Berna	Live attenuated bacterial	Oral	
Vaccinia (smallpox)	ACAM2000	Live attenuated viral	Percutaneous	
Varicella	Varivax	Live attenuated viral	SUBCUT	Minimum age 12 mo
Yellow fever	YF-Vax	Live attenuated viral	SUBCUT	Minimum age 9 mo

DT, Diphtheria-tetanus; *DTaP–Hep B–IPV,* diphtheria-tetanus-pertussis–hepatitis B–inactivated poliovirus; *DTaP–IPV,* diphtheria-tetanus-pertussis–inactivated poliovirus; *DTaP–IPV/Hib,* diphtheria-tetanus-pertussis–inactivated poliovirus/*Haemophilus influenzae* type b; *IM,* intramuscular; *SUBCUT,* subcutaneous.

TABLE 23-3

Centers for Disease Control and Prevention Recommended Immunization Schedule: Birth to 18 Years

Vaccine	Birth	1 mo	2 mo	4 mo	6 mo	12 mo	15 mo	18 mo	19-23 mo	2-3 yr	4-6 yr	7-10 yr	11-12 yr	13-18 yr
Hep B	✓	✓				✓								
Hep A								✓						
Rotavirus			✓	✓	✓									
DTaP			✓	✓	✓		✓				✓			
Hib			✓	✓	✓	✓								
PCV			✓	✓	✓	✓								
Polio			✓	✓		✓					✓			
MMR						✓					✓			
Varicella						✓					✓			
Influenza									✓ Recommended yearly					
MCV													✓	✓
HPV													✓	

DTaP, Diphtheria-tetanus-pertussis; *Hep A,* hepatitis A; *Hep B,* hepatitis B; *Hib, Haemophilus influenzae* type b; *HPV,* human papillomavirus; *MCV,* meningococcal vaccine; *MMR,* measles-mumps-rubella; *PCV,* pneumococcal conjugate vaccine.

TABLE 23-4

Centers for Disease Control and Prevention: Recommended Adult Immunization Schedule

Vaccine	19-26 yr	27-49 yr	50-59 yr	60-64 yr	≥65 yr
DTaP/Td	✓ Td booster every 10 yr with a substitute to DTaP for at least a one-time overall booster				✓
PPSV					
Influenza		✓ Recommended yearly			
Zoster				✓	

DTaP, Diphtheria-tetanus-pertussis; *PPSV,* pneumococcal polysaccharide vaccine; *Td,* tetanus-diphtheria.

disease. Once the body manufactures antibodies against the injected antigen, it has long-lasting immunity. With vaccines made from killed or inactive antigens, the risk of infection is lower. The disadvantage of using killed or inactive antigens in a vaccine is that booster shots are needed to maintain a sufficient level of antibodies to prevent disease.

Vaccine Types

Viral Vaccines

Some available vaccines (e.g., measles, mumps, rubella [MMR]; oral polio; oral rotavirus; intranasal influenza; smallpox [vaccinia]; and varicella [chickenpox]) contain live **viruses** that have been attenuated before they are given to patients. The **virions** taken are weakened so that they do not cause disease. The attenuated virus may replicate, but at a very slow rate. A person with an active immune system quickly begins to make a full complement of antibodies and antigen-induced reactions that produce immunity. The advantage of live vaccine administration is the durable and complete immunity produced. However, if a person is immunocompromised, live vaccines could carry a risk of disease and other problems. (See the table at the beginning of the chapter that presents examples of medications that cause immunosuppression; administration of vaccines to immunosuppressed patients should be avoided.)

An inactivated viral vaccine is one in which the virus products are grown in culture and the virus then is destroyed so that it cannot replicate and cause disease. Although much of the virus is destroyed, the viral capsid proteins (outer shells) remain intact and are easily recognized by the immune system. Because the capsule, or outer shell, of the antigen does not continually reinforce the response needed for the body to resist further attacks, boosters must be given to remind the body to develop antibodies in the immune system.

Bacterial Vaccines

The typhoid vaccine is an example of a live-attenuated bacterial vaccine. Some vaccines are referred to as *toxoids;* these are inactivated bacterial toxins. Although the bacterial cell has been altered so that it cannot cause disease, it still can induce an antibody response in the body.

Many people believe that immunizations are not necessary after 18 years of age. However, some vaccines, such as the tetanus toxoid, should be given to adults. Although tetanus immunizations are given to children combined with diphtheria and pertussis, tetanus booster immunizations should be given every 10 years throughout a person's lifetime. Tetanus is a disease caused by a toxin-secreting bacterium that can be contracted through scrapes and cuts caused by dirty objects.

 Tech Note!

Tuberculosis vaccine is routinely administered in many countries, such as the Philippines. Although a vaccine is available for tuberculosis, it is not used in the United States because a tuberculosis vaccine does not guarantee immunity. If a vaccine is given, antibodies are developed against the antigen; therefore, all tuberculosis tests would show positive results and a chest x-ray film would be necessary to rule out active tuberculosis.

Miscellaneous Vaccines

Although the two most common vaccines are inactivated (killed) and live-attenuated (weakened) vaccines, other, less common types of vaccines are available (Box 23-1). These vaccines are slightly different in their composition from the usual types. Unfortunately, the only two types of vaccines available are those that protect against viruses and bacterial microbes. Immunizations for diseases caused by a parasite, such as malaria, and for fungal infections have not been developed to date.

Storage of Vaccines

The Centers for Disease Control and Prevention (CDC) guidelines on the storage of vaccines have been established to ensure the vaccines' effectiveness. Most vaccines should be kept at temperatures

BOX 23-1

Less Common Vaccines and Their Specific Characteristics

Antiidiotypic Vaccines

Antiidiotypic vaccines are a newer type of vaccine based on the use of an antibody shaped like the antigen. When the antibody is administered, the body reacts as though it were the antigen. The immune system creates antibodies to fight the disease. In effect, the body is making an antibody against the injected antibody. This second antibody then can be injected to act as the vaccine, and it creates a third antibody. In the future, this method may make it possible to kill deadly viruses such as human immunodeficiency virus (HIV).

Subunit Vaccines

Subunit vaccines are small pieces of the genetic code that originate from the disease microbe. These pieces are injected into a bacterium or yeast and then grown. They are harvested and used as a vaccine to stimulate the body to produce an immune response. Because only pieces of the original virion or antigen are used, they do not carry the full extent of immunity provided by a complete antigen. Hepatitis B is a subunit vaccine that is grown in yeast cells and then given as a vaccine.

Acellular and Conjugated Vaccines

When a vaccine is disassembled or fragmented to isolate specific antigens from entire cells, it is referred to as an *acellular vaccine*. Pertussis is one type of vaccine made in this manner. Bacterial cells that have been altered and mixed with toxoids to increase their overall effectiveness are called *conjugated vaccines* (e.g., tetanus and diphtheria).

 Tech Note!

It is important to follow the manufacturer's instructions on storing vaccines. Vaccines are always kept either in the refrigerator or the freezer at the pharmacy to prevent loss of effectiveness. Never freeze refrigerate-only vaccines, because this may compromise their potency and effectiveness. A thermometer must be kept in the refrigerator and/or freezer, and the temperature must be documented daily to ensure stability.

Antitoxins and Antivenins

Antitoxins and antivenins are yet another form of antibody-based therapy that can provide protection from serious symptoms associated with an acute intoxication or envenomation. These agents contain antibodies that can neutralize dangerous toxins. For example, stepping on a rusty nail may allow the pathogen *Clostridium tetani* to enter the wound and pass into the bloodstream, where it may develop into the dangerous condition called *tetanus*. Administration of the tetanus antitoxin can protect the individual against this potentially life-threatening condition. Antivenins are given to counteract poison from creatures such as snakes and spiders. Common antitoxins include those for diphtheria, rabies, and botulism. Common antivenins include antivenin for the black widow spider (*Latrodectus mactans*) and Crotalidae polyvalent antivenin against rattlesnake venom.

 Tech Alert!

Remember these sound-alike, look-alike drugs:
cyclosporine versus cycloserine or cyclophosphamide
erlotinib versus gefitinib

between 2° and 8° C (i.e., 36° and 46° F); however, some (e.g., varicella vaccine) require freezing until the time of use. Always refer to the storage information for any vaccine product you receive to ensure proper storage and handling.

DO YOU REMEMBER THESE KEY POINTS?

- Names of the major cells and organs that make up the immune system and their functions
- The primary signs and symptoms of the various conditions discussed
- The types of immunizations currently available for children and adults
- Medications used to treat the various conditions discussed in this chapter
- The generic and trade names for the drugs discussed in this chapter
- The appropriate auxiliary labels that should be used when filling prescriptions for drugs discussed in this chapter

REVIEW QUESTIONS

Multiple Choice Questions

1. Which cells of the immune system produce antibodies?
   A. T cells
   B. Macrophages
   C. Plasma cells
   D. Eosinophils

2. This lymphoid organ is responsible for the maturation and "education" of T cells:
   A. Lymph nodes
   B. Thymus
   C. Spleen
   D. None of the above

3. Which conditions is(are) an autoimmune disorder?
   A. Type 1 diabetes mellitus (T1DM)
   B. Systemic lupus erythematosus (SLE)
   C. Rheumatoid arthritis (RA)
   D. All of the above

4. What is the brand name for adalimumab?
   A. Humira
   B. Cimzia
   C. Enbrel
   D. Simponi

5. Vaccines can protect human beings against all of the following organisms *except:*
   A. Viruses
   B. Fungi
   C. Bacteria
   D. All of the above

6. The two basic types of immunity are:
   A. Bacterial and viral
   B. Live and inactive
   C. Innate and acquired
   D. Active and passive

7. Vaccines can be altered by which of the following ways?
   A. Attenuated or weakened
   B. Inactivated or killed
   C. Attenuated or activated
   D. A and B

8. When the body comes into contact with a contagious disease, it causes:
   A. Antibodies to be produced
   B. Antigens to be produced
   C. A body rash
   D. No reaction

9. Which of these statements is(are) true about toxoids?
   A. Toxoids are bacterial toxins that have been inactivated
   B. All bacterial vaccines are toxoids
   C. Both A and B
   D. None of the above

10. Vaccines composed of small pieces of genetic code harvested from bacteria or yeast are:
    A. Acellular vaccines
    B. Conjugated vaccines
    C. Subunit vaccines
    D. Toxoid vaccines

TECHNICIAN'S CORNER

Visit the website of the Centers for Disease Control and Prevention at *www.cdc.gov* and review the most recent list of suggested immunizations for children and adults. For conditions that you are not familiar with, review the symptoms and management of that condition.

Bibliography

Abbas AK, Lichtman AHH: *Basic immunology updated edition: functions and disorders of the immune system*, ed 3, Philadelphia, 2011, Saunders.

Centers for Disease Control and Prevention (CDC): Immunization schedules. (Referenced September 6, 2014.) www.cdc.gov/vaccines/schedules.

Clinical Pharmacology Online: (Referenced September 6, 2014.) www.clinicalpharmacology-ip.com.

Damjanov I: *Pathology for the health professions*, ed 4, St Louis, 2011, Saunders.

Fishback JL: *Pathology*, ed 3, Philadelphia, 2005, Mosby.

Huether S, McCance K: *Understanding pathophysiology*, ed 5, St Louis, 2012, Mosby.

Kumar V, Abbas AK: *Robbins and Cotran pathologic basis of disease*, ed 8, Philadelphia, 2010, Saunders.

McCance KL: *Pathophysiology: the biologic basis for disease in adults and children*, ed 6, St Louis, 2010, Mosby.

Nairn R, Helbert M: *Immunology for medical students*, ed 2, St Louis, 2007, Mosby.

Page C et al: *Integrated pharmacology*, ed 3, 2006, Mosby.

Price SA et al: *Pathophysiology: clinical concepts of disease processes*, ed 6, St Louis, 2003, Mosby.

Solomon EP: *Introduction to human anatomy and physiology*, ed 3, St Louis, 2009, Saunders.

Thibodeau GA, Patton KT: *Anatomy and physiology*, ed 8, St Louis, 2012, Mosby.

Thompson JM et al: *Mosby's clinical nursing*, ed 5, St Louis, 2001, Mosby.

UpToDate Online: (Referenced September 6, 2014.) www.uptodate.com.

Therapeutic Agents for the Eyes, Ears, Nose, and Throat

Joshua J. Neumiller

OBJECTIVES

Upon completing this chapter, you should be able to do the following:

1. Describe the anatomy and physiology of the eyes, ears, nose, and throat.
2. List the primary signs and symptoms of common conditions associated with the eyes, ears, nose, and throat that are discussed in this chapter.
3. Recognize prescription and over-the-counter drugs used to treat common conditions discussed in this chapter.
4. Write the generic and trade names for the drugs discussed in this chapter.
5. List appropriate auxiliary labels when filling prescriptions for drugs discussed in this chapter.

TERMS AND DEFINITIONS

Aqueous humor The fluid found in the anterior chamber of the eye, in front of the lens

Auditory canal A 1-inch segment of tube that extends from the external ear to the middle ear

Auditory ossicles Small bones (ossicles) of the middle ear that transmit sound from the eardrum to the inner ear

Auricle The outer projecting portion of the ear

Bactericidal Able to cause bacterial cell death

Bacteriostatic Able to inhibit bacterial cell growth

Carbonic anhydrase An enzyme that converts carbonic acid into carbon dioxide and water

Cerumen Earwax

Ciliary body The part of the eye that connects the iris to the choroid

Conjunctiva The transparent protective mucous membrane that lines the underside of the eyelid

Cornea The transparent tissue covering the anterior portion of the eye

Eustachian tube A structure in the middle ear that connects with the nasopharynx (throat); it equalizes pressure between the outside air and middle ear and drains mucus

Exudate A mass of cells and fluid that has seeped out of blood vessels as a result of inflammation

Fungicidal Able to destroy or inhibit the growth of fungi

Glomerulonephritis Acute inflammation of the kidney, typically caused by an immune response

Intraocular pressure (IOP) The pressure exerted by the fluids inside the eyeball

Iris The colored part of the eye seen through the cornea; it consists of smooth muscles that regulate pupil size

Lacrimal fluid The fluid in the eye that cleans and lubricates the eyes

Larynx A hollow muscular organ that forms an air passage to the lungs and holds the vocal cords

Lens Flexible, clear tissue that focuses images

Miosis Contraction of the pupil

Mydriasis Dilation of the pupil

Myopia Nearsightedness

Ophthalmic Pertaining to the eye

Orbit The eye socket

Otic Pertaining to the ear

Ototoxicity Toxic effects on the organs of hearing or balance or on the auditory nerve

Pharynx The membrane-lined cavity behind the nose and mouth that connects them to the esophagus

Pupil The circular opening in the iris that allows light to enter

Retina The innermost layer of the eye; a complex structure considered part of the central nervous system (CNS); the retina contains photoreceptors (rods and cones) that transmit impulses to the optic nerve, in addition to the macula lutea (a yellow spot in the center of the retina)

Rheumatic fever A noncontagious acute fever marked by inflammation and pain in the joints

Sclera The white of the eyes

Sympathomimetic Producing physiological effects resembling those caused by the sympathetic nervous system

Tinnitus Ringing or buzzing in the ears

Tympanic membrane A thin membrane that separates the external ear from the middle ear; also known as the *eardrum*

Vitreous humor A gel-like substance that fills the posterior cavity of the eye between the lens and retina; it helps maintain the shape of the eye

Select Common Drugs Used for Conditions of the Eye, Ears, Nose, and Throat

Trade Name	Generic Name	Pronunciation
Products for Conditions Affecting the Eye		
Adrenergic Agonists		
OcuClear	oxymetazoline	(**ox**-ee-**met**-ah-zoe-leen)
Propine	dipivefrin	(dye-**pie**-veh-frin)
Visine	tetrahydrozoline	(tet-ra-hye-**droz**-oh-leen)
Alphagan P	brimonidine	(bri-**moe**-ni-deen)
Antihistamines		
Emadine	emedastine	(**em**-e-**das**-teen)
Mast Cell Stabilizers		
Alomide	lodoxamide	(low-**dox**-a-mide)
Alocril	nedocromil	(ne-doe-**kroe**-mil)
Alamast	pemirolast	(pem-ir-**oh**-last)
Opticrom	cromolyn	(**kroe**-moe-lin)
Nonsteroidal Antiinflammatory Drugs (NSAIDs)		
Acular	ketorolac	(**kee**-toe-**role**-ak)
Ocufen	flurbiprofen	(**flur**-bi-**pro**-fen)
Voltaren	diclofenac	(dye-**kloe**-fen-ak)
Antiinfectives		
Antibiotics		
Ciloxan	ciprofloxacin	(si-pro-**flox**-a-sin)
Genoptic	gentamicin	(**jen**-tah-**my**-sin)
Tobrex	tobramycin	(**toe**-bra-**my**-sin)
Ocuflox	ofloxacin	(oh-**flox**-a-sin)
Vigamox	moxifloxacin	(mox-i-**flox**-a-sin)
Zymar	gatifloxacin	(gat-i-**flox**-a-sin)
Antifungal		
Natacyn	natamycin	(**na**-ta-**my**-sin)
Antiviral		
Viroptic	trifluridine	(try-**floor**-eh-dean)
Beta-Adrenergic Blocking Agents		
Betagan	levobunolol	(lee-voe-**byoo**-noe-lol)
Betoptic	betaxolol	(be-**tax**-oh-lol)
Ocupress	carteolol	(**car**-tee-oh-lol)
OptiPranolol	metipranolol	(me-ti-**pran**-oh-lol)
Timoptic	timolol	(**tim**-oh-lol)
Carbonic Anhydrase Inhibitors		
Azopt	brinzolamide	(brin-**zoh**-la-mide)
Diamox	acetazolamide	(a-**seet**-ah-**zoh**-la-mide)

Select Common Drugs Used for Conditions of the Eye, Ears, Nose, and Throat—cont'd

Trade Name	Generic Name	Pronunciation
Neptazane	methazolamide	(**meth**-a-**zole**-a-mide)
Trusopt	dorzolamide	(dor-**zole**-a-mide)
Cholinergics		
Carboptic	carbachol	(**kar**-ba-kol)
Pilocar	pilocarpine	(pye-low-**kar**-peen)
Corticosteroids		
FML	fluorometholone	(**floor**-oh-**meth**-oh-lone)
Maxidex	dexamethasone	(**dex**-ah-**meth**-ah-sone)
Pred Forte	prednisolone	(pred-**niss**-oh-lone)
Zylet	loteprednol and tobramycin	(low-te-**pred**-nol)
Prostaglandin Agonists		
Lumigan	bimatoprost	(bye-**mat**-oh-prost)
Travatan	travoprost	(**trav**-oh-prost)
Xalatan	latanoprost	(la-**tan**-oh-prost)
Products for Conditions Affecting the Ear		
Anesthetic		
Auralgan	antipyrine/benzocaine	(an-tee-**pie**-reen/**ben**-zoe-kane)
Antiinfectives		
Floxin	ofloxacin	(oh-**floks**-ah-sin)
Zithromax	azithromycin	(a-**zith**-row-**my**-sin)
Amoxil	amoxicillin	(am-**ox**-i-**sil**-in)
Augmentin	amoxicillin/clavulanate	(am-**ox**-i-**sil**-in/**clav**-ue-la-nate)
Omnicef	cefdinir	(**sef**-dih-near)
Ceftin	cefuroxime	(**sef**-yoo-**rox**-eem)
Products for Conditions Affecting the Nose		
Neo-Synephrine	phenylephrine	(feh-nill-**eh**-frin)
Nasonex	mometasone	(moe-**met**-a-sone)
Rhinocort	budesonide	(byoo-**dess**-oh-nide)
Flonase	fluticasone	(floo-**tic**-ah-sone)
Products for Conditions Affecting the Throat		
Amoxil	amoxicillin	(am-**ox**-i-**sil**-in)
Augmentin	amoxicillin/clavulanate	(am-**ox**-i-**sil**-in/**clav**-ue-la-nate)

Conditions affecting the eyes, ears, nose, and throat may not seem as important as other conditions; however, the ramifications of neglecting these conditions can be severe. Not only can conditions affecting the eyes, ears, nose, and throat be uncomfortable, failure to manage conditions affecting these areas can result in long-term health consequences. In this chapter we discuss the anatomy and physiology of the eyes, ears, nose, and throat, in addition to select conditions that can affect these areas and their common treatments.

The Eyes (Ophthalmic System)

The eyes are an important sensory organ. As images are perceived, they are translated into nerve impulses that provide visual input of the surroundings to the brain. The three different levels or categories of health care personnel who specifically work in the field of eye care are opticians, optometrists, and ophthalmologists and their associated medical assistants, technicians, and nurses. Opticians are skilled in making lenses that compensate for vision loss, but they cannot prescribe medication. Optometrists are trained to perform eye examinations and may prescribe certain medications for the eye. Ophthalmologists are physicians who treat major conditions affecting the eye, including performing eye surgery.

Anatomy and Physiology of the Eye

The eye has several structures that work in unison to help protect it, maintain its shape, and facilitate vision. The eye sits in a bony socket called the **orbit**. Covering the eyes are the eyelids, which are composed of four individual layers: the outer skin, the muscles, the connective tissue, and the conjunctiva. The muscles and fibers of connective tissues are under the skin in the lid. They allow the eyelid to open and close. The **conjunctiva** is a thin, transparent mucous membrane that covers the anterior eye, the eyelids, and the **sclera** (Figure 24-1). The natural reaction of blinking protects the eye from foreign objects and allows **lacrimal fluid** (tears) to cleanse the eye. The lacrimal gland, which secretes tears into the eye, has ducts that lead into the nasal cavity. Tears contain antimicrobial enzymes that help protect the eye from infection.

The **cornea** is a bulging, transparent cover that allows light into the eye for visual acuity. It is composed of connective tissue and is covered by a thin coating of epithelium. The cornea does not contain blood vessels to provide nourishment; instead, it is nourished by aqueous humor and by oxygen from the atmosphere. The aqueous humor is found in the anterior portion of the eye, between the cornea and

the lens. Many nerve fibers in the cornea are sensitive to pain. The sclera is attached to the cornea but wraps around to the back of the eyeball (Figure 24-2). The optic nerve extends from the back of the eye through the sclera. It sends images from the eye to the brain for interpretation. From the front of the eye the sclera joins with the iris and the ciliary body. The **iris** is responsible for the color of the eye and filters light. The largest space of the eye is an area called the *posterior cavity*, which is surrounded by the lens, ciliary body, and retina. The ciliary body forms a ring around the front of the eye. The **ciliary body** is responsible for holding the **lens** in place and regulating its shape to help with focusing vision. The area between the lens and the retina is filled with a jellylike substance called the **vitreous humor**. A

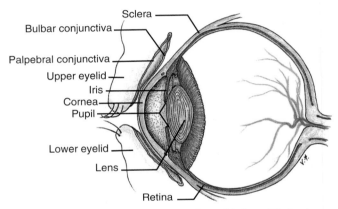

FIGURE 24-1 Anatomy of the eye. (From Potter PA, Perry AG: *Fundamentals of nursing,* ed 8, St Louis, 2013, Mosby.)

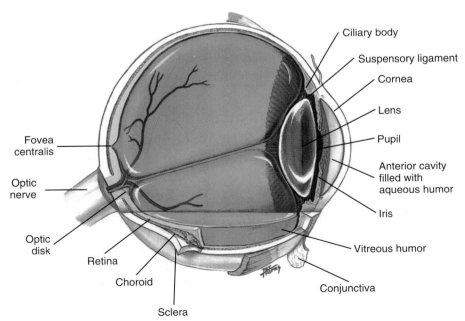

FIGURE 24-2 Cross section of the eye. (From Damjanov I: *Pathology for the health professions,* ed 4, Philadelphia, 2012, Saunders.)

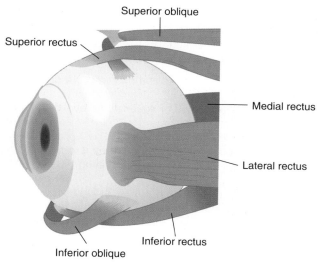

FIGURE 24-3 Eye muscles and their direction of movement. The superior rectus rotates upward and inward; the inferior rectus rotates downward and inward; the medial rectus rotates inward; the lateral rectus rotates outward; the superior oblique rotates downward and outward; the inferior oblique rotates upward and outward.

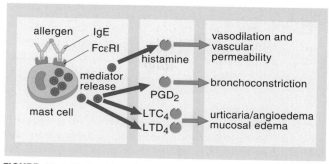

FIGURE 24-4 Mechanism of a type I hypersensitivity reaction. (From Page C et al: *Integrated pharmacology*, ed 3, St Louis, 2006, Mosby.)

function of the vitreous body is to hold the shape of the eye. The **retina** is composed of layers of neurons, nerves, pigmented epithelium, and membranous tissues. Receptor cells (known as *photoreceptors*) of the retina are responsible for vision, and the neurons provide a path for signals to travel to the brain. Six major muscles of the eye extend from the skeletal bones of the orbit. These muscles are responsible for the movement of the eye (Figure 24-3). Other important muscles include those that close and open the eyelid and dilate and constrict the pupil.

When focusing on a distant figure or trying to see in the dark, the **pupil** of the eye dilates (**mydriasis**), allowing more light to enter. When the eye is exposed to excessive light, the pupil constricts (**miosis**). **Aqueous humor** is the watery fluid that both maintains the shape of the anterior eye (i.e., between the cornea and the lens) and nourishes anterior compartment structures. Because aqueous humor is continuously synthesized, it must be released to maintain proper pressure in the anterior chamber of the eye. Excess aqueous humor drains through small ducts near the sclera and cornea, called the *canals of Schlemm.*

 Tech Note!

When we cry, the lacrimal glands are activated directly by the parasympathetic nervous system.

Vision

As discussed previously, each area of the eye has a specific function. As an image passes through the

lens, it reaches the retina at the back of the eye. Rods in the retina are responsible for sight in dim light and produce only an image in black and white; cones detect color. As the rods and cones synapse (connect) with nerve endings, the signals are sent through the optic nerve to the brain. As discussed in Chapter 15, the occipital lobe of the brain is responsible for visual interpretation.

Conditions That Affect the Eye

A variety of conditions can affect the eye. Depending on the cause, treatment can range from medication to surgery. The past several decades have seen many new developments in corrective lens treatment. For conditions such as **myopia** (nearsightedness), laser surgery is becoming a popular alternative to wearing glasses.

Many combinations of **ophthalmic** medications are available by prescription. Keeping eye solutions sterile is imperative because foreign objects instilled into the eyes can cause damage or infection. The pharmacist should instruct patients in the proper technique for administering eye drops; this is important both for effective use of the drops and also to prevent contamination of the medication (Box 24-1). Most medications should not be instilled into the eyes while the patient is wearing contact lenses. This section discusses commonly used ophthalmic medications. Table 24-1 presents a review of select nonantiinfective ophthalmic medications.

Common Conditions

Allergic Conjunctivitis

When the body comes in contact with an irritant or a foreign object, mast cells release histamine, which causes inflammation in an effort to fight the allergen (Figure 24-4). When the eyes are exposed to allergens, they become itchy, red, and watery. This condition can occur at any time; however, seasonal allergies are the most common. Seasonal allergies are the allergic reactions caused by the release of pollen from

BOX 24-1

Proper Administration of Eye Drops and Ointments

The basic steps for administering eye drops and ointments are as follows:

1. Wash hands.
2. Tilt head backward or lie down and gaze upward.
3. Gently pull lower eyelid down and away from the eye to form a pouch.
4. Place dropper directly over the eye. Do not let dropper come in contact with the eye or any other surface (e.g., fingers).
5. Look upward just before applying a drop.
6. After instilling the drop, look downward for several seconds.
7. Release lid slowly and close the eyes gently.
8. With eyes closed, use the fingertips to apply gentle pressure to the inside corner of the eye for 3 to 5 minutes (this prevents the solution from becoming part of the nasolacrimal drainage, thereby allowing the drug to enter the systemic circulation; temporary occlusion helps prevent systemic side effects and may improve drug efficacy).
9. Do not rub the eye or squeeze the eyelid and try not to blink.
10. Do not rinse the dropper.
11. If more than one type of eye drop is used, wait at least 5 minutes before administering the second agent.
12. Ointments: Follow steps 1 to 3. Then apply ointment with a sweeping motion inside the lower eyelid by squeezing the tube gently and slowly releasing the eyelid. Close the eye for 1 to 2 minutes and roll the eyeball in all directions. Remove any excess ointment from around the eye with a tissue. If using more than one kind of ointment, wait 10 minutes before applying the second ointment.

TABLE 24-1

Select Nonantiinfective Products for the Treatment of the Eye

Medication Class	Generic Name	Trade Name	Common Side Effects	Common Adult Dose
Nonsteroidal Antiinflammatory Drugs (NSAIDs)	ketorolac	Acular	• Crying	• 1 drop 4 times daily
	flurbiprofen	Ocufen	• Keratitis	• 1 drop every 30 min, starting 2 hr before procedure
	diclofenac	Voltaren	• Increased intraocular pressure	• 1 drop in affected eye 4 times daily, 24 hr after procedure, and continue for 2 wk
			• Burning/stinging	
			• Miosis	
Antihistamines: H₁-Antagonist (Some Mast Cell Stabilization)	emedastine	Emadine	• Headache	• 1 drop in affected eye up to 4 times daily
			• Hyperemia	
	azelastine	Optivar	• Itching	• 1 drop in affected eye twice daily
			• Keratitis	
			• Burning/stinging	
	ketotifen	Claritin Eye	• Conjunctivitis	• 1 drop in affected eye every 8-12 hours
			• Discharge	
			• Dry eyes	
			• Pain	
			• Eyelid disorder	
			• Photophobia	
	olopatadine	Patanol	• Cold syndrome	• 1 drop in affected eye twice daily
			• Headache	
			• Pharyngitis	
			• Taste perversion	

TABLE 24-1

Select Nonantiinfective Products for the Treatment of the Eye—cont'd

Medication Class	Generic Name	Trade Name	Common Side Effects	Common Adult Dose
Mast Cell Stabilizers	lodoxamide	Alomide	• Burning • Stinging • Headache • Blurred vision • Hyperemia	• 1-2 drops in one or both eyes 4 times daily for up to 3 months
	nedocromil	Alocril	• Headache • Unpleasant taste • Stinging • Redness • Photophobia	• 1-2 drops in each eye twice daily
	pemirolast	Alamast	• Headache • Rhinitis • Cold/flu symptoms • Dry eyes	• 1-2 drops in affected eye 4 times daily
	cromolyn	Opticrom	• Redness • Dryness • Itchy eyes • Puffy eyes	• 1-2 drops in each eye 4-6 times daily
Anticholinergics	cyclopentolate	Cyclogyl	• Pupil dilation • Paralysis of the ciliary eye muscle • Blurred vision • Dry eyes • Edema	• 1-2 drops in affected eye(s) approximately 40-50 min before procedure; repeat in 5-10 min if necessary
	atropine	Isopto Atropine		• 1-2 drops 1 hr before procedure
	scopolamine	Isopto Hyoscine	• Conjunctivitis • Irritation	• 1-2 drops in eye 1 hr before procedure
Adrenergic Agonists	oxymetazoline	OcuClear	• Redness relief • Burning • Stinging • Blurred vision	• 1-2 drops in affected eye every 6 hr as needed (prn); do not use longer than 3 days
	tetrahydrozoline	Visine		• 1-2 drops in each eye 2-4 times daily
	brimonidine	Alphagan P	• Eye pain • Stinging • Conjunctivitis • Hyperemia	• 1 drop in affected eye 3 times daily
	dipivefrin	Propine		• 1 drop in affected eye twice daily
Corticosteroids	dexamethasone	Maxidex	• Intraocular pressure increased • Conjunctival hemorrhage • Pain • Hyperemia • Cataract • Burning • Headache • Keratitis • Burning • Increased intraocular pressure • Eyelid disorders • Photophobia	• 1-2 drops in conjunctival sac every hour during the day and every other hour at night (titrate down to 3-4 times daily)
	fluorometholone	FML		• ½-inch ribbon in conjunctival sac 1-3 times daily
	prednisolone	Ocu-Pred Forte		• 1 drop every 4-6 hours
	loteprednol and tobramycin	Zylet		• 1-2 drops in affected eye every 4-6 hr

trees, grasses, and flowers. Other causes of allergies include pet dander, molds, dust mites, cigarette smoke, and other exhaust fumes that can either cause or exacerbate the condition.

Prognosis. There is no cure for allergies; however, some patients can undergo successful desensitization. Many people with allergies can minimize their symptoms with the use of medications, avoiding irritants, and limiting outdoor activities when allergen levels are high.

Non–Drug Treatment. Avoiding irritants, if possible, helps minimize allergic reactions. Staying indoors when pollen or other allergen levels are highest can be beneficial. Monthly allergy shots can be given to relieve allergy symptoms associated with the eyes.

Drug Treatment. Several agents can be used to treat allergies, such as mast cell stabilizers, antihistamines, and decongestants. Mast cell stabilizers prevent mast cells from releasing chemicals that contribute to inflammation; these are available as ophthalmic solutions and suspensions and as systemic agents. Antihistamines inhibit the release of histamine, a compound that results in the common symptoms of itching and inflammation. Inhibition of the histamine receptors diminishes the effects of seasonal allergies and other allergens. Decongestants are used to dry mucous secretions and relieve congestion caused by allergies and hay fever. Decongestants act on the specific receptors that cause constriction of the mucous membrane, thus lessening congestion. (See Chapters 19 and 27 for additional information on the treatment of allergies.) Table 24-2 provides a list of select ophthalmic decongestant, antihistaminic, and mast cell stabilizer medications.

TABLE 24-2

Select Ophthalmic Decongestants, Antihistamines, and Mast Cell Stabilizers

Generic Name	Trade Name	Availability
Decongestants		
naphazoline	All Clear AR	Over the counter (OTC)
naphazoline	AK-Con, Napha Forte	Prescription
oxymetazoline	Visine LR	OTC
phenylephrine	Neofrin, Mydfrin	Prescription
tetrahydrozoline	Visine	OTC
Antihistamines		
olopatadine	Patanol, Pataday	Prescription
emedastine	Emadine	Prescription
azelastine	Optivar	Prescription
epinastine	Elestat	Prescription
ketotifen	Claritin Eye, Zaditor	OTC
Mast Cell Stabilizers		
lodoxamide	Alomide	Prescription
nedocromil	Alocril	Prescription
cromolyn sodium	Crolom	Prescription

GENERIC NAME: lodoxamide
TRADE NAME: Alomide
INDICATION: Conjunctivitis, vernal keratitis, vernal keratoconjunctivitis
ROUTE OF ADMINISTRATION: Ophthalmic
COMMON ADULT DOSAGE: 1 to 2 drops in the affected eye(s) up to four times daily; not to be used for longer than 3 months
MECHANISM OF ACTION: Ophthalmic mast cell stabilizer (inhibits mast cell histamine release)
SIDE EFFECTS: Eye irritation, blurred vision, headache
AUXILIARY LABEL:
- For the eye.

Ophthalmic Inflammation Caused by Infection or Injury

Corticosteroids are efficacious agents used to relieve inflammation resulting from infection, allergies, or injury. They are commonly used postoperatively to treat inflammation (Figure 24-5). These agents

GENERIC NAME: emedastine
TRADE NAME: Emadine
INDICATION: Allergic conjunctivitis
ROUTE OF ADMINISTRATION: Ophthalmic
COMMON ADULT DOSAGE: 1 drop in the affected eye(s) up to four times daily
MECHANISM OF ACTION: H_1-receptor antagonist (relieves pruritus associated with allergic conjunctivitis)
SIDE EFFECTS: Eye irritation, blurred vision, headache
AUXILIARY LABEL:
- For the eye.

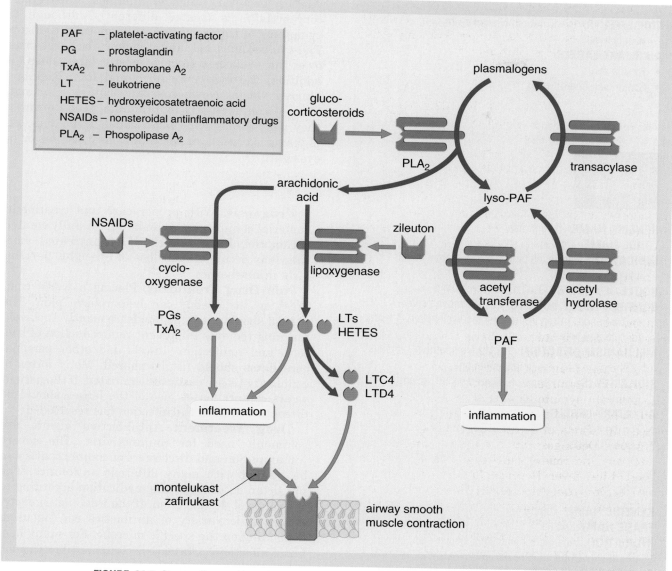

PAF   – platelet-activating factor
PG   – prostaglandin
TxA_2 – thromboxane A_2
LT   – leukotriene
HETES – hydroxyeicosatetraenoic acid
NSAIDs – nonsteroidal antiinflammatory drugs
PLA_2 – Phospolipase A_2

plasmalogens
gluco-corticosteroids
PLA_2
transacylase
arachidonic acid
lyso-PAF
NSAIDs
zileuton
cyclo-oxygenase
lipoxygenase
acetyl transferase
acetyl hydrolase
PGs TxA_2
LTs HETES
PAF
LTC4 LTD4
inflammation
inflammation
montelukast zafirlukast
airway smooth muscle contraction

FIGURE 24-5 Glucocorticosteroids reduce the production of a variety of inflammatory mediators. (From Page C et al: *Integrated pharmacology*, ed 3, St Louis, 2006, Mosby.)

should not be used any longer than necessary because they may compromise the effectiveness of the immune system, resulting in a slower rate of healing. Corticosteroid ophthalmic dosage forms include solutions, suspensions, and ointments. Side effects may include a temporary burning sensation, blurred vision, eye pain, or headaches. Most of the agents used to reduce inflammation are solutions or suspensions. Suspensions need to be shaken well before use.

Nonsteroidal antiinflammatory drugs (NSAIDs) inhibit the enzyme cyclooxygenase (COX), which is responsible for the synthesis of prostaglandins. Prostaglandins are directly related to the mechanisms responsible for inflammation and the pain associated with it. Ophthalmic NSAIDs are available only in solution.

GENERIC NAME: prednisolone
TRADE NAME: Pred-Forte (suspension)
INDICATION: Allergic conjunctivitis, postoperative ocular inflammation
ROUTE OF ADMINISTRATION: Ophthalmic
COMMON ADULT DOSAGE: 1 to 2 drops in affected eye(s) every 4 to 6 hours
MECHANISM OF ACTION: Prevents or suppresses inflammation and immune responses

SIDE EFFECTS: Eye irritation, blurred vision, watery eyes

AUXILIARY LABELS:

- For the eye.
- Shake well before using.

GENERIC NAME: flurbiprofen

TRADE NAME: Ocufen

INDICATION: Miosis inhibition, postoperative ocular inflammation

ROUTE OF ADMINISTRATION: Ophthalmic

COMMON ADULT DOSAGE: *Postoperative ocular inflammation:* 1 drop in the affected eye(s) every 4 hours for 1 to 3 weeks

MECHANISM OF ACTION: NSAID (competitively inhibits COX enzymes to reduce inflammation)

SIDE EFFECTS: Eye irritation, blurred vision, itching (pruritus)

AUXILIARY LABELS:

- For the eye.
- Use as directed.

GENERIC NAME: ketoprofen

TRADE NAME: Acular

INDICATION: Allergic conjunctivitis, ocular pain, ocular pruritus, postoperative ocular inflammation

ROUTE OF ADMINISTRATION: Ophthalmic

COMMON ADULT DOSAGE: 1 drop into affected eye(s) four times daily

MECHANISM OF ACTION: NSAID (competitively inhibits COX enzymes to reduce inflammation)

SIDE EFFECTS: Eye irritation, itching (pruritus), headache

AUXILIARY LABELS:

- For the eye.
- Use as directed.

Ophthalmic Infections

Ophthalmic infections can be caused by a variety of pathogens, including bacteria, viruses, and fungi. Table 24-3 provides an overview of select antiinfective agents for the treatment of ophthalmic infections.

Bacterial Ophthalmic Infections. Conjunctivitis is an acute inflammation of the conjunctiva caused by viruses, bacteria, fungi, or allergies. Each type of conjunctivitis is treated differently, although the symptoms of this condition are generally the same. The eye becomes red, and a yellow discharge crusts over the eyelashes (occurs mostly after sleep). In addition, the eyes may burn and itch, leading to blurred vision. Newborns can acquire a neonatal form of conjunctivitis (ophthalmia neonatorum) as they pass through the birth canal. Immediate prophylaxis is crucial, or the infant may lose his or her eyesight.

Prognosis. With proper care and treatment, bacterial conjunctivitis can be successfully treated without any lasting effects. If left untreated, scarring may occur or even loss of eyesight, particularly in newborns.

Non–Drug Treatment. Placing a warm compress on the eyelids can help relieve pain. The patient should wash the hands frequently and avoid touching the eyes to prevent reintroduction of bacteria and reinfection. Towels and other personal care items should not be shared. Many forms of conjunctivitis are easily disseminated. If the patient wears contact lenses, use of the lenses should be discontinued until the infection has resolved.

Drug Treatment. Antiinfective agents are commonly used for conjunctivitis. The severe inflammation and discomfort of conjunctivitis can be treated with many different antibiotics. The physician determines the medication according to the cause of the infection. If the infection is bacterial, a wide variety of antibiotics can be used, depending on the specific microbe. For many bacterial infections, a broad-spectrum antibiotic, such as gentamicin or ciprofloxacin, may be used.

GENERIC NAME: sulfacetamide sodium

TRADE NAME: Bleph-10 (solution, ointment)

INDICATION: Ophthalmic bacterial infections

ROUTE OF ADMINISTRATION: Ophthalmic

COMMON ADULT DOSAGE: *Solution:* 1 to 2 drops in lower eyelid every 1 to 4 hours initially; *Ointment:* Apply a thin ribbon four times daily and at bedtime

MECHANISM OF ACTION: Inhibits bacterial dihydrofolate synthetase (interferes with the synthesis of folic acid, an essential component of bacterial growth and development)

SIDE EFFECTS: Eye irritation, itching, sensitivity to light

AUXILIARY LABELS:

- For the eye.
- Use as directed.

TABLE 24-3

Select Antiinfective Agents for the Treatment of Eye Infections

Medication Class	Generic Name	Trade Name	Common Side Effects	Common Dose Range
Aminoglycoside Antibiotics	gentamicin	Genoptic	• Burning • Irritation	• 1-2 drops every 4 hr (2 drops/hr for severe infections)
	tobramycin	Tobrex	• Rash • Lid itching • Lid swelling	• 1-2 drops every 2-4 hr until improved
Fluoroquinolone Antibiotics	besifloxacin	Besivance	• Headache • Redness • Blurred vision • Pain	• 1 drop in affected eye 3 times daily for 7 days
	ciprofloxacin	Ciloxan	• White crystalline precipitate • Hyperemia • Burning • Eyelid crusting	• 1-2 drops in affected eye every 2 hr for the first 2 days, then 1-2 drops every 4 hr for the next 5 days
	ofloxacin	Ocuflox	• Blurred vision • Burning • Conjunctivitis • Photophobia • Redness • Stinging	• 1-2 drops in affected eye every 2-4 hr for the first 2 days, then use 4 times daily for an additional 5 days
	moxifloxacin	Vigamox	• Conjunctivitis • Dry eye • Hyperemia • Irritation • Decreased visual acuity	• 1 drop in affected eye 3 times daily for 7 days
	gatifloxacin	Zymar	• Edema • Dermatitis • Dry eye • Irritation • Decreased visual acuity	• 1 drop in affected eye every 2 hr while awake (max 8 times/day) on day 1, then 1 drop 2-4 times daily on days 2-7
Macrolide Antibiotics	erythromycin	Ilotycin	• Hypersensitivity • Irritation • Redness	• ½-inch ribbon 6 times daily
	azithromycin	AzaSite	• Irritation • Blurred vision • Abnormal taste • Dry eyes • Swelling	• 1 drop in affected eye twice daily for 2 days, then 1 drop daily for 5 days
Sulfonamide Antibiotics	sulfacetamide	Bleph-10	• Edema • Burning • Conjunctivitis • Hyperemia • Ulcers	• 1 to 2 drops in lower eyelid every 1 to 4 hours initially
Miscellaneous Antibiotics	polymyxin B/ trimethoprim	Polytrim	• Burning • Itching • Edema • Rash	• 1 drop in affected eye every 3 hr (max 6 doses/day) for 7-10 days
	bacitracin	BACiiM	• Blurred vision • Discomfort • Stinging	• ½-inch ribbon of ointment every 3-4 hr in the conjunctival sac for 7-10 days
Antifungals	natamycin	Natacyn	• Paresthesia • Vision changes • Burning • Edema • Hyperemia	• 1 drop in conjunctival sac every 1-2 hr; after 3-4 days, reduce to 6-8 times daily (treat for 2-3 wk)

Continued

TABLE 24-3

Select Antiinfective Agents for the Treatment of Eye Infections—cont'd

Medication Class	Generic Name	Trade Name	Common Side Effects	Common Dose Range
Antivirals	trifluridine	Viroptic	• Burning • Stinging • Edema • Increased pressure	• 1 drop in affected eye every 2 hr while awake (max 9 drops/day) until ulcer heals; then 1 drop every 4 hr for 7 days
	ganciclovir	Zirgan	• Blurred vision • Irritation • Hyperemia • Punctate keratitis	• 1 drop of gel in affected eye 5 times daily until ulcer heals; then 1 drop 3 times daily for 7 days
Immunological Agent	cyclosporine	Restasis	• Increased tear production (goal) • Burning • Hyperemia • Pain • Itching	• 1 drop in each eye every 12 hr

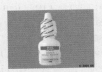

GENERIC NAME: tobramycin
TRADE NAME: Tobrex
INDICATION: Ophthalmic bacterial infections
ROUTE OF ADMINISTRATION: Ophthalmic
COMMON ADULT DOSAGE: *Solution:* Instill 1 to 2 drops every 4 hours; *Ointment:* Apply approximately 1 cm to the conjunctiva every 8 to 12 hours
MECHANISM OF ACTION: Aminoglycoside antibiotic (inhibits bacterial protein synthesis, leading to bacterial cell death)
SIDE EFFECTS: Eye irritation, itching (pruritus), sensitivity to light
AUXILIARY LABELS:
• For the eye.
• Use as directed.

MECHANISM OF ACTION: Inhibits bacterial protein synthesis
SIDE EFFECTS: Eye irritation, itching, sensitivity to light
AUXILIARY LABEL:
• For the eye.

Viral Ophthalmic Infections. The three most common viral infections of the eye are herpes simplex, keratitis, and viral conjunctivitis. The aim of antiviral therapy is to interrupt or alter the synthesis of new viruses at a specific step during replication. Many of the viruses that affect the eyes are more common in people who are immunocompromised, such as those diagnosed with acquired immunodeficiency syndrome (AIDS). Side effects of ophthalmic antiviral medications can include light sensitivity, stinging, and a mild burning sensation.

GENERIC NAME: erythromycin
TRADE NAME: Ilotycin
INDICATION: Ophthalmic bacterial infections
ROUTE OF ADMINISTRATION: Ophthalmic
COMMON ADULT DOSAGE: Instill ½-inch ribbon two to eight times daily, depending on the type and severity of the eye infection; in neonates, the ointment is applied once within 1 hour of birth for prevention of ophthalmia neonatorum

GENERIC NAME: trifluridine
TRADE NAME: Viroptic
INDICATION: Herpes simplex keratitis, keratoconjunctivitis, viral conjunctivitis
ROUTE OF ADMINISTRATION: Ophthalmic

COMMON ADULT DOSAGE: 1 drop in affected eye(s) every 2 hours while awake for a maximum of 9 drops; then treatment may decrease to 1 drop every 4 hours while awake

MECHANISM OF ACTION: Inhibits viral DNA replication

SIDE EFFECTS: Eye irritation, itching, sensitivity to light

AUXILIARY LABEL:
- For the eye.

Fungal Ophthalmic Infections. Fungal conjunctivitis is relatively rare. The primary ophthalmic agent for superficial fungal eye infections is natamycin, a **fungicidal** agent. The specific method of action of natamycin involves drug binding to the cell membrane of the fungus. When this occurs, the stability of the membrane is jeopardized, killing the fungus.

 Tech Note!
The best way to avoid conjunctivitis is to wash your hands before touching the eyes. Other possible ways to come in contact with the pathogens that cause this infection are sharing towels, pillows, and even computer keyboards.

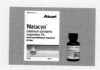

GENERIC NAME: natamycin
TRADE NAME: Natacyn
INDICATION: Blepharitis, fungal conjunctivitis, fungal keratitis
ROUTE OF ADMINISTRATION: Ophthalmic
COMMON ADULT DOSAGE: *Fungal conjunctivitis and blepharitis:* 1 drop in affected eye(s) every 4 to 6 hours; *Fungal keratitis:* 1 drop in affected eye(s) every 1 to 2 hours for 3 to 4 days, followed by 1 drop every 3 to 4 hours for a total of 14 to 21 days
MECHANISM OF ACTION: Impairs fungal cell wall membranes, leading to death of the fungus
SIDE EFFECTS: Eye irritation, itching, sensitivity to light (photophobia)
AUXILIARY LABELS:
- For the eye.
- Shake well before using.

Glaucoma

Glaucoma is a group of ophthalmic disorders characterized by high **intraocular pressure (IOP).** If left

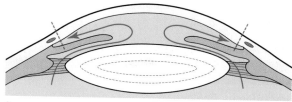

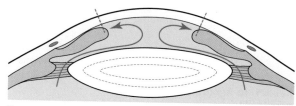

FIGURE 24-6 Glaucoma. **A,** In open-angle glaucoma the obstruction occurs in the trabecular meshwork. **B,** In closed-angle glaucoma the trabecular meshwork is covered by the root of the iris or adhesions between the iris and the cornea. (From Damjanov I: *Pathology for the health professions,* ed 4, Philadelphia, 2012, Saunders.)

untreated, glaucoma can lead to peripheral vision loss and ultimately blindness. Primary glaucoma is classified into two subtypes, open-angle glaucoma and closed-angle glaucoma. Open-angle glaucoma is characterized by a progressive, slow increase in IOP; in this form of glaucoma, the "angle" of the anterior chamber of the eye through which aqueous humor is resorbed is open. In contrast, closed-angle glaucoma is characterized by a visible obstruction of the angle, generally produced by the iris during contraction (Figure 24-6). Closed-angle glaucoma often presents suddenly, with intraocular pain, loss of vision, and redness of the eye.

Prognosis. Early diagnosis and treatment are essential for preventing irreversible vision loss. Glaucoma can be medically treated with drugs that reduce the production of aqueous humor or IOP. As mentioned, if left untreated, glaucoma can lead to blindness. Depending on the severity, a wide range of medications and treatments are available to reduce IOP.

Non–Drug Treatment. Surgery can be used to implant drainage valves for the outflow of aqueous humor. Alternatively, in some cases corrective lenses can be used for glaucoma treatment.

Drug Treatment. Treatment of glaucoma focuses on reducing IOP by increasing drainage or reducing the production of aqueous humor. Ophthalmic dosage forms include drops, suspensions, and ointments; in some cases, medicated inserts may be prescribed. Five classifications of drugs can be used to treat glaucoma: beta-adrenergic

TABLE 24-4

Select Agents for the Treatment of Glaucoma

Generic Name	Trade Name	Common Side Effects	Common Dose Range
Prostaglandin Analogues			
latanoprost	Xalatan	• Irreversible darkening of the iris	• 0.005%: 1 drop in affected eye every night
bimatoprost	Lumigan	• Change in eye color	• 0.03%: 1 drop in affected eye every night
travoprost	Travatan	• Thickening/darkening of eyelashes	• 0.004%: 1 drop in affected eye every night
		• Darkening of eyelids	
		• Hyperemia	
Cholinergic Agonists (Miotics)			
pilocarpine	Pilocar	• Headaches	• 1 drops up to 4 times daily *or* ½-inch ribbon of gel once daily at bedtime
		• Decreased night vision	
carbachol	Carboptic	• Stinging	• 1-2 drops up to 3 times daily
		• Pain	
		• Spasm	
Carbonic Anhydrase Inhibitors			
brinzolamide	Azopt	• Blurred vision	• 1 drop in affected eye 3 times daily
dorzolamide	Trusopt	• Stinging	• 1 drop in affected eye 3 times daily
		• Conjunctivitis	
		• Keratitis	
Beta-Blockers			
betaxolol	Betoptic	• Stinging/burning	• 0.5%: 1 drop in affected eye twice daily
carteolol	Ocupress	• Dry eyes	• 1%: 1 drop in affected eye twice daily
levobunolol	Betagan	• Blepharitis	• 0.5%: 1 drop in affected eye 1-2 times daily
metipranolol	OptiPranolol		• 3%: 1 drop in affected eye twice daily
timolol	Timoptic		• 0.5%: 1 drop in affected eye 1-2 times daily
Adrenergic Agents			
brimonidine	Alphagan P	• Eye pain	• 1 drop in affected eye 3 times daily
dipivefrin	Propine	• Stinging	• 1 drop in affected eye twice daily
		• Conjunctivitis	

blockers, carbonic anhydrase inhibitors, cholinergic agonists (miotics), sympathomimetics, and prostaglandin analogues. In many cases, more than one medication class is used (Table 24-4).

Tech Note!

Several prescription combination products that include medications from several drug classes are available for the treatment of glaucoma.

Beta-Adrenergic Blockers. Beta-adrenergic blockers (beta-blockers) lower IOP in open-angle glaucoma. By blocking beta-receptors, these agents prevent the activation of the beta-adrenergic response (i.e., the sympathetic, or "fight or flight," response),

which affects many body systems. Specifically, in the eye beta-adrenergic blockers are believed to reduce the production of aqueous humor by the ciliary processes to reduce IOP.

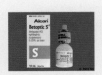

GENERIC NAME: betaxolol
TRADE NAME: Betoptic-S
INDICATION: Open-angle glaucoma
ROUTE OF ADMINISTRATION: Ophthalmic
COMMON ADULT DOSAGE: 1 to 2 drops in the affected eye(s) twice daily

MECHANISM OF ACTION: Reduces the production of aqueous humor by the ciliary processes in the eye to reduce IOP
SIDE EFFECTS: Stinging, itching, dry eyes, headache
AUXILIARY LABEL:
- For the eye.
- Shake well before using.

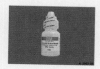

GENERIC NAME: carteolol
TRADE NAME: Ocupress
INDICATION: Open-angle glaucoma
ROUTE OF ADMINISTRATION: Ophthalmic
COMMON ADULT DOSAGE: 1 drop in the affected eye(s) twice daily
MECHANISM OF ACTION: Reduces the production of aqueous humor by the ciliary processes in the eye to reduce IOP
SIDE EFFECTS: Burning, stinging, headache
AUXILIARY LABEL:
- For the eye.

GENERIC NAME: timolol
TRADE NAME: Timoptic Ocudose, Timoptic-XE (gel-forming solution)
INDICATION: Open-angle glaucoma
ROUTE OF ADMINISTRATION: Ophthalmic
COMMON ADULT DOSAGE: 1 drop twice daily in affected eye(s); *Timoptic-XE:* 1 drop daily in affected eye(s)
MECHANISM OF ACTION: Reduces the production of aqueous humor by the ciliary processes in the eye to reduce IOP
SIDE EFFECTS: Stinging, blurred vision, headache
AUXILIARY LABEL:
- For the eye.

Carbonic Anhydrase Inhibitors. Carbonic anhydrase inhibitors inhibit the enzyme **carbonic anhydrase**, thereby decreasing the formation of aqueous humor. Directly applying these medications to the eye reduces the IOP in individuals with chronic open-

angle glaucoma. Carbonic anhydrase inhibitors also can sometimes be used in closed-angle glaucoma for a short duration to lower the IOP so that surgery can be performed. Carbonic anhydrase inhibitors can be applied locally to the eye or may be given systemically in some cases (e.g., methazolamide [Neptazane]).

GENERIC NAME: dorzolamide
TRADE NAME: Trusopt Ocumeter
INDICATION: Glaucoma
ROUTE OF ADMINISTRATION: Ophthalmic
COMMON ADULT DOSAGE: 1 drop in affected eye(s) three times daily
MECHANISM OF ACTION: Inhibits the enzyme carbonic anhydrase, thereby decreasing the formation of aqueous humor and lowering IOP
SIDE EFFECTS: Eye irritation, blurred vision
AUXILIARY LABEL:
- For the eye.

Cholinergic Agonists (Miotics). Miotics are similar to carbonic anhydrase inhibitors in the types of glaucoma they treat. These medications reduce IOP by contracting the ciliary muscle, thus increasing the outflow of aqueous humor from the eye.

GENERIC NAME: pilocarpine
TRADE NAME: Isopto-Carpine
INDICATION: Glaucoma
ROUTE OF ADMINISTRATION: Ophthalmic
COMMON ADULT DOSAGE: 1 drop in affected eye(s) up to four times daily
MECHANISM OF ACTION: Increases the outflow of aqueous humor from the eye by contracting the ciliary muscle
SIDE EFFECTS: Blurred vision, night blindness
AUXILIARY LABEL:
- For the eye.

Sympathomimetics. The name **sympathomimetic** refers to mimicking, or "acting like," the sympathetic system. Most of the agents in this class are intended specifically for people with allergies and congestion in the eyes. Sympathomimetics reduce IOP by reducing aqueous humor production and increasing its outflow. These medications are used to treat open-angle glaucoma and are often used in conjunction with other glaucoma medications to reduce IOP.

GENERIC NAME: brimonidine
TRADE NAME: Alphagan P
INDICATION: Open-angle glaucoma
ROUTE OF ADMINISTRATION: Ophthalmic
COMMON ADULT DOSAGE: 1 drop in the affected eye(s) three times daily
MECHANISM OF ACTION: Reduces IOP by reducing aqueous humor production and increasing its outflow
SIDE EFFECTS: Blurred vision, irritation, headache
AUXILIARY LABEL:
- For the eye.

Prostaglandin Analogs. Several agents are indicated to treat glaucoma under this classification, such as latanoprost, bimatoprost, and travoprost. These medications reduce IOP by increasing the outflow of aqueous humor. Ophthalmic use of prostaglandin analogs is associated with several unique adverse effects, such as discoloration of the iris due to an increase in brown pigments in the iris, and an increase in the length, thickness, and pigmentation of the eyelashes.

GENERIC NAME: latanoprost
TRADE NAME: Xalatan
INDICATION: Open-angle glaucoma
ROUTE OF ADMINISTRATION: Ophthalmic
COMMON ADULT DOSAGE: 1 drop in affected eye(s) once daily in the evening
MECHANISM OF ACTION: Reduces IOP by increasing the outflow of aqueous humor
SIDE EFFECTS: Iris discoloration, eye irritation, thickening of the eyelashes
AUXILIARY LABELS:
- For the eye.
- Possible permanent change in eye color, thickening and darkening of eyelashes, darkening of eyelids.

 Tech Note!
Xalatan should be stored in the refrigerator until opened. Once opened, it may be stored at room temperature for 6 weeks.

GENERIC NAME: bimatoprost
TRADE NAME: Lumigan
INDICATION: Open-angle glaucoma
ROUTE OF ADMINISTRATION: Ophthalmic
COMMON ADULT DOSAGE: 1 drop in affected eye(s) once daily in the evening
MECHANISM OF ACTION: Reduces IOP by increasing the outflow of aqueous humor
SIDE EFFECTS: Iris discoloration, eye irritation, thickening of the eyelashes
AUXILIARY LABELS:
- For the eye.
- Possible permanent change in eye color, thickening and darkening of eyelashes, darkening of eyelids.

 Tech Note!
A new bimatoprost formulation (Latisse) is indicated for the thickening of eyelashes. It is used to treat hypotrichosis (i.e., less than normal amount of hair) of the eyelids.

Miscellaneous Ophthalmic Agents

A variety of other miscellaneous products can be used for the treatment of ophthalmological conditions. Agents such as artificial tears are commonly purchased over the counter (OTC) for the treatment of dry eye. Their ingredients include sodium chloride, buffers to adjust for pH, and other additives to prolong their effects. The only dosage form is a solution, but they are available in various strengths and in combination with various ingredients. Another agent that can be used for severe dry eye is cyclosporine (Restasis) eye drops. Restasis helps alleviate chronic dry eyes caused by inflammation.

The Ears (Auditory System)

The human ear is responsible not only for hearing, but also for balance and maintaining equilibrium. The ear is composed of three major sections: the external ear, the middle ear, and inner ear (Figure 24-7).

Anatomy and Physiology of the Ear

External Ear

The most exterior part of the ear is called the **auricle**. This area is composed of cartilage and skin and serves as an entrance for sound waves. The auricle transmits sound waves through the external **auditory canal**. This canal leads to the **tympanic membrane** (eardrum) inside the ear. This membrane has two major functions:

- Transmission of sound waves to the middle ear
- Protection of the middle ear from foreign objects

The transmission of sound is possible because of the vibration caused when sound hits the eardrum, much the same way a drum skin vibrates and carries sound when struck with a drumstick.

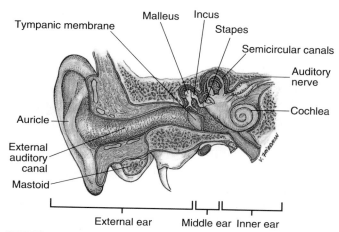

FIGURE 24-7 Anatomy of the ear. (From Potter PA, Perry AG: *Fundamentals of nursing,* ed 8, St Louis, 2013, Mosby.)

Cerumen (a waxy substance) is produced by glands inside the ear.

Middle Ear

Vibrations from the tympanic membrane are carried into the middle ear. The middle ear contains three very small, bony structures called the **auditory ossicles**: the malleus (hammer), the incus (anvil), and the stapes (stirrup). These three small bones are connected to each other and transmit the sound waves that make it to the eardrum. Another area in the middle ear is the **eustachian tube**, which leads to the nasopharynx. When a person swallows, yawns, or moves the jaw, the eustachian tube opens and relieves the change in pressure between the outside and inside atmosphere.

 Tech Note!

When a person in a car or plane is ascending altitude, the eustachian tube relieves the decreased pressure from the outside by causing a "pop" of the ear. This results in equalization of the two pressure levels.

Inner Ear

After the transmission of sound through the ossicles, the stapes (last ossicle) continues the transfer of sound into the third section of the ear, the *inner ear.* This fluid-filled area is called the labyrinth and is composed of many components that process and transmit the audible sounds via nerve impulses to the brain, where the sound is interpreted (Figure 24-8). These structures in the inner ear have separate but important functions (Box 24-2).

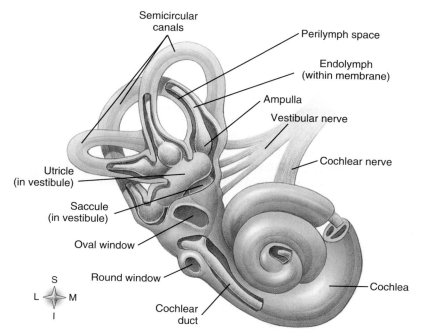

FIGURE 24-8 Anatomy of the inner ear. (From Thibodeau GA, Patton KT: *Anatomy and physiology,* ed 8, St Louis, 2012, Mosby.)

Common Conditions Affecting the Ear

Various conditions can affect the quality of hearing, including infections, swimmer's ear, earwax accumulation, damage to the eardrum, and congenital defects of the anatomy of the ear. Table 24-5 lists select products for the treatment of conditions affecting the ears. Viral ear infections cannot be treated with antibiotics. Depending on the strain of bacterial infection, certain preparations are available that are either bactericidal or bacteriostatic. **Bactericidal** agents kill the bacteria; **bacteriostatic** agents limit bacterial growth. Drugs that are bacteriostatic are used to assist the body's immune system in fighting off the bacteria.

Otitis Media

Otitis media is an infection in the middle ear and often is associated with inflammation of the eustachian tube. Otitis media is a common form of ear infection that is treated clinically (several other forms of ear infections are shown in Figure 24-9). Otitis media is associated with changes to the eardrum that can include bulging, swelling, and even perforation. Antiinfectives can be used to treat the infection. However, children who have frequent recurrent infections may require the insertion of

---

BOX 24-2

Three Main Areas of the Inner Ear and Their Functions

Cochlea
The cochlea is coiled and consists of three fluid-filled canals. The small, hairlike structures found here are connected to the acoustic nerve (i.e., the vestibulocochlear nerve [CN VIII]) that transmits impulses to the brain. As the sound waves enter, the hairs bend and create impulses that are transmitted to the acoustic nerve.

Vestibule
The vestibule is located between the cochlea and the semicircular canals and is responsible for equilibrium and balance. Small, hairlike cells are affected by gravity, and when they move, nerve impulses are transmitted to the brain, specifically to the cerebellum and midbrain areas. Thus equilibrium is maintained. This gives human beings a sense of direction and orientation.

Semicircular Canals
The three semicircular canals are filled with a fluid that helps with the transfer of messages via the acoustic nerve. Small, hairlike fibers behave as sensors, moving back and forth as the person moves forward, backward, or stops. The signals sent from two of these canals provide information to the brain about the orientation of the body when at rest, whereas the third canal sends information pertaining to the body in motion.

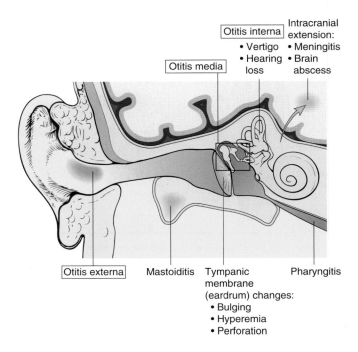

FIGURE 24-9 Infections of the ear. (From Damjanov I: *Pathology for the health professions,* ed 4, Philadelphia, 2012, Saunders.)

TABLE 24-5

Select Products for the Treatment of Conditions of the Ear

Generic Name	Trade Name	Availability	Indication
acetic acid/aluminum acetate	Domeboro	Over the counter (OTC)	Used for external ear infections and prophylaxis of swimmer's ear
benzocaine, benzethonium chloride, glycerin, PEG 300	Benzotic	Prescription	Used for pain in ear caused by swimmer's ear and infections
carbamide peroxide, glycerin, propylene glycol, sodium stannate	Debrox	OTC	Used to remove earwax
triethanolamine polypeptide oleate-condensate	Cerumenex	OTC	Used to remove earwax
isopropyl alcohol, anhydrous glycerin	Swim-EAR	OTC	Used for swimmer's ear

small tubes through the tympanic membrane to allow drainage from the middle ear and eustachian tube; this reduces the occurrence of reinfection. Common symptoms of otitis media include fever, nausea and vomiting, earache, hearing problems, and a feeling of pressure in the ear.

 Tech Note!

A classic sign that a young child may have an ear infection is constant tugging on the ears.

Prognosis. Recovery from otitis media is good with proper treatment. If serious infections are left untreated, potentially permanent damage to the ear can result.

Non–Drug Treatment. Many ear infections are self-limiting and resolve on their own after several days. Placing a warm compress on the ear can help relieve pain.

Drug Treatment. Antiinfectives are sometimes used to treat ear infections, although antibiotics are not always needed and ear infections can resolve spontaneously. Antihistamines, decongestants, and analgesics also are often used to treat the symptoms of otitis media (Table 24-6).

Cerumen Buildup

As mentioned previously, the glands near the tympanic membrane naturally produce a waxy substance referred to as *cerumen*. This is a normal process; the cerumen acts as a barrier to infection. As the amount of wax increases, the wax migrates out of the ear. If excessive wax accumulates, is not removed, or dries, it can impair an individual's ability to hear. It may be necessary for a physician to remove this waxy buildup to perform an examination or to improve hearing quality.

Prognosis. If cerumen buildup is treated appropriately, hearing improves; if it goes untreated, symptoms may include partial hearing loss, tinnitus (ringing of the ears), earache, itching, or discharge.

Non–Drug Treatment. Earwax removal is performed using an irrigation kit that includes a saline solution and an ear syringe. Using warm water and the solution, the ears are purged of excessive wax. Other treatments include using a few drops of mineral oil, glycerin, or hydrogen peroxide in the ear to soften the wax for a few days; warm water is then used to irrigate the wax out of the ear.

Drug Treatment. Several products are available to assist with earwax removal. These products work by emulsifying the ear wax to help with its removal from the ear canal.

GENERIC NAME: triethanolamine polypeptide oleate condensate

TRADE NAME: Cerumenex

INDICATION: Earwax removal

ROUTE OF ADMINISTRATION: Otic

COMMON DOSAGE: The ear canal is filled with the solution, which is allowed to sit for 15 to 30 minutes; the ear is then gently flushed to remove cerumen

MECHANISM OF ACTION: Emulsifies and disperses earwax

SIDE EFFECTS: Irritation of the ear

TABLE 24-6

Select Agents for the Treatment of Otitis Media

Medication Class	Generic Name	Trade Name	Common Oral Dose
Penicillins	amoxicillin	Amoxil	• 80-90 mg/kg/day orally (PO) divided twice daily
	amoxicillin and clavulanate	Augmentin	• 90 mg/kg/day PO divided twice daily
Cephalosporins	ceftriaxone	Rocephin	• 50 mg/kg intramuscularly (IM) as a single dose
	cefuroxime	Ceftin	• 30 mg/kg/day PO divided twice daily
	cefdinir	Omnicef	• 14 mg/kg/day PO once daily
Macrolide	azithromycin	Zithromax	• 10 mg/kg/day PO on day 1; then 5 mg/kg/day PO on days 2-5
Fluoroquinolones	ofloxacin	Floxin	• 0.3%: 5 drops in affected ear twice daily for 10 days
Analgesics	antipyrine and benzocaine	Auralgan	• Solution applied in affected ear(s) every 1-2 hr until pain and congestion are gone

BOX 24-3

Medications Associated with Ototoxicity or Tinnitus

Class	Specific Drugs
Aminoglycosides	gentamicin, tobramycin, amikacin
Macrolides	clarithromycin, erythromycin
Analgesics	aspirin, salicylates, nonsteroidal antiinflammatory drugs (NSAIDs)
Loop diuretics	furosemide, ethacrynic acid
Antineoplastics	cisplatin and platinum-containing agents
Antimalarial	quinine
Antiarrhythmic	quinidine
Glycopeptide antibiotic	vancomycin

Drug-Induced Ototoxicity

Certain medications can cause temporary or permanent hearing loss, known as **ototoxicity** (Box 24-3). This injury can present as a ringing or buzzing in the ears **(tinnitus)** and can progress to permanent ear damage if left untreated. Balance also may be affected. Specifically, aminoglycosides have been known to cause ototoxicity if given in high enough doses over a long enough period. Daily patient assessment is necessary when these drugs are prescribed; dosages should be sufficient to avoid permanent damage yet effective enough to fight bacterial infections.

Prognosis. The prognosis for drug-induced ototoxicity can be difficult to assess. Although many cases reverse themselves after drug treatment is discontinued, others cases can be permanent. Hearing loss may not occur until after several weeks of drug treatment.

Non–Drug Treatment. In most cases no treatment is possible once permanent hearing loss has occurred. In rare cases amplification may be used, depending on the cause of hearing loss and whether the drug was withdrawn soon enough.

 Tech Note!

Many ophthalmic agents, particularly antibiotics and corticosteroids, are commonly prescribed for use in the ear. This is acceptable because the ophthalmic preparations are sterile and can be used in the ear. However, otic preparations *cannot* be used in the eye because they are not sterile; in addition, the pH and other qualities of otic formulations may injure the eye.

Nose and Sinuses

Anatomy and Physiology of the Nose and Sinuses

As discussed in Chapter 19, the upper respiratory system is composed of the nose and nasal cavities, the **pharynx** (i.e., the throat), and the **larynx** (i.e., the voice box). The nose and sinuses play several physiological roles. The nasal septum separates the interior of the nose into two distinct cavities, which are lined by a mucous membrane with microscopic, hairlike structures called *cilia*. The function of the mucous membrane is to warm and moisten inhaled air before it passes into the lungs. The nose also functions as the sensory organ for the sense of smell and acts as a drainage system for tears from the eye (Figure 24-10). Because the nose and sinuses are in direct contact with the outside world, they are under constant assault by allergens and antigens that can result in allergy symptoms or infection.

Common Conditions Affecting the Nose and Sinuses

Allergic Rhinitis

Allergic rhinitis is irritation and inflammation of the mucous membranes lining the nasal passage as a result of allergen exposure. Common symptoms of allergic rhinitis include runny and itchy nose, sneezing, congestion, and postnasal drip. Postnasal drip is due to the accumulation of mucus in the back of the nose and throat. These symptoms are often treated with OTC products (Table 24-7). Additional symptoms may include coughing, watery eyes, and headache. (See Chapter 19 for a detailed review of rhinitis and its treatment.)

GENERIC NAME: triamcinolone
TRADE NAME: Nasacort Allergy 24HR
INDICATION: Allergic rhinitis
ROUTE OF ADMINISTRATION: Intranasal
COMMON ADULT DOSAGE: 2 sprays into each nostril once daily
MECHANISM OF ACTION: Corticosteroid (has antiinflammatory and vasoconstrictive effects that help treat rhinitis symptoms)
SIDE EFFECTS: Dry mouth, nasal dryness, cough, nasal irritation

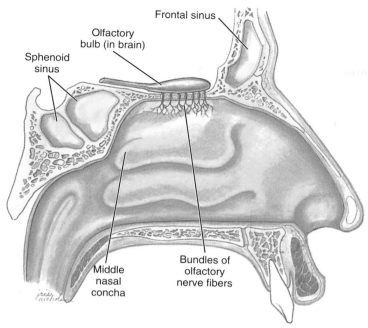

FIGURE 24-10 Location and structure of the olfactory epithelium. (From Solomon EP: *Introduction to human anatomy and physiology,* ed 3, Philadelphia, 2009, Saunders.)

TABLE 24-7

Select Over-the-Counter Products for the Treatment of Allergy Symptoms

Medication Class	Generic Name	Brand Name	Common Adult Oral Dose
Antihistamines: Oral Nonsedating*	cetirizine HCl fexofenadine	Zyrtec Allegra	• 5-10 mg orally (PO) once daily • 60 mg PO twice daily *or* • 180 mg PO once daily
Antihistamines: Oral Sedating	loratadine chlorpheniramine	Claritin Chlor-Trimeton	• 10 mg PO once daily • 4 mg PO every 4-6 hr *or* • *Extended release tablets:* 16 mg once daily
Decongestants: Oral **Decongestants: Nasal†**	diphenhydramine phenylephrine oxymetazoline	Benadryl Medi-Phenyl Afrin	• 25-50 mg PO every 4-6 hr • 10 mg PO every 4-6 hr • 2-3 sprays each nostril twice daily; do not exceed 3 days' use
	naphazoline	Privin	• 1-2 sprays every 6 hr as needed; do not exceed 3 days' use
	phenylephrine	Neo-Synephrine	• 2-3 sprays each nostril every 4 hr as needed; do not exceed 3 days' use
Mast Cell Stabilizers: Nasal **Antihistamine/Mast Cell Stabilizer: Ophthalmic**	cromolyn sodium ketotifen	Nasalcrom Zaditor	• 1 spray each nostril 3-6 times daily • 1 drop in affected eye(s) every 8-12 hr
Antihistamine/Decongestant: Ophthalmic	naphazoline tetrahydrozoline	Clear Eyes Visine	• 1-2 drops in eyes every 3-4 hr as needed • 1-2 drops in each eye 2-4 times daily

*Medications can be available combined with pseudoephedrine 120 mg and feature a "D" after the name of the decongestant product. Dosing involves a 120-mg pseudoephedrine combination pill twice day or a double strength (240 mg) combination pill once a day orally.
†Using these nasal sprays for longer than 3 days can cause rebound nasal congestion.

GENERIC NAME: fluticasone
TRADE NAME: Flonase
INDICATION: Allergic rhinitis
ROUTE OF ADMINISTRATION: Intranasal
COMMON ADULT DOSAGE: 1 or 2 sprays into each nostril once daily.
MECHANISM OF ACTION: Corticosteroid (has antiinflammatory and vasoconstrictive effects that help treat rhinitis symptoms)
SIDE EFFECTS: Headache, nosebleed, cough, nasal irritation

Bacterial Sinusitis

Acute bacterial sinusitis is an infection of the sinuses and corresponding inflammation of the nose and nasal passages that most commonly develops as a secondary infection after a viral infection of the upper respiratory tract. Symptoms of bacterial sinusitis include nasal congestion, nasal discharge, cough, sinus pressure, headache, and fever. Distinguishing between viral and bacterial sinusitis can be difficult. Because viral sinusitis improves after 7 to 10 days, a diagnosis of acute bacterial sinusitis generally is made if these symptoms have continued for longer than 10 days or if symptoms continue to worsen after 5 to 7 days.

Prognosis. The prognosis for bacterial sinusitis is good with appropriate treatment with antibiotic therapy, rest, and hydration.

Non–Drug Treatment. As noted previously, rest and fluids are an important aspect of recovery. Saline irrigation of the sinuses can reduce the need for pain medication and improve comfort, particularly in individuals who have frequent sinus infections.

Drug Treatment. After a diagnosis of bacterial sinusitis, antibiotic therapy is often implemented to fight the infection. Amoxicillin is considered first-line therapy because of its low cost and broad antimicrobial spectrum. Amoxicillin plus clavulanate (Augmentin) is also widely used. Other antibiotics that can be used include doxycycline, clarithromycin, azithromycin, and trimethoprim-sulfamethoxazole. In addition to antibiotic therapy, medications for symptom management are widely used, such as analgesics, decongestants, antihistamines, mucolytics, and intranasal glucocorticoids. See Chapter 19 for a more detailed review of these agents.

 Tech Note!
It is important that individuals who use saline irrigations to treat their sinusitis use sterile or bottled water to prepare the saline rinse. Some people have contracted amebic encephalitis from tap water rinses.

GENERIC NAME: amoxicillin plus clavulanate
TRADE NAME: Augmentin, Augmentin XR
INDICATION: Sinusitis, urinary tract infection (UTI), miscellaneous bacterial infections
ROUTE OF ADMINISTRATION: Oral
COMMON ADULT DOSAGE: *Augmentin:* 500/125 mg every 8 hours *or* 875/125 mg every 12 hours; *Augmentin XR (sinusitis):* 2 tablets every 12 hours for 10 days
MECHANISM OF ACTION: Amoxicillin is a beta-lactam antibiotic that inhibits bacterial cell wall synthesis; clavulanic acid competitively inhibits bacterial beta-lactamases to help overcome antibiotic resistance.
SIDE EFFECTS: Diarrhea, nausea, vomiting, rash
AUXILIARY LABELS:
- Take with food.
- Take until gone.

The Throat

The throat, composed of the pharynx and larynx (see Chapters 19 and 20), is the passageway into both the respiratory and gastrointestinal tracts (Figure 24-11). A variety of conditions can affect the throat, including viral or bacterial infections, sore throat associated with allergies, erosion of the esophagus due to gastric reflux, and even cancers of the larynx or pharynx.

Common Conditions Affecting the Throat

Strep Throat and Tonsillitis

Streptococcal tonsillopharyngitis (or "strep throat") is a bacterial infection of the throat associated with an abrupt onset of throat pain, fever, and **exudate** from the tonsils (Figure 24-12). The goals of antibiotic treatment are to reduce:
- The duration and severity of symptoms
- The incidence of complications (e.g., rheumatic fever)
- The transmission of the bacteria to close contacts

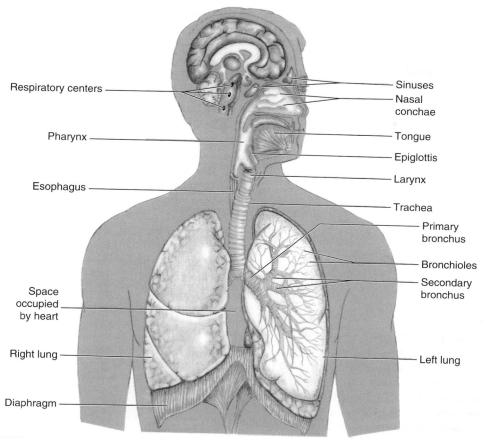

FIGURE 24-11 The respiratory system includes a series of air passageways and the paired lungs. (From Solomon EP: *Introduction to human anatomy and physiology,* ed 3, Philadelphia, 2009, Saunders.)

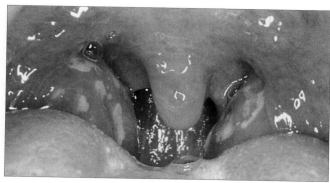

FIGURE 24-12 Streptococcal tonsillitis caused by group A beta-hemolytic *Streptococcus pyogenes,* showing intense erythema of the tonsils and a creamy, yellow exudate. (From Goering R et al: *Mims' medical microbiology,* ed 4, St Louis, 2008, Mosby.)

Prognosis. With treatment the prognosis for streptococcal infections of the throat is good. As noted previously, there is a risk of very rare complications associated with such infections, including **rheumatic fever** and **glomerulonephritis** (a form of kidney damage).

Non–Drug Treatment. As for sinusitis, adequate rest and hydration are an important component of therapy. Saltwater gargles can be used to help with symptomatic management of a sore throat.

Drug Treatment. Antibiotic options include penicillin, ampicillin, amoxicillin, cephalosporins, macrolides, and clindamycin. Analgesics, lozenges, numbing sprays, and pain strips are available OTC for the management of sore throat. (See Chapter 27 for a discussion of OTC products that can be used to treat cough and cold symptoms, including local anesthetic products for the treatment of sore throat.)

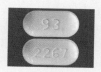

GENERIC NAME: amoxicillin
TRADE NAME: Amoxil, Moxatag (extended release)
INDICATION: Bacterial pharyngitis, bacterial tonsillitis, miscellaneous bacterial infections
ROUTE OF ADMINISTRATION: Oral

COMMON ADULT DOSAGE: *Amoxil:* 500 mg every 12 hours *or* 250 mg every 8 hours; *Moxatag:* 775 mg once daily taken within 1 hour of finishing a meal for 10 days

MECHANISM OF ACTION: Beta-lactam (penicillin) antibiotic (inhibits bacterial cell wall synthesis, leading to bacterial cell death)

SIDE EFFECTS: Nausea, vomiting, diarrhea, allergic reactions

AUXILIARY LABELS:
- [Moxatag]: Do not chew or crush.
- Take until gone.

GENERIC NAME: azithromycin

TRADE NAME: Zithromax Z-Pak, Zmax

INDICATION: Bacterial pharyngitis, bacterial tonsillitis, miscellaneous bacterial infections

ROUTE OF ADMINISTRATION: Oral

COMMON ADULT DOSAGE: 500 mg on day 1, followed by 250 mg daily for an additional 4 days

MECHANISM OF ACTION: Macrolide antibiotic (inhibits bacterial protein synthesis)

SIDE EFFECTS: Diarrhea, nausea, abdominal pain, anorexia

AUXILIARY LABELS:
- Take with or without food.
- Take until gone.

Gastroesophageal Reflux Disease

As discussed in Chapter 20, gastroesophageal reflux disease, or GERD, can occur when the upper sphincter (opening) at the top of the stomach relaxes. This allows acidic contents from the stomach to back up into the esophagus, which can result in a burning sensation in the chest or throat. Risk factors for GERD include obesity, smoking, and pregnancy, among others. If left untreated, GERD can result in significant damage to the throat. Barrett's esophagus is a disorder in which the lining of the esophagus is damaged by stomach acid. Appropriate treatment of GERD is important to prevent permanent damage.

Prognosis. With the use of medications and avoidance of foods that can make the condition worse, the outlook for GERD is quite good. Many people can make a full recovery from GERD symptoms.

Non–Drug Treatments. Avoiding foods that may bring about symptoms of GERD is an important aspect of treatment. Other non-drug approaches can include raising the head of the bed if GERD symptoms are prominent while lying down. If medication and diet are not effective, surgery is an option; however, surgery is rarely needed because of the effectiveness of medical management.

Drug Treatments. In addition to antacids, histamine-2 antagonists (H_2-antagonists) are used to treat GERD and ulcers. Agents such as cimetidine and ranitidine block H_2-receptors in the lining of the stomach. Proton pump inhibitors (PPIs) are a third type of agent used for the treatment of GERD. PPIs inhibit gastric acid secretion in the stomach lining by blocking the final enzymatic reaction before acid secretion. All three classes of these medications are available OTC, but some H_2-antagonists and PPIs require a prescription.

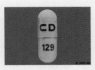

GENERIC NAME: ranitidine

TRADE NAME: Zantac (available OTC)

INDICATION: GERD, erosive esophagitis, gastric ulcer, duodenal ulcer treatment and prophylaxis (OTC for heartburn and indigestion)

ROUTE OF ADMINISTRATION: Oral; intravenous

COMMON ADULT DOSAGE: *Oral Rx dose for GERD:* 150 mg twice daily

MECHANISM OF ACTION: Competitively inhibits the binding of histamine to H_2-receptors on gastric parietal cells to reduce gastric acid secretion

SIDE EFFECTS: Constipation, nausea, abdominal pain

AUXILIARY LABEL (RX):
- May administer without regard to meals.

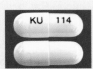

GENERIC NAME: omeprazole

TRADE NAME: Prilosec (available OTC)

INDICATION: Gastric ulcer, duodenal ulcer, GERD, erosive esophagitis; OTC for frequent heartburn occurring 2 or more days per week for up to 2 weeks

ROUTE OF ADMINISTRATION: Oral

COMMON ADULT DOSAGE: Dosage varies, depending on the severity of the condition; a common dose is 20 mg once daily; *OTC dosage:* 20 mg daily for up to 14 days

MECHANISM OF ACTION: Prevents gastric acid secretion from parietal cells of the stomach

SIDE EFFECTS: Diarrhea, nausea, headache, stomach pain, increased risk of fractures

AUXILIARY LABELS (RX):
- Take before meals.
- Do not crush or chew.

INDICATION: GERD, duodenal ulcer, gastric ulcer, NSAID-induced ulcer prophylaxis, erosive esophagitis

ROUTE OF ADMINISTRATION: Oral; intravenous

COMMON ADULT DOSAGE: Dosage varies, depending on the severity of the condition; common dose is 15-30 mg once daily

MECHANISM OF ACTION: Prevents gastric acid secretion from parietal cells of the stomach

SIDE EFFECTS: Diarrhea, nausea, headache, stomach pain, increased risk of fractures

AUXILIARY LABELS (RX):
- Take before meals.
- Do not crush or chew.

GENERIC NAME: lansoprazole
TRADE NAME: Prevacid, Prevacid 24HR (OTC)

 Tech Alert!

Remember the following sound-alike, look-alike drugs:
- Timoptic versus Viroptic
- Tobrex versus TobraDex
- prednisone versus prednisolone
- carteolol versus carvedilol

 DO YOU REMEMBER THESE KEY POINTS?

- Names of the major anatomical components of the eyes, ears, nose, and throat and their functions
- The primary signs and symptoms of the various conditions discussed
- Medications used to treat the various conditions discussed in this chapter
- The generic and trade names for the drugs discussed in this chapter
- The appropriate auxiliary labels that should be used when filling prescriptions for drugs discussed in this chapter

 REVIEW QUESTIONS

Multiple Choice Questions

1. The cornea is responsible for:
   A. Color of the eye
   B. Lubrication of the eye
   C. Protection of the eyeball
   D. Visual acuity

2. Glaucoma is a condition of the eye that results from:
   A. Narrowing of eye blood vessels
   B. Lack of aqueous humor
   C. Increased intraocular pressure
   D. Sun exposure

3. Which medication is *not* a beta-adrenergic blocker?
   A. Timoptic
   B. Betoptic
   C. Betagan
   D. Trusopt

4. Ketorolac (Ocular) is a(n):
   A. NSAID
   B. Beta-blocker
   C. Carbonic anhydrase inhibitor
   D. Prostaglandin analog

5. Miotics act by:
   A. Contraction of ciliary muscles, increasing outflow of aqueous humor
   B. Inhibition of beta sites that then relax vessels, allowing proper drainage of aqueous humor
   C. Inhibition of anhydrase, thus lessening the formation of aqueous humor
   D. The drug action is not clear

6. Natamycin is an:
   A. Antibacterial
   B. Antiviral
   C. Antifungal
   D. Antiprotozoal

7. The medical term used to describe the eardrum is:
   A. Eustachian tube
   B. Ossicle
   C. Auricle
   D. Tympanic membrane
8. The brand name of latanoprost is:
   A. Xalatan
   B. Lumigan
   C. Travatan
   D. Pilocar
9. The cavity of the middle ear contains all of the following structures *except:*
   A. Cochlea
   B. Malleus
   C. Incus
   D. Stapes
10. Cerumenex is indicated for use in the:
    A. Eye
    B. Ear
    C. Nose
    D. Throat
11. The structure in the inner ear responsible for balance is the:
    A. Semicircular canal
    B. Vestibule
    C. Cochlea
    D. A and B

12. Visine is an OTC product containing:
    A. Naphazoline
    B. Phenylephrine
    C. Tetrahydrozoline
    D. Azelastine
13. Which drug is considered first-line therapy for bacterial sinusitis?
    A. Amoxicillin
    B. Azithromycin
    C. Penicillin
    D. Ciprofloxacin
14. Which class of medications for the treatment of glaucoma is associated with the unusual side effect of darkening of the iris?
    A. Beta-blockers
    B. Miotics
    C. Prostaglandin agonists
    D. None of the above
15. Ototoxicity can be caused by:
    A. Analgesics
    B. Aminoglycosides
    C. Antineoplastics
    D. All of the above

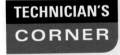
TECHNICIAN'S CORNER

Look up the following agents in *Drug Facts and Comparisons* and list the following information on each drug: generic and trade names, normal dosage, strength(s), indication, and auxiliary labels:
Xalatan
Optivar
Auralgan

Bibliography

Clinical Pharmacology Online: (Referenced September 6, 2014.) www.clinicalpharmacology-ip.com.

Damjanov I: *Pathology for the health professions*, ed 4, St Louis, 2011, Saunders.

Fishback JL: *Pathology*, ed 3, Philadelphia, 2005, Mosby.

Goering R et al: *Mims' medical microbiology*, ed 4, 2008, Mosby.

Huether S, McCance K: *Understanding pathophysiology*, ed 5, St Louis, 2012, Mosby.

McCance KL: *Pathophysiology: the biologic basis for disease in adults and children*, ed 6, St Louis, 2010, Mosby.

Page C et al: *Integrated pharmacology*, ed 3, 2006, Mosby.

Price SA et al: *Pathophysiology: clinical concepts of disease processes*, ed 6, St Louis, 2003, Mosby.

Solomon EP: *Introduction to human anatomy and physiology*, ed 3, St Louis, 2009, Saunders.

Thibodeau GA, Patton KT: *Anatomy and physiology*, ed 8, St Louis, 2012, Mosby.

Thompson JM et al: *Mosby's clinical nursing*, ed 5, St Louis, 2001, Mosby.

UpToDate Online. (Referenced September 6, 2014.) www.uptodate.com.

Therapeutic Agents for the Dermatological System

Joshua J. Neumiller

OBJECTIVES

Upon completing this chapter, you should be able to do the following:

1. Describe the anatomy and physiology of the main components of the dermatological system.
2. List the primary signs and symptoms of common conditions associated with the dermatological system.
3. Recognize prescription and over-the-counter drugs used to treat common conditions associated with the dermatological system.
4. Write the generic and trade names for the drugs discussed in this chapter.
5. List appropriate auxiliary labels when filling prescriptions for drugs discussed in this chapter.

TERMS AND DEFINITIONS

Acne vulgaris Commonly known as pimples, acne occurs when the pores of the skin are clogged with oil or bacteria

Alopecia Partial or complete absence of hair from areas of the body where it normally grows; baldness

Antiseptic A substance that slows or stops the growth of microorganisms on surfaces such as skin

Comedone A blackhead; a plug of keratin and sebum in a hair follicle that is blackened at the surface

Dermis A thick layer of connective tissue that contains collagen

Eczema A condition in which patches of skin become rough and inflamed

Emollient A preparation that softens the skin

Epidermis The outermost layer of the skin; it is composed of the stratum corneum, or horny layer, the keratinocytes (squamous cells), and the basal layer; it also contains melanin, a pigment that contributes to the color of skin and hair

Eschar A slough produced by a thermal burn, by application of a corrosive, or by gangrene

Exfoliation The peeling off of dead skin

Head louse A louse that infests the scalp and hair of the human head

Hirsutism Abnormal growth of hair on a person's face and body

Hypodermis Subcutaneous tissue

Keratolytic A drug that causes shedding of the outer layer of the skin

Melanin A dark brown to black pigment found in the hair, skin, and iris of the eye

Metastasize With regard to cancer, to spread from the place of origin as a primary tumor to distant locations in the body

Nodule A small swelling or aggregation of cells in the body

Onychomycosis A fungal infection of the fingernails or toenails

Papule A small, raised, solid pimple on the skin

Perspiration The process of sweating

Pruritus Itching

Pustule A small blister or pimple on the skin containing pus

Sebaceous glands Skin glands responsible for the secretion of oil called *sebum*

Seborrhea Excessive discharge of sebum from the sebaceous glands

Sebum An oily/waxy substance that lubricates the skin and retains water to provide moisture

Subcutaneous layer The deepest layer of the skin, consisting of fat cells and collagen; it protects the body and conserves heat

Sweat glands Glands in the dermis that are activated by an increase in body temperature to cool the body

Urticaria Red welts that arise on the surface of the skin; they are often attributable to an allergic reaction but may have nonallergic causes; also known as *hives*

Xerosis Abnormal dryness of the skin, eyes, or mucous membranes

Common Drugs Used for Conditions of the Dermatological System

Trade Name	Generic Name	Pronunciation
Antibacterials		
Sumycin	tetracycline	(**tet**-ra-**sye**-kleen)
Bacitracin	bacitracin	(bass-ih-**tray**-sin)
Bactroban	mupirocin	(myoo-**peer**-oh-sin)
Dynapen	dicloxacillin	(dye-**klox**-a-sil-in)
Ery-Tab	erythromycin	(er-**ith**-ro-**mye**-sin)
Neomycin	neomycin	(ne-oh-**mye**-sin)
Neosporin	neomycin/bacitracin/	(**nee**-oh-**mye**-sin/bas-i-tray-sin/**pol**-ee-**mix**-in)
	polymyxin b sulfate	
Antifungals		
Desenex	miconazole	(mi-**kon**-a-zole)
Lamisil	terbinafine	(**ter**-bin-a-feen)
Lotrimin	clotrimazole	(kloe-**trim**-a-zole)
Nizoral	ketoconazole	(kee-toe-**kon**-a-zole)
Tinactin	tolnaftate	(tol-**naf**-tate)
Treatment of Psoriasis		
Enbrel	etanercept	(ee-**tan**-er-sept)
Remicade	infliximab	(in-**flix**-i-mab)
Stelara	ustekinumab	(**yoo**-sti-**kin**-ue-mab)
Corticosteroids		
Triderm	triamcinolone acetonide	(trye-am-**sin**-oh-lone)
Cordran	flurandrenolide	(flur-an-**dren**-oh-lide)
Cutivate	fluticasone propionate	(floo-**tik**-a-sone)
Diprolene	betamethasone	(bay-ta-**meth**-a-sone)
Lidex	fluocinonide	(floo-oh-**sin**-oh-nide)
Temovate	clobetasol propionate	(kloe-**bay**-ta-sol)
Topicort	desoximetasone	(des-**ox**-ih-**met**-ah-sone)
Immunosuppressants		
Rheumatrex Dose Pak	methotrexate	(meth-oh-**trex**-ate)
Sandimmune, Neoral	cyclosporine	(sye-**kloe**-spor-een)
Retinoids		
Retin-A, Retin-A Micro, Avita	tretinoin	(tret-**in**-oin)
Topical Vitamin D Analogue		
Dovonex	calcipotriene	(cal-sih-poh-**try**-een)

The dermatological system, in its widest sense, involves conditions affecting the skin, scalp, hair, and nails. The skin is one of the most abused organs of the body system. It withstands damage from weather, detergents, scratches, cuts, and bruises, while continually repairing itself. The skin protects the body, regulates temperature, and acts as a sensor to outside stimuli. This chapter reviews the anatomy and physiology of the skin, hair, and nails and their functions. Common conditions that can affect the dermatological system are discussed, as are select treatments for these conditions.

Anatomy and Physiology of the Dermatological System

Skin

The skin is the largest organ of the body. It is made up of various layers that contain nerves, glands, hair, and blood vessels. The functions of the skin include protecting the body against heat, cold, light, dehydration, and infection. Nerve endings in the skin allow for the perception of pain, heat, and cold. Most of the body also is covered with hair, the follicles of which are embedded in the dermis (Figure 25-1).

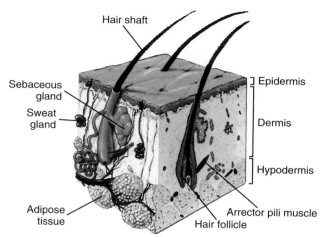

Hair shaft

Sebaceous gland

Sweat gland

Epidermis

Dermis

Hypodermis

Adipose tissue

Arrector pili muscle

Hair follicle

FIGURE 25-1 The skin consists of three layers: epidermis, dermis, and subcutaneous tissue. (From Damjanov I: *Pathology for the health professions*, ed 4, Philadelphia, 2011, Saunders.)

The top portion of the skin, the **epidermis**, can be further divided into three main layers: the horny outer layer, squamous cells, and the basal layer. The epidermis, the outermost layer, protects the layers below it. The epidermis also contains melanocytes, which produce the skin pigment **melanin**. The epidermis does not have a blood supply of its own; instead, it receives nutrition from the tissues surrounding it. Cells of the epidermis are constantly being shed and replaced. The basal layer is responsible for the production of new cells. As new skin cells are made, they push the older cells upward, and this becomes the outer layer of the epidermis. Beneath the epidermis are the dermis and the subcutaneous layers.

The **dermis** is a thick layer of connective tissue that contains collagen. The dermis is located under the epidermis (see Figure 25-1). Collagen, which is composed of interwoven, flexible fibers, helps support other structures, such as the blood vessels, glands, and nerves in the dermis. Below the dermis lies the **subcutaneous layer**, or **hypodermis**, the deepest layer; it contains fat cells that help insulate the body. Fat in the skin additionally helps cushion the body against injury and serves as an energy reserve.

Hair and Nails

Hair is primarily composed of a protein called *keratin*. The hair has roots that are embedded in the dermis, and the base contains melanocytes that are responsible for the color of hair. As a person gets older, the melanocytes stop producing the chemical melanin and the hair begins to turn gray. The hair follicle is vascularized to provide nourishment to the follicle (Figure 25-2). **Hirsutism**, which can be caused by certain medications, is an excess of hair growth,

whereas **alopecia** is the loss of hair. Alopecia can also be caused by a variety of medical conditions and medications.

Like the hair, the nails are composed of keratin, although they are much more dense than hair. The nails cover the top surface at the end of the toes and fingers. The nail root is embedded in the epidermis and provides protection to the surface of the toes and fingers. The lunula is the small white portion at the base of the nail. The cuticle is composed of keratin at the base and sides of the nail. The paronychium surrounds the nail and consists of a softer tissue (Figure 25-3).

Glands

The two types of glands in the layers of the skin are sebaceous glands and sweat glands (Figure 25-4). The **sebaceous glands**, located in the dermal layer of the skin, secrete an oily substance called *sebum*. **Sebum** lubricates the skin and retains water to keep the skin and hair from drying out. Sebum is transported by ducts to hair follicles, where this oily substance remains. Sebaceous glands can be found everywhere on the skin except the palms of the hands and soles of the feet.

Sweat glands are much smaller than sebaceous glands and are very prevalent in the soles of the feet and palms of the hands. Sweat is composed mainly of water with a low concentration of salt. When sweat glands are activated, sweat escapes through pores on the skin. As the temperature rises, the nervous system signals the glands, allowing sweat to flow onto the surface of the skin, where it evaporates and cools the skin. This process is known as **perspiration**.

Common Conditions Affecting the Dermatological System

This chapter outlines common conditions affecting the dermatological system and select treatments for the conditions discussed. Conditions affecting the skin are covered first, followed by a brief discussion of conditions of the hair and nails.

Dermatological Conditions Affecting the Skin

A variety of conditions affects the skin. Some can be effectively treated with OTC medications, but others require chronic treatment with prescription medications. Acne, sunburns, and hives are examples of common skin conditions that can be self-managed with OTC products. Serious infectious skin disorders, such as impetigo, require treatment by a physician.

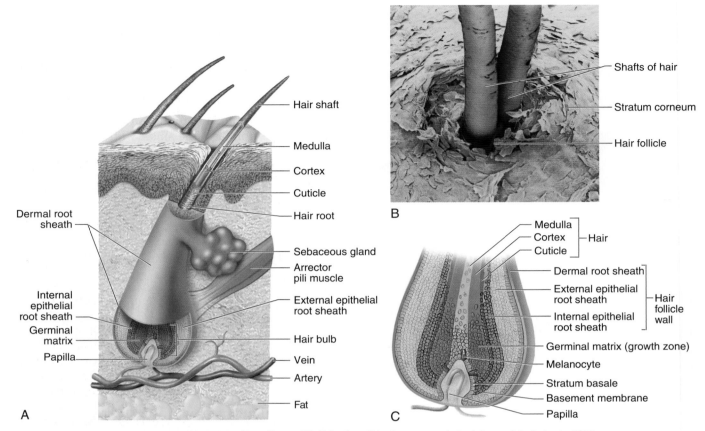

FIGURE 25-2 Hair follicle. (From Patton KT, Thibodeau GA: *Anatomy and physiology*, ed 8, St Louis, 2013, Mosby).

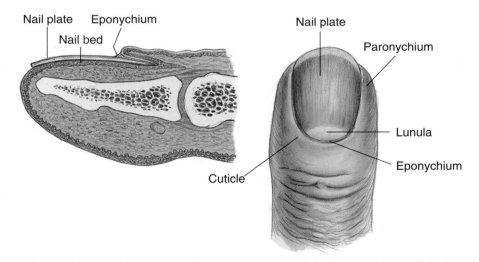

FIGURE 25-3 Nail anatomy. (Redrawn from Thompson JM et al: *Mosby's clinical nursing*, ed 5, St Louis, 2001, Mosby.)

Acne Vulgaris

Acne vulgaris (acne) is a common human skin condition characterized by areas of skin with **seborrhea**, **comedones**, **papules**, **pustules**, **nodules** and potential scarring. Acne most commonly affects skin with a high density of sebaceous glands, such as the face, chest, and back. Severe cases of acne are commonly associated with inflammation; however, acne can be present without the presence of inflammation. Acne occurs most commonly during adolescence and can occur into adulthood. Acne tends to occur during adolescence because of an increase in testosterone that occurs during puberty in both sexes.

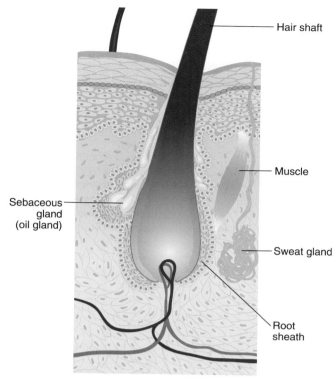

FIGURE 25-4 Glands of the skin.

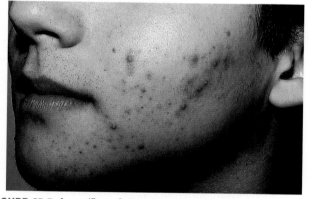

FIGURE 25-5 Acne. (From Callen JP et al: *Color atlas of dermatology,* ed 2, Philadelphia, 2000, Saunders.)

Hormones have the ability to enlarge and activate the glands of the skin. Two of the most productive glands are the sweat glands, which can become clogged, and the sebaceous glands, which produce sebum. When sebum production increases, it traps bacteria at the base of the hair follicle, and the likelihood of acne increases. The increased production of androgens during puberty leads to increased sebum production. When this occurs, the acne-causing bacteria multiply, leak from pores, and release oily chemicals onto the dermis, which can lead to inflammation (Figure 25-5).

Prognosis. The length of time before symptoms disappear varies, depending on the type of acne. Typically, as adolescents reach maturity, the frequency of outbreaks decreases, although scarring can occur in more severe cases of acne.

Non–Drug Treatment. The most effective non–drug treatment for acne is keeping the skin clean and free of bacteria by using cleansing agents that reduce sebum production and exfoliate (i.e., remove) dead skin cells. Although cleaning is clearly important, excessive cleansing can irritate the skin, worsening the condition. Various forms of light therapy can also be used to treat acne; however, the efficacy of light-based therapies for the treatment of acne vulgaris remains under investigation.

Drug Treatments. Mild acne is often treated with topical agents such as benzoyl peroxide, which helps dry the skin, and salicylic acid, which increases skin turnover. More severe inflammatory acne may require the use of topical or systemic antibiotics or topical retinoids in addition to **keratolytics.** Prescription antibiotics, such as tetracycline (orally), erythromycin (orally or topically), and clindamycin (topically), may be required. Topical retinoid agents, such as tretinoin (Retin-A Micro), increase the growth of skin around the acne areas, which causes **exfoliation** of the skin, removing dead skin cells and decreasing the formation of comedones. With retinoid treatment, the acne may seem to worsen initially but usually improves over several weeks. Oral retinoids, such as isotretinoin (Amnesteem, Claravis), are reserved for the treatment of severe acne. Retinoid therapies require that the prescriber, the pharmacy, and the patient be enrolled in a special program called iPLEDGE. The program is intended to reduce the risk of fetal exposure to the medication because systemic retinoids are known teratogens that can harm a fetus. Table 25-1 provides an overview of select agents used in the treatment of acne.

✎ ***Tech Note!***

iPLEDGE is a program aimed at preventing pregnancy during the use of isotretinoin products and at educating patients and prescribers about other potential side effects and risks of isotretinoin treatment. Visit *www.ipledgeprogram.com* to learn more about the program.

GENERIC NAME: tetracycline
TRADE NAME: Sumycin

TABLE 25-1

Select Agents for the Treatment of Acne

Medication Class	Generic Name	Trade Name	Common Adult Oral Dose
Topical Treatments			
Topical Skin Products	benzoyl peroxide	Clearasil 10%, Oxy 10%, Neutrogena 3.5%	• Apply sparingly once daily, gradually increase to 2-3 times daily
	salicylic acid	Stridex 2%, Noxzema Anti-Acne, Clean & Clear	• Apply small amount to acne in the morning and evening
	adapalene	Differin	• Apply once daily at bedtime
	dapsone	Aczone	• Apply a pea-sized amount to affected area twice daily
	azelaic acid	Azelex	• Apply thin film to the affected area twice daily
Lincosamide	clindamycin	Clindagel	• Apply to acne once daily
Macrolide	erythromycin	Akne-Mycin	• Apply over the affected area twice daily
Retinoic Acid Derivative	tretinoin	Retin-A Micro	• Apply once daily and increase concentration as tolerated
Oral Treatments			
Tetracyclines	doxycycline	Oracea	• 100 mg orally (PO) twice daily
	minocycline	Minocin	• 50-100 mg PO twice daily
	tetracycline	Sumycin	• 250-500 mg PO twice daily
Macrolide	erythromycin	Ery-Tab	• 250-500 mg PO twice daily
Sulfonamide	sulfamethoxazole/ trimethoprim	Bactrim	• 1 tablet (800 mg/160 mg) PO twice daily
Retinoic Acid Derivative	isotretinoin	Amnesteem, Claravis	• 0.5-1 mg/kg/day in 2 divided doses for 15-20 wk

INDICATION: Inflammatory acne vulgaris
ROUTE OF ADMINISTRATION: Oral
COMMON ADULT DOSAGE: 125-250 mg every 6 hours for 1 to 2 weeks, then decrease slowly to 125-500 mg daily or every other day
SIDE EFFECTS: Nausea, vomiting, anorexia, diarrhea, photosensitivity, tooth discoloration
MECHANISM OF ACTION: Inhibits bacterial protein synthesis
AUXILIARY LABELS:
• Do not take with dairy products.
• Separate from antacids or iron supplements by 4 hours.
• Take on an empty stomach.
• Take with a full glass of water.
• Avoid exposure to sunlight or tanning beds.

INDICATION: Acne vulgaris
ROUTE OF ADMINISTRATION: Topical
COMMON ADULT DOSAGE: A thin layer applied to the affected areas once daily at bedtime
MECHANISM OF ACTION: Modifies gene expression, protein synthesis, and epithelial cell growth and differentiation, leading to increased epithelial cell turnover
SIDE EFFECTS: Dry skin, itching, peeling, redness, irritation
AUXILIARY LABELS:
• For external use only.
• Keep container tightly closed.
• Avoid exposure to sunlight or tanning beds.

GENERIC NAME: tretinoin
TRADE NAME: Retin-A, Renova

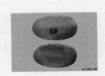

GENERIC NAME: isotretinoin
TRADE NAME: Amnesteem, Claravis, Sotret, Myorisan

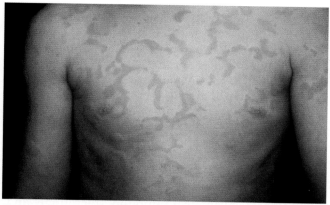

FIGURE 25-6 Urticaria. (McCance KL: *Pathophysiology: the biologic basis for disease in adults and children,* ed 6, St Louis, 2010, Mosby.)

INDICATION: Acne vulgaris, cystic acne
ROUTE OF ADMINISTRATION: Oral
COMMON ADULT DOSAGE: 0.5-1 mg/kg/day given in 2 divided doses for 15 to 20 weeks or until the total cyst count decreases by 70%
MECHANISM OF ACTION: Inhibits sebum production through a reduction in the size of sebaceous glands and possible inhibition of follicular keratinization
SIDE EFFECTS: Inflammation of the lips, irritation, pruritus, photosensitivity, rash, birth defects (pregnancy is a Black Box Warning)
AUXILIARY LABELS:
- Take with food.
- Avoid pregnancy. (Do not take this medication if you become pregnant.)

Urticaria

Urticaria is also known as hives. These superficial bumps range in size and are commonly associated with **pruritus** (Figure 25-6). Hives are commonly caused by hypersensitivity reactions to food, the environment, or drugs and can occur anywhere on the body. Topical agents can be used for hives and other noninfectious inflammatory skin rashes. Some cases of urticaria are *idiopathic,* or of unknown cause. They can disappear as rapidly as they appear.

Prognosis. Hives may dissipate within several hours, even without treatment. However, those resulting from an allergic reaction may require treatment for resolution and/or to improve the person's comfort. Removal of the allergen or cause is an important component of treatment.

Non–Drug Treatment. Applying a cold, wet compress can help alleviate the pruritus that accompanies hives.

Drug Treatment. Antihistamines are frequently used to treat the symptoms of urticaria. Topical anesthetics can also be used to alleviate symptoms of pruritus. If an antihistamine is needed, an oral one, such as oral diphenhydramine, can dramatically reduce the appearance of hives and itching; however, drowsiness is a common side effect of diphenhydramine, so patients should be cautious when using such products. (See Chapter 27 for a review of OTC antihistamine products that can be used to treat the symptoms of urticaria.)

 Tech Note!

Topical diphenhydramine products are also available OTC. Topical antihistamine use is discouraged, however, because of questionable efficacy and the possibility of sensitivity reactions after prolonged or repeated use.

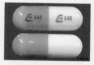

GENERIC NAME: diphenhydramine (OTC)
TRADE NAME: Benadryl
INDICATION: Hives, itching, rashes
ROUTE OF ADMINISTRATION: Oral
COMMON ADULT DOSAGE: 25 mg PO every 6 hours as needed
MECHANISM OF ACTION: Competitively inhibits the actions of histamine at H_1-receptors
SIDE EFFECTS: Drowsiness, dry mouth, dizziness, confusion, constipation, paradoxical central nervous system (CNS) stimulation
AUXILIARY LABEL:
- May cause drowsiness.

GENERIC NAME: calamine/pramoxine (OTC)
TRADE NAME: Caladryl
INDICATION: Pruritus
ROUTE OF ADMINISTRATION: Topical
COMMON ADULT DOSAGE: Applied to affected area(s) three or four times daily

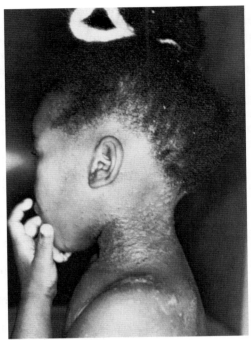

FIGURE 25-7 Lichenified, thickened, scaly skin over the neck area in childhood atopic eczema. (From Price SA, Wilson LM: *Pathophysiology: clinical concepts of disease processes,* ed 6, St Louis, 2003, Mosby.)

MECHANISM OF ACTION: Calamine (a mixture of zinc and ferrous oxide) acts as a protectant against irritants; pramoxine is a local anesthetic.
SIDE EFFECTS: Dryness; can aggravate contact dermatitis
AUXILIARY LABEL:
- Shake well before use.

Eczema

Eczema, also known as *atopic dermatitis*, is a chronic inflammatory skin condition thought to involve a genetic defect in proteins that support the epidermal barrier (Figure 25-7). It is also believed that eczema has an immune component to its pathophysiology; therefore, some of the following treatments discussed affect the immune system. Eczema is believed to affect 5% to 20% of children worldwide; the prevalence is approximately 11% in the United States. Eczema sometimes is broken down into "exogenous eczema" and "endogenous eczema." Exogenous eczema is thought to be caused by environmental irritants, whereas endogenous eczema is often linked to systemic autoimmune disorders.

Prognosis. The prognosis for eczema can vary considerably from person to person and depends on the type of eczema and the person's response to treatment. Approximately half of children with atopic eczema still experience symptoms into adulthood.

Non–Drug Treatment. A major component of management is elimination of exacerbating factors, which can include excessive bathing, low-humidity environments, stress, dry skin, or exposure to irritants. Maintaining hydration of the skin is also important. Use of thick creams or ointments can help protect against **xerosis** (dry skin).

Drug Treatment. Antihistamines are widely used to treat pruritus associated with eczema. Antiinflammatory agents, such as corticosteroids and topical calcineurin inhibitors (tacrolimus and pimecrolimus), can be used. For severe cases, agents such as oral cyclosporine and methotrexate may be used (Table 25-2). Sites of eczema can become infected through excoriation; therefore, it is not uncommon for people with eczema also to be treated with antiinfective agents for skin infections.

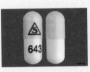

GENERIC NAME: tacrolimus
TRADE NAME: Protopic
INDICATION: Eczema, atopic dermatitis
ROUTE OF ADMINISTRATION: Topical
COMMON ADULT DOSAGE: A thin layer is applied to the affected areas twice daily.
MECHANISM OF ACTION: Inhibits calcineurin, which inhibits T-cell activation
SIDE EFFECTS: Burning, irritation, increased risk of skin infections, photosensitivity
AUXILIARY LABELS:
- Increased risk of sunburn.
- Use topically only.
- Wash hands with soap and water after application.

 Tech Note!
Tacrolimus is also available orally for prophylaxis of organ transplant rejection under the trade names Prograf and Hecoria.

GENERIC NAME: pimecrolimus
TRADE NAME: Elidel
INDICATION: Eczema, atopic dermatitis
ROUTE OF ADMINISTRATION: Topical

TABLE 25-2

Select Agents for the Treatment of Eczema

Medication Class	Generic Name	Trade Name	Common Adult Oral Dose
Topical Corticosteroids	betamethasone	Diprolene	• Apply to scalp/area twice daily
	clobetasol propionate	Temovate	• Apply to scalp/area twice daily
	fluocinolone	Synalar	• Apply thin layer to affected area 3 times/daily
	fluocinonide	Lidex	• Apply thin layer to affected area 1-2 times/daily
	flurandrenolide	Cordran	• Apply thin layer to affected area 2-3 times/daily
	fluticasone propionate	Cutivate	• Apply thin layer to affected area 1-2 times/daily
	halcinonide	Halog	• Apply thin layer to affected area 1-2 times/daily
	hydrocortisone	Aveeno Anti Itch Cream	• Apply thin layer to affected area 2-4 times/daily
	triamcinolone acetonide	Triderm	• Apply thin layer to affected area 2-4 times/daily
Topical Calcineurin Inhibitors	tacrolimus	Protopic	• Apply ointment twice a day
	pimecrolimus	Elidel	• Apply cream twice a day
Oral Calcineurin Inhibitor	cyclosporine	Gengraf, Neoral	• 3-6 mg/kg/day orally (PO) in divided doses twice daily
Immunosuppressants	methotrexate	Rheumatrex	• 0-25 mg/dose orally, intramuscularly, or subcutaneously (PO/IM/SUBCUT) once weekly
	mycophenolate	CellCept	• 2-3 g PO daily

COMMON ADULT DOSAGE: A thin layer is applied to the affected areas twice daily.

MECHANISM OF ACTION: Inhibits calcineurin, which inhibits T-cell activation

SIDE EFFECTS: Burning, irritation, increased risk of skin infections, photosensitivity

AUXILIARY LABELS:
- Increased risk of sunburn.
- Use topically only.
- Wash hands with soap and water after application.

Psoriasis

Psoriasis is a common, noninfectious inflammatory skin disorder. It has been related to genetics, especially cases with an early onset (age 40 or younger), and can last a lifetime. The onset of this painful disorder most commonly occurs between the ages of 20 and 30 or 50 and 60. The disease can range from mild to severe. This condition is not contagious, although the lesions appear inflamed. Affected areas are typically around the joints, limbs, neck, and even scalp and often appear as plaques of silvery scales that can vary greatly in size (Figure 25-8).

Prognosis. Currently no cure is available for psoriasis, and constant treatment is required to prevent outbreaks. Some can develop arthritic symptoms, but this is seen in less than one third of patients with psoriasis. For these individuals, additional medications are often prescribed, such as nonsteroidal antiinflammatory drugs (NSAIDs), sulfasalazine, methotrexate, and biological response modifiers (see Chapter 23 for a detailed description of these therapies).

Non–Drug Treatment. For mild psoriasis (covering 3% to 10% of the body), use of a high-quality moisturizer both keeps the skin moist and helps control flare-ups. **Emollients** that trap moisture work best. However, it may take time to determine which products are most effective.

Phototherapy (or UV exposure treatments) may be used to cause mild sunburn of the skin and subsequent peeling in patients with more serious disease. This is based in part on the observation that patients often notice improvements in skin lesions during the summer months. The process is done in a gradual manner over many months using UV light. Another form of light therapy

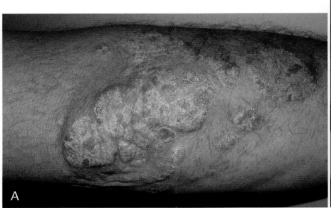
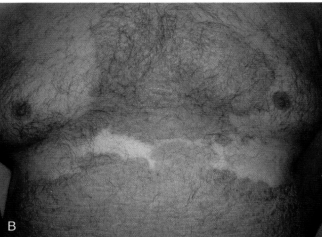

FIGURE 25-8 Psoriasis. (From Lookingbill D, Marks J: *Principles of dermatology,* ed 4, Philadelphia, 2006, Saunders.)

involves use of the excimer laser to treat mild to moderate psoriasis. These treatments require fewer sessions because only UVB wavelengths are used. Both types of light treatments are thought to be antiproliferative and antiinflammatory. The American Academy of Dermatology has published guidelines on the use of UV light for the treatment of psoriasis.

Drug Treatment. Treatment depends on the type of psoriasis, the extent of the disease, and the patient's response. Although there is no cure, measures can be taken for palliative care (i.e., care focused on pain, symptoms, and the stress of a condition). Three types of agents are used to treat psoriasis: topical agents, phototherapy, and systemic agents. Application of topical agents over the affected area or areas is usually the first line of treatment. Occlusion therapy uses moisturizers or topical medication applied to the skin, which is then wrapped with tape, fabric, or plastic. This keeps the area moist, allowing the medication to penetrate more deeply and work more effectively. This treatment should be done under the supervision of a dermatologist because it can lead to problems such as thinning of the skin. Bath soaks using agents such as Aveeno (colloidal oatmeal) can be purchased OTC and may reduce pruritus and discomfort of the skin in mild cases of psoriasis. Tar-based shampoos or preparations may be prescribed for treatment of the scalp. Calcipotriene (Dovonex) is a topical vitamin D analogue that is commonly applied to plaques to control skin turnover.

Immunosuppressants, such as topical corticosteroids, may help in refractory psoriasis. Creams may be applied after bathing to facilitate absorption, and overnight occlusive dressings may be used. The

mechanism of action of potent corticosteroids is the suppression of T-cells and other constituents that cause inflammation and an increase in cell growth; therefore, these agents must be used carefully because they impair the immune system. Biological agents such as alefacept (Amevive) may be used in patients who require systemic therapy to control skin plaques and improve skin appearance. Etanercept (Enbrel), infliximab (Remicade), and methotrexate are used in the treatment of psoriatic arthritis to prevent progression of joint damage. Table 25-3 presents a list of select agents used in the treatment of psoriasis.

GENERIC NAME: Alfacept
TRADE NAME: Amevive
INDICATION: Psoriasis
ROUTE OF ADMINISTRATION: Injection (intramuscular [IM], intravenous [IV])
COMMON ADULT DOSAGE: 15 mg IM or 7.5 mg IV once weekly for 12 weeks
MECHANISM OF ACTION: Prevents the activation of T cells to reduce inflammation
SIDE EFFECTS: Increased risk of infection, chills, cough, pharyngitis

GENERIC NAME: calcipotriene
TRADE NAME: Dovonex

TABLE 25-3

Select Agents for the Treatment of Psoriasis

Medication Class	Generic Name	Trade Name	Dosage Form	Common Adult Dose
Corticosteroids	betamethasone	Diprolene	Gel, cream, ointment, topical aerosol, lotion	• Apply to scalp/area twice daily
	clobetasol propionate	Temovate	Ointment, cream	• Apply to scalp/area twice daily
	fluocinolone	Synalar	Ointment	• Apply thin layer to affected area 3 times daily
	fluocinonide	Lidex	Cream, ointment	• Apply thin layer to affected area 1-2 times daily
	flurandrenolide	Cordran	Ointment	• Apply thin layer to affected area 2-3 times daily
	fluticasone propionate	Cutivate	Ointment	• Apply thin layer to affected area 1-2 times daily
	halcinonide	Halog	Ointment, cream	• Apply thin layer to affected area 1-2 times daily
	hydrocortisone	Aveeno Anti Itch Cream,	Cream	• Apply thin layer to affected area 2-4 times daily
	triamcinolone Acetonide	Triderm	Ointment, cream	• Apply thin layer to affected area 2-4 times daily
	desoximetasone	Topicort	Cream, gel, ointment	• Apply a thin layer to affected area twice daily
	amcinonide	Cyclocort, Amcort	Cream, lotion	• Apply thin layer to affected area 2-3 times daily
Tree Bark Extract	anthralin	Dithranol, Drithocreme	Cream, ointment, paste	• Apply once daily or as directed
Vitamin D Analogue	calcipotriene	Dovonex	Scalp solution, cream, ointment	• Apply a thin layer to affected area twice daily
Topical Retinoid	tazarotene	Tazorac	Gel, cream	• Apply a thin layer to affected area once daily
Antimetabolite/ Antipsoriatic Agent	methotrexate	Rheumatrex	Tablet	• 10-25 mg/dose orally, intramuscularly, or subcutaneously (PO/IM/SUBCUT) once weekly
Coal tar preparation	coal tar	DHS Tar, Doak Tar, Theraplex T	Shampoo, bath oil, ointment, cream, gel, lotion, paste	• Apply to affected area multiple times during the day or • Paint on scalp lesions 3-12 hr before each shower/shampoo
Monoclonal Antibodies	adalimumab	Humira	Solution for injection	• 80 mg SUBCUT once, then 40 mg every other week
	golimumab	Simponi	Solution for injection	• 50 mg SUBCUT once a month
	ustekinumab	Stelara	Solution for injection	• 45-90 mg SUBCUT at weeks 0 and 4 and then every 12 wk
Tumor Necrosis Factor (TNF) Inhibitors	etanercept	Enbrel	Solution for injection	• 50 mg SUBCUT 1-2 times weekly
	Infliximab	Remicade	Solution for injection	• 5 mg/kg intravenously (IV) at weeks 0, 2, and 6 and then every 8 wk
Calcineurin Inhibitor	cyclosporine	Sandimmune, Neoral	Capsules, oral solution	• 2.5 mg/kg/day PO divided twice daily
Psoralens	methoxsalen	Oxsoralen-Ultra	Lotion, capsules, solution	• Apply lotion before UVA light exposure (max once a week)
Oral Retinoid	acitretin	Soriatane	Capsule	• 25-50 mg PO once daily

INDICATION: Psoriasis
ROUTE OF ADMINISTRATION: Topical
COMMON ADULT DOSAGE: A thin layer is applied to affected area(s) once or twice daily.
MECHANISM OF ACTION: Synthetic analogue of vitamin D_3 (inhibits cell proliferation and induction of cell differentiation in psoriatic skin)
SIDE EFFECTS: Burning, itching, redness, swelling, dryness or peeling of the skin
AUXILIARY LABEL:
- For topical use only.

Chickenpox and Shingles

Chickenpox is a contagious disease and may cause serious complications in young children. Typical non-serious symptoms include skin blisters, fever, and an itchy rash (Figure 25-9). Some people can experience more severe effects, such as brain damage, pneumonia, infection, or (rarely) even death. If chickenpox is contracted by a pregnant female, the disease can be severe and require hospitalization. Another disorder caused by the same virus that causes chickenpox (herpes zoster) is shingles, which may appear in adulthood in a person who had childhood chickenpox. After lying dormant for several years, the virus may become activated and cause acute inflammation of the dorsal root ganglia. Symptoms include painful lesions along the nerves. Treatment for shingles includes medications such as valacyclovir (Valtrex), which can be given orally or intravenously. Acyclovir (Zovirax) also may be used over a 7-day period to reduce pain and promote healing. In 2006 a single-dose vaccine was introduced for adults older than age 60. The vaccine prevented shingles in about half the subjects tested and can reduce the pain associated with this condition. Those who should not be vaccinated include pregnant mothers or individuals who are immunocompromised. If the disease is contracted

through immunization, only a mild form results. After the injection the person may have soreness at the injection site and a mild fever. (See Chapter 23 for a more detailed description of this and other vaccines.)

GENERIC NAME: valacyclovir
TRADE NAME: Valtrex
INDICATION: Herpes, varicella
ROUTE OF ADMINISTRATION: Oral
COMMON ADULT DOSAGE: *Herpes:* 500 mg twice daily for 3 days at the first sign or symptom of lesions
MECHANISM OF ACTION: Inhibits viral DNA synthesis
SIDE EFFECTS: Headache, nausea, abdominal pain, fatigue

Burns

Burns range in severity from superficial to fourth degree; fourth-degree burns are the most severe (Box 25-1). If the degree of the burn or the size of the burn is substantial, the patient may undergo surgery to replace the damaged layers of skin (Figure 25-10). This is done by removing and grafting healthy skin from another part of the body. The new skin is thinned through a rolling process and then attached by staples to the damaged skin area. Burn hospitals require specialized solutions and medications from the pharmacy to treat patients who stay in the burn unit. First-degree burns normally can be treated at home.

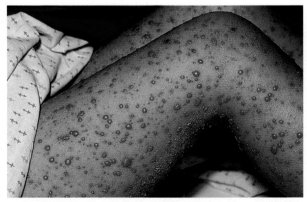

FIGURE 25-9 Chickenpox. The rash begins with macules, which turn into severe papules. Symptoms can last a few days to 2 weeks. (From Callen JP et al: *Color atlas of dermatology,* ed 2, Philadelphia, 2000, Saunders.)

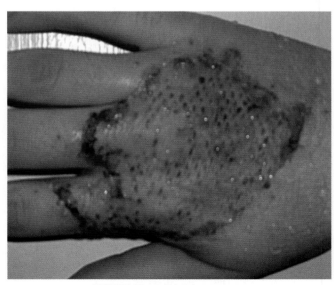

FIGURE 25-10 Third-degree burn.

BOX 25-1

Definitions of Burn Depth and Severity

Superficial: Only the outer layer (epidermis) of the skin is burned. The skin becomes red and swells, and pain is often present. Superficial burns do not blister but are painful, dry, and red and blanch with pressure. Superficial burns commonly occur with sunburn.

Partial thickness: The first layer of the skin (epidermis) burns through to the second layer (dermis). These burns can be further classified as superficial or deep. Superficial partial-thickness burns characteristically form blisters within 24 hours, are painful, red, and weeping and blanch with pressure. Deep partial-thickness burns extend into the deeper dermis and damage hair follicles and glands. Deep burns almost always blister, are patchy white to red, and do not blanch with pressure.

Full thickness: The burn extends through and destroys all layers of the dermis and often injures the subcutaneous tissue. **Eschar,** the dead and denatured dermis, is usually intact. These burns can vary in appearance from white to leathery gray to charred and black.

Fourth degree: The worst burns; the burn penetrates the deepest layers of the skin, including the muscles, tendons, and bones. Fourth-degree burns are may be life-threatening.

GENERIC NAME: silver sulfadiazine
TRADE NAME: Silvadene
INDICATION: Prevention and treatment of burn wound infections
ROUTE OF ADMINISTRATION: Topical
COMMON ADULT DOSAGE: A thin layer is applied to the affected area twice daily as directed by the physician.
MECHANISM OF ACTION: Inhibits bacteria by damaging bacterial cell membranes and cell walls
SIDE EFFECTS: Burning, rash, skin discoloration
AUXILIARY LABEL:
- For topical use only.

SPECIAL NOTE: Apply with sterile gloves.

Prognosis. Superficial and partial-thickness burns can often heal by themselves with simple care if they are small. Scarring is a common outcome of full-thickness and fourth-degree burns. The healing process can take a long time and may involve rehabilitation if tissues, muscles, and tendons are damaged. A patient with severe burns over a large surface area can be at high risk for infection, sepsis, and even death.

Non–Drug Treatment. If the burn is minor, cooling it by applying a sterile, saline-soaked gauze cooled to about 55° F can help with pain relief and limit further tissue injury. Ice should *not* be applied to the burn because this can cause additional tissue damage and pain. Any jewelry (e.g., rings) close to the affected area should be removed because jewelry may become constrictive if swelling occurs. Medical help should be sought immediately for severe burns.

Drug Treatment. Treatment can vary, depending on the type of burn. For example, in addition to thermal burns, people can experience chemical and electrical burns. Topical medications used may include silver cream (sulfadiazine [Silvadene]) and bacitracin ointment.

Warts

A common wart is caused by a virus that results in growths on the skin. Verruca plana, or flat warts, are commonly seen in children and may appear on areas such as the hands, face, and neck. Plantar warts are found on the bottom of the foot and may present with tenderness on walking. Common warts are caused by the human papillomavirus (HPV) (Figure 25-11, *A*). A physician should be seen for appropriate treatment, which may include drug treatment, liquid nitrogen (freezing) application, or surgical removal. Genital warts are different from common warts; they are caused by specific strains of HPV. Genital warts are a sexually transmitted disease (Figure 25-11, *B* and *C*). (See Chapter 22 for a more detailed discussion of sexually transmitted diseases.)

Prognosis. Warts are contagious, although some kinds resolve on their own spontaneously within several months. Other types of warts require evaluation and treatment by a physician.

Non–Drug Treatment. If no action is taken, common warts normally disappear over time. There is no non–drug treatment that is effective for common warts or genital warts. The best strategy for genital warts is prevention of sexual transmission. Gardasil (human papillomavirus vaccine) can be administered to young women and female adolescents to prevent contraction of genital warts and cervical cancer.

Drug Treatment. For common warts, OTC agents that contain salicylic acid or that freeze the wart can be used. Topical fluorouracil (Carac,

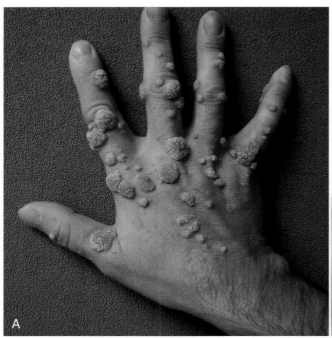
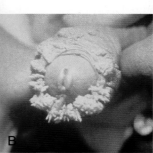
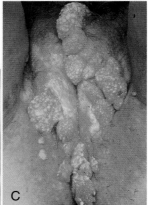

FIGURE 25-11 A, Human papillomavirus (HPV) (common warts). **B,** Genital warts, male. **C,** Genital warts, female. (**A** from Lookingbill D, Marks J: *Principles of dermatology,* ed 4, Philadelphia, 2006, Saunders; **B** and **C** courtesy New York City Health Department.)

Efudex, Fluoroplex) treats warts by interfering with skin cell growth; it is usually reserved for resistant plantar warts. Fluorouracil must be applied topically while wearing gloves or using nonmetal applicators.

GENERIC NAME: salicylic acid (OTC)
TRADE NAME: Compound W Wart Removal Gel
INDICATION: Common warts, plantar warts
ROUTE OF ADMINISTRATION: Topical
COMMON ADULT DOSAGE: Applied once or twice daily as needed (until wart is removed) for up to 12 weeks
MECHANISM OF ACTION: Removes warts by acting as a topical keratolytic agent
SIDE EFFECTS: Skin irritation
SPECIAL NOTE: Wash hands after application.

Athlete's Foot

Athlete's foot, medically known as *tinea pedis,* is most commonly caused by a fungus of the species *Trichophyton rubrum.* The name of a tinea infection depends on the site of the infection. Tinea pedis (athlete's foot) causes scaling and blisters between the

> ### 📝 Tech Note!
>
> Dermatophytosis is defined as any infection of the skin, hair, or nails caused by a dermatophyte (fungus) and characterized by redness of the skin, small popular vesicles, fissures, and scaling. Transmission of the fungus can occur through direct contact with infected lesions, with infections present on the skin of cats and dogs, and with soiled or contaminated clothing or articles such as shoes, towels, or shower stalls. Tinea pedis (athlete's foot) is a common condition affecting the toes and soles of the feet.

toes. Severe infection can cause inflammation of the skin on the entire sole and may include relentless pruritus and pain when walking. The infection can be spread by contact with shower floor surfaces or clothing, such as by sharing socks. Direct contact is required for transfer of the fungal infection (Figure 25-12).

Other types of tinea infections include:

- Tinea barbae (bearded skin)
- Tinea capitis (hair of the head)
- Tinea corpus (ringworm of the skin)
- Tinea cruris (groin, also known as "jock itch")
- Tinea manuum (hands)
- Tinea unguium (nails)

Prognosis. In most cases the prognosis for a tinea infection is good if antifungals are used and

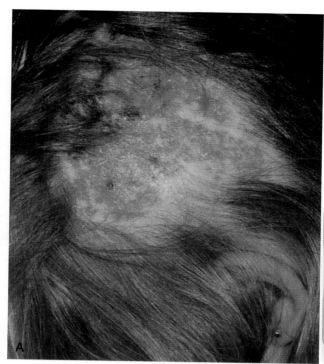
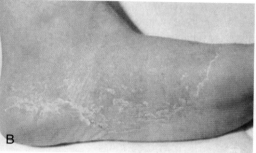

FIGURE 25-12 A, Tina capitis (head). **B,** Tina pedis (athlete's foot).

TABLE 25-4

Select Topical Agents for the Treatment of Dermatological Fungal Infections

Medication Class	Generic Name	Trade Name	Common Adult Oral Dose
Topical Antifungals	miconazole	Desenex	• Apply twice daily for 4 wk
	terbinafine	Lamisil	• Apply to affected area once daily for at least 1 wk
	clotrimazole	Lotrimin	• Apply to skin twice daily for 7 consecutive days
	ketoconazole	Nizoral	• Rub gently into affected area 1-2 times daily *or*
			• *Shampoo:* Apply once to damp skin, lather, leave on for 5 min, rinse off
	nystatin	Nystop	• Apply to the affected area 2-3 times daily

the feet are kept clean and dry. Through education on proper foot care, this condition generally can be avoided.

Non–Drug Treatment. The infection can be prevented with good hygienic practices. Keeping the feet dry and in clean, comfortable socks and shoes helps prevent athlete's foot. Exposing the feet to air whenever possible is also helpful. Avoiding walking barefoot in community showers or other places where transmission may be possible can help reduce the risk of contracting the fungus.

Drug Treatment. Most treatments involve topical agents available either OTC or by prescription. Antifungals are used to kill fungus and treat athlete's foot; OTC products usually are available in powder or spray form. More serious infections involving chronic thickening of the skin; those refractory to topical treatments often require treatment with oral antifungals. If the infection affects the nails, systemic therapy may be needed to clear the nail infection completely. Table 25-4 lists select topical antifungal agents used to treat athlete's foot and other dermatological fungal infections.

GENERIC NAME: clotrimazole (OTC)
TRADE NAME: Lotrimin AF
INDICATION: Tinea pedis and other fungal infections of the skin
ROUTE OF ADMINISTRATION: Topical
COMMON ADULT DOSAGE: A small amount of the cream is applied twice daily to the affected area.
MECHANISM OF ACTION: Azole antifungal (inhibits proper functioning of fungal cell membranes)
SIDE EFFECTS: Erythema, skin irritation, peeling, pruritus

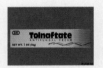

GENERIC NAME: tolnaftate (OTC)
TRADE NAME: Tinactin
INDICATION: Tinea pedis and other fungal infections of the skin
ROUTE OF ADMINISTRATION: Topical
COMMON ADULT DOSAGE: Applied to the affected area twice daily for 2 to 4 weeks
MECHANISM OF ACTION: Inhibits fungal cell growth in susceptible fungi
SIDE EFFECTS: Erythema, pruritus, inflammation, skin irritation

Impetigo

A comprehensive review of bacterial infections of the skin is beyond the scope of this chapter; however, numerous bacteria are associated with a variety of skin infections. Impetigo is one such skin infection. Impetigo is a highly contagious condition caused by streptococcal organisms, or *Staphylococcus aureus*. The bacteria can enter the body through broken skin caused by animal bites, injuries, trauma, or insect bites, although impetigo may appear in areas without a break in the skin. Potential areas that can be affected include the face, limbs, and abdomen. A thick, yellow crust characteristically is formed, sores are often itchy and oozing, and blistering is common (Figure 25-13). The infection is contagious because of the lesions' discharge.

Prognosis. The sores of impetigo heal slowly, although they rarely cause scarring. Children may have recurrences of the condition.

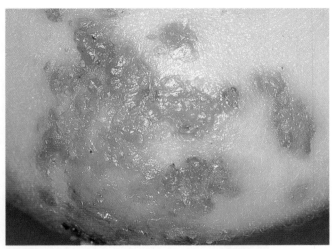

FIGURE 25-13 Impetigo. The skin shows typical yellow, crusting blisters containing pus. (From Damjanov I: *Pathology for the health professions,* ed 4, Philadelphia, 2012, Saunders.)

Non–Drug Treatment. Keeping the skin clean by washing several times daily with an antibacterial soap is recommended to remove crusted skin and oozing discharge. The condition is very contagious. Sheets, towels, and clothing should be washed frequently to help prevent the spread of infection. Isolation may be advised to reduce the transfer of bacteria to others.

Drug Treatment. Treatment includes topical antibiotics, such as mupirocin 2% ointment (Bactroban, Centany) or retapamulin 1% ointment (Altabax); these are effective for limited areas and have the advantage of having no systemic side effects. Table 25-5 lists select topical antibacterial agents that can be used to treat impetigo and other bacterial skin infections. Oral antibiotics are used for more extensive cases of impetigo or for patients who have concurrent systemic symptoms. Antibiotics used can include penicillins (e.g., dicloxacillin or Augmentin) or cephalosporins (e.g., Keflex or Ceftin) as first choices; erythromycin may be used but typically is a second-line antibiotic.

GENERIC NAME: retapamulin
TRADE NAME: Altabax
INDICATION: Impetigo
ROUTE OF ADMINISTRATION: Topical

TABLE 25-5

Select Topical Antibacterial Products

Product	Trade Names	Dosage Forms
bacitracin (OTC)	Bacitracin	Ointment
neomycin (OTC)	Neomycin	Ointment
polymyxin B sulfate, neomycin, bacitracin (OTC)	Neosporin	Ointment, cream
mupirocin 2% (Rx)	Bactroban, Centany	Ointment, cream
retapamulin 1% (Rx)	Altabax	Ointment

OTC, Over the counter; *Rx,* prescription.

COMMON ADULT DOSAGE: A thin layer is applied to affected area(s) twice daily for 5 days or as directed by the prescriber
MECHANISM OF ACTION: Inhibits bacterial protein synthesis
SIDE EFFECTS: Skin irritation, headache, diarrhea, nausea
AUXILIARY LABEL:
• For topical use only.
SPECIAL NOTE: Wash hands after application.

 Tech Note!

Prolonged use of retapamulin is not recommended because of possible overgrowth of resistant organisms. This overgrowth may lead to serious resistant infections.

Skin Cancer

Any abnormal growth of new skin tissue that results in a malignancy is known as skin cancer. Melanomas are cancerous skin growths emanating from moles and areas of the skin that may have been sunburned. The three main types of skin cancer are melanoma, squamous cell cancer, and basal cell cancer (non-melanomas) (Figure 25-14). The most aggressive and severe type of cancer is melanoma. Typically the appearance of melanomas on the skin is marked by an irregular shape, elevation off the skin, discoloring, and changes in size; these can occur anywhere on the body (Box 25-2). Melanomas start in the lower part of the epidermis, in the melanocytes (cells that color the skin). Individuals with light-colored or freckled skin, red- and blond-haired people, and Caucasians age 20 or older are at higher risk. The normal course of treatment depends on the stage or severity of the cancer. Basal cell cancer grows very slowly, occurs on the surface of the skin, and is usually due to sun damage. This type of cancer

BOX 25-2

Instructions for Detecting Possible Skin Cancers

Check yourself regularly for skin cancer using the ABCD method. This takes only a few minutes and may allow you to catch skin cancer in the early stages. Stand in front of a mirror and examine your entire body for any moles. Remember, not all moles look the same on every person; they can be different colors (red, black, brown), flat, raised, round, oval, or even irregularly shaped from the beginning. By examining yourself, you can determine whether any suspicious changes have taken place. A sudden or continuous change in the appearance of a mole is a sign that you should see your doctor. If you note such changes, see your dermatologist right away.

A—Asymmetry
Moles should appear symmetrical; this means that the two halves of the mole should look alike or be a mirror image of one another.

B—Border
The border of moles should be well defined and clear. It should not be fuzzy, blotchy, or irregular in any way.

C—Color
The color of moles must be monitored to note whether any changes occur, such as a change from light to dark in color.

D—Diameter
Melanomas are usually larger in diameter than the size of an eraser on your pencil. Anything over 6 mm should be examined by your doctor.

usually first appears on the face, and it rarely spreads to other areas. Squamous cell skin cancer normally occurs on other parts of the body (besides the face) that have been overexposed to the sun, but this type of cancer can spread to the lymph nodes and **metastasize** to other organs in the body.

Prognosis. The prognosis of any cancer depends on several factors, such as early detection, effective treatment, and a strong support system. With skin cancers the outcome is very good if the cancer is detected early, although constant awareness is necessary to catch any new areas of the skin that are changing in a suspicious way. Regularly scheduled visits with the physician play an important role in early detection.

Non–Drug Treatment. Prevention is the best treatment, including protection from harmful sun rays. The first line of treatment is surgery to remove the area of concern. Treatments include photodynamic therapy or radiation therapy. Both squamous and basal cell carcinomas are less severe and can be treated with various therapies.

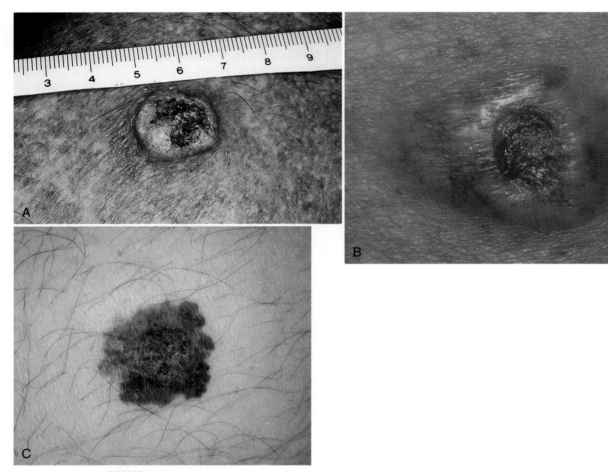

FIGURE 25-14 Types of skin cancer, **A,** Squamous cell. **B,** Basal cell. **C,** Malignant melanoma. (**A** from Noble J: *Textbook of primary care medicine,* ed 3, Philadelphia, 2001, Mosby; **B** from Goldman L, Ausiello D: *Cecil textbook of medicine,* ed 23, Philadelphia, 2003, Saunders; **C** from Townsend C et al: *Sabison textbook of surgery,* ed 18, Philadelphia, 2008, Saunders.)

Drug Treatment. If the cancer penetrates deep in the skin tissue, topical chemotherapy can be used. This type of treatment is used for large areas of cancer that cannot be surgically removed. An example is topical fluorouracil (5-FU), an antimetabolite that inhibits cancer cells from synthesizing DNA. 5-FU is used to treat basal cell and squamous cell cancers on the surface of the skin.

GENERIC NAME: fluorouracil (5-FU)
TRADE NAME: Efudex, Fluoroplex, Carac
INDICATION: Basal cell carcinoma

ROUTE OF ADMINISTRATION: Topical
COMMON ADULT DOSAGE: Applied twice daily to the skin lesion; treatment should continue for at least 3 to 6 weeks and may require treatment for as long as 10 to 12 weeks
MECHANISM OF ACTION: Antimetabolite (inhibits cancer cells synthesis of DNA)
SIDE EFFECTS: Skin irritation, dryness, photosensitivity, burning, erythema, pruritus
AUXILIARY LABELS:
- For topical use only.
- Avoid contact with eyes, nose, and mouth.
- Do not use if pregnant or breastfeeding.
- Avoid sunlight.
- Apply using gloves.

SPECIAL NOTE: Must be applied using gloves or with a nonmetal applicator; thoroughly wash hands after application.

Common Dermatological Conditions Affecting the Scalp and Hair

Head Lice

Head lice are caused by the parasite *Pediculus humanus capitis,* also known as the **head louse**. Many children come home from school with head lice. Lice can be transferred easily when children use the same hairbrush or share hats. Other ways to transmit lice include sleeping next to someone with lice and sharing clothes with someone who has lice. Symptoms include itching, sores on the head, and a tickling feeling of something moving in the hair. Several products on the market treat this infestation. Treatment of the whole family is important, even if the infestation appears to affect only one child (Figure 25-15, *A*).

Another type of lice affects the pubic area (commonly called *crabs*) and is spread through sexual contact. Other areas where lice can be found include the hair on the legs, armpits, mustache, beard, eyebrows, and eyelashes of adults (if lice are found on the eyelashes or eyebrows of children, it is considered head lice). Symptoms include pruritus and visible nits (lice eggs) or crawling lice in the genital area (Figure 25-15, *B*).

> **Prognosis.** If the infestation is treated correctly by following the directions on the treatment package, lice can be easily eliminated.
>
> **Non–Drug Treatment.** All brushes, combs, and hats must be cleaned in hot, soapy water or alcohol and should not be shared. All bed linens should be washed in hot water and dried for at least 20 minutes on the hottest setting. Items that are not washable should be dry-cleaned. All stuffed animals and blankets should be placed in a sealed plastic bag for at least 2 weeks to ensure that any lice die. Carpets and furniture should be thoroughly vacuumed. In adults, if genital lice also are present in the eyebrows or eyelashes, the lice should be removed with the fingers; medicated treatments should never be used on or around the eyes. With genital lice, sexual contact should be avoided until the infestation has been adequately treated. Physical removal of all nits is essential to adequately treat a lice infestation of any type.
>
> **Drug Treatment.** OTC agents are available, such as permethrin (Nix) topical cream rinse, Medi-Lice, Pronto, and pyrethrins and piperonyl butoxide (Tegrin LF) as shampoos. Prescription treatments include malathion (Ovide) topical and lindane (Kwell) shampoos and lotions; these are reserved for resistant cases. Lindane may cause neurotoxicity and seizures if improperly used; patient counseling on its proper use is essential for safety.
>
> A pediculicide (e.g., permethrin or pyrethrin) is used to treat pubic lice infestations; prescription therapies are reserved for resistant cases.

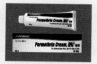

GENERIC NAME: permethrin (OTC)
TRADE NAME: Nix
INDICATION: Lice
ROUTE OF ADMINISTRATION: Topical
COMMON ADULT DOSAGE: Enough solution is used to saturate the hair and scalp; the solution is left on for 10 minutes and then rinsed out with water. Eggs (nits) are removed with the comb provided. A second treatment is performed in 7 to 10 days if needed.
MECHANISM OF ACTION: Disrupts sodium channels on the nerve cell membrane of lice, leading to paralysis and death of the parasite
SIDE EFFECTS: Itching, burning, stinging, redness, swelling
AUXILIARY LABEL:
- For topical use only.

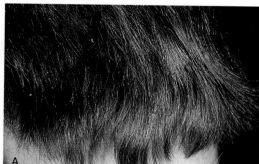
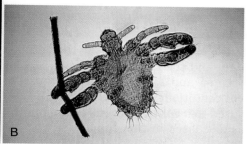

FIGURE 25-15 A, Head louse. **B,** Crab lice. (**A** from Callen JP et al: *Color atlas of dermatology,* ed 2, Philadelphia, 2000, Saunders; **B** from Auerbach PS: *Wilderness medicine,* ed 5, St Louis, 2007, Mosby.)

Common Dermatological Conditions Affecting the Nails

Onychomycosis

Nails on both the hands and feet endure daily abuse and can become damaged. Bacterial and fungal infections or trauma can occur that may discolor, deform, or cause detachment of the nail. **Onychomycosis**, a fungal infection of the nails, is the most common disease of the nails. The infection normally starts at the tip of one or more toenails. It produces thickening, discoloration, and crumbling of the nail, possibly affecting the entire nail. Infections attributable to candidal organisms are referred to as *onychomycosis*. Most infections of the nails are superficial and rarely become systemic; therefore, they typically are treated with topical agents. If a fungal infection becomes systemic, oral agents such as ketoconazole or fluconazole may be prescribed.

Prognosis. With proper treatment, the prognosis for onychomycosis is good. Although nails may require removal in severe cases, they typically grow back, and their absence does not hinder normal daily activities.

Non–Drug Treatment. People should be educated about avoiding direct contact with high-risk areas in public places (e.g., locker room floors) to avoid subsequent infections. Good hand hygiene is paramount in keeping the nails in good condition. In certain cases a combination of oral and topical agents, along with surgical removal of the affected nails, may be necessary.

Drug Treatment. The type of treatment used for onychomycosis can depend on the severity of the infection and the number of affected nails. The severity also determines the dosage form and length of treatment. Certain infections can be treated with topical antifungals, such as ciclopirox olamine 8% lacquer solution. Oral therapy may be prescribed either alone or in combination with topical treatments. Oral antifungals (e.g., terbinafine) provide higher cure rates than previously used agents such as itraconazole and griseofulvin. In severe cases, the duration of treatment can be lengthy to allow for eradication of the causative infection and for outgrowth of healthy nails. Although this chapter focuses on onychomycosis, a variety of other fungal and viral infections also can occur on the skin.

GENERIC NAME: terbinafine
TRADE NAME: Lamisil
INDICATION: Onychomycosis
ROUTE OF ADMINISTRATION: Oral
COMMON ADULT DOSAGE: 250 mg once daily for 6 weeks (fingernails) or for 12 weeks (toenails)
MECHANISM OF ACTION: Interferes with the cell membrane strength of sensitive fungi
SIDE EFFECTS: Diarrhea, abdominal pain, headache, rash
AUXILIARY LABEL:
- Take as directed.

 Tech Note!

Soap and water have always been a good way to remove bacteria from the skin; however, they do not necessarily kill all bacteria. **Antiseptics** are necessary for the health care worker because they do kill and/or inhibit the growth of germs. Unfortunately, both good and bad germs are killed when these agents are used. It is wise not to overuse antiseptics because bacteria can mutate into strains that become resistant to antiseptics that are overused. Using gloves can reduce the necessity of constant hand hygiene and also help the skin stay hydrated.

DO YOU REMEMBER THESE KEY POINTS?

- The names of the major components of the dermatological system and their functions
- The primary signs and symptoms of the various dermatological conditions discussed
- Medications used to treat the various dermatological conditions discussed in this chapter
- The generic and trade names for the drugs discussed in this chapter
- The appropriate auxiliary labels that should be used when filling prescriptions for drugs discussed in this chapter

REVIEW QUESTIONS

Multiple Choice Questions

1. The skin has many functions. Which of the following is *not* one of its main functions?
   A. Regulate body temperature
   B. Act as a sensor to a stimulus
   C. Protect the internal organs from the elements
   D. All of the above are main functions of the skin

2. _____ lubricate(s) the skin and retains water to keep the skin and hair from drying out.
   A. Sweat
   B. Sebum
   C. Pustules
   D. Retinoids

3. Which condition is associated with the development of comedones?
   A. Eczema
   B. Acne
   C. Psoriasis
   D. Tinea pedis

4. Which type of burn is the most severe?
   A. Partial-thickness
   B. Superficial
   C. Fourth-degree
   D. Full-thickness

5. Which product requires the patient and pharmacy to enroll in the iPLEDGE program due to the risk of teratogenicity?
   A. Isotretinoin
   B. Doxycycline
   C. Pimecrolimus
   D. Mycophenolate

6. The vitamin D analogue calcipotriene (Dovonex) is indicated for the treatment of:
   A. Psoriasis
   B. Acne
   C. HPV
   D. Thermal burns

7. Retapamulin (Altabax) is a topical:
   A. Antibacterial agent
   B. Antifungal agent
   C. Antiviral agent
   D. Keratolytic

8. Topical salicylic acid products are used to treat:
   A. Warts
   B. Acne
   C. Psoriasis
   D. A and B

9. Which medication could be used to treat pruritus of the skin?
   A. Tolnaftate
   B. Salicylic acid
   C. Bacitracin
   D. Caladryl

10. Impetigo can be treated with all of the following methods *except*:
    A. Keep the skin clean and dry
    B. Use both oral and topical bacterial antibiotics
    C. Use a topical antiviral
    D. Wash with antibacterial soap

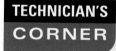

TECHNICIAN'S CORNER   Using a comprehensive drug reference (e.g., *Drug Facts and Comparisons*), look up the oral medications listed in Table 25-1 for the treatment of acne and determine what side effects are common with these medications and what warning labels, if any, should be placed on these prescriptions before they are dispensed.

Bibliography

Clinical Pharmacology Online: (Referenced September 6, 2014.) www.clinicalpharmacology-ip.com.

Damjanov I: *Pathology for the health professions*, ed 4, St Louis, 2011, Saunders.

Fishback JL: *Pathology*, ed 3, Philadelphia, 2005, Mosby.

Lookingbill D, Marks J: *Principles of dermatology*, ed 4, Philadelphia, 2006, Saunders.

McCance KL: *Pathophysiology: the biologic basis for disease in adults and children*, ed 6, St Louis, 2010, Mosby.

Patton KT et al: *Mosby's handbook of anatomy and physiology*, St Louis, 2000, Mosby.

Potter PA, Perry AG: *Fundamentals of nursing*, ed 8, St Louis, 2013, Mosby.

Price SA, Wilson LM: *Pathophysiology: clinical concepts of disease processes*, ed 6, St Louis, 2003, Mosby.

Solomon EP: *Introduction to human anatomy and physiology*, ed 3, St Louis, 2009, Mosby.

Thompson JM et al: *Mosby's clinical nursing*, ed 5, St Louis, 2001, Mosby.

UpToDate Online: (Referenced September 6, 2014.) www.uptodate.com.

26

Therapeutic Agents for the Hematological System

Joshua J. Neumiller

OBJECTIVES

Upon completing this chapter, you should be able to do the following:

1. Describe the major components of the hematological system.
2. List the primary symptoms of conditions associated with the hematological system.
3. Recognize drugs used to treat the conditions associated with the hematological system.
4. Write the generic and trade names for the drugs discussed in this chapter.
5. List appropriate auxiliary labels when filling prescriptions for drugs discussed in this chapter.

TERMS AND DEFINITIONS

Absolute neutrophil count (ANC) The number of white blood cells that are actually neutrophils

Albumin The major protein found in plasma

Anemia A decrease in the number of red blood cells or hemoglobin, which impairs the blood's ability to carry oxygen to the tissues

Bone marrow The tissue that fills the cavities in the long bones that is the source of red blood cells and many white blood cells

Colony-stimulating factor (CSF) A hormone that stimulates the bone marrow to synthesize hematopoietic cells

Cryoprecipitate Any precipitate that results from cooling; sometimes specifically used to describe a precipitate rich in coagulation Factor VIII obtained from cooling of blood plasma

Erythrocyte A cell that contains hemoglobin and can carry oxygen to the body; also known as a *red blood cell (RBC)*

Erythropoiesis The formation of erythrocytes

Erythropoietin A hormone secreted by the kidney that stimulates the production of red blood cells by stem cells in bone marrow

Granulocytopenia A reduction in the number of granulocytes, which encompass specific types of white blood cells in the blood that contain "granules"; these white blood cells include neutrophils, eosinophils, and basophils, which are all known as *granulocytes.* These are in contrast to lymphocytes, which are white blood cells devoid of granules

Hemoglobin The oxygen-carrying component of red blood cells

Hemophilia A hereditary coagulation disorder that leads to a decreased ability of the blood to clot normally

Hydrostatic pressure The pressure exerted by a fluid due to the force of gravity

Hypoxia A reduction of the oxygen supply to a tissue despite adequate perfusion of the tissue by blood

Idiopathic A term meaning "of unknown cause"

Leukemia A progressive, malignant disease of the blood-forming organs, marked by distorted proliferation and development of leukocytes and their precursors in the blood and bone marrow

Leukocyte A white blood cell

Leukopenia A reduction in the number of leukocytes (white blood cells) in the blood

Lymphoid organ A component of the system of interconnected tissues and organs by which lymph circulates throughout the body

Lymphoma Cancer of the lymphatic system

Neutropenia An abnormally low level of neutrophils in the blood

Osmosis Diffusion of fluid through a semipermeable membrane from a solution with a low solute concentration to a solution with a higher solute concentration in an effort to achieve equilibrium

Osmotic pressure The pressure exerted by the flow of water through a semipermeable membrane separating two solutions with different concentrations of solutes

Pallor A deficiency in color, particularly of the face

Phlebotomy The act or practice of opening a vein by incision or puncture to remove blood

Plasma The clear, yellowish fluid portion of blood

Plasma protein Any of the various dissolved proteins of blood plasma

Polycythemia An increase in the total cell mass of the blood

Serum The clear, yellowish fluid obtained by separating whole blood into its solid and liquid components after it has been allowed to clot; plasma minus clotting factors

Solute A substance dissolved in another substance; usually the component of a solution present in the lesser amount

Splenectomy Surgical removal of the spleen

Thrombocyte A platelet

Thrombocytopenia A decrease in the number of platelets in the blood

Von Willebrand's disease The most common inherited bleeding disorder associated with a deficiency in the clotting protein von Willebrand factor

Whole blood Blood drawn from the body from which no constituent, such as plasma or platelets, has been removed

Common Drugs Used for Conditions of the Hematological System

Trade Name	Generic Name	Pronunciation
Iron Deficiency Anemia Medications		
Feosol	ferrous sulfate	(**fare**-us **sul**-fate)
Ferrlecit	ferric gluconate	(**fer**-ik **gloo**-koe-nate)
Colony-Stimulating Factors		
Epogen	epoetin alfa	(e-**poe**-e-tin **al**-fa)
Aranesp	darbepoetin alfa	(**dar**-be-**poe**-e-tin **al**-fa)
Neupogen	filgrastim	(fil-**gras**-tim)
Neulasta	pegfilgrastim	(peg-fil-**gras**-tim)
Leukine	sargramostim	(sar-**gra**-moe-stim)
Chemotherapeutic Agents for the Treatment of Leukemia		
Cytoxan	cyclophosphamide	(sye-kloe-**foss**-fah-mide)
Cytosar	cytarabine	(sye-**tar**-a-been)
Rituxan	rituximab	(ri-**tux**-i-mab)
Gleevec	imatinib	(im-**ma**-ta-nib)
Rheumatrex	methotrexate	(meth-oh-**trex**-ate)

Anatomy and Physiology of the Hematological System

As discussed in Chapter 18, adequate blood flow is critical to delivering oxygen and nutrients to the tissues and organs of the body. Not only does the blood carry oxygen and nutrients throughout the body, it also carries wastes from the tissues and organs that it supports to organs such as the kidneys and liver for elimination. The blood additionally transports cells of the immune system (see Chapter 23) to sites of infection and injury. The following is a brief review of the components that make up whole blood and a description of the functions these components serve in the body. (See Chapter 23 for a refresher on the structure and function of the major **lymphoid organs** [i.e., thymus, spleen, and lymph nodes].)

Major Components of Blood

Plasma

Whole blood is composed of plasma and cellular components (Figure 26-1). **Plasma** is the fluid component of whole blood that is composed of water, plasma proteins, and other solutes, such as electrolytes and nutrients. Plasma accounts for approximately 50% of the volume of whole blood in a normal, healthy adult. **Serum**, which is used for some laboratory tests, is plasma that has been allowed to clot in the laboratory to remove clotting factors that can interfere with some blood tests.

Plasma Proteins

A variety of **plasma proteins** are present in the blood, such as albumin, globulins, fibrinogen, and prothrombin (see Figure 26-1). **Albumin** is critical

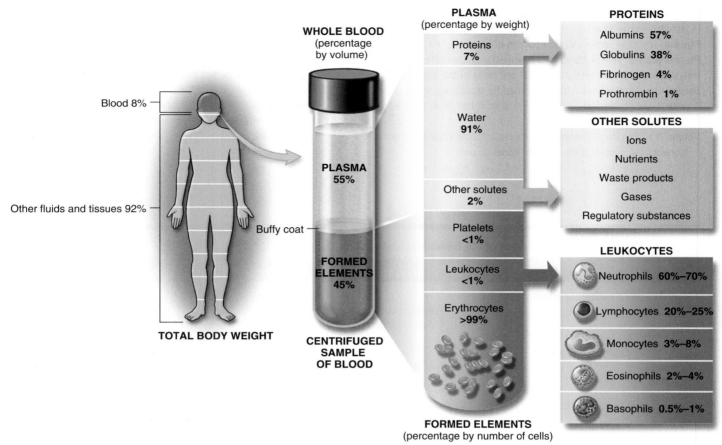

FIGURE 26-1 Composition of whole blood. Approximate values for the components of blood in a healthy adult. (From Patton KT, Thibodeau GA: *Anatomy and physiology*, ed 8, St Louis, 2013, Mosby).

for maintaining water and solute balance in the blood. Albumin is a large protein that cannot diffuse across the epithelium of the vessels, as do water and electrolytes. Thus albumin helps maintain blood volume and the transport of **solutes** between the blood and tissues (see the discussion of osmotic pressure later in the chapter). Another important function of albumin is to serve as a carrier molecule for blood components and drugs. Drug interactions between agents that bind to albumin are relatively common. Phenytoin is an example of a drug that is highly bound to albumin, and its use with other drugs that bind to albumin can lead to phenytoin toxicity. Intravenous albumin is used clinically to increase plasma volume or to increase albumin levels in people with low serum albumin levels.

Two primary forces regulate the movement of fluids and solutes into and out of the vasculature: hydrostatic pressure and osmosis. **Hydrostatic pressure** is driven by the blood pressure generated by contraction of the heart. Because of the hydrostatic pressure in the arterial capillaries, water and solutes are pushed out of the arterioles into the tissues. **Osmosis** is the movement of water down a concentration gradient. Once the blood has passed through the arterioles and returns to the venous system, **osmotic pressure** (also known as *oncotic pressure*) becomes greater than the hydrostatic pressure; therefore, water and solutes begin to move out of the tissues and back into the venous system. As mentioned previously, albumin is the major protein in the blood that maintains osmotic pressure in the vascular system. In certain cases people can produce less albumin (e.g., individuals with liver disease or malnutrition) or lose albumin from the bloodstream (e.g., in certain types of kidney disease). When this happens, osmotic pressure decreases, leading to the accumulation of fluid in the tissues and edema (Figure 26-2).

Other proteins in the plasma contribute to clotting (e.g., fibrinogen), immune function (antibodies), transport proteins, and lipoproteins (e.g., low-density lipoprotein [LDL] and high-density lipoprotein [HDL], discussed in Chapter 18).

Platelets

Platelets (also known as **thrombocytes**) are components of the blood that are essential to the process of coagulation. Platelets are not actually cells because they do not have a nucleus. Because platelets are so important to the clotting process, people are at serious risk of bleeding when platelet levels are too low **(thrombocytopenia)**. The life span of a platelet is approximately 10 days.

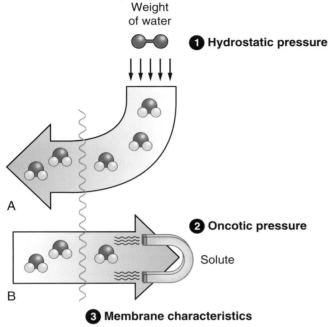

FIGURE 26-2 Hydrostatic pressure and oncotic pressure in plasma. (From Huether S, McCance K: *Understanding pathophysiology,* ed 5, St Louis, 2012, Mosby.)

Cellular Components of the Blood

A variety of cell types is found primarily in the blood. These can be divided into two main groups, leukocytes and erythrocytes (Figure 26-3). These cells (and platelets) are produced by a process known as hematopoiesis (Figure 26-4). **Leukocytes**, or white blood cells (WBCs), are cells of the immune system that help defend the body against infection. Examples of leukocytes are lymphocytes, neutrophils, and monocytes. (See Chapter 23 for a review of leukocytes and their functions in the immune system.)

Erythrocytes, or red blood cells (RBCs), are the most prevalent blood cells in the blood. The main

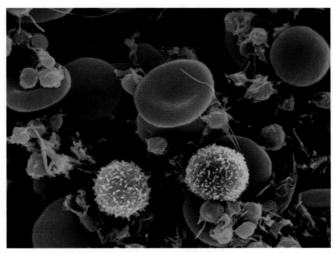

FIGURE 26-3 Blood cells. (From Huether S, McCance K: *Understanding pathophysiology,* ed 5, St Louis, 2012, Mosby.)

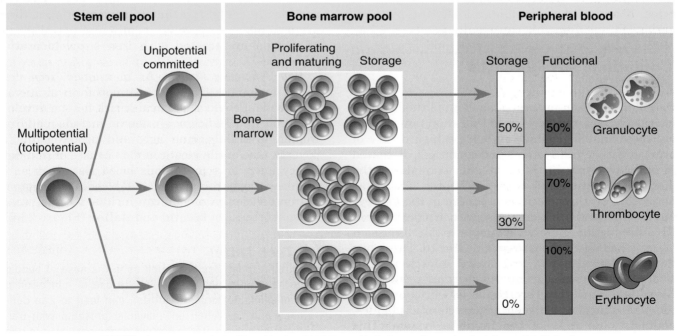

FIGURE 26-4 Hematopoiesis. (From Huether S, McCance K: *Understanding pathophysiology,* ed 5, St Louis, 2012, Mosby.)

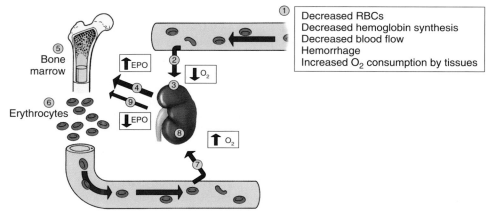

FIGURE 26-5 Role of erythropoietin in the regulation of erythropoiesis. (From Huether S, McCance K: *Understanding pathophysiology*, ed 5, St Louis, 2012, Mosby.)

function of RBCs is to carry oxygen to the tissues and organs of the body. RBC production, or **erythropoiesis**, takes place in the **bone marrow** and is driven largely by the hormone **erythropoietin**, which is produced by the kidneys (Figure 26-5). As is discussed later, erythropoietin can be used therapeutically for people with low RBC counts as a result of kidney disease or other medical conditions.

RBCs are able to effectively transport oxygen because they contain **hemoglobin**. Hemoglobin is an oxygen-carrying protein in RBCs that binds to oxygen as blood passes through the lungs. Blood is then pumped throughout the body, allowing the RBCs to deliver oxygen to the tissues. An important factor necessary for the production of hemoglobin is iron. A variety of other building blocks also is required for the proper formation of hemoglobin and erythrocytes. If any of these building blocks are deficient, various forms of anemia can result.

Conditions Affecting the Hematological System

Based on the anatomy and physiology of the hematological system, it is easy to see that conditions affecting the hematological system have a high degree of overlap with organ systems and conditions discussed in other chapters in this text. For example, in the discussion of the renal system (Chapter 22), it was noted that erythropoietin is produced in the kidneys and that people with kidney disease can have reduced RBC production. Another example is the discussion of thromboembolic diseases in Chapter 18. Thrombus formation resulting in myocardial infarction (MI), stroke (also known as a *cerebral vascular accident,* or CVA), and deep vein thrombosis (DVT) is due to a complex interplay between atherosclerotic plaques, platelets, and cells of the immune system. This chapter focuses on hematological conditions such as anemia, low cell counts (thrombocytopenia,

leukopenia, and neutropenia), and hematological cancers. A brief review of bleeding disorders and their treatment also is provided.

Common Conditions

Anemia

Anemia can be caused by a variety of factors; there are several different types and causes. In general, anemia is caused either by a reduction in the total number of RBCs available to carry oxygen or by a deficiency in the quality or quantity of hemoglobin present in RBCs. This chapter does not provide an exhaustive review of all forms of anemia; however, it presents a brief overview of iron deficiency anemia, the most common form of anemia worldwide. Although only iron deficiency anemia is discussed specifically, it is important to remember that there are a number of types of anemia and not all forms of anemia are treated with iron supplementation (Table 26-1).

Iron Deficiency Anemia. As mentioned, iron deficiency anemia is the most common form of anemia worldwide. People at particular risk for the development of iron deficiency anemia include children, women of childbearing age, and people living in poverty. One of the most common causes of iron deficiency anemia is continuous blood loss, such as in people with gastrointestinal (GI) bleeding. Symptoms of iron deficiency anemia can include fatigue, weakness, shortness of breath, and **pallor** (Figure 26-6).

 Tech Note!

Gastrointestinal bleeding, such as in the case of people who have an ulcer induced by the use of nonsteroidal antiinflammatory drugs (NSAIDs), can lead to iron deficiency anemia. When an individual presents with iron deficiency anemia, it is important for the physician to rule out unrecognized (i.e., occult) bleeding.

TABLE 26-1

Classification of Anemia

Name	Cause and/or Contributing Factors
Anemia of chronic inflammation	Increased demand for erythrocyte production due to chronic inflammation, infection, and/or malignancy
Aplastic anemia	Depressed stem cell proliferation
Folate deficiency anemia	Dietary folate deficiency
Hemolytic anemia	Destruction of mature erythrocytes due to cell lysis
Iron deficiency anemia	Lack of sufficient iron to produce hemoglobin due to chronic blood loss, dietary iron deficiency, or disruption of iron metabolism
Pernicious anemia	Vitamin B_{12} deficiency due to congenital or acquired deficiency of intrinsic factor (IF)
Sickle cell anemia	Abnormal hemoglobin synthesis and abnormal red blood cell (RBC) shape
Sideroblastic anemia	Dysfunctional iron uptake by erythroblasts and heme synthesis
Thalassemia	Impaired synthesis of hemoglobin molecule

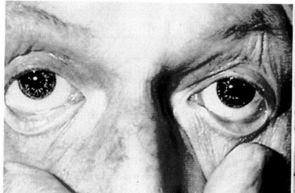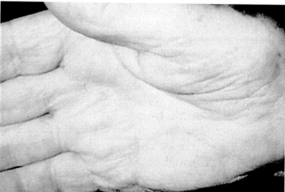

FIGURE 26-6 Pallor and iron deficiency. (From Huether S, McCance K: *Understanding pathophysiology,* ed 5, St Louis, 2012, Mosby.)

Prognosis. With appropriate identification and treatment, iron deficiency anemia usually can be treated effectively and resolved.

Non–Drug Treatment. As mentioned, the presence of iron deficiency anemia may indicate the presence of bleeding or some other metabolic contributor. The first step in the management of iron deficiency anemia should be to identify and/or rule out sources of blood loss. Unless bleeding, if present, is resolved, iron replacement therapy proves ineffective. Mild anemia may be treated with dietary changes, including an increase in iron-rich foods (e.g., spinach, beef, broccoli, liver).

Drug Treatment. Iron replacement therapy is the primary treatment for iron deficiency anemia (Table 26-2). With adequate supplementation, resolution of symptoms generally occurs within 4 weeks of treatment. The duration of supplementation depends on the extent of the deficiency and the causative factors.

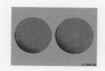

GENERIC NAME: ferrous sulfate (OTC)
TRADE NAME: Fer-Iron, Feosol
INDICATION: Iron deficiency anemia
ROUTE OF ADMINISTRATION: Oral
COMMON ADULT DOSAGE: 250-325 mg three times daily
MECHANISM OF ACTION: Iron supplement to increase iron stores and support erythropoiesis
SIDE EFFECTS: Constipation, abdominal pain, dyspepsia, stool discoloration
AUXILIARY LABEL:
- Administer with meals to minimize GI side effects.

TABLE 26-2

Iron Preparations for the Treatment of Iron Deficiency Anemia

Medication Class	Generic Name	Trade Name	Common Side Effects	Common Dose Range	Elemental Iron Content
Oral Iron Salts	ferrous sulfate	Fer-Iron, Feosol	• Nausea • Constipation • Vomiting • Dark stools	• 250-325 mg 3 times daily	60 mg/tab or 65 mg/tab
	ferrous gluconate	Ferate, Fergon		• 240 mg PO 2-4 times daily	27 mg/tab
	ferrous fumarate	Ferretts		• 325 mg PO 2-4 times daily	106 mg/tab
	iron polysaccharide	Niferex-150		• 150-300 mg PO daily in 1-2 divided doses	150 mg/tab or 50 mg/tab
Parenteral Iron	iron dextran	DexFerrum	• Injection site reactions • Hypotension • Chills • Dizziness • Nausea	• *Test dose for anaphylaxis:* 25 mg IV over 30 min • *Usual dose:* 75-100 mg IV over 1-6 hr	50 mg/mL
	ferric gluconate	Ferrlecit		• 125 mg in 100 mL NS IV over 1 hr	12.5 mg/mL
	iron sucrose	Venofer		• 100 mg in 100 mL NS IV over 15 min 1-3 times/wk	20 mg/mL

NS, Normal saline; *IV,* intravenously; *PO,* orally; *tab,* tablet.

Tech Note!

Oral iron supplements are sometimes prescribed in combination with ascorbic acid (vitamin C). The acidity of the vitamin C helps with the absorption of the iron from the gastrointestinal tract. Having the patient take oral iron with a glass of orange juice is another common strategy.

GENERIC NAME: sodium ferric gluconate complex
TRADE NAME: Ferrlecit
INDICATION: Iron deficiency anemia in people undergoing chronic dialysis and receiving epoetin alfa therapy
ROUTE OF ADMINISTRATION: Intravenous (IV)
COMMON ADULT DOSAGE: 125 mg IV during each dialysis session
MECHANISM OF ACTION: Iron supplement to increase iron stores and support erythropoiesis
SIDE EFFECTS: Injection site reaction, headache, anaphylaxis

Polycythemia

Although many conditions of the hematological system involve a deficiency in a specific cell type (e.g., thrombocytopenia, leukopenia, and neutropenia, discussed later), some forms of hematological dysfunction involve the overproduction of hematopoietic cells. **Polycythemia** is defined as excessive red cell production. People can develop either primary or secondary polycythemia. Secondary polycythemia, the most common form, occurs as a result of a physiological response to **hypoxia**. This form of polycythemia occurs when the body has difficulty oxygenating the blood, such as in people living at high altitudes, those who smoke tobacco, and those with chronic obstructive pulmonary disease (COPD). Primary polycythemia, also known as *polycythemia vera,* is a chronic condition in which the body overproduces RBCs. This overproduction is believed to be due to an increased sensitivity of stem cells in the bone marrow to the effects of erythropoietin.

Prognosis. For people with secondary polycythemia, proper treatment of the underlying condition often can result in a good prognosis. For those with polycythemia vera, the prognosis can be poor if the person does not receive appropriate treatment. With proper treatment, however, survival of 10 to 15 years is common.

Non–Drug Treatment. As mentioned previously, treatment of contributing factors is a critical component of management. Smoking cessation is recommended for those who smoke, and medical intervention for COPD and heart failure is recommended to minimize hypoxia. For individuals with polycythemia vera, **phlebotomy** frequently is used to reduce the blood volume and RBC numbers.

Drug Treatment. Drug therapy in polycythemia vera involves treatments aimed at minimizing the risk of thrombosis with myelosuppressive agents (e.g., hydroxyurea) and/or antithrombotics (e.g., anagrelide).

GENERIC NAME: anagrelide
TRADE NAME: Agrylin
INDICATION: Polycythemia vera, thrombocytosis, chronic myelogenous leukemia (CML)
ROUTE OF ADMINISTRATION: Oral
COMMON ADULT DOSAGE: Initially 0.5 mg four times daily or 1 mg twice daily; typical dosage range is 1.5-3 mg per day
MECHANISM OF ACTION: Inhibits megakaryocyte development, leading to a reduction in platelets, and also inhibits platelet aggregation
SIDE EFFECTS: Headache, diarrhea, edema, dizziness, bleeding

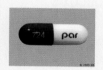

GENERIC NAME: hydroxyurea
TRADE NAME: Droxia
INDICATION: Polycythemia vera, CML, sickle cell disease, malignant melanoma, ovarian cancer
ROUTE OF ADMINISTRATION: Oral
COMMON ADULT DOSAGE: 1000-2000 mg daily divided into one to three doses
MECHANISM OF ACTION: Inhibits DNA synthesis
SIDE EFFECTS: Leukopenia, neutropenia, anemia, diarrhea, rash, fever
AUXILIARY LABEL: Wear gloves when handling capsules.

Low Cell and Platelet Counts

A variety of conditions and secondary factors can contribute to impaired hematopoiesis, resulting in conditions such as thrombocytopenia, leukopenia, and neutropenia. Agents known broadly as **colony-stimulating factors (CSFs)** sometimes are used to stimulate hematopoiesis and treat such conditions (Table 26-3).

Thrombocytopenia. *Thrombocytopenia* is simply a term used to describe a low platelet count. Thrombo-

BOX 26-1

Select Drugs Frequently Associated with Drug-Induced Thrombocytopenia

- heparin
- abciximab
- eptifibatide
- tirofiban
- quinine
- quinidine
- trimethoprim-sulfamethoxazole
- vancomycin
- linezolid
- rifampin
- piperacillin
- valproic acid
- measles-mumps-rubella (MMR) vaccine
- carbamazepine
- phenytoin

cytopenia has a variety of causes. Some of the most common causes are pregnancy (gestational thrombocytopenia), drug side effects (drug-induced thrombocytopenia [Box 26-1]), and **idiopathic** thrombocytopenia. The principal treatment goal is prevention of bleeding.

Prognosis. The prognosis for thrombocytopenia varies widely, depending on the severity of the thrombocytopenia and the underlying cause.

Non–Drug Treatment. Resolution of any contributing factors should be pursued when the underlying cause can be corrected. Transfusions to increase platelet levels may be necessary in individuals with particularly low platelet counts. Activity restrictions may be recommended in individuals with moderate to severe thrombocytopenia. Restrictions often are limited to contact sports, such as boxing and football.

Drug Treatment. In immune-mediated thrombocytopenia, steroid treatment sometimes is used to suppress the immune response. Glucocorticoid medications can be used (e.g., prednisone, dexamethasone, hydrocortisone, and methylprednisolone). Another drug, eltrombopag (Promacta), is available for patients whose condition does not respond to steroids, immunoglobulins, or **splenectomy**.

GENERIC NAME: eltrombopag
TRADE NAME: Promacta
INDICATION: Thrombocytopenia, idiopathic thrombocytopenic purpura (ITP)

TABLE 26-3

Select Colony-Stimulating Factors for the Treatment of Low Hematological Cell Counts

Medication Class	Generic Name	Trade Name	Common Side Effects	Common Dose Range
Erythropoiesis (Red Blood Cell [RBC])– Stimulating Agents	epoetin alfa	Epogen	• Fever • Headache • Itching • Nausea • Vomiting • Pain • Cough	• 50-300 units/kg intravenously or subcutaneously (IV/ SUBCUT) 3 times weekly
	darbepoetin alfa	Aranesp	• Hypertension • Edema • Abdominal pain • Shortness of breath • Cough	• 0.45–2.25 mcg/kg SUBCUT once weekly
White Blood Cell– Stimulating Agents	filgrastim	Neupogen	• Fever • Rash • Splenomegaly • Bone pain • Nose bleeds	• 5-10 mcg/kg/day SUBCUT/IV
	pegfilgrastim	Neulasta	• Edema • Headache • Bone pain • Constipation • Vomiting • Weakness	• 6 mg SUBCUT once per chemotherapy cycle
	sargramostim	Leukine	• Fever • Headache • Hypertension • Edema • Rash • Hyperglycemia • Diarrhea	• 250 mcg/m^2/day SUBCUT/IV

ROUTE OF ADMINISTRATION: Oral
COMMON ADULT DOSAGE: 25-50 mg once daily
MECHANISM OF ACTION: Thrombopoietin receptor
  agonist (increases platelet production)
SIDE EFFECTS: Thrombosis, nausea, vomiting, dyspepsia
AUXILIARY LABELS:
• Take on an empty stomach.
• Take at least 1 hour before or 2 hours after meals.

Neutropenia. **Neutropenia** can occur in conjunction with a variety of other conditions (e.g., aplastic anemia, leukemia, vitamin B$_{12}$, folate deficiency), during chemotherapy treatment, and as an isolated condition. When a patient is assessed for neutropenia, the **absolute neutrophil count (ANC)** often is used to define the neutropenia as mild, moderate, or severe.

Two other terms often are used interchangeably with the term *neutropenia,* but these are actually slightly different conditions:

• **Leukopenia:** A low total WBC count (granulocytes and lymphocytes); almost all people with leukopenia also have neutropenia.
• **Granulocytopenia:** A reduced number of circulating granulocytes (neutrophils, eosinophils, and basophils). Because neutrophils are the predominant granulocyte cell type, people with granulocytopenia almost always also have neutropenia.

The primary concern in a patient with neutropenia is an increased risk of infection. However, neutropenia also can be a symptom of an underlying condition requiring identification and treatment.

Prognosis. Recurrent infection is the primary risk associated with neutropenia. The prognosis depends largely on the degree of neutropenia and the cause.

Non–Drug Treatment. Overall treatment depends on the cause and degree of neutropenia.

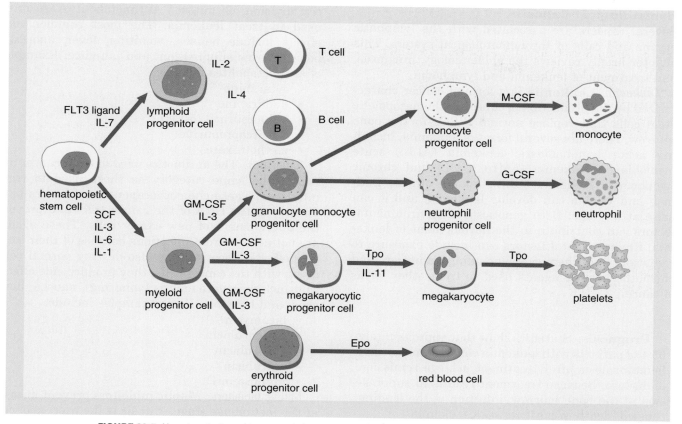

FIGURE 26-7 Hematopoiesis and hematopoietic growth factors. (From Page C et al: *Integrated pharmacology,* ed 3, St Louis, 2006, Mosby.)

Non–drug treatment for patients with chronic neutropenia includes avoidance of infection. A critical component of care is regular dental care to prevent gingivitis and associated infection.

Drug Treatment. The primary drugs used in the treatment of neutropenia are recombinant growth factors or CSFs. These agents can be used prophylactically for chemotherapy-induced neutropenia and for therapeutic use in people with preexisting neutropenia. Current therapies are either granulocyte colony-stimulating factors (G-CSF) or granulocyte-macrophage colony-stimulating factors (GM-CSF) (see Table 26-3). Figure 26-7 shows where these growth factors act in the differentiation of hematopoietic cells.

INDICATION: Chemotherapy-induced neutropenia, febrile neutropenia, neutropenia
ROUTE OF ADMINISTRATION: Subcutaneous injection
COMMON ADULT DOSAGE: 5-10 mcg/kg daily
MECHANISM OF ACTION: Recombinant G-CSF (stimulates the production of neutrophils in the bone marrow)
SIDE EFFECTS: Bone pain, hypotension, hyperuricemia
AUXILIARY LABEL:
• Do not shake prior to administration.

GENERIC NAME: sargramostim
TRADE NAME: Leukine
INDICATION: Chemotherapy-induced neutropenia, febrile neutropenia, neutropenia
ROUTE OF ADMINISTRATION: Intravenous; subcutaneous
COMMON ADULT DOSAGE: 250 mcg/m²/day
MECHANISM OF ACTION: Recombinant GM-CSF (stimulates the production of neutrophils, eosinophils, and monocytes within the bone marrow)
SIDE EFFECTS: Bone pain, hypotension, peripheral edema

GENERIC NAME: filgrastim
TRADE NAME: Neupogen

Hematological Cancers

Several cancers are associated with the lymphatic organs and cells of the hematological system. This chapter briefly reviews the epidemiology, prognosis, and treatment of leukemia and lymphoma.

Leukemia. **Leukemia** is a form of cancer characterized by the production of cancerous hematopoietic stem cells that replace normal WBCs in the bone marrow. There are several forms of leukemia, including acute lymphoblastic leukemia (ALL), acute myeloblastic leukemia (AML), CML, and chronic lymphocytic leukemia (CLL), among others. Both men and women can develop leukemia, and it can arise at any age. Both genetics and environmental factors can contribute to the development of leukemia. Environmental factors can include exposure to radiation and chemicals, including radiation and chemotherapeutic agents used to treat other forms of cancer.

Prognosis. Statistics show that approximately 65% of patients with leukemia who resume normal hematopoiesis after treatment achieve remission of disease. Because treatment results in suppression of the bone marrow, infection is the leading cause of death in patients with leukemia.

Non–Drug Treatment. As noted previously, morbidity and mortality from infection are the leading causes of death in people treated for leukemia. Important elements of non–drug therapy include precautions against the transmission of infectious disease. In line with suppression of the bone marrow, individuals receiving chemotherapy for leukemia are also at increased risk for bleeding, and sometimes the use of blood products (e.g., RBCs, platelets) is required to treat or prevent bleeding events.

Drug Treatment. Drug therapy is directed at elimination of cancerous hematopoietic cells in the bone marrow. Table 26-4 presents select chemotherapeutic agents used to treat leukemia (and other hematological cancers). Although this chapter focuses on hematological cancers, many of the same chemotherapeutic agents are used for a variety of forms of cancer. Several key categories of chemotherapeutic agents and how they work are described briefly.

Antimetabolite Agents. DNA and RNA are nucleic acids, which are made up of individual nucleotides. Nucleotides contain purine or pyrimidine bases. These bases are part of the nucleotides that are used in the DNA synthesis. The structure of antimetabolites is similar these bases, but because they are not identical, antimetabolites prevent the completion of cell division, or mitosis. Antimetabolites are often used to treat leukemia. The most common side effects include nausea, vomiting, fever, anorexia, bone marrow suppression, and jaundice. Examples of antimetabolites include:

- cytarabine
- fludarabine
- 5-fluorouracil (5-FU)
- 6-mercaptopurine
- methotrexate

Antibiotics. The antibiotics used to treat cancer are not in the same category as those used to treat infections. These chemotherapeutic antibiotics bind directly to the DNA of the cancer cells and prevent the development of new cancer cells. These agents are not used to treat infections because of their toxic side effects. Because they also destroy normal cells along with the cancer cells, they produce side effects that include severe emesis (vomiting), nausea, diarrhea, and hair loss. Some examples include:

- bleomycin
- daunorubicin
- doxorubicin
- idarubicin
- mitomycin-C

Mitotic Inhibitors. Mitotic inhibitors prevent mitosis at the metaphase stage. Mitosis is the process of cell division that all cells must perform (Figure 26-8). The agents used to prevent this cellular reproduction are a group of alkaloids derived from plants. Diseases such as Hodgkin's disease and various cancers that may not respond to other medications are often treated with mitotic inhibitors. Side effects may include appetite loss, back pain, diarrhea, hair loss, increased sweating, nausea, vomiting, voice changes, and discoloration of the skin. These agents include:

- etoposide
- vinblastine
- vincristine
- vinorelbine

Alkylating Agents. The two major types of alkylating agents are the nitrogen mustards and nitrosoureas. Although their structures are similar, their methods of action and side effects are different. Because alkylation is a normal reaction that takes place in the DNA between chemical compounds, these agents are able to bind to certain bases of the DNA. New bonds (created by alkylation) are made between components; when this occurs, the rapidly dividing cancer cells are damaged and unable to further proliferate. Diseases most often treated with these agents include Hodgkin's disease, retinoblastoma, lymphocytic leukemia, and inoperable cancers.

Nitrogen Mustards. Nitrogen mustards were some of the first chemotherapeutic agents used to treat cancer. These agents were used in chemical warfare in World War I. On examination of soldiers exposed

TABLE 26-4

Select Chemotherapeutic Agents Used in the Treatment of Hematological Cancers

Medication Class	Generic Name	Trade Name	Select Common Side Effects	Common Dose Range*
Alkylating Agents	chlorambucil	Leukeran	• Fever • Edema • Rash • Amenorrhea • Sterility • Neutropenia	• 30 mg/m² orally (PO) per day on specific cycle days
	cyclophosphamide	Cytoxan	• Alopecia • Sterility • Nausea • Vomiting • Hemorrhagic cystitis • Urinary fibrosis	• 200 mg/m² intravenously (IV) on specific cycle days
	carboplatin	Paraplatin	• Pain • Electrolyte imbalance • Vomiting • Myelosuppression • Renal complications	• 315 mg/m² daily IV infusion
Purine Nucleoside Analogues	fludarabine	Fludara	• Edema • Fever • Rash • Nausea • Anorexia • Bleeding • Cough	• 25 mg/m² IV on specific cycle days
	pentostatin	Nipent	• Fever • Rash • Nausea • Anemia • Weakness	• 4 mg/m² IV every 2 wk
	cladribine	Leustatin	• Flulike symptoms • Rash • Injection site reactions • Infection	• 0.09 mg/kg/day IV infusion
	mercaptopurine	Purinethol	• Anemia • Bleeding • Hepatotoxicity • Anorexia	• 1.5-5 mg/kg/day PO
Pyrimidine Analogue	cytarabine	Cytosar-U	• Fever • Rash • Nausea	• 100 mg/m²/dose IV
Monoclonal Antibodies	rituximab	Rituxan	• Infusion reaction • Neuropathy • Nausea • Rash • Fever • Fatigue • Tumor lysis syndrome	• 375-500 mg/m²/dose IV
	alemtuzumab	Campath	• Fever • Hypotension • Nausea • Rash • Vomiting • Injection site reaction	• 30 mg/dose IV infusion

Continued

TABLE 26-4

Select Chemotherapeutic Agents Used in the Treatment of Hematological Cancers—cont'd

Medication Class	Generic Name	Trade Name	Select Common Side Effects	Common Dose Range*
Anthracyclines	daunorubicin idarubicin	Cerubidine Idamycin	• Cardiac toxicity • Alopecia • Urine discoloration • Nausea • Injection site reaction • Vomiting	• 45 mg/m²/day IV bolus • 12 mg/m²/day IV slow infusion
Topoisomerase II Inhibitor	etoposide	Toposar	• Alopecia • Nausea • Anorexia • Neuropathy	• 75 mg/m²/day IV over 1 hr
Vinca Alkaloids	vindesine	Eldisine	• Flulike symptoms • Nausea • Loss of reflexes	• 3-4 mg/m²/week IV
	vincristine	Vincasar PFS	• Alopecia • Constipation • Pain • Peripheral neuropathy • Hearing loss	• 2 mg/dose IV at specified cycle days
Tyrosine Kinase Inhibitors	dasatinib	Sprycel	• Nausea • Anemia • Arthralgia • Headache • Rash	• 140 mg PO once daily for cycle
	imatinib	Gleevec		• 400 mg PO once daily for cycle
	nilotinib	Tasigna		• 300 mg PO twice daily for cycle
Retinoic Acid Derivative	tretinoin	Vesanoid	• Edema • Chest discomfort • Headache • Fever • Liver toxicity	• 45 mg/m²/day PO in 2 divided doses
Antimetabolites	methotrexate	Rheumatrex	• Headache • Rigidity • Infections	• 12 mg/dose intrathecal
	hydroxyurea	Hydrea	• Edema • Fever • Nausea • Drowsiness	• 50 mg/kg/dose PO 4 times daily

*Doses can vary by patient and indication for use.

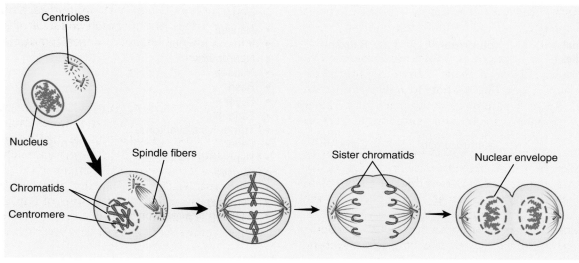

FIGURE 26-8 Mitosis.

to these agents, it was discovered that nitrogen mustards reduced the number of WBCs. Because of this effect on WBCs, they were used to treat leukemia, which is marked by a high WBC count. Although effective, the first nitrogen mustards had severe side effects; they have been replaced with agents that are derived from the same chemical structure but better tolerated. Side effects may include low blood counts, nausea, vomiting, mouth sores, hair loss, darkening of veins used for infusion, and loss of fertility. Examples of nitrogen mustard agents include:

- chlorambucil
- cyclophosphamide
- ifosfamide

 Tech Note!

When preparing chemotherapeutic agents, the technician must wear special chemotherapy gloves or must double-glove to protect the skin. Gowns and masks are also advised if the technician is preparing agents that must be compounded, reconstituted, or admixed. Such agents are prepared in a special laminar flow hood to prevent unwanted exposure. If a chemotherapeutic agent spills on the gloves, the top gloves can be removed and discarded into an appropriate container for hazardous waste, and a new pair of gloves can be worn. Always follow the appropriate procedures for the type of agent handled.

Nitrosoureas. These agents can cross the blood-brain barrier that surrounds the central nervous system. Because of this ability, they can be used to treat cancers in the brain. Side effects of these agents may include nausea, vomiting, intense flushing of the skin, reddening of the eyes, headache, and rash. The following drugs are nitrosoureas:

- carmustine
- lomustine

Other Antineoplastic Agents. Various other chemotherapeutic agents are commonly used to treat cancer. Antiandrogens, for example, are used to treat prostate cancer. Also known as *immunotherapy*, biological therapy is a type of cancer treatment that uses natural substances or substances produced in the laboratory. Some of these substances stimulate the body's own immune system to resist cancer. In addition, they can stop or slow the growth of cancer cells and prevent cancer from spreading. Certain cancers are affected by this type of therapy. These drugs often are used in conjunction with other forms of chemotherapy and radiation therapy. Biological therapy also can be used to treat diseases other than cancer; for example, rituximab can be used in the treatment of rheumatoid arthritis.

Lymphoma. **Lymphomas**, as the name suggests, are cancers associated with the lymphatic system.

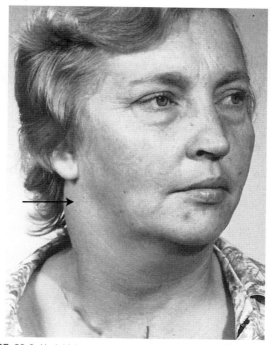

FIGURE 26-9 Hodgkin's lymphoma and enlarged cervical lymph node. (From Huether S, McCance K: *Understanding pathophysiology,* ed 5, St Louis, 2012, Mosby.)

Lymphomas initially develop in the lymph nodes or spleen. (For a review of the anatomy and physiology of the lymphatic system, see Chapter 23.) The inflammation associated with the development of lymphomas often leads to enlargement of the lymph nodes, which can be an early symptom of the cancer (Figure 26-9). A major risk factor for the development of lymphoma is the presence of a disorder associated with immunodeficiency (e.g., acquired immunodeficiency syndrome [AIDS]). Another risk factor that has been identified is exposure to herbicides, pesticides, and organic solvents. Viruses, such as the Epstein-Barr virus, also have been associated with the development of certain types of lymphoma. The two broad categories of lymphoma are Hodgkin's disease and non-Hodgkin's lymphomas. Although the signs and symptoms of these two forms of lymphoma overlap, they are treated differently and have different prognoses.

Prognosis. The prognosis for lymphoma varies widely based on the type and stage (Table 26-5).

Non–Drug Treatment. As with leukemia, supportive measures for lymphoma, such as prevention and aggressive treatment of infection, are important. Radiation therapy also can be used, depending on the type and stage of lymphoma.

Drug Treatment. A variety of chemotherapeutic agents can be used to treat hematological

TABLE 26-5

Stages of Cancer

Stage	Description
Stage I	Defined by small tumors located in one part of the body. Many cancers of this type are very treatable because the cancer is small and localized. This type of cancer may be cured by surgery and a small dose of radiation therapy.
Stage II	Slightly more serious than stage I cancer. Stage II tumors are larger but have not spread to the surrounding tissues and lymph nodes. The tumor can still be extracted surgically, and radiation can help ensure that the cancer does not return.
Stage III	The cancer has begun to move from the local organ to the surrounding lymph nodes. Once this occurs, treatment and cure become more difficult. Treatment typically involves surgery to remove the tumor and radiation and chemotherapy to kill the cancer cells that have moved to the lymph nodes and surrounding tissues.
Stage IV	Metastatic cancer, the most advanced form of cancer. This type of cancer is characterized by large tumors that have spread to surrounding organs. Once cancer has metastasized, it generally cannot be completely removed by surgery.

cancers, and the treatments used vary, depending on the type and stage of cancer (see Table 26-4). Combination therapies are frequently used. For example, for the treatment of Hodgkin's disease, standard combinations can be used, such as MOPP (nitrogen *m*ustard + *O*ncovorin + *p*rednisone + *p*rocarbazine) or ABVD (*A*driamycin + *b*leomycin + *v*inblastine + *d*acarbazine).

Bleeding Disorders

Bleeding disorders generally are associated with a defect in one or more clotting factors involved in the coagulation process (Figure 26-10). Bleeding disorders can be drug induced, genetic (hemophilia, von Willebrand's disease), or due to other disease processes (e.g., liver disease or vasculitis). Drug-induced bleeding is relatively common and can be associated with antiplatelet agents (e.g., aspirin and clopidogrel), anticoagulants (e.g., warfarin), and NSAIDs.

 Tech Note!

Warfarin (Coumadin) is the most common drug associated with adverse drug events leading to emergency department visits and hospitalization. Extreme care should be taken when preparing warfarin prescriptions to ensure patients receive the correct dosage and instructions for use. In addition, the pharmacist should ensure that people using warfarin understand that they should avoid taking aspirin and other NSAIDs due to the risk of bleeding. These patients should also be consistent in their intake of foods rich in vitamin K, such as spinach and liver, because of these foods may affect the anticoagulant effect of warfarin.

Hemophilia is a hereditary coagulation disorder associated with intermittent bleeding episodes. Hemophilia is associated with either a deficiency or lack of either antihemophilic Factor VIII (known as *hemophilia A*) or Factor IX (Figure 26-11). The treatment of hemophilia involves prophylactic blood infusions or the use of recombinant Factor VIII or Factor IX products.

Von Willebrand's disease is the most common inherited coagulation disorder and is associated with decreased activity of von Willebrand's factor. Von Willebrand's factor is important for facilitating platelet binding in the vasculature. Treatment involves strategies to increase the availability of von Willebrand's factor and include the use of **cryoprecipitate**, Factor VIII concentrates, desmopressin (DDAVP), fresh frozen plasma, and estrogen therapy.

GENERIC NAME: desmopressin
TRADE NAME: DDAVP
INDICATION: Bleeding prophylaxis, hemophilia A, hemorrhage, surgical bleeding, von Willebrand's disease
ROUTE OF ADMINISTRATION: Intravenous (IV); subcutaneous (SUBCUT); intranasal
COMMON ADULT DOSAGE: *IV/SUBCUT:* 0.3 mcg/kg; *Intranasal:* 1 spray (150 mcg) in each nostril
MECHANISM OF ACTION: Increases plasma Factor VIII and von Willebrand's factor
SIDE EFFECTS: Facial flushing, headache, hyponatremia

 Tech Alert!

Remember the following sound-alike, look-alike drugs:
   Coumadin versus Cardura
   Neulasta versus Lunesta
   Neupogen versus Neumega

I. Subendothelial exposure

- Occurs after endothelial sloughing
- Platelets begin to fill endothelial gaps
- Promoted by thromboxane A_2 (TXA$_2$)
- Inhibited by prostacyclin I_2 (PGI$_2$)
- Platelet function depends on many factors, especially calcium

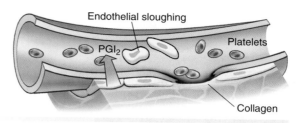

II. Adhesion

- Adhesion is initiated by loss of endothelial cells (or rupture or erosion of atherosclerotic plaque), which exposes adhesive glycoproteins such as collagen and von Willebrand factor (vWF) in the subendothelium. vWF and, perhaps, other adhesive glycoproteins in the plasma deposit on the damaged area. Platelets adhere to the subendothelium through receptors that bind to the adhesive glycoproteins (GPIb, GPIa/IIa, GPIIb/IIIa).

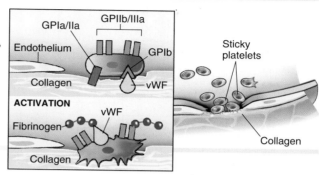

III. Activation

- After platelets adhere they undergo an activation process that leads to a conformational change in GPIIb/IIIa receptors, resulting in their ability to bind adhesive proteins, including fibrinogen and von Willebrand factor
- Changes in platelet shape
- Formation of pseudopods
- Activation of arachidonic pathway

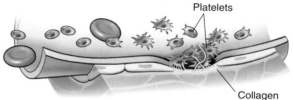

IV. Aggregation

- Induced by release of TXA$_2$
- Adhesive glycoproteins bind simultaneously to GPIIb/IIIa on two different platelets
- Stabilization of the platelet plug (blood clot) occurs by activation of coagulation factors, thrombin, and fibrin
- Heparin neutralizing factor enhances clot formation

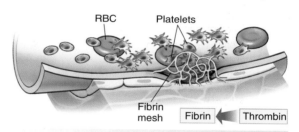

V. Platelet plug formation

- RBCs and platelets enmeshed in fibrin

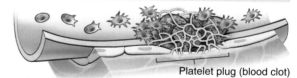

VI. Clot retraction and clot dissolution

- Clot retraction, using large number of platelets, joins the edges of the injured vessel
- Clot dissolution is regulated by thrombin and plasminogen activators

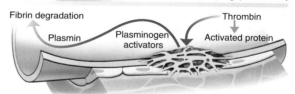

FIGURE 26-10 Blood vessel damage, blood clot, and clot dissolution. (From Huether S, McCance K: *Understanding pathophysiology,* ed 5, St Louis, 2012, Mosby.)

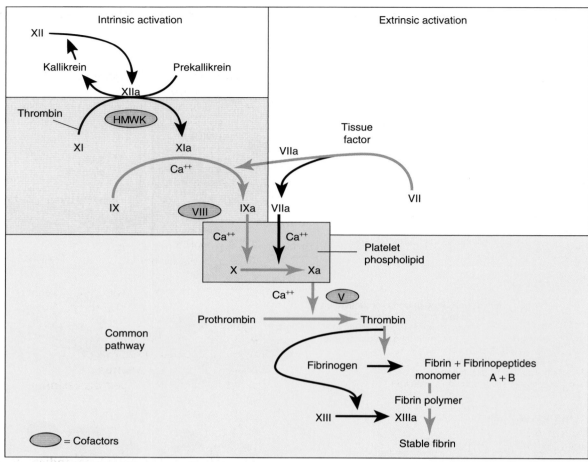

FIGURE 26-11 Activation of Factor X by the steps in the extrinsic and intrinsic coagulation pathways. (From Price SA et al: *Pathophysiology: clinical concepts of disease processes,* ed 6, St Louis, 2003, Mosby.)

DO YOU REMEMBER THESE KEY POINTS?

- Names of the major components of the hematological system and their functions
- The primary symptoms of the various hematological conditions discussed
- Medications used to treat the various hematological conditions discussed

- The generic and trade names for the drugs discussed in this chapter
- The appropriate auxiliary labels that should be used when filling prescriptions for drugs discussed in this chapter

REVIEW QUESTIONS

Multiple Choice Questions

1. _____ is the movement of water down a concentration gradient.
   A. Hydrostatic pressure
   B. Osmosis
   C. Diuresis
   D. Plasmosis

2. Plasma that has been allowed to clot in the laboratory to remove clotting factors that can interfere with some blood tests is known as _____.
   A. Serum
   B. Whole blood
   C. Erythrocytes
   D. Fibrinogen

3. A condition associated with abnormally low platelets in the blood is known as:
   A. Leukocytosis
   B. Leukopenia
   C. Thrombocytopenia
   D. Neutropenia
4. Which hormone is produced in the kidney and stimulates the bone marrow to produce red blood cells?
   A. Prothrombin
   B. Fibrinogen
   C. Leukine
   D. Erythropoietin
5. What is the brand name for sodium ferric gluconate complex?
   A. Epogen
   B. Neulasta
   C. Ferrlecit
   D. Feosol
6. _____ is defined as excessive red blood cell production.
   A. Polycythemia
   B. Thrombocytopenia
   C. Anemia
   D. None of the above
7. Which medication is approved for the treatment of polycythemia vera?
   A. Epoetin alfa
   B. Darbepoetin alfa
   C. Anagrelide
   D. Sargramostim
8. Which condition(s) is(are) associated with the development of neutropenia?
   A. Aplastic anemia
   B. Leukemia
   C. Vitamin B_{12} deficiency
   D. All of the above

9. MOPP is a combination therapy for the treatment of:
   A. Hodgkin's disease
   B. Leukemia
   C. Non-Hodgkin's lymphoma
   D. Hemophilia
10. Which drug is *not* believed to contribute to drug-induced bleeding?
    A. Ibuprofen
    B. Warfarin
    C. Clopidogrel
    D Acetaminophen
11. Which condition is associated with a deficiency or a lack of either Factor VIII or Factor IX?
    A. Hemophilia
    B. Von Willebrand's disease
    C. Thrombocytopenia
    D. Hodgkin's disease
12. _____ is associated with the destruction of mature erythrocytes due to cell lysis.
    A. Aplastic anemia
    B. Pernicious anemia
    C. Hemolytic anemia
    D. Iron deficiency anemia
13. The brand name for pegfilgrastim is:
    A. Aranesp
    B. Leukine
    C. Neulasta
    D. Neupogen
14. Eltrombopag (Promacta) is indicated for the treatment of:
    A. Thrombocytopenia
    B. Hemophilia
    C. Neutropenia
    D. Leukopenia
15. Which medications is(are) *not* associated with drug-induced thrombocytopenia?
    A. Heparin
    B. Quinine
    C. Vancomycin
    D. All of the above are associated with drug-induced thrombocytopenia.

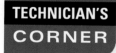

TECHNICIAN'S CORNER Using an online drug information reference, perform a search of medications associated with the development of anemia as a drug side effect. If a person were picking up a refill for one of these medications and also was purchasing an OTC iron supplement, what (if anything) would you do?

Bibliography

Clinical Pharmacology Online. (Referenced September 6, 2014.) www.clinicalpharmacology-ip.com.

Damjanov I: *Pathology for the health professions*, ed 4, St Louis, 2011, Saunders.

Fishback JL: *Pathology*, ed 3, Philadelphia, 2005, Mosby.

Huether S, McCance K: *Understanding pathophysiology*, ed 5, St Louis, 2012, Mosby.

McCance KL: *Pathophysiology: the biologic basis for disease in adults and children*, ed 6, St Louis, 2010, Mosby.

Page C et al: *Integrated pharmacology*, ed 3, St Louis, 2006, Mosby.

Price SA et al: *Pathophysiology: clinical concepts of disease processes*, ed 6, St Louis, 2003, Mosby.

Solomon EP: *Introduction to human anatomy and physiology*, ed 3, St Louis, 2009, Mosby.

Thibodeau GA, Patton KT: *Anatomy and physiology*, ed 8, St Louis, 2012, Mosby.

Thompson JM et al: *Mosby's clinical nursing*, ed 5, St Louis, 2001, Mosby.

UpToDate Online. (Referenced September 6, 2014.) www.uptodate.com.

Over-the-Counter (OTC) Medications

Joshua J. Neumiller

OBJECTIVES

Upon completing this chapter, you should be able to do the following:

1. Describe the most common conditions treated with over-the-counter (OTC) products.
2. Recognize OTC drugs used to treat the conditions discussed in this chapter.
3. Describe the U.S. Food and Drug Administration's regulations concerning the manufacture of OTC products.
4. Write the generic and trade names for the OTC drugs discussed in this chapter.
5. Recognize common dosage forms and safety considerations for the OTC products discussed in this chapter.

TERMS AND DEFINITIONS

Analgesic A drug that relieves pain by reducing the perception of pain

Antiinflammatory A drug that reduces swelling, redness, and pain and that promotes healing

Antipyretic A drug that reduces fever

Antitussive A drug that can decrease the coughing reflex

Behind-the-counter drug A medication that does not require a prescription but is kept "behind the counter" and can be purchased only at a pharmacy

Circadian rhythm A daily cycle of activity in living organisms; the term can pertain to sleep/wake cycles

Expectorant A chemical that aids in the removal of mucous secretions from the respiratory system; it loosens and thins sputum and bronchial secretions for ease of expectoration

Legend drug A medication regulated by law; a prescription is required to obtain it

Nutraceutical A food or naturally occurring supplement thought to have a beneficial effect on human health

Over-the-counter (OTC) medication A medication that does not require a prescription and may be purchased by customers at any retail outlet

Pruritus Itching of the skin

Common Select Over-the-Counter (OTC) Medications

Trade Name	Generic Name	Pronunciation
Fever/Pain Product		
Tylenol	acetaminophen (APAP)	(a-**seet**-a-**min**-oh-fen)
Fever/Pain/Inflammation Products		
Ecotrin	aspirin (ASA)	(**as**-pir-in)
Motrin, Advil	ibuprofen (IBU)	(**eye**-bue-**proe**-fen)
Aleve	naproxen	(na-**prox**-en)

Continued

Common Select Over-the-Counter (OTC) Medications—cont'd

Trade Name	Generic Name	Pronunciation
Sleep Aids		
Benadryl	diphenhydramine	(**dye**-fen-**hye**-dra-meen)
Unisom	doxylamine	(dox-**il**-a-meen)
Circadin	melatonin	(meh-lah-**toe**-nin)
Cold/Cough Products		
Robitussin	guaifenesin	(gwye-**fen**-e-sin
Benadryl	diphenhydramine	(**dye**-fen-**hye**-dra-meen)
Sudafed*	pseudoephedrine	(soo-doe-e-**fed**-rin)
Nasal Product		
Neo-Synephrine	phenylephrine	(feh-nill-**eh**-frin)
Sore Throat Product		
Chloraseptic	benzocaine	(**ben**-zoe-kane)
Stomach Products		
Pepcid AC	famotidine	(fam-**oh**-ti-deen)
Prilosec OTC	omeprazole	(oh-**mep**-ra-zole)
Zantac 150, Zantac 75	ranitidine	(ra-**ni**-ti-deen)
Tums	calcium carbonate	(**kal**-see-um **kar**-bo-nate)
Prevacid 24HR	lansoprazole	(lan-**soe**-pra-zol)
Intestinal Products		
Metamucil	psyllium	(sil-**ee**-um)
Imodium AD	loperamide	(loe-**per**-a-mide)
Senokot	senna	(**seh**-nah)
Dulcolax	bisacodyl	(bis-**ak**-oh-dil)
Miscellaneous Products		
Compound W	salicylic acid	(**sal**-i-**sil**-ik **a**-sid)
Monistat	miconazole	(my-**caw**-nah-zole)
Cortizone-10	hydrocortisone	(**hye**-droe-**kor**-ti-sone)

*Pseudoephedrine does not require a prescription, but it is a behind-the-counter drug.

If you walk into your corner drugstore, you will see the massive number of **over-the-counter (OTC) medications** available for purchase (Figure 27-1). No prescriptions are necessary for the purchase of OTC products, and customers are not required to obtain advice from the pharmacy staff about the appropriate use of OTC products. Just as certain food staples are kept on hand in the kitchen, so have certain OTC medications become common staples of home medicine cabinets. For example, a basic shopping list might include items such as flour, sugar, eggs, acetaminophen (Tylenol), cough syrup, and ibuprofen (Motrin).

Since the mid-1980s, the number of OTC drugs available to consumers has increased sharply. The following statistics from the Consumer Healthcare

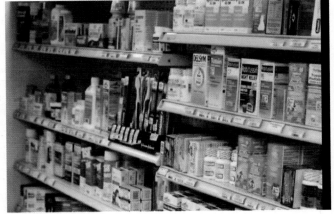

FIGURE 27-1 More than 100,000 OTC products can be created from different combinations of only 1000 ingredients. (CPHA, 2001)

Products Association provide useful data on the use and sale of OTC items, the reduction in health care costs possible from the use of OTC drugs, and the future of OTC medications.

- Since 1976, 106 ingredients, dosages, or indications have been switched from prescription to OTC status.
- Ninety-three percent of U.S. adults prefer to treat their minor ailments with OTC medicines before seeking professional care.
- Forty percent of adults in the United States have avoided taking sick days from work because they used an OTC medicine.
- Using OTC medications to treat common upper respiratory infections saves the U.S. health care system and economy $4.75 billion each year.
- Most Americans (92%) believe that OTC medicines are entirely safe and effective.

In this chapter common conditions treated with OTC medications are explored, as are the most common OTC products used to treat those conditions. Common dosage forms are discussed, and an overview of the regulations established by the U.S. Food and Drug Administration (FDA) pertaining to OTC products is presented.

Although federal law requires that pharmacists counsel Medicaid patients receiving new prescriptions and individual states have additional counseling requirements, OTC medications do not fall under these categories, unless a prescription is written for the OTC item. However, in patient counseling, it is important that the pharmacist ask about OTC medication use because many of these agents can interact with both prescription medications and certain medical conditions. The ability to buy drugs off the shelf can translate into substantial savings for consumers, which is only one of many reasons individuals use OTC products. Consumers also use OTC products for the following reasons.

- They want to save money, and OTC medications generally are less expensive than prescription drugs. The individual also saves money by avoiding physicians' appointments, which involve the cost of the office visit and missed time at work.
- Consumers want to be involved in their own treatment, and OTC medications give them this capability.
- OTC medications are more easily obtainable than prescriptions because they do not require a prescription, and stores that carry OTC medications usually have longer business hours than traditional pharmacies.

However, when patients decide to treat themselves by purchasing an OTC medication, important factors should be taken into account. First, there is a wide variety of drugs from which to choose; therefore, correctly identifying the cause of the symptom or problem is the first step. If the self-diagnosis is wrong, the OTC medication may mask an important underlying condition. For example, if a person with diarrhea purchases an antidiarrheal medication, the diarrhea may stop for a short time, but the underlying cause could be something more serious that may require diagnosis and treatment by a physician. For this reason, it is important to educate consumers on the need to follow the instructions on OTC products, including the appropriate duration of treatment with OTC medicines.

Many OTC medications list specific age groups that should not take the medication. Parents should consult with their child's pediatrician before giving any OTC medication to a child, especially one younger than 4 years. In addition to these considerations, children with colds may develop ear infections and other conditions that warrant seeing a pediatrician for appropriate prescription treatment. The following are some important considerations that consumers should address before buying and using OTC medications.

- Various OTC medications have identical ingredients; however, consumers often purchase a more expensive name brand, not realizing that they are obtaining the same medication as the less expensive generic form.
- Manufacturers may swap "like ingredients." The label shows the ingredient change or reformulation. Consumers often overlook this if they do not read labels carefully. Consequently, consumers may be unaware that they are using a formulation different from what they used previously.
- A person who is on a special diet, has allergies, has diabetes, or is taking other medications that may interact with OTC drugs should use caution in selecting an OTC product.
- Extra care should be taken when purchasing OTC medications for infants or young children; consumers should know and follow guidelines related to the safety of agents based on the child's age. This includes topical agents.
- When trying a new agent, individuals should watch carefully for any adverse reactions that may occur. They should seek advice from their pharmacist or physician if they experience anything out of the ordinary while taking an OTC product.
- Many if not most OTC and prescription medications cannot be taken if a woman is pregnant or nursing. Those who are pregnant or breastfeeding should always seek professional advice before taking an OTC product.

Food and Drug Administration Regulations

Similar to prescription medications, OTC drugs are regulated by the FDA. However, FDA regulations pertaining to OTC products are quite different from those for prescription products. Although the FDA requires that all new drugs undergo a new drug application (NDA) process before approval, drugs deemed "generally recognized as safe and effective (GRASE)" are exempted from this regulation. Historically, many drug products were available as OTC products before the NDA process. To efficiently handle the OTC products already available, the FDA implemented the OTC monograph system so that classes of OTC products could be reviewed by expert panels for designation as GRASE. Because more than 300,000 OTC products are marketed, the FDA reviews the active ingredients and labeling requirements of drug classes instead of individual drug products. The resulting OTC drug monographs are published in the *Federal Register* and outline acceptable ingredients, doses, formulations, and labeling. For products that are not covered by an OTC monograph because of their active ingredient or ingredients and labeling requirements, approval via the traditional NDA system is necessary. New products that conform to a final OTC monograph can be marketed without further FDA review.

How a Prescription Drug Becomes an Over-the-Counter Drug

An "Rx to OTC switch" takes place through one of two processes: (1) under the OTC drug review or (2) through submission of additional information by the manufacturer to the original product NDA. One of the FDA's main considerations is whether enough information is available to prove that the medication can be safely taken without a health care provider's prescription and oversight of treatment. Another factor considered is evidence that the product's labeling can be read, understood, and followed by the consumer without the guidance of a health care provider. The amount of research done before a new OTC drug is released is extensive. The FDA must approve all new drugs entering the marketplace and has strict guidelines (as discussed in Chapter 2). The same standards of safety and effectiveness placed on **legend drugs** (those requiring a prescription) are used to approve OTC drugs. To meet the criteria for designation as an OTC product, drug companies must perform comprehensive studies on the drug's labeling to determine whether consumers can easily and safely take the medication in question. In addition, if a prospective OTC drug has a lower dosage than a prescription dose, studies must be conducted to evaluate the effectiveness of the drug at the lower dosage. If the agent meets all the criteria, it is approved as an OTC medication. If the agent has been approved already as a prescription drug and the manufacturer wants it to be offered also as an OTC drug, it does not require further testing. Many drugs sold OTC are also marketed as legend drugs. The difference often is the strength of the drug and in some cases the indications for use. For instance, ibuprofen is available OTC in 200 mg tablets for the relief of fever or mild pain or inflammation; however, if 400, 600, or 800 mg is needed, a prescription is required. Notable agents recently making the Rx to OTC switch include nonsedating antihistamines for the treatment of seasonal allergies (e.g., Zyrtec, Allegra), proton pump inhibitors for the treatment of GERD (Prilosec OTC and Prevacid 24HR), and polyethylene glycol (MiraLax) for the management of constipation.

Common Conditions Treated with OTC Drugs

As stated previously, thousands of OTC medications are available, considering the brands, generic versions, combinations, various strengths, and dosage forms. Table 27-1 lists some of the most common OTC medications, the symptoms they treat, and the most popular routes of administration. As new medications enter the market as OTC drugs, consumers can choose even more routes of administration.

OTC Pain Relievers and Antipyretics

Analgesic and **antipyretic** agents help reduce or relieve pain (analgesic) and fever (antipyretic). Aspirin (acetylsalicylic acid [ASA]) has the added benefit of being an **antiinflammatory** agent when used at sufficient doses. As noted in Chapter 18, aspirin also decreases the clotting ability of platelets and is used extensively for primary and secondary prevention of heart attack and stroke.

 Tech Note!

Reye's syndrome is a rare condition that can affect children and teenagers who have an active case of certain viral illnesses (e.g., chickenpox or influenza) and take products containing aspirin. The symptoms include vomiting, lethargy, delirium, and coma. Permanent brain damage can occur, and the condition can be fatal. Although the fatality rate is less than 20%, it is safer to prevent the possibility of such adverse effects by instructing these patients or their caregivers to avoid using aspirin and aspirin-containing products (aspirin can often be a "hidden" component of OTC products).

Other OTC pain relievers are widely used for the treatment of arthritis, headaches, and miscellaneous

TABLE 27-1

Common Categories of OTC Products

Type of Drug	Symptom Treated	Route of Administration
Analgesics	Pain	Oral, topical, rectal
Antiinflammatories	Inflammation/arthritis pain	Oral, topical
Antipyretics	Fever	Oral, rectal
Antihistamines	Allergies	Oral, intranasal
Decongestants	Congestion	Oral, intranasal
Headache products	Pain	Oral
Sleep aids	Insomnia	Oral
Expectorants	Productive cough	Oral
Cough suppressants	Dry cough	Oral
Sore throat products	Pain	Oral
Sunscreens	Sunburn prophylaxis	Topical
Sunburn products	Pain/inflammation	Topical
Antacids	Indigestion	Oral
Antidiarrheals	Diarrhea	Oral, rectal
Laxatives	Constipation	Oral, rectal
Acne products	Pimples	Topical
Antibiotics	Topical infection treatment/prophylaxis	Topical
Antifungals	Dry, flaking skin and pain caused by fungus	Topical
Cold sore preparations	Painful canker sores	Topical
Wart removal products	Wart growth	Topical

TABLE 27-2

Select OTC Pain Medications

Medication Class	Generic Name	Trade Name	Common Adult Oral Dose
Salicylate	aspirin	Bayer Aspirin, Ecotrin	• 325-650 mg orally (PO) or rectally (PR) every 4 hr as needed (max 4 g/day)
Analgesic	acetaminophen	Tylenol	• 325-650 mg PO or PR every 4-6 hr as needed; not to exceed 1 g/dose or 3 g/day or 3000 mg/day*
Nonsteroidal Antiinflammatory Drugs (NSAIDs)	ibuprofen	Advil	• 200-400 mg PO every 4-6 hr as needed
	naproxen	Aleve	• 220-440 mg PO in first hour, then 220 mg PO every 8-12 hr (max 660 mg/day)

*Makers of Tylenol Extra Strength recommend a limit of 3 g per day, but FDA maintains 4 g per day maximum. http://www.fda.gov/Drugs/DrugSafety/ucm239821.htm

aches and pains. Nonsteroidal antiinflammatory drugs (NSAIDs), such as ibuprofen and naproxen, are staples of most medicine cabinets in the United States and are effective analgesics, antipyretics, and antiinflammatory agents. Acetaminophen (Tylenol) is another widely used OTC product that acts as both an analgesic and antipyretic. Table 27-2 lists select OTC products for the treatment of pain and fever.

 Tech Note!
A potential and common side effect of NSAIDs is an increase in blood pressure. For patients reporting a recent increase in their blood pressure, it is always a good idea to ask them about the use of OTC NSAIDs to determine whether the change could be related to the use of these products.

 Tech Note!
Acetaminophen is a common component of many OTC products such as Tylenol, combination cough and cold preparations, and prescription pain relievers. Patients may not realize that many of the products they take contain acetaminophen; this puts them at risk for liver toxicity if they take too much on a daily basis.

OTC Allergy Treatments

A variety of OTC products is available for the treatment of allergy symptoms (Table 27-3). These products can contain several agents, such as decongestants, antihistamines, and analgesics. (See Chapter 19 for

TABLE 27-3

Select OTC Products for the Treatment of Allergy Symptoms

Medication Class	Generic Name	Trade Name	Common Adult Oral Dose
Antihistamines: Oral Nonsedating*	cetirizine HCl	Zyrtec	• 5-10 mg orally (PO) once daily
	fexofenadine	Allegra	• 60 mg PO twice daily or 180 mg PO once daily
Antihistamines: Oral Sedating	loratadine	Claritin	• 10 mg PO once daily
	chlorpheniramine	Chlor-Trimeton	• 4 mg PO ever 4-6 hr *or* • *Extended-release tablets:* 16 mg once daily
Decongestant: Oral Decongestants: Nasal†	diphenhydramine	Benadryl	• 25-50 mg PO every 4-6 hr
	phenylephrine	Medi-Phenyl	• 10 mg PO every 4-6 hr
	oxymetazoline	Afrin	• 2-3 sprays each nostril twice daily; not to be used for longer than 3 days
	phenylephrine	Neo-Synephrine	• 2-3 sprays each nostril every 4 hr as needed; not to be used for longer than 3 days
Mast Cell Stabilizer: Nasal	cromolyn sodium	Nasalcrom	• 1 spray each nostril 3-6 times daily
Antihistamine/Mast Cell Stabilizer: Ophthalmic	ketotifen	Zaditor	• 1 drop into the affected eye(s) every 8-12 hr
Antihistamine/Decongestant: Ophthalmic	naphazoline	Clear Eyes	• 1-2 drops into eyes every 3-4 hr as needed
	tetrahydrozoline	Visine	• 1-2 drops in each eye 2-4 times daily

*Medications may be combined with pseudoephedrine 120 mg and feature a "D" after the name of the decongestant product. Dosing involves a 120 mg pseudoephedrine combination pill twice day or a double-strength (240 mg) combination pill once a day orally.
†Using these nasal sprays longer than 3 days can cause rebound nasal congestion.

a detailed discussion of decongestants, antihistamines, and expectorants for the treatment of allergies.) Briefly, decongestants are indicated for stuffiness and congestion of the nasal passages and sinuses. Because they cause vasoconstriction, decongestants open these passages and allow the release of mucus to reduce congestion. Antihistamines are used to minimize symptoms of **pruritus** (itching), hives, sneezing, and itchy, runny eyes; they block histamine (H_1-receptors), which causes allergic reactions. Many different types of these agents are available OTC. First-generation agents include diphenhydramine (Benadryl) and chlorpheniramine (Chlor-Trimeton). Cetirizine (Zyrtec) is considered a weakly-sedating antihistamine because it causes slightly less drowsiness than first-generation agents. Loratadine (Claritin) does not typically cause drowsiness. OTC antihistamines normally are effective for mild allergic symptoms, but people with severe allergies may require prescription medications.

OTC Products for the Treatment of Cough and Cold Symptoms

The cold and flu section is one of the largest areas of the pharmacy. Many manufacturers offer the same types of ingredients in different proportions and combinations (Table 27-4). For congested coughs, **expectorants** can help expectorate phlegm. For dry coughs

that do not produce phlegm, an **antitussive** agent commonly is used to reduce the coughing.

Sore, scratchy, and dry throats usually arise from a cold or flu. They can be treated with many different agents available as OTC medications. If a sore throat continues without relief for more than a couple of days and is accompanied by a productive cough, the person should see a physician so that infection can be ruled out. A sore throat can be a symptom of a streptococcal bacterial infection, also known as strep throat. Strep throat is managed with prescription antibiotics. In addition to taking antibiotics, the patient may relieve throat pain with various OTC syrups, sprays, and analgesics. The components typically used in these products include menthol, alcohol, and topical anesthetics, such as benzocaine.

OTC Products for Insomnia

Many people suffer from insomnia. Many OTC medications contain an antihistamine to treat insomnia (e.g., diphenhydramine, doxylamine) (Table 27-5). Some OTC combination products also contain acetaminophen or magnesium salicylate to assist with nighttime pain relief if the insomnia is thought to be pain related. OTC sleep aids are intended to be used for transient insomnia and not for chronic use. Melatonin is a **nutraceutical** widely used for sleep problems. It is an endogenous hormone secreted by the

TABLE 27-4

Select OTC Products for the Treatment of Cough and Cold Symptoms*

Medication Class	Generic Name	Trade Name	Common Adult Oral Dose
Antipyretic (Fever) and Analgesics	acetaminophen	Tylenol	• 325-650 mg orally (PO) or rectally (PR) every 4-6 hr as needed; not to exceed 1 g/dose or 3 g/day[†]
	ibuprofen	Advil	• 200-400 mg PO every 4-6 hr as needed
Cough Suppressant (antitussive)	dextromethorphan	Delsym	• *Immediate release:* 10-20 mg PO every 4 hr as needed *or* • 30 mg every 6-8 hr as needed • *Extended release* (Delsym): 60 mg every 12 hr as needed
Expectorant	guaifenesin	Mucinex	• 200-400 mg PO every 4 hr (max 2400 mg/day)
Systemic Decongestant Local Anesthetics	phenylephrine benzocaine, menthol	Medi-Phenyl Chloraseptic Sore Throat Lozenges	• 10 mg PO every 4-6 hr • 1 lozenge (10-15 mg) dissolved slowly in mouth; may repeat every 2 hr
	pectin	Halls Lozenges	• 1-2 lozenges dissolved in mouth over time; may repeat every 2 hr
	phenol	Chloraseptic Spray	• 5 sprays on the affected area; may repeat every 2 hr
	benzocaine, glycerin	Cepacol Dual Relief Spray	• 1 spray to affected area, wait longer than 1 min and spit; may repeat 4 times daily
Antihistamine: Sedating	diphenhydramine	Benadryl	• 25-50 mg PO every 4-6 hr

*Refer to other sections and tables for other options and more information on antihistamines, decongestants, sleep, and pain/analgesia medications. Many cough and cold products are available in combination form.
[†]Makers of Tylenol Extra Strength recommend a limit of 3 g per day, but FDA maintains 4 g per day maximum. http://www.fda.gov/Drugs/DrugSafety/ucm239821.htm

TABLE 27-5

Select OTC Products for the Treatment of Insomnia*

Medication Class	Generic Name	Trade Name	Common Adult Oral Dose
Hormone/Nutritional Supplement Histamine Antagonist (First Generation)/Ethanolamine Derivatives	melatonin doxylamine	Bio-Melatonin, Circadin Unisom Sleep-Tabs	• 1-3 mg orally (PO) • 25-50 mg PO once daily 30 min before bedtime
	diphenhydramine	Benadryl, Sleep-Eze, Tylenol PM	• 25-50 mg PO once daily 30 min before bedtime

*The U.S. Food and Drug Administration (FDA) recommends developing healthy sleep habits before trying medications.

pineal gland that plays a role in the regulation of **circadian rhythms**.

Although a prescription is not needed for an OTC sleep aid, it is still a good idea for people to discuss the use of these products with their pharmacist, physician, or other health care provider. OTC sleep aids generally are intended to be used for no longer than 2 weeks; therefore, people experiencing prolonged difficulties with sleep should seek evaluation by a physician. It is also important to stress the importance of nonpharmacological approaches that may help treat insomnia, such as sleeping on a regular schedule, avoiding caffeine and daytime naps, exercising, and managing stress.

Tech Note!

Diphenhydramine is renowned for causing next-day drowsiness, often accompanied by confusion, particularly in older adults. Diphenhydramine use also has been associated with an increased risk of falls in older individuals, so it should be used with caution in these patients.

Gastroesophageal Reflux Disease and Indigestion

Several classes of OTC medications are available to treat indigestion and gastroesophageal reflux disease (GERD) (Table 27-6). Histamine-2 antagonists (H_2-antagonists) are used to reduce acid secretion to help diminish symptoms of heartburn and/or acid reflux. Proton pump inhibitors (PPIs) also work to decrease acid secretion, and antacid agents can be used to increase the pH level in the stomach, which ultimately helps reduce heartburn. (See Chapter 20 to review the mechanisms of action of these medication classes.)

 Tech Note!

Chronic heartburn symptoms may be due to an ulcer caused by *Helicobacter pylori*, a bacterium associated with gastric ulcers that can cause the symptoms of heartburn. If the problem persists for longer than 2 weeks, the person should seek medical evaluation for an ulcer.

Antacids generally are reserved for short-term relief of heartburn, whereas PPIs and H_2-receptor antagonists can be used for maintenance therapy with a prescription. Occasional side effects associated with antacid use can include constipation, diarrhea, and stomach cramps. Drug-drug interactions are possible with antacid products. For example, antacids containing calcium (e.g., Tums) may reduce the absorption and effectiveness of certain antibiotics, such as tetracycline and quinolone antibiotics. Antacids can also affect the absorption of levothyroxine, a thyroid hormone. Antacids, PPIs, and H_2-receptor antagonists can also interact with drugs that require a highly acidic environment for proper absorption. As noted previously with OTC analgesics, it is important to question patients about their use of OTC products for the treatment of heartburn because of the potential for drug interactions with these products.

 Tech Note!

Because calcium absorption is acid dependent, long-term use of a PPI has been linked to an increased risk of bone fracture due to decreased calcium absorption.

OTC Agents for Other Gastrointestinal Conditions

Table 27-7 presents remedies for intestinal discomfort and pain resulting from constipation, diarrhea,

TABLE 27-6

Select OTC Products for Treatment of Gastroesophageal Reflux Disease and Indigestion

Generic Name	Trade Name	Common Dosage Range
Antacids		
Neutralize existing stomach acid		
sodium bicarbonate	Alka-Seltzer	• 325 mg-2 g orally (PO) 1-4 times daily
calcium carbonate	Tums	• 1-2 tablets or 5-10 mL PO every 2 hr (max 7000 mg/day)
magnesium hydroxide	Milk of Magnesia	• 2-4 tablets or 5-15 mL PO as needed (prn) up to 4 times daily
H_2-Blockers		
Block the action of histamine that causes secretion of stomach acid		
ranitidine	Zantac 150	• 75-150 mg PO 30-60 min before ingesting heartburn-causing agents (max 300 mg/day)
cimetidine	Tagamet HB	• 200 mg PO 1-2 times daily 30 min before ingesting heartburn-causing agents
famotidine	Pepcid AC	• 10-20 mg PO 1-2 times daily 15-60 min before ingesting heartburn-causing agents
Proton Pump Inhibitors		
Inactivate the acid pumps throughout cells in the stomach		
omeprazole	Prilosec OTC	• 20 mg PO once daily for 14 days
lansoprazole	Prevacid 24HR	• 15 mg PO once daily for 14 days

TABLE 27-7

Select OTC Products for Treatment of Gastrointestinal Conditions Such as Constipation and Diarrhea

Medication Class	Generic Name	Trade Name	Common Dose Range	Onset
Fiber/Bulk Laxative	psyllium	Metamucil	• 2.4-7.2 g per day divided into multiple doses	12-72 hr
Stool Softener	docusate sodium	Colace	• 50-500 mg/day orally (PO) in 1-4 divided dose	12-72 hr
Hyperosmolar Agent Stimulants	sorbitol	Neosorb	• 15-30 mL PO 1-2 times daily	1-2 days
	bisacodyl	Dulcolax	• 5-15 mg PO once daily	6 hr
	senna	Senokot	• 2-4 tabs PO 1-2 times daily	6-12 hr
Saline Laxatives	magnesium citrate	Citroma	• 150-300 mL PO 1-2 times daily	0.5-3 hr
	magnesium hydroxide	Milk of Magnesia	• 15-30 mL PO 1-2 times daily	0.5-6 hr
Lubricant Laxative	mineral oil	Kondremul	• 15-45 mL PO once daily	6-8 hr
Suppositories	glycerin	Sani-Supp	• 1 supp rectally (PR) as needed (prn) once daily	15-60 min
Enemas	bisacodyl	Dulcolax	• 1 supp PR prn once daily	15-60 min
	sodium phosphate	Fleet	• 1 unit PR as a single dose	5-15 min
	mineral oil	Fleet Mineral Oil Enema	• 118 mL PR as a single dose	6-8 hr
Antidiarrheals	loperamide	Imodium	• 4 mg PO initially, then 2 mg after each stool (max 16 mg/day)	1 hr
	bismuth subsalicylate	Pepto-Bismol	• 524 mg PO every 30-60 min prn, up to 8 doses daily	1 hr

or gas (flatulence). Laxatives and stool softeners are commonly purchased OTC. (See Chapter 20 for a review of the treatment of constipation and diarrhea.) For the treatment of gas, simethicone (Gas-X) is the most commonly used agent. Beano, which contains the enzyme alpha-galactosidase, can be taken along with foods that contain gas-producing carbohydrates. Beano neutralizes the production of gas, which is created as a by-product of bacteria that live in the intestines as foods are digested.

 Tech Note!

Psyllium is the only agent that can be used for both constipation and diarrhea because it works as a bulk-forming agent. Therefore, psyllium is often referred to as a "bowel stabilizer" and can be useful for people with diarrhea and those who cycle between episodes of diarrhea and constipation.

Miscellaneous OTC Products for Skin-Related Conditions

Several OTC agents are available to treat a variety of skin conditions (Table 27-8). Minor cuts and scrapes can be treated with topical antiinfective agents, such as Neosporin. Acne, common among teenagers, is treated primarily with benzoyl peroxide. Hives can occur as an allergic reaction and are commonly treated with antihistamines or topical hydrocortisone products. Athlete's foot and jock itch are fungal conditions that can be treated with several types of nonprescription topical antifungals, which are readily available OTC in a variety of dosage forms. Common warts can be treated effectively with salicylic acid and other topical agents.

Considerations for Special Populations

As the population ages and lives longer, the number of older adults purchasing OTC medications increases. Compared with legend drugs, more OTC drugs are available in different dosage forms, strengths, and combinations. Some older adults buy OTC medications because they lack or have inadequate insurance coverage, and they may choose the wrong medication. Often an appropriate medication is not available in OTC form. It is important for pharmacists to question all customers with a new prescription about their OTC drug and herbal use, but this is particularly important for older adults because of the number of products they often use. In some instances OTC and herbal products can interact with prescription medications (e.g., OTC NSAIDs interact with warfarin, increasing the risk of bleeding). It is important to explain to people that just because a product is available OTC does not mean it is 100% safe for everybody.

TABLE 27-8

Select Miscellaneous Topical OTC Products Used to Treat a Variety of Skin Conditions

Skin Condition	Generic Name	Trade Name	Dosage Form
Cuts/scrapes	bacitracin	Bacitracin	Ointment
	neomycin	Neomycin	Ointment
	polymyxin B sulfate, neomycin, bacitracin	Neosporin	Ointment, cream
Acne	benzoyl peroxide	Clearasil Max Strength	Cream
		Oxy 10 Cover	Cream
		Oxy 5	Lotion
		Clean & Clear	Lotion
Hives, inflammation	diphenhydramine	Benadryl	Lotion, cream
	hydrocortisone	Cortizone-10	Cream, ointment
Athlete's foot	miconazole	Lotrimin AF, Zeasorb-AF	Powder
	tolnaftate	Tinactin	Liquid, powder, aerosol, cream
	terbinafine	Lamisil	Cream, topical solution
Warts	salicylic acid	Freezone	Liquid
		Compound W	Gel, liquid
		Wart-Off	Solution

Another group of people at particular risk for receiving an inappropriate medication, the wrong dose, or the wrong drug product are infants and young children. Most products are dosed based on the age and weight of the child. However, because a parent does not need a prescription to obtain these medications, they have been used in excess many times. Problems have arisen from parents having difficulty measuring the proper dose of medicine for their child and from blatant misuse of the product. For example, diphenhydramine is often given inappropriately to help children sleep rather than for its intended purpose. In response to concerns about inappropriate use of OTC cough and cold products in children, the FDA has recommended that these products not be used to treat infants and children under 2 years of age because of serious and potentially life-threatening side effects. For use of these products in children over age 2, the FDA has established several recommendations for parents to follow.

- Check the "active ingredients" section of the Drug Facts label to make sure the product contains ingredients that treat the symptoms the child is experiencing.
- If giving more than one OTC cough and cold medicine to a child, be very careful not to duplicate the types of drugs used.
- Carefully follow the directions on the Drug Facts label.

- Use only the measuring spoons or cups that come with the medicine or those made especially for measuring drugs.
- Choose OTC cough and cold medicines with childproof safety caps, when available, and store the medicines out of reach of children.
- Understand that OTC cough and cold medicines are intended only to treat the child's symptoms.
- Do not use OTC cough and cold medicines to sedate a child or to make children sleepy.
- If any questions arise about using cough or cold medicines in children age 2 or older, call a physician, pharmacist, or other health care professional.

Restricted OTC Products

Certain drugs are kept behind the counter in the United States to regulate access to these products (Table 27-9). Although they are referred to as **behind-the-counter drugs**, they do not belong to a specific OTC "class" of drugs under FDA rules, unlike in other countries such as England and Canada. Also, under the 2005 Combat Methamphetamine Epidemic Act (see Chapter 2), any products containing pseudoephedrine must be kept behind the pharmacy counter, and information about individuals purchasing pseudoephedrine products must be logged and maintained.

TABLE 27-9

Current Medications Available Behind the Counter in the United States

Brand Name	Generic Name	Conditions
Sudafed	pseudoephedrine	Log book containing purchaser's name, address, identification, and signature; date and time of sale; and name and quantity of product sold to be maintained for at least 2 years Limited amount may be purchased for 1-day and 1-month intervals

 DO YOU REMEMBER THESE KEY POINTS?

- The most common conditions treated with OTC products
- Brand and generic names of common OTC drugs used to treat the conditions discussed in this chapter

- Regulations concerning the manufacture of OTC products as established by the FDA
- Common dosage forms and safety considerations for the OTC products discussed in this chapter

REVIEW QUESTIONS

Multiple Choice Questions

1. Because a drug is available as an OTC product, it is 100% safe and effective for all patients.
   - **A.** True
   - **B.** False

2. All of the following medications are H_2-antagonists *except*:
   - **A.** Cimetidine (Tagamet)
   - **B.** Famotidine (Pepcid)
   - **C.** Loperamide (Imodium)
   - **D.** Ranitidine (Zantac)

3. Which class of drugs is *not* available OTC for the management of GERD?
   - **A.** Proton pump inhibitors
   - **B.** H_2-receptor antagonists
   - **C.** Sucralfate
   - **D.** Antacids

4. The FDA recommends that children under the age of _____ should *not* use OTC cough and cold products.
   - **A.** 1 year
   - **B.** 2 years
   - **C.** 4 years
   - **D.** 5 years

5. Which OTC product is widely used for the primary and secondary prevention of heart attacks?
   - **A.** Acetaminophen
   - **B.** Aspirin
   - **C.** Ibuprofen
   - **D.** Nitroglycerin

6. Which drug does *not* have antiinflammatory properties?
   - **A.** Aspirin
   - **B.** Ibuprofen (Advil)
   - **C.** Acetaminophen (Tylenol)
   - **D.** Naproxen sodium (Aleve)

7. Which agent can be used to help with both constipation and diarrhea?
   - **A.** Psyllium
   - **B.** Loperamide
   - **C.** Calcium carbonate
   - **D.** Docusate

8. Which class of OTC products is commonly associated with an increase in blood pressure?
   - **A.** NSAIDs
   - **B.** Stimulant laxatives
   - **C.** Hydrocortisone cream
   - **D.** Cromolyn sodium

9. What is the generic name for the active ingredient of Prilosec OTC?
   - **A.** Pantoprazole
   - **B.** Omeprazole
   - **C.** Aripiprazole
   - **D.** Fluconazole

10. The OTC product most commonly used as an antihistamine is:
    - **A.** Aspirin
    - **B.** Ibuprofen
    - **C.** Diphenhydramine
    - **D.** Polyethelene glycol

11. What is the generic name for the active ingredient of Benadryl?
    A. Ibuprofen
    B. Doxylamine
    C. Acetaminophen
    D. Diphenhydramine
12. Which statement is true about melatonin?
    A. It is an OTC treatment for diarrhea.
    B. It is an endogenous hormone.
    C. It is an endogenous neurotransmitter.
    D. It is an OTC treatment for athlete's foot.
13. OTC agents such as Tums and Milk of Magnesia can reduce the effectiveness of:
    A. Quinolones
    B. Tetracyclines
    C. Insulin
    D. Both A and B

14. OTC ibuprofen is used for:
    A. Fever
    B. Inflammation
    C. Pain
    D. All of the above
15. What is the main ingredient in expectorant OTC medications?
    A. Guaifenesin
    B. Diphenhydramine
    C. Naphazoline
    D. None of the above

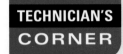

TECHNICIAN'S CORNER

Using a drug information resource, determine which OTC products contain the following:
acetaminophen
ibuprofen
aspirin
If customers are purchasing multiple OTC products containing the same product, it is always a good idea to notify the pharmacist.

Bibliography

Clinical Pharmacology Online: (Referenced August 30, 2014.) www.clinicalpharmacology-ip.com.

Consumer Healthcare Products Association. (Referenced August 30, 2014.) www.chpa-info.org.

UpToDate Online: (Referenced August 30, 2014.) www.uptodate.com.

U.S. Food and Drug Administration: Drug applications for over-the-counter drugs. (Referenced August 21, 2012). www.fda.gov/drugs/developmentapprovalapplications/over-the-counterdrugs/default.htm.

U.S. Food and Drug Administration: Now available without a prescription. (Referenced August 21, 2012). www.fda.gov/drugs/resourcesforyou/comsumers/ucm143547.htm.

U.S. Food and Drug Administration. Public Health Advisory: FDA recommends that over-the-counter (OTC) cough and cold products not be used for infants and children under 2 years of age. (Referenced August 23, 2012). www.fda.gov/drugs/drugsafety/postmarketdrugsafetyinformationforpateintsandproviders/drugsafetyinformationforhealthcareprofessionals/publichealthadvisories/ucm051137.htm.

Complementary and Alternative Medicine (CAM)

Joshua J. Neumiller

OBJECTIVES

Upon completing this chapter, you should be able to do the following:

1. Define complementary and alternative medicine (CAM) and describe CAM therapies currently in use.
2. Recognize the most common herbal products used in the United States and recognize conditions they are used to treat.
3. Understand potential risks, such as side effects and drug-herbal interactions, that can occur with herbal product use.

4. Write the common and scientific names for the herbal products discussed in this chapter.
5. Recognize other CAM practices, including those pertaining to mind and body medicine and manipulative practices.

TERMS AND DEFINITIONS

Alternative medicine Any range of medical therapies not regarded as orthodox by Western medicine

Ayurveda A holistic traditional medical system, originating in India, that emphasizes the prevention of disease

Biofeedback The use of electronic monitoring of an automatic bodily function to train someone to acquire voluntary control of that function

Chiropractic medicine Manual manipulation of the joints and muscles

Complementary medicine A range of medical therapies that fall beyond the scope of Western medicine and that may be used in a complementary fashion with traditional medicine practices

Diagnosis A physician's recognition of a condition or disease based on its outward signs and symptoms and/or confirming tests or procedures

Herb Any plant that is valued for its aromatic, medicinal, flavorful, or other properties

Homeopathy A system of therapy based on the belief that dilutions of medicinal substances that cause a specific symptom can be used to treat an illness that yields the same symptoms; homeopathic remedies are regulated by the U.S. Food and Drug Administration (FDA) under the Food, Drug, and Cosmetic Act

Prophylaxis Treatment or measure to prevent disease

Synthetic medicine A medication made in a laboratory from chemical processes

Traditional Chinese medicine CAM whole medical system including a range of traditional medicine practices originating in China

Select Common Herbal Products

Common Name	Scientific Name	Select Common Uses
Garlic	*Allium sativum*	Hypertension, hypercholesterolemia, antimicrobial
Echinacea	*Echinacea angustifolia, Echinacea pallida, Echinacea purpurea*	Immunostimulant, treatment of common cold and other respiratory infections
Saw palmetto	*Serenoa repens*	Benign prostatic hyperplasia (BPH)
Ginkgo	*Ginkgo biloba*	Dementia, peripheral vascular disease, intermittent claudication
Soy	*Glycine max*	Hyperlipidemia, menopausal symptoms, osteoporosis prevention, cardiovascular disease prevention
Cranberry	*Vaccinium macrocarpon*	Urinary tract infections (UTIs)
Ginseng	*Panax quinquefolius*	Stimulant, diabetes, digestive aid
Black cohosh	*Actaea racemosa*	Menopausal symptoms, premenstrual syndrome (PMS)
St. John's wort	*Hypericum perforatum*	Depression, anxiety
Milk thistle	*Silybum marianum*	Antioxidant, toxin-induced liver damage

This chapter presents information on complementary and alternative medicine (CAM), including the origins of various nontraditional therapies from Eastern and Western cultures. The fact is that many people use CAM in pursuit of better health. The 2007 National Health Interview Survey (NHIS) reported that approximately 38% of adults use CAM. Because the use of CAM is so prevalent, it is important to have a general understanding of these practices. A review of herbal remedies is presented, with monographs for 10 select top-selling herbal products. Common uses and known interactions of these herbs are explained.

What Is Complementary and Alternative Medicine?

Defining CAM can be difficult because the field is very broad and constantly evolving. To understand the meaning of CAM, it is useful first to define traditional medicine. Traditional medical treatment often includes the use of medication prescribed by physicians, consisting of common agents or treatments for medical conditions. This includes physician visits, possibly followed by radiographic examinations, laboratory tests, or other tests, to enable the physician to make a **diagnosis**. Traditional medicine involves the use of legend (prescription) and over-the-counter (OTC) medications. Follow-up visits aim to ensure the success of the treatment, and regular visits monitor the patient's condition.

The alternative approach might consist of visits to a practitioner of **chiropractic medicine** (chiropractor), a homeopathic physician (**homeopathy**), or other practitioner, followed by treatments used in those specific areas of study (Table 28-1). These treatments might include the use of herbs, acupuncture, acupressure, yoga, and tai chi. Many alternative approaches have been in practice for thousands of years, whereas traditional medicine has existed for only a few hundred years. Nevertheless, traditional medicine is the standard for the Western world today.

CAM, by definition, is complementary and alternative medicine. **Alternative medicine** includes a range of medical therapies not regarded as orthodox by Western medicine that are used in place of conventional medicine. **Complementary medicine** refers to the use of these same alternative therapies along with conventional medicine. An example of this would be using acupressure or acupuncture together with prescription pain medication to help control pain.

As noted previously, CAM therapies are widely used. Therefore, it is important for pharmacy technicians to understand these practices because many patients and customers use CAM. An important point for the pharmacy profession is the fact that herbal therapies are widely used and are often sold in large quantities in the pharmacy. Because CAM use is so prevalent, a division of the National Institutes of Health (NIH) is dedicated to the study of CAM. The National Center for Complementary and Alternative Medicine (NCCAM) was formed in the early 1990s with three primary goals: (1) to perform research on alternative treatments, (2) to train individuals interested in learning CAM techniques, and (3) to provide the consumer with information on the various CAM therapies available. The importance of CAM in the current medical arena is highlighted by

TABLE 28-1

Select Examples of Complementary and Alternative Medicine Treatments

Type of Treatment	Description
Acupressure	Acupressure is based on the same principles as acupuncture. Instead of using needles to unblock pathways carrying energy, the practitioner uses his or her hands to apply pressure to specific points on the body.
Acupuncture	Acupuncture is based on the meridians in the body. These lines are believed to carry energy to specific parts of the body. When they become blocked, illness or pain can occur. The practitioner relieves blocked pathways with the use of needles.
Aromatherapy	Through the sense of smell, various blends of fragrances result in relief of certain ailments. Aromatic herbs, perfumes, and oils are frequently used.
Ayurveda	Ayurveda is based on the spiritual side of the body and all that affects the body, including the environment, emotional stability, and physical health. Practitioners find ways to change what is necessary to enable the patient to be more in tune with the outside world. This includes various postures, meditation, and massage. Changing habits is a large part of this treatment.
Biofeedback	Biofeedback is a learned technique that enables self-control of various physiological responses of the body. This includes voluntary systems and involuntary systems of the body. A practitioner teaches it only until the patient is proficient in using the technique on his or her own.
Traditional Chinese medicine	Chinese medicine is based on the body spirits of the yin and yang, which are acknowledged as having similar elements, yet are different in order. Therefore, each is treated differently. Diagnosis is based on the person's dreams, tastes, sensations, smell, and other senses. Various types of treatments are used, including herbal remedies and acupuncture.
Chiropractic medicine	Chiropractic treatment is based on the belief that the realignment of the body, specifically the spine, can remedy certain conditions. Periodic adjustments usually are required to align the spine and various joints throughout the body. In this way, pressure or pain is relieved.
Herbal remedies	The medicinal purposes of herbs have been learned through historical literature and by word of mouth. Herbal therapies are available for the treatment of a variety of ailments and are frequently sold in pharmacies and health food stores. Physicians and other health care providers often recommend herbal therapies; herbals are a common component of complementary medicine.
Homeopathy	Homeopathy is the traditional belief that "like cures like." Various types of toxins are mixed in extreme dilutions to the point where they are often undetectable by scientific means. This minute amount of "toxin" from which the patient is suffering allows the patient's body to fight the illness.

the fact that more than half of the medical schools in the United States currently offer classes on CAM, which can include courses on dietary supplement therapy (e.g., vitamins and minerals), herbal medicine, acupuncture, and homeopathy.

Types of CAM

As discussed previously, CAM is constantly changing and adapting; as a result, many types of CAM have become available. The NCCAM website is a great resource for researching these therapies. This chapter briefly reviews some of the more common CAM practices, but it is by no means a comprehensive review. Although there are no formal CAM categories, many resources, including NCCAM, group CAM practices into broad categories. In this chapter, CAM practices that fall in the following broad categories are discussed: natural products, mind and body medicine, and manipulative practices. Although these categories are not formally defined (and some CAM may fit into more than one category), they are useful for discussing the various types of CAM.

Natural Products

Natural products constitute a broad category of CAM that includes the use of **herbs** (herbal remedies), vitamins, minerals, and other natural products, such as probiotics. Although by this definition the use of vitamins is considered CAM, the use of daily multivitamins and other such supplementation generally is not considered CAM. The use of herbal products is one of the most common forms of CAM. According to the 2007 NHIS, nearly 18% of adults in the United States take a nonvitamin and nonmineral natural product. Accordingly, this section focuses on herbal remedies and includes a discussion of 10 select, commonly used herbal products.

TABLE 28-2

Common Uses and Cautionary Notes for Select Herbal Products

Herb	Species	Uses	Cautions
Black cohosh	*Cimicifuga racemosa**	Menopause, premenstrual syndrome	• Should not be used if pregnant. • May cause liver toxicity.
Chamomile	*Matricaria recutita**	Gastrointestinal upset, skin conditions	• Should not be used if pregnant. • Safe if used in small quantities and short term.
Garlic	*Allium sativum*	Antiinfective, antibiotic	• Safe if used in small quantities.
Ginkgo	*Ginkgo biloba*	Increases circulation	• Should not be used if pregnant.
Ginseng	*Panax quinquefolius*	Stress relief	• Safe if used in small quantities.
Milk thistle	*Silybum marianum*	Common cold	• Studies are not complete because of the many different species and parts of herbaceous plant used.
St. John's wort	*Hypericum perforatum*	Antidepressant	• Safe if used in small quantities.

*Various species are used; some side effects may differ, depending on the species.

 Tech Note!
Herbal medicines account for some of the first attempts to improve human health. The mummified prehistoric "ice man" discovered in the Italian Alps in 1991 was found to be in possession of medicinal herbs!

Herbal Products

Although herbal remedies have been in existence for thousands of years, herbal therapies have gained increasing popularity in recent years. The herbal remedy market is expected to grow even more in the coming years because of many factors, such as the increasing age of the population and the rising costs associated with traditional health care and medications. Because many herbals are sold in the pharmacy, it is important for technicians to familiarize themselves with the most popular herbal products on the market (Table 28-2). Many people do not report herbal use to their health care providers. These patients believe it is not important because herbal products are "natural" and therefore not harmful. However, many reports of harmful interactions between natural products, legend drugs, and OTC medications have been documented (Table 28-3).

Many of the drugs used in traditional medicine today are medications originally derived from plant sources. Chemicals that have undergone efficacy and safety testing for the treatment of certain medical conditions or ailments are often then manufactured as **synthetic medicines** in a laboratory. For this reason, most Western medicine discovered from plants does not incorporate the whole plant or even part of the plant. Although herbs and herbal supplements are subjected to regulations enforced by the U.S. Food and Drug Administration (FDA), they are not regulated in the same way as drugs because they are considered dietary supplements. (See Chapter 27 for a discussion of OTC and dietary supplement regulation.)

Because many herbs have been used in different cultures for thousands of years, they often have many different names. For example, Echinacea is also known as black sampson, sampson root, narrow-leafed purple coneflower, and red sunflower. A knowledge of the family name of the herb is important in case of possible unwanted interactions or reactions. For instance, if someone is allergic to an herbal product, then any herbal drug from the same family may cause an allergic response. Knowing the species of the herb is also important because species can vary even if they are closely related. Some studies have been completed on only one of many species of herbs used to prepare herbal supplements. Several herbal textbooks can be referenced to determine the family of an herb. Another great reference for herbal product information is the Natural Medicines Comprehensive Database.

Garlic. Oral garlic (Figure 28-1) is used for its antihyperlipidemic, antihypertensive, and antifungal effects. However, the level of evidence supporting the use of garlic for all the conditions it is used to treat varies considerably. Garlic is considered safe when used orally at appropriate doses; it was used safely in clinical studies lasting up to 7 years without reports of significant toxicity.

Scientific Name: Allium sativum

Also Known As: Ail, Ajo, Da Suan, Lasuna, Rason, stinking rose

TABLE 28-3

Select Examples of Herb-Drug Interactions

Herbal Drug	Drug	Potential Interaction
Black cohosh	Estrogens, esterified	May increase estrogen activity.
Echinacea	Ketoconazole	May have additive hepatoxic effects.
	Tacrolimus	May decrease effects of tacrolimus.
Garlic	Chlorzoxazone	May decrease effectiveness of chlorzoxazone.
	Nimodipine	May increase antihypertensive effect.
	Quinapril	May increase antihypertensive effect.
	Reserpine	May increase antihypertensive effects.
	Terazosin	May decrease effects of terazosin.
Ginkgo biloba	NSAIDs	May increase risk of bleeding.
	Chlorothiazide	May increase blood pressure.
	Clopidogrel	May increase risk of bleeding.
	Ethosuximide	May decrease effectiveness of ethosuximide blood concentrations.
	Imipramine	May decrease seizure threshold.
	Warfarin	May increase risk of bleeding.
Ginseng	Digoxin	May increase serum digoxin levels.
	Estrogen, esterified	May increase hormonal effects.
	Nimodipine	May worsen hypertension.
	Oxymorphone	May decrease opioid analgesic effectiveness.
	Quinapril	May worsen hypertension.
	Terazosin	May decrease effectiveness of terazosin.
	Warfarin	May decrease effectiveness of warfarin.
St. John's wort	Amoxapine	May increase risk of serotonin syndrome.
	Chlorpropamide	May increase risk of hypoglycemia.
	Cyclosporine	May decrease cyclosporine effectiveness.
	Dapsone	May decrease dapsone blood concentration.
	Desipramine	May increase desipramine's pharmacological effects and risk of toxicity.
	Duloxetine	May increase adverse effects.
	Estrogen, esterified	May decrease levels of esterified estrogens.
	Fluoxetine	May increase fluoxetine's pharmacological effects and risk of toxicity.
	Imipramine	May increase imipramine's pharmacological effects and risk of toxicity.
	Lamivudine and many antiviral drugs for HIV	May decrease blood concentration and effectiveness in treating HIV.
	Methocarbamol	May increase CNS depression.
	Oxytetracycline	May increase risk of photosensitivity.
	Paroxetine	May increase paroxetine's pharmacological effects and risk of toxicity.
	Piroxicam	May increase risk of phototoxicity.
	Quinine	May decrease quinine levels.
	Reserpine	May increase CNS depression.
	Sulfisoxazole	May cause photosensitization.
	Theophylline	May decrease metabolism of theophylline.
	Venlafaxine	May increase sedative effect of venlafaxine.
	Warfarin	May decrease the effects of warfarin.
	Yohimbine	May increase blood pressure and risk of hypertensive crises.

CNS, Central nervous system; *HIV,* human immunodeficiency virus; *NSAIDs,* nonsteroidal antiinflammatory drugs.

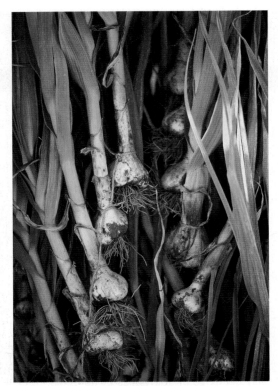

FIGURE 28-1 Garlic. (Courtesy Martin Wall Photography, 2011.)

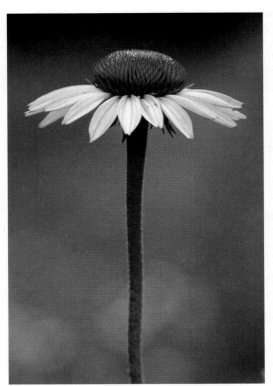

FIGURE 28-2 Purple coneflower. (Courtesy Martin Wall Photography, 2011.)

Possibly Effective to Treat: Atherosclerosis, hypertension, ringworm (garlic gel), athlete's foot (garlic gel)

Potential Side Effects: Gastrointestinal (GI) irritation, heartburn, flatulence, nausea, vomiting, breath and body odor

Echinacea. Echinacea, often also referred to as purple coneflower (Figure 28-2), is commonly used orally for treating and preventing the common cold and other upper respiratory conditions. Echinacea, which is well characterized as an immunostimulant, is also used to treat a variety of other infections. This herb is considered safe when used orally at appropriate doses in the short term. Although studies lasting up to 12 weeks have demonstrated safety with several formulations of Echinacea, safety data for long-term use is lacking.

Scientific Names: Echinacea angustifolia, Echinacea pallida, Echinacea purpurea

Also Known As: Purple coneflower, American coneflower, comb flower, red sunflower, snakeroot

Possibly Effective to Treat: Common cold, vaginal candidiasis

Potential Side Effects: Nausea, diarrhea, heartburn, headache, dizziness, insomnia

Saw Palmetto. Saw palmetto (Figure 28-3) is widely used as an herbal treatment for benign prostatic hyperplasia (BPH) but is also used orally as a mild diuretic, sedative, antiseptic, and antiinflammatory agent. It is the ripe fruit of the plant that is

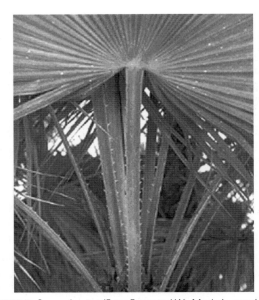

FIGURE 28-3 Saw palmetto. (From Freeman LW: *Mosby's complementary and alternative medicine: a research-based approach*, ed 3, St Louis, 2009, Mosby.)

used medicinally. Saw palmetto has been used safely in clinical studies lasting up to 1 year, but it is considered unsafe to use during pregnancy because of its hormonal activity.

Scientific Names: Serenoa repens, Serenoa serrulata, Sabal serrulata

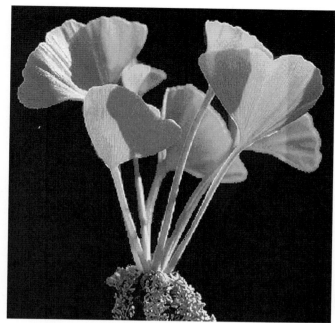

FIGURE 28-4 Ginkgo biloba. (From Freeman LW: *Mosby's complementary and alternative medicine: a research-based approach,* ed 3, St Louis, 2009, Mosby.)

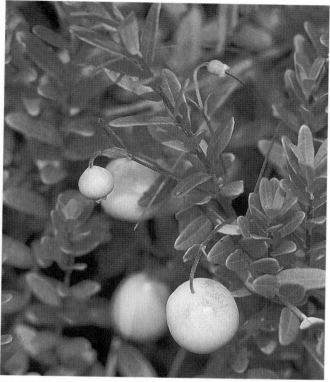

FIGURE 28-5 Cranberry. (From Freeman LW: *Mosby's complementary and alternative medicine: a research-based approach,* ed 3, St Louis, 2009, Mosby.)

Also Known As: American dwarf palm tree, cabbage palm, Ju-Zhong, Sabal, Sabal Fructus, saw palmetto berry

Possibly Effective to Treat: BPH

Potential Side Effects: Dizziness, headache, nausea, constipation, diarrhea

Ginkgo Biloba. Ginkgo biloba, also known as ginkgo, is widely used for conditions of the memory, such as Alzheimer's disease and vascular dementia (Figure 28-4). The applicable parts of ginkgo are the leaf and the seed; an extract made from the ginkgo leaf is the most common form used. Standardized extracts have been used safely in clinical trials lasting several weeks to 6 years.

Scientific Name: Ginkgo biloba

Also Known As: Fossil tree, ginkgo folium, Japanese silver apricot, kew tree, maidenhair tree, Yinhsing

Possibly Effective to Treat: Age-related memory impairment, dementia, diabetic retinopathy, glaucoma, peripheral vascular disease (PVD), premenstrual syndrome (PMS), Raynaud's syndrome, vertigo

Potential Side Effects: Headache, dizziness, palpitations, constipation, rash

Soy. Soy is widely used as a milk substitute in food products for individuals with lactose intolerance and in infant feeding formulas. As an oral herbal product, soy is used for a variety of conditions ranging from high cholesterol to prevention of cardiovascular disease. Soy products in doses up to 60 g per day have been safely used in studies lasting up to 16 weeks.

Scientific Name: Glycine max

Also Known As: Isoflavones, isolated soy protein, plant estrogen, soybean, soy isoflavone, soy fiber, soy protein isolate, texturized vegetable protein

Possibly Effective to Treat: Diabetes, nephropathy, diarrhea, hyperlipidemia, menopausal symptoms, osteoporosis

Potential Side Effects: Constipation, diarrhea, bloating, nausea

Cranberry. The cranberry fruit (Figure 28-5) is most widely used for the treatment and/or prevention of urinary tract infections (UTIs). Cranberry can be taken as a juice product (e.g., Ocean Spray cranberry juice cocktail) or as cranberry capsules. Cranberry juice is widely used as a beverage, and the use of cranberry is considered quite safe.

Scientific Name: Vaccinium macrocarpon

Also Known As: Agrio, craneberry, Da Guo Yue Jie, Tsuru-Kokemomo

Possibly Effective to Treat: UTIs

Potential Side Effects: GI upset and diarrhea with very large doses (3 to 4 L of juice per day)

Ginseng. Ginseng root is used for a variety of conditions, such as diabetes, respiratory tract infections, and even attention deficit/hyperactivity disorder (ADHD). Additionally, ginseng often is used for overall wellness and as an antiinflammatory.

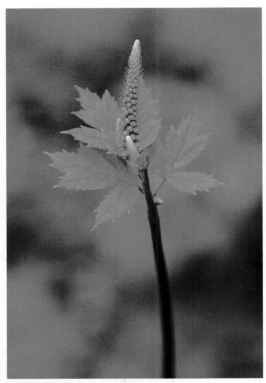

FIGURE 28-6 Black cohosh. (Courtesy Martin Wall Photography, 2011.)

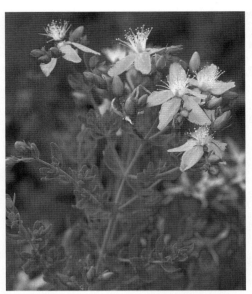

FIGURE 28-7 St. John's wort. (From Freeman LW: *Mosby's complementary and alternative medicine: a research-based approach,* ed 3, St Louis, 2009, Mosby.)

Scientific Name: Panax quinquefolius

Also Known As: Red berry, Ren Shen, Sang, Shang, Shi Yang Seng, Xi Yang Shen

Possibly Effective to Treat: Diabetes, respiratory tract infections

Potential Side Effects: Headache, insomnia, GI discomfort

Black Cohosh. Black cohosh (Figure 28-6), is used primarily for hot flashes associated with menopause. Although short-term studies have concluded that black cohosh is safe, some studies have shown that liver toxicity may occur; therefore, a cautionary statement must be included on the label of this agent. Black cohosh must not be confused with herbs with similar-sounding names, such as blue and white cohosh. These are not used for the same purpose and have different interactions with other medications.

Scientific Name: Actaea racemosa

Also Known As: Black snakeroot, bugbane, bugwort, cohosh negro, phytoestrogen, rattle root, rattle weed, Sheng Ma, squaw root

Possibly Effective to Treat: Menopausal symptoms

Potential Side Effects: GI upset, rash, headache, dizziness, weight gain, breast tenderness

St. John's Wort. St. John's wort (Figure 28-7) is frequently used for neuropsychiatric conditions such as depression and anxiety. The parts of the plant that are used are the flowers and leaves. Interestingly, several active constituents have been isolated from St. John's wort, including melatonin. St. John's wort is believed to have serotonergic effects, which may account for its beneficial effects for depression and anxiety.

Scientific Name: Hypericum perforatum

Also Known As: Goatweed, hard hay, *Hypericum,* Klamath weed, Saynt Johannes wort, Tipton weed

Likely Effective to Treat: Depression

Possibly Effective to Treat: Menopausal symptoms, wound healing

Potential Side Effects: Insomnia, vivid dreams, restlessness, GI discomfort, dizziness, headache

Milk Thistle. The milk thistle seed is the most commonly used part of the plant. One of the most common reasons people take milk thistle is for toxic liver damage caused by chemicals. It also has been used intravenously for the treatment of mushroom poisoning. Preliminary clinical research suggests that milk thistle may be beneficial in improving liver function in people with alcoholic liver disease; however, this has yet to be proven.

Scientific Name: Silybum marianum

Also Known As: Holy thistle, lady's thistle, Marian thistle, silibinin, *Silybum,* silymarin, St. Mary thistle

Possibly Effective to Treat: Allergic rhinitis, diabetes, dyspepsia

Potential Side Effects: Diarrhea, nausea, flatulence, bloating, anorexia

Herbal Preparations

How herbs are prepared can determine the strength of the active ingredients. Herbs that are brewed for teas are usually more potent than those prepared in capsule form. Teas can be prepared by various methods. *Infusions* are made by pouring hot water onto herbs and letting them steep for several minutes;

TABLE 28-4

Examples of Various Herbal Preparations

Dosage Form	Route of Administration	Ingredients	Use, Strength, Onset of Action
Syrups, diluted; tinctures	Internal	Alcohol, glycerin	Usually a potent form.
Tablets, capsules	Internal	Powdered	Slower to act; broken down in the stomach.
Teas	Internal	Syrups, sweeteners	May be better tasting with sweeteners added; teas may be stronger than tablets or capsules.
Aromatic solutions, baths	External	Scented water	Used to treat skin conditions and burns.
Oils	External	Extracted oil from herbs	Used for sore muscles and skin conditions.
Compresses, salves	External	Compresses made from teas, salves from herbal oils	For compresses, a cloth soaked in herbal tea is applied to skin site; used for conditions such as bruises and cramps.

decoctions are produced by simmering herbs in water for 15 to 20 minutes; and *cold infusions* are made by allowing herbs to soak in cold water over many hours. Various methods are used, depending on the type of herb being prepared (Table 28-4). As noted previously, some medical schools are including studies of herbal remedies and their preparation because of their prevalence and possible benefits when used in combination with traditional medicine.

 Tech Note!

As the popularity of alternative therapies increases, the medical community must meet the responsibility of staying up-to-date with information about such therapies. Increased use of herbal remedies may have a great impact on medication interactions because herbal remedies have a direct effect on other drugs prescribed or purchased over the counter. The pharmacy technician must know the most common interactions between common herbal remedies and legend drugs. In this way, the technician is able to assist the pharmacist in identifying individuals who may want or need counseling.

Mind and Body Medicine

Mind and body CAM practices are based on the interactions between the brain, mind, body, and behavior. The intent of these CAM practices is to use the power of the mind to positively affect physical function and health. A variety of forms of CAM fall into this category; specific information on meditation, yoga, acupuncture, and acupressure is provided in the following sections.

 Tech Note!

Hippocrates, widely referred to as the father of Western medicine, noted the moral and spiritual aspects of healing. He believed that attitude, environmental factors, and natural remedies all were integral components of medical treatment.

Meditation

Meditation is a well-known mind-body form of CAM that has many types and variations. Most forms of meditation originated in ancient religious and spiritual traditions. To practice meditation, the individual learns to focus his or her attention to achieve a state of greater calmness, psychological balance, and physical relaxation.

Yoga

Yoga is a form of mind-body practice that originated in ancient Indian philosophy (Figure 28-8). A variety of styles of yoga has evolved. Yoga often is used to maintain physical health and flexibility, and it incorporates elements of physical posturing, breathing techniques, and meditation. The 2007 NHIS identified yoga as one of the top 10 complementary health practices used by adults in the United States; approximately 6% of respondents reported using yoga for health purposes in the previous 12 months. Hatha yoga is the most commonly practiced form of yoga in the United States and Europe. Hatha yoga incorporates the use of postures *(asanas)* and breathing exercises *(pranayama)*. Because yoga can help maintain flexibility, posture, and balance, it is used by

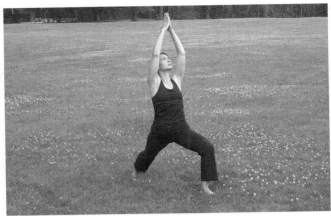

FIGURE 28-8 Standing pose for alignment and balance. (From Deutsch JE, Anderson EZ: *Complementary therapies for physical therapy: a clinical decision-making approach*, Philadelphia, 2008, Saunders.)

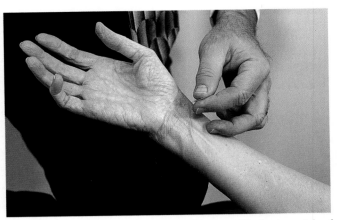

FIGURE 28-9 Acupuncture. (From Potter PA, Perry AG: *Fundamentals of nursing*, ed 8, St Louis, 2013, Mosby.)

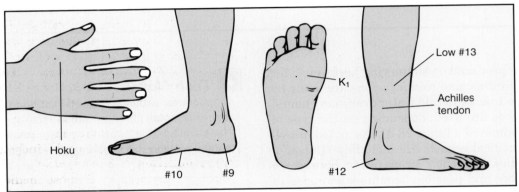

FIGURE 28-10 Acupressure points. (From Potter PA, Perry AG: *Fundamentals of nursing*, ed 8, St Louis, 2013, Mosby.)

people with a variety of health conditions associated with aging.

Acupuncture

Acupuncture has been used for thousands of years, and extensive studies have been done in the Eastern and Western worlds. Acupuncture is used as a complementary treatment for conditions such as chronic pain, depression, addiction, and other ailments. It is based on the Chinese belief that the body is composed of energy channels. When these channels become blocked, sickness may result. The use of needles at specific points throughout the body is thought to release these channels, bringing the body into harmony once again (Figure 28-9).

Acupressure

Acupressure is closely related to acupuncture because it also uses specific energy points across the body. Instead of using needles, pressure is applied by hand to the specific point to unblock the channels (Figure 28-10). Insurance companies are beginning to pay for acupuncture and acupressure treatment if

recommended by a physician for the treatment of pain. Acupressure classes are available, in which a person can learn how to perform the technique on his or her own body.

Manipulative and Body-Based Practices

Manipulative and body-based CAM practices focus on alignment and proper functioning of various structures and systems of the body. Such structures and systems that may be the focus of these forms of CAM are the bones and joints, soft tissue, circulatory system, and lymphatic systems. The two most common forms of CAM that fall in this category include spinal manipulation and massage therapy.

 Tech Note!

Spinal manipulation has been dated back to the ancient Greeks. Massage therapy dates back thousands of years and has been referenced in ancient writings originating from China, Japan, India, Egypt, Greece, and Rome.

Spinal Manipulation

Chiropractic therapy is an orthopedic approach to treating pain resulting from misalignment of the bones and joints. Certain changes in the skeletal structure are believed to interfere with the nervous system and other organ systems. The treatment given to a patient by a chiropractic physician is referred to as *manipulation*. Treatment can include hands-on adjustments of the spine or joints and application of massage and heat therapy. Research has proved that some forms of manipulation can be helpful, specifically manipulation of the lower back. Although use of chiropractic therapy is increasing, various forms of treatment are controversial. Some physicians promote the use of manipulation of certain parts of the skeletal structure, whereas other physicians believe it may be harmful. Skepticism about the ability of manipulation to treat many common illnesses abounds, and studies are being conducted to determine exactly which therapy works and why it is effective. Practitioners must attend an accredited school to attain the degree Doctor of Chiropractic (DC). Many insurance companies cover chiropractic treatment based on physician referrals.

Massage Therapy

Massage therapy encompasses a large variety of different techniques. It generally involves use of the hands and fingers, but the practitioner may also use his or her forearms, elbows, or feet (Figure 28-11). Massage is used to manipulate muscles and other soft tissues of the body. It is used for a variety of health-related purposes, such as to relieve pain, rehabilitate physical injuries, induce relaxation, and reduce anxiety and stress. As for spinal manipula-tion, insurance plans often cover massage therapy, particularly for musculoskeletal conditions, with a proper medical referral.

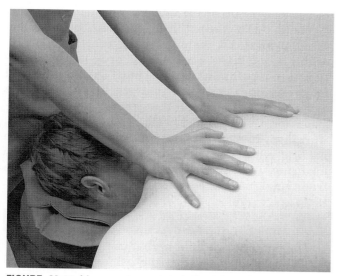

FIGURE 28-11 Massage is most typically delivered with the hands, although the forearms, elbows, or feet also may be used. (From Freeman LW: *Mosby's complementary and alternative medicine: a research-based approach*, ed 3, St Louis, 2009, Mosby.)

Other CAM Practices

In addition to the small sample of CAM practices briefly described in this chapter, a multitude of CAM therapies is available. Whole medical systems, which are complete systems of medical theory and practice, such as **traditional Chinese medicine** and **ayurveda**, are also considered CAM. Traditional Chinese medicine has been a well-known art based on more than 4000 years of trial and error. Although herbal remedies might come to mind readily when the topic of Chinese medicine is discussed, it involves much more than the use of herbs. The heart of Chinese practice is yin and yang, which represent male and female entities, respectively. The ancient Chinese belief contends that although men and women are made of the same substances, their spirits are different; therefore, appropriate treatment is different. Practitioners conduct examinations by asking the patient about dreams, strange tastes, or smells experienced. Also, a visual examination of the skin and voice tone is performed. Once the diagnosis is complete, the practitioner may prescribe the necessary treatment, which could include a variety of herbs, minerals, and/or vegetables. Herbs and other remedies are used in Chinese medicine to cure the body of the original illness and for disease **prophylaxis**. Chinese medicine is still in use today; many health care providers, including pharmacists, take classes based on Chinese knowledge of herbs and their medicinal uses.

Ayurveda is an ancient Indian approach to medicine that is still practiced today. Dating back thousands of years, ayurveda is based on the person knowing and understanding the spiritual self. This knowledge encompasses the body and all that affects it. With insight into the various effects of outside influences on the body's spirit, it is possible to make assumptions. A person can predict whether something will have a positive effect or a negative effect on the body. For example, certain colors, sounds, clothing, and other environmental stimuli are taken into consideration. The types of foods and herbs consumed also play a role in the overall health of the individual. These assumptions are then applied to physical and spiritual activities. Based on the individual's personality type, practitioners suggest ways to alter the diet and/or lifestyle to cure and prevent illnesses. This type of treatment is practiced today in many parts of the world. Medical schools teaching this approach are located in India. Courses in Indian medicine are also offered in various medical schools in the United States.

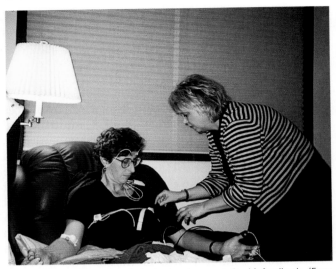

FIGURE 28-12 Example of electrode placement for biofeedback. (From Potter PA, Perry AG: *Fundamentals of nursing*, ed 8, St Louis, 2013, Elsevier.)

Biofeedback is another form of CAM that is used for treatment of stress, hypertension, and other conditions. Biofeedback uses the patient's mental ability to alter his or her own vital signs, such as blood pressure, heart rate, and even gastrointestinal activity. The body is divided into two types of movement, voluntary and involuntary. Voluntary movements include the musculoskeletal system and involve purposeful actions such as walking, sitting, standing, and bending. People have control over these functions daily; therefore, adjusting behavior does not take much conscious effort. With biofeedback, a person is taught how to mentally access and alter involuntary body functions, such as heartbeat, breathing, and digestion. These functions do not normally require conscious thought. Biofeedback usually is taught by an instructor who uses electrical leads that provide a readout of data. Patients are connected to monitors that allow them to see what their bodies are experiencing (Figure 28-12). For example, the instructor might have the patient alter the heart rate to a certain level through concentration. Gradually, the person is able to adjust body functions as needed without the use of a monitor. Biofeedback is a way of connecting the mind to the body. Patients need to practice these techniques frequently to achieve their full benefit. Biofeedback can be used as an alternative to or in addition to medication for conditions such as anxiety, low back pain, neuromuscular dysfunction, and tension headaches. Biofeedback therapy is partially reimbursed by many insurance companies with a physician's approval. Once the technique of biofeedback has been perfected, it can be done at any time without supervision.

The term *homeopathy*, translated from Greek, simply means "like suffering." The premise of homeopathy is the belief that "like cures like." Homeopathy is also sometimes referred to as the law of similars. The belief is that consuming a small amount of the substance that caused a person's disease or condition enables the body to fight the disease. Homeopathy became well known in the late 1700s through the efforts of Samuel Hahnemann, a German physician. After ingesting a small amount of quinine, he exhibited symptoms of malaria, the disease that quinine cured. Over time he perfected the necessary minute amount of quinine that was needed to instigate a cure rather than illness. Homeopathy was first used in the United States in the 1800s and became a popular treatment. Although homeopathy has remained a well-accepted form of treatment in parts of Europe, it is generally considered an alternative treatment in the United States.

Thousands of homeopathic remedies are available, but only one remedy is correct for each illness; therefore, homeopathic physicians must know what will work for the patient. Unlike with herbs and other alternative treatments, the FDA oversees the manufacture of homeopathic drugs. Under FDA guidelines, a homeopathic drug must meet standards for strength, quality, purity, and other parameters established in the *Homeopathic Pharmacopeia*, which contains monographs on ingredients used in homeopathic medicine. All homeopathic agents must be manufactured using good manufacturing practices (GMP). Additionally, if the homeopathic drug is a prescription, it must contain the same label as that indicated for prescription drugs. If sold over the counter, the agent must comply with the general labeling provisions for OTC products (e.g., indications for use, warnings, and directions for use). Although more medical schools are offering classes on homeopathic medicine, it is still somewhat controversial in the traditional medical community.

DO YOU REMEMBER THESE KEY POINTS?

- The definition of complementary and alternative medicine (CAM) and examples of CAM therapies currently in use
- The most common herbal products used in the United States and the conditions they are most commonly used to treat

- The potential risks of herbal use
- The common and scientific names for the herbal products discussed in this chapter

REVIEW QUESTIONS

Multiple Choice Questions

1. Homeopathy is known as the law of similars, which can be best described as:
   - A. Taking a similar drug that works but at a much reduced cost
   - B. Taking a drug that is similar to legend drugs but does not require a prescription
   - C. Taking a drug that causes the same illness as the one you are trying to cure
   - D. Taking a drug that causes a similar reaction to traditional agents

2. *Silybum marianum* is known commonly as _____ and is used most commonly to treat _____.
   - A. Ginger, motion sickness
   - B. St. John's wort, depression
   - C. Milk thistle, liver conditions
   - D. Garlic, infections

3. Which herbal product is commonly used to treat depression?
   - A. Echinacea
   - B. Ginkgo biloba
   - C. St. John's wort
   - D. Milk thistle

4. Which herbal product is used to treat menopausal symptoms?
   - A. Saw palmetto
   - B. Ginkgo biloba
   - C. St. John's wort
   - D. Black cohosh

5. Which herbal product is used to treat conditions associated with impaired memory?
   - A. Saw palmetto
   - B. Ginkgo biloba
   - C. Soy
   - D. Black cohosh

6. Which herbal product is commonly used to treat the symptoms of BPH?
   - A. Saw palmetto
   - B. Ginkgo biloba
   - C. Soy
   - D. Milk thistle

7. Which herbal product is commonly taken to help treat and prevent urinary tract infections (UTIs)?
   - A. Ginkgo biloba
   - B. St. John's wort
   - C. Cranberry
   - D. Garlic

8. Which herbal product is commonly used as an immunostimulant to prevent the common cold?
   - A. Echinacea
   - B. Ginkgo biloba
   - C. Black cohosh
   - D. Milk thistle

9. _____ is closely related to acupuncture, but uses pressure instead of needles to unblock energy channels.
   - A. Massage therapy
   - B. Acupressure
   - C. Biofeedback
   - D. Yoga

10. The one drug classification that has unwanted interactions with many herbal drugs is:
   - A. Antiulcer agents
   - B. Anticoagulants
   - C. Vitamins
   - D. Analgesics

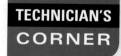
TECHNICIAN'S CORNER

Using an appropriate drug/herbal medication reference, research the typical uses, preparations, and potential side effects of the following herbal products not specifically discussed in this chapter:
- Melatonin
- Valerian
- Kava kava

Bibliography

Clinical Pharmacology Online. (Referenced August 30, 2014.) www.clinicalpharmacology-ip.com.

Deutsch JE, Anderson EZ: *Complementary therapies for physical therapy: a clinical decision making approach*, Philadelphia, 2008, Saunders.

Freeman LW: *Mosby's complementary and alternative medicine: a research-based approach*, ed 3, 2009, Mosby.

National Center for Complementary and Alternative Medicine (NCCAM), National Institutes of Health: (Referenced August 30, 2014.) http://nccam.nih.gov

Natural Medicines Comprehensive Database: (Referenced August 30, 2014.) www.naturalmedicinesdatabase.com.

Potter P, Perry A: *Fundamentals of nursing*, ed 8, St Louis, 2013, Mosby.

Skidmore L: *Mosby's handbook of herbs and natural supplements*, ed 4, Philadelphia, 2010, Elsevier.

UpToDate Online. (Referenced August 30, 2014.) www.uptodate.com.

Review for the Pharmacy Certification Board (PTCB) Examination

In 1995, the Pharmacy Certification Board (PTCB) was created to develop a voluntary pharmacy technician certification program that would be nationally recognized. The PTCB developed an exam that allowed pharmacy technicians to show that they had the skills and knowledge to perform their jobs correctly. This exam was named the Pharmacy Technician Certification Exam (PTCE). The PTCE is a computer-based, closed-book exam administered at Pearson VUE test centers nationwide. It consists of a total of 90 questions, 10 of which are not scored. The 10 unscored questions are used to provide information for future exams. The questions are written to assess the knowledge and skills deemed necessary to perform the work of the pharmacy technician. The PTCE assesses knowledge based on nine knowledge domains: (1) Pharmacology for Technicians (which constitutes 13.75% of the PTCE); (2) Pharmacy Law and Regulations (which constitutes 12.5% of the PTCE); (3) Sterile and Non-sterile Compounding (which constitutes 8.75% of the PTCE); (4) Medication Safety (which constitutes 12.5% of the PTCE); (5) Pharmacy Quality Assurance (which constitutes 7.5% of the PTCE); (6) Medication Order Entry and Fill Process (which constitutes 17.5% of the PTCE); (7) Pharmacy Inventory Management (which constitutes 8.75% of the PTCE); (8) Pharmacy Billing and Reimbursement (which constitutes 8.75% of the PTCE); and (9) Pharmacy Information Systems Usage and Application (which constitutes 10% of the PTCE). Candidates must meet certain criteria to sit for this exam; they must have a high school diploma or a graduate equivalency diploma (GED), and they must submit the appropriate application form, fee, and supporting documents. If a candidate has been convicted of a drug- or pharmacy-related felony or has had any felony convictions during the 5 years before applying for the PTCE, he or she would not qualify to take the exam.

In 2005 the Institute for the Certification of Pharmacy Technicians (ICPT) began offering a similar exam, known as the Exam for the Certification of Pharmacy Technicians (ExCPT). This is an on-demand, computer-based, timed exam that lasts 2 hours and 10 minutes. It consists of 120 multiple choice questions, 20 of which are pretested for possible use on future exams. The questions on the ExCPT are categorized into three areas: Regulations and Technician Duties (25%), Drugs and Therapy (23%), and Dispensing Process (52%).

To maintain both of these certificates, the pharmacy technician must recertify every 2 years by completing 20 hours of continuing education, including at least 1 hour related to pharmacy law.

The following practice examination consists of 90 questions that represent the same topics and proportions as those found on the PTCB exam.

1. Which of the following is the DEA number for Dr. James Stephens?
   A. BS8293501
   B. BS5836727
   C. BJ5836727
   D. BJS8293501
2. A prescriber calls in for a refill for Lyrica; which medication is to be refilled?
   A. Propranolol
   B. Gabapentin
   C. Pregabalin
   D. Prednisone
3. How would the label for an albuterol inhaler read with the directions of 1 puff q4-6h prn SOB?
   A. Spray 1 puff 4-6 times a day per nostril for shortness of breath.
   B. Inhale 1 puff every 4-6 hours per nostril for shortness of breath.
   C. Spray 1 puff 4 times a day as needed for shortness of breath.
   D. Inhale 1 puff every 4-6 hours as needed for shortness of breath.

4. Which of the following OTC medications is sold behind the counter, and only a controlled amount can be purchased per month?
   A. Allegra-D
   B. Robitussin DM
   C. Zyrtec
   D. Benadryl

5. Which of the following is a Schedule II medication?
   A. Tylenol #3
   B. Ambien
   C. Codeine
   D. Xanax

6. Which of the following has no accepted medical use in the United States?
   A. Schedule I
   B. Schedule II
   C. Schedule III
   D. Schedule IV

7. If an order is written for vancomycin 1500 mg q4h, how much vancomycin will the patient receive in a 24-hour period?
   A. 1.5 g
   B. 3 g
   C. 6 g
   D. 9 g

8. How may 1-L bags should be sent to the unit to last a patient 24 hours if the infusion is ordered to be given at a rate of 150 mL/hr?
   A. 1
   B. 2
   C. 3
   D. 4

9. Which of the following is an antihistamine?
   A. Lorazepam
   B. Loratadine
   C. Lopressor
   D. Levothyroxine

10. Schedule III medications are refilled:
    A. As needed for a year
    B. Every 30 days for a year
    C. Up to 5 times in a 6-month period
    D. Up to 6 times per year

11. Androderm is available in which dosage form?
    A. Injection
    B. Topical patch
    C. Topical lotion
    D. Oral tablets

12. An order is sent to the pharmacy for 40 mEq of KCl. You have a vial with a concentration of 2 mEq/mL. What volume of KCl is needed to fill the order?
    A. 80 mL
    B. 60 mL
    C. 40 mL
    D. 20 mL

13. How many doses of cefazolin 2 g are available in a bulk vial of 10 g cefazolin?
    A. 1 dose
    B. 2 doses
    C. 5 doses
    D. 10 doses

14. A prescription is written for amoxicillin 250 mg/5 mL, 1 tsp tid for 10 days. What size bottle is to be given to fulfill the prescription?
    A. 150 mL
    B. 50 mL
    C. 75 mL
    D. 200 mL

15. If a prescription is written for Keflex 250 mg suspension qid for 7 days, what size bottle is to be given if Keflex 500 mg/5 mL is available?
    A. 50 mL
    B. 75 mL
    C. 100 mL
    D. 150 mL

16. Erythromycin eye drops are ordered to be given 1 gtt ou bid prn. What is the correct size bottle to be given to fill a prescription for a 30-day supply?
    A. 5 mL
    B. 20 mL
    C. 25 mL
    D. 30 mL

17. Which volume of the *United States Pharmacopeia* would a pharmacist use to look up a specific law affecting pharmacy practice?
    A. Volume I
    B. Volume II
    C. Volume III
    D. Volume IV

18. The last two digits of an NDC number represent:
    A. Drug
    B. Manufacturer
    C. Quantity
    D. Dose

19. The technician is asked to measure out 1.5 mL; what size syringe should be used for best accuracy?
    A. 1 mL
    B. 3 mL
    C. 5 mL
    D. 10 mL

20. A patient calls in for a refill of his hypertension medicine; which of the following should be refilled?
    A. Lyrica
    B. Zyrtec
    C. Lipitor
    D. Lopressor

21. An order for Regular insulin states that it is to be given 50 units qac for 30 days. How many vials are to be dispensed if the insulin is available in a 10-mL vial at a concentration of 100 units/mL?
    A. 1
    B. 2
    C. 4
    D. 5

22. The Roman numeral for 238 is:
    A. CCXXXVIII
    B. LLVVVXIII
    C. XXVVVLIII
    D. XLVIII

23. A patient asks you about the possible side effects of a medication; you:
    A. Search the Internet for the answer
    B. Advise the patient to contact her physician
    C. Refer the patient to the pharmacist
    D. Advise the patient to contact the manufacturer

24. How many milliliters are in 3 ounces?
    A. 60 mL
    B. 90 mL
    C. 120 mL
    D. 180 mL

25. A prescription is written for Lexapro 7.5 mg bid. If Lexapro 5 mg is dispensed, what quantity is needed to fill a 30-day supply?
    A. 90 tablets
    B. 30 tablets
    C. 45 tablets
    D. 60 tablets

26. An order is written for 0.75 g of ceftriaxone. In stock you have a bulk bottle with a concentration of 250 mg/mL. What is the volume needed to fill this order?
    A. 2 mL
    B. 6 mL
    C. 3 mL
    D. 5 mL

27. Which of the following is *not* an agent for treating neuropathic pain?
    A. Lidoderm
    B. Elavil
    C. Lyrica
    D. Valium

28. Which of the following is classified as an SSRI antidepressant?
    A. Pristiq
    B. Prozac
    C. Serzone
    D. Pamelor

29. Which medication is used to treat anxiety?
    A. Buspirone
    B. Carbamazepine
    C. Risperidone
    D. Quetiapine

30. Which of the following is *not* used to treat ADHD?
    A. Atomoxetine
    B. Methylphenidate
    C. Lisdexamfetamine
    D. Chlorpromazine

31. A 1-L bag contains how many grams of dextrose 70%?
    A. 70 g
    B. 700 g
    C. 7000 g
    D. 7 g

32. Which medication is used to lower cholesterol?
    A. Metoprolol
    B. Bumetanide
    C. Atorvastatin
    D. Candesartan

33. Which is *not* a common side effect of beta-2 agonists?
    A. Anxiety
    B. Rapid heartbeat
    C. Tremors
    D. Coughing

34. Methylprednisolone is available in all of the following dosage forms *except*:
    A. Capsules
    B. Tablets
    C. Injection
    D. Dosepak

35. A physician writes a prescription for prednisone 5 mg to be taken as follows: 20 mg bid, decrease by 5 mg every 2 days until gone. How many tablets should be dispensed?
    A. 20 tablets
    B. 40 tablets
    C. 16 tablets
    D. 8 tablets

36. Which of the following antihistamines is also commonly used as a sleep aid?
    A. Loratadine
    B. Cetirizine
    C. Diphenhydramine
    D. Levocetirizine

37. Adequate intake of which element is essential for preventing and treating osteoporosis?
    A. Potassium
    B. Calcium
    C. Magnesium
    D. Zinc

38. Which of the following is *not* a skeletal muscle relaxer?
    A. Lioresal
    B. Carisoprodol
    C. Diazepam
    D. Meloxicam
39. What is the most serious side effect of opioid analgesics?
    A. Respiratory depression
    B. Sedation
    C. Nausea
    D. Constipation
40. Tobramycin 240 mg is ordered to be given q6h. What is the volume needed for a 24-hour period if the concentration in stock is 40 mg/mL?
    A. 6 mL
    B. 12 mL
    C. 24 mL
    D. 48 mL
41. What is the strength of codeine found in Tylenol #3?
    A. 3 mg
    B. 30 mg
    C. 15 mg
    D. 60 mg
42. Which hypoglycemic is the only biguanide?
    A. Nateglinide
    B. Saxagliptin
    C. Metformin
    D. Acarbose
43. Which is a long-acting insulin?
    A. Glulisine
    B. Regular
    C. Lispro
    D. Glargine
44. What class of medications is used to treat hypertension?
    A. Beta-blockers
    B. Monoamine oxidase inhibitors
    C. Proton pump inhibitors
    D. Analgesics
45. Antiemetics are also known as:
    A. Antidiarrheals
    B. Antinausea agents
    C. Laxatives
    D. Antacids
46. A patient comes into the pharmacy with a prescription to treat her conjunctivitis. The prescription is most likely written for which of the following medications?
    A. Restasis
    B. Cortisporin
    C. Zaditor
    D. Azopt
47. Which of the following medications is *not* used for hormone therapy in women?
    A. Activella
    B. Prempro
    C. Proscar
    D. Menest
48. A prescription is dropped off for Amoxil 500 mg, 1 tsp tid × 10 days. You have Amoxil 250 mg/5 mL in stock. What volume is needed to fill the prescription?
    A. 50 mL
    B. 100 mL
    C. 200 mL
    D. 300 mL
49. Which vitamin is also known as thiamine?
    A. Vitamin B_1
    B. Vitamin B_2
    C. Vitamin B_3
    D. Vitamin B_{12}
50. Which of the following is the study of the manufacture of medications for effective delivery into the body?
    A. Pharmacokinetics
    B. Bioavailability
    C. Biopharmaceutics
    D. Pharmacodynamics
51. Which of the following is a semisolid medication dosage form that is applied to the skin or mucous membranes?
    A. Cream
    B. Ointment
    C. Lotion
    D. Paste
52. Which of the following is a disadvantage of the extended-release dosage form?
    A. The drug is delivered in a slow, controlled, and consistent manner so that the same amount of medication is absorbed throughout a given period.
    B. Patients are more likely to take their medications properly, and are less likely to experience side effects, if they can take the medications less often.
    C. The risk of side effects is reduced because the medication is delivered in smaller amounts over a long period.
    D. There may be a delay between the time the patient takes the medication and the time it takes effect.
53. Which route of administration involves injecting a drug into a joint?
    A. Intraarticular
    B. Intrapleural
    C. Intraarterial
    D. Intratracheal

54. A prescription is written for enalapril 7.5 mg daily. If you have 5-mg tablets in stock, how many tablets are needed for a daily dose?
    A. ½ tablet
    B. 2½ tablets
    C. 3 tablets
    D. 1½ tablets

55. What is the Arabic number for CIX?
    A. 59
    B. 109
    C. 111
    D. 61

56. A patient weighs 215 lb. How much does the patient weigh in kilograms?
    A. 97.7 kg
    B. 473 kg
    C. 236.5 kg
    D. 215 kg

57. You purchase Tylenol elixir over the counter. According to the directions, you are to give 1½ teaspoons. What is the volume to be given in milliliters?
    A. 2.5 mL
    B. 5 mL
    C. 7.5 mL
    D. 10 mL

58. A physician orders tobramycin 2 mg/kg/day for a 68-lb child. If you have in stock a 40 mg/mL vial, how many milligrams will the child receive per day?
    A. 74.8 mg
    B. 299.2 mg
    C. 15.5 mg
    D. 61.8 mg

59. A physician orders dextrose 20% in 750 mL. You have dextrose 10% and dextrose 50% in stock. How much of each do you need to make the ordered solution?
    A. 187.5 mL of dextrose 10% and 562.5 mL of dextrose 50%
    B. 450 mL of dextrose 10% and 300 mL of dextrose 50%
    C. 562.5 mL of dextrose 10% and 187.5 mL of dextrose 50%
    D. 300 mL of dextrose 10% and 450 mL of dextrose 50%

60. A 2-L bag contains how many grams of dextrose 70%?
    A. 140 g
    B. 1400 g
    C. 14,000 g
    D. 14 g

61. Compounded preparations should contain at least _____, but no more than _____, of the labeled active ingredient unless a stricter guideline applies.
    A. 80%; 120%
    B. 99%; 101%
    C. 90%; 110%
    D. 95%; 105%

62. Inert ingredients are also known as:
    A. Active ingredients
    B. Therapeutic ingredients
    C. Inactive ingredients
    D. None of the above

63. Which of the following IV containers include less than or equal to 100 mL of fluid?
    A. Large-volume parenterals
    B. Piggybacks
    C. Minibags
    D. Flexible plastic bags

64. Which of the following is *not* a risk of IV therapy?
    A. Infection
    B. Phlebitis
    C. Allergic reactions
    D. Rapid onset of action

65. Which medications must *always* be compounded in a vertical laminar flow hood?
    A. TPNs
    B. Antibiotics
    C. Antivirals
    D. Chemotherapeutic drugs

66. What is the most common source of contamination of pharmacy-prepared sterile products?
    A. Airborne
    B. Cross-contamination
    C. Touch
    D. None of the above

67. Which medication is never dispensed in a child-resistant vial?
    A. Penicillin
    B. Enalapril
    C. Lorazepam
    D. Nitroglycerin

68. What type of equipment is used to protect workers from exposure to hazardous drugs?
    A. Horizontal laminar flow workbench
    B. Biological safety cabinet
    C. Temperature-controlled walk-in vault
    D. Vertical laminar flow workbench

69. Total parenteral nutrition contains all of the following *except*:
    A. Carbohydrates
    B. Vitamins
    C. Antibiotics
    D. Electrolytes

70. Medications that could be added to a TPN solution include all of the following *except*:
    A. Antibiotics
    B. H₂-blockers
    C. Insulin
    D. Octreotide

71. NaCl is an abbreviation for:
    A. Potassium chloride
    B. Sodium chloride
    C. Nitrogen chloride
    D. Phosphate chloride

72. Vitamin B₁₂ is also called:
    A. Niacin
    B. Thiamine
    C. Cyanocobalamin
    D. Riboflavin

73. Retinol is also known as:
    A. Vitamin A
    B. Vitamin C
    C. Vitamin E
    D. Vitamin K

74. Mg is the symbol for which element?
    A. Manganese
    B. Sodium chloride
    C. Riboflavin
    D. Magnesium

75. Which of the following is *not* considered a prescribing error?
    A. Incorrect dose
    B. Incorrect duration of therapy
    C. Incorrect administration time
    D. Incorrect number of doses

76. Which of the following is *not* a high-alert medication as defined by the ISMP?
    A. Heparin
    B. Lomotil
    C. Insulin
    D. Succinylcholine

77. A prescription is called in for Zestril; which medication is to be filled?
    A. Enalapril
    B. Fosinopril
    C. Lisinopril
    D. Ramipril

78. Which of the following is classified as a loop diuretic?
    A. Spironolactone
    B. Metolazone
    C. Hydrochlorothiazide
    D. Furosemide

79. A dry, bothersome cough is a common side effect of which class of medication?
    A. ACE inhibitors
    B. Beta-blockers
    C. Calcium channel blockers
    D. Vasodilators

80. Which of the following is a class IB antiarrhythmic agent?
    A. Mexiletine
    B. Quinidine
    C. Flecainide
    D. Dofetilide

81. The term *prophylaxis* means:
    A. To treat a condition once it has been diagnosed
    B. A weak cardiovascular system
    C. A preventive treatment
    D. To cure to a condition

82. Theophylline is a methylxanthine that comes in all of the following dosage forms *except*:
    A. Injection
    B. Inhaler
    C. Tablet
    D. Elixir

83. The generic name for Advair is:
    A. Albuterol
    B. Ipratropium/albuterol
    C. Formoterol/budesonide
    D. Salmeterol/fluticasone

84. A medication is to be given qac; when should this medication be given?
    A. Before meals
    B. After meals
    C. Every morning with breakfast
    D. Every evening with supper

85. A medication is to be given daily at 1700; what time is the medication due?
    A. 7:00 AM
    B. 7:00 PM
    C. 5:00 PM
    D. 3:00 PM

86. A prescriber writes an order for a medication to be given every 8 hours times 5 doses. If the first dose is given at 0600, what time will the last dose be given?
    A. 10:00 PM
    B. 6:00 AM
    C. 2:00 PM
    D. 6:00 PM

87. Tobramycin 120 mg is ordered to be given q6h. The bulk bottle in stock is 10 mL at a concentration of 40 mg/mL. How many vial(s) is(are) needed to make a 24-hour supply?
    A. 1
    B. 2
    C. 3
    D. 4

88. A nonproductive cough without chest congestion can be treated with a(n):
    A. Expectorant
    B. Antihistamine
    C. Corticosteroid
    D. Antitussive

0

89. Which of the following is an example of a combination opioid analgesic?
    A. Dilaudid
    B. Ultram
    C. Ultracet
    D. Subutex
90. Which insulin has an onset of action of about 15 minutes?
    A. Apidra
    B. Levemir
    C. Lantus
    D. B and C

Answer Key

1. B. BS5836727 (Chapter 2)
2. C. Pregabalin (Chapter 17)
3. D. Inhale 1 puff every 4 to 6 hours as needed for shortness of breath (Chapter 4)
4. A. Allegra-D (Chapter 5)
5. C. Codeine (Chapter 2)
6. A. Schedule I (Chapter 2)
7. D. 9 g (Chapter 6)
8. D. 4 (Chapter 6)
9. B. Loratadine (Chapter 19)
10. C. Up to 5 times in a 6-month period (Chapter 2)
11. B. Topical patch (Chapter 5)
12. D. 20 mL (Chapter 6)
13. C. 5 doses (Chapter 6)
14. B. 150 mL (Chapter 6)
15. B. 75 mL (Chapter 6)
16. C. 10 mL (Chapter 6)
17. C. Volume III (Chapter 7)
18. C. Quantity (Chapter 8)
19. B. 3 mL (Chapter 6)
20. D. Lopressor (Chapter 16)
21. D. 5 (Chapter 6)
22. A. CCXXXVIII (Chapter 6)
23. C. Refer the patient to the pharmacist (Chapter 3)
24. B. 90 mL (Chapter 6)
25. A. 90 tablets (Chapter 6)
26. C. 3 mL (Chapter 6)
27. D. Valium (Chapter 17)
28. B. Prozac (Chapter 15)
29. A. Buspirone (Chapter 15)
30. D. Chlorpromazine (Chapter 15)
31. B. 700 g (Chapter 6)
32. C. Atorvastatin (Chapter 16)
33. D. Coughing (Chapter 16)
34. A. Capsules (Chapter 16)
35. B. 40 tablets (Chapter 6)
36. C. Diphenhydramine (Chapter 15)
37. B. Calcium (Chapter 16)
38. D. Meloxicam (Chapter 17)
39. A. Respiratory depression (Chapter 1)
40. C. 24 mL (Chapter 6)
41. B. 30 mg (Chapter 1)
42. C. Metformin (Chapter 16)
43. D. Glargine (Chapter 16)
44. A. Beta-blockers (Chapter 16)
45. B. Antinausea agents (Chapter 20)
46. B. Cortisporin (Chapter 24)
47. C. Proscar (Chapter 22)
48. D. 300 mL (Chapter 6)
49. A. Vitamin B_1 (Chapter 28)
50. C. Biopharmaceutics (Chapter 5)
51. B. Ointment (Chapter 5)
52. D. There may be a delay between the time the patient takes the medication and the time it takes effect (Chapter 5)
53. A. Intraarticular (Chapter 5)
54. D. 1½ tablets (Chapter 6)
55. B. 109 (Chapter 6)
56. A. 97.7 kg (Chapter 6)
57. C. 7.5 mL (Chapter 6)
58. D. 61.8 mg (Chapter 6)
59. C. 562.5 mL of dextrose 10% and 187.5 mL of dextrose 50% (Chapter 6)
60. B. 1400 g (Chapter 6)
61. C. 90%; 110% (Chapter 6)
62. C. Inactive ingredients (Chapter 3)
63. B. Piggybacks (Chapter 12)
64. D. Rapid onset of action (Chapter 12)
65. D. Chemotherapy (Chapter 12)
66. C. Touch (Chapter 12)
67. D. Nitroglycerin (Chapter 16)
68. B. Biological safety cabinet (Chapter 12)
69. C. Antibiotics (Chapter 12)
70. A. Antibiotics (Chapter 12)
71. B. Sodium chloride (Chapter 12)
72. C. Cyanocobalamin (Chapter 28)
73. A. Vitamin A (Chapter 28)
74. D. Magnesium (Chapter 28)
75. C. Incorrect administration time (Chapter 3)
76. B. Lomotil (Chapter 5)
77. C. Lisinopril (Chapter 16)
78. D. Furosemide (Chapter 16)
79. A. ACE inhibitors (Chapter 16)
80. A. Mexiletine (Chapter 16)
81. C. A preventive treatment (Chapter 19)
82. B. Inhaler (Chapter 19)
83. D. Salmeterol/fluticasone (Chapter 19)
84. A. Before meals (Chapter 4)
85. C. 5:00 PM (Chapter 6)
86. C. 2:00 PM (Chapter 6)
87. B. 2 (Chapter 6)
88. D. Antitussive (Chapter 19)
89. C. Ultracet (Chapter 15)
90. A. Apidra (Chapter 16)

If students find that they need further review for the PTCE, as well as more practice questions and examinations, they should purchase the book Mizner, James J: *Mosby's Review for the Pharmacy Technician Certification Examination*, ed 3, St Louis, 2014, Mosby (ISBN: 978-0-323-11337-3).

Appendix B

Top 200 Prescription Drugs

	Brand Name	Generic Name	Drug Classification*	Indication or Use
1	Abilify	aripiprazole	Antipsychotic	Schizophrenia
2	AcipHex	rabeprazole	PPI	GERD
3	ActoPlus Met	pioglitazone/metformin	Biguanide/thiazolidinedione	Type 2 diabetes mellitus
4	Actos	pioglitazone	Thiazolidinedione	Type 2 diabetes mellitus
5	Adderall XR	dextroamphetamine/amphetamine	Amphetamine	ADHD
6	Advair Diskus	fluticasone/salmeterol	Beta-2 agonist/corticosteroid	Asthma, COPD
7	Aggrenox	aspirin/dipyridamole	Antiplatelet	Thrombotic stroke prevention
8	Alphagan P	brimonidine tartrate	Alpha-agonist	Glaucoma
9	Altace	ramipril	ACE inhibitor	Hypertension
10	Ambien	zolpidem	Gamma-aminobutyric acid agonist	Insomnia
11	Amoxil	amoxicillin	Penicillin antibiotic	Bacterial infection
12	Androgel	testosterone topical	Androgen	Hypogonadism
13	Aricept	donepezil	Alzheimer's disease; dementia	Alzheimer's disease
14	Arimidex	anastrozole	Hormonal oncologic	Cancer
15	Armour Thyroid	thyroid	Thyroid	Hypothyroidism
16	Asacol	mesalamine	Inflammatory bowel disease	Ulcerative colitis
17	Asmanex Twisthaler	mometasone	Corticosteroid	Asthma
18	Astelin	azelastine	Histamine-1 (H_1) receptor inhibitor	Respiratory allergies
19	Atacand	candesartan cilexetil	ARB	Hypertension
20	Ativan	lorazepam	Benzodiazepine	Anxiety
21	Augmentin	amoxicillin/clavulanate	Penicillin combination antibiotic	Bacterial infection
22	Avalide	irbesartan/hydrochlorothiazide	ARB/thiazide combination	Hypertension
23	Avapro	irbesartan	ARB	Hypertension
24	Avelox	moxifloxacin	Quinolone antibiotic	Bacterial infection
25	Avodart	dutasteride	5-alpha reductase inhibitor	BPH
26	Bactrim or Septra	trimethoprim/sulfamethoxazole	Sulfa antibiotic	Bacterial infection
27	Bactroban	mupirocin	Topical antibacterial	Skin infection
28	Beconase AQ	beclomethasone	Corticosteroid	Allergic rhinitis
29	Benicar	olmesartan	ARB	Hypertension
30	Benicar HCT	olmesartan/hydrochlorothiazide	ARB/thiazide combination	Hypertension
31	BenzaClin	clindamycin/benzoyl peroxide	Topical antibiotic	Acne
32	Boniva	ibandronate	Bisphosphonate	Osteoporosis
33	Byetta	exenatide	GLP-1 receptor agonist	Type 2 diabetes mellitus
34	Bystolic	nebivolol	Beta-blocker	Hypertension
35	Caduet	amlodipine/atorvastatin	CCB/HMG-CoA reductase inhibitor combination	Hypertension and hyperlipidemia
36	Catapres-TTS	clonidine	Alpha-agonist	Hypertension

Continued

	Brand Name	Generic Name	Drug Classification*	Indication or Use
37	Celebrex	celecoxib	COX-2 inhibitor	Inflammation
38	Celexa	citalopram	SSRI	Depression
39	Chantix	varenicline	Partial cholinergic nicotinic agonist	Smoking cessation
40	Cheratussin AC	codeine/guaifenesin	Antitussive and expectorant combination	Expectorant and cough suppressant
41	Cialis	tadalafil	PDE-5 inhibitor	Erectile dysfunction
42	Cipro	ciprofloxacin	Quinolone antibiotic	Bacterial infection
43	Ciprodex Otic	ciprofloxacin/ dexamethasone	Quinolone/corticosteroid	Bacterial external ear infection
44	Cleocin	clindamycin	Antibacterial	Bacterial infection
45	Combivent	ipratropium/albuterol	Anticholinergic/beta-2 agonist	Asthma
46	Concerta	methylphenidate	Central nervous system stimulant	ADHD
47	Coreg	carvedilol	Beta-blocker	Hypertension
48	Cosopt	dorzolamide/timolol	Beta-blocker/carbonic anhydrase inhibitor	Glaucoma
49	Coumadin	warfarin	Vitamin K antagonist	Anticoagulation
50	Cozaar	losartan	ARB	Hypertension
51	Crestor	rosuvastatin	HMG-CoA reductase inhibitor	Hyperlipidemia
52	Cymbalta	duloxetine	SNRI	Depression
53	Deltasone	prednisone	Corticosteroid	Inflammation
54	Depakote ER	divalproex sodium	Neurologic	Bipolar disorder, migraine headache, seizure disorder
55	Desyrel	trazodone	Serotonin reuptake inhibitor	Insomnia, depression
56	Detrol LA	tolterodine	GU antispasmodic	Incontinence
57	Differin	adapalene	Retinoid	Acne vulgaris
58	Diflucan	fluconazole	Antifungal	Fungal infection
59	Dilantin	phenytoin	Hydantoin	Status epilepticus
60	Diovan	valsartan	ARB	Hypertension
61	Diovan HCT	valsartan/ hydrochlorothiazide	ARB/thiazide combination	Hypertension
62	Dyazide	triamterene/ hydrochlorothiazide	Potassium-sparing/thiazide diuretic combination	Hypertension
63	Effexor	venlafaxine	SNRI	Depression
64	Elavil	amitriptyline	TCA	Depression
65	Enablex	darifenacin	GU antispasmodic	Overactive bladder
66	EpiPen	epinephrine	Catecholamine	Anaphylaxis
67	Esidrix	hydrochlorothiazide	Thiazide diuretic	Hypertension
68	Evista	raloxifene	SERM	Osteoporosis
69	Flexeril	cyclobenzaprine	Muscle relaxant	Skeletal muscle relaxant
70	Flomax	tamsulosin	Alpha-blocker	BPH
71	Flonase	fluticasone	Corticosteroid	Allergic rhinitis
72	Flovent HFA	fluticasone	Corticosteroid	Asthma
73	Fluzone	influenza vaccine	Influenza vaccine	Influenza
74	Focalin XR	dexmethylphenidate	Central nervous system stimulant	ADHD
75	Folic acid	vitamin B_9	Vitamin	Dietary supplement
76	Fosamax	alendronate	Biphosphonate	Osteoporosis
77	Fosamax Plus D	alendronate with vitamin D	Biphosphonate	Osteoporosis
78	Geodon	ziprasidone	Antipsychotic	Schizophrenia
79	Gianvi	drospirenone/ethinyl estradiol	Monophasic oral contraceptive	Oral contraceptive
80	Glucophage	metformin	Biguanide	Type 2 diabetes mellitus
81	Glucotrol	glipizide	Sulfonylurea	Type 2 diabetes mellitus

	Brand Name	Generic Name	Drug Classification*	Indication or Use
82	GlycoLax	polyethylene glycol 3350	Osmotic laxative	Constipation
83	Humalog	insulin lispro	Insulin	Diabetes mellitus
84	Humulin N	insulin NPH	Insulin	Diabetes mellitus
85	Hyzaar	losartan/ hydrochlorothiazide	ARB/thiazide combination	Hypertension
86	Imitrex	sumatriptan	Serotonin 5-HT$_1$ receptor agonist	Migraine headache
87	Januvia	sitagliptin	DPP-4 inhibitor	Type 2 diabetes mellitus
88	K-Dur, Klor-Con, Klor-Con M, Micro K	potassium chloride	Electrolyte	Potassium supplement
89	Kariva	desogestrel/ethinyl estradiol	Monophasic oral contraceptive	Oral contraceptive
90	Keflex	cephalexin	Cephalosporin antibiotic	Bacterial infection
91	Keppra	levetiracetam	Antiepileptic	Seizure
92	Klonopin	clonazepam	Benzodiazepine	Seizure
93	Lamictal	lamotrigine	Antiepileptic	Bipolar disorder
94	Lanoxin	digoxin	Cardiac glycoside	Arrhythmia, myocardial infarction
95	Lantus	insulin glargine	Insulin	Diabetes mellitus
96	Lasix	furosemide	Loop diuretic	Hypertension
97	Lescol XL	fluvastatin	HMG-CoA reductase inhibitor	Hyperlipidemia
98	Levaquin	levofloxacin	Quinolone antibiotic	Bacterial infection
99	Levitra	vardenafil	PDE-5 inhibitor	PDE-5 inhibitor
100	Lexapro	escitalopram	SSRI	Depression
101	Lidoderm	lidocaine	Analgesic	Neuralgia
102	Lipitor	atorvastatin	HMG-CoA reductase inhibitor	Hyperlipidemia
103	Loestrin Fe24	norethindrone/ethinyl estradiol	Monophasic oral contraceptive	Oral contraceptive
104	Lopressor	metoprolol tartrate	Beta-blocker	Hypertension
105	Lovaza	omega-3-acid ethyl esters	Esterified fish oils	Hypertriglyceridemia
106	Lovenox	enoxaparin	Low-molecular-weight heparin	DVT prophylaxis
107	Lumigan	bimatoprost	Prostaglandin analogues	Glaucoma
108	Lunesta	eszopiclone	Nonbenzodiazepine hypnotic	Insomnia
109	Lyrica	pregabalin	Neurologic	Neuropathic pain
110	Maxzide	triamterene/ hydrochlorothiazide	Potassium-sparing/thiazide diuretic	Hypertension
111	Medrol	methylprednisolone	Corticosteroid	Inflammation
112	Mevacor	lovastatin	HMG-CoA reductase inhibitor	Hyperlipidemia
113	Micardis	telmisartan	ARB	Hypertension
114	Micardis HCT	telmisartan/ hydrochlorothiazide	ARB/thiazide combination	Hypertension
115	Micronase or DiaBeta	glyburide	Sulfonylurea	Type 2 diabetes mellitus
116	Mirapex	pramipexole	Dopamine agonist	Parkinson's disease
117	Mobic	meloxicam	NSAID	Osteoarthritis
118	Motrin[†]	ibuprofen	NSAID	Inflammation
119	Namenda	memantine	NMDA receptor agonist	Alzheimer's disease
120	Naprosyn	naproxen	NSAID	Inflammation
121	Nasacort AQ	triamcinolone	Corticosteroid	Allergic rhinitis
122	Nasonex	mometasone furoate	Corticosteroid	Allergic rhinitis
123	Neurontin	gabapentin	Neurologic	Seizure
124	Nexium[†]	esomeprazole	PPI	GERD
125	Niaspan	niacin	Nicotinic acid	Hyperlipidemia
126	Norvasc	amlodipine besylate	CCB	Hypertension

Continued

	Brand Name	Generic Name	Drug Classification*	Indication or Use
127	NuvaRing	etonogestrel/ethinyl estradiol	Estrogen/progestin	Contraceptive
128	Omnicef	cefdinir	Cephalosporin antibiotic	Bacterial infection
129	Ortho-Tri-Cyclen Lo	ethinyl estradiol/ norgestimate	Triphasic oral contraceptive	Oral contraceptive
130	Oxycontin	oxycodone	Opioid	Analgesic
131	Patanol	olopatadine	Allergy	Allergic conjunctivitis
132	Paxil	paroxetine	SSRI	Depression
133	Penicillin VK	penicillin	Penicillin antibiotic	Bacterial infection
134	Pepcid†	famotidine	H_2 blocker	GERD
135	Phenergan	promethazine	Antihistamine	Antiemetic
136	Plavix	clopidogrel	Antiplatelet	Thrombotic event prevention
137	Pravachol	pravastatin	HMG-CoA reductase inhibitor	Hyperlipidemia
138	Premarin	conjugated estrogens	Estrogen	Vasomotor symptoms
139	Prevacid†	lansoprazole	PPI	GERD
140	Prilosec†	omeprazole	PPI	GERD
141	ProAir HFA, Proventil HFA, Ventolin HFA	albuterol	Bronchodilator	Asthma
142	Prometrium	progesterone	Progestin	Amenorrhea
143	Propecia	finasteride	5-alpha-reductase inhibitor	Male pattern baldness
144	Protonix	pantoprazole	PPI	GERD
145	Provigil	modafinil	Sympathomimetic-like amine	Narcolepsy
146	Prozac	fluoxetine	SSRI	Depression
147	Pulmicort Respules	budesonide	Corticosteroid	Asthma
148	Relpax	eletriptan	5HT receptor agonist	Migraine headache
149	Requip	ropinirole	Dopamine agonist	Parkinson disease
150	Restasis	cyclosporine	Calcineurin inhibitor immunosuppressant	Ocular dryness
151	Rhinocort AQ	budesonide	Corticosteroid	Asthma
152	Risperdal	risperidone	Antipsychotic	Schizophrenia
153	Seroquel	quetiapine fumarate	Antipsychotic	Schizophrenia
154	Singulair	montelukast	Leukotriene receptor antagonist	Asthma
155	Skelaxin	metaxalone	Muscle relaxant	Musculoskeletal pain
156	Soma	carisoprodol	Muscle relaxant	Skeletal muscle relaxant
157	Spiriva Handihaler	tiotropium	Anticholinergic	COPD
158	Strattera	atomoxetine	Norepinephrine reuptake inhibitor	ADHD
159	Suboxone	buprenorphine/ naloxone	Opioid agonist/antagonist	Opioid maintenance
160	Sular	nisoldipine	CCB	Hypertension
161	Symbicort	budesonide/formoterol	Corticosteroid/beta-2 agonist	Asthma
162	Synthroid	levothyroxine sodium	Thyroid	Hypothyroidism
163	Tenormin	atenolol	Beta-blocker	Hypertension
164	Tessalon Perles	benzonatate	Antitussive	Cough
165	Topamax	topiramate	Antiepileptic	Seizure
166	Toprol XL	metoprolol succinate	Beta-blocker	Hypertension
167	Travatan	travoprost	Prostaglandin analog	Glaucoma
168	Tricor	fenofibrate	Fibrate	Hyperlipidemia
169	Triesence or Trivaris	triamcinolone	Corticosteroid	Ocular inflammation
170	Trileptal	oxcarbazepine	Antiepileptic	Partial seizure
171	TriNessa	norgestimate/ethinyl estradiol	Triphasic oral contraceptive	Oral contraceptive
172	Tri-Sprintec	norgestimate/ethinyl estradiol	Triphasic oral contraceptive	Oral contraceptive
173	Tussionex	chlorpheniramine/ hydrocodone	Antihistamine/antitussive combination	Upper respiratory symptoms

	Brand Name	Generic Name	Drug Classification*	Indication or Use
174	Tylenol with codeine	acetaminophen/codeine	Opioid combination	Analgesic
175	Ultram	tramadol	Opioid	Analgesic
176	Uroxatral	alfuzosin	Alpha-blocker	BPH
177	Vagifem	estradiol	Estrogen	Vulvovaginal atrophy
178	Valium	diazepam	Benzodiazepine	Anxiety
179	Vasotec	enalapril	ACE inhibitor	Hypertension
180	VESIcare	solifenacin	Antispasmodic	Overactive bladder
181	Viagra	sildenafil	PDE-5 inhibitor	Erectile dysfunction
182	Vibramycin	doxycycline hyclate	Tetracycline antibiotic	Bacterial infection
183	Vicodin	hydrocodone/acetaminophen	Opioid combination	Analgesic
184	Vigamox	moxifloxacin	Quinolone antibiotic	Bacterial conjunctivitis
185	Vitamin D†	ergocalciferol	Vitamin	Vitamin D deficiency
186	Vytorin	ezetimibe/simvastatin	HMG-CoA reductase combination	Hypercholesterolemia
187	Vyvanse	lisdexamfetamine	Central nervous system stimulant	ADHD
188	Wellbutrin XL	bupropion	antidepressant	Depression
189	Xalatan	latanoprost	Prostaglandin analog	Glaucoma
190	Xanax	alprazolam	Benzodiazepine	Anxiety
191	Xopenex HFA	levalbuterol	Beta-2 agonist	Bronchospasm
192	Zantac†	ranitidine	H_2 blocker	GERD
193	Zestoretic	lisinopril/hydrochlorothiazide	ACE inhibitor/thiazide combination	Hypertension
194	Zestril or Prinivil	lisinopril	ACE inhibitor	Hypertension
195	Zetia	ezetimibe	Cholesterol absorption inhibitor	Hyperlipidemia
196	Zithromax	azithromycin	Macrolide antibiotic	Bacterial infection
197	Zocor	simvastatin	HMG-CoA reductase inhibitor	Hyperlipidemia
198	Zoloft	sertraline	SSRI	Depression
199	Zyloprim	allopurinol	Xanthine oxidase inhibitor	Gout
200	Zyprexa	olanzapine	Antipsychotic	Schizophrenia, bipolar disease

Modified from Mizner JJ: *Mosby's review for the Pharmacy Technician Certification Examination*, ed 3, St Louis, 2014, Mosby.
*According to Epocrates.
†Prescription.
ACE, Angiotensin-converting enzyme; *ADHD,* attention deficit/hyperactivity disorder; *ARB,* angiotensin II–receptor blocker; *BPH,* benign prostatic hypertrophy; *CCB,* calcium channel blocker; *COPD,* chronic obstructive pulmonary disease; *COX,* cyclooxygenase; *DPP-4,* dipeptidyl peptidase 4; *DVT,* deep vein thrombosis; *GERD,* gastroesophageal reflux disease; *GLP,* glucagon-like peptide; *GU,* genitourinary; *HMG-CoA,* 3-hydroxy-3-methyl-glutaryl/coenzyme A; *NMDA,* N-methyl-D-aspartate; *NSAID,* nonsteroidal antiinflammatory drug; *PDE-5,* phosphodiesterase type 5; *PPI,* proton pump inhibitor; *SERM,* selective estrogen receptor modulator; *SNRI,* serotonin-norepinephrine reuptake inhibitor; *SSRI,* selective serotonin reuptake inhibitor; *TCA,* tricyclic antidepressant.

Appendix C

Top 30 Herbal Remedies

Common Name	Scientific Name	Common Reported Uses
Aloe vera (leaf)	*Aloe* spp.	Wound and burn healing
American ginseng (root)	*Panax quinquefolius*	Energy, stress, immune system support
Bilberry (berry)	*Vaccinium myrtillus*	Eye and vascular support
Black cohosh (root)	*Cimicifuga racemosa*	Menopause, premenstrual syndrome (PMS)
Cascara sagrada (aged bark)	*Rhamnus purshiana*	Laxative
Cat's claw (root, bark)	*Uncaria tomentosa*	Antiinflammatory, immune system support
Chondroitin	Nutraceutical	Osteoarthritis
Dong quai (root)	*Angelica sinensis*	Energy (females), menopause, dysmenorrhea, PMS
Echinacea (flower, root)	*Echinacea purpurea, Echinacea angustifolia*	Support of common cold, immunostimulant
Evening primrose (seed oil)	*Oenothera biennis*	PMS, menopause
Feverfew (leaf)	*Tanacetum parthenium*	Antiinflammatory, migraine prevention
Fish oils	Nutraceutical	Lower triglycerides, heart health
Garlic (bulb)	*Allium sativum*	Antimicrobial, lower cholesterol
Ginger (root)	*Zingiber officinale*	Antiemetic, gastrointestinal distress, dyspepsia
Ginkgo (root)	*Ginkgo biloba*	Support of memory, increased blood flow to brain, prevention of dementia
Ginseng	*Panax quinquefolius, Panax ginseng*	Increase physical endurance and concentration, lessen fatigue
Glucosamine	Nutraceutical	Osteoarthritis
Goldenseal (root)	*Hydrastis canadensis*	Chest congestion, cystitis
Grape seed (seed, skin)	*Vitis vinifera*	Support circulation
Green tea (leaf)	*Camellia sinensis*	Cancer prevention, antioxidant, lower cholesterol, weight maintenance
Isoflavones (soy)	Nutraceutical	Cancer prevention, decrease bone loss, hot flashes
Kava (root)	*Piper methysticum*	Anxiety, sedation
Melatonin	Nutraceutical	Insomnia
Milk thistle (seed)	*Silybum marianum*	Antioxidant, liver support
Saw palmetto (berry)	*Serenoa repens*	Benign prostatic hyperplasia
Siberian ginseng (root)	*Eleutherococcus senticosus*	Athletic performance, stress, immune builder
St. John's wort (flowering buds)	*Hypericum perforatum*	Depression, anxiety
Valerian (root)	*Valeriana officinalis*	Sedative, muscle spasms
Wild yam (tuber)	*Dioscorea villosa*	Female vitality

A

Abortifacient Any treatment that causes abortion of a fetus

Absolute neutrophil count (ANC) The number of white blood cells that are actually neutrophils

Absorption (gastrointestinal) The processes by which nutrients, fluids, and medications are moved from the gastrointestinal tract into the bloodstream

Accreditation Council for Pharmacy Education (ACPE) A national agency for the accreditation of professional degree programs in pharmacy and providers of continuing pharmacy education

Acidification (urinary) The conversion of urine to a more acidic content

Acidosis The increase in the blood's acidity that results from an accumulation of acid or a loss of bicarbonate; the pH of the blood is decreased

Acne vulgaris A condition in which the pores of the skin are clogged with oil or bacteria; commonly known as *pimples*

Acromegaly A condition caused by excessive growth hormone production during adulthood

Act A statutory proposal passed by Congress or any legislature that is a "bill" until it is enacted and becomes law

Addison's disease A condition that causes a decrease in the levels of adrenocortical hormones (e.g., mineralocorticoids and glucocorticoids), resulting in symptoms such as muscle weakness and weight loss

Adjudication The process by which a prescription is submitted electronically to a third-party payer to obtain reimbursement for the pharmacy for the medication dispensed

Adrenal cortex The portion of the adrenal gland that secretes such steroids as mineralocorticoids, glucocorticoids, and sex steroids

Adrenal medulla The portion of the adrenal gland that synthesizes and secretes the catecholamines norepinephrine and epinephrine

Adulteration The mishandling of medication that can lead to contamination/impurity, falsification of contents, or loss of drug quality or potency; adulteration may cause injury or illness in the consumer

Albumin The major protein found in plasma

Aldosterone The principal mineralocorticoid in the body that maintains sodium and potassium homeostasis by stimulating the kidneys to conserve sodium and excrete potassium; a steroid hormone secreted by the adrenal cortex that regulates the salt and water balance in the body

Alkalosis The increase in the blood's alkalinity that results from an accumulation of alkali or a reduction of acid content; the pH of blood is increased

Allergen A substance that causes an allergic reaction

Alligation A mathematical method of solving problems that involves the mixing of two solutions or two solids of different percentage weights to achieve a desired third strength

Alopecia The partial or complete absence of hair from areas of the body where it normally grows; baldness

Alternative medicine Any range of medical therapies not regarded as orthodox by Western medicine

Alveoli Tiny air sacs in the lungs where the exchange of oxygen and carbon dioxide takes place

Alzheimer's disease A progressive form of dementia that affects memory, thinking, and behavior

Amendment A change in the original act or law

American Association of Pharmacy Technicians (AAPT) The first pharmacy technician association, founded in 1979

American Pharmacists Association (APhA) The oldest pharmacy association, founded in 1852

American Society of Health-System Pharmacists (ASHP) An association of pharmacists, pharmacy students, and technicians practicing in hospitals and health care systems, including home health care; the ASHP has a long history of advocating patient safety and establishing best practices to improve medication use; it was founded in 1942

American Society of Health-System Pharmacists (ASHP) Model Curriculum for Pharmacy Technician Education and Training A model that provides details on how to meet the ASHP goals for pharmacy technician training programs

Amino acids Molecules that are the building blocks of proteins

Analgesic A drug that relieves pain by reducing the perception of pain

Anaphylaxis An extreme, potentially life-threatening allergic reaction

Androgen Male hormone

Anemia A decrease in the number of red blood cells or hemoglobin, which impairs the blood's ability to carry oxygen to the tissues

Aneurysm A balloonlike bulge or dilation of an artery resulting from weakening of the arterial wall

Angina Chest pain resulting from an inadequate supply of oxygen to the heart muscle

Angiotensin II A peptide hormone that causes vasoconstriction and a subsequent increase in blood pressure

Anion A negatively charged ion

Antibodies Complex molecules (immunoglobulins) that are made in response to the presence of an antigen (e.g., a protein of bacteria or other infecting organism) and that neutralize the effect of the foreign substance

Anticholinergic A term meaning inhibiting the physiological action of acetylcholine

Anticoagulant An agent used to prevent the formation of blood clots

Antiemetics A drug effective in the treatment of nausea and vomiting

Antigen A substance that prompts the production of antibodies, resulting in an immune response

Antigen-presenting cell (APC) A cell of the immune system that presents antigens to lymphocytes to activate an immune response

Antihistamine A drug or other compound that inhibits the effects of histamine; antihistamines are used especially in the treatment of allergies

Antihyperlipidemics A diverse group of pharmaceuticals used in the treatment of hyperlipidemia

Antiinflammatory A drug that reduces swelling, redness, and pain and that promotes healing

Antipyretic A drug that reduces fever

Antiseptic A substance that slows or stops the growth of microorganisms on surfaces such as the skin

Antitussive A drug that can reduce the coughing reflex of the central nervous system

Aorta The great arterial trunk that carries blood from the heart to be distributed to tissues of the body

Aphasia A communication disorder resulting from damage or injury to language parts of the brain; it is more common in older adults, particularly those who have had a stroke

Apothecary The Latin term for pharmacist; also, a place where drugs are sold

Apothecary system A system of measurement once used in the practice of pharmacy to measure both volume and weight; it has been mostly replaced by the metric system

Aqueous humor The fluid found in the anterior chamber of the eye, in front of the lens

Arrhythmia An abnormal or irregular heart rhythm

Artery A vessel that carries oxygenated blood from the heart to the tissues of the body

Arthroplasty Surgical reconstruction or replacement of a joint

ASAP order As soon as possible but not an emergency

Aseptic technique A technique used in the sterile compounding of hazardous and nonhazardous materials to minimize the introduction of microbes or unwanted debris that could cause contamination of the preparation; the procedures used to eliminate the possibility of a drug becoming contaminated with microbes or particles

Aspiration The drawing of a foreign substance into the respiratory tract during inhalation

Atherosclerosis A process of progressive thickening and hardening of the walls of medium-sized and large arteries as a result of fat deposits on their inner lining

Atrium The entry chamber on both sides of the heart

Attention deficit/hyperactivity disorder (ADHD) A physiological brain disorder that affects the ability to engage in quiet, passive activities or to focus one's attention; it is attributable to an imbalance of neurotransmitters in the brain

Attenuated A term describing an altered or weakened live vaccine made from the disease organism against which the vaccine protects

Attitude A mental disposition or feeling a technician adopts with regard to customers, coworkers, or duties at work

Auditory canal A 1-inch segment of tube that extends from the external ear to the middle ear

Auditory ossicles The small bones of the middle ear that transmit sound from the eardrum to the inner ear

Auricle The outer projecting portion of the ear

Automated dispensing system (ADS) Computerized cabinets that control inventory on nursing floors, in emergency departments, and in surgical suites and other patient care areas; electronic systems used to dispense medications

Autonomic nervous system A branch of the nervous system that carries out "automatic" bodily functions; it is composed of the sympathetic and parasympathetic systems

Auxiliary label A label that provides supplementary information about proper and safe administration, use, or storage of a medication

Average wholesale price (AWP) The average price at which a drug is sold; the data are compiled from information provided from manufacturers, distributors, and pharmacies; the AWP is often used in calculations related to medication reimbursement

Avoirdupois system A system of measurement previously used in pharmacy for the determination of weight in ounces and pounds; has been mostly replaced by the metric system

Ayurveda A holistic traditional medical system originating in India; in the system the prevention of disease is emphasized

B

Bactericidal Leading to bacterial cell death

Bacteriostatic A term meaning inhibiting bacterial cell growth

Bank Identification Number (BIN) A six-digit number on a prescription drug card that is used for routing and identification to process a prescription claim

Barbiturate A drug derived from barbituric acid; a barbiturate acts as a central nervous system depressant; barbiturates are often used in the treatment of seizures and as sedative and hypnotic agents

Behind-the-counter (BTC) drugs A group of medications that is kept behind the pharmacy counter and that requires a pharmacist's intervention before the medication can be sold to a patient; BTC medications are not considered prescription medications; they are nonprescription drugs that are kept behind the pharmacy counter, and only limited amounts may be sold or a pharmacist's permission may be required for purchase

Benign A condition, tumor, or growth that is not cancerous and therefore does not metastasize (spread)

Benign prostatic hyperplasia (BPH) Enlargement of the prostate

Beyond-use date (BUD) Defined by USP Chapter <797> as the date or time after which a compounded sterile preparation (CSP) shall not be administered, stored, or transported; the BUD is determined from the date the preparation is compounded

Bioavailability The degree to which a drug or other substance becomes available to the target tissue after administration

Bioequivalence The relationship between two drugs that have the same dosage and dosage form and similar bioavailability; generic versions of a medication must show bioequivalence to the original approved brand product as a requirement for drug approval

Biofeedback The use of electronic monitoring of an automatic bodily function to train a person to acquire voluntary control of that function

Biological response modifier (BRM) An agent used to modify the body's immune response

Biological safety cabinet (BSC) A hood that should be used for hazardous sterile preparations in the clean room

Blister pack See *bubble pack*

Blood-brain barrier (BBB) A barrier that exists in the brain as a result of special permeability characteristics of the capillaries that supply brain cells; these capillaries prevent certain solutes or chemicals from being transferred from the blood to the brain

Bloodletting The practice of draining blood; it was believed to release illness

Blood pressure The pressure of the blood in the arteries.

Board of pharmacy (BOP) A state-managed agency (board) that licenses pharmacists and may either register or license pharmacy technicians to work in a pharmacy

Bone fracture A break or rupture of a bone

Bone marrow The fatty network of connective tissue that fills the cavities in the long bones; it is the source of red blood cells and many white blood cells

Boxed warning A drug warning placed in the prescribing information or package insert of a product that indicates a significant risk of potentially dangerous side effects. It is the strongest warning the U.S. Food and Drug Administration (FDA) can give. It is common in the pharmacy profession to call these warnings "Black Box Warnings" because of their appearance on a drug label; the warning is often enclosed in a black outlined box to draw attention to the content

Bradykinesia Slowed movement

Brainstem A section of the brain consisting of the medulla oblongata, pons, and midbrain; the brainstem connects the forebrain and cerebrum to the spinal cord

Brand name The name a company assigns to a commercial drug product for marketing and identification purposes. Most proprietary names are trademarked and belong to originator products. The named products are often protected, for a time, by patents; also known as the *proprietary name* or *trade name*

Bronchi Any of the major air passages of the lungs that diverge from the windpipe

Bronchioles Any of the small branches into which a bronchus divides in the respiratory tract

Bubble pack A preformed card with 28-, 30-, and 31-day depressions that can hold medications; they are sealed with a foil card backboard and usually used for long-term care medications

Bulk repackaging The process by which the pharmacy transfers a medication manually or by means of an automated system from a manufacturer's original container to another type of container unrelated to dispensing a prescriber's order

C

Caduceus Often confused as the symbol of the medical field; it is a staff with two entwined snakes and two wings at the top

Calcitonin A thyroid hormone that helps to regulate blood concentrations of calcium and phosphate and promotes the formation of bone

Calibration The markings on a measuring device

Cancellous bone A meshwork of spongy bone typically found at the core of vertebral bones in the spine and the ends of long bones; also called *spongy bone*

Capillary An extremely small vessel that connects the ends of the smallest arteries (arterioles) to the smallest veins (venules), where the exchange of nutrients, waste products, oxygen, and carbon dioxide occurs

Carbohydrates Chemical compounds that contain carbon, hydrogen, and oxygen (e.g., sugars, glycogen, starches, and cellulose)

Carbonic anhydrase An enzyme that converts carbonic acid into carbon dioxide and water

Cardiac muscle A type of muscle tissue found only in the heart

Cardiac output The amount of blood the heart pumps through the circulatory system in a minute

Catecholamines Hormones produced in the brainstem, nervous system, and adrenal glands; they help the body respond to stress and prepare the body for the "fight or flight" response; they also are important in the regulation of the heart rate, blood pressure, and nervous system functions

Cation A positively charged ion

Central nervous system (CNS) The division of the nervous system made up of the brain and spinal cord; the CNS coordinates sensory and motor control of bodily functions

Cerebellum A structure posterior to the pons and medulla oblongata that is responsible for posture, balance, and voluntary muscle movement

Certified pharmacy technician A technician who has passed the national certification examination; the technician can use the abbreviation CPhT after his or her name

Cerumen Earwax

Chain pharmacy A corporate-owned group of pharmacies that share a brand name and central management and usually have standardized business methods and practices

Channel In communications, a written message, spoken words, or body language

Chemical structure The makeup of a chemical, including factors such as the elements, shape, bonding types, and molecular configurations; the nature of a chemical's structure has much to do with the chemical's stability, reactivity, and physical and chemical properties

Chiropractic medicine A system of medical practice that involves manual manipulation of the joints and muscles

Chloasma Hyperpigmentation of the skin that is limited or confined to a certain area

Chronic kidney disease (CKD) A condition in which the kidneys' ability to function properly is diminished

Chyme The soupy mixture (semifluid consistency) of food after it has mixed with stomach acids and digestive enzymes as it passes into the duodenum (first part of the small intestine)

Cilia Short, microscopic, hairlike structures

Ciliary body The part of the eye that connects the iris to the choroid

Circadian rhythms A daily cycle of activity observed in living organisms; the term can pertain to sleep/wake cycles

Civilian Health and Medical Program of the Department of Veterans Affairs (CHAMPVA) A program for veterans with permanent service-related disabilities and their dependents and spouses and children of veterans who died from service-connected disability; also known as the Veterans Health Administration (VHA)

Clean room A contained and controlled environment in the pharmacy that has a low level of environmental pollutants such as dust, airborne microbes, aerosol particles, and chemical vapors; the clean room is used for preparing sterile medication products

Closed-door pharmacy A pharmacy to which medications are called in from institutions such as long-term care facilities, and the medications are then delivered; closed door pharmacies are not open to the public

Closed formulary A system in which medication use is tightly restricted to medications provided on the formulary list; medications that are not listed as preapproved drugs per the health plan provider or pharmacy benefits manager are not reimbursed except under extenuating circumstances and with proper documentation

Coagulation Solidification, or a change from a fluid state to a solid state, as in the formation of a blood clot

Coinsurance A type of insurance in which the policyholder pays a share of the payment made against a claim

Collecting duct The duct system of the kidneys in which a series of tubules connect the nephrons to the ureter

Colony-stimulating factor (CSF) A hormone that stimulates the bone marrow to synthesize hematopoietic cells

Comedone A plug of keratin and sebum in a hair follicle that is blackened at the surface; commonly called a *blackhead*

Communication The ability to express oneself in such a way that one is readily and clearly understood

Community pharmacy Pharmacies that serve patients in their communities; consumers can walk in and purchase a prescription or OTC drug; also known as *outpatient pharmacies* or retail pharmacies

Comorbidity A concomitant but not necessarily related medical condition that exists simultaneously with another condition

Compact bone The type of rigid bone that constitutes most of the skeleton; also known as *cortical bone*

Compassion A feeling of wanting to help someone who is sick or in trouble

Competency The capability or proficiency to perform a function

Complementary medicine A range of medical therapies that fall beyond the scope of Western medicine but that may be used in a complementary fashion with traditional medicine practices

Compounded sterile preparations (CSPs) Substances prepared in a sterile environment with nonsterile ingredients or devices that must be sterilized before they are used

Compounding The act of mixing, reconstituting, and packaging a drug

Compounding record (CR) Documentation of nonsterile compounding

Computerized physician order entry (CPOE) A computerized order entry

Confidentiality The practice of keeping privileged customer information from being disclosed without the customer's consent

Conjunctiva The transparent protective mucous membrane that lines the underside of the eyelid

Continuing education (CE) Courses taken beyond the basic technical education, usually required for license or certification renewal

Controlled substance Any drug or other substance categorized as Schedule I through V and regulated by the Drug Enforcement Administration

Conversion factor A fraction used to convert one unit into another without changing the value of the number

Copayment The portion of the prescription bill that the patient is responsible for paying

Cornea The transparent tissue covering the anterior portion of the eye

Coronary artery Either of two arteries that supply the tissues of the heart; one arises one from the left side of the aorta and the other from the right side of the aorta

Crash carts Moveable carts containing trays of medications, administration sets, oxygen, and other materials that are used in life-threatening situations such as cardiac arrest; also known as *code carts*

Cream A hydrophilic base

Cretinism A condition in which the development of the brain and body is inhibited by a congenital lack of thyroid hormone secretion

Cryoprecipitate Any precipitate that results from cooling; a term sometimes specifically used to describe a precipitate rich in coagulation Factor VIII obtained from cooling of blood plasma

Cyclooxygenase (COX) Either of two related enzymes that control the production of prostaglandins

Cytokine A protein that signals cells of the immune system

D

Deductible The amount paid by a policyholder out of pocket before the insurance company pays a claim

Depot An area of the body where a substance can accumulate or be stored for later distribution

Dermis A thick layer of connective tissue that contains collagen

Diagnosis A physician's recognition of a condition or disease based on its outward signs and symptoms and/or confirming tests or procedures

Dialysate The fluid into which material passes by way of the membrane in dialysis

Dialysis The passage of a solute through a semipermeable membrane to remove toxic materials and to maintain fluid, electrolyte, and pH levels of the body system when the kidneys are malfunctioning

Diaphragm A dome-shaped, muscular partition separating the thorax from the abdomen that plays a major role in breathing

Diastole The period when the heart is in a state of relaxation and dilation

Digestion The mechanical, chemical, and enzymatic action of breaking down food into molecules that can be used in metabolism

Diluent/solvent An inert product, either liquid or solid, that is added to a preparation to reduce the strength of the original product

Dilution The process of adding a diluent or solvent to a compound, resulting in a product of increased volume or weight and lower concentration

Diplomacy The skill of dealing with others without causing bad feelings

Direct manufacturer ordering A process in which pharmacies may join a group purchasing organization (GPO) and contract directly with the manufacturer to obtain better pricing

Dispense as written (DAW) codes A numerical set of codes, created by the National Council for Prescription Drug Programs (NCPDP), that is used when filling prescriptions; the code can affect reimbursement amounts by insurance companies

Distribution The movement of a medication throughout blood, organs, and tissues after administration

Diuretic An agent that increases urine output and excretion of water from the body

Dogma A principle or set of principles laid down by an authority as incontrovertibly true

Drip rate/drop rate The number of drops (gtt) administered over a specific time via an intravenous infusion (e.g., gtt/min)

Drop factor The size of the drops produced by tubing used to administer a medication; the size is measured in gtt/mL, and the drop factor is indicated on the tubing package

Drug classification Categorization of a drug based on its various characteristics, including chemical structure, action, and/or therapeutic or anatomical use

Drug diversion The intentional misuse of a drug intended for medical purposes; the Drug Enforcement Administration usually defines diversion as the recreational use of a prescription or scheduled drug; diversion can also refer to the channeling of the prescription drug supply away from legal distribution and to the illegal street market

Drug Enforcement Administration (DEA) The agency of the U.S. Department of Justice that enforces U.S. laws and regulations related to controlled substances

Drug Enforcement Administration (DEA) number An alphanumeric number consisting of two letters and seven numbers that is assigned to prescribers authorized by the DEA to prescribe controlled substances

Drug Facts and Comparisons A reference book found in pharmacies that contains detailed information on medications

Drug Topics Red Book A reference book listing National Drug Code (NDC) numbers, manufacturers, and average wholesale pricing of drug products; pharmacies often include this type of product and pricing information on their online database systems, which are provided by companies such as First Data-Bank and Gold Standard

Drug utilization evaluation (DUE) A program for ensuring that prescribed drugs are used appropriately; an authorized, structured, ongoing review of health care provider prescribing, pharmacist dispensing, and patient use of medication; the primary goal of any DUE program is an increase in medication-related efficacy and safety; formerly known as drug utilization review

Dysarthria A speech deficiency that interferes with the normal control of the speech mechanism

Dyspnea Difficult or labored breathing

E

Eczema A medical condition in which patches of skin become rough and inflamed

Edema A condition characterized by an excess of watery fluid that collects in the cavities or tissues of the body

Electronic medication administration record (eMAR) Technology that automatically documents the administration of medication into certified electronic health record (EHR) systems; the report serves as a legal record of medications administered to a patient at a facility by a health care professional

Elimination The final elimination of a drug or other substance from the body via normal body processes, such as kidney elimination (urine), biliary excretion (bile to stool), sweat, respiration, or saliva

Elixir A base solution that is a mixture of alcohol and water

Embolus A clump of material, often a blood clot, that travels from one part of the body to another and then obstructs a blood vessel; it may consist of any material, including bacteria or air

Emesis A medical term for vomiting

Emollient A preparation that softens the skin

Emulsion A mixture of two or more liquids that do not usually blend together, which are mixed using a stabilizing agent; the process of making an emulsion is called *emulsification*

Endocardium The thin membrane that lines the interior of the heart; the inner layer of the heart wall

Endocrine glands Glands in the body that produce hormones that enter the bloodstream to reach their target site or act at target sites near the site of hormone release

Endocrinologist A physician who specializes in the treatment of conditions involving the endocrine system

Endometrium The mucous membrane lining the inner wall or layer of the uterus

Enteral A route of administration by way of the intestine, such as orally, rectally, or sublingually

Enzyme A protein that accelerates a reaction by reducing the amount of energy required to initiate a reaction

Epicardium The outer layer of the heart wall; the inner layer of the pericardium

Epidermis The outermost layer of the skin, composed of the stratum corneum, or horny layer; the keratinocytes (squamous cells); and the basal layer; it also contains melanin, a pigment that contributes to the color of skin and hair

Epilepsy A brain disorder marked by repeated seizures over time

e-Prescribing The computer-to-computer transfer of prescription data between pharmacies, prescribers, and payers

Erectile dysfunction (ED) The inability to maintain an erection sufficient for satisfying sexual activity

Erythrocyte A cell that contains hemoglobin and can carry oxygen to the body; also known as a *red blood cell* (RBC)

Erythropoiesis The formation of erythrocytes

Erythropoietin A hormone secreted by the kidney that stimulates the production of red blood cells by stem cells in the bone marrow

Eschar A slough produced by a thermal burn, by a corrosive application, or by gangrene

Essential hypertension The most common form of hypertension; it occurs in the absence of any evident cause

Estrogen Any of a group of anabolic sex hormones that promote the development and maintenance of female sexual characteristics

Ethics The values and morals used within a profession

Etiquette An unwritten guideline or rule of behavior

Euphoria A feeling or state of intense excitement and happiness

Eustachian tube A tubular structure in the middle ear that connects with the nasopharynx (throat); it functions to equalize pressure between the outside air and middle ear and to drain mucus

Excipient An inert substance added to a drug to form a suitable consistency for dosing

Excretion Elimination of waste products and other remnants of metabolism, primarily through stools and urine

Exfoliation The peeling off of dead skin

Exocrine glands Glands that produce hormones that are sent to the target organ or tissue via a tube or duct

Exophthalmos Prominence (protrusion) of the eyeball out of the orbit; bilateral presentation commonly is caused by an increase in thyroid hormone

Expectorant A chemical that aids in the removal of mucous secretions from the respiratory system by loosening and thinning sputum and bronchial secretions for ease of expectoration

Expiration The act of breathing out; exhalation

Extrapyramidal symptoms Symptoms often produced by antipsychotic medications; they include parkinsonism, dystonia, and tremors

Exudate A mass of cells and fluid that has seeped out of blood vessels as a result of inflammation

F

Fallopian tube A narrow tube that connects the ovary to the uterus

Fascicles A bundle of structures, such as muscle fibers

FDA See *Food and Drug Administration (FDA)*

Federal legend The statement found on the labeling of all prescription medications: "Federal law prohibits the dispensing of this *drug* without a prescription"

Fertilization The process by which sperm unites with an ovum

Fibrates A class of antihyperlipidemic drugs primarily effective at lowering triglycerides

First-pass effect The process by which a portion of the dose is metabolized before the drug has a chance to be distributed systemically

Fistula A permanent abnormal passageway between two organs in the body or between an organ and the exterior of the body

Floor stock Drugs that are not labeled for a specific patient or maintained at a nursing station or other department of the institution (excluding the pharmacy) for administration to a patient of the facility

Flow rate/infusion rate The amount of intravenous solution administered over a specified period (e.g., mL/min, mL/hr, gtt/min); volume/time

Food and Drug Administration (FDA) The agency in the U.S. Department of Health and Human Services responsible for ensuring the safety, efficacy, and security of human and veterinary drugs, biological products, medical devices, the national food supply, cosmetics, and radioactive products

Formulary A list of drugs that have been approved for use in hospitals by the pharmacy and therapeutics committee of the institution and are the standard stock carried by the pharmacy and other departments; also, a list of drugs covered by an insurance company

Formulation record A document similar to a recipe used in preparation of nonsterile compounds

Franchise A form of business organization in which a firm that already has a successful product or service (the franchisor) enters into a continuing contractual relationship with other businesses (franchisees) operating under the franchisor's trade name and usually with the franchisor's guidance, in exchange for a fee

Fungicidal Able to destroy or inhibit the growth of fungi

G

Gametes Sex cells, or ova and sperm

Gastroparesis Delayed gastric emptying

Gauge The size of a needle opening

Generic name The name assigned to a medication; the nonproprietary name of a drug

Gigantism A condition associated with excessive production of growth hormone during childhood or adolescence that results in excessive height and growth of body tissues

Glomerulonephritis Acute inflammation of the kidney typically caused by an immune response

Glucometer A device used to test blood sugar levels in people with diabetes mellitus

Goiter A condition in which the thyroid gland is enlarged because of a lack of iodine; it can be either a simple goiter or a toxic goiter (i.e., resulting from a tumor)

Good manufacturing practices (GMP) Federal guidelines that must be followed by all entities that prepare and package medication or medical devices

Gout A painful form of arthritis characterized by defective metabolism of uric acid

Granulocytopenia A reduction in the number of granulocytes (i.e., specific types of white blood cells [WBCs] that contain "granules"); these include neutrophils, eosinophils, and basophils; all are known as *granulocytes*

Graves disease A condition caused by hypersecretion of thyroid hormones; symptoms include diffuse goiter, exophthalmos, and skin changes

H

Half-life (1) The amount of time it takes a chemical to be decreased by one half; (2) the time required for half the amount of a substance, such as a drug in a living system, to be eliminated or disintegrated by natural processes; (3) the time required for the concentration of a substance in a body fluid (blood plasma) to decrease by half

Hashimoto's thyroiditis An autoimmune disease that leads to hypothyroidism

Hazardous drug Any drug that has been proven to have dangerous effects during animal or human testing; it may cause cancer or harm to certain organs or pregnant women

Hazardous waste Any waste that meets the Resource Conservation and Recovery Act (RCRA) definition of ignitability, corrosiveness, reactivity, or toxicity

Head louse A louse that infests the scalp and hair of the human head

Health care–associated infection (HAI) An infection that patients acquire during the course of receiving treatments for other conditions in an institutional setting

Health Insurance Portability and Accountability Act of 1996 (HIPAA) A federal law that protects patients' rights, establishes national standards for electronic health care communication, and ensures the security and privacy of health data

Health maintenance organization (HMO) An insurance plan that that allows coverage for in-network only physicians and services and uses the primary care physician (or provider) as the "gatekeeper" for a patient's health care; patients often have co-pays to defray the costs of medical care and prescription drugs

Heart failure Inability of the heart to keep up with the demands on it; specifically, failure of the heart to pump blood with normal efficiency

Help desk A 24/7 toll-free hotline to an insurance company that pharmacists can use to ask specific questions about insurance claims and coverage, in addition to pharmacy-specific inquiries

Hematopoiesis The formation of blood cells

Hemoglobin The oxygen-carrying component of red blood cells

Hemophilia A hereditary blood coagulation disorder that leads to a decreased ability to clot normally

Hemorrhagic stroke A stroke caused by the rupture of a blood vessel in the brain

Herb Any plant that is valued for its aromatic, medicinal, flavorful, or other properties

Herbals A substance made from or using herbs

High-density lipoprotein (HDL) A lipoprotein of blood plasma that is composed of a high proportion of protein with little triglyceride and cholesterol; it is associated with a decreased probability of developing atherosclerosis

Hippocratic Oath An oath taken by physicians concerning the ethics and practice of medicine

Hirsutism Abnormal growth of hair on a person's face and body

Homeopathy A system of therapy based on the belief that dilutions of medicinal substances that cause a specific symptom can be used to treat an illness that yields the same symptoms; homeopathic remedies are regulated by the FDA under the Food, Drug, and Cosmetic Act

Homeostasis The equilibrium pertaining to the balance of the body with respect to fluid levels, pH level, osmotic pressures, and concentrations of various substances; the tendency of the body to maintain stability (e.g., body temperature)

Horizontal laminar flow hood An environment for the preparation of compounded sterile preparations in which air originating from the back of the hood moves forward across the hood and into the room

Hormones Chemical substances produced and secreted by an endocrine duct into the bloodstream that result in a physiological response at a specific target tissue

Household system A system of measurement commonly used in the United States; volumes are measured using household utensils

Humoral immunity The immune response mediated by antibodies

Hydrophilic Water loving; any substance that easily mixes in water

Hydrophobic Water hating; any substance that does not mix or dissolve in water

Hydrostatic pressure The pressure exerted by a fluid due to the force of gravity

Hyperalimentation Parenteral (intravenous) nutrition for patients who are unable to eat solids or liquids; also known as *total parenteral nutrition* (TPN)

Hyperglycemia An elevated concentration of glucose in the blood

Hypertension High blood pressure

Hyperthyroidism Excessive secretion of thyroid hormone

Hypocalcemia A low concentration of calcium in the blood

Hypodermis Subcutaneous tissue

Hypoglycemia An excessively low concentration of glucose in the blood

Hypokalemia A low concentration of potassium in the blood

Hypopituitary dwarfism Short stature due to a deficiency in growth hormone during childhood

Hypotension Low blood pressure

Hypoxia Reduction of the oxygen supply to a tissue despite adequate perfusion of the tissue by blood

I

Idiopathic Of unknown cause

Immunity A type of resistance to infection caused by an immune response from the body after exposure to antigens or administration of a vaccine

Immunization The act of conferring immunity, such as with vaccination

Immunoglobulin An antibody

Inert ingredient An ingredient that has little or no effect on body functions

Infection control Policies and procedures put in place to minimize the risk of spreading infections in hospitals or other health care facilities

Inflammation A localized physical condition associated with red, swollen, hot, and often painful tissue

Influenza A respiratory tract infection caused by an influenza virus

Ingestion The act of taking in food, liquid, or other substances (e.g., medications)

Innate immunity Natural immunity

Inpatient pharmacy A pharmacy in a hospital or institutional setting

Inscription The name, dosage form, strength, and quantity of the medication prescribed

Insomnia Difficulty falling or staying asleep

Inspiration The act of breathing in; inhalation

Instill To place into; instillation instructions are commonly used for ophthalmic or otic drugs

Institute for Healthcare Improvement (IHI) A nonprofit organization committed to the improvement of health care by promoting promising concepts through safety, efficiency, and other patient-centered goals

Institute of Medicine (IOM) Established under the National Academies and a part of the National Academy of Sciences, this nonprofit organization provides scientifically informed analysis and guidance regarding health and health policy; projects include studies of drug safety systems within the United States and recommendations for patient safety

Institute for Safe Medication Practices (ISMP) A nonprofit organization devoted entirely to promoting safe medication use and preventing medication errors; the organization gathers information on drug errors and suggests new, safer standards to prevent such errors

Institutional pharmacy A pharmacy in which patients receive care on site, such as in hospitals, extended-living homes, long-term care, and hospice facilities; institutional pharmacies are also found in government-supported hospitals run by the Veterans Health Administration, Indian Health Service, and the Bureau of Prisons

Insulin resistance Resistance of the tissues of the body (skeletal muscle and fat) to the effects of insulin; insulin resistance is associated with the development of type 2 diabetes mellitus

International System of Units (SI) A system of measurement based on seven base units with prefixes that change units by multiples of 10; the prefixes for the modern metric system are taken from the French Système International d'Unités and were adopted to provide a single worldwide system of weights and measures

International time A 24-hour method of keeping time in which hours are not distinguished between AM and PM, but rather are counted continuously throughout the day

Interstitial space A small, narrow space between tissues

Intraocular pressure The pressure exerted by the fluids inside the eyeball

Inventory The amount of product a pharmacy has for sale

Investigational drug A drug that has not been approved by the FDA for marketing but is in clinical trials; the term can also pertain to an FDA-approved drug for which the manufacturers are seeking approval of a new indication for use

Ion An atom or molecule with a net electric charge (positive or negative)

Iris The colored part of the eye seen through the cornea; it consists of smooth muscles that regulate pupil size

Ischemic stroke An stroke caused by blockage of a blood vessel in the brain

J

Just-in-time ordering A system in which a product is ordered just before it is used

Juvenile rheumatoid arthritis (JRA) Rheumatoid arthritis that affects children

K

Keratolytic A drug that causes shedding of the outer layer of the skin

L

Lacrimal fluid The fluid within the eyes that cleans and lubricates them

Laminar flow hood An environment for the preparation of sterile products

Larynx The hollow muscular organ that forms an air passage to the lungs and holds the vocal cords

Laudanum A mixture of opium and alcohol used to treat dozens of illnesses through the 1800s

Leech A type of segmented worm with suckers that attaches to the skin of a host; leeches engorge themselves on the host's blood

Legend drugs Drugs that require a prescription; these drugs carry the federal legend: "Federal law prohibits the dispensing of this medication without a prescription"

Lens The flexible, clear tissue that focuses images

Leukemia A progressive, malignant disease of the blood-forming organs, marked by distorted proliferation and development of leukocytes and their precursors in the blood and bone marrow

Leukocyte A white blood cell (WBC)

Leukopenia A reduction in the number of leukocytes (white blood cells) in the blood

Licensed pharmacy technician A pharmacy technician who is licensed by the state board; licensing ensures that an individual has at least the minimum level of competency required by the profession

Ligament Fibrous connective tissue that connects to bones

Lithotripsy Treatment with ultrasound shock waves to break a kidney stone into small particles

Low-density lipoprotein (LDL) A molecule that is a combination of lipid (fat) and protein

Lumen The channel inside a tube, such as a blood vessel

Lymph node A structure that consists of many small, oval nodules that filter lymphatic fluid and fight infection; the site of lymphocyte, monocyte, and plasma cell production

Lymphocyte A mononuclear leukocyte found in the blood, lymph, and lymphoid tissues; lymphocytes are white blood cells that, unlike granulocytes, do not have "granules"

Lymphoid organ The system of interconnected tissues and organs by which lymph circulates throughout the body

Lymphoma Cancer of the lymphatic system

M

Maggots Fly larvae that feed on dead tissue; they are used in medicine to clean wounds that do not respond to routine antibiotics

Mammary gland The milk-producing gland of women

Managed care An organized health care delivery system designed to improve both the quality and accessibility of health care, including pharmaceutical care, while containing costs

Markup The amount (usually a percentage) added to a wholesale price to make a profit

Medicaid A federal- and state-operated insurance program that covers health care costs and prescription drugs for low-income children, adults, and elderly and those with disabilities

Medicare A government-managed insurance program composed of several coverage plans for health care services and supplies; it is funded by both federal and state entities, and individuals must meet specific requirements to be eligible; individuals must be 65 years or older, or younger than 65 with long-term disabilities, or suffer from end-stage renal disease

Medicare Modernization Act (MMA) A law that provides for prescription drug coverage for those covered by Medicare

Medication error Any preventable event that may cause or lead to inappropriate medication use or patient harm

Medication error prevention Methods used by pharmacy, medicine, nursing, and other allied health professionals to prevent medication errors

Medication order A prescription written for administration in a hospital or institutional setting

Medication reconciliation The process of comparing a patient's medication orders with all the medications the patient was taking before admission to the hospital

Medicine The science and art dealing with the maintenance of health and the prevention, alleviation, or cure of disease

Medigap plan Supplemental insurance provided through private insurance companies to help cover costs not reimbursed by the Medicare plan, such as coinsurance, copays, and deductibles

MedMARx A national, Internet-accessible database that hospitals and health care systems use to track adverse drug reactions and medication errors

MedWatch A program established by the FDA for reporting drug and medical product safety alerts and label changes; the program also provides a voluntary adverse event reporting system for medications, medical products, and devices

Melanin A dark brown to black pigment found in the hair, skin, and iris of the eye

Menopause The cessation of menstruation; a natural phenomenon in which a woman passes from a reproductive state to a nonreproductive state

Menses The time of menstruation

Metabolism The processes by which the body breaks down or converts medications to active or inactive substances; the primary site of drug metabolism in humans is the liver; however, select drugs are metabolized through other processes

Metastasis The process by which cancer spreads from the place of origin (e.g., a primary tumor) to distant locations in the body

Metric system The approved system of measurement for pharmacy in the United States based on multiples of 10; the basic units of measurement are the gram (g) for weight, the liter (L) for volume, and the meter (m) for length

Micturition Urination

Miosis Contraction (constriction) of the pupil of the eye

Misbranding Labeling of a product that is false or misleading; label information must include the directions for use; safe and/ or unsafe dosages; manufacturer, packer, or distributor; quantity; and weight

Monocyte A phagocytic leukocyte

Monograph Comprehensive information on a medication's actions in that class of drugs; it also lists generic and trade names, ingredients, dosages, side effects, adverse effects, how the patient should take the medication, and foods or other drugs (e.g., OTC medications, herbals) to avoid while taking the medication

Morals Beliefs concerning or relating to what is right or wrong in human behavior

Mortar and pestle A bowl and tool with a rounded knob used to grind substances into fine powder or to mix liquids

Motor nerve A nerve carrying impulses from the brain or spinal cord to a muscle or gland

Multiple sclerosis (MS) A chronic autoimmune disorder that affects nerves in the CNS, leading to impaired motor function

Muscle fiber Muscle cell

Myasthenia gravis A neuromuscular disorder that leads to weakness of the skeletal muscles

Mydriasis Dilation of the pupil

Myocardial infarction (MI) The death of myocardial tissue as the result of a sudden deprivation of oxygenated blood flow, often because of a blood clot plugging a coronary artery; also known as a *heart attack*

Myocardium The middle muscular layer of the heart wall; it consists of cardiac muscle tissue

Myopia Nearsightedness

Myxedema A condition associated with a decrease in overall thyroid function in adults; also known as *hypothyroidism*

N

Narcotic A nonspecific term used to describe a drug (e.g., opium) that in moderate doses dulls the senses, relieves pain, and induces profound sleep but that in excessive doses causes stupor, coma, or convulsions, and may lead to addiction; from the standpoint of U.S. law, opium, opiates (derivatives of opium), and opioids, in addition to cocaine and coca leaves, are narcotics

National Association of Boards of Pharmacy (NABP) A national organization for members of state boards of pharmacy

National Coordinating Council for Medication Error Reporting and Prevention (NCC MERP) An independent council of more than 25 organizations, founded by the United States Pharmacopeia (USP), that addresses interdisciplinary causes of medication errors and strategies for prevention

National Drug Code (NDC) number A unique 10- or 11-digit number given to all drugs for identification purposes; in health and drug databases, the NDC has three segments (the first four digits identify the drug manufacturer, the next four identify specifics about the product, and the last two identify the drug packaging); placeholder zeros are inserted in the proper order in the code to standardize data transmissions

National Healthcareer Association (NHA) A certifying organization for a variety of health care careers, including the National Board for Certification of Pharmacy Technicians (NBCPT) and the Institute for the Certification of Pharmacy Technicians (ICPT)

National Pharmacy Technician Association (NPTA) A pharmacy association primarily for technicians that was founded in 1999

National Provider Identifier (NPI) A unique, 10-digit identification number for covered health care providers that is issued by the Centers for Medicare and Medicaid Services (CMS) to standardize health data transmissions

Negative feedback A self-regulating mechanism in which the output of a system has input or control on the process; the stimulus results in reactions that reduce the effects of the stimulus

Negligence A legal concept that describes an action taken without the forethought that should have been used by a reasonable person of similar competency

Nephron The filtering unit of the kidneys

Neuromuscular junction The junction between a nerve fiber and the muscle it supplies

Neuron The basic building block and cell of the nervous system

Neutropenia An abnormally low level of neutrophils in the blood

Nicotinic acid A member of the vitamin B complex; also known as *niacin*

Nitrate A medicine used to treat heart conditions such as angina

NKA No known allergies

NKDA No known drug allergy

Nocturia Urination at night

Nodule A small swelling or aggregation of cells in the body

Non-formulary drugs A list of drugs that are not included in the list of preferred medications that a committee of pharmacists and doctors deems to be the safest, most effective, and most economical; they are drugs not included in the drug list approved for reimbursement by the health care plans unless specific exceptions are filed and accepted by the institutional protocols

Non-proprietary (generic) name A short name coined for a drug or chemical not subject to proprietary (trademark) rights and recommended or recognized by an official body

Nonsterile compounding A process of compounding two or more medications in a nonsterile environment (no clean room or hood required)

Nonverbal communication The act of giving or exchanging information without using any spoken words

Nosocomial infection An infection that originates in the hospital or institutional setting

Nutraceutical A food or naturally occurring supplement thought to have a beneficial effect on human health

O

Occupational Safety and Health Administration (OSHA) A federal agency that oversees safety in the workplace; OSHA is responsible for establishing the Safety Data Sheet (SDS) requirements

Ointment A hydrophobic product, such as petroleum jelly

Oleaginous base An ingredient used in compounding that does not dissolve in water

Omnibus Budget Reconciliation Act of 1990 (OBRA '90) A law that changed reimbursement limits and mandated drug utilization evaluation, pharmacy patient consultation, and educational outreach programs

Onychomycosis A fungal infection of the fingernails or toenails

Oocyte (ova) The female reproductive germ cell, more commonly known as an egg

Oogenesis The production or development of an egg

Open formulary A formulary list that is essentially unrestricted in the types of drugs offered or that can be prescribed and reimbursed under the health provider plan or pharmacy benefit plan

Ophthalmic   Pertaining to the eye

Opioid   Any agent that binds to opioid receptors

Opioid analgesics   An analgesic medication that activates opioid receptors

Opium   An analgesic made from the poppy plant

Orbit   The eye socket

Orthostatic hypotension   A temporary lowering of blood pressure, usually related to suddenly standing up

Osmosis   Diffusion of fluid through a semipermeable membrane from a solution with a low solute concentration to a solution with a higher solute concentration in an effort to achieve equilibrium

Osmotic pressure   The pressure exerted by the flow of water through a semipermeable membrane separating two solutions with different concentrations of solutes

Osteoarthritis   A condition marked by degeneration of joint cartilage and the underlying bone

Osteoporosis   A medical condition in which the bones become brittle and fragile from loss of bone density and poor microarchitecture

Otic   Pertaining to the ear

Ototoxicity   Toxic effects on the organs of hearing or balance or on the auditory nerve

Outpatient pharmacies   Pharmacies that serve patients in community or ambulatory settings

Ovaries   The female reproductive organs in which ova or eggs are produced

Over the counter (OTC) medication   A medication that can be purchased without a prescription; nonlegend medications; it may be purchased by customers at any retail outlet

Ovulation   The release of an egg from the ovary

P

Package insert   The official prescribing information for a prescription drug; the medication information sheet provided by the manufacturer that includes side effects, dosage forms, indications, and other important information

Palliative   A substance that brings relief but does not cure

Pallor   Deficiency in color, particularly of the face

Pancreas   The endocrine gland that produces both insulin and glucagon

Papule   A small, raised, solid pimple on the skin

PAR   See *periodic automatic replacement (PAR) level*

Parasympathetic nervous system (PSNS)   The division of the autonomic nervous system that functions during restful situations

Parenteral medication   A medication that bypasses the digestive system but is intended for systemic action; the term most commonly describes medications given by injection, such as intravenously or intramuscularly

Parkinson's disease   A movement disorder with the classic symptoms of tremor, rigidity, bradykinesia, and postural instability

Patient profile   An electronic or written record listing important patient personal and health information, including comprehensive information on the medications the patient takes, disease states, and any food or drug allergies the patient may have

Pelvic inflammatory disease (PID)   Inflammation of the female genital tract, accompanied by fever and lower abdominal pain

Perception   The way a person thinks about or understands someone or something

Pericardium   The fluid-filled membrane that surrounds the heart; also called the *pericardial sac*

Periodic automatic replacement (PAR) level   A minimum set amount of stock that must be kept on hand

Peripheral nervous system (PNS)   The division of the nervous system outside the brain and spinal cord

Peripheral neuropathy   Damage to nerves of the peripheral nervous system

Peripheral parenteral administration   Injection of a medication into the veins on the periphery of the body rather than a central vein or artery

Peripheral parenteral nutrition (PPN)   Intravenous nutrition administered through the veins on the periphery of the body rather than a central vein or artery

Peripheral resistance   Vascular resistance to the flow of blood in peripheral arterial vessels

Peristalsis   The contraction and relaxation of the tubular muscles of the esophagus, stomach, and intestines that move substances from the mouth to the anus

Peritonitis   Inflammation of the peritoneum, typically caused by bacterial infection

Perspiration   The process of sweating

Phagocyte   A cell of the immune system that engulfs cells, debris, and antigens

Pharmacist   A health care professional who dispenses drugs and counsels patients on the use of medications and any interactions the drugs may have with food or other drugs

Pharmacokinetics   The study of the absorption, metabolism, distribution, and elimination of drugs

Pharmacy   A place where drugs are sold

Pharmacy benefit management (PBM)   The development and management of broad and cost-efficient prescription drug benefits for a large group of patient populations

Pharmacy clerk   A person who assists the pharmacist at the front counter of the pharmacy; the person who accepts payment for medications

Pharmacy technician   A person who assists a pharmacist by filling prescriptions and performing other nondiscretionary tasks

Pharmacy Technician Certification Board (PTCB)   A national board for the certification of pharmacy technicians; the PTCB provides a national exam for pharmacy technicians

Pharmacy Technician Educators Council (PTEC)   A U.S. organization that promotes teachers' strategies and instructions for pharmacy technician education

Pharmacy and therapeutics committee (P&T committee)   A medical staff composed of physicians, pharmacists, pharmacy technicians, nurses, and dieticians, who provide necessary information and advice to the institution or insurer on whether a drug should be added to a formulary

Pharynx   The membrane-lined cavity behind the nose and mouth that connects them to the esophagus

Phlebotomy   The process of opening a vein by incision or puncture to remove blood

Physicians' Desk Reference (PDR)   One of the many reference books on medications; it compiles and publishes select manufacturer-provided package inserts and prescribing information useful for health professionals

Plasma   The clear, yellowish fluid portion of blood

Plasma cell   A cell of the immune system that secretes antibodies

Plasma protein   Any of the various dissolved proteins of blood plasma

Pleural cavity   The cavity in the thorax that contains the lungs and heart

Point of sale (POS)   A system that allows inventory to be tracked as it is used

Polycythemia   An increase in the total cell mass of the blood

Polyneuropathy   A neurological disorder that occurs when many nerves throughout the body malfunction; it can be associated with painful neuropathy

Precipitate   To separate from solution or suspension; a solid that emerges from a liquid solution

Preferred provider organization (PPO)   An insurance plan in which patients choose a provider from a specified list, resulting in reduced costs for medical services

Pregnancy Category A system used by the FDA to describe five levels of assessment of the fetal effects caused by a drug; a required section of current prescription drug labeling; introduced in 1979, the system is currently under reevaluation for usefulness and inclusion on the prescription label

Prescription An order for medication issued by a physician, dentist, or other properly licensed practitioner, such as a physician assistant or nurse practitioner

Prime vendor A large distributor of medications and retail products that contracts with the pharmacy to deliver the bulk of the pharmacy's medications in exchange for lower prices (e.g., McKesson, Cardinal Health, and AmerisourceBergen)

Prior authorization Insurance-required approval for a restricted, non-formulary, or noncovered medication before a prescription medication can be filled

prn An abbreviation for a Latin term *(pro re nata)* meaning "as needed"

Prodrug An inactive substance that is converted to a drug in the body by the action of enzymes or other chemicals

Professionalism Conforming to the right principles of conduct (work ethics) as accepted by others in the profession

Progesterone An anabolic sex hormone that stimulates the uterus to prepare for pregnancy

Prophylactic Treatment given before an event or exposure to prevent the occurrence of a condition or symptom

Prophylaxis To prevent disease

Prostaglandin A mediator responsible for inflammation features such as swelling, pain, stiffness, redness, and warmth

Prostate A gland surrounding the neck of the bladder in males that produces a fluid component of semen

Protected health information (PHI) A patient's personal health data; under HIPAA, this information is protected from sharing or distribution without permission

Protocol A set of standards and guidelines within which a facility operates

Pruritus Itching of the skin

Psychosis A mental illness characterized by loss of contact with reality; psychosis may be a true mental illness, may be due to an underlying medical condition (e.g., dementia, drug withdrawal syndromes), or may be induced by substances such as medications, recreational drugs, or poisons

Pulmonary artery One of the two vessels formed as terminal branches of the pulmonary trunk that convey unaerated blood to the lungs

Punch method Manual filling of capsules with powdered medication that has been premixed

Pupil The circular opening in the iris that allows light to enter

Pustule A small blister or pimple on the skin containing pus

Pyxis An automated dispensing system often used in hospitals

R

Reconstitute To add a diluent (e.g., saline or sterile water) to a powder

Reconstitution To mix a liquid and a powder to form a suspension or solution

Refill Permission by a prescriber to replenish a prescription

Registered pharmacy technician A pharmacy technician who is registered through the state board of pharmacy; the registration process helps maintain a list of those working in pharmacies and may require a background check through the legal system; the registration process does not guarantee the level of the registrant's knowledge or skills

Renal artery One of the pair of arteries that branch from the abdominal aorta; each kidney has one renal artery

Renal osteodystrophy A condition resulting from chronic kidney disease (CKD) and renal failure; it is marked by elevated serum phosphorus levels, low or normal serum calcium levels, and stimulation of parathyroid function, resulting in bone disease

Renal vein The vein in which filtered blood from the kidneys is sent back into the body's circulatory system; each kidney has one renal vein

Renin An enzyme secreted by and stored in the kidneys that promotes the production of the protein angiotensin

Repackaging The act of reducing the amount of medication taken from a bulk bottle

Resorption The process or action by which something is reabsorbed (e.g., bone resorption in the development of osteoporosis)

Retail price The wholesale price plus markup

Retina The innermost layer of the eye; a complex structure considered part of the CNS; the retina contains photoreceptors (rods and cones), which transmit impulses to the optic nerve, and the macula lutea (a yellow spot in the center of the retina)

Reye's syndrome A life-threatening metabolic disorder in young children of uncertain cause that sometimes is precipitated by aspirin use

Rheumatic fever A noncontagious, acute fever marked by inflammation and pain in the joints

Rheumatoid arthritis (RA) A progressive degenerative and crippling autoimmune disease of the joints

Risk evaluation and mitigation strategy (REMS) A strategy to manage a known or potential serious risk associated with a drug or biological product

S

Safety Data Sheets (SDSs) Documents that provide chemical product information; an SDS includes the product name, composition (chemicals in the product), hazards, toxicology, and other information regarding the proper steps to take with spills, accidental exposure, handling, and storage of the product; filing of an SDS in the pharmacy or workplace is usually a requirement to meet Occupational Safety and Health Administration (OSHA) standards; formerly known as Material Safety Data Sheets

Satellite pharmacy A specialty pharmacy located away from the central pharmacy, such as with an operating room (OR), emergency department (ED), or a neonatal pharmacy; it typically is staffed by a pharmacist and a pharmacy technician

Schizophrenia A group of mental disorders characterized by inappropriate emotions and unrealistic thinking

Sclera The white of the eyes

Sebaceous glands The skin glands responsible for the secretion of oil called *sebum*

Seborrhea Excessive discharge of sebum from the sebaceous glands

Sebum An oily/waxy substance that lubricates the skin and retains water to provide moisture

Secondary hypertension Hypertension that results from an underlying identifiable cause

Serum The clear, yellowish fluid obtained by separating whole blood into its solid and liquid components after it has been allowed to clot; plasma minus clotting factors

Shaman A person who holds a high place of honor in a tribe as a healer and spiritual mediator

Signatura (signa or sig) The directions on a prescription that explain how the patient is to take the prescribed medication; a Latin expression meaning to "write on label"

Skeletal muscle Muscle connected to the skeleton to form part of the mechanical system that moves the limbs and other parts of the body

Skeletal system The hard structure (bones and cartilages) that provides a frame for the body

Society for the Education of Pharmacy Technicians (SEPhT) A national pharmacy technician organization that promotes the education and training of pharmacy technicians; it provides links to medication safety and quality practices for technicians

Sole proprietorship An unincorporated business owned by one person

Solute The ingredient dissolved into a solution

Solution A water base in which the ingredient or ingredients are dissolved completely

Solvent The greater part of a solution that dissolves a solute

Somatic nervous system The motor neurons of the peripheral nervous system that control voluntary actions of the skeletal muscles and provide sensory input (touch, hearing, sight)

Sperm (spermatozoa) Male reproductive germ cells

Spermatogenesis The development of sperm in the testes

Spermicide An agent that kills sperm

Spleen The lymphatic organ involved in the production and removal of blood cells and storage of lymphocytes

Splenectomy Surgical removal of the spleen

Spongy bone The meshwork of spongy bone typically found at the core of vertebral bones in the spine and the ends of long bones, also known as *cancellous bone*

Sputum The fluid (mucus) expectorated from the lungs and bronchial tissues

Staff of Asclepius The symbol of the medical profession; it is a wingless staff with one snake wrapped around it

Standard operating procedures (SOPs) Written guidelines and criteria that list specific steps for various competencies

Standard Precautions (Universal Precautions) A set of standards that lowers the possibility of contamination and lowers the risk of transmission of infectious disease; Standard Precautions are used throughout a health care facility, including to prepare medications

Standing order Written protocols for drugs or treatment that is to be used in a specific situation

Stat order A medication order that must be filled immediately; that is, as quickly as is safely possible to prepare the dose, usually within 5 to 15 minutes

Statins An informal term for HMG-CoA reductase inhibitors, which are used for the treatment of hyperlipidemia, primarily to lower LDL cholesterol

Stent A tube designed to be inserted into a vessel or passageway to keep it open

Sterile preparation A preparation that contains no living microorganisms

Stress incontinence Involuntary emission of urine when pressure in the abdomen suddenly increases

Strip pack A strip of heat-sealed packets, each holding one tablet or capsule, that is used in the bulk repackaging process

Stroke The sudden death of some brain cells due to lack of oxygen when blood flow to the brain is impaired by blockage (ischemic stroke) or rupture (hemorrhagic stroke) of an artery to the brain

Subchondral bone The bone located below the cartilage, particularly within a joint

Subcutaneous layer The deepest layer of the skin, which consists of fat cells and collagen; it protects the body and conserves heat

Subscription The part of the prescription that provides specific instructions to the pharmacist on how to compound the prescription

Superscription The heading of a prescription, represented by the Latin symbol Rx, meaning "take thou" or "you take"; the symbol has come to represent prescription or pharmacy

SureMed An automated dispensing system often used in hospitals

Surface area The amount of an object's surface that is in contact with its surroundings

Suspension A solution in which the powder does not dissolve into the base and must be shaken before use

Sweat glands Glands in the dermis that are activated in response to increased body temperature to cool the body

Sympathetic nervous system A division of the autonomic nervous system that functions during stressful situations; the "fight or flight" part of the autonomic nervous system

Sympathomimetic Producing physiological effects resembling those caused by the sympathetic nervous system

Syndrome A set of conditions that occur together

Synovium A thin membrane in synovial (freely moving) joints that lines the joint capsule and secretes synovial fluid

Synthetic medicine A medication made in a laboratory from chemical processes

Syrup A sugar-based liquid

Systemic Pertaining to the entire organism; widespread rather than local

Systemic lupus erythematosus (SLE) An autoimmune inflammatory disease of connective tissue that has variable features, including fever, weakness, fatigability, and other systemic manifestations

Systole The period when the heart contracts; the period specifically during which the left ventricle of the heart contracts

T

Tachycardia A rapid heart rate, usually defined as faster than 100 beats per minute

Tact The ability to do or say things without offending or upsetting other people

Tardive dyskinesia A type of dyskinesia (unwanted, involuntary rhythmic movements) considered a potential side effect of dopamine antagonists such as phenothiazines or other medications (e.g., metoclopramide); the symptoms may continue even after discontinuation of the offending drug

Telepharmacy The provision of pharmaceutical care through the use of telecommunications and information technologies to patients at a distance

Tendon A flexible but inelastic cord of strong, fibrous collagen tissue that attaches a muscle to a bone

Teratogen Any agent causing abnormal embryonic or fetal development

Testes The male reproductive organs that produce sperm

Testosterone An anabolic sex hormone produced in the testes that stimulates the development of male sexual characteristics

The Joint Commission (TJC) An independent, nonprofit organization that accredits hospitals and other health care organizations in the United States; accreditation is required to accept Medicare and Medicaid payment

Therapeutic alliance A trust relationship between a health care professional and a patient that incorporates the patient's perceptions of the acceptability of interventions and mutually agreed upon goals for treatment

Thrombin An enzyme formed in coagulating blood from prothrombin; thrombin reacts with fibrinogen and converts it to fibrin, which is essential in the formation of blood clots; thrombin levels tested by performing a prothrombin time or partial thromboplastin time blood test

Thrombocyte A platelet

Thrombocytopenia A decrease in the number of platelets in the blood

Thrombolytic A medication used to break up a thrombus or blood clot

Thrombosis The formation or presence of a blood clot in a blood vessel.

Thyroxine (T_4) A thyroid hormone derived from tyrosine (amino acid); it influences the metabolic rate

Tinnitus Ringing or buzzing in the ears

Tort An act that causes harm or injury to a person intentionally or because of negligence

Total parenteral nutrition (TPN) Large-volume intravenous nutrition administered through the central vein (subclavian vein), which allows for a higher concentration of solutions

Toxoid A type of vaccine in which a toxin has been rendered harmless but still invokes an antigenic response, improving immunity against the active toxin at some future date

Traditional Chinese medicine (TCM) A complementary and alternative medicine (CAM) system that includes a range of traditional medicine practices originating in China

Transient ischemic attack (TIA) A neurological event that produces the signs and symptoms of a stroke, which go away within a short period

Transplant rejection An immune response after tissue/organ transplant

Treatment authorization request (TAR) The process used by Medicare and Medicaid for assistive technology devices that cost more than $100; durable medical equipment (e.g., wheelchairs, walkers) also requires a TAR; similar to a preauthorization form

Trephining The practice of making an opening in the head to allow disease to leave the body

TRICARE A health benefit program for active-duty and retired personnel in all seven uniformed services. It also covers dependants of military personnel who were killed while on active duty; formerly CHAMPUS

Triglyceride The major form of fat stored by the body; a triglyceride consists of three molecules of fatty acid combined with a molecule of the alcohol glycerol

Triiodothyronine (T$_3$) A thyroid hormone that helps regulate growth and development and controls metabolism and body temperature; mainly produced through the metabolism of thyroxine

Triturate To grind or crush powder (e.g., a tablet) into fine particles

Troche A flat, disklike tablet that dissolves between the gum and cheek

Tubular reabsorption The conservation of protein, glucose, bicarbonate, and water from the glomerular filtrate by the tubules

Tubular secretion A function of the nephron in which ions, toxins, and water are secreted into the collecting duct to be excreted

Tympanic membrane A thin membrane that separates the external ear from the middle ear; also known as the *eardrum*

Type 1 diabetes mellitus (T1DM) A form of diabetes mellitus associated with an absolute deficiency of insulin production by the pancreas; people with T1DM require insulin therapy

Type 2 diabetes mellitus (T2DM) A form of diabetes mellitus associated with insulin resistance and a relative deficiency of insulin. People with T2DM can be treated with oral drugs, noninsulin injectable medications, and insulin

U

Unit dose A single dose of a drug; individualized packaged doses used in institutional practice settings

United States Pharmacopeia (USP) An independent, nonprofit organization that establishes documentation on product quality standards, drug quality and information, and health care information on medications, over-the-counter products, dietary supplements, and food ingredients to ensure the appropriate purity, quality, and strength; Chapter 797 (Pharmaceutical Compounding—Sterile Preparations) in the USP-NF is a set of enforceable sterile compounding standards and describes the guidelines, procedures, and compliance requirements for compounding sterile preparations; it also establishes the standards that apply to all settings in which sterile preparations are compounded

United States Pharmacopeia–National Formulary (USP-NF) A publication of the USP that contains standards for medications, dosage forms, drug substances, excipients, medical devices, and dietary supplements

Ureteroscopy Examination of the upper urinary tract, usually performed with an endoscope passed through the urethra

Urethritis Inflammation of the urethra

Urge incontinence Incontinence of urine due to involuntary bladder contractions that result in an urgent need to urinate

Uric acid The water-insoluble end-product of purine metabolism; deposition of uric acid as crystals in the joints and kidneys causes gout

Urolithiasis A condition in which solid mineral deposits form stones in the urinary tract

Urticaria Red welts that arise on the surface of the skin; they often are caused by an allergic reaction but may have non-allergic causes; also known as *hives*

Uterus The female organ in the lower abdomen where gestation of a fetus occurs

V

Vaccine A biological preparation that improves immunity to a particular disease by invoking an immune response and a "memory" of the response for future protection

Vasoconstriction Narrowing of the blood vessels that results from contraction of the muscular walls of the vessels

Vasodilation Widening of the vasculature, leading to increased blood flow

Vasopressin An alternate term for antidiuretic hormone (ADH)

Vein A vessel that carries deoxygenated blood to or toward the heart

Vena cava One of the two large veins that carry deoxygenated blood from the upper (superior vena cava) and lower (inferior vena cava) parts of the body to the right atrium of the heart

Ventricle One of the two lower chambers of the heart

Verbal communication The sharing of information through the use of speech

Vertical laminar flow hood An environment for the preparation of chemotherapeutic and hazardous agents in which air originating from the roof of the hood moves downward (over the agent) and is captured in a vent on the floor of the hood

Virion A virus particle

Virus A microscopic, nonliving organism that replicates exclusively inside the host's cell using parts of the cell, including DNA, ribosomes, and proteins

Vitreous humor A gel-like substance that fills the posterior cavity of the eye, between the lens and retina; it helps maintain the shape of the eye

Volume The amount of liquid in a container

Von Willebrand's disease The most common inherited bleeding disorder; it is associated with a deficiency in the clotting protein, von Willebrand's factor

W

Whole blood Blood drawn from the body from which no constituent, such as plasma or platelets, has been removed

Wholesale cost The purchase price of a product (e.g., medicine), which is marked up for resale

Wholesalers Companies that stock a variety of drug manufacturers' medications and normally have a "just in time" turnaround for ordered drugs; this means that drugs ordered today will arrive tomorrow.

Workers' compensation Government-required and government-enforced medical coverage for workers injured on the job, paid for by the employer. The programs are managed by each state in accordance with the state's workers' compensation laws

X

Xerosis Abnormal dryness of the skin, eyes, or mucous membranes

Page numbers followed by "f" indicate figures, "t" indicate tables, and "b" indicate boxes.